FOR
REFERENCE ONLY

# Obstetrics and Gynaecology

An evidence-based text for MRCOG

# Obstetrics and Gynaecology

An evidence-based text for MRCOG

SECOND EDITION

**David M Luesley** MA, MD, FRCOG
Professor of Gynaecological Oncology, University of Birmingham; and
Clinical Director, Pan-Birmingham Gynaecological Cancer Centre,
Birmingham, UK

**Philip N Baker** DM, BMedSci, BM, BS, FRCOG
Dean of the Faculty of Medicine and Dentistry, University of Alberta,
Edmonton, Canada

**SECTION EDITORS**

**Linda Cardozo** MD FRCOG
Professor of Urogynaecology; King's College Hospital, London

**James Drife** MD FRCOG FRCPEd FRCSEd FCOGSA FFSRH
Emeritus Professor, Department of Obstetrics and Gynaecology, Leeds General
Infirmary, Leeds

**Lucy Kean** DM FRCOG
Consultant Obstetrician (Subspecialist in Maternal and Fetal Medicine)
University Hospitals, City Campus, Nottingham

**Mark D Kilby** MD FRCOG
Professor in Maternal and Fetal Medicine, Division of Reproduction and Child Health
Birmingham Women's Hospital, University of Birmingham, Birmingham

**Henry C Kitchener** MD FRCOG FRCS (Glasgow)
Professor of Gynaecological Oncology and Head, Academic Unit of Obstetrics
and Gynaecology, University of Manchester, Manchester

**William L Ledger** MA DPhill (Oxon) MB ChB FRCOG
Head of Section of Reproductive and Developmental Medicine; and Professor of
Obstetrics and Gynaecology, Royal Hallamshire Hospital, Sheffield

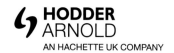

**HODDER**
ARNOLD
AN HACHETTE UK COMPANY

First published in Great Britain in 2004 by Arnold

This second edition published in 2010 by
Hodder Arnold, an imprint of Hodder Education, an Hachette UK Company,
338 Euston Road, London NW1 3BH
Error! Hyperlink reference not valid.
**http://www.hodderarnold.com**

Whilst the advice and information in this book are believed to be true and accurate at the date of going
to press, neither the authors nor the publisher can accept any legal responsibility or liability for any
errors or omissions that may be made. In particular     but without limiting the generality of the
preceding disclaimer every effort has been made to check drug dosages; however it is still possible
that errors have been missed. Furthermore, dosage schedules are constantly being revised and new
side-effects recognized. For these reasons the reader is strongly urged to consult the drug companies’
printed instructions before administering any of the drugs recommended in this book.

*British Library Cataloguing in Publication Data*
A catalogue record for this book is available from the British Library

*Library of Congress Cataloging-in-Publication Data*
A catalog record for this book is available from the Library of Congress

ISBN    978 0 340 99013 1
ISBN [ISE] 978 0 340 99052 0     International Students’ Edition, restricted territorial availability


2 3 4 5 6 7 8 9 10

Commissioning Editor: Gavin Jamieson
Project Editor: Joanna Silman
Production Controller: Joanna Walker
Cover Designer: Helen Towson
Indexer: Laurence Errington
Cover images © Science Photo Library


Typeset in 10/12 Minion-Regular by MPS Limited, A Macmillan Company

What do you think about this book? Or any other Hodder Arnold title?
Please visit our website: www.hodderarnold.com

Printed and bound in India by Replica Press.

To my daughters, Alice and Megan (DL)
To my elder daughter, Charlotte (PB)

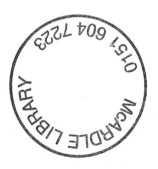

# Contents

## PART ONE    INTRODUCTORY/GENERAL      Part Editor: James Drife

## PART TWO    OBSTETRICS      Part Editor: Philip Baker

# Contributors

**Philip N. Baker** DM, BMedSci, BM, BS, FRCOG
Dean of the Faculty of Medicine & Dentistry, University of Alberta, Edmonton, Canada

**Linda Cardozo** MD FRCOG
Professor of Urogynaecology, King's College Hospital, London

**Ying Cheong**
Senior Lecturer, Subspecialist in Reproductive Medicine and Surgery, Southampton Fertility Unit, University of Southampton School of Medicine, Southampton

**Arri Coomarasamy** MD MRCOG
Subspecialist in Reproductive Medicine and Surgery, and Consultant Gynaecologist, University of Birmingham

**Sarah M Creighton** MD FRCOG
Consultant Gynaecologist, University College London Hospital, UCL Institute of Women's Health, London

**Hilary OD Critchley** BSc MBChB MD FRCOG FRANZCOG FFRSH FMedSci
Professor of Reproductive Medicine, Honorary Consultant Obstetrician and Gynaecologist, University of Edinburgh, Centre for Reproductive Biology, Edinburgh

**Margaret E. Cruickshank** MB ChB MD FRCOG
Senior Lecturer in Gynaecological Oncology, Department of Obstetrics and Gynaecology, Aberdeen Maternity Hospital, Aberdeen

**Andrew Currie** BM DCH FRCPCH FRCP Ed
Consultant Neonatologist, Leicester Royal Infirmary, University Hospitals of Leicester NHS Trust, Leicester

**Rebecca Deans** MBBS MMed MRANZCOG
Fellow in Paediatric and Adolescent Gynaecology, University College London Hospital, London; and Conjoint Lecturer, University of New South Wales, Sydney, Australia

**Gabrielle Downey**
Consultant Obstetrician and Lead Colposcopist at City Hospital, Dudley Road, Birmingham

**James Drife** MD FRCOG FRCPEd FRCSEd Hon FCOGSA
Professor, Department of Obstetrics and Gynaecology, General Infirmary, Leeds

**Diana Fothergill** BSc Med Sci Hons MB ChB FRCOG
Consultant Obstetrician and Gynaecologist, The Jessop Wing, Sheffield Teaching Hospitals NHS Trust, Sheffield

**Harold Gee** MD FRCOG
Consultant Obstetrician, Director of Postgraduate Education, Medical Director, RCOG Examiner, Birmingham Women's Hospital, Birmingham

**Joanna C. Gillham** BSc MB BS MRCOG
Clinical Research Fellow, Maternal and Fetal Health Research Centre, Academic Unit of Obstetrics and Gynaecology and Reproductive Health Care, St Mary's Hospital, Manchester

**Barry W. Hancock** MD FRCP FRCR OBE
Emeritus Professor of Medical Oncology and former Director of Trophoblastic Disease Centre, Weston Park Hospital, Sheffield

**Richard Hayman** BSc MB BS MRCOG DM
Consultant in Obstetrics and Gynaecology, Gloucester Royal Hospital, Gloucester

**Susan J. Houghton** MB ChB MRCOG
Consultant Obstetrician and Gynaecologist, Good Hope Hospital, Sutton Coldfield

**Kulsum Jaffer** BSc MBBS FRCOG FFSRH
Consultant in Sexual and Reproductive Health, Heart of Birmingham Teaching Primary Care Trust, St Patrick's Centre, Birmingham

**Tracey A. Johnston** MD MRCOG
Birmingham Woman's Health NHS Foundation Trust, Birmingham

**Griff Jones** BSc MB BS MRCOG FRCSC
Consultant Obstetrician and Gynaecologist, Winchester District Memorial Hospital, Winchester, Ontario, Canada

**Lucy Kean** DM FRCOG
Consultant Obstetrician Subspecialist in Maternal and Fetal Medicine, University Hospitals, City Campus, Nottingham

**Louise Kenny** MB ChB hons PhD MRCOG
Consultant Obstetrician and Gynaecologist and Professor of Obstetrics, The Anu Research Centre, University College Cork, Cork University Maternity Hospital, Cork

**Yakoub Khalaf**
Guy's and St Thomas' Hospital Foundation Trust, Guy's Hospital, London

**Mark D. Kilby** MD MRCOG
Professor in Maternal and Fetal Medicine, Division of Reproduction and Child Health, Birmingham Women's Hospital, Birmingham

**Henry C. Kitchener** MD FRCOG FRCS Glasgow
Professor of Gynaecological Oncology and Head, Academic Unit of Obstetrics and Gynaecology, University of Manchester, Manchester

**Ellen Knox** MD MRCOG
Subspeciality Trainee in Maternal and Fetal Medicine, Birmingham Women's Hospital, Birmingham, UK

**Sailesh Kumar** MB BS MMed O&G FRCS MRCOG FRANZCOG DPhil Oxon
Honorary Senior Lecturer and Consultant in Maternal and Fetal Medicine, Centre for Fetal Care, Imperial College London, Queen Charlotte's and Chelsea Hospital, London

**William L. Ledger** MA DPhil Oxon MB ChB FRCOG
Head of Section of Reproductive and Developmental Medicine; and Professor of Obstetrics and Gynaecology, Royal Hallamshire Hospital, Sheffield

**David M. Levy** FRCA
Consultant Obstetric Anaesthetist, Anaesthetics Directorate, Nottingham University Hospitals, Queens Medical Centre Campus, Nottingham

**Murray Luckas** MD MRCOG
Consultant Obstetrician and Gynaecologist, Leighton Hospital, Crewe

**David M. Luesley** MA MD FRCOG
Lawson Tait Professor of Gynaecological Oncology, School of Cancer Sciences, University of Birmingham; and Clinical Director, Pan-Birmingham Gynaecological Cancer Centre, City Hospital, Birmingham

**Sheila McLean** LLB MLitt PhD LLD (Abertay, Edin) FRSE FRCGP FRCP Edin FRSA
International Bar Association Professor of Law and Ethics in Medicine, University of Glasgow, Glasgow

**Ismaiel Mahfouz** MSc MRCOG
Senior Clinical Research Fellow, Urogynaecology Unit, King's College Hospital, London, UK

**Melanie C Mann** FRCOG FFFP Dip GUM
Consultant in Contraception and Reproductive Health, Worcestershire PCT, Arrowside Unit, Alexandra Hospital, Redditch, Worcestershire

**Bill Martin**
Consultant in Maternal and Fetal Medicine, Birmingham Women's Hospital, Birmingham

**Pierre L Martin-Hirsch** MRCOG
Consultant Gynaecological Oncologist, Central Lancashire Teaching Hospitals, Preston

**Mostafa Metwally** MD MRCOG
Subspecialist in Reproductive Medicine and Surgery. Clinical Research Fellow in Reproductive Medicine, The Academic Unit of Reproductive and Developmental Medicine, Royal Hallamshire Hospital, Sheffield

**Michele P Mohajer** BM BS FRCOG MD
Consultant in Maternal and Fetal Medicine, Royal Shrewsbury Hospital, Shrewsbury

**Dimitrios Nikolaou** MD MRCOG
Consultant Gynaecologist, Specialist in Reproductive Medicine and Surgery, Director, Ovarian Ageing and Fertility program, Department of Obstetrics and Gynaecology, Chelsea and Westminster Hospital, Imperial College School of Medicine, London

**Michele P Mohajer** BM BS FRCOG MD
Consultant in Feto-Maternal Medicine, Royal Shrewsbury Hospital NHS Trust, Shrewsbury

**Catherine Nelson-Piercy** MA FRCP
Consultant Obstetric Physician, Guy's and St Thomas' Hospitals, London

**David Nunns** MD MRCOG
Consultant Gynaecological Oncologist, Nottingham City Hospital, Nottingham

**Michael Paterson** MB ChB MD FRCOG FRCS (Ed)
Consultant Gynaecologist, Royal Hallamshire Hospital, Sheffield

**Richard Porter** MA MSc FRCOG
Consultant Obstetrician and Gynaecologist, Royal United Hospital, Bath

**Angie Rantell** BSC HONS RN
Senior Urogynaecology Nurse Specialist, King's College Hospital, London

**Charles Redman** MB ChB FRCOG FRCS (Ed)
Consultant Gynaecologist, City General, North Staffordshire Hospital, Stoke-on-Trent

**Fiona M Reid** MD MRCOG
Consultant Urogynaecologist, The Warrell Unit, St Mary's Hospital, Manchester

**Arasee Renganathan** MB BS MRCOG
Research Fellow, Urogynaecology Department, King's College Hospital, London, UK

**Karina Reynolds** MD FRCS MRCOG
Consultant in Gynaecological Oncology, Gynaecological Cancer Centre, Barts Hospital, London

**Devender Roberts**
Consultant in Maternal and Fetal Medicine, Liverpool Women's Hospital, Crown Street, Liverpool

**Dudley Robinson** MBBS MD MRCOG
Consultant Urogynaecologist/Honorary Senior Lecturer, Department of Obstetrics and Gynaecology, King's College Hospital, London

**Jane Rufford** MRCOG
Locum Consultant Gynaecologist, Department of Obstetrics and Gynaecology, King's College Hospital, London

**Andrew Shennan** MB BS MD FRCOG
Professor of Obstetrics, Maternal and Fetal Research Unit, St Thomas' Hospital, London

**Anthony RB Smith** MD FRCOG
Consultant Gynaecologist, The Warrell Unit, St Mary's Hospital, Manchester

**John AD Spencer** MB BS BSc AKC FRCOG FHEA
Consultant Obstetrician and Gynaecologist, Portland Hospital, London

**Sushma Srikrishna** MRCOG
Subspeciality Trainee in Urogynaecology, Department of Urogynaecology, King's College Hospital, London

**Sudha Sundar** MPHIL MRCOG
Senior Lecturer/HON NHS Consultant Academic Department of Gynaecological Oncology, Pan Birmingham Gynaecological Cancer Centre, City Hospital, Birmingham

**Myles Taylor** BA MRCOG PhD
Consultant Obstetrician and Gynaecologist, Royal Devon and Exeter NHS Foundation Trust, Child and Women's Health, Exeter

**Jane Thomas** MB ChB MSc and MRCOG
Former Director, National Collaborating Centre for Women's and Children's Health, and Honorary Consultant Obstetrician and Gynaecologist, Nuffield Department of Obstetrics and Gynaecology, Oxford

**Peter J Thompson** MB BS MRCOG
Consultant Obstetrician, Birmingham Women's Hospital, Birmingham

**John Tidy** MD FRCOG
Consultant Gynaecological Oncologist, The Jessop Wing, Sheffield

**Clare Tower** MBCHB PHD MRCOG
Clinical Lecturer/Subspeciality Trainee in Maternal and Fetal Medicine, Maternal and Fetal Health Research Centre, St Mary's Hospital, Manchester

**Elias Tzakas** MBBS MRCOG
Mitera Hospital, Athens, Greece

**Aarti Umranikar** MRCOG MFFP
Senior Registrar in Obstetrics and Gynaecology, Princess Anne Hospital, Southampton

**Linda Watkins** MBChB MRCOG
Consultant Obstetrician, Liverpool Woman's Hospital, Liverpool

**Christine P West** MD FRCOG
Consultant Obstetrician and Gynaecologist, Royal Infirmary of Edinburgh

# Preface

There are many demands made on modern medical practitioners. First, to provide high-quality patient-focused care that should be based upon the best evidence available. Next, to compare the care delivered with agreed standards with the objective of continuing to improve the process. There is also a duty to work towards filling the gaps in the evidence base through properly constructed and conducted research. Not least, there is a responsibility to disseminate new ideas and information through teaching and educational programmes.

With the first edition of this book we deviated somewhat from the established textbook model to recognize the importance of a solid evidence-based foundation for obstetrical and gynaecological practice, moving away in certain instances from traditional or 'enteric-based' practice. The aim was to base each section, where applicable, on evidence and to include a critique of such evidence. This second edition retains that key feature; and our contributors have revised and updated their chapters in line with current evidence and clinical practice.

We have developed a simple template to link MRCOG syllabus criteria with the evidence that underlies practice. It will be obvious to most readers that the strength of evidence varies widely and in some instances it can hardly be recognized at all. Our contributors have worked hard to provide both balance and breadth to the sections that they have addressed Sections are broken down into separate chapters, but we feel that a sense of continuity has been imparted to a recognized area of obstetric or gynaecological care. Contributors were chosen because of their expertise, but also because they are currently involved in the shaping of care and therefore have a first-hand feel for the evidence. The members of the editorial team have worked closely with each other and the contributors to try to maintain the original template-format emphasis on evidence and its strength, with continued close reference to the MRCOG syllabus. We not only feel that the final product will help trainees come to appreciate and understand the core knowledge of their chosen discipline, but also hope it will fire their enthusiasm to seek more information and continue to strive for excellence in all aspects of their professional careers.

Textbooks do not make good doctors, but good doctors must practise from a sound basis of knowledge, and this text aims to provide in some measure the foundation of core knowledge required of a practising obstetrician and gynaecologist.

David M. Luesley and Philip N. Baker

# Acknowledgements

The editors and contributors are grateful for the contribution of the following authors who wrote chapters for the first edition of this book but have not been involved in this new edition:

James Balmforth, Sandie Bohin, Ian J Etherington, Griff Jones, Justin Konje, Hany AMA Lashen, Alec McEwan, Enda McVeigh, Lawrence J Mascarenhas and David Somerset

# List of abbreviations used

| | | | |
|---|---|---|---|
| 5-FU | 5-fluorouracil | BMI | body mass index |
| 7-DHCO | 7-dehydrocholesterol | BMJ | British Medical Journal |
| AAA | arterio-arterial anastamatoses | BMPs | bone morphogenic proteins |
| ABC | airway, breathing, circulation | BNF | British National Formulary |
| AC | abdominal circumference | BP | blood pressure |
| ACE | angiotensin II converting enzyme | bpm | beats per minute |
| ACE | angiotensin-converting enzyme | BPP | biophysical profile |
| AChE | acetylcholinesterase | BPS | bladder pain syndrome |
| ACHOIS | Australian Carbohydrate Intolerance Study in Pregnant Women | BSAC | British Society for Antimicrobial Chemotherapy |
| ACTG | AIDS Clinical Trial Group | BSO | bilateral salpingo-oopherectomy |
| ACTH | adrenocorticotrophic hormone | BV | bacterial vaginosis |
| AEDF | absent end-diastolic flow | bvm | bag–valve–mask |
| AEDs | anti-epileptic drugs | CAH | chronic active hepatitis |
| AFC | antral follicular counts | CAH | congenital adrenal hyperplasia |
| AFE | amniotic fluid embolism | CAIS | complete androgen insensitivity syndrome |
| AFI | amniotic fluid index | | |
| AFLP | acute fatty liver of pregnancy | CASA | computer-assisted sperm analysis |
| AFP | alpha-fetoprotein | CBT | cognitive behavioural therapy |
| AFS | American Fertility Society | CCAML | congenital cystic adenomatous malformation of the lung |
| AFV | amniotic fluid volume | | |
| AHA | American Heart Association | CDSR | Cochrane Database of Systematic Reviews |
| AIDS | acquired immunodeficiency syndrome | | |
| | | CEE | conjugated equine oestrogens |
| AIS | adenocarcinoma-in-situ | CEMACH | Confidential Enquiry into Maternal and Child Health |
| ALF | acute liver failure | | |
| ALOs | actinomyces-like organisms | CEPOD | confidential enquiries into perioperative deaths |
| ALT | alanine transaminase | | |
| AMH | anti-Müllerian hormone | CESDI | confidential enquiry into stillbirth and deaths in infancy |
| ANA | antinuclear antibody | | |
| APC | activated protein C | CFU | colony-forming units |
| APH | antepartum haemorrhage | CHC | combined hormonal contraception |
| aPL | antiphospholipid | CHD | coronary heart disease |
| APS | antiphospholipid syndrome | CHM | complete hydatidiform mole |
| APTT | activated partial thromboplastin time | CI | confidence interval |
| ARBs | angiotensin II type 1 receptor blockers (angiotensin receptor antogonists) | CIGN | cervical intraepithelial glandular neoplasia |
| | | CIN | cervical intraepithelial neoplasia |
| ARM | artificial rupture of membranes | CIS | carcinoma-in-situ |
| ART | anti-retroviral therapy | CKD | chronic kidney disease |
| ASA | American Society of Anesthesiologists | CLASP | collaborative low-dose aspirin study in pregnancy |
| ASRM | American Society of Reproductive Medicine | | |
| | | CMA | Canadian Medical Association |
| AST | aspartate aminotransferase (aspartate transaminase) | CMACE | Centre for Maternal and Child Enquiries |
| | | CMV | cytomegalovirus |
| ATP | adenosine triphosphate | CNS | central nervous system |
| AUM | ambulatory urodynamic monitoring | CNST | Clinical Negligence Scheme for Trusts |
| AVMs | arteriovenous malformations | | |
| β-hCG | beta-human chorionic gonadotrophin | COCP | combined oral contraceptive pill |
| b-IFN | beta-interferon | COMET | Comparative Obstetric Mobile Epidural Trial |
| BAD | British Association of Dermatologists | | |
| BASHH | British Association for Sexual Health and HIV | COS | controlled ovarian stimulation |
| | | COX-2 | cyclo-oxygenase-2 |
| BCG | bacille Calmette Guérin | CPAP | continuous positive airway pressure |
| BFLUTS | Bristol Female Urinary Tract Symptoms | | |
| BMD | bone mineral density | | |

| | | | |
|---|---|---|---|
| CPD | cephalo-pelvic disproportion | ENG | etonogestrel |
| CPR | cardiopulmonary resuscitation | EOA | early ovarian ageing |
| CPS | Crown Prosecution Service | ER | extended-release |
| CRP | C-reactive protein | ER | oestrogen receptors |
| CRS | congenital rubella syndrome | ERCP | endoscopic retrograde cholangiopancreatography |
| CS | caesarean section | | |
| CSE | combined spinal–epidural | ERCS | elective repeat caesarean section |
| CSF | cerebrospinal fluid | ERPC | evacuation of products of conception |
| CSII | continuous subcutaneous insulin infusion | ERT | oestrogen replacement therapy |
| | | ESHRE | European Society of Human Reproduction and Embryology |
| CSM | Committee on Safety of Medicines | | |
| CT | computed tomography | ESR | erythrocyte sedimentation rate |
| CTG | cardiotocography | ESSIC | European Society for the Study of Bladder Pain Syndrome/Interstitial Cystitis |
| CTPA | computed tomography pulmonary angiogram | | |
| | | ET | embryo transfer |
| CVA | cerebrovascular accidents | FA | fertility awareness |
| CVP | central venous pressure | FAI | free androgen index |
| CVS | chorionic villus sampling | FAS | fetal alcohol syndrome |
| CXR | chest x-ray | FBC | full blood count |
| D&C | dilatation and curettage | FBS | fetal blood sampling |
| D&E | dilatation and evacuation | FDPs | fibrin degradation products |
| DARE | Database of Reviews of Effectiveness | FDV | Qfirst desire to void |
| DC | dichorionic | fFN | fetal fibronectin |
| DC/DA | dichorionic diamniotic | FFP | fresh frozen plasma |
| DES | diethylstilbestrol | FGM | female genital mutilation |
| DHEA | dehydroepiandrosterone | FGR | fetal growth restriction |
| DHT | dihydrotestosterone | FHM | Fundal height measurement |
| DI | donor insemination | FIGO | Federation of Gynaecology and Obstetrics |
| DIC | disseminated intravascular coagulation | | |
| | | FIGO | International Federation of Gynaecology and Obstetrics |
| DIC | disseminated intravascular coagulopathy | | |
| | | FISH | fluorescence in-situ hybridization |
| DKA | diabetic ketoacidosis | FMC | fetal movement counting |
| DMPA | depot medroxy progesterone acetate | FME | forensic medical examiner, previously known as a police surgeon |
| DMSO | dimethyl sulphoxide | | |
| DSD | disorders of sex development | FSE | fetal scalp electrode |
| dsDNA | double-stranded DNA | FSH | follicle stimulating hormone |
| DUB | dysfunctional uterine bleeding | FVL | Factor V Leiden |
| DVP | deepest vertical pool | GABA-A | gamma-aminobutyric acid type A |
| DVT | deep venous thrombosis | GAG | glycosaminoglycan |
| E3 | oestriol | GBS | Group B streptococcal |
| E3G | oestrone-3-glucuronide | GCIG | Gynaecologic Cancer Intergroup |
| EAS | external anal sphincter | GDM | gestational diabetes mellitus |
| EBV | Epstein–Barr virus | GnRH | gonadotrophin-releasing hormone |
| EC | emergency contraception | GP | general practitioner |
| ECG | electrocardiogram | GRIT | Growth Restriction Intervention Trial |
| ECMO | extracorporeal membrane oxygenation | GTD | gestational trophoblastic disease |
| | | GTN | gestational trophoblastic neoplasia |
| ECV | external cephalic version | GTN | glyceryl trinitrate |
| EDD | estimated date of delivery | GUM | genitourinary medicine |
| EDF | end-diastolic flow | HAART | highly active anti-retroviral therapy |
| EEG | electroencephalogram | HAPO | hyperglycemia and adverse pregnancy outcomes |
| EFM | electronic fetal monitoring | | |
| eGFR | estimated glomerular filtration rate | Hb | haemoglobin |
| EIA | enzyme immunoassay | HBV | hepatitis B virus |
| EMG | electromyography | hCG | human chorionic gonadotrophin |
| ENA | extractable nuclear antigens | | |

| | | | |
|---|---|---|---|
| HCM | hypertrophic cardiomyopathy | ISSVD | International Society for the Study of Vulvar Diseases |
| HCV | hepatitis C virus | ITP | idiopathic thrombocytopenic pupura |
| HDL | high-density lipoprotein | ITT analysis | intention to treat |
| HDU | high dependency unit | IUCD | intrauterine contraceptive device |
| HELLP syndrome | haemolysis, increased liver enzymes and low platelets | IUD | intrauterine death |
| HFEA | Human Fertilisation and Embryology Authority | IUD or Cu-IUD | intrauterine device |
| | | IUFD | intrauterine fetal death |
| HHC | hyperhomocystinaemia | IUGR | intrauterine growth restriction |
| HIE | hypoxic–ischaemic encephalopathy | IUI | intrauterine insemination |
| HIT | heparin-induced thrombocytopenia | IUP | intrauterine pregnancy |
| HIV | human immunodeficiency virus | IUS | intrauterine system |
| HLA | human leukocyte antigen | IVC | inferior vena caval |
| HMB | heavy menstrual bleeding | IVF | in-vitro fertilization |
| hMG | human menopausal gonadotrophins | IVF-ET | IVF and embryo transfer |
| | | IVS | intravaginal slingplasty |
| HNPCC | hereditary non-polyposis colorectal cancer | IVU or IVP | intravenous urogram |
| | | JVP | jugular venous pressure |
| HPL | human placental lactogen | KCl | potassium chloride |
| HPV | human papilloma virus | LAGB | laparoscopic adjustable gastric banding |
| HRT | hormone replacement therapy | LAM | lactational amenorrhoea method |
| HSDD | hypoactive sexual desire disorder | LARC | long active reversible contraption |
| HSV | herpes simplex virus | LAVH | laparoscopically assisted vaginal hysterectomy |
| HSV-1 | herpes simplex type 1 virus | | |
| HSV-2 | herpes simplex type 2 virus | LDL | low-density lipoprotein |
| HTA | Health Technology Assessment Database | LH | luteinizing hormone |
| HTA | Human Tissue Authority | LHCRG | luteinizing hormone/hCG receptor |
| HUS | haemolytic uraemic syndrome | LMP | last menstrual period |
| IBD | inflammatory bowel disease | LMWH | low molecular weight heparin |
| IBIS | International Breast Cancer Intervention Study | LMWH | low-molecular-weight heparin |
| | | LN | lymph node |
| IBS | irritable bowel syndrome | LNG | levonorgestrel |
| ICIQ | International Consultation on Incontinence Questionnaire | LNG-IUS | levonorgestrel-releasing intrauterine system |
| ICON | International Collaborative Ovarian Neoplasm collaborators | LOD | laparoscopic ovarian drilling |
| | | LP | lichen planus |
| ICP | intracranial pressure | LS | lichen sclerosus |
| ICS | International Continence Society | LSCS | lower segment caesarean section |
| ICSI | intracytoplasmic sperm injection | LSIL | low-grade squamous intraepithelial lesions |
| ICU | intensive care unit | | |
| IDU | injecting drug users | LUNA | laparoscopic uterine nerve ablation |
| IE | infective endocarditis | LUTS | lower urinary tract symptoms |
| Ig | immunoglobulin | MAP | mean arterial pressure |
| IGF-1 | insulin-like growth factor 1 | MAR | mixed antibody reaction |
| IGFBP1 | insulin-like growth factor binding protein 1 | MAS | meconium aspiration syndrome |
| | | MC | monochorionic |
| IgG | immunoglobulin G | MC/DA | monochorionic diamniotic |
| IgM | immunoglobulin M | MCA | middle cerebral artery |
| IHCP | intrahepatic cholestasis of pregnancy | MCH | mean corpuscular haemoglobin |
| IIQ | Incontinence Impact Questionnaire | MCHC | mean cell Hb concentration |
| ILCOR | International Liaison Committee on Resuscitation | MCHC | mean corpuscular haemoglobin concentration |
| | | MCV | mean cell volume |
| IOL | induction of labour | MCV | mean corpuscular volume |
| IPPV | intermittent positive pressure ventilation | MDKD | multicystic dysplastic kidney disease |
| IQR | interquartile range | MDMA | 3,4-methylenedioxymethamphetamine |
| ISD | intrinsic sphincter deficiency | | |

| | | | |
|---|---|---|---|
| MDT | multidisciplinary team | OSATS | objective structured assessment of techinical skill |
| MEA | microwave endometrial ablation | | |
| MFPR | multi-fetal pregnancy reduction | PAIS | partial androgen insensitivity syndrome |
| MG | myasthenia gravis | | |
| MHRA | Medicines and Healthcare products Regulatory Agency | PAPP-A | pregnancy-associated plasma protein-A |
| MIN | multicentric intraepithelial neoplasia | PAT | pregnancy-associated thrombocytopenia |
| MIS | Müllerian inhibiting substance | | |
| MLS | Maternal Lifestyles Study | PBC | primary biliary cirrhosis |
| MMF | mycophenolate mofetil | PCA | patient-controlled analgesia |
| MMPs | matrix metalloproteinases | PCEA | patient-controlled epidural analgesia |
| MMR | maternal mortality rate | PCOS | polycystic ovary syndrome |
| MMT | methadone maintenance treatment | PCR | polymerase chain reaction |
| MoM | multiple of the normal median | PCRH | placental corticotrophin-releasing hormone |
| MPA | medroxyprogesterone acetate | | |
| MPD | maximum pool depth | PDL | primary dysfunctional labour |
| MR | magnetic resonance | PDS | polydioxanone suture |
| MRC | Medical Research Council | PE | pulmonary embolism |
| MRI | magnetic resonance imaging | PECOT | population, exposure, comparison, outcome and time |
| MRSA | methacillin resistant staphylococcus aureus | | |
| | | PEEP | positive end-expiratory pressure |
| MS | multiple sclerosis | PEFR | peak expiratory flow rate |
| MSAFP | maternal serum alpha-fetoprotein | PEP | post-exposure prophylaxis |
| MSM | men who have sex with men | PEPSE | post-exposure prophylaxis for HIV following sexual exposure |
| MSU | midstream urine | | |
| MUP | motor nerve unit potential | PET | positron emission tomography |
| MVA | manual vacuum aspiration | PET | pre-eclampsia |
| N2O/O2 | nitrous oxide and oxygen | PFMT | pelvic floor muscle training |
| NAAT | nucleic acid amplification tests | PFR | peak flow rate |
| NAS | neonatal abstinence syndrome | PG | prostaglandin |
| NCEPOD | National Confidential Enquiry into Patient Outcome and Death | PGD | pre-implantation genetic diagnosis |
| | | PGM | pro-thrombin gene mutation |
| NCSP | National Chlamydia Screening Programme | PID | pelvic inflammatory disease |
| | | PIH | pregnancy-induced hypertension |
| NET-EN | norethisterone enantate | PIVKA | prothrombin induced by vitamin K absence |
| NFP | natural family planning | | |
| NHS | National Health Service | PLGF | placental growth factors |
| NHSCSP | National Health Service Cervical Screening Programme | PMB | post-menopausal bleeding |
| | | PMDD | premenstrual dysphoric disorder |
| NICE | National Institute for Health and Clinical Excellence | PMR | perinatal mortality rate |
| | | PMS | premenstrual syndrome |
| NICU | neonatal intensive care unit | PMSG | pregnant mare serum gonadotrophins |
| NIH | National Institute of Health | | |
| NMG | neonatal myasthenia gravis | PND | perinatal death notification |
| NNT | number needed to treat | POF | premature ovarian failure |
| NPSA | National Patient Safety Agency | POI | progestogen only implants |
| NSAID | Non-steroidal anti-inflammatory drugs | POIC | progestogen only injectable contraception |
| NSC | National Screening Committee | POP-Q | Pelvic Organ Prolapse Quantification |
| NST | non-stress test | POPs | progestogen only pills |
| NT | nuchal translucency | PPH | postpartum haemorrhage |
| NTDs | neural tube defects | PPIUS | Patient Perception of Intensity of Urgency Scale |
| OAA | Obstetric Anaesthetists' Association | | |
| OAB | overactive bladder | PPROM | preterm premature rupture of membranes |
| OCP | oral contraceptive pill | | |
| OGTT | glucose tolerance test | PR | progesterone receptors |
| OHSS | ovarian hyperstimulation syndrome | PROM | pre-labour rupture of membranes |
| OR | odds ratio | PSN | presacral neurectomy |

| | | | |
|---|---|---|---|
| PT | pro-thrombin time | TCRE | transcervical resection of the endometrium |
| PTL | preterm labour | TDF | testes-determining factor |
| PTNS | posterior tibial nerve stimulation | TED | thromboembolic deterrent |
| PTSD | post-traumatic stress disorder | TENS | transcutaneous electrical nerve stimulation |
| PTU | propylthiouracil | | |
| PUVA | psoralens and ultraviolet A | TGF-B | transformin growth factor-B |
| QF-PCR | quantitative fluorescence polymerase chain reaction | TIBC | total iron-binding capacity |
| | | TMN | tumour, nodes, metastases |
| RA | rheumatoid arthritis | TPHA | *T. pallidum* haemagglutination assay |
| RCOG | Royal College of Obstetricians and Gynaecologist | TRH | thyrotropin-releasing hormone |
| RCT | randomized controlled trial | TSH | thyroid-stimulating hormone |
| REDF | reversed end-diastolic flow | TTN | transient tachypnoea of the newborn |
| REM | rapid eye movement | TTP | thrombotic thrombocytopenic purpura |
| rFSH | recombinant FSH | | |
| Rh | Rhesus | TTTS | twin–twin transfusion syndrome |
| RMI | risk of malignancy index | TVS | transvaginal ultrasound scanning |
| RPR | rapid plasma reagin | TVT | tension-free vaginal tape |
| RR | relative risk | UADWs | umbilical artery Doppler waveforms |
| RRSO | risk-reducing salpingo-oopherectomy | UAE | uterine artery embolization |
| | | UDCA | ursodeoxycholic acid |
| RT-PCR | reverse transcriptase–polymerase chain reaction | UDI | urogenital distress inventory |
| | | uE3 | unconjugated oestriol |
| RVVC | recurrent vulvovaginal candidiasis | UICC | Union Internationale Contre le Cancer |
| SANDS | Stillbirth and Neonatal Death Society | | |
| SARC | sexual assault referral centres | UKCTOCS | United Kingdom Collaborative Trial of Ovarian Cancer Screening, |
| SCBU | special care baby unit | | |
| SCC | squamous cell carcinoma | UKFOCSS | United Kingdom Familial Ovarian Cancer Screening Study |
| SCI | spinal cord injury | | |
| SDV | strong desire to void | UKMEC | UK Medical Eligibility Criteria |
| sEMG | surface electromyographic | UKOSS | UK Obstetric Surveillance System |
| SERM | selective oestrogen receptor modulators | UKOSS | United Kingdom Obstetric Surveillance System |
| sFLT | soluble fms-like tyrosine kinase-1 | | |
| SGA | small for gestational age | UPP | urethral pressure profilometry |
| SGOT | serum glutamic-oxaloacetic transaminase | UPSI | unprotected sexual intercourse |
| | | USI | urodynamic stress incontinence |
| SGPT | serum glutamic pyruvic transaminase | UTI | urinary tract infection |
| SHBG | sex hormone binding globulin | VaIN | vaginal intraepithelial neoplasia |
| SIDS | sudden infant death syndrome | VBAC | vaginal birth after caesarean section |
| SLE | systemic lupus erythematosus | VCU | videocystourethrogram |
| SMR | severe mental retardation | VDRL | Venereal Disease Research Laboratory |
| SSRIs | selective serotonin reuptake inhibitors | VIN | vulval intraepithelial neoplasia |
| STANÔ | ST analysis | VLP | virus-like particles |
| STD | sexually transmitted disease | VTE | venous thrombo-embolism |
| STI | sexually transmitted infections | VVA | veno-venous anastomatoses |
| STV | short-term variability | VVC | vulvovaginal candidiasis |
| SUDEP | sudden unexpected death in epilepsy | vWD | von Willebrand's disease |
| SUZI | subzonal sperm injection | vWF | von Willebrand factor |
| SVT | supraventricular tachycardia | VZIG | varicella zoster IgG |
| T3 | triiodothyronine | VZIG | VZV immunoglobulin |
| T4 | thyroxine | VZV | varicella zoster virus |
| TAH/BSO | total abdominal hysterectomy and bilateral salpingo-oopherectomy | WHO | World Health Organization |
| | | WHOMEC | WHO Medical Eligibility Criteria |
| TAP | transversus abdominis plane | WY | woman years |
| TB | tuberculosis | ZD | zona drilling |
| TBA | thermal balloon ablation | ZDV | zidovudine |
| TBG | thyroid-binding globulin | ZIFT | zygote intrafallopian transfer |

# How to use this book

The following features are used throughout the book to highlight the key information and to clearly identify the evidence-base.

## MRCOG standards

An MRCOG standards box appears at the start of every chapter listing the relevant standards and/ or theoretical and practical skills relating to the topic. Where there are no standards specified in the MRCOG curriculum, we have given a summary of best practice.

## EBM

Evidence-based medicine boxes are included to provide a rapid summary of the evidence relating to the interventions and treatments discussed in each chapter. Where evidence is limited, this is also stated.

## KEY POINTS

Key points boxes are at the end of chapters to summarize the main points in a section.

## Evidence scoring

It is one of the key principles of this book that doctors assess the quality and applicability of available evidence. The evidence considered by the authors has been graded according to the structure below, in accord with the system used in Guidelines published by the RCOG.

Classification of evidence levels

A   systematic review or meta-analysis

B   one or more well designed randomised controlled trials

C   non-randomised controlled trials, cohort study etc.

D   retrospective, uncontrolled

E   'expert opinion'

# PART ONE

# Introductory/General

# Evidence-based medicine and medical informatics

*Jane Thomas*

## INTRODUCTION

This chapter outlines what evidence-based medicine is and how to practise it and some key epidemiological and statistical concepts that will help you to understand the terms used within this book, in clinical research and in the MRCOG examination.

In order to keep up to date, doctors need to be able to evaluate research evidence critically and integrate it into their practice. Evidence-based medicine is the conscientious, explicit and judicious use of current best evidence in making decisions about health care. The 'best evidence' is patient-centred clinical research on the precision of diagnostic tests, the power of prognostic markers and the effectiveness and safety of therapeutic interventions. Individual clinical expertise is the proficiency and judgement that individual clinicians acquire through clinical experience and clinical practice. Evidence and expertise need to be incorporated into decision making whilst taking into account patient preferences, concerns and expectations.[1] The concept of evidence-based medicine fits into the model of lifelong learning and clinical accountability of clinical governance.

The volume of published medical research and the average time a doctor has available for reading mean it is not possible for clinicians to read all the research literature published.[1] However, developments in information technology and the Internet have made practising evidence-based medicine technically feasible. The practice of evidence-based medicine comprises five steps:

1. defining a clinical question,
2. finding the best evidence,
3. appraising the evidence for its validity (closeness to the truth), impact (size of effect) and applicability (usefulness in clinical practice),
4. integrating the findings of the critical appraisal with clinical expertise and patient values,
5. reviewing (auditing) clinical practice and the efficiency of the above steps.

## STEP 1. SETTING THE CLINICAL QUESTION

Generating an answerable clinical question that is precise and specific is the basis of evidence-based medicine. The development of a search strategy will flow from this. Focused clinical questions include four components – 'PICO':[1,2]

- **P** – the population: a description of the patients, such as their age, parity, clinical problem and the healthcare setting;
- **I** – the intervention(s) (or exposure): these are the main actions, such as treatment, diagnostic test or risk factor;
- **C** – the comparison group: for example, placebo or alternative treatment;
- **O** – the outcome: for example, the change in health expected as a result of the intervention.

The type of studies that will be sought is determined by the type of clinical question. For example, for a question about therapy, the highest level of evidence is based on randomized controlled trials (RCTs); for a question about aetiology, cohort or case control may be more appropriate. For observational studies, the intervention is often an exposure and additional factors (length of follow up or time) may be included. This is sometimes a population, exposure, comparison, outcome and time (PECOT) question.[3]

An example of a vague clinical question is: 'Should we use antibiotic prophylaxis at caesarean section?'. This question could be focused in a number of ways.

- *Population.* Are you interested in all caesarean sections, or a specific subgroup, such as emergency or repeat caesarean section?
- *Intervention.* Antibiotic prophylaxis. Do you want to specify the antibiotic? Are you interested in the dose/ duration of use?
- *Comparison.* Is this compared to no antibiotics or another intervention or another antibiotic – or a different dose or treatment schedule?
- *Outcomes.* What do you anticipate the antibiotics will do? Will they reduce post-operative wound infection, or other outcomes such as endometritis or urinary tract infection (UTI), or other measures of febrile or infective morbidity such as length of hospital stay? Are there adverse effects?

An example of a focused question is: 'For women having emergency caesarean section, does co-amoxiclav reduce the post-operative endometritis compared with amoxicillin?'. This is a question about treatment, so we would look for the following study designs:

- systematic reviews (with or without meta-analysis) of RCTs,
- randomized controlled trials,
- well-designed controlled studies without randomization.

## STEP 2. FINDING THE BEST EVIDENCE

Research evidence is often categorized into either primary (RCT, cohort, case–control, cross-sectional or case series) or secondary (systematic review with or without meta-analysis, guidelines). If you are attempting to find out what is the right thing to do, one option would be to conduct a systematic review and to identify all the relevant primary research, appraise the quality of the research and summarize the results.[4] However, this would not be a practical solution every time you had a clinical question, nor would it be a good use of resources to repeat a review that has already been done. During the last decade, the number of guidelines and systematic reviews increased exponentially. It is necessary to know where to find good-quality, synthesized information and how to distinguish between the good and not so good. Reviews and clinical guidelines are made up of primary research, so it is important that you are able to appraise both the methods of the review and the studies on which it is based, so that you can judge whether or not it is a valid review or guideline.

### Clinical guidelines

Clinical guidelines are systematically produced statements to assist practitioners and patients in making decisions about specific clinical situations. Only guidelines that use well-recognized and accepted methodology should be considered. The key features of such guidelines are:

- a multidisciplinary working group,
- a well-described systematic review of the literature,
- graded recommendations with explicit links to the evidence,
- quality control, e.g. input by an independent advisory board or by independent peer review.

Often, guidelines are not published in peer-reviewed journals and therefore will not be indexed in either MEDLINE or EMBASE. Searching for guidelines on the following databases via the Internet will allow you to access those for which the methodological quality can be appraised:

- NHS evidence ‹www.library.nhs.uk/guidelinesFinder/›
- National Guidelines Clearinghouse: ‹www.guideline.gov/›
- OMNI: ‹www.intute.ac.uk/› (click advanced search, specify Medicine including dentistry in the subject area and Practice Guidelines in Resource Type)
- Canadian Medical Association (CMA) Infobase: ‹www. cma.ca/cpgs/›
- Guidelines and Guidelines in Practice: ‹www.eguidelines. co.uk›
- Turning Research Into Practice (TRIP): ‹www. tripdatabase.com/›
- Royal College of Obstetricians and Gynaecologists (RCOG): ‹www.rcog.org.uk›

The RCOG website provides a guide to searching for evidence[3] and a number of National Institute for Health and Clinical Excellence (NICE) evidence-based guidelines. *Green Top Guidelines* can also be found on the site. Further information on appraising guidelines is available.[1,5–8]

### Searching for systematic reviews

If no relevant guidelines can be found, the next stage is to search for other forms of pre-synthesized evidence, e.g. systematic reviews (of RCTs) with or without meta-analysis. A systematic review (as opposed to a traditional review) involves clearly defined questions, extensive search of the literature, appraising the quality of studies located by the search with explicit criteria, and analysing the research findings using appropriate methods. Data from each of the individual studies may be pooled and analysed using a technique known as 'meta-analysis'. The best resource for systematic reviews (and RCTs) is the Cochrane Library, which contains the following components for searching for systematic reviews:

- Cochrane Database of Systematic Reviews (CDSR)
- Database of Reviews of Effectiveness (DARE)
- Health Technology Assessment Database (HTA) (this includes UK and international HTA assessments).

Clinical evidence is another source of reviews of systematic reviews: ‹http://clinicalevidence.bmj.com/ceweb/index. jsp›. Fellows and Members of the RCOG can also access

Evidence Based Medicine Reviews, the British Medical Journal (BMJ), MEDLINE from 1993, Best Evidence from 1991, and the Cochrane Library.

## Searching for primary research evidence

There are numerous different library databases; different databases index different journals and may be general or topic specific. There is a variety of interfaces for the electronic databases, for example OVID, Silverplatter or Pubmed; most are available online. MEDLINE is produced by the US National Library of Medicine and is widely available free of charge. EMBASE has a greater European emphasis in terms of the journals it indexes and has a high level of pharmacologic content. Much of the nursing and midwifery research is not indexed by MEDLINE or EMBASE. To find such research, databases such as MIDIRS, BNI and CINAHL should be searched. Psychological literature is indexed on Psychinfo or Psychlit.

Citation searching ISI Web of Science will locate research papers that have referenced papers you intend to include in your research.

There are methodological filters that identify study designs, for example RCTs; these are designed to make your search more precise, although this may be at the expense of sensitivity, i.e. a high proportion of citations retrieved by your search may be relevant, but it might not include all relevant citations on the topic if these have not been indexed in a way that the filters would pick up. For further information about and examples of filters, visit CASPfew Filters at ‹wwwlib.jr2.ox.ac.uk/caspfew/filters/›.

## Developing a search strategy

Developing a search strategy usually involves combining free text and controlled text terms. Using the components of your clinical question (population, intervention, comparison, outcomes and study design), make a list of the synonyms, abbreviations and spelling variations (e.g. labor or labour) that might have been used by the authors to describe the concept. If you already know of relevant papers, scan them for more possible search terms. This list can be your free text terms.

The next stage is to list useful controlled text terms or subject headings. In MEDLINE, these are known as MeSH (Medical Subject Headings). In most databases, they will be found in the thesaurus or index. If you know of a relevant paper, check the subject headings under which it is indexed.

Having developed a focused four-part question (population, intervention, comparison, outcome – PICO), create a separate search strategy for each component. The next stage is to combine these searches. Combination is achieved by 'Boolean Logic' and works in a manner similar to combining numbers in algebra. Boolean Logic uses the terms 'and', 'or' and 'not' to create a set of results that should contain papers relevant to the clinical question.

For example, combining cervical *and* cancer will retrieve all the papers that contain both terms. Combining cervical *or* cancer will retrieve all papers in which either one or both terms are found. To find papers relating to post-operative infection, it would be necessary to combine both the lists of controlled and free text terms above with *or*. Combining induction *not* labour will retrieve all papers that contain the word induction, but do not also include the term labour. Care should be used when combining terms with *not*, as it will exclude any papers that discuss both the term of interest and the one to be excluded.

All databases also have useful search commands and symbols; however, these vary among databases. If you are conducting a systematic review or hope to publish the findings of your review, you need to keep your search strategies and record how many articles were found and which were included or excluded.

## STEP 3. APPRAISING THE EVIDENCE

Critical appraisal is the process of deciding if the research you have found can help you in answering your clinical question. The first filter is: 'Does this paper address my clinical question?' (i.e. are the population, intervention, comparisons and outcomes the same or similar to those in your question?).[1]

The second stage is to look at the study design (the methods section of a paper). The acceptable study design is determined by your clinical question. For questions about therapy, RCTs or systematic reviews of RCTs provide the least biased estimate of effectiveness; for diagnostic test accuracy, studies that compare the 'new' test to a 'gold standard' test are needed; for questions about prognosis, studies that follow up groups of patients for a specified period of time (cohort studies) are needed. A systematic review summarizes the results from a body of research, usually RCTs. Quality assessment is an essential part of the process of systematic review. If the 'constituent studies' are flawed, the conclusions of systematic reviews may also not be valid.[1,4]

### Bias

Bias is a systematic difference between groups that distorts the comparison between groups so that the 'true' effect is either exaggerated or reduced. The quality of a study is the degree to which the study design, conduct and analysis have minimized bias. External validity examines the extent to which the results of a study are applicable to other clinical circumstances, i.e. its generalizability. Internal validity examines the extent to which systematic error (or bias) is minimized within the study. The biases include:

- **selection bias** – the difference in the patient characteristics (such as prognosis) between comparison groups,

- **performance bias** – differences in the provision of care apart from the treatment under evaluation,
- **detection bias** – differences in the measurement or assessment of outcomes,
- **attrition bias** – the occurrence and handling of patient withdrawals or attrition.

Different study types are prone to different biases; therefore, there are different validity checklists for different studies based on the conduct, design and analysis.[1] Appraising the quality of a study is dependent on how the study is reported. To ensure more consistency of study reporting in journals, a number of reporting standards have been introduced in the last decade, for example the CONSORT statement for reporting RCTs,[9] QUOROM updated to PRISMA for systematic reviews of RCTs,[10] and STARD for diagnostic tests.[11]

## Understanding RCTs

For the MRCOG, you need to understand the design of an RCT; therefore, the rest of this section deals only with appraising RCTs. The RCT is the 'gold standard' method for evaluating the effectiveness of therapeutic interventions as it gives the least biased estimate of effect of treatment interventions. A confounder is a factor (such as disease severity) that may influence the choice of treatment and the outcome of care.

Confounding is one reason for the tendency of non-randomized trials to overestimate treatment effects when compared with RCTs. With a well-conducted RCT, randomization will create groups that are comparable with respect to any known or unknown potential confounding factors (providing the sample size is sufficiently large).

There are two common methods used to assess the quality of RCTs: a component approach (assess answers to each question – or quality domain) or assigning a 'score' to answers to each question and creating a composite quality score. Using different quality scores can impact on the conclusions of a review and introduce a 'quality score bias'. There are more than 39 different quality scores for RCTs alone. Many of the items assessed within individual composite scores examine features of trials not known to be associated with bias. The information needed to appraise the research methods should be outlined in the methods section. The key questions to ask when appraising an RCT are outlined below, with an explanation of why these are important.[1] The first four questions relate to study validity, the fifth to interpreting the results.

## 1. Was the assignment of treatment randomized?

The process of randomization requires that those recruiting to a trial or participating in the trial cannot predict which group they will be allocated to. The process of randomization involves two stages:

1. generation of an unpredictable allocation sequence (random number),
2. concealment of this sequence from those enrolling participants in the trials.

Failure to secure the concealment of the sequence may allow selective enrolment depending on prognostic factors. A trial in which it is possible to predict the treatment allocation is more likely to be biased. The 'gold standard' for randomization used in large multi-centre trials is 'central computer' randomization. The use of sealed envelopes may be subverted (for example, by holding the envelope up to the light); methods that could be predictable are date of birth, alternate days and hospital number.

## 2. Were the groups similar at the start of the trial?

The aim of randomization is the creation of groups that are comparable with respect to any known or unknown potential confounding factors (providing the sample size is sufficiently large). Randomization reduces bias in those selected for treatment and guarantees treatment assignment is not based on patients' prognosis. RCTs will have eligibility criteria, but within this trials report the characteristics of the patients according to the treatment received in Table 1 of the results section. The characteristics (such as age, parity) of the two groups should not be different.

## 3. Were the groups treated equally?

Apart from the intervention being studied, the groups should be treated identically – differences in treatment between groups may occur if treatment allocation is known. This is called performance bias and can be minimized by standardization of care protocol and by 'blinding'. RCTs may blind patients and therapists. Therapists may not treat both patient groups in a similar manner or patients may behave differently if they know which group they are in.

*Detection (or measurement) bias* applies to the measurement or assessment of the outcome. This should be standardized across all patients. Again, knowledge of treatment allocation may influence assessors. For an objective outcome (such as death), this may be less important, but for outcomes that are subjective, interpretation may differ if the assessor has prior knowledge of allocation. This bias can be minimized by using objective outcomes and by ensuring those assessing outcomes are not aware of treatment allocation. This approach is used in surgical RCTs: the surgeon undertaking the treatment has to be aware of the treatment allocation, identical surgical dressings are used for all patients, and the assessment of recovery is carried out by another person who is not aware of treatment allocation.

## 4. Are all the patients accounted for at the conclusion?

The process of randomization gives us comparable groups at the start of a trial, but results are only valid if we can account for all these patients at the end of the trial. Therefore, once randomized, a patient should be included in the analysis of that group even if he or she discontinues therapy, crosses over or never receives treatment. Loss of patients to follow up or exclusion of patients from the analysis can lead to bias. Some losses may occur even in the best quality studies, but this should not differ between groups, should be of similar types of patients and should not exceed the outcome event rate. Loss to follow-up of more than 20 per cent of recruits poses a serious threat to the validity of a study.

Intention to treat (ITT analysis) of RCTs ensures that comparisons of effects of care are made only between patients in the groups to which they were originally randomly allocated. ITT analysis includes all patients regardless of the treatment actually received or subsequent withdrawal or deviation from the protocol. Some treatments may result in large numbers of drop-outs, for example if side effects are unpleasant. Failure to account for these when examining interventions may cause false conclusions to be reached. These attritional issues are central to the generalizability of a treatment's final effect in clinical practice.

## 5. Are these findings important?

The analysis of RCTs is often a simple comparison of percentages. The difference in the event rate (outcome of interest) in the treatment group compared to that in the comparison group is:

> Control event rate (%) – experimental event rate (%)
> = absolute risk reduction or risk difference (%)

If an effect is seen in a trial, the final question is: 'Could this difference have arisen by chance?'. In general, it is accepted that there is a 5 per cent chance of our concluding that there is a difference when in fact there is not – a 5 per cent chance of making a type 1 error – and hence we use a 95 per cent confidence interval (95% CI). Also, by convention we accept an 80 per cent chance that we will detect a difference if one exists (this is the 'power' of a study). Increasing the number of patients in a study will reduce the chance of either error or increase the certainty of our estimates. The chance of these errors is also related to the size of difference we want to detect (we will need a larger study to detect a small difference between the two groups) and the frequency of the event (evaluating a very rare outcome such as occurs in 1:1000 people will need more people than an outcome that occurs in 1:100 or 1:10 people).

Confidence intervals can be calculated for this risk difference. The CI estimates the range of values likely to include the 'true' value. Usually, we use 95 per cent CIs.

Finally, if you have a result that suggests a significant difference in outcome between two groups, you may want to consider what this means in practice. An alternative way of expressing this difference is the 'number needed to treat' (NNT). The NNT is simply 1 divided by the absolute risk reduction.

## STEP 4. INTEGRATING THE EVIDENCE

If you have found valid research with important findings that address your clinical question, the next step is to consider if these results apply to your individual patient.[1] Two questions to consider are:

1 Is your patient so different from those in the trial that the results cannot help you?
2 Do the findings fit with your patient's preferences and values?

One of the consistent findings of health services research is the gap between research evidence and practice.[12] It is a challenge for clinicians to keep up to date, but perhaps even harder is the challenge to alter established patterns of care. This can be a challenge for individuals, but also for the organizations they work in. If the change required is complex or involves change in the organization and/or patients' attitudes, it is harder to achieve. There is no single strategy for getting research into practice that is sufficient on its own or significantly better than alternative strategies. Therefore a number of approaches are needed.

Research evidence is more likely to influence practice if it confirms our preconceptions.[13] In interpreting research evidence, we also need to be aware of our own biases; we may be less questioning of research evidence that affirms our own beliefs or practice, while scrutinizing more closely the evidence that challenges them.[12]

## STEP 5. AUDIT

This includes two concepts of audit.

1 Audit of your practice of evidence-based medicine – keeping a record of your clinical questions and findings and evaluating how you could do this more efficiently.
2 Clinical audit – measuring whether you are putting the research evidence into practice.

Clinical audit is a process that seeks to improve patient care and outcomes through systematic review of care against explicit criteria and the implementation of change.[14] Whereas research is concerned with discovering the right thing to do, audit is concerned with ensuring that the right thing is done. A recent review of the evidence has concluded that audit is an effective method of improving the quality of care.[15]

The same review also describes the audit methods associated with successful audit projects.

Audit may evaluate the structure (organization or provision) of services, the process of care or the outcome of care against an agreed standard. For example, research evidence suggests that the outcome for patients with ovarian cancer is better if they are operated on by an appropriately trained gynaecologist and managed within the framework of a multidisciplinary team. An audit of the referral and management of patients with ovarian cancer can provide an overview of service provision in this area.

*Process measures* are clinical practices that have been evaluated in research and been shown to have an influence on outcome. For example, the use of antenatal steroids has improved perinatal outcome; evaluation of this process of care would entail measuring the proportion of appropriate cases that received antenatal steroids.

An *outcome measure* is the physical or behavioural response to an intervention, for example the health status (dead or alive), cure following surgery for stress incontinence, level of knowledge or satisfaction (e.g. users' views on the care they have received). Outcomes can be desirable, for example improvement in the patient's condition or quality of life, or undesirable, e.g. side effects of a treatment. The assessment of outcomes such as cancer survival rates is fundamental to measuring quality of care. Outcomes are not a direct measure of the care provided (e.g. social and health inequalities may contribute to variation in mortality rates); therefore, mechanisms to account for these differences are required (e.g. case-mix adjustment for co-morbidity). Outcomes may be delayed, and not all patients who experience substandard care will have a poor outcome. Outcome measures such as mortality and morbidity are nevertheless important, and this is a major justification for regular monitoring. 'Critical incident' or 'adverse event' reporting involves the identification of patients who have experienced an adverse event (e.g. Confidential Enquiries Maternal and Child Health (CEMACH), now part of the Centre for Maternal and Child Enquiries (CMACE), and National Confidential Enquiry into Patient Outcome and Deaths (NCEPOD)).

## Undertaking audit

Audit can be considered to have five principal steps (commonly referred to as the audit cycle):

1  selection of a topic,
2  identification of an appropriate standard,
3  data collection to assess performance against the pre-specified standard,
4  implementation of changes to improve care, if necessary,
5  data collection for a second, or subsequent, time to determine whether care has improved.

Audit projects require a multidisciplinary approach, with involvement of stakeholders (including consumers or users

of the service provided) and the local audit department at the planning stage. Good planning and resources are also necessary to ensure their success.

It is essential to establish clear aims and objectives when choosing what to audit, so that the audit is focused towards addressing specific issues within the selected topic. A key consideration is: 'How will we use the results of this audit to change or improve practice?' Priority should be given to common health problems, areas associated with high rates of mortality, morbidity or disability, and those for which good research evidence is available to inform practice or aspects of care that use considerable resources. It is important to involve those who will be implementing change at this stage of the audit process.

In audit, review criteria are generally used for assessing care. The criterion is the reference point against which current practice is measured. The first four steps above should be the starting point for developing criteria. Review criteria should be explicit rather than implicit and need to lead to valid judgements about the quality of care, and relate to aspects of care that are important to patients or impact on clinical outcomes.

The standard/target level of performance is defined as 'the percentage of events that should comply with the criterion' (e.g. the proportion of women delivered by caesarean section who received thromboprophylaxis, or the proportion of women with dysfunctional uterine bleeding who were offered transcervical resection of the endometrium (TCRE) or endometrial ablation). 'Benchmarking' is defined as the 'process of defining a level of care set as a goal to be attained'. There is insufficient evidence to determine whether it is necessary to set target levels of performance in audit.

## Data collection

Data collection in criterion-based audit is generally undertaken to determine the proportion of cases in which care is in accordance with the criteria. In practice, the following points need to be considered.

Consideration needs to be given to which data items are needed in order to answer the audit question. For example, if undertaking an audit on caesarean section rates, collecting information on the number of caesarean sections alone will not give sufficient information to measure the caesarean section rate. Data on the number of other births that took place are also required. Definitions need to be clear so that there is no confusion about what is being collected. For example, if collecting data on rupture of membranes, it may need to be specified whether this is spontaneous or artificial.

Data collectors should always be aware of their responsibilities to the Data Protection Act and any locally agreed guidelines. Under the current Data Protection Act, it is an offence to collect personal details of patients such as names, addresses or other items that are potentially identifiable for the individual without consent. Data storage needs to be secure and safe. There seems to be consensus that clinical audit is part of direct patient care and therefore consent to the use of data for audit can be implied through consent to treatment provided patients are informed that their data may be used in this way. It is rarely acceptable to use patient identifiers such as names and addresses; however, some form of pseudoanonymized identifiers should be used. Audit project protocols should be submitted to the local Research and Development Committee and Ethics Committees to seek approval, if necessary. Guidance on how to do this can be obtained from the respective bodies.

Routinely collected data can be used if all the data items required are available. It will be necessary to check the definitions for data items that are used within the routine database to ensure its usefulness for the aims of the audit. Also, the completeness and coverage of the routine source need to be known. Where the data source is clinical records, the training of data abstractors and the use of a standard proforma can improve the accuracy and reliability of data collection. The use of multiple sources of data may also be helpful; however, this can also be problematic, as it will require linking of data from different sources with common unique identifiers.

## Questionnaires

Questionnaires are often used as a tool for data collection. Questions may be open or closed. Generally, questionnaire design using open questions (e.g. 'What was the indication for caesarean section?', followed by space for free text response) is easier, but analysis of these data is difficult, as there will be a range of responses and interpretation can be problematic. Open questions may be more difficult and time consuming to answer and can lead to non-response resulting in loss of data.

Questionnaires can be composed entirely of closed questions (i.e. with all possible answers predetermined). More time needs to be spent in developing this type of questionnaire, but the analysis is generally easier. The following is an example of this.[16]

Which of the following statements most accurately describes the urgency of this caesarean section?

- Immediate threat to the life of the fetus and the mother.
- Maternal or fetal compromise that is not immediately life threatening.
- No maternal or fetal compromise but needs early delivery.
- Delivery timed to suit the woman and staff.

Closed questions assume that all possible answers to the question are known but not the distribution of responses. Time and consideration need to be given to the options available for response, because, if a desired response is not available, the question may just be missed out and it may put people off completing the rest of the questionnaire. The 'other' category can be used with the option 'please specify', which gives an opportunity for the respondent to write in a response. However, if this is used, thought must be given *a priori* as to how these free text responses will be coded and analysed. In some situations, not having an 'other' category may lead to the question not being answered at all, which means data will be lost.

If questionnaires are developed for a specific project, they need to be piloted and refined to ensure their validity and reliability before use as a tool for data collection. While those who developed the questionnaire understand the questions being asked, the aim of piloting is to check that those who have to fill in the questionnaire are able to understand and respond with ease. Questionnaires that are not user friendly are associated with lower response rates, the quality of data collected will be poor, and hence the results will be of little value.

## Who collects the data?

Thought also needs to be given to who is going to collect the data, as well as to the time and resources that will be involved. In small audit projects, it may be feasible for the principal investigators to go through clinical notes for data abstraction. However, for larger projects, e.g. a prospective audit on induction of labour practices within a maternity unit, it may be more appropriate for those involved in the care of the women giving birth (e.g. midwives or obstetricians) to fill in standard data collection sheets. Where available, audit support staff should be involved.

## Analysing the data

Data that are collected on paper forms are usually entered onto electronic databases or spreadsheets, such as Microsoft Access, Epi Info or Excel, for cleaning and analysis. Data entry may be done by Optical Character Recognition (OCR) software, Optical Mark Readers (OMR) or manually. Optical character recognition is most accurate for questionnaire data using tick boxes, but less accurate for free text responses. The method of data entry needs to be taken into account when designing the questionnaire or data collection sheet. For manual data entry, accuracy is improved if double data entry is used. However, this can be a time-consuming exercise. If the facilities and resources are available, electronic collection of data can be considered. In this case, data are entered immediately at source into a computer and saved onto disks. While this is quick and requires minimal storage space, it can be difficult to handle unexpected responses. As information is entered directly into a computer, it cannot be verified or double-entered.

Consideration also needs to be given to the coding of responses on the database. For ease of analysis of closed questions, it is generally better to have numeric codes for responses. For example, yes/no responses can be coded to take the value 0 for no and 1 for yes. Missing data will also need to be coded, for example with the number 9. The code

General

assigned for missing data should be distinguished from the code used when the response is 'not known' (if this was an option on the questionnaire). It is advisable to incorporate consistency checks as data are being entered to minimize errors.

Simple statistics are often all that is required. Statistical methods are used to summarize data for presentation in the form of summary statistics (means, medians or percentages) and graphs. Statistical tests are used to find out the likelihood that the data obtained have arisen by chance, and how likely it is that a real difference exists between two groups. Before data collection has started, it is essential to know what data items will be collected, whether comparisons will be made, and the statistical methods that will be used to make these comparisons.[17]

Data items that have categorical responses (e.g. yes/no or A/B/C/D) can be expressed as percentages. Some data items are collected as continuous variables, for example mother's age, height and weight. These can either be categorized into relevant categories and then expressed as percentages or, if they are normally distributed (bell-shaped curve), the mean and standard deviations may be reported. If they are not normally distributed, a median and range can be used. These summary statistics (percentages and means) are useful for describing the process, outcome or service provision that was measured.

Comparisons of percentages between different groups can be made using a $\chi^2$ test. T tests can be used to compare means between two groups, assuming these are normally distributed. Non-parametric statistical methods can be used for data that are non-normally distributed. These comparisons are useful in order to determine if there are any real differences in the observed findings, for example when comparing audit results obtained at different time points or in different settings. In some situations, a sample size calculation may be necessary to ensure that the audit is large enough to detect a clinically significant difference between groups if one exists. In this situation, it is important to consult a statistician during the planning stages of the audit project. These simple statistics can be easily done on Microsoft Excel spreadsheets and Access databases. Other useful statistical software packages include Epi Info, SAS, SPSS, STATA and Minitab.

## Implementation of findings

Data analysis and interpretation will lead to the identification of areas of clinical practice that need to change. Several methods may be needed to ensure this change takes place, but simple strategies such as feeding back findings are sometimes effective. Change does not always occur in audit, and consideration of the reasons for failure may take place after the second data collection. Resistance to change among local professionals or in the organizational environment or team should be considered. Patients themselves may have preferences for care that make change difficult.

## GLOSSARY OF TERMS

**Auditable standard** An agreed standard against which practice can be assessed.

**Case–control study** The study reviews exposures or risk factors, comparing the exposure in people who have the outcome of interest, for example the disease or condition (i.e. the cases), with patients from the same population who do not have the outcome (i.e. controls).

**Cohort study** The study involves the identification of two groups (cohorts) of patients, one of which has received the exposure of interest and one of which has not. These groups are followed forward to see if they develop the outcome (i.e. the disease or condition) of interest.

**Confounder** A factor that may offer an alternative explanation for the observed association between an exposure and the outcome of interest.

**Cross-sectional study** The observation of a defined population at a single point in time or time interval. Exposure and outcome are determined simultaneously.

**Denominator data** Data describing the population within which a study group has been identified (e.g. in a hospital study of caesarean section the denominator data refer to every birth that occurred within the unit during the audited period, irrespective of the type of delivery that was undertaken).

**Mean** This is the summary statistic used when the data follow a normal distribution. It is the sum of all the values divided by the number of values. The standard deviation gives a measure of the spread of individual values about the mean.

**Median** If the data are arranged in an increasing order, the middle value is the median. The range is the difference between the largest and smallest values. The interquartile range (IQR) is the difference between the bottom quarter and top quarter of the data. This is the summary statistic used when the data are not normally distributed.

**Meta-analysis** An overview of a group of studies that uses quantitative methods to produce a summary of the results.

**Number needed to treat** This is the number of patients who need to be treated to prevent one outcome.

**Odds ratio** This describes the odds that a case (a person with the condition) has been exposed to a risk factor relative to the odds that a control (a person without the condition) has been exposed to the risk. The crude odds ratio describes the association without taking into consideration the possible effect of any confounders. Adjusted odds ratios describe the association having been adjusted for the effect of confounders.

**Positive predictive value** This describes the percentage of people who have a positive test who really have the condition. The predictive value is dependent upon the prevalence of the disease in the population being tested, i.e. if the disease is rare, the predictive value is low, due to the greater influence of false-positive tests.

**Randomized, controlled trial** A group of patients is randomized into an experimental group and a control group. These groups are followed up for the variables and outcomes of interest. This study is similar to a cohort study, but the exposure is randomly assigned. Randomization should ensure that both groups are equivalent in all aspects except for the exposure of interest.

**Risk difference** The difference in risk of developing the outcome of interest between the exposed and control groups.

**Risk ratio** Risk is a proportion or percentage. The risk ratio is the ratio of risk of developing the outcome of interest in an exposed group compared with the risk of developing the same outcome in the control group. It is used in RCTs and cohort studies.

**Sensitivity** The ability of a test to detect those who have the disease, i.e. the proportion (percentage) of people with the condition who are detected as having it by the test.

**Specificity** The ability of the test to identify those without the disease, i.e. the proportion of people without the condition who are correctly reassured by a negative test.

**Systematic review** A literature review that aims to minimize bias and random errors by using a system that is documented in a materials and methods section, and which may or may not include meta-analysis.

## Key References

1. Straus SE, Richardson WS, Paul Glasziou, Haynes RB. *Evidence-based Medicine: How to Practice and Teach EBM*, 3rd edn. Oxford: Churchill Livingstone: 2005.
2. EPIQ (Effective Practice, Informatics and Quality Improvement). Professor Rod Jackson, Head of the Section of Epidemiology and Biostatistics, University of Auckland: available from ‹http://fmhs.auckland.ac.nz/soph/depts/epi/epiq/ebp.aspx›.
3. Royal College of Obstetricians and Gynaecologists. Searching for Evidence. Clinical Governance Advice No. 3. London: RCOG Press, 2001.
4. Khan KS, Kuntz R, Kleijnen J, Antes G. Systematic reviews to support evidence based medicine. *How to Review and Apply Findings of Healthcare Research*. London: Royal Society of Medicine Press, 2003.
5. Guyatt GH for the GRADE Working Group. Rating quality of evidence and strength of recommendations GRADE: an emerging consensus on rating quality of evidence and strength of recommendations. *BMJ* 2008; **336**: 924–6.
6. Guyatt GH for the GRADE Working Group. Rating quality of evidence and strength of recommendations: What is "quality of evidence" and why is it important to clinicians? *BMJ* 2008; **336**: 995–8.
7. Guyatt GH *et al.* for the GRADE Working Group. Rating quality of evidence and strength of recommendations: Going from evidence to recommendations. *BMJ* 2008; **336**: 1049–51.
8. NHS Evidence – National Library of Guidelines Appraisal of guidelines research and evaluation. Available from: http:// library.nhs.uk/guidelinesFinder/Page.aspx? pagename=APPRAISAL
9. Schulz KF, Altman DG, Moher D for the CONSORT Group. CONSORT 2010 Statement. Updated guidelines for reporting parallel group randomized trials. *BMJ* 2010; **340**: c332.
10. Moher D, Liberati A, Tetzlaff J, Altman DG for the PRISMA Group. Preferred reporting items for systematic reviews and meta-analyses: the PRISMA statement. *BMJ* 2009; **339**: 332–6.
11. Bossuyt PM, Reitsma JB, Bruns DE *et al.* Towards complete and accurate reporting of studies of diagnostic accuracy: the STARD initiative. Standards for Reporting of Diagnostic Accuracy. *BMJ* 2003; **326**: 41–4.
12. Grol R, Grimshaw J. From best evidence to best practice: effective implementation of change in patients' care. *Lancet* 2003; **362**: 1225–30.
13. Kaptchuk EJ. Effect of interpretive bias on research evidence. *BMJ* 2003; **326**: 1453–5.
14. Royal College of Obstetricians and Gynaecologists. *Understanding Audit.* Clinical Governance Advice No. 5. London: RCOG Press, 2003.
15. NHS, National Institute for Clinical Excellence, Commission for Health Improvement, Royal College of Nursing, University of Leicester. *Review of the Evidence. Principles for Best Practice in Clinical Audit.* London: National Institute for Clinical Excellence, 2002.
16. Thomas J, Paranjothy S; Royal College of Obstetricians and Gynaecologists: Clinical Effectiveness Support Unit. *The National Sentinel Caesarean Section Audit Report.* London: RCOG Press, 2001.
17. Brocklehurst P, Gates S. Statistics. In: O'Brien PMS, Broughton PF (eds). *Introduction to Research Methodology for Specialists and Trainees.* London: RCOG Press, 1999: 147–60.

# The general principles of surgery

*Fiona M Reid and Anthony RB Smith*

## INTRODUCTION

'Choose well, cut well, get well'. Surgery has three phases. In the pre-operative phase the correct operation should be chosen for a patient, who should be in an optimal condition. A well-trained, competent surgeon should then perform the surgery in a safe environment. During the post-operative phase, the patient should be monitored, encouraged and advised. Each phase is equally important. These are the basic principles of surgery, and this chapter examines how they may be achieved.

## THE PRE-OPERATIVE PHASE

There is always more than one treatment option and it is the role of a gynaecologist to counsel the patient about the appropriate options. The process of selecting the best procedure for a patient is inseparable from that of obtaining informed consent. A booklet of guidelines to obtaining consent is available from the General Medical Council or on the internet at ‹www.gmc-uk.org/standards›.

When counselling patients about treatment options, effective communication is imperative. This may necessitate the use of written material or visual aids. It may require the use of interpreters for foreign or sign language. Preferably, interpreters should be independent professionals and not family members who could have a vested interest in a particular treatment.

Patients should be informed of the advantages and disadvantages of each procedure, the success rates, failure rates, side effects and common complications. Risk should be quantified rather than being described subjectively with terms such as 'slight' or 'rare'.

Increasingly, the adequacy of consent is assessed legally by the concept of 'material risk'. A risk is material if:

*In the circumstances of the case, a reasonable person in the patient's position, if warned of the risk, would be likely to attach significance to it or if the medical practitioner is, or should reasonably be aware that the*

*particular patient if warned of the risk, would be likely to attach significance to it.*[1]

In practice, this implies that even rare complications that are serious or that carry significance to an individual's social life or employment should be addressed.

Patients should have adequate time to reflect on the information they have been given prior to making a decision. It should not be assumed that a patient understands the general risks of surgery, such as anaesthetic complications.

The General Medical Council's guidelines on informed consent state that ultimately it is the responsibility of the person performing the procedure to ensure informed consent has been obtained.

### Optimizing pre-operative health

Although most gynaecological surgery is performed on relatively healthy women, it is imperative that all patients undergoing surgery are in their optimum condition. Smokers should be encouraged to stop at least 24 hours before surgery to reduce the level of carboxyhaemoglobin in the blood and minimize the cardiovascular effect of nicotine.[2] Screening for sexually transmitted diseases or bacterial vaginosis prior to pelvic procedures should be considered.[3]

Basic pre-operative screening involves a detailed history and a general examination. Routine screening blood tests have not been shown to influence cancellations or perioperative complications, and the majority of abnormal results could have been predicted from the history and examination.[4] A study by Golub *et al.*[5] in the USA demonstrated that avoiding batteries of routine pre-operative tests could save US$397 per patient.

Ideally, pre-operative investigations should be specific to each individual. Even routine sickle testing of at-risk adults has been challenged because patients with sickle cell disease would already have been detected as children due to chronic haemolytic anaemia. Also, no sickling complications have been reported in sickle cell trait patients for the past 15 years.[6]

The morbidity and mortality of surgery and anaesthesia are increased in patients with co-existing disease (Table 2.1).[7]

**Table 2.1** Medical conditions most commonly associated with increased surgical morbidity

| Ischaemic heart disease |
| Congestive cardiac failure |
| Arterial hypertension |
| Chronic respiratory disease |
| Diabetes mellitus |
| Cardiac arrhythmia |
| Anaemia |

**Table 2.2** The American Society of Anesthesiologists' (ASA) physical status classification system

| ASA 1 | Normal healthy patient |
|---|---|
| ASA 2 | Patient with mild controlled systemic disease which does not affect normal activity |
| ASA 3 | Patient with severe systemic disease which limits activity |
| ASA 4 | Patient with severe systemic disease which is incapacitating and is a constant threat to life |
| ASA 5 | Moribund patient not expected to survive 24 hours with or without operation |

Elective surgery should be delayed for six months after a myocardial infarct because 35 per cent will re-infarct before three months and this risk falls to 4 per cent after six months.[8] Of the deaths reported in the National Confidential Enquiries into Perioperative Deaths (NCEPOD) Report 2001, 60 per cent of patients had ischaemic heart disease.[9] The history is as important as the investigations: a pre-operative electrocardiogram (ECG) on patients with proven ischaemia will be normal in 20–50 per cent of cases.[10]

Protocols should be available on the ward for the management of common conditions such as diabetes mellitus.

It is the surgeon's responsibility to liaise with the anaesthetist and other specialties if patients have concurrent illness. At times it can be difficult to convey the complexity of a patient's condition, and the American Society of Anesthesiologists (ASA) scoring system[11] can be a useful communication tool (Table 2.2).

Venous thrombosis embolism (VTE) is one of the most serious complications of surgery, and all units should have clear protocols for thromboprophylaxis. NICE guidance CG46 2007[12] recommends that the risk of thromboembolism should be assessed in all patients. Risk factors are shown in Table 2.3. Risk assessment is summarized in Table 2.4 and prophylaxis should be prescribed according to risk (Table 2.5). The incidence of deep venous thrombosis (DVT) without prophylaxis in gynaecological surgery is estimated to be 16 per cent (95 per cent CI 13–19).[12]

**Table 2.3** Patient-related risk factors of venous thromboembolism

| Active cancer or cancer treatment |
| Active heart disease or respiratory failure |
| Acute medical illness |
| Age over 60 years |
| Antiphospholipid syndrome |
| Behçet's disease |
| Central venous catheter in situ |
| Continuous travel more than 3 hours approximately 4 weeks before surgery |
| Immobility (e.g. greater than 3 days bed rest) |
| Inflammatory bowel disease |
| Myeloproliferative disease |
| Nephrotic syndrome |
| Obesity (BMI>30) |
| Paraproteinaemia |
| Paroxysmal nocturnal haemoglobinuria |
| Personal or family history of VTE |
| Pregnancy or puerperium |
| Recent myocardial infarct or stroke |
| Severe infection |
| Use of oral contraception or HRT |
| Varicose veins associated with phlebitis |
| Inherited thrombophilias |

**Table 2.4** Stratification of risk factors for venous thromboembolism

| Risk | Patient group |
|---|---|
| Low | Minor surgery (<60 min); no risk factors other than age >60 years |
| Medium | Minor surgery (<60 min); age <60 years with one or more risk factors |
| | Major surgery; age <60 years; no additional risk factors |
| High | Minor surgery; age >60 years with additional risk factors |
| | Major surgery; age <60 years with additional risk factors |
| | Major surgery; age >60 years; No additional risk factors |

The Department of Health has recommended that all patients undergoing elective surgery should be screened pre-operatively for methicillin-resistant staphylococcus aureus (MRSA).[13,14] All patients with positive skin screen for MRSA should undergo skin decolonization therapy with recommended skin wash. For procedures that require

**Table 2.5** Recommended prophylaxis thrombo

| Low risk | Medium risk | High risk |
|---|---|---|
| Early mobilization | Early mobilization | Early mobilization |
| AND | AND | AND |
| Knee length graduated compression stockings | Knee length graduated compression stockings | Knee length graduated compression stockings |
| Immediately pre-op | Immediately pre-op | Immediately pre-op |
| Continue until discharge | Continue until discharge | Continue until discharge |
| | AND | AND |
| | Intermittent pneumatic compression if operation >60 minutes | Intermittent pneumatic compression if operation >60 minutes |
| | AND | AND |
| | LMWH starting 6 p.m. evening before theatre if possible | LMWH (consider higher dose) starting 6 p.m. evening before theatre if possible |
| | Continue until discharge | Continue until discharge |

antibiotic prophylaxis, patients with current or previous MRSA colonization should receive teicoplanin or vancomycin intravenously.

## KEY POINTS

### Consent

- Selecting the best procedure is inseparable from gaining informed consent.
- It is the operator's responsibility to ensure that informed consent has been obtained.
- Effective communication is imperative: interpreters or visual aids may be necessary.
- Patients should receive detailed information on benefits and risks.
- Patients should have adequate time to reflect on this information.

### Optimizing pre-operative health

- Smoking should be stopped 24 hours before surgery.
- Combined oral contraceptives should be stopped one month before major surgery.
- Pre-operative screening should be by history and examination; routine blood tests are rarely helpful.
- Routine surgery should be delayed for six months after myocardial infarction.
- If there is concurrent illness, liaison with the anaesthetist and other specialists is essential.
- All units should have clear protocols for thromboprophylaxis.
- All patients undergoing elective surgery should be screened for MRSA.

## INTRAOPERATIVE CARE

A full knowledge of abdominal and pelvic anatomy is essential for gynaecological surgery. In cases in which the anatomy is distorted, the surgeon should attempt to restore normal anatomy and work from first principles. Tissue planes should be utilized and tissues should be handled gently. Many gynaecologists gain most of their early surgical experience in the obstetric theatre, where speed tends to be valued above all else. Technique should be valued above speed.

Adequate access is essential. A senior surgeon called to a difficult case often first improves access. This includes good bowel packing.

Asepsis is obviously important; however, some aseptic practices are traditions and are not based on evidence. Pre-operative shaving, for example, is aesthetic to the surgeon and allows for the painless removal of the dressing post-operatively, but it does not appear to alter wound infection rates.[15] The use of a single dose of prophylactic antibiotics to prevent wound infection or septicaemia is now widely accepted.[16] However, prolonged courses of antibiotics or use of unnecessary antibiotics should be avoided due to the risk of *Clostridium difficile* infection.

NICE has recently published guidance stating that antimicrobial prophylaxis against infective endocarditis is not required in patients undergoing urological, gynaecological and obstetric procedures where infection is not already present.[17] If infection is present then patients at high risk of endocarditis should receive antibiotics to cover the organisms which cause infective endocarditis. Patients considered to be at risk of infective endocarditis are shown in Table 2.6.

**Table 2.6** Adults at risk of infective endocarditis

| |
|---|
| Acquired valvular heart disease |
| Valve replacement |
| Structural congenital heart disease, including surgically corrected defects, but excluding isolated atrial septal defects, fully repaired ventricular septal defects or fully repaired patent ductus arteriosus, and closed devices that are judged to be epithelialized |
| Hypertrophic cardiomyopathy |
| Previous infective endocarditis |

Facemasks in general abdominal surgery and certainly in laparoscopic procedures do not appear to affect infection rates. However, eye protection or face shields to protect the surgeon's mucous membranes from the patient's bodily fluids are sensible. Without serum testing, it is impossible to know if a patient has hepatitis or human immunodeficiency virus (HIV) and therefore all patients are a potential risk. All healthcare workers should be immunized against hepatitis B. Cotton gowns provide protection of one's nakedness only!

Drains may be used if clinically indicated and not as an alternative to good haemostasis. There is no robust evidence to support their use. A drain is probably advisable when a urinary tract injury has been repaired, in case of urinary leakage. Possible complications of drains include trauma during insertion, blockage, infection, erosion of adjacent tissue and retention of a foreign body.

# TECHNICAL EQUIPMENT FOR SURGERY

Surgeons should have an understanding of the principles of the equipment they use.

Diathermy involves the passage of electrical current through the patient's body. Electrocution does not occur because the frequency of current used in diathermy is much higher than that of mains electricity. Mains electricity is a low-frequency alternating current (50 Hz in the UK). Low-frequency currents cause depolarization and neuromuscular stimulation. Diathermy utilizes a very high frequency (400 kHz to 10 MHz) alternating current. It does not cause depolarization but it does excite ions, and this causes heat, particularly when in a high-density form.

In monopolar diathermy, the active electrodes and the return electrode are some distance apart. In bipolar diathermy, the two electrodes are only millimetres apart.

Factors that influence the diathermy effect are current density, the resistance of the tissue, the waveform and the duration of activation.

At high current density, heat is produced. The size of the electrode influences current density. At the tip of an active electrode, the current density is high, and therefore heat is generated. The return electrode's surface area is large, so the current density is low and no heating occurs.

The resistance of tissues is indirectly proportional to their water content: higher water content reduces resistance. Tissues with high resistance require a higher output (watts), from the diathermy generator, to generate heat.

Cutting is achieved by using a low voltage but a high frequency current that is constantly flowing. The current is concentrated in a very small area and the high energy level causes so much ion excitation that the cells explode, releasing steam. If coagulation is required, an intermittent high-voltage current is used, with current flowing for only 6 per cent of the time. Thus, a cutting current is inherently safer because of the lower voltage reducing the risk of inadvertent current discharge.

The safety of diathermy systems is continually improving. Initially, grounded generators were used, whereby current could return to ground via the path of least resistance. Since 1968, solid-state isolated generators have been used. These avoid burns at other sites such as drip stands because current will not flow unless current is returning to the generator. However, return electrode burns can still occur if the pad is not attached completely. Systems of contact quality monitoring have been available since the 1980s to prevent return electrode burns.

There are some specific hazards related to electrosurgery in laparoscopic procedures.

Direct coupling is the inadvertent flow of current from one instrument to another and may be secondary to insulation failure. Insulation failure can result from damaged equipment or the use of excessive voltage with coagulation current. Capacitance coupling can occur if a capacitor is created. Two conductors separated by an insulator form a capacitor, for example an insulated laparoscopic instrument passing through a metal port. The current stored in the capacitor can discharge into the patient, causing burns. The higher the current passing through the instrument, the greater will be the capacitance current. Plastic ports do not eliminate the risk of capacitance coupling because the patient's bowel or omentum can act as the second conductor. Capacitance coupling can be avoided with active electrode monitoring systems.

Other causes of diathermy burns are careless technique, not checking the dial setting before use, the use of spirit-based

## KEY POINTS

### Intraoperative care
- Technique should be valued above speed.
- Adequate access is essential.
- Asepsis is important, but some practices are not evidence based.
- Single-dose antibiotic prophylaxis is now widely accepted.
- All patients are a potential risk and all healthcare workers should be immunized against hepatitis B.
- Drains should be used only when clinically indicated.
- Surgeons should understand the principles of the equipment they use: this applies particularly to diathermy.

skin preparation near diathermy, or someone other than the surgeon activating the current flow.

More detailed explanations of the principles of diathermy are available at an interactive website: ‹www.valleylabeducation.org›.

# Minimal access surgery

*Diseases that harm call for treatments that harm less.*

William Osler (1849–1919)

The most common endoscopic techniques used in gynaecology are laparoscopy and hysteroscopy.

## Laparoscopy

The possible benefits of laparoscopy are shown in Table 2.7. Many of these purported benefits have not undergone robust analysis. In a randomized trial of open versus laparoscopic colposuspension, in which the patients were blinded to the type of surgery, there was no significant difference in the length of hospital stay, but the laparoscopic group returned to normal activities significantly earlier than the open group.[18]

Many complications specific to laparoscopic surgery are related to the method of entry into the peritoneal cavity. The risk is as great for a diagnostic laparoscopy as it is for a major operative laparoscopic procedure.[19] The risk of bowel injury is 0.4–3 per 1000 and of vascular injury 0.2–1 per 1000 laparoscopies.[20] Bowel adhesions to the anterior abdominal wall occur in 0.5 per cent of patients with no previous surgery, increasing to 20 per cent if they have had a previous pfannenstiel incision and to 50 per cent if they have had a midline incision.[21] To minimize this risk, safe entry techniques have been recommended (Table 2.8). Open laparoscopy has been advocated, particularly by general surgeons, because it appears to reduce the risk of vascular injury, but it does not reduce the risk of bowel

**Table 2.7** Benefits of laparoscopy

| Patients |
| --- |
| Less pain[17] |
| Less blood loss[17,18] |
| Less scarring |
| Quicker recovery[17] |
| **Surgeon** |
| Safer 'closed/no touch surgery' |
| Better display of anatomy |
| **Healthcare providers** |
| Reduced in-patient stay |
| Reduced social cost |

**Table 2.8** A safe entry technique for laparoscopy

| |
| --- |
| The patient should be lying flat |
| Ensure the bladder is empty and check the abdomen for masses |
| Make the primary incision at the base of the umbilicus |
| Insert the Veress needle through the base of the umbilicus, sensing a double click |
| Insert 2–3 mL of saline through the Veress: it should run in freely |
| Aspirate back: nothing should be aspirated |
| Fill with $CO_2$ to a pressure of 25 mmHg |
| Repeat the saline test |
| Insert the primary trocar |

injury. Microlaparoscopy at Palmers point can also be used. Published recommendations on safe entry are formed from expert opinion [E],[20] not clinical trials, because the number of subjects required to perform trials to investigate entry techniques is prohibitively large.

## Hysteroscopy

This common procedure has specific safety issues. Distension media for hysteroscopy include carbon dioxide, normal saline or glycine. Water is not used as a distension medium because it is hypo-osmolar and, once absorbed, causes haemolysis.

If intrauterine electrosurgery is to be performed using monopolar equipment, the solution must be non-conductive so that the electrical current is not dissipated. Solutions containing electrolytes can be used with recently developed bipolar electrosurgery equipment.

The complications of hysteroscopy include uterine perforation and fluid absorption. Uterine perforation can be associated with damage to the bowel or intraperitoneal haemorrhage. A high index of suspicion and early recourse to diagnostic laparoscopy are advisable.

Fluid may be absorbed at the time of hysteroscopy. If excessive, it can result in hyponatraemia and hypo-osmolality, clinically characterized by nausea, vomiting, seizures, coma and even death. The amount of fluid absorbed is dependent on the volume infused and the infusion pressure. Owing to the short duration of a diagnostic procedure, excessive fluid retention is unlikely to be a problem.

Large-volume fluid absorption is most likely when large vessels are opened at endometrial resection. The main precaution to avoid excessive absorption is accurate measurement of the fluid deficit throughout the procedure.

Fluid absorption increases significantly when the intra-uterine pressure exceeds the mean arterial pressure (MAP). When gravity (the height of the bag) is used to drive the fluid, the lowest pressure (height) to distend the cavity should be used. It should not exceed the MAP. If the giving set contains a drip chamber, the height of the fluid is taken from the drip chamber, but if this fills, the pressure is calculated from the fluid level in the bag.

## KEY POINTS

### Laparoscopy

- Many of the purported benefits have not undergone robust analysis.
- Many of the complications relate to the method of entry into the peritoneal cavity: safe entry techniques, formed from expert opinion, have been published [E].

### Hysteroscopy

- Non-conducting distension media must be used for intra-uterine electrosurgery with monopolar equipment.
- Uterine perforation may occur: a high index of suspicion is needed, with early recourse to laparoscopy.
- Excessive fluid absorption may lead to seizures and even death.
- Accurate measurement of fluid deficit is needed throughout the procedure.

## Local anaesthetic

Two common complications to consider when using local anaesthetic are systemic toxicity and delayed haemorrhage if it is combined with adrenaline. The duration of action and safe dosages are shown in Table 2.9.

Initial symptoms of toxicity are peri-oral paraesthesiae, tinnitus or visual disturbance. These may be followed by convulsions or cardiotoxicity, arrhythmia, complete heart block or cardiac arrest.

## Sedation

A trained doctor should administer sedation. This doctor should be responsible only for administering the sedation and for cardiorespiratory monitoring. He or she should not perform the surgery.

The objective is to produce a level of sedation at which the patient is relaxed, calm and rational, and verbal communication is continuously possible. Sedation can result in unconsciousness or general anaesthesia. Facilities must be available to manage an anaesthetized patient.

All patients should be monitored with a pulse oximeter during sedation. Reversal agents should be avoided as their

**Table 2.9** Properties of local anaesthetic agents

| Agent | Duration of action (hours) | Maxium dosage (mg/kg) | |
|---|---|---|---|
| | | Plain solution | With adrenaline |
| Lignocaine | 1–3 | 3 | 7 |
| Bupivacaine | 1–4 | 2 | 2 |
| Prilocaine | 1–3 | 4 | 8 |

half-life may be shorter than the sedative, leading to delayed respiratory depression. Patients should be observed for at least 2 hours prior to discharge.

## KEY POINTS

### Local anaesthetic

- Common complications of local anaesthetic are systemic toxicity and (if combined with adrenaline) delayed haemorrhage.
- Sedation should be administered by a trained doctor who is not performing the surgery.
- Facilities must be available to manage an anaesthetized patient.
- Patients should be observed for at least 2 hours prior to discharge.

# POST-OPERATIVE CARE

This can be divided into three phases:

1 immediate: theatre recovery;
2 early: until discharge from hospital;
3 late: home.

## Theatre recovery

Airways, breathing and circulation (ABC) are the important parameters immediately after the operation. All staff should maintain life support skills. Up-to-date resuscitation guidelines are available on the internet (‹www.resus.org.uk›). Patients should be stable when they leave the recovery area. This includes the relief of pain.

## Ward care

A doctor should review post-operative patients at least daily. A useful acronym for daily post-operative assessments is SOAP (subjective, objective, assessment, plan) (Table 2.10).

Adequate analgesia should be prescribed. Units can rationalize prescribing using guidelines, for example an analgesic ladder – paracetamol, non-steroidal anti-inflammatory

**Table 2.10** Daily post-operative assessment

| SOAP |
|---|
| Subjective: how does the patient feel? |
| Objective: blood pressure, temperature and fluid balance |
| Assessment: physical examination |
| Plan: plan of care for the next 24 hours |

drugs (NSAIDs), patient-controlled analgesia (PCA)/opioid and epidural.

Fluid balance is important. Most gynaecological patients will tolerate a 'standard fluid recipe' of 2500 mL per day. Careless prescribing can lead to hyponatraemia or pulmonary oedema. Evidence-based practice of post-operative fluid management is sparse and equivocal. Agreement exists that the daily requirements of sodium and potassium are 1 mmol/kg. However, the effects of stress hormones associated with surgery are poorly understood, and electrolytes should be checked every 24–48 hours if a patient remains on intravenous fluids, to guide fluid prescription.

Oliguria is a urine output of less than 20 mL/h in each of 2 consecutive hours. Oliguria due to hypovolaemia may result from:

- active haemorrhage,
- unreplaced blood loss,
- ileus: fluid loss into the gastrointestinal tract,
- loss of plasma into the abdomen,
- oedema.

If fluid balance is difficult, it may require central venous pressure monitoring and transfer to a high dependency unit (HDU) or intensive care unit (ICU). The National CEPOD 2001 enquiry found that 16 per cent of patients were not admitted to ICU/HDU, despite there being a demonstrable need.[9]

Fluids for volume expansion should be blood or colloids. In the management of critically ill patients in intensive care, the TRICC study found that the group managed with a conservative transfusion strategy (Hb 7–9 g/dL) did significantly better than a group given a liberal transfusion management (Hb 10–12 g/dL) in terms of in-hospital mortality, adverse cardiac events, rate of organ dysfunction and overall transfusion rates [D].[22] Further up-to-date guidance on all aspects of blood transfusion can be found at ‹www.transfusionguidelines.org.uk›.

## DISCHARGE

Discharge should be planned. The patient should be aware of normal recovery rates, and be given advice about when to return to work, social activities and sexual intercourse. However, this information is usually based on traditional practice rather than evidence.

The general practitioner (GP) should be informed of the patient's treatment. An effective way to inform GPs is to give a brief discharge letter to the patient to take to the GP, followed by a formal letter. It may be necessary for social services, Macmillan nurses or district nurses to be involved in discharge procedures.

The need for follow-up visits is dependent on the surgery performed. The advantages and disadvantages are listed in Table 2.11.

**Table 2.11** Follow-up clinics

| Advantages |
| --- |
| Audit |
| Proactive detection of complications |
| Provide ongoing treatment |
| Completeness of treatment episode |

| Disadvantages |
| --- |
| Delay in reviewing complication |
| Anxiety waiting for results |
| Time spent seeing well people |
| Cost to the health service |
| Cost to the patient in travel and time off work |

## KEY POINTS

### Postoperative care

**Immediate**
- All staff should maintain life support skills.

**Early**
- A doctor should review patients at least daily.
- Analgesia and fluid balance are important.

**Discharge**
- Patients should be given full advice about recovery rates and activities.
- The GP and, if necessary, other services should be promptly informed.
- Not all procedures require routine follow up.

## DAY CASE SURGERY

There are special considerations to be accounted for in day case surgery, including patient selection and discharge arrangements.

Day surgery units should have clear protocols for patient selection to ensure patient safety and minimize cancellations (Table 2.12): patients should be generally fit and ambulant; they should be able to climb one flight of stairs; they should not be grossly obese (BMI >35).[23]

Day surgery units should have written criteria for patients' discharge.[24,25] Patients should have stable vital signs, be orientated in time and place and able to tolerate oral fluids; they should be able to dress and walk unaided; they must have a responsible and physically able adult to collect them and care for them overnight; they should have adequate analgesia and be aware of the action to take in the event of complications. A contact telephone number should be given for advice after discharge.

**Table 2.12** Common conditions that require further assessment

| |
|---|
| Uncontrolled hypertension, BP >170/100 mmHg |
| Cardiac failure |
| MI/TIA/CVA in past six months |
| Severe asthma/respiratory disease |
| Diabetes – IDDM or poorly controlled NIDDM (BG >11 mmol/L) |
| Renal or hepatic disease |
| Alcoholism or narcotic addiction |
| Advanced multiple sclerosis or myasthenia |
| Severe cervical spondylosis |
| Severe psychiatric disease |
| Drugs: MAOIs, digoxin, steroids, anticoagulants, GTN, diuretics and anti-dysrhythmics |

- BG, blood glucose; BP, blood pressure; CVA, cerebrovascular accident; GTN, glyceryl trinitrate; IDDM, insulin-dependent diabetes mellitus; MAOIs, monoamine oxidase inhibitors; MI, myocardial infarction; NIDDM, non-insulin-dependent diabetes mellitus; TIA, transient ischaemic attack.

## KEY POINTS

There should be:
- clear protocols for patient selection
- written criteria for discharge.

## RISK MANAGEMENT

Risk management is the process of examining procedures to prevent accidents and assessing incidents to prevent recurrence. Some of the most serious mistakes occur from the most simple system errors.

The introduction of simple protocols can avoid common mistakes such as retained swabs and ensure that the correct operation is performed on the correct patient.

The positive impact of a simple surgical check list was demonstrated in a large multinational study. Data on clinical processes and outcomes were collected on 3733 patients undergoing non-cardiac surgery in eight different countries. Following the introduction of a 19-item Surgical Safety Checklist, data were collected on 3955 patients. The death rate was 1.5 per cent before the checklist was introduced and declined to 0.8 per cent afterwards ($p = 0.003$). Inpatient complications occurred in 11 per cent of patients at baseline and in 7 per cent after introduction of the checklist ($p < 0.001$) [C].[26]

Examining 'near misses' is as important as examining actual 'incidents'. Hospitals should have a reporting procedure that is accessible to all staff.

## KEY POINTS

**Risk management**
- Risk can be reduced by simple protocols.
- There should be reporting systems for incidents and 'near-misses'

## CONCLUSIONS

Technicians can perform procedures, while surgeons should orchestrate care.

Surgeons have a responsibility to ensure they are adequately trained, have counselled the patient pre-operatively and are performing the correct operation, and to provide post-operative care.

Audit is important to review practice and should be part of a surgeon's remit. Surgeons must be provided with the time and resources required to audit their practice. League tables of surgical care will only be informative when all aspects of care are included in the assessment. The National Confidential Enquiry into Perioperative Deaths is a national surgical audit that can be found at ‹www.ncepod.org.uk›.

## ACKNOWLEDGEMENT

This chapter was written for the first edition of the book by Fiona M. Reid and Anthony R.B. Smith. It has been updated for this second edition by Fiona M. Reid.

## Key References

1. Rogers vs Whitaker. *CRL* 1992: 479.
2. Jones R. Smoking before surgery: the case for stopping. *BMJ* 1985; **290**: 1763–4.
3. Department of Health. *National Strategy for Sexual Health and HIV*. London: Department of Health, 2001.
4. Johnson H, Knee-Iloi S, Butler T *et al.* Are routine pre-operative laboratory screening tests necessary to evaluate ambulatory surgical patients? *Surgery* 1988; **104**: 639–45.
5. Golub R, Cantu R, Sorrento J *et al.* Efficacy of preadmission testing in ambulatory surgical patients. *Am J Surg* 1992; **163**: 565–71.
6. Wong E-M, Tillyer M, Saunders P. Pre-operative screening for sickle cell trait in adult day surgery; is it necessary? *Ambulatory Surg* 1996; **4**: 41–5.
7. Campling A, Devlin H, Hoile R, Lunn J. *The Report of the National Confidential Enquiry into Perioperative Deaths, 1991/1992*. London: NCEPOD, 1993.
8. Portal R. Elective surgery after myocardial infarction. *BMJ* 1982; **284**: 843–4.
9. National Confidential Enquiry into Perioperative Deaths. Changing the way we operate: National Confidential

Enquiry into Perioperative Deaths. London: NCEPOD, 2001.

10. Jones R. Influence of coexisting disease. In: Kirk R, Mansfield A, Cochrane J (eds). *Clinical Surgery in General*. London: Churchill Livingstone, 1996: 67–83.

11. Robinson P, Hall G. Preoperative assessment. In: *How to Survive in Anaesthesia*. London: BMJ Publishing Group, 1997: 98.

12. NICE. Venous thromboembolism – Reducing the risk of venous thromboembolism (deep vein thrombosis and pulmonary embolism) in inpatients undergoing surgery. NICE guideline CG46 April 2007.

13. Department of Health. Screening for MRSA colonisation – a strategy for NHS Trusts: a summary of best practice. Nov 2006 www.dh.gov.uk/en/publicationsandstatistics/Publications/Publications PolicyAndGuidance/DH_063188.

14. Department of Health. MRSA operational guidance July 2008 DoH www.dh.gov.uk/en/Publicationsandstatistics/Lettersandcirculars/Dearcolleagueletters/DH_086687.

15. Leaper D. Surgical access, incisions and the management of wounds. In: Kirk R, Mansfield A, Cochrane J (eds). *Clinical Surgery in General*. London: Churchill Livingstone, 1996: 201–7.

16. Pollock A. Surgical prophylaxis – the emerging picture. *Lancet* 1988; **1**: 225–30.

17. NICE. Antimicrobial prophylaxis against infective endocarditis. Available from: www.nice.org.uk/CG064

18. Carey M, Rosamilla G, Maher C *et al.* Laparoscopic versus open colposuspension: a prospective multicentre randomised single blind trial. *Neuro Urodyn* 2000; **19**: 389–90.

19. Fatthy H, El Hao M, Samaha I, Abdallah K. Modified Burch colposuspension: laparoscopy versus laparotomy. *J Am Assoc Gynecol Laparoscopists* 2001; **8**: 99–106.

20. Preventing entry related gynaecological laparoscopic injuries. RCOG Green-top guideline No. 49 May 2008.

21. Audebert A, Gomel V. Role of microlaparoscopy in the diagnosis of peritoneal and visceral adhesions and the prevention of bowel injury associated with blind trocar insertion. *Fertil Steril* 2000; **73**: 631–5.

22. Hebert PC, Wells G, Martin C *et al.* A Canadian survey of transfusion practices in critically ill patients. Transfusion Requirements in Critical Care Investigators and the Canadian Critical Care Trials Group. *Crit Care Med* 1998; **26**: 482–7.

23. Millar J, Rudkin G, Hitchcock M. *Practical Anaesthesia and Analgesia for Day Surgery*. Oxford: BIOS Scientific Publishers, 1997.

24. Korttila K. Recovery from outpatient anaesthesia. *Anaesthesia* 1995; **50**(Suppl.): 22–8.

25. Chung F. Discharge criteria – a new trend. *Can J Anaesth* 1995; **42**: 1056–8.

26. Haynes A, Weiser G, Berry W *et al.* A surgical checklist to reduce morbidity and mortality in a global population. *N Engl J Med* 2009; **360**: 491–9.

# Communication and counselling

*Richard Porter*

## INTRODUCTION

Humans communicate in myriad ways. Doctors do not always give the impression of being entirely alert to this. It is possible to be a proficient diagnostician or a highly competent surgeon, or both, and to be a poor communicator with patients. But I would argue that it is not possible to be a good doctor in the modern world without being a good communicator. After all, communication with patients is what principally distinguishes us from veterinary surgeons – with all due respect to veterinary surgeons.

This chapter does not presume to list the methods used in medical schools to improve patient–doctor communication. Medical school (undergraduate) curricula have developed teaching programmes that focus on this topic, and there is a body of academic research that underpins the strategies used by clinicians in eliciting and imparting information from and to patients as effectively as possible. Primary care training rightly regards the teaching of communication skills as one of the most important parts of the introduction of a trainee to general practice. However, in specialist training in obstetrics and gynaecology, one might be forgiven for thinking that there is a belief that the lessons have been adequately learned in medical school, so little formal teaching is given on the topic in many training schemes.

This is, however, being addressed. Recent changes in the examination for membership of the Royal College of Obstetricians and Gynaecologists have introduced OSCE stations that incorporate contact with actors, who indeed give feedback on the standards of the doctors. This is a welcome shift in emphasis, and will no doubt be followed up with many well-designed initiatives – for which there is clearly a real need.

However, it is important to remember that doctors do not only communicate with patients and their relatives. This chapter is an attempt to apply a sideways and personal look at the broader area of communication in clinical practice: communication between doctor and patient, between doctor and doctor, and between doctors and other professionals – in other words, the wider picture.

## COMMUNICATION WITH PATIENTS (AND THEIR RELATIVES AND FRIENDS)

In obstetrics and gynaecology, good communication with patients generally requires:

- *Respect for the patient as an individual.* Even if she holds opinions and beliefs that may not be the same as ours.
- *Respect for women.* In cultures where this is not automatic, it is frequently observed that communication is at a lamentably low level, even when women interact with other women doctors. At its most extreme, women will simply avoid contact with medical services, with dire consequences for health outcomes, such as maternal and perinatal mortality. If an obstetrician/gynaecologist does not respect patients as women, it is difficult to understand why such a doctor remains in this specialty.
- *The ability of the doctor to understand the patient, and the patient to understand the doctor.* Language barriers are not a justification for substandard clinical care on either a medico-legal or a moral level.[1] We may require the use of interpreters, but we must remember that the problem may not just be with the words used. Even when a doctor and a patient ostensibly speak the same language, they may not be using the words in the same way, and this can be a cause of major and potentially dangerous misunderstanding.

- *The ability to listen.* This is not an open-ended commitment: some patients will want to tell us far more than we need, want or have time to hear. But achieving the right balance is essential, and sometimes very challenging.
- *Flexibility.* Any doctor who says that he or she takes a history in the same way under all circumstances is being either extraordinarily naïve or economical with the truth. A good doctor is constantly looking for nuances in the nature of the communication with the patient that will show the way forward in that contact.

## Verbal communication with patients

Assuming that you and the patient are speaking (literally) more or less the same language:

- *Are you using a vocabulary that is appropriate to her?* I well remember watching a brilliant researcher explaining in detail to a totally bemused mother the physics of Doppler wave forms. This was in response to her anxious question – while being scanned at 34 weeks gestation – 'Whassat doing then?'. This was (to be honest) hilarious to watch – but a tragic illustration of the limitations of intelligence.
- *Are you going too fast?* How often do we see colleagues checking with patients, after imparting manageable (bite-sized?) chunks of information, whether or not they have understood? Not nearly often enough, I would predict. If we wait until the end of a long discussion, with masses of pieces of information, can we be surprised if the patient surrenders and says that she has understood – just to make us go away? In fact, I cherish the lesson I learnt from a patient who, after I had explained that she needed her urodynamics repeating (I assumed that she knew what I was talking about because she had had the test before), was asked by the sister when leaving the room, 'So, did you understand all that?', and said loudly (she was a bit deaf), 'Not a word dear'.
- *Are you 'talking down' to her?* In this new era of patients accessing information on the Internet, few things are more likely to raise hackles than giving the impression that you assume that they are ignorant.
- *Are you giving her more information than she wants?* This is one of the most difficult areas in current practice (see Obtaining consent, p.24). How much is enough, and how much too much? In oncology care, this is a particularly important issue, and is beyond the scope of this chapter. The problem is compounded by perceptions about a litigious environment. Yet we must recognize that we have a duty of care to our patients, and that may mean that we should make judgements about the appropriateness or otherwise of imparting every iota of information.
- *Do you recognize the cultural sensitivities influencing her decisions?* In our multi-cultural society, we are becoming better at not trampling on the sensitivities of, for example, women who have religious reasons for not wanting to see men in a medical context, but it is still incumbent upon us to be alert to the possibility of unexpected beliefs and taboos.

## Non-verbal communication with patients

A patient is more often than not in a state of some unease when meeting a doctor, and she will be responding to far more than what is said or not said. The nature of the space where the meeting takes place, the smells of the environment, the extraneous noises – all will influence both her perception of the event and the way in which she takes the information on board. A doctor cannot often immediately influence these factors, but can certainly add to or detract from the experience by means of non-verbal communication. Much of this is a matter of common courtesy, but it is easy to let our standards slip on occasion – and patients notice it, you can be sure. Surely the guiding principle here is that you should act towards your patients exactly as you would wish to be acted towards yourself – and the use of the word 'act' is not accidental, for every contact with a patient is to a degree a theatrical event.

The following are some examples.

- *How do you greet the patient?* Do you stand up? Do you have your back to her when she comes in? Do you shake her hand? Do you invite her to sit? I suspect that we have all seen 'eminent' doctors greet a patient by continuing to talk to medical students. What sort of an impression does that give?
- *What is your facial expression?* A smile, a furrowed brow, a scowl, a dead-pan expression – all will convey some message to the patient. Is the message the one you want to convey? The problem can, of course, get slightly out of hand: the phoney facial expression is just as unsettling as the unthinking one. Think of a politician delivering an unpalatable message with a sanctimonious look. None of us would like to be compared to politicians, I assume.
- *Do you look her in the eye when talking to her, or do you stare at the floor?* This again may reflect your cultural background, or even perhaps your innate modesty, but it may lead to unintended inferences by the patient. Would you propose marriage while looking at the floor? (Of course some might: I am reminded of the schoolmaster who did so by asking his intended if she wanted his surname on her gravestone. Tastes differ…)
- *How do you sit during a consultation?* Are you leaning forward in an attentive pose, or slouching in the chair? Body language is powerful, and can be deeply unsettling for your patient.
- *When you stand (e.g. in a bedside consultation), how far away are you?* Are you too close for the patient's comfort, or are you so far that you give the impression that you regard the patient as another life form? Remember that differences in height – e.g. when you stand over a patient who is lying on a bed – can result in, to put it mildly, unintended distortions in communication.

- *Have you ensured that she is at her ease?* Is she embarrassed (more than is usual) by her state of undress? As ever, the question is: would you or your nearest and dearest want to be treated like this?

I have no doubt that every reader of this chapter can add other examples of good and bad practice that they have encountered in their professional lives. None of us succeeds at all times in making good communication with patients and their families and friends, but we should at least strive to stand back at times and analyse our performance, and to continue to improve.

## Communication with a complaining or angry patient

I personally know of no more challenging area of communication, and this is clearly not an area where 'dry runs' are particularly easy to construct. However, for better or for worse, these situations are becoming more common as patients and their families become more vocal. Good communication can make the difference between a problem that is resolved there and then and one that lingers, often with complex ramifications. The principles of communication are essentially the same as above, but the application of the principles may prove exceedingly difficult. Staying calm may prove to be the most difficult part of the equation.

## COMMUNICATION WITH OTHER STAFF

Although communication with patients is of paramount importance, the issue of communication with other professionals is also crucial. In hospital medicine, there is no such thing as a single-handed department, and dysfunction all too easily follows from poor inter-professional communication.

Any trainee who has worked in a department where rivalries pollute the atmosphere will know how destructive that can be. Many of these problems themselves arise from poor communication skills, but poor communication will surely follow from these rivalries.

The areas of importance are discussed below.

### Doctor–doctor communication

Juniors need to communicate with other more senior doctors (and vice versa), and doctors of the same grade with each other. Now that trainers are themselves being more commonly trained to train, and in the increasingly informal atmosphere in which we work in hospital practice, it should follow that this 'vertical downward' communication will be better handled. This is also assisted by the reduction in 'patronage' over the last few years, which makes for a far more healthy training environment. However, that is beyond the scope of this chapter.

Yet, strangely perhaps, few if any trainees have been taught how to communicate 'upwards' with their trainers. Does this need to be taught? I would suggest that it does. Consider the 2 a.m. phone call to the consultant on call. Does the trainee have any idea what this feels like for the recipient of the call, roused from sleep? Possibly the best advice I received about this was the suggestion that the caller should be taught immediately to communicate the status of the call. Was it a call that: (a) required the consultant's presence, (b) required the consultant's advice, or (c) was merely to inform the consultant? This is an example of learned communication that hugely enhances the transfer of information, almost certainly to the advantage of the patient.

The most formal type of doctor–doctor communication is case presentation. This is a skill and, like many others in postgraduate training, it is currently barely, if at all, taught. Yet without this skill there can be serious difficulties within the clinical team.

The simplest advice is, I believe, the best: present cases in three parts – the synopsis, the detail and the summary (or, in other words, tell them what you are going to say, tell them what you want to say and then remind them what you have just told them).

All trainees should practise these skills as often as possible, and should learn to teach them to the next generation.

### Doctor–midwife/nurse communication

The other area of inter-professional communication – doctor–midwife/nurse communication – is just as important. Gone, thankfully, are the days of the presumed superiority of doctors. Instead we now respect the professional contributions of each other for what they are: interdependent and worthy of mutual respect. Nevertheless, all have to work to maintain the best possible level of communication at all times. Examples of departments where communication has failed abound – and the overall departmental dysfunction that ensues is massive, detrimental to patient care and wholly unnecessary. Like any relationship, this one will have ups and downs. The mark of maturity is when the system can tolerate these, and learn from them.

### Written communication

The two areas are clinical records and letters to other professionals. The skills required are similar, but different in detail.

### Clinical records

The quality of clinical records is of vital importance. Well-constructed clinical records communicate with other professionals and protect patients. They also may protect the writer from future medico-legal attack. Poor quality clinical records, by contrast, confuse other professionals and endanger patients. Records should be (as far as possible for those of us whose handwriting is only marginally more decipherable than Egyptian hieroglyphs) legible. They must also be dated, timed and signed (identifiably), if referring to an in-patient. There should be no exceptions to this.

The thicker clinical records become, the less useful they are as modes of information transfer. Thought must therefore be given to what and how much you write. Write only what is necessary and sufficient. Historically, midwives have written more than is necessary, and doctors far less than is necessary. Fortunately, that gap has recently narrowed considerably. Nevertheless, all those involved in medico-legal practice express continuing concern about the quality of note keeping.

### Letters

A generation ago, letters between doctors were more stylish, idiosyncratic and interesting. Unfortunately, they were also far less useful in transferring medical information. We live in an era in which letters are increasingly computer generated. Whether these letters are more effective in transferring information is yet to be determined, but I would suggest that the best letters are a compromise. If they are too short, they will be easily read, but they may omit relevant and necessary detail. If they are needlessly long, they risk losing the attention of the reader and remaining unread. Your letter should be relevant to the recipient. I remain astonished by some letters in clinical practice, written by highly intelligent clinicians, which seem not to recognize what the aim of the exercise is (it is communication, not intellectual gratification). You must also remember that letters are crucially important medico-legal documents: you must ensure that what is typed is what you intended.

## OBTAINING CONSENT

This is an area in which communication skills are sorely tested. How much information is required to enable a patient to give truly informed consent? All surgery could, for example, lead to death, but is it necessary to include that in the discussion? As it stands, it is probably fair to say that today's practice will appear wrong within a short time. Even the test of 'how much would you like to know if it were you signing the consent form?' is probably an unreliable yardstick. The sensitive clinician will increasingly

need to enter into the discussion with an open mind and sensitive antennae, as well as (in UK practice) familiarity with the General Medical Council requirements in this field.[2]

## COUNSELLING

As obstetricians and gynaecologists, we become involved in counselling in several types of difficult circumstances (e.g. malignant disease, prenatal screening dilemmas, preconception counselling). As stated above, counselling is the application of the full range of communication skills in a specific area of professional expertise. There is no added magic in the process.

## CONCLUSIONS

This is an area where common sense rules. Integrity and respect for others are 'all' that is required. Always ask yourself if you, or your closest relatives, would want to be communicated with in this manner. It really is that simple.

### KEY POINTS

**The guiding principles are:**
- Strive not to give any opinion that is not based on evidence.
- Admit ignorance – or absence of professional knowledge – where that pertains.
- Empathy and sympathy are welcome, but professional objectivity is highly valued.
- Involve whatever other professionals are necessary – our patients no longer expect omniscience from us; indeed, they probably distrust those who seem to claim it.

### Key References

1. General Medical Council. Good Medical Practice. London: GMC, 2006. Available from: www.gmc-uk.org/static/documents/content/GMC_GMP_0911.pdf
2. General Medical Council. Consent: patients and doctors making decisions together. London: GMC, 2008. Available from: www.gmc-uk.org/static/documents/content/Consent_2008.pdf

# The law, medicine and women's rights

*Sheila McLean*

## INTRODUCTION

It is probably true to say that the relationship between law and medicine in the past has sometimes been characterized by confrontation, even hostility. Increasingly, however, doctors are turning to the law themselves as a way of obtaining guidance as to what is and what is not permissible in their practice. Thus, rather than law being seen simply as a mechanism for judging allegations of negligence, it has taken on the role of standard setter, particularly in some areas of medicine, such as obstetrics and gynaecology.

This change has arisen largely as a consequence of medicine's capacities in managing pregnancy. The ability to monitor fetal development in particular has radically altered the way in which physicians perceive their role in respect of the pregnant woman, and has in some cases led to legal action. It has been said that, in the past, women told their doctors about their pregnancies, but now doctors tell women. The ability to visualize the fetus in the womb means that it becomes endowed, however subconsciously, with the characteristics of a child much earlier in pregnancy than would previously have been the case. The temptation therefore is to treat the fetus as a separate and unique patient. As Harrison says:

> *The fetus has come a long way – from biblical 'seed' and mystical 'homunculus' to an individual with medical problems that can be diagnosed and treated. Although he cannot make an appointment and seldom even complains, this patient will at times need a physician.*[1]

In some countries, this has led to a growing recognition of the alleged 'rights' of the fetus, which may on occasion conflict with the rights and interests of the pregnant woman. So common is this problem that it has been given a descriptive name of its own – maternal/fetal conflict – yet, as Hubbard says:

> *It makes no sense, biologically or socially, to pit fetal and maternal 'rights' against one another. Indeed, legal 'rights' do not offer a proper framework for assessing the situation of a pregnant woman and her fetus. As long as they are connected, nothing can happen to one that does not affect the other.*[2]

However, one thing must be made clear at the outset. In law, the fetus has no rights, and therefore to talk about fetal rights is misleading. Nonetheless, it is generally conceded that the embryo or fetus of the human species is worthy of some respect.[3] To say this, however, is quite different from asserting that it is a rights holder and worthy of equal consideration with the pregnant woman.

Most pregnant women will have no difficulty in behaving throughout their pregnancy in ways which maximize the potential health and safe delivery of their child. But not all women feel this way, or act this way, and this may be for reasons which appear to third parties unintelligible – even downright offensive or callous. However, the fact that women are free, autonomous actors means that their decisions – however unpalatable – must be given respect. This is not always easy for clinicians to accept, particularly when the woman's behaviour threatens the survival of an otherwise viable fetus. Indeed, a number of cases have reached courts in which doctors have asked that the choices of women should be overturned in the interests of fetal survival, as well as, sometimes, in the interests of saving the woman's life.

However, the basic legal position is clear. If a woman is otherwise legally competent, then her wishes must be respected, even if the result is her death or the death of an otherwise viable fetus. No matter how harsh this sounds, it is the law, and there are good reasons for the law to adopt this position. While recognizing that this may be problematic for those caring for the pregnant woman, the fact of pregnancy does not reduce the rights of women to make autonomous, self-regarding decisions. The interests of the embryo or fetus are not completely ignored by the law, however. The general principle underpinning the law is to offer benefit to the embryo or fetus wherever possible (without, for example, breaching the rights of others). Once born alive, children are entitled to sue for damage they sustained prenatally (even pre-conception). This is based on the assumption that where a benefit should accrue, it is for the law to ensure that it does. But this is not to say that the law recognizes the fetus as a rights holder before birth. Rather, it accepts that the injury arises at the moment the fetus becomes a child, and therefore is entitled to have rights attributed to it.

## A BRIEF ANALYSIS OF CASE LAW

It is in the grey areas that problems have arisen, and an analysis of some of the leading cases will help to explore both the content of and the rationale for the law's attitude. Although the law is clear that the fetus has no rights, this does not mean that women's autonomous decisions about the management of their pregnancy and labour have always been respected. The first case to arise in the UK was that of *Re S.*[4] in 1992. In this case, a woman refused a caesarean section on religious grounds. Her doctors believed that both her life and the life of her fetus were at risk and sought court authority to proceed with the caesarean section, even in the face of her objections. A judge heard the case as a matter of urgency (the hearing took about 20 minutes) and authorized the carrying out of the operation.

Perhaps unsurprisingly, this judgement was widely criticized for a number of reasons. First, the speed of the hearing was felt to prevent the nuances of the case being properly considered. Sir Stephen Brown's judgement, which is extremely brief, merely comments that:

*The consultant is emphatic. He says it is absolutely the case that the baby cannot be born alive if a Caesarean operation is not carried out. He has described the medical condition. I am not going to go into it in detail because of the pressure of time.*[5]

Second, it is most unusual to interfere with people's religious commitments in this way and, given the passing of the Human Rights Act 1998, it is fairly certain that this judgement would not be compatible with the terms of the Act. Article 9 of the European Convention on Human Rights requires states to permit freedom of thought, conscience and religion, with the implication that this also includes the freedom to act on religious commitments. Manifestly, this right would be limited if, for example, X's freedom of religion threatened the life of Y. However, since the fetus – even at full term – is not a person for legal purposes, then this is not directly relevant. Equally, it is possible that Article 8 of the Convention – the right to respect for private and family life – could be called into play in such situations. This article of the Convention is generally described as being the one that most clearly supports autonomy.

Third, the woman was at no time represented at the hearing, which would also fall foul of Article 6 of the Convention on Human Rights; the right to a fair hearing. Finally, proceeding to surgery against the expressed wishes of a competent woman effectively means that she was the victim of an assault on her person (again in breach of the Convention, Article 5 – the right to liberty and security of the person) in the interests, in large part, of saving her fetus. Of course, the court was also concerned with the danger to the life of the woman, but as courts have said on numerous occasions, a person is free to decline even life-saving treatment, no matter the reason for that choice, as long as they are competent.[6]

Subsequent cases, such as *St George's Healthcare NHS Trust v S, R v Collins and others, ex parte S,*[7] showed the lengths to which doctors and the law were prepared to go in forcing women to accept medical treatment deemed to be essential to save the fetus. S was diagnosed as suffering from severe pre-eclampsia, and was advised that an early delivery would be needed. She understood that both she and the fetus might die if surgery was not undertaken, but nonetheless refused it. On 26 April 1997 an order had been made which dispensed with her consent to the treatment. She had also been made subject to an order under the Mental Health Act 1983 to be admitted for 'assessment'. No treatment for her alleged depression was offered. S continued to record her extreme objections to the caesarean section. During her time in hospital, '… it was still believed by the psychiatrist who had played a significant part in the decision to admit her to hospital under s 2 that her capacity to consent was intact'.[8] It has already been indicated that a competent adult is free to refuse consent to life-saving treatment. As Lord Mustill said in the case of *Airedale NHS Trust v Bland*:[9]

*If the patient is capable of making a decision on whether to permit treatment and decides not to permit it his choice must be obeyed, even if on any objective view it is contrary to his best interests. A doctor has no right to proceed in the face of objection, even if it is plain to all, including the patient, that adverse consequences and even death will or may ensue.*[10]

Given that the psychiatrist was willing to state that her competence was not in issue, the decision of the lower court to authorize the section flies in the face of the general rule of law, and was ultimately criticized by the Court of Appeal. However, one earlier case had suggested that the only situation in which the law might be different was where '… the choice may lead to the death of a viable fetus',[11] although the jurisprudential basis for this exception is unclear. As the court in *St George's NHS Trust v S* noted, it is not sufficient simply to ignore the interests of the fetus. But as was also said, in this case there was no conflict between the interests of the mother and the fetus, because '… the procedures to be adopted to preserve the mother and her unborn child did not involve a preference for one rather than the other'.[12]

In addition, the court hazarded a look into the future, noting that it may soon be the case that relatively minor medical intervention on an adult might save the life of an unborn fetus. In contemplating a refusal of consent in such a case, the court said:

*The refusal would rightly be described as unreasonable, the benefit to another human life would be beyond value, and the motives of the doctor admirable. If, however, the adult were compelled to agree, or rendered helpless to resist, the principle of autonomy would be extinguished.*[13]

Finally, in the context of obstetrical intervention, it is worth restating the words of Butler-Sloss LJ in the case of

*Re MB*.[14] In this case she made an obiter explanation of the law as it currently stands:

> *The fetus up to the moment of birth does not have any separate interests capable of being taken into account when a court has to consider an application for a declaration in respect of a caesarean section operation. The law does not have the jurisdiction to declare that such medical intervention is lawful to protect the interests of the unborn child even at the point of birth.*[15]

Thus, even if we disapprove of the decisions of pregnant women, it is essential to ensure that her autonomy is respected where she is legally competent. Legal competence (or its absence) is now statutorily defined by the Adults with Incapacity (Scotland) Act 2000 and the Mental Capacity Act 2005. The issue of competence is, of course, central to the management of any disputes that arise between pregnant women and those caring for them. The Royal College of Obstetricians and Gynaecologists' Ethics Committee advises healthcare professionals as follows:

> *If the patient's capacity is seriously in doubt, it should be assessed as a matter of priority by a medical practitioner experienced in such assessments (such as a consultant psychiatrist). If, following assessment, there remains a serious doubt about the patient's competence, legal advice should be sought.*

It would seem, therefore, taking each of these cases into account, that the law is now clear that a competent refusal by a pregnant woman of treatment designed to save the life or preserve the health of her fetus (and/or herself) must be respected. This conclusion doubtless will sit uncomfortably with those whose mission is to save life, particularly given the tendency to view the fetus as a separate entity from the woman. However, there are, as I have suggested, good reasons for the law to adopt this position, which – it should be noted – does not prevent those caring for pregnant women from using persuasion (not coercion) in advising women as to the clinically optimal path.

The principle of autonomy permeates our law and our ethics. It is a principle that can be freely exercised as part of our citizenship, subject only to the caveat that it may be restricted when its exercise threatens others. But as courts agreed in the case of *Paton v Trustees of BPAS*[16] – a case in which a man attempted to prevent his wife from terminating a pregnancy – and in *Re F (in utero)*[17] – a case in which an attempt was made to make a fetus a ward of court – the fetus does not have independent legal standing, and its interests cannot serve to outweigh the right of a woman to make autonomous decisions. This conclusion was further reinforced in the case of *Vo v France*. In the case of *Re F*, Balcombe LJ made it clear that it was not for the courts to make decisions that would fly in the face of this conclusion. As he said:

> *If the law is to be extended in this manner, so as to impose control over the mother of an unborn child, where such control may be necessary for the benefit of that child, then under our system of parliamentary democracy it is for Parliament to decide whether such controls can be imposed and, if so, subject to what limitations or conditions.*[18]

That Parliament has declined to do this is a reflection of the interest which we all have in protecting autonomy, even when to do so is emotionally difficult. Just as it is not for judges to change the law, neither is it for doctors to do so.

But it is not just the protection of the abstract concept of autonomy which mandates the current legal response. In jurisdictions beyond those of the United Kingdom, decisions – often generated by doctors and handed down by courts – have served to demonstrate clearly the dangers of attributing rights to fetuses either during pregnancy or at the point of delivery. Medical recognition of the potential harm that can be caused by pregnant women to developing embryos and fetuses in the course of the pregnancy has in some countries resulted in the aggressive 'policing' of pregnancy; an egregious invasion of liberty. All too often, it appears that fetal interests have relatively easily been taken to trump women's rights. In the USA, for example, Kolder *et al*.[19] found that of 21 applications for court orders by public hospitals, 86 per cent were successful. Interestingly – and arguably ominously – 81 per cent of the women affected were black, Hispanic or Asian and 24 per cent did not have English as a first language. In addition, 46 per cent of heads of maternal medicine thought that women should be detained when they refused to follow medical advice and thereby endangered their fetuses.

In addition, as Sherman notes:

> *Pregnant drug abusers have been jailed to keep them free of illegal substances that might harm fetuses. And laws have been expanded so that pregnant women who do ingest drugs harmful to the fetus can be charged with or investigated for child abuse.*[20]

While removing the availability of illicit substances might ultimately serve the long-term interests of the women (as well as benefiting the fetus), women in the United States have also been incarcerated because of their use of legal substances, such as alcohol. Moreover, those women addicted to illicit drugs are sometimes unable to gain access to programmes that might assist them in beating their addiction; locking them up or otherwise coercing them in the interests of their embryos/fetuses seems like a heavy-handed way of avoiding the need to address the fundamental problem head on.

In other cases, medical opinion that a natural delivery was too risky has been used to mandate coercion, but of course medical judgements can be wrong. In *Jefferson v Griffin Spaulding County Hosp. Auth.*,[21] for example, a court upheld an order for a forced caesarean section, although in fact the woman delivered naturally. Yet at the time the order was sought, doctors had claimed that vaginal delivery carried a 99 per cent chance of fetal death and a 50 per cent chance of maternal death.

The consequences of coercion are perhaps most poignantly demonstrated by the US case of *In re AC*.[22] It was in fact on this case that the UK judge in *Re S*[23] depended for his authorization of the forced intervention. Interestingly, he appeared to have failed to observe that *AC* had already been overturned on appeal.[24]

The facts of the case make tragic reading. Angela Carder was a young woman who had suffered from leukaemia as a child. Her condition had gone into remission; she married and became pregnant, but in the course of the pregnancy the leukaemia returned aggressively. It was clear that Angela Carder would die. At about 26½ weeks into the pregnancy, her doctors summoned a judge to the hospital and sought authority to carry out a caesarean section on Mrs Carder, despite her clear refusal to consent. When the case was first heard, the order was granted and the operation proceeded in the face of Mrs Carder's objections. Neither she nor the child survived, and indeed the section was listed as a contributing cause of death on the death certificate. In a trenchant criticism of this judgement, the distinguished American academic George Annas described what had happened as follows:

> They [the judges] treated a live woman as though she were already dead, forced her to undergo an abortion and then justified their brutal and unprincipled opinion on the basis that she was almost dead and her fetus's interests in life outweighed any interest that she might have in her own life and health.[25]

## Why not intervene?

Despite the temptations to manage pregnancy and childbirth with substantial, if not primary, concern for the welfare of the developing embryo or fetus, it should be clear from consideration of the cases that unthinkingly adopting such a position is potentially dangerous. In respect of intervening in lifestyle choices during pregnancy, it seems clear that the women in the cases discussed were treated differently from other competent adults solely on the basis of their biological capacities. The fact that we generally wish to protect the fetus does not give us a right to do so at the expense of the woman. Equally, since many of the harms likely to be caused will occur in the early stages of pregnancy – when the woman may not even know that she is pregnant – the logical conclusion of this would be that every fertile, sexually active woman would need to behave at all times as if she were pregnant, or run the risk of being accused of harming her fetus, and perhaps even – in the USA at least – of being deprived of her liberty. Equally, as Draper says, 'it is one thing to show what a woman ought to do in relation to her unborn child and quite another thing to say that this obligation ought to be enforced'.[26]

Although some authors have suggested that the way forward is through a 'careful balancing of the offspring's welfare and the pregnant woman's interest in liberty and

bodily integrity …',[27] such a balancing act is arguably at best inappropriate and at worst doomed to failure. The very act of 'balancing' automatically implies that there are relevant things to be balanced. It has already been agreed that the embryo or fetus of the human species is worthy of some respect, but this is not equivalent to saying that such respect is capable of being weighed in the scales against an existing person. Even in cases where a born person's life is threatened by the failure of another to undergo medical treatment in their aid, the law is unable to compel submission to treatment. This was clearly seen in one US case. In this case, the defendant refused to consent to a treatment that could have saved the life of the plaintiff. As the judge in that case said:

> Morally, this decision rests with the defendant, and in the view of the court, the refusal of the defendant is morally indefensible. For our law to compel the defendant to submit to an intrusion of his body would change every concept and principle upon which our society is founded. To do so would defeat the sanctity of the individual …[28]

## MATERNAL/FETAL CONFLICT

As has been said, the circumstances described above have come to be called maternal/fetal conflict. I have argued elsewhere[29] that this categorization is inherently flawed, not least because it describes the pregnant woman as a 'mother' (which she is not yet) and assumes that conflict is possible. Arguably, conflict implies hostility and yet it is not obvious that a fetus can be hostile to the pregnant woman, nor that the pregnant woman's decisions are taken out of hostility for the fetus. Nonetheless, this term has now become an accepted part of the language. Leaving aside these concerns, then, it is worth briefly analysing the implications of this purported conflict which is highly emotive because, as Lew says:

> Conflicts between a woman's needs and those of her fetus are vexing because they pit powerful cultural norms against one another; the ideal of autonomy and the ideal of maternal self-sacrifice. Parents who make sacrifices for their children should be encouraged, even lauded, but the law should not require such sacrifices. Self-sacrifice is a gift. Forcing a pregnant woman to sacrifice her health for her fetus is simply slavery.[30]

Nor can it be presumed that it is always possible to measure the risk taken by the woman versus the risk to the fetus of non-intervention. A caesarean section carries risk (albeit that risk is lower given today's standards of medical treatment), but even if the risk is minimal, and the potential benefits to the fetus are considerable, we still do insult to the fundamental principles of law and ethics by compelling women to rescue their fetuses. No such ethical or legal principle is widely recognized and, as has been said, 'even where there is a duty to rescue, the law never requires rescues which jeopardize life and limb'.[31]

# CONCLUSION

The developing capacities of modern medicine have served both to enhance the care of pregnant women and to confront women and those caring for them with new dilemmas. During pregnancy, the widespread use of prenatal screening makes the actualization of reproductive choice both more complex and more intangible. At the point of labour and birth, the clinical ability to rescue poses real tensions in cases where competent women wish to assert their own autonomy at the potential expense of both themselves and their fetuses. The consequences, as Gregg has said, are that:

*Women's bodies increasingly have become medicalized as fertility testing, techniques of 'assisted conception', prenatal diagnosis, fetal monitoring, induced labor and Cesarean sections have become normal, if not expected, interventions in woman's procreative processes. Procreative technologies can enhance both the range of choices for women and the possibility of greater social control of women's choices.*[32]

It is clear that, often encouraged by healthcare professionals, courts in particular have become increasingly intrusive into women's decision-making in the course of their pregnancy and at the point of birth. Medicine and the law make powerful allies in this venture, yet their collusion is a direct disavowal of the rights that we otherwise respect. The position in the UK now seems to have been clarified after a decade of highly dubious decisions, at least as far as forced caesarean sections are concerned, and the current legal position is endorsed by the Ethics Committee of the Royal College of Obstetricians and Gynaecologists. It is to be hoped that, where the woman and physician share a relationship based in trust and the free exchange of relevant information, problematic cases will arise infrequently and, in the United Kingdom at least, this has proved to be the case. However, the impetus that triggered the call for courts to intervene in these decisions has not disappeared. The motivation of those caring for pregnant women is all too intelligible. However, no matter its source – religion, professionalism or whatever – it does violence to other principles which have long been deemed essential to the proper functioning of society. All too often, the motivation for intervention is worthy, but it is no less a matter of concern for that. As Ikenotos has said:

*To the extent that the state invokes the* parens patriae *power to prevent harm to the fetus, the state subordinates the interests of the woman to those of the fetus. To the extent that the state regulates pregnant women to promote public health, safety, and morals – an exercise of the police power – it subordinates the interests of the*

*woman to those of the rest of society. In either case, when the state regulates women as childbearers, it legislates the ideology of motherhood.*[33]

It is not necessary to adopt a particular woman-centred philosophy, such as feminism, to understand the damage done to respect for persons by treating pregnant women without regard for their views. To be sure, the commitment to respecting autonomy does not prevent healthcare professionals from making an attempt to inform women as to the risks they run both for themselves and for their fetuses if certain decisions are made, and to persuade them to think again. However, attempts to enforce the 'right' decision (clinically at least) by resort to the law mark a departure, which should be resisted, from the traditional relationship between doctor and patient. Such a relationship is ideally based on trust, not coercion; on respect, not condemnation. The ability to visualize and assess the development of an embryo or fetus, and to visualize and monitor in the womb, while often immensely helpful to pregnant women, is a technical, not an ethical, issue, and provides insufficient justification to invade the rights of a live, competent individual, however painful that conclusion may be.

## KEY POINTS

- The law is no longer simply a mechanism for judging allegations of negligence, but has taken on the role of standard setter.
- Modern fetal imaging technology has increased the temptation to treat the fetus as a separate patient with unique 'rights'.
- Although the human fetus is worthy of respect, it does not, in law, have rights.
- Occasionally, a woman's decision or behaviour may threaten the survival of an otherwise viable fetus. The law says that if the woman is otherwise legally competent, her wishes must be respected.
- Children are entitled to sue for damage which they sustained prenatally, but this is still not the same as saying that the fetus has rights before birth.
- There have been cases of legally enforced obstetric intervention in the UK but the law has now been made clear: a competent refusal by a pregnant woman of treatment designed to save the life of her fetus (and/or herself) must be respected.
- In the USA, ominously, court-ordered treatment has mainly involved disadvantaged ethnic groups or women who did not have English as their first language.
- Pregnant women should not be treated differently from other competent adults.
- The concept of 'maternal/fetal conflict', in a legal context, is inherently flawed and is best avoided.
- The law and medicine make powerful allies. Attempts by the law to enforce the 'right' clinical decision are a departure from basic legal principles and should be resisted.

## Key References

1. Harrison MR. Unborn: historical perspective of the fetus as patient. *Pharos* 1982; **19**: 23–4.

2. Hubbard R. Legal and policy implications of recent advances in prenatal diagnosis and therapy. *Women's Rights Law Report* 1982; **7**: 202–15.

3. See, for example, Review of the Guidance on the Research Use of Fetuses and Fetal Material (Polkinghorne Report) Cm 762/1989, para. 2.4. 'Central to our understanding is the acceptance of a special status for the living human fetus at every stage of its development which we wish to characterise as a profound respect based on its potential to develop into a fully-formed human being.'

4. Butterworth's Medico-Legal Reports No. 79, p. 69 (1992).

5. Butterworth's Medico-Legal Reports No. 9, p. 70 (1992).

6. See, for example, Re C (adult: refusal of medical treatment) 1994. All England Law Reports No. 1, p. 819: F v West Berkshire Health Authority (Mental health Act Commission intervening) Butterworth's Medico-Legal Reports No. 4, p. 1 (1989).

7. Butterworth's Medico-Legal Reports No. 44, p. 160 (1998).

8. Butterworth's Medico-Legal Reports No. 44, p. 169 (1998).

9. Butterworth's Medico-Legal Reports No. 12, p. 64 (1993).

10. Butterworth's Medico-Legal Reports No. 12, p. 136 (1993).

11. Per Lord Donaldson in Re T (adult: refusal of medical treatment) Butterworth's Medico-Legal Reports No. 9, p. 46 (1992).

12. Butterworth's Medico-Legal Reports No. 9, p. 176 (1992).

13. *id.*

14. Butterworth's Medico-Legal Reports No. 38, p. 175 (1997).

15. Butterworth's Medico-Legal Reports No. 38, p. 186 (1997).

16. All England Law Reports No. 2, p. 987 (1978).

17. All England Law Reports No. 2, p. 193 (1988).

18. All England Law Reports No. 2, p. 200 (1988).

19. Kolder V, Gallagher J, Parsons MT. Court-ordered obstetrical interventions. *N Engl J Med* 1987; **316**: 1192–6.

20. Sherman R. A pyrrhic victory, a court battle: forced Caesarian. *Natl Law J* 1989; **16**: 3.

21. 274 S.E. 2d 457 (Ga 1981).

22. 533 A.2d 611 (D.C. 1987).

23. 533 A.2d 611 (D.C. 1987). Note 4, supra.

24. In re A.C. 573 A.2d 1235 (D.C. 1990).

25. Annas G. She's going to die: the case of Angela C. Volume 18, No 1, Hastings Center Report, 1988, Volume 23, p. 25.

26. Draper H. Women, forced Caesareans and antenatal responsibilities. Working Paper No. 1. Feminist Legal Research Unit, University of Liverpool, 1, 1992, p. 13.

27. Robertson J, Schulman J. Pregnancy and prenatal harm to offspring: the case of mothers with PKU. Volume 17, No. 4, Hastings Center Report, 1987, Volume 23, p. 32.

28. McFall v Shimp (1978) 127 Pitts Leg J 14.

29. McLean SAM. Moral status (who or what counts?). In: Bewley S, Ward RH (eds), *Ethics in Obstetrics and Gynaecology*. London: RCOG Press, 1994, pp. 26–33.

30. Lew JB. Terminally ill and pregnant: state denial of a woman's right to refuse a Caesarean section. *Buffalo Law Rev* 1990; **38**: 619, 621–2.

31. Lew JB. Terminally ill and pregnant: state denial of a woman's right to refuse a Caesarean section. *Buffalo Law Rev* 1990; **38** note 30, supra, p. 641.

32. Gregg R. 'Choice' as a double-edged sword: information, guilt and mother-blaming in a high-tech age. *Women Health* 1993; **20**: 53.

33. Ikenotos LC. Code of perfect pregnancy. *Ohio State Law J* 1992; **53**: 1205, 1284–5.

# PART TWO

# Obstetrics

# SECTION A
## Antenatal complications: maternal

# Routine antenatal care: an overview

*John A D Spencer*

## INTRODUCTION

The antenatal period offers many opportunities to provide targeted health services. Antenatal care became associated with general health evaluation in the UK as a result of the increasing recognition that factors such as nutrition, social conditions and birth spacing influence pregnancy outcome.

The concept of antenatal admission to hospital is attributed to Ballantyne, who was apparently concerned about fetal deformity and stillbirth 100 years ago in Edinburgh. However, it was after the First World War that serious interest in maternal well-being began to influence antenatal care. In 1944 the Royal College of Obstetricians and Gynaecologists (RCOG) reported on a National Maternity Service. The National Health Service (NHS) began in 1948 and from then on the pattern of antenatal care – monthly visits to a clinic until 32 weeks, then fortnightly and then weekly visits (see below) – continued broadly unchanged for over 40 years.

A new era in antenatal care began with *Changing Childbirth*, the report of an Expert Maternity Group, published in 1993. At this time, more than 98 per cent of deliveries were in hospital. The main recommendations of the Expert Maternity Group were the need for more choice, better communication and continuity of care. These were accepted as government policy, and so began the first re-organization of antenatal care since its development within the NHS.

The RCOG responded quickly by organizing a 2-day Study Group in conjunction with the Royal College of Midwives and the Royal College of General Practitioners. The papers and discussion were published in 1994 (The Future of the Maternity Services) together with recommendations. However, the era of guidelines was dawning and, in 1998, the RCOG set up a multidisciplinary working group to formulate a National Antenatal Care Guideline for normal pregnancy (1998–2001). Before this group concluded its work, the establishment of NICE, the National Institute for Clinical Excellence (now called the National Institute for Health and Clinical Excellence), raised clinical guideline development to a different level of organization. The RCOG successfully bid to host the first National Collaborating Centre (the National Collaborating Centre for Women's and Children's Health) and a reformed Guideline Development Group took over formulation of the first National Antenatal Care Guideline.[1] The first publication (Antenatal Care: routine care for the healthy pregnancy woman) was in 2003 and an update was published in 2008.[2]

There have been other significant developments since the previous edition of this chapter. A UK National Screening Committee[3] was established to review available evidence and provide advice on screening. In 2004, the government published a national service framework for children, young people and maternity services[4] which set out standards for service configuration. These were updated in 2007 in the policy document entitled Maternity Matters.[5] More recently, the NHS Library for Health[6] was set up to act as a single reference point for practitioners; in April 2009 this transferred to NICE and became known as NHS Evidence.

This chapter was originally based on the (unpublished) work of the RCOG National Antenatal Care Guideline Working Group (1998–2001). This revision highlights changes that are contained in the recent NICE guideline. The focus remains women-centred care and informed, evidence-based, decision making.

## DEFINITION

Antenatal care embraces:

- maternal health checks,
- evaluation of fetal health and development,
- disease screening,
- analysis of risk for the development of complications, and
- provision of advice and education – antenatal care is intended to facilitate preparation for childbirth and, to some extent, subsequent childcare.

It remains accepted that maternity services should be centred on the woman and her needs. Each woman requires sufficient help and information to enable her to make an informed decision about her care. This process of empowerment relies on good communication, which remains a key factor not only between health professionals and the woman, but also between different health professionals providing the service. This is essential so that effective team working can provide safe and supportive continuity of care.

Recent developments are reported in the first revision of the national guideline.[2] These include increased emphasis on evidence-based advice, awareness of vitamin-D deficiency, universal screening for sickle cell diseases and thalassaemias, recommendation of early testing by the 'combined test' for Down's syndrome screening, and universal screening for gestation diabetes.

## COMPONENTS OF ANTENATAL CARE

Table 5.1 lists a number of specific observations and measurements made during pregnancy, along with the reason for the task and the application of the method used. It immediately shows the complexity of routine antenatal care, and the overlapping nature of many of the perceived reasons for providing such care.

Antenatal care routinely begins late in the first trimester, at a time when the incidence of miscarriage rapidly declines. Fetal development is largely complete by 12 weeks and fetal normality is no longer assumed. Strategies of testing which aim to identify major fetal anomalies begin at the time of

**Table 5.1** Components of routine antenatal care in the UK

| What and why | When and where | How and who |
|---|---|---|
| **Prenatal advice**<br><br><br>Assessment of maternal health<br><br>Education | Before conception | GP, public awareness, dietician |
| **Diagnosis of pregnancy** | Amenorrhoea | Kit, self-testing |
| **First visit**<br><br>Education<br>Identify urgent referral<br>Routine referral to Maternity Services | GP surgery or clinic | GP or midwife |
| **Early/booking scan**<br>Confirm dates<br>Identify multiple pregnancy | 8–14 weeks | Ultrasound scan |
| **Booking history**<br>Assess maternal health<br>Assess risk<br>Education | 10–14 weeks<br>Home or clinic | Midwife |
| **Blood pressure**<br><br><br>Identify hypertension/ PET | Booking/early pregnancy and regular intervals | Blood pressure and proteinuria<br><br>Midwife or healthcare assistant |
| **Midstream urine culture**<br>Identify urinary tract infection | Booking/early Pregnancy<br>Booking and regular intervals | Midwife<br><br>Midwife |
| **Down's syndrome test**<br>NT/combined/integrated | 10–13 weeks (not universally available) | Scan and blood tests |
| **Booking blood tests**<br>Infection screen<br>Maternal health screen | 10–13 weeks | Blood test |
| **Serum screen for Down's syndrome**<br>(if late booking) | 15–20 weeks | Blood test |
| **Anomaly scan**<br>Fetal anatomy | 18–22 weeks | Ultrasound scan |
| **Glucose challenge test**<br><br>Gestational diabetes | 24–28 weeks | Glucose tolerance test |

**Table 5.1** *continued*

| What and why | When and where | How and who |
|---|---|---|
| **Abdominal palpation**<br><br>Uterine size and fetal growth | 20–36 weeks, regularly | Symphysis fundal distance |
| **Fetal movements**<br><br><br>Fetal hypoxia (chronic) | 26–42 weeks | Fetal movements, self-assessment |
| **Blood tests**<br><br>Maternal health screen<br>Fetal risk of Rhesus isoimmunization<br>Advice on minor symptoms | 28 and 34 weeks | Blood test |
| **Abdominal palpation**<br>Fetal lie and presentation | 36 weeks | Midwife |
| **Induction of labour**<br>Cervical assessment | 41 weeks | Midwife |

- PET, pre-eclampsia; NT, nuchal translucency.

booking (ideally 10 weeks) with the first (viability) scan and continue until around 20 weeks. Once neonatal viability is reached (24 weeks), antenatal care focuses more on monitoring maternal and fetal well-being to ensure that deviation from normality is recognized. Blood pressure measurement is the most important maternal observation and is, itself, a diagnostic test as raised blood pressure defines hypertension. Other observations during pregnancy do not give such a clear-cut indication of the problem being looked for.

## Screening

### Definition of screening

To be effective, screening should lead to identification of a problem in order to allow appropriate intervention. Most tests during pregnancy are considered screening tests and a positive result does not mean the condition is present. Rather, a positive result indicates increased risk of the problem being present. The reason for this distinction is that screening tests have a false-positive rate which means that a proportion of test results are positive when the condition is not present. The effectiveness of a screening test will depend upon whether all the cases with the condition being tested for give a positive result, otherwise some cases will be missed (false-negative result). The detection rate of

a screening test describes the proportion of the problem (affected cases) in the population that is actually picked up by the test. It is represented by the proportion of all positive results that are 'true' (ratio of true positives divided by true positives plus false negatives). False-positive results may lead to intervention when the condition is not present.

## Information from observations

Recording outpatient cardiotocograph (CTG) traces is an example of an observation commonly used as a test (in this case of fetal well-being) for which benefit has not been shown. However, all practising clinicians are aware of cases in which an outpatient CTG, usually performed in response to maternal concern about fetal activity, has identified chronic fetal hypoxia and resulted in urgent delivery. Thus, as with other observations, confusion has arisen between the true meaning of the observation made versus the clinical predictive value expected – or hoped for. Some observations continue to be used as 'tests' even though the evidence about their routine use either does not exist or does not show benefit.[7,8] Presumably it is believed that not performing such tests would result in greater harm than occurs from the known false positives and false negatives. Many observations have not been studied appropriately to confirm or refute this. Another assumption is that normal observations provide reassurance. This may be the case in the short term, but some studies have shown that 'normal' results may be falsely reassuring.

## Maternal health (lifestyle considerations)

### Social circumstances

Improvements in the standard of living, and general social circumstances, have reduced the need for antenatal care to focus on poor nutrition and poverty. However, poor circumstances still interfere with access to antenatal care, and women with this background still present late for antenatal care. Socially excluded women and their babies are at much higher risk than women in more comfortable circumstances.

### Smoking and alcohol

Advice to give up smoking is based on good evidence that doing so is effective [A] (see also Chapter 6.12, Drug and alcohol abuse and Chapter 6.13, Smoking). If women cease smoking, fewer complications develop during pregnancy. There is less chance of placental abruption, preterm delivery and fetal cleft lip/palate. The association between maternal smoking and low birth weight is well known. Strategies to reduce maternal smoking during pregnancy have been well studied; there is NICE public health guidance now available.[9] The evidence concerning cannabis in pregnancy is insufficient, but it is considered good practice to advise women to discontinue its use during pregnancy.

Alcohol passes across the placenta but there is no good evidence of harm. Although the safe level of alcohol is not known, fetal alcohol syndrome is rare. New advice is that women should avoid alcohol during the first three months of pregnancy because there may be an increased risk of miscarriage. Women are advised to limit alcohol consumption during pregnancy [C] to a maximum of four units per week. Getting drunk may be harmful to the fetus.

## Medication

Few medications, either prescribed or over-the-counter, and complimentary therapies have been established as safe during pregnancy.

## Supplements and vitamins

Folate supplementation (400 µg up to three months before conception) is recommended [A] on the basis of strong evidence that the incidence of neural tube defects is reduced (The Cochrane Library). Vitamin A supplements (especially doses above 700 µg) might be teratogenic and should be avoided, as should liver and liver products which may contain high levels. There is new advice on vitamin $D^2$ and certain groups at greatest risk of deficiency are advised to consider 10 µg/day (as in the Healthy Start multivitamin supplement). These groups include women who are of South Asian, African, Caribbean and Middle Eastern origin. Other risk groups are women with limited exposure to sunlight, whose diet is low in foods containing vitamin D and women with a pre-pregnancy BMI above 30 kg/m$^2$.

## Food hygiene

Attention to food hygiene is advised in order to avoid food poisoning and the specific effects of some microorganisms on the pregnancy. Washing salads and fruit (*Toxoplasma*), thorough cooking of meat (*Listeria* and *Salmonella*) and avoiding unpasteurized milk, soft cheese, pâté (*Listeria*) and raw eggs (*Salmonella*) are particularly important. Avoiding cat litter (*Toxoplasma*) and washing hands after gardening (*Toxoplasma*, *Listeria*) are also recommended.

## Physical exertion

To continue in employment after 33 weeks of pregnancy, a woman requires a doctor's certificate to indicate that she is fit to do so. Physically demanding work has been associated with poor outcomes, such as preterm birth, pre-eclampsia and low birth weight.[10] Maintenance of normal exercise is encouraged [C] during pregnancy (The Cochrane Library). Sexual intercourse in late pregnancy has not been found to be associated with an increased risk of preterm delivery [A].

## Travel

The use of compression stockings is an effective method of reducing the risk of venous thromboembolism related to long-haul air travel. The correct use of seat belts for car travel should be explained (above and below the bump). Before travelling abroad, flying, vaccinations and travel insurance should be discussed with a midwife or doctor.

## Minor symptoms of pregnancy

A number of minor and physiological changes to body function occur during pregnancy. These sometimes cause anxiety and need to be differentiated from more serious conditions.

## Gastrointestinal

Early effects of pregnancy on the gastrointestinal system are well recognized. Nausea and vomiting are common and are not associated with adverse outcome. These symptoms usually resolve by 20 weeks and may be helped by an antihistamine if persistent. Hyperemesis gravidarum needs to be identified and requires referral for inpatient assessment and management. Later in pregnancy, 'heartburn' (gastric reflux) and oesophagitis result from relaxation of the gastric sphincter associated with increasing abdominal pressure. Antacids can be helpful, and meals can be smaller and more frequent. Constipation is also common, due to the relaxant effects of progesterone. Fibre supplements and osmotic laxatives, such as lactulose, may help.

## Cardiovascular

Headaches and occasional fainting can occur as the body adapts to the increasing blood volume and fall in vascular resistance. Persistent headache in the late second and third trimesters may be an indication of pre-eclampsia. Palpitations are not common, but short episodes associated with posture change are unlikely to be serious. The supine position should be avoided in the third trimester to prevent supine aorto-caval hypotension. Varicose veins are common, as are haemorrhoids. There are no preventative measures. Support tights may help the symptoms of varicose veins, and frequent short periods of rest, lying laterally, may help.

## Respiratory

Dyspnoea of pregnancy may increase during pregnancy, but does not usually cause concern. Significant breathlessness should always be checked in order to exclude infection, asthma, heart failure or pulmonary emboli.

## Musculoskeletal

Carpal tunnel syndrome and ulnar nerve compression often cause hand symptoms late in pregnancy, associated with oedema. Analgesia and advice on posture are appropriate. Splinting is not usually required. Backache often develops during the third trimester and should be managed by advice on posture. Pubic symphysis diastasis may require strong analgesia. Referral to physiotherapy is not usually beneficial. Leg cramps are common and may indicate overheating of the legs at night. A deep vein thrombosis must be excluded if calf pain persists. Oedema of the lower legs is common.

## Genitourinary

Frequency of micturition is common as term approaches, due to pressure of the fetal head on the bladder. Dysuria is an indication for a urine culture. Vaginal discharge is common and usually mucoid. It should not be watery. However, profuse discharge often creates a feeling described as 'being wet', which needs to be distinguished from liquor leakage. Vulval irritation is commonly the result of *Candida* infection and requires appropriate treatment. Vulval ulceration should be checked if there is vulval pain. Herpes is an indication for referral to an obstetrician to discuss mode of delivery.

## Skin

Minor rashes and irritations are common, but pruritus is a symptom of cholestasis, and liver function tests should be checked.

## First antenatal visit (GP or midwife)

This is often a time for confirmation of pregnancy, but general practitioners (GPs) rarely perform pregnancy testing now and women should purchase a testing kit from the chemist. The first day of the last menstrual period, assuming a regular monthly cycle, is used to calculate the estimated date of delivery (EDD) by adding nine calendar months plus 7 days. Uncertainty about dates or early pregnancy complications are indications for an early ultrasound scan. Antenatal care requires certainty about the EDD in order to determine the timing of routine tests and check-ups. Booking should, ideally, be by 10 weeks gestation.

## Urgent referral to maternity services

The main reasons for recommending an early first visit are to check maternal health (see above) and exclude the need for early referral to an obstetrician, usually for prenatal testing. Indications for prenatal testing include sickle cell disease or haemoglobinopathy such as beta-thalassaemia. In such cases the option of chorionic villus sampling (CVS) should be discussed and offered. One reason for early testing by 12 weeks is so that suction termination of pregnancy is available if appropriate. If a woman has no intention of terminating an abnormal pregnancy, testing may still be offered for the purpose of obtaining information to reassure her or help her prepare for the delivery of an affected child. However, the risk of miscarriage after CVS may mean that testing is declined, especially if termination is not an option. Such discussions are ideally carried out in a prenatal clinic,

before conception, when appropriate blood testing and counselling can occur. Women with some medical conditions, such as diabetes and other conditions requiring medication, should also be referred early.

## Routine referral to maternity services

According to the local protocol, the woman is usually directed to a midwife for 'booking' into the local system. The choice of place for delivery and the type of antenatal care available are highly dependent upon local arrangements. Increasingly, a booking history is taken at home, or in the GP surgery. If the GP has identified a pre-existing medical condition, such as insulin-dependent diabetes, asthma, epilepsy or thyroid disease, referral may be directly to a specialist clinic. In some circumstances, midwifery booking can precede attendance at the consultant clinic.

## Early pregnancy/booking scan

It is common practice to arrange an ultrasound scan during the late first or early second trimester. This is important for the serum-screening programme for Down's syndrome, which requires an accurate assessment of gestation. The scan is usually arranged before 14 weeks (assessed by dates). Occasionally, gross anomalies will be identified, but the idea of routine scanning in the first trimester for fetal abnormalities is still under research.

## Booking (midwife)

### History and risk assessment

The primary purpose of the booking history is to identify potential risk factors related to the woman's current or past health. A thorough history, including family history, is essential. Many obstetric units use a family history of diabetes in a first-degree relative as an indication to screen later in pregnancy. Past obstetric history will indicate whether specific risks need to be anticipated. A decision about subsequent care will be governed by the result of this assessment (Table 5.2). A previous normal pregnancy, labour and delivery indicates minimal risk, provided the woman is still under 35 years of age. A pregnancy considered to be at minimal risk is suitable for total midwifery care and may be a candidate for home birth or delivery in a midwife-led unit if these options are available. Currently, however, an evidence base is lacking for risk assessment and the use of selection criteria for booking.[11] There is new advice regarding the need to note, and communicate, any relevant history of mental disorder.[2]

### Maternal examination

Assessment of maternal health at booking is guided by the history. General examination needs to note height (short stature is less than 1.50 m) and weight. Obesity should be

**Table 5.2** Examples of common risk factors at booking and arising during pregnancy

| Risk | Suggested action |
|---|---|
| *Maternal health* | |
| Maternal age | |
|   <16 years | Social worker referral |
|   >35 years | Prenatal diagnosis (obstetric clinic) |
| Short stature (e.g. European <1.5 m) | Discuss trial of labour (consultant unit referral) |
| Obesity (BMI >30 kg/m$^2$) | Dietary advice |
| Smoking | Reduce |
| Pre-existing medical condition and long-term medical treatment | Refer to specialist obstetric clinic |
| Hepatitis or HIV positive | Refer to specialist clinic |
| *Past medical history* | |
| Family history of genetic disorder | Refer to specialist clinic |
| Genital tract surgery or abnormality | |
|   Myomectomy | Obstetric opinion about delivery |
|   Cervical cone biopsy and late termination | Refer by 12 weeks if cervical suture to be considered |
|   Anal sphincter surgery | Consider elective casearean section |
| *Past obstetric history* | |
| Five or more previous births | Refer to obstetric unit |
| Three or more miscarriages | Refer to obstetric unit |
| Serious complication during: | Refer to obstetric unit |
| Pregnancy | |
|   Preterm | |
|   Haemorrhage | |
|   Hypertension | |
|   Stillbirth | |
| Delivery | |
|   Casearean | |
|   Third-degree tear | |
| Postpartum | |
|   Haemorrhage | |
|   Infection | |
|   Large baby | |
|   Shoulder dystocia | |
| Neonatal admission | |
| Neonatal loss | |
| *Present pregnancy* | |
| Hyperemesis gravidarum | Admit |
| Multiple pregnancy | Refer to obstetric unit |
| Anaemia (Hb <9 g/dL) | May need transfusion |
| Any minor symptom persisting | Urgent referral or next clinic as appropriate |
|   Significant breathlessness | |
|   Abdominal pain | |
|   Calf pain/swelling | |
|   Headache | |
|   Vaginal leakage | |
| Hypertension (BP >140/90 mmHg) | Urgent referral to obstetric unit |
| Haemorrhage after 24 weeks | Admit to obstetric unit |
| Transverse lie after 36 weeks | Admit to obstetric unit |
| Concern about fetal movements | Urgent referral to obstetric unit |
| Not delivered at 41 weeks | Refer to next obstetric clinic |

- BMI, body mass index; BP, blood pressure; Hb, haemoglobin; HIV, human immunodeficiency virus.

assessed by body mass index (>29) and is an indication for dietary advice. There is no indication for repeated weighing during pregnancy unless it is part of dietary management. Auscultation of the heart and lungs is not considered necessary in the absence of a relevant medical history.[12] Abdominal examination should look for scars from previous surgery. Breast and pelvic examination are not routine in the absence of complications.

A urine sample should be sent for culture to identify asymptomatic bacteriuria [B]. Treatment is effective and should be offered [A]. A history of previous genital tract infection or preterm labour is an indication to culture for pathogenic vaginal flora. Carrier status for group B beta-haemolytic *Streptococcus* is usually an opportunistic finding, and there are insufficient data to recommend routine screening.[13]

## Blood pressure

### Hypertension

Hypertension – blood pressure (BP) of 140/90 mmHg or above – at booking requires referral to an obstetrician for advice and management; the management of chronic hypertension is discussed in Chapter 6.1, Chronic hypertension. (Indeed, the fall in blood pressure in early pregnancy leads some practitioners to regard 130/80 as the upper limit of normal at a booking assessment.) Pregnancy-induced hypertension (PIH) is a benign rise in BP after 20 weeks gestation (see Chapter 7.6, Pre-eclampsia and non-proteinuric pregnancy-induced hypertension).

Identification of pre-eclampsia requires regular BP checks, use of urinalysis and measurement of plasma urate (see Chapter 7.6, Pre-eclampsia and non-proteinuric PIH). Oedema no longer forms part of the definition of this condition as it occurs commonly in pregnancy. Risk factors for pre-eclampsia include maternal age of 40 or more, nulliparity, pregnancy interval of 10 years of more, family history, previous history, BMI of 30 kg/m$^2$ or more, pre-existing vascular disease such as hypertension, pre-existing renal disease and multiple pregnancy. Symptoms include severe headache, problems with vision, severe pain in the epigastrium, vomiting and/or sudden swelling of the case, hands or feet.

Traditional patterns of antenatal care advocated around 13 visits with BP testing at 12, 16, 20, 24, 28, 30, 32, 34, 36 weeks and then weekly until delivery. Even with this strategy, some cases of pre-eclampsia are missed; the woman may present with symptoms such as headache, epigastric pain, visual disturbance or even eclampsia itself. Recently, models of care with fewer check-ups have been tried, and have shown no increase in adverse outcome (see below). The present recommendation for uncomplicated low risk pregnancy care is ten visits if nulliparous, and seven if parous. Urine should be tested for protein whenever BP is measured. Persistent proteinuria is an indication for urgent referral to an obstetric unit.

## Booking blood tests

### Full blood count

Haemoglobin is measured [B] to assess anaemia (World Health Organization definition <11 g/dL), which, if severe (<7 g/dL), is a risk for maternal morbidity. Referral to an obstetrician is appropriate. Iron deficiency can be confirmed by measuring ferritin. Low values for mean corpuscular volume (MCV), mean corpuscular haemoglobin (MCH) and mean corpuscular haemoglobin concentration (MCHC) are suggestive, but may not occur in the presence of folate deficiency. Alpha-thalassaemia trait may not be distinguishable from mild iron deficiency. Routine iron supplementation has been shown to maintain normal ferritin levels and reduce the likelihood of anaemia, although no benefits during pregnancy have been shown [A]. Thrombocytopenia (platelet count <100 × 10$^9$/L) is also a reason for referral to an obstetrician.

Blood should be retested at 28 weeks. The normal lower limit of the UK range for pregnancy is 11 g/100 mL at booking and 10.5 g/100 mL at 28 weeks. Anaemia complicating pregnancy is discussed further in Chapter 7.1, Anaemia.

Screening for sickle cell diseases and thalassaemias should be offered to all women as early as possible and, ideally, before 10 weeks of pregnancy. If the prevalence of sickle cell diseases is low (1.5 cases per 10 000 pregnancies or less) then the Family Origin Questionnaire[14] can be used. Where the prevalence is high then a blood test should be offered. A mean corpuscular haemoglobin (MCH) below 27 pgm is also an indication for laboratory screening.

### Blood group and red cell antibodies

Rhesus status, blood group and red blood cell antibodies should be determined in early pregnancy [A]. The presence of red cell antibodies (up to 5 per cent of the population) is a risk factor for haemolytic disease of the newborn. Rhesus-negative blood group is a risk for isoimmunization secondary to contact with rhesus-positive red cells from the fetus. Prophylactic administration of anti-D (currently 1250 IU) is given after potential sensitizing events (delivery, miscarriage, antepartum haemorrhage) and routinely at 28 and 34 weeks of pregnancy [A] in non-sensitized women (The Cochrane Library). The presence of atypical red cell antibodies is a reason for referral to an obstetrician (see Chapter 17, Fetal hydrops).

### Maternal infection screening

All women should be offered screening for asymptomatic bacteriuria by midstream urine early in pregnancy because treatment reduces the risk of pyelonephritis. Screening for bacterial vaginosis does not reduce adverse outcomes, particularly preterm birth. Information about the risk of chlamydia should be given routinely but is not recommended as part of routine screening. Routine screening for cytomegalovirus, toxplasmosis and hepatitis C is not recommended. There is insufficient evidence to support routine screening for varicella (chicken pox) and human parvovirus B19. A history of possible exposure is an indication for referral to an obstetric unit.

Rubella antibodies indicate immunity to infection and therefore negate any risk of congenital rubella syndrome. Seronegative women are identified in order to offer postnatal vaccination. If testing is late (second or third trimester), a positive result may reflect infection in the first trimester of pregnancy. Syphilis,[15] hepatitis B[16] and human immunodeficiency virus (HIV) screening[17] is advocated because effective treatments are available, either during or after pregnancy. Referral to an obstetric unit is required.

## Down's syndrome

Routine screening tests and counselling for anomaly screening are discussed in Chapter 10.1, Biochemical screening. Down's syndrome screening should, ideally, be performed before 14 weeks using the 'combined test' (nuchal translucency by ultrasound scan, beta-hCG, pregnancy associated plasma protein A). The fetal anomaly scan is not appropriate as a diagnostic tool for Down's syndrome.

It should be self-evident that appropriate education and counselling about all tests is required during early pregnancy. In particular, the idea of screening for fetal abnormalities with tests that are not diagnostic requires an understanding of the implications of false-negative and false-positive results.

## Fetal anomaly scan

An ultrasound scan of the fetus is offered between 18 and 21 weeks to check for major anomalies. This has become known as 'the 20-week scan'. The RCOG[18] has issued guidance with regard to the standard of this scan. About 2 per cent of pregnancies have an abnormality. Women should be made aware of the limitations of the examination and factors that limit its success (maternal obesity and fetal position). Fetal echocardiography involving the four-chamber view of the fetal heart and outflow tracts is a new recommendation. The detection rate varies between 15 and 80 per cent according to the anomaly present and its severity (see Chapter 10.2, Ultrasound screening).

The finding of a low-lying placenta is common at the time of the fetal anomaly scan and will have resolved by term. However, a repeat transabdominal scan at 32 weeks should be offered if the placenta is noted to extend over the internal os.

The finding of two or more soft markers on routine scan is an indication for specialist opinion.

## Gestational diabetes

Impaired glucose tolerance occurs in pregnancy, and may be sufficient to merit the term 'gestational diabetes mellitus' (GDM). Screening at booking should use risk factors such as BMI above 30 kg/m$^2$, previous macrosomic baby weighing 4.5 kg or more, previous history, and family history of a first-degree relative with diabetes, family origin from a high prevalence area.[19] A number of proposals have been made regarding diagnosis, with advocates for the use of a 75 or 100 g carbohydrate oral tolerance test (or 'challenge'). After a normal fasting result (upper limit 5.3–5.8 mmol/L), cut-off values of blood glucose at 2 hours are 8.6 or 9.2 mmol/L[20] (see also Chapter 7.5).

## Uterine palpation

### Fetal growth monitoring

Fetal growth monitoring is intended to identify cases where the fetus is small or large. Fetal growth restriction (FGR) carries a risk of hypoxia in labour, due to placental insufficiency. A large fetus is at risk of shoulder dystocia. Clinical palpation of the abdomen and measurement of the symphysis–fundal distance are equally effective at predicting the extremes of fetal size at the end of pregnancy. Nevertheless, symphysis–fundal distance should be recorded at each antenatal visit after 24 weeks. Charts exist by which symphysis–fundal measurements can be compared with

population data. Use of the value obtained at 20 weeks may help in the interpretation of values later in pregnancy.

## Indications for an ultrasound scan

Clinical concern about fetal size or growth is an indication for an ultrasound scan. The risk factors for FGR should be evaluated by an obstetrician. Routine assessment of fetal growth by ultrasound scan in the third trimester of low-risk pregnancies is not effective in identifying differences in pregnancy outcome and is not recommended [A]. Similarly, routine use of Doppler ultrasound examination of the umbilical artery is not recommended [A].

## Abnormal fetal lie and presentation

Ascertainment of a longitudinal lie and cephalic presentation should be ascertained by abdominal palpation at around 36 weeks gestation, although no testing of this has been reported. Breech presentation prior to 36 weeks is not uncommon. The management of breech presentation after 36 weeks is discussed in Chapter 35, Breech presentation. Suspected malpresentation of the fetus is an indication for an ultrasound scan. Transverse lie is an indication for admission to an obstetric unit for further investigation and planned delivery. Breech presentation at 36 weeks is an indication for external cephalic version unless contraindicated by labour, previous caesarean section, fetal compromise, ruptured membranes, vaginal bleeding or a medical condition.

## Fetal movements

Normal fetal activity during the third trimester is an indication of adequate fetal oxygenation. A large trial using movement charts[7] found no reduction in late pregnancy stillbirths when the further management was by CTG. There are a large number of 'false-positive' alarms, but the technique is simple. Routine formal fetal movement counting is not recommended. However, women who are concerned about inadequate fetal movements will report for further investigation. The appropriate strategy appears to be lacking. A normal CTG may be falsely reassuring although one trial showed a reduction in stillbirths at the expense of increased operative intervention.[21] Further research is required. Biological variations in fetal activity, including the now well-described fetal 'rest–activity' behavioural cycle, need to be taken into account when interpreting concerns about fetal activity.

## Routine induction of labour

By 40 weeks gestation, less than 60 per cent of women have delivered. Routine induction of labour is not indicated before 41 weeks. By 42 weeks, less than 20 per cent of women remain undelivered, and evidence suggests a rise in the rate of stillbirths. Further evidence has shown that routine induction of labour is less costly and results in a lower caesarean section rate than conservative management with monitoring [A] (see Chapter 25, Induction of labour).

Women whose pregnancy passes beyond 41 weeks should routinely be offered induction of labour. This should be preceded by vaginal examination and a membrane sweep. If induction is declined then monitoring after reaching 42 weeks is indicated. This is usually an ultrasound scan, to check liquor volume, and twice weekly CTG monitoring of the FHR.

## ORGANIZATION OF ANTENATAL CARE

### Traditional model

Early formalization of antenatal care after the Second World War recommended a minimum of monthly check-ups until 28 weeks, fortnighy check-ups until 36 weeks and then weekly visits until labour. The first visit to the GP would ideally be by 12 weeks. Subsequent care would be according to a risk evaluation performed at the booking clinic. Full (hospital) care, shared care (between hospital and GP) and community care (between community midwife and GP) were the usual options. Community care was often linked to deliveries booked into a 'GP unit', either separate from or co-located with a consultant delivery unit.

### New models

One of the earliest changes in recent years was a small reduction in the number of antenatal visits without evidence of an adverse effect (Table 5.3). Most studies suggest extending the intervals between check-ups. While there is a suggestion that fewer visits may be associated with a reduction in women's satisfaction with the care received, more women would choose the same care again.[22] Other changes in the

**Table 5.3** Recommended schedule of antenatal care[2]

| Weeks of pregnancy | Nulliparous | Multiparous |
|---|---|---|
| 10 (booking) | √ | √ |
| 16 weeks (review results) | √ | √ |
| 18 – 20 week scan | √ | √ |
| 25 weeks | √ | x |
| 28 weeks | √ | √ |
| 31 weeks | √ | x |
| 34 weeks | √ | √ |
| 36 weeks | √ | √ |
| 38 weeks | √ | √ |
| 40 weeks | √ | x |
| 41 weeks (plan induction) | √ | √ |

provision of antenatal care during recent years include the recognition and acceptance that uncomplicated pregnancies, and those without risk, do not need to be seen by a consultant obstetrician [A]. Continuity of care provided by a group of midwives is associated with lower intervention rates and beneficial psychosocial outcomes. It is recommended that women carry their own pregnancy record [A].

Increasingly, antenatal care for women with uncomplicated pregnancies is being provided in the community which has resulted in a reduction in the number of women attending hospital antenatal clinics. The quality of care provided to women with complications has increased as a result of the greater time available.

### KEY POINTS

- Antenatal care has undergone significant change in the last 18 years, with an emphasis on empowerment of women, better communication, use of evidence, care outside hospital provided by midwives.
- Minor symptoms of pregnancy should be treated and should be differentiated from symptoms of serious disease.
- Antenatal care involves checking maternal health and fetal well-being, assessing risk factors, screening for disease and abnormalities and providing education and advice.
- Screening raises false-negative and false-positive results. Some observations have not been fully evaluated with regard to their use and is a test in this respect.
- Women are advised about lifestyle matters such as smoking and alcohol use. Social circumstances are important, and women who live in difficult circumstances and book late (or not at all) are at greatest risk.
- At the first visit, women who require urgent referral should be identified.
- An early ultrasound scan for dating can be very helpful.
- Booking involves a detailed history, measurement of weight and height and urine analysis.
- Blood pressure checks are important, but even frequent measurements cannot prevent some unexpected cases of symptomatic pre-eclampsia.
- Full blood count, blood grouping and rhesus status and blood screening for some infections are all recommended.
- The combined test for Down's syndrome is recommended. A fetal anomaly scan is recommended. Full counselling is essential.
- Screening for haemoglobinopathies and gestation diabetes risk incorporates the use of risk factors.
- Abdominal palpation will detect the extremes of abnormal fetal growth. The lie and presentation should be checked at 36 weeks.
- Self-reporting of fetal movements as a test of fetal well-being is simple but has a high false-positive rate.
- Routine induction of labour at 41 weeks is not justified, but at 42 weeks results in lower rates of caesarean section and stillbirth.

## ACKNOWLEDGEMENTS

The author wishes to acknowledge assistance for the previous edition of this chapter from the Clinical Evidence Support Unit, Royal College of Obstetricians and Gynaecologists (Dr Jane Thomas, Director) while he was chairman of the RCOG Multiprofessional Evidence-based Guideline Group looking at Antenatal Care for the Healthy Woman. The group was discontinued in 2002, when production of this guideline was taken over by the National Institute for Clinical Evidence.

## Key References

1. ‹www.nice.org.uk/aboutnice/howwework/developing-niceclinicalguidelines/nationalcollaboratingcentres/nationalcollaboratingcentreforwomenandchildrenshealth/p43.jsp›
2. ‹www.nice.org.uk/Guidance/CG62›
3. ‹www.library.nhs.uk/SCREENING/SearchResults.aspx?catID=1328›
4. ‹www.dh.gov.uk/en/Healthcare/NationalServiceFrame works/Children/DH_4089111›
5. ‹www.dh.gov.uk/en/Publicationsandstatistics/Publications/PublicationsPolicyAndGuidance/DH_073312›
6. ‹www.library.nhs.uk/Default.aspx›
7. Grant A, Elbourne D, Valentin L, Alexander S. Routine formal fetal movement counting and risk of antepartum late death in normally formed singletons. *Lancet* 1989; **2**: 345–9.
8. Spencer JAD. Assessment of fetal well-being in late pregnancy. In: Edmonds DK (ed.). *Dewhurst's Textbook of Obstetrics and Gynaecology for Postgraduates.* Oxford: Blackwell Science, 1999, 119–33.
9. ‹www.nice.org.uk/PH010›
10. Mozurkewich E, Luke B, Avni M, Wolf F. Working conditions and adverse pregnancy outcome: a meta-analysis. *Obstet Gynecol* 2000; **95**: 623–35.
11. Campbell R. Review and assessment of selection criteria used when booking pregnant women at different places of birth. *Br J Obstet Gynaecol* 1999; **106**: 550–6.
12. Hall MH. Prepregnancy and antenatal care. In: Chamberlain G, Steer P (eds). *Turnbull's Obstetrics.* London: Churchill Livingstone, 2001, 105–16.
13. ACOG Committee Opinion (Number 173). Prevention of early-onset group B streptococcal disease in newborns. Committee on Obstetric Practice, American College of Obstetricians and Gynecologists. *Int J Gynecol Obstet* 1996; **54**: 197–205.
14. ‹www.sickleandthal.org.uk/Documents/F_Origin_Questionnaire.pdf›
15. Public Health Laboratory Service. *Antenatal Syphilis Screening in the UK: a Systematic Review and National Options Appraisal with Recommendations.* Report to the National Screening Committee. London: 1998.
16. Department of Health. *Screening of Pregnant Women for Hepatitis B and Immunisation of Babies at Risk.* Health Services Circular Number 127. London: HMSO, 1998.
17. NHS Executive. *Reducing Mother to Baby Transmission of HIV.* Health Services Circular Number 183. London: HMSO, 1999.
18. Royal College of Obstetricians and Gynaecologists. *Ultrasound Screening for Fetal Abnormalities.* RCOG Working Party. London: RCOG Press, 1997.
19. ‹www.nice.org.uk/CG063›
20. Metzger BE and the organizing committee of the Third International Workshop Conference on Gestational Diabetes Mellitus. Summary and recommendations. *Diabetes* 1991; **40**: 197–201.
21. Neldam S. Fetal movements as an indicator of fetal well-being. *Dan Med Bull* 1983; **30**: 274–8.
22. Carroli G, Villar J, Piaggio G *et al.* WHO systematic review of randomised controlled trials of routine antenatal care. *Lancet* 2001; **348**: 213–18.

# 6.1 Chronic hypertension

*Andrew Shennan*

## INTRODUCTION

Pre-existing hypertension will affect between 1 and 2 per cent of women of reproductive age. Some of these women will be on long-term treatment that may have implications for pregnancy. It is not unusual for hypertension unrelated to the pregnancy to be first diagnosed when these women attend their antenatal clinics. In addition, women who have underlying hypertension are at increased risk of developing pre-eclampsia and its sequelae. Women who present with hypertension in pregnancy must have other causes considered, and an understanding of the aetiology and management is essential to the obstetrician.

## DEFINITION

Chronic hypertension is defined as the presence of persistent hypertension, of whatever cause, before the 20th week of pregnancy (in the absence of a hydatidiform mole), or persistent hypertension beyond 6 weeks post-partum.

As hypertension is a continuous variable, there is no standard definition to indicate the point at which adverse events occur. In non-pregnant individuals, there is a steady and linear increased risk of future cardiovascular morbid events, directly proportional to both systolic and diastolic blood pressures. Generally, a sustained blood pressure greater than 140/90 mmHg is deemed hypertensive, but the significance of this will depend on the clinical situation, such as the individual's age and other risk factors, such as smoking and hyperlipidaemia. Anti-hypertensive treatment is known to reduce the risk of later coronary heart disease (by approximately 16 per cent) and stroke (by 38 per cent) [A].

## AETIOLOGY

Overall, approximately 95 per cent of hypertension is known as primary or essential hypertension; 5 per cent is secondary, usually related to underlying renal or adrenal disease. However, the incidence of secondary hypertension is increased in the age group of women attending the antenatal clinic. Renal disease may be directly due to glomerulonephritis or tubulo-interstitial disease, such as that due to reflux pyelonephritis or stones. Renal artery stenosis can also cause renal hypertension. Endocrine causes include Cushing's syndrome, Conn's syndrome, phaeochromocytoma and thyroid disease.

## MANAGEMENT

### Preconception, assessment and counselling

A woman who is found to be hypertensive prior to pregnancy can be advised about appropriate anti-hypertensive therapy suitable for pregnancy and about other life modifications that can be made prior to conception. It is known that a high body mass index (BMI) is associated with increased blood pressure, and that weight loss may reduce hypertension [C]. In addition, it has also been shown that both salt and alcohol intake are associated with high blood pressure, and moderation of both is advised in hypertensive individuals [C]. Generally speaking, hypertensive individuals are asymptomatic, but a careful history needs to be taken in order to identify any relevant symptoms and to exclude possible genetic causes of renal disease, such as autosomal dominant polycystic kidneys.

The type of anti-hypertensive taken should be considered, and it is generally recommended that both diuretics and angiotensin-converting enzyme (ACE) inhibitors be changed to alternative anti-hypertensive agents [D].

A physical examination should include calculation of the BMI as well as fundoscopy to look for evidence of arterial disease. Although rare, possible causes of secondary hypertension should be sought. Bruits in the renal artery or a systolic murmur in association with delayed femoral pulses could indicate coarctation of the aorta. On abdominal examination, polycystic kidneys may be palpable. Retinal changes associated with hypertension include mild vessel tortuousity, silver wiring and arteriovenous nipping. If severe, retinal haemorrhages may be seen in association with hard exudates, cotton-wool spots and papilloedema.

Women who are found to be hypertensive pre-pregnancy or in early pregnancy should have circulating levels of urea and electrolytes checked, urine analysis and a 24-hour urine collection for protein and creatinine clearance performed. Women with severe hypertension or proteinuria should have a chest x-ray, electrocardiogram (ECG) and antinuclear antibody testing. If there is a long history of severe hypertension, cardiac function should be assessed with an echocardiogram. Investigations of lupus anticoagulant and anticardiolipin antibodies should be performed if there is a history of thromboembolic events or recurrent pregnancy loss.

Glomerulonephritis, polycystic kidney or chronic pyelonephritis may be suggested by haematuria and microscopic proteinuria identified on dipstick testing of the urine. High sodium will be apparent in those individuals with primary hyperaldosteronism (Conn's syndrome). Low sodium can be caused by high doses of diuretics. Potassium is usually low in Conn's syndrome or high in those with renal failure. Some ACE inhibitors or potassium-sparing diuretics can cause hypocalcaemia.

A raised urea or creatinine may indicate renal impairment and a renal cause of hypertension. Chronic renal failure can also result in low serum calcium, although primary hyperparathyroidism can be associated with hypertension and this results in elevated calcium levels.

Young women with chronic hypertension usually require referral for more detailed investigation, which may include baseline ECG and serum lipids to ascertain future risk. Women who have paroxysmal or severe hypertension, particularly associated with sweating or palpitations, need a 24-hour collection for catecholamine metabolites to exclude a phaeochromocytoma. In those cases in which Cushing's syndrome is considered, a 24-hour collection of urinary free cortisol may be taken. Determinations of plasma aldosterone or cortisol and adrenocorticotrophic hormone (ACTH) concentrations are occasionally helpful in identifying particularly uncommon causes of secondary hypertension. If indicated by biochemistry results, renal imaging or angiography may also be performed.

## THERAPEUTIC CONSIDERATIONS OF PRE-EXISTING MEDICATIONS

### Diuretics

Thiazide diuretics are still used (although usually in older patients) as a primary treatment of hypertension in non-pregnant individuals as they are both cheap and easy to use with a once-daily dose (see also Chapter 8, Medication in pregnancy). It is generally believed that diuretics should be avoided in pregnancy as they act by increasing renal excretion of sodium and water, which will reduce blood volume, and this is unlikely to be a desirable physiological effect in pregnancy [E].[1] However, direct evidence of harm is limited.

### Angiotensin-converting enzyme inhibitors and angiotensin receptor antagonists

These anti-hypertensives act on the rennin–angiotensin–aldosterone system and are increasingly used in individuals with uncomplicated hypertension. However, they are associated with renal toxicity in the fetus[2] and should be avoided in pregnancy [D]. If possible, it is desirable to change to another medication pre-pregnancy or as soon as pregnancy is diagnosed [D].

### Other antihypertensive agents

There have been some reports that beta-blockers are associated with intrauterine growth restriction [B].[3]

For this reason, they are usually avoided if an appropriate alternative can be used. Other anti-hypertensives, calcium channel blockers, centrally acting drugs such as methyldopa and labetalol (a combined alpha and beta blocker) have all been used in pregnancy. There is no significant advantage of one over another and individuals can continue this therapy into pregnancy, if necessary. The drug with the longest, most established safety profile is methyldopa; both neonatal and longer-term outcome data have been assessed and no detrimental effects have been demonstrated with its use [B].[4] As methyldopa can cause depression and tiredness and, very occasionally, liver dysfunction, new anti-hypertensives such as labetalol are increasingly being used [E].

## MATERNAL AND FETAL ASSESSMENT

Once pregnant, the woman with underlying chronic hypertension should be closely monitored for the development of pre-eclampsia. More than one in five women with chronic hypertension have been shown to develop pre-eclampsia [D].[5,6] Uterine artery Doppler velocity waveforms have been used to assess risk in these individuals.[7] It is important to ensure that women have a strict antenatal schedule and that blood pressure and urine analysis are checked at least every 2 weeks [E]. Even women who do not develop overt signs of pre-eclampsia appear to be at increased risk.[8] The risks include a higher rate of intrauterine growth restriction, and women with chronic hypertension should have regular checks for growth with ultrasound for fetal biometry, liquor assessment and umbilical artery Doppler studies, to 34 weeks gestation.

In the chronically hypertensive woman, as in the normotensive woman, pregnancy is associated with a physiological rise in blood pressure, but a sudden and profound increase should alert the clinician to the possibility of pre-eclampsia. For this reason, as blood pressure measurement cannot be relied upon to identify pre-eclampsia, urinalysis is particularly important. Measurement of platelets and uric acid may help identify those individuals who are going to develop the clinical manifestations of pre-eclampsia, as abnormalities may predate proteinuria by some weeks [C].

The second most common complication is a placental abruption (see Chapter 23, Antepartum haemorrhage); the incidence of placental abruptions is 2–10 per cent in women with chronic hypertension.

## MANAGEMENT OF MATERNAL HYPERTENSION

The aim is to maintain blood pressure below 150/100 mmHg; however, the diastolic blood pressure should remain above 80 mmHg. In women with evidence of end organ damage, the blood pressure threshold should be less than 140/90 mmHg. There is considerable debate as to whether women who have moderate hypertension (140/90–160/100 mmHg) should have antihypertensive treatment. There are 24 randomized control trials evaluating antihypertensives in moderate hypertension in pregnancy. However, the total number of women studied is less than 4000. Treatment is associated with a reduction in severe hypertension (by approximately one-half) [A].[9] However, there is no significant difference in the incidence of pre-eclampsia or change in perinatal mortality, preterm birth rate or small for gestational age [A].

Different drugs have been compared in 17 randomized, control trials with just over 1000 women, and it was shown that no one drug has a clear advantage over another. Therefore, it remains unclear whether antihypertensive drug therapy for mild to moderate hypertension during pregnancy is worthwhile [A]. Certain investigators have suggested, through careful analysis of data from these trials, that the babies of those individuals who are treated may be slightly smaller [D].[10] This has led some practitioners to advocate cessation of anti-hypertensive treatment in pregnancy for women with mild/moderate hypertension [E].[11] If therapy is discontinued, blood pressure should be rigorously monitored (day case assessment units may be the optimal environment for this), and treatment will need to be re-instigated in a substantial minority of women.

Severe hypertension (blood pressure 160/110 mmHg) requires immediate treatment to prevent the risk of stroke and to reduce other morbidity (see Chapter 7.6, Pre-eclampsia and non-proteinuric pregnancy-induced hypertension) [C].[12]

Women with severe chronic hypertension should be carefully monitored for at least 48 hours after delivery as they are at risk of developing renal failure, pulmonary oedema and hypertensive encephalopathy.

Antihypertensive therapy should be continued in the immediate puerperium and then reviewed 2 weeks post-natally. Methyldopa should be discontinued within 2 days of birth and the previous antihypertensive treatment the woman was receiving prior to pregnancy recommenced.

Chronic hypertension is a risk factor for pre-eclampsia, but the converse is also true: nearly half the women with pre-eclampsia will develop chronic hypertension in later life.[13]

- The treatment of moderate hypertension in pregnancy is associated with a significant reduction in severe hypertension.
- Anti-hypertensive treatment in pregnancy does not influence the perinatal mortality rate or the subsequent development of pre-eclampsia.

Antenatal complications: maternal

## KEY POINTS

- Diuretics and ACE inhibitors should be stopped or changed pre-pregnancy or at early gestation.
- Women with hypertension first diagnosed in early pregnancy should be investigated for secondary causes.
- Chronic hypertension is associated with an increased risk of pre-eclampsia.
- Superimposed pre-eclampsia may be diagnosed by identifying proteinuria on urinalysis; raised uric acid levels or falling platelet counts may be the first indication of risk.

## Key References

1. Sibai BM, Grossman RA, Grossman HG. Effects of diuretics on plasma volume in pregnancies with long-term hypertension. *Am J Obstet Gynecol* 1984; **150**: 831–5.
2. Thorpe-Beeston JG, Armar NA, Dancy M *et al.* Pregnancy and ACE inhibitors. *Br J Obstet Gynaecol* 1993; **1000**: 692–3.
3. Butters L, Kennedy S, Rubin PC. Atenolol in essential hypertension in pregnancy. *BMJ* 1990; **301**: 587–9.
4. Cockburn J, Moar VA, Ounsted M, Redman CW. Final report of study on hypertension in pregnancy: the effects of specific treatment on the growth and development in children. *Lancet* 1982; **1**: 647–9.
5. Chappell LC, Enye S, Seed P *et al.* Adverse perinatal outcomes and risk factors for preeclampsia in women with chronic hypertension: a prospective study. *Hypertension* 2008; **51**: 1002-9.
6. Sibai BM, Lindheimer M, Hauth J *et al.* Risk factors for preeclampsia, abruptio placentae, and adverse neonatal outcomes among women with chronic hypertension. National Institute of Child Health and Human Development Network of Maternal–Fetal Medicine Units. *N Engl J Med* 1998; **339**: 667–71.
7. Frusca T, Soregaroli M, Zanelli S *et al.* Role of uterine artery Doppler investigation in pregnant women with chronic hypertension. *Eur J Obstet Gynecol Reprod Biol* 1998; **79**: 47–50.
8. McCowan LM, Buist RG, North RA, Gamble G. Perinatal morbidity in chronic hypertension. *Br J Obstet Gynaecol* 1996; **103**: 123–9.
9. Abalos E, Duley L, Steyn DW, Henderson-Smart DJ. Antihypertensive drug therapy for mild to moderate hypertension during pregnancy. *Cochrane Database Syst Rev* 2001; **2**: CD002252.
10. Magee LA, Ornstein MP, von Dadelszen P. Management of hypertension in pregnancy. *BMJ* 1999; **318**: 1332–6.
11. Sibai BM. Diagnosis and management of chronic hypertension in pregnancy. *Obstet Gynecol* 1991; **78**: 451–61.
12. Sibai BM. Treatment of hypertension in pregnant women. *N Engl J Med* 1996; **335**: 257–65.
13. Bellamy L, Casas JP, Hingorami AD, Williams DJ. Pre-eclampsia and risk of cardiovascular disease and cancer in later life: systematic review and meta-analysis. *BMJ* 2007; **335**: 974.

# 6.2 Diabetes mellitus

*Clare L Tower*

---

## MRCOG standards

### Knowledge criteria

Understand the epidemiology, aetiology, pathophysiology, clinical characteristics, prognostic features and management of disorders of carbohydrate metabolism:

- type 1 and type 2 diabetes,
- maternal, fetal and neonatal complications,
- diabetic ketoacidosis,
- diet,
- drugs (insulins and hypoglycaemic agents).

### Clinical competency

Diagnose, investigate and manage, with direct supervision, insulin-dependent diabetes and impaired glucose tolerance.

## INTRODUCTION

Diabetes is the most common medical condition encountered during pregnancy, with between 0.5 and 5 per cent of pregnancies being complicated by either pre-existing or gestational diabetes.[1,2] Both type 1 and type 2 diabetes are increasing in incidence and are both associated with a higher risk of a poor obstetric outcome. In 1990, the St Vincent Declaration set a series of targets to improve the outcome of pregnant women with diabetes, with the aim that the risks should approximate to those of the non-diabetic populations. Unfortunately, the recent CEMACH report on diabetes in pregnancy found that current care falls well short of this target.[2]

## PHYSIOLOGICAL CHANGES IN PREGNANCY

Pregnant women have considerably altered carbohydrate metabolism. There is hyperplasia of the pancreatic islet cells which leads to a doubling in insulin production between the first and the third trimesters. Although there is an initial increase in insulin sensitivity during the first trimester, the release of insulin-resistant hormones (human placental lactogen, glucagons, progesterone and corticotrophin releasing hormone) from the placenta results in progressive glucose intolerance (insulin resistance) with advancing gestation. In addition to the increased glucose uptake of the fetus, there is increased peripheral uptake, increased glycogenesis and reduced hepatic gluconeogenesis. The renal tubular threshold for glucose falls, such that glycosuria is common. Overall, fasting glucose levels fall by 10–20 per cent and postprandial levels are higher.

## PATHOGENESIS

There are two forms of pre-existing diabetes, type 1 and type 2. The prevalence of diabetes in women of reproductive age is 1.2 per cent and is increasing.[3] Overall, for adults in the UK, 90 per cent have type 2 diabetes and 10 per cent type 1. However, in pregnant women, this pattern is reversed, with 27 per cent having type 2 diabetes, and 73 per cent having type 1.[2]

### Type 1 diabetes

Type 1 diabetes mellitus (juvenile onset) is an auto-immune disease that usually presents in childhood or young adulthood. Autoimmune destruction of the pancreatic islet cells results in insulin deficiency and causes symptoms of thirst, polyuria, blurred vision, weight loss and, if untreated, progression to life-threatening diabetic ketoacidosis. There is a genetic component and it is associated with HLA-DR3 and HLA-DR 4. It is not associated with obesity. The baby of an affected mother has a 2 per cent risk of developing diabetes, while the child of an affected father faces an 8 per cent risk. If both parents have type 1 diabetes, there is a 30 per cent risk to their offspring.

## Type 2 diabetes

Type 2 disease (maturity onset) is a disease of peripheral insulin resistance rather than deficiency. Although it more commonly occurs over the age of 40 years, it often occurs at a younger age (25 years and upwards) in those of South Asian and Afro-Caribbean origin. The incidence increases with age and body weight and there is a stronger genetic component than in type 1. Hyperglycaemia is commonly present for a prolonged period prior to diagnosis and although these patients sometimes require insulin treatment, they do not become ketotic if it is withdrawn. At present, type 2 diabetes accounts for the minority of pregnant women with diabetes. However, this is expected to rise with increasing maternal obesity, age and social deprivation.[2] The risks to the affected offspring are higher than in type 1 diabetes. Offspring of an affected mother or father have a 15 per cent risk, and if both parents are affected the risk is 75 per cent.

Women with type 1 or type 2 diabetes are at risk of microvascular and macrovascular complications, resulting in a reduced life expectancy. The recent CEMACH report confirmed that all women with pre-existing diabetes (type 1 and type 2) have uniformly poorer outcomes than women without diabetes.[2]

## Pre-conception

Optimizing pre-conception care in women with diabetes has been shown to improve outcome. Despite this, the CEMACH report found that only 35 per cent of pregnant women with diabetes received adequate pre-conceptional counselling and care.[4]

### Type 1

Pre-conceptual counselling guidelines are outlined in Table 6.2.1. The risk of major congenital malformations, in particular cardiac and neural tube defects, increases with poor control of blood glucose during the first 8 weeks of pregnancy. Levels of glycosylated haemoglobin, $HbA_{1C}$, are used to reflect long-term glycaemic control. If significantly raised, to greater than 8.5–9.5 per cent, malformation rates of around 20 per cent have been reported, and these risks fall if levels of $HbA_{1C}$ can be reduced.[2,5] Therefore, women should be advised that optimizing diabetic control pre-pregnancy will improve outcome of pregnancy. Good glycaemic control will also reduce the risks of miscarriage, stillbirth and neonatal death. Recent NICE guidelines suggest that women should be advised that although good control of diabetes improves risk, it does not eliminate it.[6] The guidelines also suggest that women should aim for an $HbA_{1C}$ of 6.1 per cent [C]. Women with an $HbA_{1C}$ greater than 10 per cent should be advised to avoid pregnancy until better control is achieved.[6] Goals should be set with the

**Table 6.2.1** Pre-conceptual counselling

| |
|---|
| Multidisciplinary |
| Optimize glycaemic control – aim for $HbA_{1C}$ 6.1 per cent or less |
| Discuss hypoglycaemia |
| Review diet and weight loss |
| Discuss complications of pregnancy |
| Prescribe folic acid 5 mg |
| Review renal function and blood pressure |
| Retinal assessment |
| Review other medications, e.g. ACE inhibitors, statins |
| Smoking cessation |

woman, involving other members of the multidisciplinary team. More rigorous control will increase the risks of hypoglycaemia, thus this should be discussed, and women and their families should be aware of the treatments for this (see below).

Other aspects of the women's diabetes should also be reviewed, such as blood pressure, renal function and retinal assessment. The use of any medications that are contraindicated in pregnancy should be assessed and changed if a suitable alternative exists. Typical drugs falling into this category are statins, angiotensin II converting enzyme (ACE) inhibitors and angiotensin II type 1 receptor blockers (ARBs). Renal function should be checked and women with creatinine levels greater than 120 µmol/L should be referred to a renal physician. Women who have significant retinopathy or nephropathy should be advised that pregnancy may accelerate these pathological processes. The opportunity should also be taken to counsel about diet, weight control and smoking cessation. Women should be prescribed 5 mg of folic acid to be taken pre-conception and for the first 12 weeks of pregnancy [D,E]. The risks of other complications of pregnancy, including pre-eclampsia, birth trauma, fetal macrosomia and the increased risk of caesarean section, should also be discussed.

### Type 2

It is estimated that there may be around half a million individuals in the UK with undiagnosed diabetes, usually type 2. Therefore, type 2 diabetes is often unrecognized prior to pregnancy and may be misdiagnosed as gestational diabetes during pregnancy. Recent data suggest that women with type 2 diabetes have a similar increase in risk of congenital abnormality to those with type 1, at around double that of women without diabetes.[5] Therefore, much of the pre-conception advice is the same as that for type 1 diabetes. This group of women are more likely to be overweight and should be helped to reduce their weight if their body mass index is greater than 27 kg/m$^2$ [C][6]. Women taking oral hypoglycaemic agents should have their medication reviewed. Metformin is probably safe to take in pregnancy so can be continued, but current advice is that other oral hypoglycaemics should be changed. Some women may achieve better control by converting to insulin, and this should be discussed with the woman.

## ANTENATAL CARE

The risks and complications of pregnancy in a woman with diabetes are summarized in Table 6.2.2. The aim of antenatal care is to target and reduce these risks. There is no doubt that pregnant women with diabetes are best managed in a joint clinic involving diabetologists, obstetricians, dieticians, specialist midwives and nurses. Unfortunately, the CEMACH survey found that a third of maternity in England, Northern Ireland and Wales did not provide such specialist services.[2] Women should be booked for care early in pregnancy, preferably before 10 weeks. An early ultrasound scan will enable viability and dating to be confirmed. At this early appointment, a full clinical history and medication review should be conducted. If retinal or renal assessment has not occurred during the preceding 12 months, these should be arranged.

In common with all women, women with diabetes should be offered screening for Down's syndrome. The recommended first trimester test which reaches the current required criteria of a detection rate of 75 per cent and a false positive rate of less than 3 per cent is the combined test, consisting of nuchal translucency, β-hCG,

**Table 6.2.2** Complications of pregnancy associated with diabetes

| Fetal risks | Maternal risks |
| --- | --- |
| Miscarriage | Hypoglycaemia |
| Congenital anomaly | Diabetic ketoacidosis |
| Stillbirth | Operative delivery |
| Prematurity | Worsening of retinal disease |
| Risk of diabetes | Worsening of pre-existing renal impairment |
| Macrosomia | Pre-eclampsia |
| Shoulder dystocia and birth injury | |
| Respiratory distress | |
| Neonatal hypoglycaemia and poor feeding | |

pregnancy-associated plasma protein A (PAPP-A). If women present too late, or the nuchal translucency is unobtainable or not available, they should be offered the triple (β-hCG, unconjugated oestriol (uE3), β-fetoprotein (AFP)) or quadruple test (triple + inhibin A) in the second trimester. The nuchal translucency measurement is unaffected by diabetes. However, diabetes is associated with lower levels of AFP and uE3 in the second trimester, hence risk adjustments need to be made. Recent data have also suggested that first trimester PAPP-A and β-hCG may be reduced, although the data are conflicting. Maternal weight and poor diabetic control are two factors that may also reduce the levels of these markers, thus explaining the differences between these studies.

## MEDICATIONS

Good glycaemic control is the key to improving the outcome of pregnancy in women with diabetes. This can be achieved using a combination of diet, insulin and, less commonly, with oral hypoglycaemic agents.

### Oral hypoglycaemic agents

Oral hypoglycaemic agents are often used in patients with type 2 diabetes. The main classes of these drugs are shown in Table 6.2.3. With the exception of metformin and glibenclamide, there are little available data regarding the safety of most of these drugs in pregnancy, or whether they cross the placenta. Metformin is increasingly used in women with polycystic ovarian syndrome as it reduces the risk of first trimester miscarriage and reduces the risk of developing gestational diabetes. Metformin is known to cross the placenta, but two systematic reviews of its use in early pregnancy have not shown any increase in the risk of congenital malformations.[7,8] Glibenclamide may cross the placenta in small amounts and some small observational studies suggest that it may reduce morbidity and mortality in developing countries in which insulin use is impractical and expensive. Of the other sulphonylureas, chlorpropamide and tolbutamide, although probably not associated with congenital malformations, may be associated with prolonged neonatal hypoglycaemia and seizures. There are very few data relating to the newer classes of drugs, and it is largely unknown whether drugs such as nateglinide are able to cross the placenta.

Current recommended practice is for women who conceive on oral hypoglycaemic agents to be switched to insulin therapy as soon as they are pregnant. However, there is growing interest in the use of metformin and glibenclamide in the management of type 2 diabetes or gestational diabetes. These drugs are cheaper, easier and more convenient, have fewer risks of hypoglycaemia and may have beneficial

**Table 6.2.3** Oral hypoglycaemic agents

| Sulphonylureas |
|---|
| Chlorpropamide |
| Glibenclamide |
| Gliclazide |
| Glimepiride |
| Glipizide |
| Gliquidone |
| Tolbutamide |
| **Biguanides** |
| Metformin |
| **α-glucosidase inhibitors** |
| Acarbose |
| **Thiazolidinediones** |
| Pioglitazone |
| Rosiglitazone |
| **Drugs stimulating insulin release** |
| Nateglinide |
| Repaglinide |

effects on long-term prognosis. A randomized controlled trial (RCT) of glibenclamide compared to insulin for the treatment of gestational diabetes found no significant differences in the major outcomes of macrosomia, blood glucose, neonatal hypoglycaemia or admissions to neonatal intensive care.[9] An RCT comparing metformin with insulin in gestational diabetes (MIG trial) has recently confirmed the safety and benefit of metformin treatment in women with gestational diabetes after 20 weeks gestation.[10] Current NICE recommendations are that metformin may be considered as an alternative to insulin therapy in pregnant women with type 2 diabetes.[6] Individual risks and benefits should be considered and the patient involved in the decision. However, this remains the exception rather than the rule in current practice.

# Insulin

Insulin is the current recommended treatment for the majority of pregnant women with diabetes.[6] Initially, insulin available for human use was cow or pig insulin. However, the majority of insulins in current use are recombinant insulins or their analogues. These analogues have a modified amino acid structure to improve absorption profile such that risks of hypoglycaemia are less and more stable blood glucose levels are achieved. There are four main types of insulin available for use, categorized by duration of action (summarized in Table 6.2.4). The newer long acting insulin analogues may be associated with fewer hypoglycaemic episodes as they provide steady background levels without peaks. Insulin regimes vary with the individual, but will typically consist of a long-acting basal insulin, given once or twice a day, with additional boluses given via a pen to cover meal times. Some insulin preparations contain a combination of two types of insulin, for example Mixtard 30, which contains a short-acting insulin together with intermediate NPH insulin (thus are biphasic), given twice a day. Commonly, type 2 diabetics may be able to achieve good control following conversion from oral agents with these preparations.

Continuous subcutaneous insulin infusion (CSII) pumps were initially introduced in the 1970s, are growing in popularity and are particularly useful in patients with unstable diabetes and troublesome hypoglycaemia. The pumps consist of a cannula that is inserted into the subcutaneous abdominal tissue (site changed every 3 days) through which a continuous basal level of fast-acting insulin is administered. Additional boluses are also given through the pump for meal times. In general, studies have shown CSII is associated with improved $HbA_{1C}$ and lower hypoglycaemia rates.

Although there is now a large body of data relating to the short-acting insulin analogues in pregnancy such as Lispro and Aspart, there are no studies of glulisine, glargine and detemir. Thus, current NICE recommendations are that the latter preparations are avoided during pregnancy. [E].[6] Lispro and Aspart may offer some benefits in terms of fewer hypoglycaemic episodes and better control, but until

**Table 6.2.4** Types of insulin

| Type | Examples | Onset | Peak | Duration |
|---|---|---|---|---|
| Rapid acting | Lispro (Humalog) | 15 min | 30–90 min | 5 hours |
| | Aspart (NovoRapid) | | | |
| | Glulisine (Apidra) | | | |
| Short acting | Regular | 30 min | 2–4 hours | 4–8 hours |
| Intermediate acting | NPH (isophane), lente | 2–6 hours | 4–14 hours | 14–20 hours |
| Long acting | Ultralente | 6–14 hours | Small (or none) 10–16 hours | 20–24 hours |
| | Glargine | 1–2 hours | none | 24 hours |
| | Detemir | | | |

sufficiently powered studies are available, use of these drugs should be determined on an individual basis.[6] However, they may be recommended for many patients as they reduce the risks of hypoglycaemia.

# GLYCAEMIC CONTROL

Fetal macrosomia, defined by either a birth weight greater than 4 kg, or a birth weight centile greater than 90, is associated with increased rates of caesarean section, and birth injury such as shoulder dystocia, fractures and brachial plexus injury. Most macrosomic infants are uniformly or symmetrically large (70 per cent), and this pattern also occurs in women without diabetes. Asymmetrically large infants in whom the thoracic and abdominal circumference is greater than the head circumference are at greater risk of shoulder dystocia. Over the last few years, data have suggested that obtaining good glycaemic control (see Table 6.2.5), as indicated by a satisfactory $HbA_{1C}$ level (84 per cent had levels less than 7 per cent), does not reduce the risk of macrosomia.[11] In contrast, observational studies have demonstrated that postprandial blood glucose measurements in the third trimester correlated with macrosomia [B]. The risks of respiratory distress and preterm labour also increase with worsening glycaemic control [C]. Women with diabetes also have an increased risk of stillbirth. The recent CEMACH report found that women whose babies had congenital malformations, or suffered a stillbirth or neonatal death, had worse glycaemic control (as monitored by higher $HbA_{1C}$ levels) throughout pregnancy [D].[4]

**Table 6.2.5** Glycaemic control – recommended levels[6]

| Pre-conception |
| --- |
| $HbA_{1C}$ <7 per cent |
| **First trimester** |
| $HbA_{1C}$ <7 per cent |
| Pre-prandial blood glucose 3.5–5.9 mmol/L |
| Post-prandial blood glucose <7.8 mmol/L |
| **Second and third trimester** |
| Use of $HbA_{1C}$ not recommended |
| Pre-prandial blood glucose 3.5–5.9 mmol/L |
| Post-prandial blood glucose <7.8 mmol/L |
| **Monitoring** |
| Fasting levels and 1 hour after every meal |
| Women taking insulin should also test before bedtime |
| Women with type 1 diabetes should be offered ketone testing strips for use if they become hyperglycaemic or feel unwell |
| Medical review on a regular basis (1–2 weekly) |

Glycosylated haemoglobin represents blood glucose levels in the preceding 4–12 weeks, and does not reflect subtle changes in blood glucose, in particular postprandial levels. Furthermore, it falls in response to the physiological changes in late pregnancy, and the timescale may not be appropriate in pregnant women. Two small randomized controlled trials of pre-prandial and postprandial blood glucose monitoring have found improved outcomes in women in the postprandial group [B].[12,13] Therefore, NICE currently recommends the use of 1 hour postprandial blood glucose measurements of less than 7.8 mmol/L during pregnancy, and states that there is no evidence for the use of $HbA_{1C}$ in the second and third trimesters of pregnancy, hence it should not be routinely used.[6] Pre-prandial glucose levels should be between 3.5 and 5.9 mmol/L. Typically, insulin requirements will increase with gestation, and obtaining good control necessitates frequent review by a diabetic team at 1–2 weekly intervals.

## Hypoglycaemia

Tighter glycaemic control in pregnancy is associated with an increase in the risk of hypoglycaemia. This is compounded by the fact that pregnant women also have an altered hormonal response to hypoglycaemia and reduced awareness.[14,15] Pregnancy-related nausea and vomiting can worsen this. One study of 84 women found that 71 per cent of women suffered a hypoglycaemic episode requiring assistance, and that this peaked at between 10 and 15 weeks.[16] The recent CEMACH report found that women with type 1 diabetes are much more likely to suffer recurrent hypoglycaemia (61 per cent) than those with type 2 (21 per cent).[4] It is therefore vital that pregnant women who are taking insulin, and their families, are fully educated about the symptoms and treatment of hypoglycaemia. NICE defines hypoglycaemia as a blood glucose of <3.5 mmol/L, and this level of blood glucose should be treated even if the patient is asymptomatic. If the patient is conscious, this should be by consuming 10–15 g of glucose (approximates to four teaspoons of sugar, half a can of juice or three glucose tablets). Alternatives include a glucose gel (two tubes of HypoStop/Glucogel) which can be rubbed on the inside of the cheek. This should be followed by a slower releasing carbohydrate such as bread or a sandwich. If unconscious, a family member can administer glucagon (0.5–1 mg) intramuscularly. This has a rapid onset and lasts approximately 90 minutes. For these reasons, it is recommended that patients carry information identifying them as having diabetes. Patients in hospital can be given 150 mL of 10 per cent dextrose intravenously. Once a patient is conscious, they should be given oral therapy as above. If after 10 minutes the blood glucose remains less than 5 mmol/L, the treatment should be repeated. Insulin doses with the next meal should not be withheld but may require modification.

Antenatal complications: maternal

## Diabetic ketoacidosis

Diabetic ketoacidosis (DKA) occurs when there is insufficient insulin to metabolize blood glucose. This can be caused by failure to appreciate the increasing insulin requirements in pregnancy, missed insulin doses, concurrent illness such as infection, steroid therapy and stress. It is defined as a plasma glucose over 12 mmol/L, an arterial pH of less than 7.3, with ketonuria or ketonaemia, and is associated with poor maternal and fetal outcome. CTG abnormalities are typical in the third trimester and resolve with treatment of the hyperglycaemia. Treatment should involve the diabetic teams, treatment of the precipitating cause and will usually require intravenous insulin via a sliding scale. A continuous CTG may be necessary, but should be given careful consideration. CTG abnormalities are to be expected in a woman with DKA, and it would be unsafe to perform an emergency caesarean until the woman is stable from metabolic and haemodynamic perspectives. Severe hyperglycaemia requiring intensive treatment is defined as persistent premeal blood glucose values of greater than 12 mmol/L on two consecutive occasions, or a random level of more than 15 mmol/L. Involvement of diabetologists is recommended as it is important to ensure that the hyperglycaemia is at variance to the patients' usual level of control.

## ADMINISTRATION OF CORTICOSTEROIDS

Corticosteroids, given to reduce neonatal morbidity and mortality associated with prematurity, almost always have an adverse effect on glucose tolerance, resulting in an increased insulin requirement. This can be achieved by increasing subcutaneous doses, or by the use of intravenous insulin via a sliding scale.[6] The peaks in blood glucose usually occur between 9 and 15 hours after the first dose and 8–15 hours after the second dose. Diabetes should not be considered a contraindication to the use of antenatal steroids.

## COMPLICATIONS OF DIABETES

The longer the duration of the diabetes, the higher the chance of a patient having pre-existing vasculopathy, renal dysfunction, neuropathy and diabetic retinopathy. The presence of these complications increases the risks of pre-eclampsia and fetal growth restriction. Pregnancy is associated with progression of pre-existing retinopathy, and this is more likely with increased severity of the pre-existing disease, duration of diabetes, poor glycaemic control and rapid improvements in control [C]. However, NICE consider that the benefits of improved glycaemic control overall outweigh the risks of progression of diabetic retinopathy [E].[6] The presence of hypertension also worsens progression of retinopathy, thus it has been suggested that, in women with these complications, blood pressure should be kept at 120–130/70–80 mmHg. Betablockers should be avoided as antihypertensives due to their possible adverse effects of glucose metabolism. Thus, NICE currently recommends that retinal assessment with pupil dilation should be conducted at booking and at 28 weeks if the booking assessment is normal. If retinopathy is present, a further assessment at 16–20 weeks is necessary.[6] There is evidence that some diabetic retinopathy may regress after delivery, but women with retinopathy should undergo further retinal assessment by six months postpartum.

Diabetic nephropathy is considered as a continuous spectrum from microalbuminuria, proteinuria and impaired renal function to end stage renal disease in which there is increasing serum urea and creatinine. Overall, with the exception of women with pre-existing renal failure, nephropathy does not deteriorate with pregnancy. However, there is an increased risk of growth restriction, pre-eclampsia and preterm birth. Thus increased surveillance is required in these women. Although low dose aspirin and uterine artery Doppler assessments have been used in other high risk pregnancies, there is currently no specific evidence to support their use in women with these diabetic complications.

## Congenital anomalies

The recent CEMACH enquiry found the prevalence of confirmed major anomalies to be 41.8/1000 total births in pregnant women with diabetes.[4] The most common are cardiac abnormalities in which there is a 3–5-fold increased relative risk for women with diabetes. Although caudal regression (sacral agenesis) is the most well known associated abnormality (200-fold increased risk), the prevalence is low. Diabetes conveys a 2–10-fold increased risk of neural tube defects. Thus, all women with diabetes should have a detailed fetal anatomy scan at 20 weeks, which should include the four chamber cardiac view and the outflow tracts. NICE currently do not recommend specialist fetal echocardiography for women with diabetes.[6]

## Fetal monitoring

All fetal monitoring in the third trimester of pregnancy is aimed at reducing the two most significant late pregnancy complications of diabetes, macrosomia and the risks of shoulder dystocia, and stillbirth. The CEMACH report found that the stillbirth rate after 24 weeks was 26.8 per 1000 live births and stillbirths, compared to the national background rate of 5.7 per 1000.[4] The stillbirth rate varied with gestation, with 17.2 per cent occurring at 24–27 weeks, 13.8 per cent at 28–31, 41.4 per cent at 32–36 weeks and 27.6 per cent at 31–41 weeks [D]. Monitoring strategies aimed at reducing these risks comprise of regular ultra-sound scans and CTGs, but there is no good evidence for the use of any of these in the care of women with diabetes. Furthermore, interpretation must consider the effects of diabetes on the monitoring. Diabetes may reduce the variability and increase the baseline fetal heart rate. There may also be fewer movements and thus less accelerations. Therefore, patterns of change may be a better indicator of deterioration in fetal well-being. Most units conduct regular ultrasound scans for growth, liquor volume and Doppler in women with diabetes at 2–4-weekly intervals, guided by findings and control of blood glucose. Growth velocity and, in particular, crossing centiles are of use in identifying the development of macrosomia and growth restriction.

## Mode and timing of delivery

The CEMACH enquiry found high rates of induction of labour and caesarean section in women with diabetes.[4] The induction of labour rate was 39 per cent, compared to a background rate of 21 per cent, and the caesarean section rate was 67 per cent [D]. Higher rates of caesarean sections and shoulder dystocia have also been described in large cohorts in other populations. There is now some evidence to suggest that induction of labour at 38 weeks may reduce the risks of shoulder dystocia in macrosomic infants of women with diabetes. An RCT compared induction with expectant management in women requiring insulin (most had gestational diabetes) and found that expectant management did not reduce caesarean section rates and increased the rates of large babies and shoulder dystocia [B].[17] A further case controlled trial from Israel compared induction at 38–39 weeks with expectant management in type 1 diabetes. The rate of shoulder dystocia was lower in the induction group [C].[18] Interestingly, there is also retrospective data suggesting that induction is associated with a reduction in caesarean section rates in women with diabetes [D]. Thus current NICE guidance is that women with diabetes and a normally grown baby should be offered delivery (induction or caesarean section if indicated) after 38 completed weeks.[6] Women with an ultrasound diagnosis of macrosomia should be informed of the risks and benefits of induction of labour, vaginal birth and caesarean section.[6] One retrospective case controlled study suggested that caesarean section was safer with estimated fetal weights greater than 4.25 kg, thus some advocate this fetal weight as a cut-off [D].

## Intrapartum care

Good control of maternal blood glucose during labour in women with diabetes is important due to the association between hyperglycaemia and neonatal hypoglycaemia. Some infants produce high levels of insulin antenatally in response to high levels of glucose crossing the placenta. After delivery, there is withdrawal of the maternal glucose but a persistent high level of neonatal insulin production, resulting in neonatal hypoglycaemia. More recently, data have suggested that short term control of maternal blood glucose, i.e. during labour, may impact on neonatal hypoglycaemia. Several studies have shown that a maternal blood glucose of greater than 7.1 mmol/L is associated with neonatal hypoglycaemia [C]. Furthermore, maternal hyperglycaemia is also associated with 'perinatal asphyxia' and 'fetal distress' [C]. Thus, current guidance is that maternal blood glucose should be kept between 4 and 7 mmol/L during labour and delivery.[6] However, there are no studies investigating the best method of achieving this. Blood glucose should be tested hourly and women not maintaining their blood glucose within this range should be commenced on an intravenous insulin and dextrose infusion via a sliding scale. Sliding scales should be developed together with local Diabetologists, but an example is given in Table 6.2.6. This may be considered at the onset of labour for women with type 1 diabetes, particularly if their oral intake is reduced. It will also be required for women delivered by elective caesarean section. However, some women, particularly those with a CSII pump, may manage the required level of control without the use of a sliding scale. Care should be taken with the use of sliding scales, and the intravenous infusions regularly checked (preferably hourly), as severe clinical incidents and death have occurred when infusions have become blocked or run too fast.

Induction of labour in women with diabetes is conducted in the same way as women without diabetes (syntocinon infusions should be administered in saline), and NICE guidelines state that diabetes alone is not a contraindication to allowing a vaginal birth after a caesarean section.[6]

There are very few studies of the use of analgesia during labour and delivery. Thus NICE guidelines state that analgesia for women with diabetes should be managed in the usual way.[6] However, prolonged diabetes and hyperglycaemia may be associated with delayed gastric emptying, thus increasing risks for women requiring a general anaesthetic. General anaesthesia also increases risks of hypoglycaemia and reduces awareness, thus these women should have blood glucose monitoring every 30 minutes until fully conscious. Since women with other co-morbidities, such as autonomic neuropathy or obesity, face additional risks, these women should be offered an anaesthetic review during the third trimester.

## Postpartum care

With delivery of the placenta, insulin requirements dramatically decrease, thus all women will require a reduction in insulin dose, even when managed with the insulin sliding scale. Consultant diabetologist involvement is very important at this time, and especially when the patient is converted back to subcutaneous insulin. Advice varies regarding the subcutaneous insulin dose following

**Table 6.2.6** Example sliding scale for use during labour in pregnant women taking insulin

| Hourly blood glucose (mmol/L) | Insulin rate (units per hour = mL per hour) | Other action |
|---|---|---|
| 3.0 or less | 0 | Repeat glucose test, give glucose[a] if <3.1, check all lines and infusion pumps, call consultant |
| 3.1–3.9 | 0.5 | Repeat glucose test, give glucose if <4.0 and symptomatic[a] if hypo confirmed, check all lines and infusion pumps |
| 4.0–6.9 | 1 | |
| 7.0–7.9 | 2 | |
| 8.0–8.9 | 3 | |
| 9.0–10.9 | 4 | Call consultant |
| 11.0–16 | 6 | Stop dextrose, start 0.9 per cent saline, call consultant |
| More than 16 | 8 | Stop dextrose, start 0.9 per cent saline, call consultant |

[a]Treat hypoglycaemia with three glucose tablets, 60 mL lucozade or 150 mL of intravenous 10 per cent dextrose.

- Serious clinical incidents including death have occurred with sliding scale insulin regimens. Please follow protocol precisely.
- Setting up the insulin sliding scale should always be done in consultation with the consultant physician. Some patients required higher or lower insulin infusion rates, especially if they are receiving high dose of insulin (>60 units/day).
- The insulin infusion rate should be reduced immediately after delivery – the consultant physician will advise.
- The aim is to keep blood glucose concentration between 4 and 7 mmol/L.
- If blood glucose levels do not fall into the 4–7 mmol/L range after 3 hours of i.v. insulin, contact either the consultant physician, the diabetes specialist midwife or the on call medical team.
- Set up the following infusions that can be given through the same venflon using a Y connector:
  - IVAC drip – 10 per cent dextrose 500 ml at –83 mL/hour.
  - Infusion syringe pump – 50 units actrapid insulin in 50 mL of normal saline.
- It is very important that the lines and pumps are checked hourly, AND if there is unexplained hyper- or hypoglycaemia – failure of either IVAC pump or line can cause unexplained dangerous hyper- or hypoglycaemia.
- The rate of the insulin pump is adjusted based on hourly blood glucose measurements

Taken from St Mary's Hospital guidelines, Central Manchester University Hospitals NHS Foundation Trust, Dr Martin Rutter and Dr Mike Maresh.

delivery for women with pre-existing diabetes. Some suggest changing insulin regimes to the pre-pregnancy dosing, others suggest a halving of insulin doses. Our local practice is to reduce the insulin dose to 50 per cent of the pre-pregnancy dose for the first 12–36 hours and then to increase the dose gradually to the pre-pregnancy dose or to whatever dose is required to achieve capillary blood glucose values of 5–9 mmol/L in the immediate postpartum period. Seven-times daily capillary blood glucose monitoring is recommended to aid insulin dose adjustment for the first 2–3 days following delivery. Hypoglycaemia is a major risk for women with type 1 diabetes at this time, especially in overweight or obese women who experience a large increase in their insulin requirements during pregnancy. Women who have undergone caesarean section will require continuation of the sliding scale until normal eating is resumed. Women with type 2 diabetes can change from insulin back to their oral hypoglycaemic agents.

## Breastfeeding

Small cohort studies have demonstrated that breastfeeding increases the frequency of hypoglycaemia in insulin-dependent diabetics [C]. Thus women should be advised to have a snack before or during breastfeeding. Oral hypoglycaemic agents cross into breast milk in small quantities. NICE currently recommends that women with pre-existing type 2 diabetes can safely take metformin and glibenclamide while breastfeeding, but that other oral hypoglycaemic agents should probably be avoided.[6] There are limited data regarding the use of other prenatally prescribed drugs, such as angiotensin converting enzyme inhibitors, statins and angiotensin receptor antagonists, and breastfeeding. These drugs are probably present in breast milk in small amounts. Current guidance is that drugs avoided in the antenatal period should also be avoided during breastfeeding.[6] However, a risk–benefit analysis should be conducted on an individual patient basis.

## Contraception and follow up

Women with pre-existing diabetes should be referred back to their routine diabetic care team, usually following a 6 week postnatal review. Contraception should be discussed, as future pregnancies should be planned and the NICE postnatal care guidelines suggest that this should be within 1 week of delivery. The recent CEMACH report found that women with a poor obstetric outcome were less likely to receive such advice.[4] Low-dose oestrogen containing pills have little impact on diabetic control, and progesterone-only pills can be used in women with type 1 diabetes providing there is good control of blood glucose and plasma lipids. Contraceptive choices should be discussed with individual women, with careful consideration of their risk factors.

In particular, caution should be taken in women with risk factors for vascular disease. Women should also be made aware of the importance of preconception care when planning future pregnancies.

## KEY POINTS

- Insulin requirements usually increase during pregnancy.
- Women with diabetes have poorer pregnancy outcomes than women without diabetes.
- Good glycaemic control pre-conception and in the first 8 weeks reduces the risk of congenital abnormalities (HbA1c of 6.1 per cent).
- Pregnant women with diabetes should be managed in a joint obstetric/diabetic clinic involving the input of obstetricians, diabetologists, dieticians, specialist nurses and midwives.
- Pre-prandial blood glucose should be 3.5-5.9 mmol/L.
- Post-prandial levels should be less than 7.8 mmol/L.
- Post-prandial bood glucose levels, rather than levels of HbA1c, should be used to monitor glycaemic control in the second and third trimesters as these are associated with a better outcome.
- Tight glycaemic control results in a higher incidence of hypoglycaemia.
- Diabetic ketoacidosis is associated with poor maternal and fetal outcome.
- Women with diabetes should be offered monitoring of fetal growth and well-being, although there is no good evidence that these monitoring strategies reduce the risks of stillbirth and macrosomia.
- Women with diabetes should be offered delivery after 38-39 weeks, as there is evidence that this reduces risk shoulder dystocia and caesarean section.
- Women with macrosomia should have the risks and benefits of different modes of delivery discussed with them.
- Maternal blood glucose should be kept between 4 and 7 mmol/L during labour and delivery to reduce the risks of neonatal hypoglycaemia. This may require an insulin/dextrose infusion.
- Insulin requirements fall rapidly postnatally.
- Breastfeeding is associated with hypoglycaemia.
- All women should receive postnatal advice regarding contraception and planning their next pregnancy.

## Key References

1. DOH. National Service Framework for Diabetes: Standards. London: Department of Health, 2002.

2. CEMACH. Confidential Enquiry into Maternal and Child Health. Diabetes in Pregnancy: Are we providing the best care? Findings of a National Enquiry: England, Wales and Northern Ireland. London: CEMACH, 2007.

3. Shelton N. Health Survey for England 2006: The Information Centre, Joint Health Surveys Unit, National Centre for Social Research, Department of Epidemiology and Public Health at the Royal Free and University College Medical School, 2008.

4. CEMACH. Confidential Enquiry into Maternal and Child Health 2005. Pregnancy in women with type 1 and type 2 diabetes in 2002–3. England, Wales and Northern Ireland. London, 2005.

5. Macintosh MC, Fleming KM, Bailey JA *et al*. Perinatal mortality and congenital anomalies in babies of women with type 1 or type 2 diabetes in England, Wales, and Northern Ireland: population based study. *BMJ* 2006; **333**: 177.

6. NICE. Diabetes in Pregnancy. Management of diabetes and its complications from pre-conception to the postnatal period. London, 2008.

7. Hawthorne G. Metformin use and diabetic pregnancy – has its time come? *Diabet Med* 2006; **23**: 223–7.

8. Gilbert C, Valois M, Koren G. Pregnancy outcome after first-trimester exposure to metformin: a meta-analysis. *Fertil Steril* 2006; **86**: 658–63.

9. Langer O, Conway DL, Berkus MD *et al*. A comparison of glyburide and insulin in women with gestational diabetes mellitus. *N Engl J Med* 2000; **343**: 1134–8.

10. Rowan JA, Hague WM, Gao W *et al*. Metformin versus insulin for the treatment of gestational diabetes. *N Engl J Med* 2008; **358**: 2003–15.

11. Evers IM, de Valk HW, Mol BW *et al*. Macrosomia despite good glycaemic control in Type I diabetic pregnancy; results of a nationwide study in The Netherlands. *Diabetologia* 2002; **45**: 1484–9.

12. Manderson JG, Patterson CC, Hadden DR *et al*. Preprandial versus postprandial blood glucose monitoring in type 1 diabetic pregnancy: a randomized controlled clinical trial. *Am J Obstet Gynecol* 2003; **189**: 507–12.

13. de Veciana M, Major CA, Morgan MA *et al*. Postprandial versus preprandial blood glucose monitoring in women with gestational diabetes mellitus requiring insulin therapy. *N Engl J Med* 1995; **333**: 1237–41.

14. Rosenn BM, Miodovnik M, Khoury JC, Siddiqi TA. Counterregulatory hormonal responses to hypoglycemia during pregnancy. *Obstet Gynecol* 1996; **87**: 568–74.

15. Diamond MP, Reece EA, Caprio S *et al*. Impairment of counterregulatory hormone responses to hypoglycemia in pregnant women with insulin-dependent diabetes mellitus. *Am J Obstet Gynecol* 1992; **166**: 70–7.

16. Rosenn BM, Miodovnik M, Holcberg G *et al.* Hypoglycemia: the price of intensive insulin therapy for pregnant women with insulin-dependent diabetes mellitus. *Obstet Gynecol* 1995; **85**: 417–22.

17. Kjos SL, Henry OA, Montoro M *et al.* Insulin-requiring diabetes in pregnancy: a randomized trial of active induction of labor and expectant management. *Am J Obstet Gynecol* 1993; **169**: 611–15.

18. Lurie S, Insler V, Hagay ZJ. Induction of labor at 38 to 39 weeks of gestation reduces the incidence of shoulder dystocia in gestational diabetic patients class A2. *Am J Perinatol* 1996; **13**: 293–6.

# 6.3 Cardiac disease

*Catherine Nelson-Piercy*

## INTRODUCTION

Cardiac disease in pregnancy is rare in the UK, but common in developing countries. This chapter covers the most important conditions relevant to pregnancy, including pulmonary hypertension, aortic dissection, ischaemic heart disease, mitral stenosis and mechanical heart valves. Peripartum cardiomyopathy is included as it is specific to the pregnant or postpartum state.

## PHYSIOLOGICAL CHANGES IN PREGNANCY

Cardiac output increases by 40 per cent, reaching a maximum by the mid-second trimester. There is peripheral vasodilatation, an increase in heart rate and a fall in systemic and pulmonary vascular resistance. Labour and delivery are associated with further increases in cardiac output. Palpitations, extrasystoles and ejection systolic murmurs are common in pregnancy but rarely represent underlying pathology. The electrocardiogram (ECG) changes associated with normal pregnancy include atrial and ventricular ectopics, a 'left shift' in the QRS axis, a small Q wave and inverted T wave in lead III, and ST segment depression and T wave inversion in the inferior and lateral leads.

## INCIDENCE

Although cardiac disease in pregnancy is rare (<1 per cent) in the UK, cardiac disease is the most common cause of maternal death.[1] Ischaemic heart disease is becoming more common in pregnancy, and deaths in pregnancy and the puerperium from myocardial infarction and ischaemic heart disease are increasing.[1] Congenital heart disease is encountered more frequently as those who have received corrective surgery as children reach child-bearing age. Rheumatic heart disease is less common in the UK, but is encountered increasingly in women from developing countries.

## AETIOLOGY

The aetiology of heart disease may be divided into congenital and acquired causes. The most common congenital heart diseases encountered in pregnancy are ventricular and atrial septal defects (ASD, VSD) and patent ductus arteriosus. These are mostly diagnosed before pregnancy and are usually either haemodynamically insignificant or corrected. Acquired causes of cardiac disease include ischaemic heart disease, rheumatic heart disease, cardiomyopathies, and aneurysms and dissection of the aorta or its branches.

**Table 6.3.1** New York Heart Association (NYHA) functional classification

| NYHA | Symptoms |
|------|----------|
| I | No symptoms and no limitation in ordinary physical activity |
| II | Mild symptoms and slight limitation during ordinary activity |
| III | Marked limitation in activity due to symptoms, even during less than ordinary activity. Only comfortable at rest. |
| IV | Severe limitations. Experiences symptoms even at rest |

## GENERAL PRINCIPLES

When assessing or counselling a pregnant or potentially pregnant woman with heart disease, it is important to remember that the outcome and safety of pregnancy are related to the presence and severity of pulmonary hypertension, the presence of cyanosis, the haemodynamic significance of the lesion and the functional class [D].[2] The functional class is determined by the level of activity that leads to dyspnoea (see Table 6.3.1). In addition, women with previous cardiac events including transient ischaemic attacks, arrhythmia, pulmonary oedema or heart failure, and those with left-sided lesions (e.g. aortic or mitral stenosis) or myocardial dysfunction, are at risk in pregnancy.[3] Women with congenital heart disease are at increased risk of having a baby with congenital heart disease, and should therefore be offered detailed fetal scanning for cardiac anomalies. During pregnancy, women with heart disease require multidisciplinary team care,[2] with regular antenatal visits and judicious monitoring to avoid or treat expediently any anaemia, infection or hypertension. There should be early involvement of obstetric anaesthetists and a carefully documented plan for delivery.[2]

## PULMONARY HYPERTENSION

The most common forms of pulmonary hypertension encountered in women of child-bearing age are idiopathic pulmonary arterial hypertension, Eisenmenger's syndrome (when pulmonary hypertension develops secondary to a large left-to-right shunt such as a VSD, and the shunt is reversed to become right to left, with consequent cyanosis), secondary to chronic pulmonary thromboembolic disease, secondary to connective tissue disorders particularly scleroderma, sickle cell disease and secondary to cardiac lesions causing raised pulmonary capillary wedge pressure such as mitral stenosis. Pulmonary hypertension from any cause is dangerous and maternal mortality is 40 per cent [D],[4] although this may be decreasing.[5] The danger relates to fixed pulmonary vascular resistance and an inability to increase

pulmonary blood flow, with refractory hypoxaemia. Most pregnancy-associated deaths can be attributed to thromboembolism, hypovolaemia or pre-eclampsia.

## Management

Women with pulmonary hypertension should be advised to avoid pregnancy or, in the event of unplanned pregnancy, to have a therapeutic termination [D].[5,6] If such advice is declined, multidisciplinary care and elective admission for bed rest, oxygen and thromboprophylaxis are recommended [D].[4] Therapies such as endothelin antagonists (e.g. Bosentan) and sildenafil should be continued in pregnancy, not withstanding the possible fetal risks associated with the former. Some centres have successfully used nebulized or intravenous prostacyclin.[2,5]

> **EBM**
>
> - Most published evidence relating to pulmonary hypertension comes from retrospective cohorts and case series.
> - All the literature supports a high risk of maternal death sufficient to make this condition one of the absolute contraindications to pregnancy.
> - There is no evidence that monitoring the pulmonary artery pressure prepartum or intrapartum improves outcome.

## AORTIC DISSECTION

Aortic dissection is a common cause of cardiac death in pregnancy,[1] and pregnancy increases the risk of aortic dissection. Most cases occur in late pregnancy at or near term or in the early puerperium. Certain conditions predispose to aortic dissection. These include bicuspid aortic valve, aortic coarctation, Turner's syndrome, Ehlers Danlos syndrome (vascular type IV) and Marfan's syndrome.[7] Marfan's is an autosomal dominant condition with typical skeletal and other features including tall stature, a high arched palate, scoliosis and lens dislocation. Progressive aortic root dilatation and an aortic root dimension >4 cm are associated with increased risk [D].[8] Conversely, in women with minimal cardiac involvement and an aortic root <4 cm, pregnancy outcome is good [C]. Overall, pregnancy is associated with a 5-fold increased risk of aortic complications in women with Marfan's syndrome.[9]

## Management

Acute aortic dissection should be suspected if a woman in late pregnancy presents with severe chest or interscapular pain, particularly if associated with systolic hypertension, different blood pressures in each arm, an early diastolic murmur of aortic regurgitation or any of the above listed predisposing factors. Urgent imaging with CT, MRI or echo is indicated and, if the diagnosis is confirmed, cardiac surgery referral is mandatory. Women with Marfan's with aortic roots >4.5 cm should be advised to delay pregnancy until after aortic root repair. Recommendations include monthly echocardiograms, beta-blockers for those with hypertension or aortic root dilatation, vaginal delivery for those with stable aortic root measurements, but elective caesarean section with epidural if there is an enlarged or dilating aortic root [D].[8]

---

**EBM**

- Most published evidence relating to Marfan's syndrome comes from retrospective cohorts and case series.
- The literature supports a higher risk of aortic rupture and maternal death if the aortic root is >4 cm.

---

## MITRAL STENOSIS

Mitral stenosis is increasingly encountered in migrant women, who may or may not have had the diagnosis made prior to pregnancy.[10] A history of previous mitral valvotomy does not preclude restenosis. Mitral stenosis is the most common rheumatic heart disease and is important in pregnancy because women may deteriorate secondary to tachycardia, arrhythmias or the increased cardiac output. The commonest complication is pulmonary oedema secondary to increased left atrial pressure and precipitated by increased heart rate or increased volume (such as occurs during the third stage of labour) [C].[10] The risk is increased with severe mitral stenosis, moderate or severe symptoms prior to pregnancy, and in those diagnosed late in pregnancy [C].[11]

### Management

Women with severe mitral stenosis should be advised to delay pregnancy until after balloon, open or closed mitral valvotomy or mitral valve replacement. Beta-blockers decrease heart rate and the risk of pulmonary oedema [D],[10] but if medical therapy fails or for those with severe mitral stenosis, balloon mitral valvotomy may be safely and successfully used in pregnancy [D].[10] Women with mitral stenosis should avoid the supine and lithotomy positions as much as possible for labour and delivery. Fluid overload must be avoided [E]. Pulmonary oedema should be treated in the usual way with oxygen and diuretics.

---

**EBM**

- Most published evidence relating to mitral stenosis comes from retrospective cohorts and case series.
- The literature supports a higher risk of pulmonary oedema in severe mitral stenosis.
- Beta-blockers, diuretics and balloon valvotomy are safe in pregnancy.

---

## MECHANICAL HEART VALVES

The problem for women with metal heart valve replacements is that they require life-long anticoagulation, and this must be continued in pregnancy because of the increased risk of thrombosis. Warfarin is associated with warfarin embryopathy[12] and increased risks of miscarriage, stillbirth and fetal intracerebral haemorrhage.[13] Heparin, even in full anticoagulant doses, is associated with increased risks of valve thrombosis and embolic events [C].[12,13]

### Management

The safest option for some mothers is to continue warfarin throughout pregnancy [C].[12,13] Other management strategies include replacing the warfarin with high-dose unfractionated or low-molecular-weight heparin (LMWH), either from 6 to 12 weeks gestation to avoid warfarin embryopathy or throughout pregnancy.[14] Since the risk of thrombosis is less with the newer bileaflet valves (e.g. Carbomedics), and valves in the aortic position, it may be that high doses of heparin throughout pregnancy are appropriate in women with these valves [E]. If heparin or LMWH is used, doses should be adjusted according to APTT or anti-Xa levels and low-dose aspirin is usually also given.[14] Whichever management option is chosen, warfarin should be discontinued and substituted with heparin for 10 days prior to delivery to allow clearance of warfarin from the fetal circulation. For delivery itself, heparin therapy is interrupted, but restarted post-partum. Warfarin is recommened 5–7 days post-partum [E]. In the event of bleeding or the need for urgent delivery in a fully anticoagulated patient, warfarin may be reversed with fresh frozen plasma (FFP) and vitamin K, and heparin with protamine sulphate.

---

**EBM**

- Most published evidence relating to mechanical heart valves comes from retrospective cohorts and case series of women with older generation valves, such as Starr-Edwards and Bjork Shiley valves.
- The literature supports a lower risk of thromboembolic events if warfarin is continued throughout pregnancy.

Antenatal complications: maternal

If heparin is used, this should be in full anticoagulant doses, adjusted according to regular monitoring.

## ISCHAEMIC HEART DISEASE

Ischaemic heart disease in pregnancy is becoming more common as maternal age and obesity increase.[1,15] The risk of myocardial infarction is increased in women over 35 years old, multigravid women, in those who smoke and in women with diabetes, obesity, hypertension and hypercholesterolaemia [C].[15] Acute coronary syndromes may be diagnosed as in the non-pregnant patient with troponin levels, which are not altered by pregnancy, and ECG changes. Infarction most commonly occurs in the post-partum period. The maternal death rate is about 10 per cent.[15] In pregnancy, other underlying aetiologies for myocardial infarction, such as coronary artery thrombosis or dissection, should be considered [C].[1]

### Management

Management of acute MI is as for the non-pregnant woman [D]. Coronary angiography should not be withheld in pregnant patients. Percutaneous coronary intervention may provide a better alternative to thrombolysis in these situations as it is associated with less bleeding risk and also allows management of spontaneous dissections with stent implantation. However, stent implantation may be associated with an increased risk of coronary dissection in a vulnerable vessel [D]. For secondary prevention in women with known ischaemic heart disease, both aspirin and beta-blockers are safe in pregnancy [A]. Statins should be discontinued prior to and for the duration of pregnancy [E].

## ENDOCARDITIS PROPHYLAXIS

The current UK recommendations from the National Institute for Clinical Excellence (NICE) 2008 are that antibiotic prophylaxis against infective endocarditis (IE) is not required for childbirth. The British Society for Antimicrobial Chemotherapy (BSAC) 2006, and the American Heart Association (AHA) have recommended cover only for patients deemed to be at high risk of developing IE (such as women with previous IE) and for those who have the poorest outcome if they develop IE (such as those with cyanotic congenital heart disease) (see below under Published guidelines). If antibiotic prophylaxis is used, it should be with amoxycillin 2 g i.v. plus gentamicin 120 mg i.v. at the onset of labour or ruptured membranes or prior to caesarean section, followed by amoxycillin 500 mg orally (or i.m./i.v. depending on the patient's condition) 6 hours

later. For women who are penicillin allergic, vancomycin 1 g i.v. or teicoplanin 400 mg i.v. may be used instead of amoxycillin.[16]

## HYPERTROPHIC CARDIOMYOPATHY

Most cases of hypertrophic cardiomyopathy (HCM) are familial, inherited as autosomal dominant. Women may be asymptomatic, especially if diagnosed because of family screening, or may experience syncope or 'angina-like' chest pain. The danger relates to left ventricular outflow tract obstruction that may be precipitated by hypotension or hypovolaemia. Provided these are avoided, pregnancy is usually well tolerated. Beta-blockers should be continued in pregnancy or initiated for symptomatic women [D].[17]

## PERIPARTUM CARDIOMYOPATHY

This pregnancy-specific condition is defined as the development of cardiac failure between the last month of pregnancy and five months postpartum, the absence of an identifiable cause, the absence of recognizable heart disease prior to the last month of pregnancy and left ventricular systolic dysfunction demonstrated by classic echocardiographic criteria [C].[18] Risk factors include multiple pregnancy, hypertension, multiparity, increased age and Afro-Caribbean race [D].[2]

Diagnosis should be suspected in puerperal women or those in late pregnancy with breathlessness and signs of heart failure. It is confirmed with echocardiography showing left ventricular dysfunction and often dilatation of all four chambers of the heart. Treatment is as for other causes of heart failure, with oxygen, diuretics, vasodilators, angiotensin-converting enzyme (ACE) inhibitors if postpartum and inotropes if required. Prognosis and recurrence depend on the normalization of left ventricular size and function within six months of delivery [C].[2,18]

## ARRHYTHMIAS

A sinus tachycardia requires investigation for possible underlying pathology such as blood loss, infection, heart failure, thyrotoxicosis or pulmonary embolus, but no treatment is required if such causes are excluded. The most common arrhythmia encountered in pregnancy is supraventricular tachycardia (SVT). An SVT that does not respond to vagal manoeuvres may be safely terminated in pregnancy with adenosine [D] or intravenous verapamil.

## KEY POINTS

- Heart disease is a common cause of maternal mortality in the UK.
- Eisenmenger's syndrome, other causes of pulmonary hypertension, severe mitral stenosis, Marfan's syndrome with aortic root dilatation and severe cardiomyopathy are contraindications to pregnancy.
- The safest option for some women with mechanical heart valves is to continue warfarin in pregnancy, notwithstanding the associated fetal risks.
- Antibiotic prophylaxis against endocarditis is no longer recommended peripartum in women with heart disease.

## Published Guidelines

NICE Clinical Guideline. Prophylaxis against infective endocarditis. March 2008 http://www.nice.org.uk/nicemedia/pdf/CG64NICEguidance.pdf

## Key References

1. Lewis G (ed). The Confidential Enquiry into Maternal and Child Health (CEMACH). Saving Mothers' Lives: reviewing maternal deaths to make motherhood safer 2003-2005. The Seventh Report on Confidential Enquiries into Maternal Deaths in the UK. London: CEMACH, Dec 2007.
2. Steer P, Gatzoulis M, Baker P (eds) *Cardiac Disease in Pregnancy*. London: RCOG Press, 2006.
3. Siu SC, Sermer M, Colman JM *et al.* Prospective multicenter study of pregnancy outcomes in women with heart disease. *Circulation* 2001; **104**: 515–21.
4. Yentis SM, Steer PJ, Plaat F. Eisenmenger's syndrome in pregnancy: maternal and fetal mortality in the 1990s. *Br J Obstet Gynaecol* 1998; **105**: 921–2.
5. Bédard E, Dimopoulos K, Gatzoulis MA. Has there been any progress made on pregnancy outcomes among women with pulmonary arterial hypertension? *Eur Heart J* 2009; **30**: 256–65.
6. Thorne SA, Nelson-Piercy C, MacGregor A. Risks of contraception and pregnancy in heart disease. *Heart* 2006; **92**: 1520–25.
7. Immer FF, Bansi AG, Immer-Bansi AS *et al.* Aortic dissection in pregnancy: analysis of risk factors and outcome. *Ann Thorac Surg* 2003; **76**: 309–14.
8. Lipscomb KJ, Clayton Smith J, Clarke B *et al.* Outcome of pregnancy in women with Marfan's syndrome. *Br J Obstet Gynaecol* 1997; **104**: 201–6.
9. Pacini L, Digne F, Boumendil A *et al.* Maternal complication of pregnancy in Marfan syndrome. *Int J Cardiol* 2009; **136**: 156–61.
10. Tsiaras S, Poppas A. Mitral valve disease in pregnancy: outcomes and management. *Obstet Med* 2009; **2**: 6–10.
11. Silversides CK, Colman JM, Sermer M, Siu SC. Cardiac risk in pregnant women with rheumatic mitral stenosis. *Am J Cardiol* 2003; **91**: 1382–5.
12. Chan WS, Anand S, Ginsberg JS. Anticoagulation of pregnant women with mechanical heart valves. *Arch Intern Med* 2000; **160**: 191–6.
13. Sadler L, McCowan L, White H *et al.* Pregnancy outcomes and cardiac complications in women with mechanical, bioprosthetic and homograft valves. *Br J Obstet Gynaecol* 2000; **107**: 245–53.
14. Oran B, Lee-Parritz A, Ansell J. Low molecular weight heparin for the prophylaxis of thromboembolism in women with prosthetic mechanical heart valves during pregnancy. *Thromb Haemostat* 2004; **92**: 747–51.
15. Ladner HE, Danielsen B, Gilbert WM. Acute myocardial infarction in pregnancy and the puerperium: a population-based study. *Obstet Gynecol* 2005; **105**: 480–4.
16. Dajani AS, Taubert KA, Wilson W *et al.* Prevention of bacterial endocarditis. Recommendations by the American Heart Association. *J Am Med Assoc* 1997; **277**: 1794–801.
17. Oakley CM, Warnes CA. *Heart disease in pregnancy*, 2nd edn. Oxford: Wiley Blackwell, 2007.
18. Pearson GD, Veille JC, Rahimtoola S *et al.* Peripartum cardiomyopathy. National Heart, Lung and Blood Institute and Office of Rare Diseases (NIH). Workshop Recommendations and Review. *J Am Med Assoc* 2000; **283**: 1183–8.

# 6.4 Thyroid disease

*Andrew Shennan*

## INTRODUCTION: PHYSIOLOGY OF THYROID FUNCTION

### Maternal physiology

Thyroid disease occurs in more than 1 per cent of the population and is the most common pre-existing endocrine disorder in pregnant women. A fundamental understanding of thyroid function in pregnancy is essential. Thyroid-stimulating hormone (TSH) is released from the anterior pituitary in 1–2-hourly cycles. It increases both the synthesis and release of thyroxine (T4) and triiodothyronine (T3). The T3 and T4 are mostly protein bound – to thyroid-binding globulin (TBG), albumin and transthyretin. Although the concentration of TBG is low, the binding affinity is high, and TBG binds 75 per cent of thyroid hormones. The unbound thyroid hormones have biological activity; only 0.04 per cent of T4 and 0.05 per cent of T3 are free.

Iodide is essential for the synthesis of thyroid hormones, and the thyroid gland actively traps iodine, ultimately releasing thyroglobulin molecules. Each molecule carries three or four molecules of T4. Circulating T3 is produced principally by peripheral deiodination of T4, by deiodinase enzyme, and is three times more potent than T4. Although the production of T3 is lower than that of T4, more T3 is available as a free, inactive compound.

In pregnancy, there is altered TBG production as a result of increased oestrogen synthesis. Levels of TBG increase in the first 2 weeks of pregnancy, and triple to reach a plateau by 20 weeks, due to glycosylation that is oestrogen driven. The half-life extends from 15 minutes to 3 days in this time. The increase in TBG leads to an increase in the serum concentrations of total T4 and T3, but there are no changes in the amount of free circulating (unbound) thyroid hormones, although these must be interpreted with pregnancy-specific reference ranges. There is iodine deficiency in pregnancy as a result of loss through increased glomerular filtration. This results in increased uptake by the thyroid gland, which can result in enlargement and the appearance of a goitre. Fetal thyroid activity also depletes the maternal iodide pool from the second trimester, probably via diffusion along a concentration gradient.

As human chorionic gonadotrophin (hCG) and TSH share a common alpha subunit and have similar beta subunits, TSH receptors are prone to stimulation by hCG. In conditions such as molar pregnancy, hyperemesis gravidarum and multiple pregnancy, increased thyroid activity has been noted, associated with high levels of hCG. Even in normal pregnancy, a fall in TSH levels is associated with peak hCG concentrations, and there is a correlation between levels of T4 and hCG. In pregnancy, there is also placental conversion of T4 to T3. Low levels of T4 will increase this activity, producing more active thyroid hormone. Deiodination also occurs in trophoblasic and placental tissue, preventing excess thyroid hormone exposure to the baby and perhaps explaining the fall in T4 found in the mother in later pregnancy.[1]

## Fetal thyroid function

During the first trimester, the fetus requires maternal T4 for normal fetal brain development. It is likely that T4 crosses the placenta in small amounts before 12 weeks gestation to facilitate this (otherwise, T3, T4 and TSH do not cross the placenta). From 10 weeks gestation, the fetal thyroid gland produces both T4 and T3. From this point onwards, the fetal thyroid axis is independent and there is little relationship between maternal and fetal levels. Fetal levels reach those of the adult by 36 weeks gestation. Although fetal TSH concentrations are greater than maternal TSH levels, T3 is lower in the fetus, probably as a result of little peripheral conversion and a good placental barrier.

Both thyrotropin-releasing hormone (TRH) and iodine freely cross the placenta. (TRH has unsuccessfully been investigated as a method of stimulating thyroid function to enhance fetal lung maturity.)

Congenital hyperthyroidism can occur through TSH receptor stimulating antibodies which cross the placenta. Very rarely, mutations of the TSH receptor result in either congenital hyperthyroidism or hypothyroidism.

## Thyroid function tests in pregnancy

In pregnancy, it is important to measure free T4 and T3 and to base management decisions principally on these levels [C]; TSH levels are often suppressed, and can only be detected with new, ultrasensitive assays.

As T4 levels fall during pregnancy, the lower limit of normal for free T4 is below that of non-pregnant women. As there is more conversion of T4 to T3, low levels of T4 are not necessarily indicative of hypothyroidism.[2]

Thyroid hormones are involved in the metabolism of alpha-fetoprotein (aFP), and there has been some concern that aFP measurements may be unreliable. However, in women suspected of having thyroid disease, the available evidence suggests aFP measurements can still be used for Down's serum screening [D].

## AETIOLOGY AND MANAGEMENT OF THYROID DISEASE

## Iodine

Women in areas of iodine deficiency may have goitres and reduced reproductive success.[3] In iodine deficiency, the maternal thyroid gland has a greater affinity for iodine than the placenta and the fetuses are thus prone to cretinism – the leading preventable cause of mental retardation worldwide.

The fetal cochlea, cerebral neocortex and basal ganglia are particularly sensitive to iodine deficiency.[4] Iodine administration prior to conception and up to the second trimester will improve neurological outcome by protecting the fetal brain. Iodination of water, salt or flour, or even annual injections for reproductive age women, can easily achieve this.

Although the introduction of iodine supplementation in certain areas of the developing world has reduced both the miscarriage and stillbirth rates, high levels of iodine intake can cause fetal hyperthyroidism. Therefore, some cough medicines and eye drops containing iodine should be avoided, as should radiological procedures utilizing iodinated contrast dyes. Similarly, amiodarone, which is rich in iodine, should be avoided in pregnancy unless absolutely necessary for life-threatening arrhythmias. In these cases, neonatal assessment must be made regarding thyroid function. Radioactive iodine, which destroys the fetal thyroid, must never be used, even in early pregnancy, as damage can occur before there is active fetal tissue.

## Hyperemesis gravidarum

In women with hyperemesis, T4 levels may be elevated with suppression of TSH. These changes probably result from high levels of hCG, which stimulate the TSH receptors[5] and occur in approximately 40 per cent of hyperemesis cases (particularly in those with more severe disease). This usually resolves by 20 weeks gestation. The clinical signs of thyrotoxicosis are generally absent and, as the condition improves, T4 levels only remain elevated if true hyperthyroidism ensues.

Antithyroid medication should not be used in hyperemesis as the thyroid abnormality is biochemical and self-limiting and is not related to an overactive thyroid [D]. When used, this type of medication is generally ineffective or required in unacceptably high doses.

## Hyperthyroidism

Hyperthyroidism occurs in approximately 1 in 500 pregnancies and is usually due to Graves' disease (autoimmune thyrotoxicosis). Less than 5 per cent of cases result from a toxic nodule, thyroiditis or a carcinoma. If pregnant women present with hyperthyroidism, hyperemesis or a molar pregnancy must be considered.

Graves' disease is associated with a hyperplastic goitre and often with exophthalmos. Disease severity is correlated to immunoglobulin G (IgG) thyrotropin receptor stimulating antibody levels. The disease typically remits in the last two trimesters,[6] and in approximately a third of cases treatment may be discontinued, although a flare may occur following delivery. First trimester disease may be exacerbated by high hCG levels.

Typical signs of thyroidism are difficult to elicit in pregnancy, but poor weight gain in the presence of a good appetite or a tachycardia >100 beats per minute (bpm) that is unresponsive to a Valsalva manoeuvre may indicate the disease. Onycholysis does reflect disease activity, unlike the eye signs and pretibial myxoedema. Unfortunately, many other symptoms, such as fatigue and heat intolerance, are common in pregnancy and are not useful.

It is essential to maintain euthyroidism in pregnancy, as uncontrolled disease is associated with maternal and fetal complications, including thyroid storm, heart failure and maternal hypertension. Observational studies have reported increased rates of premature labour, growth restriction and stillbirth. Treatment is similar to that for non-pregnant women, although radioactive iodine must not be given [D]. Surgery may be considered if medical treatment fails or there is a clinical suspicion of cancer or compressive symptoms due to a goitre.

Medical treatment involves blocking thyroid hormone synthesis. Propylthiouracil (PTU) and carbimazole both reduce the titre of TSH receptor antibodies, directly influencing the aetiology of Graves' disease. PTU was previously the preferred therapy, as it not only inhibits T4 synthesis by blocking the incorporation of iodine into tyrosine, but also inhibits the peripheral conversion of T4 to T3. However, both drugs probably cross the placenta in the same proportion and there is no need to change from carbimazole to PTU [D]. Both drugs are equally beneficial and the dose of either can be titrated against maternal well-being and biochemical status [D].[7] Neither PTU nor carbimazole is thought to be teratogenic, and the relationship previously found between aplasia cutis of the scalp and these drugs is unlikely to exist. Antithyroid drugs can cause agranulocytosis and so a sore throat should be thoroughly investigated.

It is recommended that thyroid function tests be performed every 4–6 weeks. When Graves' disease is stable, beta-blockers can be used to control the symptoms of tachycardia or tremor, and propranolol is the recommended therapy [D].

As both PTU and carbimazole cross the placenta, both may influence the fetus.[8] The minimal dose required in the mother should therefore be used, and it is usual to aim for free T4 levels at the upper limit of normal [E]. Even if the fetus does become hypothyroid, neurodevelopmental status is preserved, although careful control can still lead to neonatal hypothyroidism and even neonatal goitre. The goitres are generally small, clinically unimportant and tend to resolve within 2 weeks. No long-term fetal side effects of antithyroid drugs have been demonstrated, although the studies performed have been small and retrospective.

Both drugs are expressed in breast milk, but have little effect on thyroid function.

## Fetal hyperthyroidism

When maternal thyrotropin receptor stimulating antibodies cross the placenta, they can cause fetal or neonatal thyrotoxicosis. The fetal thyroid is capable of responding

to these antibodies after 20 weeks gestation, and potential effects should be monitored in the second half of pregnancy. Assessment should include maternal perception of fetal movements, standard growth assessments (symphyseal–fundal height) and measurement of the fetal heart rate, which, if >160 bpm, may be indicative of fetal thyrotoxicosis. An ultrasound scan can be used to exclude a fetal goitre or clinically undetected fetal growth restriction. In suspected cases, cordocentesis for free T4 and TSH determination can be performed and is preferable to amniocentesis [D].

Premature delivery is associated with fetal hyperthyroidism. Hydrops fetalis and death can occur and a fetal goitre can cause polyhydramnios and an obstructed delivery. The condition is also associated with craniosynostosis and intellectual impairment. The fetus can be effectively treated in one of two ways, either by maternal administration of antithyroid agents, which cross the placenta, or by delivery. The fetal heart rate can be used to titrate the dose of antithyroid drugs. The mother can be treated with T4 to offset any hypothyroid effects, as T4 will not cross the placenta [C]. As thyroid TSH receptor stimulating antibodies have a long half-life (3 weeks), they can cause neonatal hyperthyroidism. The symptoms may therefore only present in the baby after a week and tend to be non-specific, such as poor weight gain, feeding and sleeping. A goitre may also cause problems with breathing and feeding. Fetal/neonatal hyperthyroidism is responsible for substantial mortality.

Women who have had Graves' disease treated by surgery may be euthyroid, but still have active antibodies. Therefore, TSH receptor antibodies should be measured in these women and in women with active Graves' disease. As long as antibody levels are low, involvement of the fetus is unlikely. If antibody levels are high, fetal/neonatal thyroid function should be checked, both in cord samples and in peripheral samples taken approximately a week after delivery.

## Hypothyroidism

Hypothyroidism occurs in nearly 1 per cent of pregnant women and is usually due to autoimmune Hashimoto's thyroiditis or idiopathic myxoedema; the condition can also occur following treatment of hyperthyroidism. Direct pituitary causes are rare.

In pregnancies complicated by hypothyroidism, babies are normally grown and do not seem to have an increased risk of congenital anomalies. Large studies have not yet confirmed this apparent lack of adverse events. Aberrant thyroid function has been implicated in the aetiology of recurrent miscarriage, but the evidence for this is weak, and the current Royal College of Obstetricians and Gynaecologists' (RCOG) guidelines suggest abandoning routine testing of thyroid function in the investigation of recurrent miscarriage.

There is a reduced intelligence quotient (IQ) in babies of women with hypothyroidism that is not adequately treated, or that goes unrecognized. The insult is likely to occur in the first trimester, and therefore pre-conceptual optimization of T4 therapy is important [D].[9,10] Referral to a physician interested in the field would seem prudent.

As hypothyroidism is associated with subfertility, it is rare to make a new diagnosis in pregnancy. The classical symptoms of hypothyroidism, such as tiredness, constipation, anaemia, weight gain, carpal tunnel syndrome and hair changes, are common in pregnancy and cannot be relied upon to discriminate onset or worsening of the disease. The management is therefore based principally on biochemical measures. Thyroxine is titrated against biochemical results and is safe in pregnancy and lactation [C]. As long as the patient is clinically euthyroid, thyroid function tests should be performed every 2–3 months. More frequent measurements are made if the clinical or biochemical condition is deranged [E]. Most pregnant women do not need any increase in therapy [C].[11] Some authors have advocated a routine increase in the first trimester, but as there have been some reports of adverse events with thyroxine therapy, such as miscarriage, it would seem prudent to titrate therapy to biochemistry.[12] A low free T4 level indicates a need for increased therapy, rather than a raised TSH [D].[13]

## Fetal hypothyroidism

Although Hashimoto's hypothyroidism results in the autoantibodies crossing the placenta, it does not affect fetal thyroid development. However, very rarely, TSH receptor blocking antibodies can cause a transient hypothyroidism in either a fetus or baby.

## Postpartum thyroiditis

Postpartum thyroiditis can occur up to a year following delivery and can manifest as high or low T4 levels. The incidence varies widely and, when diagnosed biochemically, has been reported as to be as low as 2 per cent in New York and as high as 17 per cent in Wales. Most women will not have clinically apparent disease, and may present with depression or be diagnosed as having Hashimoto's hypothyroidism as they tend to present to general practitioners, who may be unaware of the condition. Women on long-term T4 treatment following an onset soon after pregnancy should have this diagnosis considered.

The condition is thought to be autoimmune and presents postpartum following a return to normal immunity after delivery. Ninety per cent of women will have thyroid antiperoxidase antibodies (compared with 10 per cent of the normal population). Histology from thyroid biopsies suggests a chronic thyroiditis with lymphocytic infiltration but not fibrosis (which is a typical feature of Hashimoto's thyroiditis).

The disease may present initially between 1 and 3 months postpartum with thyrotoxicosis and later with hypothyroidism. Radioactive iodine or technetium uptake tests can help distinguish between postpartum thyroiditis (low uptake) and Graves' (high uptake), but lactation should not continue during testing [D]. If symptomatic with hyperthyroidism, beta-blockers can be used; antithyroid drugs are inappropriate, as T4 production is not increased [D]. Hyperthyroidism is due to destruction of thyroid follicles and the release of preformed hormones. The destruction of thyroid follicles ultimately leads to the hypothyroid phase, which is more likely to be associated with symptoms such as tiredness and cold intolerance and even a goitre. At this stage, the differential diagnosis includes Hashimoto's thyroiditis and Sheehan's syndrome. A course of T4 may be necessary. If the symptoms of hypothyroidism are due to Hashimoto's thyroiditis, withdrawing treatment will result in relapse, but cessation of T4 is probably the only way to avoid unnecessary long-term treatment.

The period of hypothyroid state is variable, and permanent hypothyroidism can result (approximately 5 per cent of antibody-positive postpartum thyroiditis sufferers). The condition will recur in 70 per cent of future pregnancies and women with postpartum thyroiditis should be followed up to ensure that permanent hypothyroidism does not occur [E]. This would usually involve annual TSH and T4 measurement.

## THYROID CANCER IN PREGNANCY

Thyroid cancer is two to three times more common in women than men, and 50 per cent of cases occur within the reproductive age group. Pregnancy itself does not appear to influence the survival rates of women diagnosed with thyroid cancer. It is recommended that pregnancy should be delayed after treatment with radioactive iodine, probably for a period of a year [D], in view of the higher incidence of congenital anomalies that follow this treatment.

If a pregnant woman presents with a thyroid nodule, thyroid function tests and an ultrasound are indicated. Thyrotoxicosis occurring with cystic nodules is unlikely to be malignant, but other nodules should be investigated with a fine-needle aspirate. Cellular cytology from a fine-needle aspirate may suggest an underlying malignancy, and serial ultrasound should be performed. Removal of nodules that are increasing in size should be considered. A thyroidectomy can be performed, usually in the second trimester of pregnancy. If radioactive iodine is required, this should not be administered during breastfeeding [D].

Thyroid globulin concentration cannot be used to detect a relapse of thyroid cancer in pregnancy, as it is already elevated. Women on suppressive doses of T4 may continue this therapy, with the usual aim of reducing TSH to undetectable levels.

## KEY POINTS

- Management decisions should be based on free T4 and T3 measurements in pregnancy; T4 is found at the lower limits of normal in pregnancy and trimester-specific reference ranges should be used for all assessments of thyroid function in pregnancy.
- Management of hypothyroidism should be optimized prior to conception, and pregnant women may need to alter their dose of thyroxine from early pregnancy.
- Forty per cent of women with hyperemesis gravidarum have elevated T4 (and suppressed TSH); they do not require antithyroid treatment. This will usually resolve by 20 weeks gestation.
- Graves' disease is the most common cause of hyperthyroidism, and euthyroidism should be maintained in pregnancy with antithyroid drugs. Thyroid status should be checked every 4-6 weeks. Treatment can be reduced in the third trimester to prevent fetal hyperthyroidism, then restored postnatally.
- Women with hypothyroidism should be euthyroid prior to conception to avoid intellectual impairment in the baby. The fetus requires maternal thyroxine in early pregnancy.

## Key References

1. Koopdonk-Kool JM, de Vijlder JJM, Veenboer GHM et al. Type II and type III deiodinase activity in human placenta as a function of gestational age. *J Clin Endocrinol Metab* 1996; **81**: 2154–8.
2. Kortaba DD, Garner P, Perkins SL. Changes in serum free thyroxine, free tri-iodothyronine and thyroid stimulating hormone reference intervals in normal term pregnancy. *J Obstet Gynecol* 1995; **15**: 5–8.
3. Dillon JC, Milliez J. Reproductive failure in women living in iodine deficient areas of West Africa. *Br J Obstet Gynaecol* 2000; **107**: 631–6.
4. Cao XY, Jiang XM, Dou ZH et al. Timing of vulnerability of the brain to iodine deficiency in endemic cretinism. *N Engl J Med* 1994; **331**: 1739–44.
5. Kimura M, Amino N, Tamaki H. Gestational thyrotoxicosis and hyperemesis gravidarum: possible role of HCG with higher stimulating activity. *Clin Endocrinol* 1993; **38**: 345–50.
6. Kung AWC, Jones BM. A change from stimulatory to blocking antibody activity in Graves' disease during pregnancy. *J Clin Endocrinol Metab* 1998; **83**: 514–18.
7. Wing DA, Miller LK, Cunnings PP et al. A comparison of propylthiouracil versus methimazole in the treatment of hyperthyroidism in pregnancy. *Am J Obstet Gynecol* 1994; **170**: 90–95.
8. Momotani N, Noh JY, Ishikawa N, Ito K. Effects of propylthiouracil and methimazole on fetal thyroid status in mothers with Graves' hyperthyroidism. *J Clin Endocrinol Metab* 1997; **82**: 3633–6.
9. Haddow JE, Palomaki GE, Allan WC et al. Maternal thyroid deficiency during pregnancy and subsequent neuropsychological development of the child. *N Engl J Med* 1999; **341**: 549–55.
10. Pop VJ, Kuijpens JL, van Baar AI et al. Low maternal free thyroxine concentrations during early pregnancy are associated with impaired psychomotor development in infancy. *Clin Endocrinol* 1999; **50**: 149–55.
11. Girling JC, de Swiet M. Thyroxine dosage during pregnancy in women with primary hypothyroidism. *Br J Obstet Gynaecol* 1992; **99**: 368–70.
12. Anselmo J, Cao D, Karrison T et al. Fetal loss associated with excess thyroid hormone exposure. *JAMA* 2004; **292**: 691–5.
13. Hypothyroidism in the pregnant woman. *Drug Ther Bull* 2006; **44**: 53–6.

# 6.5 Haematological conditions

*Joanna C Gillham*

## MRCOG standards

### Relevant standards

- Conduct pre-pregnancy counselling to a level expected in independent primary care.
- Conduct booking visit, including assessment of intercurrent disease.
- Diagnose and plan management with appropriate consultation in the following conditions: maternal haemoglobinopathy and coagulation defects.

In addition, we would suggest the following.

### Theoretical skills

- Revise the normal mechanism of coagulation in the vascular system.
- Understand how this changes in normal pregnancy.
- Know the common inherited coagulation disorders.

### Practical skills

- Be able to diagnose and treat a thromboembolic event in pregnancy.
- Be competent in the management of the antepartum, intrapartum and postpartum periods for a patient with previous venous thromboembolism or inherited thrombophilia.
- Be able to conduct prenatal counselling and subsequent pregnancy management of those patients with inherited bleeding disorders.
- Be able to conduct prenatal counselling and subsequent management of those patients with haemoglobinopathies – sickle cell disease, thalassaemia.

## ANAEMIA

Acquired anaemias are discussed in Chapter 7.1, Anaemia. This chapter deals with the pre-existing anaemias.

## Aplastic/hypoplastic anaemia

This is secondary to a failure of the bone marrow to produce erythrocytes. It may be pre-existing or develop during pregnancy (and can be recurrent). It is thought that the pregnancy further depresses the bone marrow and exacerbates the condition. In the past, termination of pregnancy was recommended, but supportive measures have improved and, as long as the maternal condition is satisfactory, the pregnancy should be allowed to proceed. Pure red cell aplasia is rare but can be managed with transfusion.

## Haemolytic anaemias

These disorders are rare, but the outlook in pregnancy is generally good. Management depends on the underlying pathology. In inherited conditions (congenital spherocytosis, pyruvate kinase deficiency, etc.), treatment is with transfusion. Many of these patients will have had a splenectomy, and penicillin prophylaxis should be given. Iron overload should be screened for, because of the chronic haemolysis, and cardiac assessment performed as necessary. In autoimmune haemolytic anaemias, the prognosis has improved significantly with the use of steroids and immunosuppressants. Close monitoring is required to ensure rapidly developing profound anaemia is avoided. Any underlying cause should be treated optimally (e.g. systemic lupus erythematosus, SLE).

## HAEMOGLOBINOPATHIES

The haemoglobinopathies are inherited disorders of haemoglobin synthesis (thalassaemias) or structure (sickle cell syndromes) that are responsible for significant morbidity and mortality on a worldwide scale. They have distinct ethnic preponderance, but, secondary to the increased mobility of the world's population and interethnic mixing, these conditions are no longer unusual within the UK, although the prevalence varies enormously from region to region.

There are two pairs of globin chains in each haemoglobin molecule. There are three normal haemoglobins, all of which have one pair of alpha-globin chains and one pair of gamma-chains (HbF), beta-chains (HbA) or delta-chains (HbA2). As alpha-chains are essential for all three types of haemoglobin, alpha-chain production is under the control of four genes, two inherited from the mother and two from the father. The majority of adult haemoglobin (0.95 per cent) is HbA, and beta-chain production is under the control of two genes, one from the mother and one from the father.

Thalassaemia is caused by a quantitative defect of globin gene production, which leads to instability of haemoglobin and ineffective red blood cell production. If all four alpha-globin genes are defective (and therefore there is no alpha-globin chain production), the outcome is Hb Bart's hydrops, which results in fetal hydrops and is incompatible with survival. One defective gene results in alpha-thal+ trait, and two defective genes result in either alpha-thalo trait (both defective genes from one parent) or homozygous alpha-thal+ trait (one defective gene from each parent). In all three of these situations, the patient is asymptomatic. If three defective genes are inherited (one from one parent and two from the other), this results in HbH disease, which causes a moderate haemolytic anaemia.

In contrast, if one beta-globin gene is defective, this causes beta-thalassaemia trait or minor, which is associated with mild anaemia. If both beta-globin genes are defective, no beta-globin chains are produced, and this results in beta-thalassaemia major, the majority of affected individuals being transfusion-dependent for life, with all the consequences of iron overload.

The sickle cell syndromes are associated with a qualitative globin gene defect. It is the structure of the globin chains rather than the production that is abnormal. Many different forms exist, but the most common and clinically most important is HbS, in which there is a single amino acid substitution (from glutamic acid to valine) in the beta-globin chain which renders it insoluble in the deoxygenated state. This alters the shape of the red blood cell into a sickle shape, hence the name. These sickled red cells are permanently removed from the circulation (haemolytic anaemia). The life expectancy of a normal red blood cell is 120 days and of a sickled cell 5–30 days. Sickle cell trait (HbAS) is much more common than sickle cell disease (HbSS). Other haemoglobin variants exist (e.g. HbC, HbE), but are less common. If both partners carry a haemoglobin variant (i.e. trait), there is a 1:4 chance of the child inheriting both the abnormal genes, and thus sickle cell disease. This risk increases to 1:2 if one partner has two abnormal genes (i.e. disease) and the other has trait.

## Screening

The implications of the major haemoglobinopathies (beta-thalassaemia major and sickle cell disease) are such that the introduction of universal antenatal and neonatal screening occurred in 2005, as selective screening proved to be ineffective [E]. As the major haemoglobinopathies are autosomal recessive conditions, with carrier status having little implication for health, many people are completely unaware that they are carriers. Neonatal screening has been incorporated into universal blood spot screening, as there is a proven reduction in morbidity and mortality in sickle cell disease with early diagnosis and prophylactic treatment [C].[1]

Screening for the thalassaemias is by examining the red cell indices and the HbA2 levels. With thalassaemia traits, there is a reduced mean corpuscular volume (MCV <75 fL), reduced mean corpuscular haemoglobin (MCH <27 pg), and a normal or near-normal mean corpuscular haemoglobin concentration (MCHC). MCH is the most accurate marker. In addition, in beta-thalassaemia trait there is an elevated HbA2 (>3.5 per cent). In alpha-thalassaemia traits, the changes may be minimal in alpha-thal+ trait. DNA analysis is required to confirm the diagnosis. Screening for sickle cell variants is carried out by HPLC or electrophoresis. Anything other than HbAA is regarded as a variant (e.g. HbAS, AC, SC, etc.).

If a woman is found to be a haemoglobinopathy carrier, her partner should be screened as early as possible and, if there is a risk of the fetus having a major haemoglobinopathy, urgent expert counselling should be given to allow the couple to make an informed choice regarding prenatal diagnosis and termination of pregnancy [E]. Ideally, this screening and counselling should be done pre-pregnancy. Prenatal diagnosis is carried out by DNA analysis with chorionic villi and fetal blood preferable to amniotic fluid (less free fetal DNA is present). The optimal method of prenatal diagnosis is chorionic villus sampling in the first trimester [E], which also allows surgical termination of pregnancy, if the parents so desire, should the fetus be affected.

Some mixed haemoglobinopathies can have increased maternal risk as well as sickle cell anaemia (HbSS) and B thalassaemia major, intermedia and HbH disease. These are HbSC disease, HbS/β thalassaemia, HbS/Dpunjab, HbS/Oarab, HbSE and HbS/Lepore.

## Thalassaemias in pregnancy

### Alpha-Thalassaemias

Those with trait may become anaemic during pregnancy, and iron and folate supplementation should be given, although parenteral iron should be avoided. Those with HbH disease have a chronic haemolytic anaemia and require 5 mg folic acid daily. They are often not iron deficient because of the chronic haemolysis, and transfusion is often indicated to treat the anaemia. It must be remembered that the maternal complications when a fetus has Hb Bart's hydrops include early-onset severe pre-eclampsia, and intrapartum problems secondary to the delivery of a grossly hydropic fetus and placenta, including primary postpartum haemorrhage.

### Beta-Thalassaemia

Those with trait are often anaemic. These women should take 5 mg folic acid daily, and oral iron supplements if the ferritin is low (never parenteral iron). If the anaemia does not respond, transfusion may be indicated.

Pregnancy is rare in transfusion-dependent beta-thalassaemia major, although with aggressive iron chelation programmes the rate is increasing. Some women with beta-thalassaemia major are not truly transfusion dependent, and pregnancies have been reported. In all cases of beta-thalassaemia major, iron overload is a major concern, particularly in terms of myocardial function, and a cardiology assessment should be performed. Iron supplementation should always be avoided, and the anaemia treated with transfusion. Folate supplementation (5 mg/day) is required. All women with beta-thalassaemia major should be looked after in pregnancy by a team consisting of a haematologist and an obstetrician with the relevant expertise [E].

The risks of thalassaemia major in pregnancy are outlined in Table 6.5.1.[2]

**Table 6.5.1** Risks of thalassaemia major in pregnancy

| General | In pregnancy |
| --- | --- |
| Chronic anaemia | Partner screening if not known |
| Iron overload | Discuss prenatal diagnosis if required |
| Hepatic dysfunction | Infection |
| Endocrine dysfunction | ? blood antibodies with risk of haemolytic disease |
| Increased risk of infection | Thromboembolic disease |
| Cardiomyopathy | Increased transfusion needs |
| Osteoporosis | Folate supplementation 5 mg/day |
| Transfusion transmitted infections | Fetal growth surveillance |

## KEY POINTS

### Thalassaemias
- These are inherited disorders of haemoglobin synthesis.
- Normal-structure haemoglobin has one pair of alpha-globin chains and one pair of alpha-, beta- or gamma-globin chains.
- The majority of adult haemoglobin is HbA – alpha- and beta-globin.
- If two defective alpha-globin chains are present = alpha-thalassaemia trait.
- If three defective alpha-globin genes are present = HbH disease.
- If four defective alpha-globin genes are present = Hb Bart's hydrops – incompatible with survival.
- Screening is by examining the red cell indices and the HbA2 levels.
- Thalassaemia traits possess ↓ MCV, ↓ MCH and a normal or near-normal MCHC.

## Sickle cell variants in pregnancy

Those with trait are not at increased risk of adverse maternal or fetal outcome other than the risks to the mother if severe hypoxia develops – of which the anaesthetist should be aware and general anaesthesia avoided if possible – and the risks to the fetus of inheriting major disease if the father also has trait.

## Sickle cell disease in pregnancy

It is very unusual to diagnose sickle cell disease during pregnancy, as the vast majority of affected individuals are aware of the diagnosis from childhood. However, milder forms of sickle cell disease (e.g. HbSC) may be diagnosed for the first time in pregnancy. The clinical features of sickle cell disease include:

- chronic haemolytic anaemia
- painful crises
- hyposplenism
- increased risk of infection
- avascular bone necrosis
- increased risk of cerebrovascular accidents (CVA)
- chest syndrome.

During pregnancy, crises may become more frequent and close attention must be paid to optimal management. The frequency of crises is higher in HbSS (up to 50 per cent) compared with HbSC (27 per cent).[3] Increased risks for women with sickle cell disease are outlined in Table 6.5.2.[3]

**Table 6.5.2** Increased risks for women with sickle cell disease

| General | In pregnancy |
| --- | --- |
| Chronic haemolytic anaemia | Miscarriage |
| Painful crises | Need for partner testing and possibly prenatal diagnosis |
| Hyposplenisn | Infection – particularly urinary tract |
| Increased risk of infection | Intrauterine growth restriction |
| Iron overload | Pre-eclampsia |
| Avascular bone necrosis | Haemolytic disease of the new born |
| Increased risk of cerebro-vascular accident | Fetal death *in utero* |
| Sickle chest syndrome | Prematurity |
| Pulmonary hypertension | Thromboembolic disease |
| Retinal disease | Perinatal mortality Maternal mortality |

Ideally, women should be seen in a joint clinic by an obstetrician and a haematologist with expertise in haemoglobinopathies [E]. Pre-pregnancy counselling is optimal, but often women present when already pregnant. Partner screening and counselling regarding prenatal diagnosis should be given if these aspects have not already been addressed. Iron chelation should be stopped prior to conception, as the agents used are contraindicated in pregnancy. A ferritin level should be checked and, if elevated or there is a history of significant iron overload, an echocardiograph and cardiac assessment should be performed to exclude cardiomyopathy. The need for folic acid supplementation (5 mg/day) and penicillin prophylaxis throughout pregnancy should be emphasized. Renal and hepatic function should be assessed regularly, as both can be compromised. Haemoglobin and HbS level should be monitored regularly, and a programme of top-up or exchange transfusion implemented as indicated. These patients have often had multiple transfusions in the past, and may have multiple blood group antibodies that can cause problems with cross-matching. Venous access can also be significantly compromised. Any signs of infection should be treated aggressively, and dehydration and exposure to cold avoided, as in the non-pregnant state.

In the event of a crisis or chest syndrome, good oxygenation and hydration are essential, as well as adequate pain relief. The patient must be kept warm and any infection promptly treated. In severe cases, top-up transfusion or even exchange transfusion may be required. Careful consideration should be given to the use of thromboprophylaxis.

From the fetal perspective, regular assessment of fetal growth and placental function is indicated with ultrasound and Doppler assessment. Caesarean section should only be performed for obstetric indications, and general anaesthesia should be avoided if possible.

In labour, intravenous fluids must be given to avoid dehydration, and oxygen used to prevent hypoxia. Attention should be paid to analgesia, and continuous electronic fetal monitoring is recommended. Consideration should be given to the use of thromboprophylaxis; the use of prophylactic antibiotics remains controversial.

## Haemoglobinopathies

- Universal antenatal and neonatal screening for the inherited haemoglobinopathies is being considered as selective screening is not effective.
- Neonatal screening for inherited haemoglobinopathies reduces morbidity and mortality by early diagnosis and prompt treatment.
- If a woman is found to be a haemoglobinopathy carrier, her partner should be screened to allow pre-pregnancy genetic counselling, if necessary, or prenatal diagnosis and the option of a termination of pregnancy.
- Pregnant women with any haemoglobinopathy (if not trait) should be looked after by a haematologist and an obstetrician with relevant expertise.

### KEY POINTS

**Sickle cell syndrome**

- This is an inherited disease of haemoglobin structure.
- In sickle cell, HbS is secondary to a single amino acid substitution in the beta-globin chain.
- HbS is insoluble in the deoxygenated form – altering the red blood cell shape to a sickle.
- Sickle cell syndrome is inherited as an autosomal recessive disease.
- Screening is via electrophoresis.
- In sickle cell trait, there is no increased maternal or fetal adverse outcome, unless there is severe hypoxia in the mother or the risk of disease to the fetus should the father be a haemoglobinopathy carrier.
- Women with sickle cell syndrome have an increased risk of adverse outcome in pregnancy.

### KEY POINTS

**Sickle cell disease in pregnancy**

- The women should be seen in a joint obstetric/haematology clinic.
- Pre-pregnancy counselling is the gold standard.
- If not, partner screening and counselling regarding prenatal diagnosis are required.
- Folic acid supplementation (5 mg/day) and penicillin prophylaxis should be continued for the duration of the pregnancy.
- Haemoglobin, ferritin and HbS levels and renal and hepatic function tests need to be assessed monthly.
- Top-up or exchange transfusion may be warranted antenatally.
- Any signs of infection or dehydration should be managed aggressively.
- Ultrasound scans for fetal assessment are required from 28 weeks of pregnancy.
- Caesarean section should be for routine obstetric reasons and general anaesthesia avoided if at all possible.

## PLATELET DISORDERS

Multinucleated cells in the bone marrow (megakaryocytes) produce platelets. They have a critical role in normal haemostasis and in thrombotic disorders, and circulate for 7–10 days. Bleeding can result from abnormal platelet function or a reduced count of normal platelets.[4] The normal platelet count is $150–350 \times 10^9$/L. The maternal platelet count decreases between 20 and

40 weeks gestation by approximately 12 per cent.[5] Platelets are removed by the spleen, and an elevated platelet count is found in those patients who have had a splenectomy. There are other, rare, causes of increased platelet counts that are not usually seen in pregnancy. The main concern is that of an increased risk of thromboembolic disease, which can be minimized by low-dose aspirin (75 mg or 150 mg/day).

## Thrombocytopenia

Thrombocytopenia, defined as a platelet count of $<150 \times 10^9$/L, occurs in up to 7–10 per cent[6] per cent of pregnancies. A falsely low platelet count may occur due to platelet agglutination in a blood sample, caused by the anticoagulant EDTA. Thus, thrombocytopenia should be confirmed by examination of a peripheral blood film. If clumping is seen, a citrated sample should be sent; if this gives a normal platelet count, all samples should be sent in citrate rather than EDTA, and no other action is required. Patients with severe thrombocytopenia often have petechiae and mucocutaneous bleeding, resulting from small, unsealed endothelial lesions. By contrast, patients with the inherited bleeding disorders do not have petechiae or excessive bleeding from small cuts as their platelet adhesion and aggregation tend to be sufficient.[4]

If mild thrombocytopenia is discovered, a repeat full blood count (FBC) is required in one month to ensure there has been no further fall. If the platelet count is falling, or on initial testing is found to be $<100 \times 10^9$/L, the following tests should be performed.

- FBC, clotting profile, renal and liver function tests, urate.
- Examination of peripheral blood film.
- Lupus anticoagulant, anticardiolipin antibodies, antinuclear antibodies.
- Virology screen.
- Platelet autoantibodies. Because of the complexity of platelet membranes, the precise identification and measurement of such antibodies have been difficult. These antibodies can be present in both gestational and immune thrombocytopenia.
- Bone marrow aspiration may need to be considered in severe thrombocytopenia.

### Causes of thrombocytopenia in pregnancy

- Pregnancy-associated thrombocytopenia (PAT) – 74 per cent.[7]
- Hypertensive disorders of pregnancy – 21 per cent.
- Immune disorders – 4 per cent.
- Others (disseminated intravascular coagulation (DIC), thrombotic thrombocytopenic purpura (TTP), HELLP syndrome, acute fatty liver) – 2 per cent.

### Pregnancy-associated thrombocytopenia

Up to 74 per cent of pregnant women develop PAT. This is a benign, symptomless condition. The mother is at no increased risk of haemorrhagic problems and there is no effect on the fetus, and no treatment is required. Resolution tends to occur within 6 weeks of delivery. The platelet count will be normal at the booking visit if this is in the first or early second trimester. The platelet count usually remains above $100 \times 10^9$/L. If the platelet count is lower than this initially, continues decreasing rapidly or the thrombocytopenia occurs early on in the pregnancy, other diagnoses must be considered.[4] If the woman books late in pregnancy and is already thrombocytopenic, idiopathic thrombocytopenic pupura (ITP) often cannot be excluded and, because of the fetal implications, should be treated as such until the diagnosis can be clarified, often after delivery.

### Familial thrombocytopenia

This is an autosomal dominant condition that causes profound thrombocytopenia, with platelet counts of around $20 \times 10^9$/L, although spontaneous bleeding is rare. There is no effective drug therapy and management is supportive when required. The fetus has a 50 per cent chance of being affected, and the same measures apply regarding delivery as with ITP (see below).

### Storage pool disease

In this condition, the platelet count is normal but platelet function is abnormal, and a significant bleeding history as well as a family history is usually present. It is unlikely that this diagnosis will be made during pregnancy, and most cases seen are already known about and under the care of a haematologist. Diagnosis is confirmed by platelet function tests and management is supportive. The condition is autosomal dominant, and the fetus therefore has a 50 per cent risk of being affected. Traumatic delivery should thus be avoided.

## AUTOIMMUNE DISEASE

### Idiopathic immune thrombocytopenic purpura

This is isolated thrombocytopenia with no clinically apparent associated disorders. The diagnosis is largely after exclusion of the other causes of thrombocytopenia. It is the most common autoimmune disorder, affecting 1–3 in 1000 pregnancies, and the platelet count may well be decreased at the initial booking visit. Antibodies, usually IgG, are directed against the platelet membrane. Often patients are asymptomatic and pregnancy does not always (but can) exacerbate the disease. If the platelet count is $>50 \times 10^9$/L, no treatment is necessary. Major bleeding is rarely seen unless the platelet count is $<10 \times 10^9$/L. Patients with clinical bleeding or a count $<50 \times 10^9$/L are treated with oral corticosteroids; 70–90 per cent of women will respond within 3 weeks. Corticosteroids act by inhibiting platelet antibody production and increasing bone marrow platelet production. Patients who fail to respond to steroids are treated with intravenous immune globulin, which prolongs the clearance time of circulating immune complexes. The length of effect is variable, but in the order of 2–3 weeks. Steroids should always be tried in the first instance, as immune globulin is a blood product, requires hospital admission for administration as a day case and is very expensive. Splenectomy in pregnancy is rarely required. Platelet transfusions are used only in the acute situation, to deal with haemorrhage or to cover delivery. The decision to use platelet transfusions should be made in conjunction with a consultant haematologist.

Maternal antibodies may cross the placenta and affect the fetus, causing thrombocytopenia; 4–10 per cent of neonates are at risk of having severe thrombocytopenia at birth or during the first week of life.[4] The maternal platelet count does not correlate with the fetal platelet count, and it is not predictive of any adverse fetal outcome.[8] Administration of corticosteroids or immune globulin does not affect the fetal platelet count. In labour, fetal blood sampling and invasive fetal monitoring should be avoided, as should ventouse extraction, because of the risk of cephalhaematoma. If an instrumental delivery is unavoidable, low cavity forceps only should be used by an experienced operator, but traumatic delivery must be avoided [D]. There appears to be no benefit conferred by delivery by caesarean section [D]. The management of the baby in the neonatal period is most important; platelet counts and paediatric assessments are indicated (the nadir of the neonatal platelet count occurs on day 4–7).

---

## KEY POINTS

**Idiopathic thrombocytopenic pupura**
- Antibodies are directed against the platelet membrane.
- Prevalence: 1-3/1000.
- Treatment: corticosteroids, intravenous immune globulin, splenectomy, platelet transfusion.
- Fetal effect: fetal/neonatal thrombocytopenia.

---

## Acquired Glanzman's disease

Rarely, in some cases of ITP, the circulating immune complexes can bind to the platelets and inhibit their function. In this situation, the haemorrhagic history is in excess of that expected from the platelet count, and patients may give a history of excessive bruising or bleeding, even with a platelet count of $>50 \times 10^9$/L (i.e. platelet function is inadequate). Diagnosis is by platelet function tests and bleeding time, and treatment consists of immune suppression with steroids, etc., as well as supportive measures in the form of platelet transfusion when required. Close liaison with the haematology department is advised.

## Antiphospholipid syndrome/systemic lupus erythematosus

The thrombocytopenia found in these conditions can be profound. The presence of IgG antibodies prolongs the partial thromboplastin time and, very rarely, the prothrombin time. Paradoxically, these patients are at a greater risk of thrombosis than of bleeding. Treatment is with aspirin and heparin. The fetus is not at risk of thrombocytopenia (see Chapter 6.7, Autoimmune conditions, for further details).

## Pre-eclampsia

Pre-eclampsia is associated with the activation of the coagulation system. Thrombocytopenia in varying degrees is found in 30 per cent or more of patients.

Between 4 and 12 per cent of women with pre-eclampsia may have haemolysis, increased liver enzymes and low platelets (HELLP syndrome) (see Chapter 7.6, Pre-eclampsia and non-proteinuric pregnancy-induced hypertension, for further details).

## Infection

Many infectious diseases, for example viruses – human immunodeficiency virus (HIV), cytomegalovirus (CMV) and Epstein–Barr virus (EBV) – mycoplasma, bacterial infection and malaria, can be associated with thrombocytopenia. There are no fetal effects of the thrombocytopenia; however, the underlying disease may have further implications (see Chapter 7.4, Infection, for further details).

## Drugs

Heparin, quinine, rifampicin and trimethoprim are some of the drugs that can cause thrombocytopenia. This usually resolves fairly quickly on stopping the causative agent.

## THE HAEMOSTATIC MECHANISM

The factors involved in the cessation of bleeding are:

1 *Haemostasis.* There is obliteration of the injured vessel, with vasoconstrictors released from platelets and external pressure from haematoma formation or contraction of the surrounding smooth muscle. There is an additional contribution via platelet aggregation.

2 *Coagulation*

    a. Stage 1. Intrinsic mechanism – activation of factors XII, XI and IX by vessel wall damage; then factor VIII activation in the presence of calcium causes activation of factor X. Extrinsic mechanism – tissue damage releases factors III and VII, causing activation of factor X.

    b. Stage 2. Activated factor X, with factor V and calcium, convert factor II (prothrombim) to thrombin.

    c. Stage 3. Thrombin converts factor I (fibrinogen) to a fibrin monomer, which forms a fibrin polymer and eventually fibrin.

## MATERNAL PHYSIOLOGICAL CHANGES IN PREGNANCY

(The changes in the blood volume and red cell mass in a normal pregnancy are discussed in Chapter 7.1, Anaemia.) The total white cell count increases in pregnancy, with counts as high as $16 \times 10^9$/L observed in the third trimester. Counts up to $30 \times 10^9$/L have been observed in a normal labour. Lymphocytes and monocytes remain at pre-pregnancy levels; the rise is in polymorphonuclear leukocytes.

Pregnancy is a pro-thrombotic physiological state. There is a marked increase in the level of fibrinogen and factor VIII. Factors V, VII, X, XII and von Willebrand factor (vWF) also increase, but to a lesser extent. There is little increase in factor IX. The anticoagulants antithrombin III and protein C remain at a steady level, and protein S level is decreased by 40 per cent. Acquired activated protein C resistance is present and fibrinolysis is inhibited with decreased plasminogen activator inhibitor.

---

### KEY POINTS

**Haematological changes in normal pregnancy**
- ↑ white cell count
- ↑ factors V, VII, VIII, IX, X, XII, fibrinogen, vWF
- ↑ antithrombin III, protein C
- ↑ protein S, plasminogen activator inhibitor
- ↑ platelets

---

## VENOUS THROMBOEMBOLIC DISEASE

The major predisposing factors to venous thromboembolic (VTE) disease are the activation of blood coagulation, venous stasis and endothelial injury (Virchow's triad). The risk of VTE is increased with pregnancy to approximately 1/1000 pregnancies,[9] and is greater in the postpartum compared to the antepartum period. The pregnancy-associated increase in clotting factors is discussed above. With advancing gestation, the enlarging uterus diminishes the venous return from the legs, with increasing venous stasis ensuing. These factors, often combined with antenatal immobilization, prolonged labour, dehydration, excessive blood loss and possible surgery, explain the risk of VTE being increased approximately 5-fold with pregnancy and the puerperium. Other general risk factors are prolonged immobilization, malignancy, chronic inflammatory disease, oestrogens and the combined oral contraceptive pill/hormone replacement therapy (HRT), nephrotic syndrome, major surgery, particularly orthopaedic and pelvic, antiphospholipid syndrome and sepsis. The presentation of VTE is complicated in that the symptoms of lower limb oedema and dyspnoea are common complaints of the normal pregnant woman. Any clinical suspicion of VTE must be investigated immediately to avoid the risks and costs of inappropriate anticoagulation [C]. VTE disease is the leading cause of maternal mortality in the UK,[10] with the majority of deaths from pulmonary embolism following caesarean section, and occurring after the first week of the puerperium, hence after discharge from hospital. All those involved with the care of these women should be alert to this fact.[10] Many of the guidelines for the management of VTE in the non-pregnant patient are based on level A evidence.

Pregnancy is a risk factor for VTE and is associated with a 10-fold increase compared with the risk for non-pregnant women (see Table 6.5.3). Some women are at an even higher risk during pregnancy because they have one or more additional risk factors.[9,11,12]

For a woman with a previous VTE and no known thrombophilia, the risk of recurrence in pregnancy is increased to 2–3 per cent from about 0.1 per cent. However, the risk is higher if the woman has a thrombophilia or if the previous VTE was in an unusual site or was unprovoked [D].[11] Ideally, before pregnancy a woman with a previous VTE should have a careful history taken and undergo screening for both inherited and acquired thrombophilias.[11]

Women with a previous VTE and no thrombophilia should, as a minimum, be offered prophylaxis with low molecular weight heparin for 6 weeks after delivery. Whether they need antenatal coagulation is more controversial. If the previous VTE was associated with a temporary risk factor, e.g. surgery, antenatal anticoagulation is not required [E].[13]

Women with no thrombophilia but who have a previous VTE associated with oestrogen (e.g. on the oral contraceptive pill), additional risk factors (e.g. obesity), previous recurrent VTE, a family history of a VTE in a first degree relative or a previous VTE in an unusual site (e.g. axilliary vein), should be offered thromboprophylaxis with low molecular weight heparin (LMWH) [E].[11]

**Table 6.5.3** Risk factors for venous thromboembolic disease in pregnancy and puerperium

| Pre-existing | | New onset or transient | |
| --- | --- | --- | --- |
| **Previous VTE** | **Thrombophilia** | **Surgical procedure in pregnancy or puerperium** | **Ovarian hyperstimulation syndrome** |
| Antithrombin III deficiency | Protein C or S deficiency | Hyperemesis | Severe infection |
| Factor V Leiden | | Severe dehydration | Immobility >4 days bed rest |
| Prothrombin gene variant | Some medical disorders, e.g. nephrotic syndrome | Excessive blood loss | Pre-eclampsia |
| Anti-phospholipid syndrome (lupus ± anti cardiolipin antibodies, | Inflammatory disorders, e.g. inflammatory bowel disease | Long haul travel | Prolonged labour |
| Age >35 | Sickle cell disease | Midcavity instrumental delivery | Caesarean section |
| BMI >30 | Gross varicose veins | Immobility after delivery | |
| Parity >4 | Myeloproliferative disorders | | |

Women with a previous VTE and who are found to have a thrombophilia (see section below) should be offered thromboprophylaxis with LMWH antenatally and at least 6 weeks post-natally.

Women who have no previous history of VTE but who are found to have a thrombophilia may require antenatal or post-natal LMWH, depending on the specific thrombophilia (see below) and the presence/absence of other risk factors.

# THROMBOPROPHYLAXIS IN NORMAL PREGNANCY

In general, women with three or more risk factors from Table 6.5.3, should be considered for antenatal LMWH and for postpartum LMWH for at least 3–5 days.

A woman with two or more risk factors should be considered for prophylactic LMWH for 3–5 days after a vaginal delivery.

Delivery by caesarean section increases the risk of VTE by 2–8 times. The highest risk is with an emergency procedure under a general anaesthetic. In 1995, the Royal College of Obstetricians and Gynaecologists (RCOG) issued guidelines with regard to thromboprophylaxis following caesarean section.[14] These are broad guidelines and in reality most units have a local protocol. Increasingly, many units are giving all patients who are delivered by caesarean section (both elective and emergency) thromboprophylaxis. The most recent Confidential Enquiry into Maternal Deaths in the UK[10] has reported a decrease in the number of deaths from VTE following caesarean section, which they attribute to more widespread use of thromboprophylaxis since the introduction of the RCOG guidelines. However, the Confidential Enquiry recommended more widespread use of thromboprophylaxis, even after normal delivery.

## Antenatal thromboprophylaxis

The agent of choice for antenatal thromboprophylaxis is LMWH. The risk of heparin-induced thrombocytopenia and osteoporosis is reduced compared to unfractionated heparin. The platelet count should be measured 1 week after commencing LMWH. Providing a patient has normal renal function, monitoring of anti-Xa levels is not required for prophylaxis doses.[11]

Warfarin should be avoided, especially between 6 and 12 weeks pregnancy, as it is associated with up to a 5 per cent risk of teratogenicity. After this gestation, it is associated with increased risks of miscarriage, fetal and maternal haemorrhage, neurological problems and fetal death *in utero*.[15] It is safe to breastfeed on warfarin. There is an increased risk of postpartum haemorrhage.

## Intrapartum thromboprophylaxis

If a patient is in labour or thinks she may be (and has previously been on antenatal prophylactic LMWH) then she should be advised not to inject any further heparin until assessment at the hospital. Depending on the indication, if a woman is on treatment doses of LMWH antenatally, she may have her anticoagulation lowered around delivery. Again, depending on the indication, if on prophylactic antenatal LMWH, she may stop her anticoagulation during labour. To minimize the risk of epidural haematoma, regional techniques should be avoided until 12 hours following a prophylactic dose of LMWH. When a patient is on a therapeutic dose of LMWH, regional techniques should be avoided until 24 hours after the last dose of LMWH.[16]

If prophylactic dose heparin is required postnatal, it should be ensured that administration is at least 4 hours after removal of an epidural catheter. An epidural catheter should not be removed within 12 hours of an LMWH injection.

There is an increased risk of wound haematoma of 2 per cent following caesarean section with LMWH usage.[11] The skin should be closed by staples or interrupted sutures to allow drainage of any haematoma.

In postnatal prophylactic LMWH, patients with a body weight of >90 kg should receive the standard dose but this is increased to twice daily dosing.

## KEY POINTS

- At the beginning of pregnancy, a risk factor assessment for VTE should be performed and the woman then counselled accordingly. The management plan should be reassessed if any new problems arise or if she is admitted into hospital.
- Women with a previous VTE should be screened for inherited and acquired thrombophilias. This should ideally be prior to pregnancy and if not, then at first presentation in pregnancy.
- If a woman has had a previous VTE associated with a temporary risk factor that has resolved and if she has no underlying thrombophilia, LMWH should be offered for 6 weeks postpartum. The need for antenatal prophylaxis is more controversial and may not be required.
- If the patient has a positive thrombophilia screen but has recurrent VTE, VTE in a first degree relative, previous VTE in an unusual site or a previous VTE that was related to oestrogen, antenatal thromboprophylaxis with LMWH is required in the antenatal period. Antenatal prophylaxis should begin as soon as practical – often as soon as an ultrasound scan confirms a viable intra-uterine pregnancy.
- Women with a previous VTE and any positive testing for thrombophilia should be offered thromboprophylaxis with LMWH antenatally and for at least 6 weeks postpartum.
- Women who have a body weight of >90 kg need increased LMWH for prophylaxis and twice daily dosing. Similarly, if the body weight is <50 kg, the dose of LMWH may need to be reduced.
- Women with three or more risk factors (see Table 6.5.3) should be considered for thromboprophylaxis with LMWH antenatally and for 3–5 days postpartum.
- Regional anaesthesia is appropriate if the last injection of LMWH (if at prophylactic doses) was more than 12 hours previously.

# THROMBOEMBOLIC DISEASE IN PREGNANCY AND THE PUERPERIUM – ACUTE MANAGEMENT

The subjective clinical assessment of VTE in pregnancy is more difficult than in the non-pregnant women. Clinicians should always remember that VTE is up to ten times more common in the pregnant woman than in the non-pregnant woman of the same age.[17] The puerperium is the highest risk time, but a VTE can occur at any point in pregnancy and so a low threshold should be employed for definitive testing.

## Deep vein thrombosis

### Symptoms and signs
The majority of deep vein thromboses (DVTs) occurring during pregnancy are in the left leg. Symptoms include pain in affected calf/leg, swelling, fever, erythema and increased heat of the affected leg. A positive Homan's sign is unreliable.

### Investigation
In clinically suspected VTE, treatment with low-molecular-weight heparin should be given until the diagnosis is excluded by objective testing [A].[18]

1  *D-dimers.* VTE is associated with increased levels of blood D-dimer, and this is often now used as a screening test in non-pregnant individuals. However, elevations in D-dimer level are found in uncomplicated pregnancy, with levels increasing with advancing gestation. A positive D-dimer screen is of no prognostic significance in VTE in pregnancy, but a low level of D-dimer in pregnancy suggests there is no VTE.
2  *Duplex ultrasound.* This has a high sensitivity and specificity in proximal DVTs and is non-invasive. It is unreliable for calf DVT as it has a much lower sensitivity. If the initial ultrasound scan is negative and there is a low level of clinical suspicion, anticoagulant treatment can be stopped. If the ultrasound is negative and there is a high level of clinical suspicion, the patient should be anticoagulated and the ultrasound repeated in a week, or venography performed [E].[18] Isolated below-knee DVT is uncommon in pregnancy, but if identified, treatment should be given.
3  *Venography.* This adequately visualizes calf and deep veins. Disadvantages include the use of radiation, an allergic reaction to the dye used and a 5 per cent risk of causing thrombosis.

### Management
Graduated compression stockings (TEDS) should be worn in the acute period and it is recommended that they should be worn on the affected leg for two years after the event to reduce the incidence of post-thrombotic syndrome [A].[14,18] Compliance is often a problem in pregnancy, mainly secondary to poor fit of the stockings; therefore careful measurement and fitting are essential. Hot weather and not having enough pairs also affect compliance.

Before commencing anticoagulant treatment, blood should be taken for an FBC, clotting, renal and liver function tests, and there should be a thrombophilia screen to screen for both inherited and acquired thrombophilia.[18]

Low-molecular-weight heparin (LMWH) by subcutaneous injection is the treatment of choice in both the pregnant and non-pregnant population. A recent Cochrane review concluded that LMWH was at least as effective as unfractionated heparin in preventing recurrent VTE, and significantly reduced the occurrence of major haemorrhage during the initial treatment and overall mortality at the end of follow-up [A].[19] Treatment for VTE occurring in relation to pregnancy should continue for at least 6–12 weeks after delivery or six months after the initial episode – whichever is the longer [C].[20]

Heparin does not cross the placenta, is not teratogenic and does not cause an anticoagulant effect in the fetus. Complications of long-term heparin treatment are osteopenia, thrombocytopenia and allergic skin reactions at the site of injection.

Osteopenia is less common with LMWHs compared to unfractionated heparins, although it can still occur, especially if other risk factors are present. Early heparin-induced thrombocytopenia (HIT) occurs 1–5 days after the start of therapy and is usually mild. Late heparin-induced thrombocytopenia is due to IgG-mediated platelet activation and usually occurs 5–15 days after commencement. This can produce a rapid fall in the platelet count and is highly prothrombotic. HIT should be screened for by checking the maternal platelet count weekly for the first 4 weeks of treatment. HIT is less common with LMWH compared to unfractionated heparin. Most cases respond rapidly to changing LMWH to danaparoid. If an allergic response develops at the injection sites, changing the brand of heparin (and thus the vehicle) may lead to resolution.

Therapeutic doses of LMWH should be given in two subcutaneous divided doses with dosage titrated against the women's booking or most recent weight.[18] Routine measurement of peak anti-Xa levels in a pregnant patient for treatment of acute VTE is not recommended in women except at extremes of body weight (<50 kg or >90 kg) or if renal impairment is present. The factor Xa levels should be performed immediately pre-dose and 2 hours post-dose.[18]

Consideration should be given to the use of a temporary inferior vena caval filter in the perinatal period for women with iliac vein VTE, to reduce the risk of PE or in women with a proven DVT and who had recurrent PE despite adequate anti-coagulation.[18]

Any woman on heparin during pregnancy must have a carefully documented care plan for labour and delivery. Induction of labour is often employed to facilitate dose adjustment in a planned way, and to try to minimize exposure to heparin because of the potential bone effects. Women should be advised that if there are any signs of labour, they should omit their heparin until they are seen and assessed. When full therapeutic doses are employed, a decision must be made antenatally as to whether the risk of VTE is such that the heparin cannot be stopped, in which case the dose should be reduced to a prophylactic level for the duration of labour. In this case, regional anaesthetic blockade is contraindicated.

It should be remembered that in an emergency, protamine sulphate can be used to reverse the effects of heparin, but usually only achieves 60 per cent reversal.

Warfarin is an oral coumarin, and is the most commonly used anticoagulant. It acts in the liver by inhibiting the synthesis of four vitamin K-dependent coagulant proteins (factors II, VII, IX, X) and at least two vitamin K-dependent anticoagulant factors, proteins C and S. Warfarin crosses the placenta freely and is teratogenic, causing chondrodysplasia punctata (nasal hypoplasia, saddle nose, frontal bossing, short stature, mental retardation, cataract and optic atrophy; see Chapter 8, Medication in pregnancy). The teratogenic effects are avoided if warfarin is stopped prior to 6 weeks gestation, and patients on long-term warfarin should be fully counselled regarding this and have direct access to either the haematology department or obstetric unit to be converted to heparin as soon as they have a positive pregnancy test. Warfarin also causes anticoagulation in the fetus, with risks of gross retroplacental or intracerebral bleeding, and microcephaly has been described in these fetuses. There is no agent available which can rapidly reverse the effects of warfarin, and reversal by stopping therapy and giving vitamin K takes up to 5 days. Women on warfarin are converted to heparin towards the end of pregnancy to allow more control of the haemorrhagic risk associated with delivery in the anticoagulated patient. Certain patients, those with metal heart valves or heparin allergy, may still require treatment with warfarin in pregnancy despite the risks, although with close heparin monitoring, patients with metal heart valves have been managed successfully throughout pregnancy on LMWH, and newer anticoagulants with less risk to the fetus may be available soon.

Warfarin is not excreted in significant quantities in breast milk, and is thus safe in breastfeeding mothers. Postpartum warfarin should be avoided until at least day 3, and for longer if the patient is at an increased risk of a postpartum haemorrhage.

## KEY POINTS

### Deep vein thrombosis
- Symptoms and signs: pain, swelling, fever, erythema, positive Homan's sign.
- The majority in pregnancy are in the left leg.
- Investigation: D-dimer, duplex ultrasound, venography.
- Treatment: TEDS, LMWH (twice daily dosing).

Routine measurement of peak anti-Xa levels in pregnant patients for treatment of acute VTE is not recommended in women except at extremes of body weight (<50 kg or >90 kg). Measurement of factor Xa levels should be performed immediately pre-dose and 2 hours post dose.

- Treatment until 6 weeks postpartum or three months after VTE - whichever is the longer.

# PULMONARY EMBOLISM

This can occur with or without preceding DVT. Symptoms range from minimal disturbance to sudden collapse and death, depending on the size, number and site of the emboli.

## Signs and symptoms

These include dyspnoea, chest pain, cough, haemoptysis, pyrexia, tachycardia, tachypnoea, cyanosis, raised jugular venous pressure (JVP), pleural rub, pleural effusion and right ventricular failure.

## Investigations

- Arterial blood gas analysis – hypoxia and hypercapnia.
- Electrocardiogram (ECG): inverted T waves and atrial arrhythmia are suggestive. In pregnancy, normal ECG findings can be a right axis deviation and T wave inversion and a Q wave in lead III, which in the non-pregnant patient would be suggestive of a pulmonary embolism (PE).
- Chest x-ray (CXR): an abnormal CXR is found in 69–80 per cent of patients with a PE.
- Ventilation-perfusion scan: in cases of suspected PE, both a V/Q scan and a bilateral Doppler ultrasound of the leg veins should be performed [E].[18] This is a sensitive but not specific test. Interpretation of a V/Q scan is given as a probability rating. Anticoagulation should be continued when the V/Q scan reports a medium or high probability of a PE. If the scan reports a low probability and Doppler studies of the leg are positive, anticoagulation should be continued. If the leg Doppler studies are also negative, yet there is a high degree of clinical suspicion, continuation of treatment with repeat testing in 1 week should be considered [E].[7]
- Computed tomography pulmonary angiogram (CTPA) is the gold standard for the diagnosis of PE and is necessary if other pulmonary pathology is present or if a VQ is inconclusive.
- Women with a suspected PE should be advised that V/Q scanning carries a slightly increased risk of childhood cancer compared with CTPA (1/280 000 versus less than 1/1 000 000) but carries a lower risk of maternal breast cancer (lifetime risk increased by up to 13.6 per cent with CTPA, background risk of 1/200 for study population) [D,E].[18]

## Treatment

- Collapsed, shocked patients need to be assessed by a team of experienced, multidisciplinary clinicians (medical, haematological and obstetric) to decide on a individual basis whether a women receives intravenous unfractionated heparin, thrombolytic therapy or a thoracotomy and surgical embolectomy. Intravenous unfractionated heparin is the preferred treatment in massive PE with cardiovascular compromise.[18] If unfractionated heparin is administered, the platelet count needs to be checked at least every other day until day 14 or until the unfractionated heparin is stopped.
- For smaller, minimally symptomatic clots, LMWH may be used in the acute phase, and certainly in the further treatment for the PE after this phase. The initial drug dosage is based on the patient's early pregnancy weight.
- Warfarin has a minimal place in the treatment of the pregnant woman for acute VTE, but is suitable in the postpartum period.
- Inferior vena caval (IVC) filters are reserved for those cases with recurrent PE despite adequate anticoagulation or for patients who cannot receive anticoagulation.
- There is limited information on the use of thrombolysis for a PE in the pregnant woman. Streptokinase is most commonly used and does not cross the placenta. The major side effect can be severe genital tract bleeding, and its use should therefore be reserved for those patients who are haemodynamically unstable.
- Surgical embolectomy: a specialist clinician should follow up women who have experienced a thrombosis during pregnancy. Once they are at least 6 weeks postpartum, and have discontinued anticoagulant therapy, a thrombophilia screen should be performed if this has not already been done.

---

**KEY POINTS**

### Pulmonary embolism

- Symptoms and signs: chest pain, dyspnoea, haemoptysis, pyrexia, tachycardia, tachypnoea, cyanosis, ↑ JVP, pleural rub/effusion, right ventricular failure.
- Investigation: arterial blood gas, ECG, CXR, V/Q scan, spiral CT, pulmonary angiogram.
- Treatment: acute phase and a large PE - intravenous unfractionated heparin.
- With smaller, minimal symptom PE or in longer term treatment - LMWH.
- Other treatment: IVC filter, thrombolysis, surgical embolectomy.

---

## Management of venous thromboembolism

- Any clinical suspicion of VTE must be investigated as soon as possible.
- While awaiting investigation, appropriate thromboprophylaxis should be commenced.
- In DVT investigation, if clinical suspicion is high and initial Doppler negative, repeat or more invasive testing should be considered.

- TEDS should be worn for two years after a VTE event.
- LMWH by subcutaneous injection is the treatment of choice in DVT in both the pregnant and non-pregnant population.
- If a PE is suspected, a V/Q scan and bilateral leg Doppler ultrasound studies should be performed.
- During pregnancy and the puerperium, management of the woman should be at an obstetric medicine or a joint haematology/obstetric clinic.

# THE THROMBOPHILIAS

A thrombophilia is defined as a predisposition to thrombosis, secondary to any persistent or identifiable hypercoagulable state. This can be inherited or acquired.

Thrombophilia is present in at least 15 per cent of the western population and can be identified in up to 50 per cent of those with a history of VTE.[21] Protein C, protein S, anti-thrombin III, Factor V Leiden (FVL) and the prothrombin gene mutation (PGM) 20210 are now the most common causes of hypercoagubility. Others include hyperhomocystinaemia (HHC), elevated factor VII and the antiphospholipid syndrome.

There is a well-established association between antiphospholipid antibodies and pregnancy loss, but available data also suggest additional associations for the other thrombophilias. The contribution of thrombophilia to preeclampsia and fetal growth restriction is less well established.

## Protein C deficiency

Protein C circulates in an inactive state. Thrombin 'activates' this vitamin K-dependent protein, and activated protein C with its cofactor protein S inactivates the clotting factors Va and VIIIa. Protein C deficiency is present in approximately 1 in 500 people with an autosomal dominant pattern of inheritance. In patients with protein C deficiency, thrombosis occurs in 25 per cent of pregnancies without anticoagulation. Two-thirds of these are in the postpartum period.

## Protein S deficiency

Protein S is a vitamin K-dependent protein, which is a cofactor for activated protein C. Protein S levels decrease in pregnancy, and are reduced in women using the combined oral contraceptive pill and HRT. A definitive diagnosis of protein S deficiency cannot therefore be made until these influences have been removed, which may take several weeks. The prevalence of protein S deficiency in the general population is unknown.

## Antithrombin III deficiency

Antithrombin III inactivates thrombin and factors IXa, Xa, XIa and XIIa, and is a naturally occurring anticoagulant.

Its activity is amplified by heparin. Deficiency occurs in 1 in 5000 people and its inheritance is autosomal dominant. The risk of thrombosis is up to 70 per cent in untreated patients, thus anticoagulation is recommended.

## Factor V Leiden

Activated protein C (APC) resistance has numerous underlying causes, but the vast majority of patients with APC resistance were found to have the same point mutation in the gene for clotting factor V – the Factor V Leiden mutation. Other causes of APC resistance are increased levels of factor VIII or the presence of antiphospholipid antibodies. In Caucasian populations, FVL is the most common inherited thrombophilia, with a reported prevalence of between 2 and 15 per cent. It is less common in people of African and Asian origin. Depending on patient selection, FVL is found in 20–50 per cent of patients presenting with a first episode of venous thrombosis.[20] Overall, only a small proportion of those who carry the mutation develop a thrombosis, but it is associated with a 20-fold increased risk of thrombosis during pregnancy. At present, routine screening is not advocated, and selective screening should be confined to those with a personal or family history of VTE.

## Prothrombin G20210A mutation

The G→A transition at the nucleotide 20210 in the prothrombin gene is associated with elevated plasma prothrombin levels and up to a five times increased risk of venous thrombosis. The prevalence in Northern Europe is around 2 per cent in the healthy population and 6 per cent in unselected cases with a first episode of VTE.[20] It is inherited in an autosomal dominant pattern.

## Hyperhomocysteinaemia

Homocysteine is produced solely from the metabolism of the essential amino acid methionine. Inherited HHC results from genetic defects affecting this pathway. Acquired HHC may be secondary to folate, vitamin $B_6$ and $B_{12}$ deficiencies and antifolate medication such as methotrexate.[22] A fasting value of homocysteine >15 μmol/L is considered to be a raised level. This is associated with both arterial and venous thrombosis.

## Antiphospholipid syndrome

This is a thrombophilia characterized by either positive anticardiolipin antibodies or the lupus anticoagulant. It can be primary (no associated autoimmune disease) or secondary. In the latter case, it may be secondary to autoimmune conditions (SLE, rheumatoid arthritis), drugs (antibiotics, procainamide), or viral infections (HIV, hepatitis C, syphilis). Clinical manifestations include arterial and venous thrombosis, recurrent pregnancy loss, thrombocytopenia, livedo reticularis and neurological symptoms.

## Testing for thrombophilia

Testing of unselected patients is inappropriate and there should be clear guidelines as to which patients should be tested [E]. Some tests for heritable thrombophilia are affected by pregnancy, the post-thrombotic state and by anticoagulant use, thus careful timing of investigation and interpretation of results are required.[20]

### Initial assessment

This should include a detailed personal and family history, ideally with any history of VTE objectively confirmed. Any additional risk factors should be identified. A comprehensive thrombophilia screen encompasses the following.

- Activated partial thromboplastin time (APTT)/ pro-thrombin time (PT)/thrombin clotting time.
- Functional assays to determine antithrombin III and protein C levels, antiphospholipid antibodies.
- Immunoreactive assays for protein S antigen.
- The modified APC:SR test can be used to identify causes of APC resistance other than FVL.
- PCR-based testing for PGM and FVL.

## Management of pregnancy

### Preconception

Thrombophilia clinics looking after young women must have close liaison with the obstetric unit. Women with identified heritable thrombophilias should be given information about the perceived risk of pregnancy-associated venous thrombosis. Women on long-term anticoagulant therapy (warfarin) need to understand the risk of fetal complications.

### Antenatal

The management of pregnant women with known thrombophilic defects and no prior venous thromboembolism remains controversial, because of the lack of knowledge of the natural history of the various thrombophilias. Women on long-term anticoagulation and women with antithrombin III deficiency (whether or not they have had a previous VTE) are considered at high risk of pregnancy-associated VTE. Women with a previous history of VTE and who have a thrombophilic defect are at a moderate risk, as are those without prior VTE history, but with a protein C deficiency, homozygous for FVL or PGM. The general consensus is that these groups should receive both antepartum and postpartum thromboprophylaxis [E]. Those at a perceived slight increased risk are women with no personal history of VTE but who have been screened for thrombophilia because they have a family history (protein S deficiency, heterozygous for FVL or PGM). In general, this group of women do not require LMWH antenatally, but consideration should be given to prophylaxis post-delivery [E].[20] Some would advocate low-dose aspirin in the antenatal period.[21] If a patient does not want to continue injections throughout the puerperium, she may change to warfarin. Generally, oral anticoagulants may be introduced on the first or second postpartum day and the heparin withdrawn when the INR is in the recommended range (Table 6.5.4).

**Table 6.5.4** Management of known thrombophilic defects

| Previous venous thromboembolic disease | Inherited/acquired Thrombophilia | Risk of venous thromboembolic disease during pregnancy | Antenatal prophylaxis | Postnatal prophylaxis |
|---|---|---|---|---|
| Yes | Any +ve thrombophilia testing | – | Yes – LMWH | Yes – LMWH |
| No | Anti-throbim III deficiency | 40–68% | Yes – LMWH | Yes – LMWH |
| No | Protein C deficiency | 0–22% | Yes – LMWH | Yes – LMWH |
| No | Homozygous factor V Leiden | Approximately 10% | Yes – LMWH | Yes – LMWH |
| No | Homozygous prothrombin gene | Uncertain | Yes – LMWH | Yes – LMWH |
| No | Prothrombin gene + factor V leiden | Uncertain | Yes - LMWH | Yes – LMWH |
| No | Protein S deficiency | Uncertain | No – ? consider aspirin | ? – consider |
| No | Heterozygous factor V Leiden | 3% | No – ? consider aspirin | ? – consider |
| No | Heterozygous prothrombin gene | 1–4% | No – ? consider aspirin | ? – consider |
| Yes | Any other thrombophilic defect – e.g. APS | 30% | Yes – LMWH | Yes – LMWH |

- APS, antiphospholipid syndrome; LMWH, low-molecular-weight heparin.

## Thrombophilia and pregnancy outcome

Maternal thrombophilias are now recognized to be associated with pregnancy complications, including recurrent miscarriage, intrauterine growth restriction, pre-eclampsia, placental abruption and intrauterine fetal death. The proposed pathophysiology is logical, namely that the thrombophilia encourages placental thrombosis, causing placental infarction, which ultimately affects placental function. In view of this, many women with recurrent pregnancy loss, history of intrauterine death, severe, recurrent or early onset pre-eclampsia or IUGR are screened for an underlying thrombophilia.

A systematic review in 2006[23] reported the thrombophilic associations with adverse pregnancy outcome (see Table 6.5.5).

**Table 6.5.5** Thrombophilic associations with adverse pregnancy outcomes

| Pregnancy outcome – ↑ risk of | Thrombophilia association |
| --- | --- |
| Early pregnancy loss | Lupus anticoagulant, anti-cardiolipin antibodies, homozygous factor V Leiden, heterozygous prothrombin G20210A, hyperhomocysteinaemia |
| Late pregnancy loss >24 weeks | Protein S deficiency, lupus anticoagulant, heterozygous for factor V Leiden or prothrombin gene 20210A |
| Pre-eclampsia | Anti-cardiolipin antibodies, hyperhomocysteinaemia, heterozygous for factor V Leiden or prothrombin gene G20210A, homozygous for methyl-tetrahydrofolate reductase |
| Placental abruption | Heterozygous for factor V Leiden or prothrombin gene 20210A or hyper-homocysteinaemia |
| Fetal growth restriction | Homozygous factor V Leiden, heterozygous prothrombin G20210A |

### KEY POINTS

**Pregnancy outcome and inherited thrombophilia**

There is an increased association with:

- recurrent miscarriage
- FGR
- pre-eclampsia
- placental abruption
- intrauterine fetal death.

There is no good evidence available regarding the management of the pregnant women with a previous VTE or with an inherited thrombophilia. Guidelines are based on expert opinion.

# INHERITED BLEEDING DISORDERS

## Haemophilia

The haemophilias are inherited deficiencies of factor VIII or factor IX. The genes for both factors are located on the X chromosome, thus the haemophilias are X-linked conditions. The daughters of a man with haemophilia are obligate carriers, while his sons are unaffected. The daughters of a haemophilia carrier have a 50 per cent risk of also being carriers, while 50 per cent of the male offspring of a carrier will be affected (the other 50 per cent inheriting no abnormal genes). Genetic counselling should be available before, during and after the process of haemophilia screening [E], and a fully documented pedigree study should be carried out for each family. The haemophilias are categorized according to plasma levels of factor VIII or IX coagulant into mild (5 per cent to 40 per cent), moderate (1–5 per cent) and severe (<1 per cent).[24,25] Severity breeds true in the same kindred. Up to one-third of newly diagnosed infants with haemophilia have no family history and are the result of a spontaneous mutation, often in the mother (90 per cent).

Non-invasive prenatal diagnosis can commence with fetal sexing either from free fetal DNA in the maternal blood in the first trimester, or from ultrasound diagnosis. Knowledge of fetal gender allows invasive testing to be avoided and management of labour and delivery can be planned.

Invasive prenatal diagnosis by chorionic villus sampling in the first trimester (and amniocentesis in the second trimester) is available if the genetic mutation is known (there are >200 known mutations in the factor VIII and IX genes that result in haemophilia). This can also sex the fetus. Alternatively, direct fetal blood sampling may be carried out at 18 weeks or more gestation for clotting factor assay. This procedure is more technically difficult and is reserved for those cases in whom it is not possible to carry out DNA-based family studies in time or because such studies were carried out and were not informative. The maternal clotting factor level should be checked prior to any invasive procedure and prophylactic treatment arranged if the level is <50 IU/dL.

As carriers have one affected gene, it is often assumed that their factor levels will be 50 per cent of normal, but because of lyonization (random inactivation of one of each pair of X chromosomes), levels vary from 10 to 120 IU/dL. Those with levels <30 IU/dL may have a significant bleeding history, and are at risk of significant haemorrhage when challenged. Bleeding episodes of both haemophilias are treated with intravenous injection of the relevant coagulation factor concentrate. In the past, this consisted of pooled plasma of blood donors, and many haemophiliacs were thus exposed to HIV and the hepatitis viruses. Recombinant (i.e. synthetic) factors are now available, but are expensive. However, the government has now funded the use of recombinant factors in all children and new patients, including carriers who require prophylaxis for periods of high risk. This removal of the risk of virally transmitted disease, plus the use of prophylactic factor replacement from childhood and advances in other therapies, have significantly altered the outlook for children with haemophilia and their families, and less than 50 per cent of those at risk now avail themselves of prenatal diagnosis.

## Haemophilia A

Haemophilia A is a deficiency of factor VIII and accounts for 80–85 per cent of haemophilia cases and affects 1:5000 live male births. Most cases are caused by the intron 22 inversion, and prenatal diagnosis is often available if requested. The woman's factor VIII should be assessed; if it is low, she may be at risk of bleeding at the time of the invasive procedure and thus require cover with either desmopressin (DDAVP – see below) or recombinant factor VIII.

### Antenatal

Management of these cases should always be co-ordinated by a team with the relevant expertise, and preferably in association with a recognized haemophilia centre [E]. Clear guidelines should be documented for the management of the remainder of pregnancy and labour and delivery in the form of a care plan. The maternal factor VIII level should be checked in each trimester. The levels of factor VIII and vWF normally increase in pregnancy and, if normal levels are attained, the woman is at no increased risk of haemorrhage either during pregnancy or at the time of delivery, and therefore regional blockade is not contraindicated. For those women who do not attain normalization of factor VIII levels during pregnancy, cover is required for delivery or invasive procedures. Recombinant factor VIII, or DDAVP (desmopressin) if they are responders, can be used. DDAVP can increase factor VIII levels. This is a synthetic analogue of antidiuretic hormone, and should only be used under the supervision of a haematologist familiar with its use in pregnancy. It is given intravenously or intranasally, a method that is useful in the prevention and treatment of secondary postpartum haemorrhage or prolonged/heavy postnatal bleeding. A test dose should be ideally given pre-conceptually to assess the patient's response, as this can vary. DDAVP has anti-diuretic effects and therefore during use, fluid intake should be restricted to 1.5 L in 24 hours.

### Intrapartum

On admission in labour, it is necessary to establish the most recent factor VIII level and read the care plan that has been prepared antenatally. If the factor VIII level is normal in the third trimester, no special maternal precautions are indicated. If it is low, DDAVP or recombinant factor VIII should be given as per the care plan (see Table 6.5.6).[26] This should ideally be given under the supervision of a haemophilia centre and there is therefore an argument to deliver these women in an obstetric unit that has direct access to a haemophilia centre [E]. Once adequate factor VIII levels are attained, no other special precautions are necessary – i.e. there is no contraindication to epidural, etc. If haemophilia is suspected in the fetus, it is wise to avoid fetal scalp electrodes and fetal blood sampling. With regard to mode of delivery, there is no place for elective caesarean section unless obstetric indications dictate this [D]. Delivery should be achieved by the least traumatic route possible.

### Postpartum

At the time of delivery, cord blood should be sent for all male newborns for an urgent factor VIII level unless haemophilia has been excluded by prenatal diagnosis.[25] If haemophilia is diagnosed, a dose of recombinant factor VIII is given to the neonate to minimize the risk of intracranial haemorrhage [E]. This may be difficult to achieve in smaller units, and again consideration should be given to delivering these cases in a unit attached to a haemophilia centre [E]. Intramuscular injections should be avoided

**Table 6.5.6** Management of bleeding disorders

| Condition | Intrapartum/immediate post partum | Post partum |
|---|---|---|
| Carriers of haemophilia | Recombinant factor VIII or IX<br>Factor VIII or IX concentrate<br>Desmopressin ($\uparrow$ factor VIII only)<br>Tranexamic acid | Tranexamic acid<br>Intranasal desmopressin |
| Von Willebrand disease | Concentrate containing VWF<br>Desmopressin (type 1 and some type 2)<br>Platelets (type 2b)<br>Tranexamic acid | Tranexamic acid<br>Intranasal desmopressin |
| Factor XI deficiency | Factor XI concentrate<br>Recombinant factor VIII<br>Fresh frozen plasma<br>Tranexamic acid | Tranexamic acid |

until the haemophilia status is known, and vitamin K can be given orally. If the diagnosis is confirmed, referral to the appropriate paediatric haemophilia centre should be made and follow up arranged prior to discharge home.

From the maternal perspective, Factor VIII levels fall dramatically back to the pre-pregnancy levels within 48 hours of delivery, and there is thus an increased risk of secondary postpartum haemorrhage, particularly in low-level carriers. The use of intranasal DDAVP has been described above and can be used safely in breastfeeding mothers. Tranexamic acid, 1 g three times daily, is also useful in minimizing postnatal bleeding. In some cases, recombinant factor replacement may need to be continued for several days after delivery.

## Haemophilia B (Christmas disease)

This is factor IX deficiency, and most of the above counselling, diagnosis and management decisions are the same as for haemophilia A. The exceptions are that factor IX levels do not significantly rise in pregnancy, and therefore haemophilia B carriers are much more likely to require factor replacement to cover delivery, and DDAVP does not increase factor IX levels.

---

### EBM: Haemophilia

- If a fetus is suspected of having haemophilia, no advantage is conferred by delivery by elective caesarean section.
- Avoid instrumental delivery if possible; if necessary, preference is for the use of forceps rather than the ventouse.
- Regional analgesia/anaesthesia may well be appropriate.

---

## FACTOR XI DISEASE

Factor XI is a serine protease inhibitor. There is a poor correlation between the plasma level of factor XI and the bleeding tendency. Factor XI does not increase in pregnancy. Despite this, many women with known factor XI deficiency do not experience any problems during pregnancy and delivery, without any factor replacement. However, in view of its unpredictable nature, delivery should be in a centre where fresh frozen plasma can be given immediately if required. There is a plasma-derived concentrate of factor XI available. Care needs to be taken with the use of this concentrate, as it contains a number of other proteins and can contribute a thrombotic risk.

## Other factor deficiencies

Deficiencies of most of the clotting factors have been described, and the clinical problems can range from insignificant to severe/life-threatening with respect to labour and delivery. In these rare cases, there should be close collaboration with the relevant expert centres.

## VON WILLEBRAND'S DISEASE

Von Willebrand factor is a plasma protein that has two main functions: stabilization of factor VIII and adherence of platelets to injured vessel walls. Von Willebrand's disease (vWD) is the most common inherited bleeding disorder (prevalence 0.8–1.3 per cent). Both sexes are affected by vWD as the vWF gene is on chromosome 12, and these patients have defective factor VIII and vWF.

There are three different types of vWD. Types 1 and 2 are inherited with an autosomal dominant inheritance pattern, and type 3, the most severe, has an autosomal recessive inheritance pattern. Type I vWD is the most common and mildest form, present in approximately 75 per cent of patients. It is associated with a quantitative deficiency of vWF; in type 2 the defect is qualitative (i.e. functional). In type 2b, there is an associated thrombocytopenia. In these cases there is often a family history of mucocutaneous bleeding, and a personal history of a bleeding tendency – epistaxis, menorrhagia, inappropriate bleeding after dental/surgical procedures. Type 3 vWD is associated with a negligible amount of vWF (both quantity and function) and therefore a significant reduction in factor VIII activity. In these cases the bleeding history is severe, similar to haemophilia.

Laboratory diagnosis measures ristocetin cofactor activity (which assesses vWF activity), as well as vWF antigen and factor VIII (a von Willebrand screen). As stress, tissue trauma and pregnancy all increase vWF and factor VIII levels, it can be difficult to confirm the diagnosis in pregnancy if this has not already been established. Also, during pregnancy, secondary to these increases, the bleeding tendency in type 1 improves, although there is no clinical improvement in type 2 despite an increase in the blood parameters. There is no improvement in type 3 with pregnancy.[27] As with haemophilia, because of the rapid decrease in factor VIII and vWF following delivery, the major haemorrhagic risk is postpartum. In type 1 vWD, DDAVP therapy can be useful. It indirectly stimulates the release of vWF from endothelial cells, causing increased levels of vWF for 4–6 hours. The released vWF binds factor VIII in the liver and increases the levels of circulating factor VIII/vWF complex.[25]

## Antenatal

Before conception, ideally the vWD subtype should be ascertained and the patient's response to DDAVP should be evaluated.[27] DDAVP response can be undertaken in the second trimester if this has not previously been determined. Genetic counselling should be undertaken pre-pregnancy. Antenatal diagnosis of vWD is usually not required or requested as the bleeding tendency is relatively mild, and the majority of cases of type 3 are asymptomatic carriers, unless there has already been an affected child born to the couple. The potential risks of pregnancy and delivery should be discussed with regard to the haemorrhagic risk.

The majority of cases are type 1, and most will normalize during pregnancy with no haemostatic support being required until the postnatal period, if at all. Routine monitoring of the clotting level and platelets should be carried out at booking, 28 weeks, 34 weeks and before any invasive procedures. Other types require specific counselling regarding haemostatic support and factor replacement. As with the haemophilias, these women should be cared for in association with a haemophilia centre [E], and care patterns are similar to those described above. A von Willebrand screen should be performed in each trimester, and a clear plan documented for care in labour and delivery, as well as the postnatal period.

## Labour and delivery

In type 1 vWD, regional anaesthesia can be considered safe if the von Willebrand screen has normalized (the vast majority of cases). This should be avoided in other types of vWD unless the appropriate factor support has been given, as in type 2 the von Willebrand screen can appear normal but the bleeding diathesis remains. Close collaboration with the haematology department and consultant anaesthetist is required. In view of the genetic inheritance, the fetus may be at an increased risk of haemorrhage, and although there is little evidence available in the literature with regard to vWD, the same conditions should apply as with the haemophilias – i.e. avoid fetal blood sampling and invasive monitoring in labour, and avoid episiotomies and instrumental vaginal delivery. As with the haemophilias, caesarean section should be performed for obstetric reasons only.[28] Primary and secondary postpartum haemorrhages are increased compared to both the normal pregnancy population and haemophilia carriers,[27] as the factor VIII and vWF both decrease rapidly following delivery to pre-pregnancy levels. Active third stage management is recommended to reduce the risk of primary postpartum haemorrhage.

## Postpartum

If factor replacement has been necessary for delivery, it should be continued postnatally until the risk of haemorrhage has decreased, unless the patient is a known DDAVP responder, in which case this can be administered intravenously or intranasally.

For those in whom factor replacement was not used, prophylactic intranasal DDAVP and oral tranexamic acid can be used as an outpatient to minimize the risk of PPH.

Type 3 vWD can be diagnosed from cord blood after birth, and should be done if the neonate is known to be at increased risk (this applies to very few cases). It is almost impossible to diagnose the more common, milder forms of vWD in a neonate as the levels of vWF rise significantly during birth, and therefore can mask these forms of the disease. However, there is no urgency to make the diagnosis at birth, as the risk of bleeding in the neonatal period is very low.

## KEY POINTS

### Bleeding disorders
- Haemophilia A: deficiency of factor VIII.
- Haemophilia B: deficiency of factor IX.
- Both are X-linked recessive disease, with females being carriers.
- Pre-pregnancy counselling is important.
- Non-invasive prenatal sexing is available: free fetal DNA in maternal circulation or second trimester ultrasound assessment.
- Invasive prenatal testing is available: chorionic villus sampling, amniocentesis, cordocentesis.
- Maternal factor levels should be checked at booking, and at 28 and 34 weeks gestation.
- Intrapartum investigations should include full blood count, clotting profile, group and save of serum. Intravenous access should be established.
- If the fetus is at risk of a bleeding disorder: avoid intramuscular injection, fetal blood sampling and fetal scalp electrodes.
- If a coagulation screen is normal and the levels of the relevant factor activity are >50 IU/dL, regional anaesthesia should not be contraindicated.
- In women with levels of factor activity <50 IU/dL or there is a severe form of inherited bleeding disorders (e.g. type 2 and 3 vWD and homozygote factor XI deficiency), the use of regional anaesthesia is generally not recommended – advance multi-disciplinary care plans are essential.
- Normal vaginal delivery should be the mode of choice if no other obstetric indication for abdominal delivery is present. Delivery should be achieved by the least traumatic method, e.g. a low forceps delivery would be considered less traumatic than a caesarean section with a deeply engaged head. Forceps should be used if an assisted delivery is required.
- Factor levels should be monitored post delivery and prophylaxis given to maintain VWF and factor VII levels >50 IU/dL for at least 3 or 5 days following a caesarean section.
- The incidence of both primary and secondary PPH is increased among haemophilia carriers (22 and 11 per cent respectively), vWD (16-29 and 20-29 per cent respectively) women with factor XI deficiency (16 and 20 per cent respectively).[26]
- A cord blood sample should be collected from neonates at risk of moderate or severe inherited bleeding disorders. Until the coagulation status is known, intramuscular injections should be avoided and vitamin K given orally.
- Clotting factors in neonates only reach adult levels at six months of age, thus mild forms of inherited bleeding disorders cannot reliably be diagnosed at birth.

## MALIGNANCY

Haematological malignancies are discussed in Chapter 7.3, Malignancy. It must be noted that after patients have received radiotherapy or chemotherapy, there is an anxiety that this may cause increased genetic mutation and abnormality should they subsequently become pregnant. These subtle defects, if they are indeed present, cannot be diagnosed prenatally, and therefore referral for chorionic villus sampling or amniocentesis on this basis is futile.

## ACKNOWLEDGEMENT

Grateful thanks to Tracey Johnston for her contribution to this chapter.

## Key References

1. SMAC Report. *Sickle Cell, Thalassaemia and other Haemoglobinopathies*. London: Department of Health, 1993.
2. Johnston TA. Haemoglobinopathies in pregnancy. Review. *Obstet Gynecol* 2005; **7**: 149–57.
3. Howard RJ, Tuck SM, Pearson TC. Pregnancy in sickle cell disease in the UK: results of a multicentre survey of the effect of prophylactic blood transfusion on maternal and fetal outcome. *Br J Obstet Gynaecol* 1995: **102**: 947–51.
4. George JN. Platelets. *Lancet* 2000; **355**: 1531–9.
5. Kaplan C, Forestier F, Dreyfus M *et al.* Maternal thrombocytopenia during pregnancy: diagnosis and aetiology. *Semin Thromb Hemost* 1995; **21**: 85–94.
6. Karim R, Sacher RA. Thrombocytopenia in pregnancy. *Curr Hematol Rep* 2004; **3**: 128–33.
7. Federici L, Serraj K, Maloisel F, Andreas E. Thrombocytopenia during pregnancy: from etiologic diagnosis to therapeutic management. *Presse Med* 2008; **37**: 1299–307.
8. Shehata N, Burrows R, Kelton JG. Gestational thrombocytopenia. *Clin Obstet Gynecol* 1999; **42**: 327–34.
9. McColl MD, Ramsey JE, Tait RC *et al.* Risk factors for pregnancy associated venous thromboembolism. *Thromb Haemost* 1997; **78**: 1183–8.
10. The National Institute for Clinical Excellence, The Scottish Executive Health Department, The Department of Health, Social Services and Public Safety, Northern Ireland. *Why Mothers Die 1997–1999. The Confidential Enquiry into Maternal Deaths in the United Kingdom.* London: RCOG, 2001.
11. Thromboprophylaxis during pregnancy, labour and after vaginal delivery. Green top guidelines no 37. London: RCOG, January 2004.
12. Simpson EL, Lawrenson RA, Nightingale AL, Farmer RDT. Venous thromboembolism in pregnancy and the puerperium: incidence and additional risk factors from a London perinatal database. *BJOG* 2001; **108**: 56–60.
13. Brill-Edwards P, Ginsbery JS, for the Recurrence of Clot in Pregnancy (ROCIT) study group. Safety of withholding heparin in women with a previous episode of venous thromboembolism. *N Engl J Med* 2000; **343**: 1439–44.
14. Greer IA, Thomsom AJ. *Thromboembolic Disease in Pregnancy and the Puerperium*. Clinical Green Top Guidelines. London: RCOG, 2001.
15. Chan WS, Anand S, Ginsberg JS. Anticoagulation of pregnant women with mechanical heart valves: a systematic review of the literature. *Arch Intern Med* 2000; **160**: 191–6.
16. Horlocker TT, Wedel DJ. Spinal and epidural blockade and pre-operative low, molecular weight heparin: smooth sailing on the titanic. *Anaesth Analg* 1998; **86**: 1153–6.
17. Rodger MA, Walker M, Wells PS. Diagnosis and treatment of venous thromboembolism in pregnancy. *Best Prac Res Clin Haematol* 2009; **16**: 279–96.
18. Thromboembolic Disease in Pregnancy and the Puerperium: Acute Management. Green top guideline 28. London: RCOG, February 2007.
19. Van den Belt AGM, Prins MH, Lensing AWA *et al.* Fixed dose subcutaneous low molecular weight heparins versus adjusted dose unfractionated heparin for venous thromboembolism. *Cochrane Database Syst Rev* 2004; (**4**): CD001100.
20. Walker ID, Greaves M, Preston FE (on behalf of The British Society of Haematologists). Guideline – Investigation and management of heritable thrombophilia. *Br J Haematol* 2001; **114**: 512–28.
21. Pabinger I, Vormittag R. Thrombophilia and pregnancy outcomes. *J Thromb Haemost* 2005; **3**: 1603–10.
22. Girling J. Thromboembolism and thrombophilia. *Curr Obstet Gynaecol* 2001; **11**: 15–22.
23. Robertson L, Wu O, Langhorne P *et al.* Thrombophilia in pregnancy: a systematic review. *Br J Haematol* 2006; **132**: 171–96.
24. Walker MC, Ferguson SE, Allen VM. Heparin for pregnant women with acquired or inherited thrombophilias. *Cochrane Database Syst Rev* 2003; (**2**): CD003580.
25. Kulkarni R, Lusher J. Perinatal management of newborns with haemophilia. *Br J Haematol* 2001; **112**: 264–74.
26. Chi C, Kadir R. Management of women with inherited bleeding disorders in pregnancy. *TOG* 2007; **9**: 27–33.
27. Giangrande PL. Management of pregnancy in carriers of haemophilia. *Haemophilia* 1998; **4**: 779–84.
28. Fausett B, Silver RM. Congenital disorders of platelet function. *Clin Obstet Gynecol* 1999; **42**: 390–405.

# 6.6 Renal disease

*Catherine Nelson-Piercy*

---

## MRCOG standards

### Relevant standards

To understand and demonstrate appropriate knowledge skills and attitudes in relation to pregnant women with kidney disease.

### Theoretical skills

Understand the epidemiology, aetiology, pathophysiology, clinical characteristics, prognostic features and management of women with kidney disease.

### Practical skills

Be able to manage independently:

• urinary tract infection.

Be able to manage under direct supervision pregnant women with:

• hydronephrosis,
• reflux nephropathy,
• renal transplant,
• acute renal failure.

## INTRODUCTION

Urinary tract infection is a common cause of maternal morbidity and a potential cause of perinatal morbidity and mortality via preterm labour. Renal disease is an important predisposing factor for pre-eclampsia and fetal growth restriction (FGR). The combination of hypertension and proteinuria at booking (provided this is in the first or early second trimester) suggests pre-existing renal disease and should prompt further investigation. A serum creatinine is mandatory in such cases to exclude pre-existing renal impairment.

The number of women with renal transplants considering pregnancy is increasing and success rates are high, but case selection is required. Acute renal failure in pregnancy is rare, but renal impairment and oliguria commonly accompany obstetric conditions, particularly haemorrhage and pre-eclampsia.

## PHYSIOLOGICAL CHANGES IN PREGNANCY

There is dilatation of the ureters and renal calyces in pregnancy. This must be remembered when interpreting ultrasound scans of the renal and urinary tract systems in pregnancy. Both renal plasma flow and glomerular filtration increase dramatically in pregnancy.[1] This results in an increased urinary protein excretion and increased creatinine clearance.[1] Thus, in the second trimester, the upper limit for serum creatinine falls to around 65 μmol/L with a mean of 54 μmol/L,[1] and throughout pregnancy the upper limit for proteinuria is taken as 300 mg/24 hours.

## URINARY TRACT INFECTION

### Incidence

Urinary tract infection (UTI) is more common in pregnancy because of the physiological dilatation of the upper renal tract. The incidence of asymptomatic bacteriuria in pregnancy ranges from 4 to 7 per cent, and up to 40 per cent of the women affected will develop symptomatic UTI in pregnancy. Cystitis complicates about 1 per cent of pregnancies, and 1–2 per cent of pregnant women develop pyelonephritis. Women who have a history of previous UTI are at increased risk of UTI in pregnancy, as are those with diabetes, those receiving steroids or immunosuppression, those with polycystic kidneys, reflux nephropathy, congenital abnormalities of the renal tract (e.g. duplex kidney or ureter), neuropathic bladder (e.g. spina bifida or multiple sclerosis) or urinary tract calculi.

## Presentation

A midstream urine (MSU) specimen performed as part of routine antenatal screening may reveal asymptomatic bacteriuria. Additional MSUs are indicated in pregnancy in those women at increased risk as described above, and those with symptoms of UTI. Typical clinical features are urinary frequency, dysuria, haematuria, proteinuria and suprapubic pain. Fever, loin and/or abdominal pain, vomiting and rigors suggest pyelonephritis.

## Diagnosis

Much dipstick proteinuria in pregnancy is erroneously attributed to UTI. Indeed, a diagnosis of pre-eclampsia may not be considered if it is assumed that proteinuria is due to UTI (see Chapter 7.6, Pre-eclampsia and non-proteinuric pregnancy-induced hypertension). Dipsticks for nitrites and leukocyte esterase may be used to help exclude UTI, but their positive predictive value is low and therefore any positive dipstick should be followed up with an MSU. A clinical diagnosis should always be confirmed with culture of an MSU sample. Bacteriuria is considered significant if there are more than 100 000 organisms per millilitre of urine. Urine culture resulting in a non-significant or mixed growth should be repeated on a fresh MSU specimen.

## Management

All bacteriuria in pregnancy requires treatment to prevent pyelonephritis and preterm delivery (Cochrane guideline A) (Table 6.6.1). Treatment for 3 days is sufficient for asymptomatic bacteriuria [E].[2] Regular urine cultures should be taken following treatment to ensure eradication of the organism. About 15 per cent of women will have recurrent bacteriuria during the pregnancy and will require a second course of antibiotics. The choice of antibiotic depends on the sensitivities of the causative organism, but in suspected pyelonephritis, treatment should begin before the results of culture are available. Penicillins (amoxycillin) and cephalosporins are safe and appropriate antibiotics in pregnancy. Augmentin (co-amoxiclav) increases the risk of necrotizing enterocolitis in the neonate. Cefadroxil 500 mg bd is effective against the majority of urinary pathogens. Nitrofurantoin should be avoided in the third trimester as it may cause haemolytic anaemia in the neonate and trimethoprim should be avoided in the first trimester because of its antifolate action. For acute cystitis, a 7-day course of antibiotics is recommended and antibiotics should be continued for 10–14 days for pyelonephritis [E].[2]

In pyelonephritis with vomiting or pyrexia, antibiotics should be given intravenously until the pyrexia settles; intravenous fluids may also be required. Renal function should be checked. Ultrasound examination of the renal tract is indicated in those with pyelonephritis or two or more proven UTIs. This is to exclude hydronephrosis,

**Table 6.6.1** Suggested treatment regimens for urinary tract infection (UTI) in pregnancy

| **Oral antibiotics** |
| --- |
| Amoxycillin 500 mg tds |
| Cefadroxil 500 mg bd |
| Cephalexin 250 mg tds |
| Nitrofurantoin 100 mg tds (not third trimester) |
| Trimethoprim 200 mg bd (not first trimester) |
| **Intravenous antibiotics for pyelonephritis** |
| Cefuroxime 750 mg–1.5 g tds |
| Amoxycillin 1 g tds |
| Gentamicin 5–7 mg/kg daily as one dose and then further doses as determined by serum gentamicin concentrations. (for organisms resistant to, or women allergic to, penicillins and cephalosporins) |
| **Duration of treatment** |
| Asymptomatic bacteriuria: 3 days |
| Acute cystitis: 7 days |
| Pyelonephritis: 10–14 days |
| **Prophylaxis of UTI** |
| Cephalexin 250 mg od |
| Amoxycillin 250 mg od |

congenital abnormalities and renal calculi. Continuous prophylactic antibiotics are only usually recommended for those with two or more confirmed (with a positive culture) UTIs and one of the above risk factors.

## RENAL IMPAIRMENT

### Aetiology

In women of child-bearing age, the most common causes of renal impairment are reflux nephropathy, diabetes, systemic lupus erythematosus (SLE), other forms of glomerulonephritis and adult polycystic kidney disease. Conventionally, chronic kidney disease (CKD) is classified as CKD 1–5 depending on the degree of renal impairment[1] (Table 6.6.2). However, it must be remembered that the estimated glomerular filtration rate (eGFR) is not validated for use in pregnancy and so the serum creatinine level should be used. However, the serum creatinine is also dependent on the

**Table 6.6.2** Stages of chronic kidney disease

| Stage | GFR (mL/min/1.73 m²) |
|-------|----------------------|
| 1     | >90                  |
| 2     | 60–89                |
| 3     | 30–59                |
| 4     | 15–29                |
| 5     | <15 or dialysis      |

muscle mass, so a figure that represents moderate impairment in an 85 kg woman may represent severe impairment for a 50 kg woman. It has been estimated that around 1 in 750 pregnancies are complicated by CKD stages 3–5.

## Presentation

If renal disease is not diagnosed pre-pregnancy, it is usually first recognized because of hypertension and proteinuria and/or haematuria in early pregnancy, prompting blood tests for urea and creatinine. However, a common caveat is to attribute hypertension and proteinuria to underlying renal disease rather than to the much more common pre-eclampsia, which may rarely present before 20 weeks gestation. If there is no record of blood pressure or urinalysis in the first trimester to allow the hypertension and proteinuria to be designated 'new onset', a differentiation between pre-eclampsia and renal disease is more difficult.

## Effect of pregnancy on renal impairment

In general, those with mild impairment (creatinine <125 µmol/L) tolerate pregnancy well and do not usually suffer deterioration in renal function as a result of the pregnancy. The serum creatinine will follow a trend similar to that in normal pregnancy, i.e. it will fall to a nadir in the second trimester and then rise again but remain below non-pregnant levels in the third trimester. Conversely, those with severe impairment of renal function (creatinine >180 µmol/L) are at increased risk of permanent loss of function during and after the pregnancy (50 per cent will have a permanent decline in function) and even end-stage renal failure (35 per cent within one year) [C].[1]

## Effect of renal impairment on pregnancy outcome

All women with renal impairment are at increased risk of pre-eclampsia, FGR and spontaneous and iatrogenic preterm delivery [C].[1,3] Again, outcome depends on the level of impairment and the level of any pre-existing hypertension [C].[3–6] Those with severe renal impairment (creatinine >250 µmol/L) and hypertension have a less than 50 per cent chance of successful pregnancy, often developing severe, early-onset pre-eclampsia with marked fetal growth restriction. Even in the absence of pre-eclampsia or uteroplacental dysfunction, one may be faced with the need to deliver a woman with rapidly worsening renal function in order to avoid dialysis, resulting in a pre-viable or extremely preterm infant. For these reasons, it is usual to counsel women with severe renal impairment against pregnancy [C].[3–5] Women with severe renal impairment may also develop polyhydramnios and the risk of cord prolapse. This is probably the result of fetal polyuria in response to the high osmotic load from increased maternal urea. Those with nephrotic syndrome and heavy proteinuria also develop worsening hypoalbuminaemia in pregnancy, with the associated risks of pulmonary oedema and venous thrombosis.

## Management

This should begin with pre-pregnancy counselling and should involve multidisciplinary care by clinicians with expertise in the management of these high-risk pregnancies.[3] It is important to document baseline (pre-pregnancy and early pregnancy) values for creatinine, uric acid, albumin and protein excretion. Some increase in proteinuria is inevitable in pregnancy and does not necessarily indicate superimposed pre-eclampsia or worsening renal disease. Deterioration in renal function at any stage in pregnancy should prompt a search for reversible causes such as UTI or dehydration.

Tight control of any hypertension is important to minimize the risk of deterioration in renal function. Blood pressure should be maintained below 140/90 mmHg.[3] The choice of anti-hypertensive agents is no different in women with renal disease [E]. Many renal patients, especially those with significant proteinuria, are receiving angiotensin-converting enzyme (ACE) inhibitors or angiotensin receptor antagonists (ARBs). These should be discontinued prior to pregnancy as they are teratogenic [C].[7] Diuretics are also usually discontinued and their use restricted to severe hypoalbuminaemia and insipient pulmonary oedema [D].

Not only are women with renal disease at high risk of pre-eclampsia, but it is also often difficult to diagnose in the presence of pre-existing hypertension and proteinuira. Admission should be considered with worsening hypertension, increasing serum creatinine, and large increases in proteinuria. Useful additional features to support a diagnosis of pre-eclampsia include FGR, thrombocytopenia and abnormal liver function. The use of prophylactic low-dose (75 mg/day) aspirin is appropriate to decrease the risk of pre-eclampsia in those with renal impairment and hypertension [A].[8] Serial scans for fetal growth and liquor volume, and serial haematology and biochemistry are essential in the monitoring of these pregnancies [D].[3,9]

If renal impairment is discovered for the first time in pregnancy, and is not readily attributable to pre-eclampsia, investigation should include blood glucose (for diabetes), antinuclear antibodies (for SLE)[9] and a renal tract ultrasound (e.g. for polycystic kidneys or to demonstrate small kidneys suggestive of chronic renal failure) [D].

Postpartum, continued close monitoring is necessary to ensure the renal function returns to pre-pregnancy levels. ACE inhibitors may be safely used in breastfeeding women. Those with newly suspected underlying renal disease should be referred to a nephrologist.

## EBM: Renal impairment

- The risks of obstetric complications such as pre-eclampsia, FGR and iatrogenic preterm delivery increase with increasing baseline serum creatinine.
- The chances of successful pregnancy decrease with increasing baseline serum creatinine.
- The risks of temporary and permanent deterioration in renal function increase with increased baseline serum creatinine.
- Women with severe renal impairment (creatinine >250 μmol/L) are usually advised against pregnancy.

## RENAL TRANSPLANTS

The rates of successful pregnancy outcome in women with well-functioning renal transplants are similar to those of the general population. Women are usually advised to delay pregnancy for 1–2 years after transplantation to allow graft function to stabilize and immunosuppression to reach maintenance levels [E]. The risks in pregnancy are the same as for women with renal impairment (see above) and relate to the pre-pregnancy level of function of the allograft and the presence of hypertension [C].[10]

In addition, these women are immunosuppressed and therefore more prone to infection. There are substantial data regarding the safety of immunosuppressive drugs in pregnancy. Prednisolone [C], azathioprine [C], cyclosporin[10] [C] and tacrolimus [C] are all considered safe. However, women receiving cyclosporin or tacrolimus are generally advised not to breastfeed. This may not be justified [E]. Mycophenolate mofetil (MMF) has caused toxicity in animal studies and is thought to be teratogenic in humans.[10] Women can usually be switched from MMF to azathioprine prior to pregnancy.

## DIALYSIS

Because women with end-stage renal failure have markedly reduced fertility, pregnancy on dialysis is unusual. The chances of a successful pregnancy outcome are sufficiently low, and the attendant risks sufficiently high, to counsel women on dialysis against pregnancy [E].[3] Anaemia and

haemorrhage are common, and the risks of miscarriage, fetal death, pre-eclampsia, preterm labour, preterm rupture of the membranes, polyhydramnios and placental abruption are increased [C].[11] Women who decide to continue with pregnancy require increasing dialysis in order to maintain the pre-dialysis urea, 15–20 mmol/L [C].[3,11] The incidence of poor obstetric outcome is similar with both haemodialysis and peritoneal dialysis.

## ACUTE RENAL FAILURE IN PREGNANCY

Acute renal failure is rare in pregnancy, the most common causes being pre-eclampsia and related syndromes, haemorrhage, infections, drugs, particularly non-steroidal anti-inflammatory drugs, and obstruction due to ureteric damage or stones. Conversely, mild degrees of renal impairment are more common, and again are usually related to pre-eclampsia or blood loss. Acute renal failure most commonly complicates the early postpartum period. It is characterized by oliguria, a rising urea and creatinine, a metabolic acidosis and hyperkalaemia. In the obstetric situation, there may be an associated coagulopathy. An isolated rise in urea (without concomitant rise in creatinine) is often observed following antenatal corticosteroid administration. A rare cause of renal failure, that is most commonly encountered postpartum, is haemolytic uraemic syndrome (HUS). The hallmark of this condition is a microangiopathic haemolytic anaemia (diagnosed with a blood film) associated with renal failure and thrombocytopenia.

### Pre-eclampsia and renal failure

Oliguria is an almost universal finding in pre-eclampsia and is excerbated by Syntocinon and caesarean section. It does not alone indicate renal failure, but should prompt measurement of serum urea and creatinine. Renal failure is more common in acute fatty liver[12] (see Chapter 6.8, Liver and gastrointestinal disease), HELLP syndrome (7 per cent) [C][13] and eclampsia (6 per cent) than in 'straightforward' pre-eclampsia. HELLP syndrome is the most common cause (50 per cent) of acute renal failure in the context of pre-eclampsia.

The management of acute renal failure depends on the cause: blood volume replacement for haemorrhage, delivery for pre-eclampsia, cessation of nephrotoxic drugs. Postpartum management is largely conservative and supportive. Accurate assessment of fluid balance with the use of a central venous pressure (CVP) line is important. Provided blood loss and volume depletion have been excluded as causes (CVP high or normal), fluids are only given to replace insensible losses and the previous hour's urine output. Iatrogenic fluid overload must be avoided in pre-eclampsia because these women are often hypoalbuminaemic and particularly susceptible to pulmonary oedema. Overzealous fluid administration is far more dangerous than oliguria. Dialysis may rarely become necessary, but a need for long-term renal replacement therapy is extremely unusual.

---

## KEY POINTS

- UTIs are common in pregnancy, and bacteriuria requires treatment to prevent pyelonephritis and preterm labour.
- The risks of complications, such as pre-eclampsia and FGR, and deterioration in renal function are high and the chances of successful pregnancy lower in women with severe renal impairment.
- Women with well-functioning renal allografts generally have successful pregnancies, but should be advised to delay pregnancy until about two years after transplantation.
- Women on dialysis have a low chance of successful pregnancy.
- Acute renal failure is rare, but may complicate haemorrhage and pre-eclampsia.

## Published Guidelines

Smaill F, Vazquez JC. Antibiotics for asymptomatic bacteriuria in pregnancy. *Cochrane Database Syst Rev* 2007; (**2**): CD000490.

## Key References

1. Williams D, Davison J. Chronic kidney disease in pregnancy. *BMJ* 2008; **336**: 211–15.
2. Cattell WR. Urinary tract infection in women. *J R Coll Phys Lond* 1997; **31**: 130–33.
3. Davison J, Nelson-Piercy C, Kehoe S, Baker P (eds). *Renal Disease in Pregnancy*. Report of RCOG Study Group. London: RCOG, 2008.
4. Epstein FH. Pregnancy and renal disease. *N Engl J Med* 1996; **335**: 277–8.
5. Jones DC, Hayslett JP. Outcome of pregnancy in women with moderate or severe renal insufficiency. *N Engl J Med* 1996; **335**: 226–32.
6. Jungers P, Chauveau D. Pregnancy in renal disease. *Kidney Int* 1997; **52**: 871–85.
7. Cooper WO, Hernandez-Diaz S, Arbogast PG *et al.* Major congenital malformations after first-trimester exposure to ACE inhibitors. *N Engl J Med* 2006; **354**: 2443–51.
8. Duley L, Henderson-Smart DJ, Knight M, King JF. Antiplatelet agents for preventing pre-eclampsia and its complications (Cochrane Review). *Cochrane Database Syst Rev* 2004; (**1**): CD004659. Review. Update in: *Cochrane Database Syst Rev* 2007; (**2**): CD004659.
9. Germain S, Nelson-Piercy C. Lupus nephritis and renal disease in pregnancy. *Lupus* 2006; **15**: 148–55.
10. Armenti VT, Constantinescu S, Moritz MJ, Davison JM. Pregnancy after transplantation. *Transplant Rev* 2008; **22**: 223–40.
11. Hou SH. Pregnancy in women with chronic renal insufficiency and end stage renal disease. *Am J Kidney Dis* 1999; **33**: 235–52.
12. Knight M, Nelson-Piercy C, Kurinczuk JJ *et al.* A prospective national study of acute fatty liver of pregnancy in the UK. *Gut* 2008; **57**: 951–6.
13. Drakeley AJ, Le Roux PA, Anthony J, Penny J. Acute renal failure complicating severe preeclampsia requiring admission to an obstetric intensive care unit. *Am J Obstet Gynecol* 2002; **186**: 253–6.

# 6.7 Autoimmune conditions

*Catherine Nelson-Piercy*

## MRCOG standards

### Relevant standard

To understand and demonstrate appropriate knowledge skills and attitudes in relation to pregnant women with connective tissue disease.

### Theoretical skills

To understand the epidemiology, aetiology, pathophysiology, clinical characteristics, prognostic features and management of women with connective tissue disease. To understand the use of immunosuppressant drugs in pregnancy.

### Practical skills

Be able to manage under direct supervision pregnant women with:

- SLE,
- rheumatoid arthritis,
- antiphospholipid syndrome.

## INTRODUCTION

This chapter covers the autoimmune connective tissue diseases, including rheumatoid arthritis (RA), systemic lupus erythematosus (SLE) and antiphospholipid syndrome (APS), Sjogren's syndrome and scleroderma. Autoimmune thrombocytopenia is discussed in Chapter 6.5, Haematological conditions; myasthenia gravis in Chapter 6.10, Neurological conditions; and autoimmune thyroid disease in Chapter 6.4, Thyroid disease.

Changes in the immune system in pregnancy result in relative suppressed cell-mediated immunity and enhanced humoral immunity. These changes revert postpartum when there is a sudden reduction of oestrogen, progesterone and cortisol levels. The postpartum period is therefore a time of theoretical susceptibility to autoimmune disorders. This means that some autoimmune conditions such as RA improve in pregnancy and may flare, worsen or present *de novo* in the postpartum period. In pregnancy, many of the issues for women with connective tissue disease relate to the safety of the drugs used to control their disease and to the degree of any systemic involvement of their disease.

## RHEUMATOID ARTHRITIS

This is a chronic, inflammatory, symmetrical arthritis causing joint pain, stiffness and deformity. Systemic features include rheumatoid nodules, pulmonary granulomas, vasculitis, Sjogren's syndrome (see below) and scleritis. Haematological abnormalities include a normocytic anaemia and raised erythrocyte sedimentation rate (ESR). Rheumatoid arthritis is usually associated with rheumatoid factor and 30 per cent of cases are antinuclear antibody (ANA) positive. Up to 20–30 per cent are Ro/La positive (see below) and 5–10 per cent are antiphospholipid (aPL) antibody positive (see below), although APS is rare. Pregnancy is associated with a decrease in T-cell immunity that is reversed postpartum.[1] This may explain why three-quarters of women with RA experience improvement in their symptoms during pregnancy and why those who improve usually flare postpartum.[2] Rheumatoid arthritis has no adverse effect upon pregnancy outcome. Limitation of hip abduction is rarely severe enough to preclude vaginal delivery, and atlanto-axial subluxation is a rare complication of general anaesthesia for caesarean section. Severe joint deformity and disability may rarely necessitate the need for help with care of the infant.

### Management

Assessment of disease activity is usually clinical. The ESR is raised in normal pregnancy and does not therefore provide a reliable marker of disease activity. As arthritis often improves in pregnancy, some reduction in analgesia may be possible.

## DRUGS FOR AUTOIMMUNE CONDITIONS

Paracetamol is safe in pregnancy and may be instituted or continued in maximal doses if required. The commonly used drugs for connective tissue disease are summarized in Table 6.7.1.[3]

Non-steroidal anti-inflammatory drugs (NSAIDs), such as ibuprofen and diclofenac, are often used in women with RA and SLE as well as over-the-counter analgesics in the general population. They are normally avoided in pregnancy because they are detrimental to the fetal kidney, causing oligohydramnios, and they may cause premature closure of the ductus arteriosus, leading to pulmonary hypertension and fetal haemorrhage, in large doses. Neither aspirin nor the other NSAIDs are teratogenic, so it is not necessary to discontinue these drugs prior to conception [C]. However, there is an association between NSAIDs and infertility due to luteinized unruptured follicle syndrome.[4] They should therefore be withdrawn if there is a history of infertility [D]. Occasionally, they are used in pregnancy when alternatives, such as paracetamol, codeine or corticosteroids, are inadequate or inappropriate. In such cases, they should be discontinued by 32 weeks gestation, as the effects on the fetal renal function and the ductus are reversible prior to delivery.[3] The selective cyclo-oxygenase-2 (COX-2) inhibitors are also contraindicated in pregnancy.

Corticosteroids are the first-line anti-inflammatory drugs in pregnancy.[3] They are used for many connective tissue diseases, not only for the arthritis manifestations, but also to treat vasculits, skin involvement, renal lupus and thrombocytopenia. There is no evidence to support the premise that steroids will prevent flare, either antenatal or postnatal, but they remain the mainstay of management for these disorders in pregnancy. They must never be withheld because of erroneous fears concerning their effects on the fetus. Many women are understandably reluctant to use any drugs, but particularly steroids, in pregnancy and therefore, if they are used, this must be with adequate counselling regarding their safety in pregnancy to ensure concordance with therapy [E]. Any possible small risk of teratogenesis (there are some data suggesting a small increased risk of oral clefting with first trimester exposure[5]) is dwarfed by the beneficial effects to the fetus of controlling the maternal disease process [C]. Caution is needed because the use of steroids in pregnancy is associated with an increased risk of infections and gestational diabetes. Large doses of steroids are associated with an increased risk of preterm rupture of the membranes.

Azathioprine is also safe in pregnancy. The fetal liver lacks the enzyme that converts azathioprine to its active metabolites. Azathioprine is used as a 'steroid-sparing' agent and there are reassuring data regarding a lack of adverse effects on babies born to mothers receiving this drug for renal transplants, inflammatory bowel disease and connective tissue diseases [C].[3] A study has shown that there are no detectable levels of the metabolites of azathioprine in the blood of neonates who were fully breastfed by women receiving azathioprine [D].[6]

Anti-malarials, such as hydroxychloroquine, are safe in pregnancy [C].[3] Discontinuation of this drug is associated with a risk of SLE flare.

Sulphasalazine is safe in pregnancy and breastfeeding. It is a dihydrofolate reductase inhibitor and therefore associated with an increased risk of neural tube, oral cleft and cardiovascular defects. Therefore, folate supplementation (5 mg per day) is advised [B].

Gold and D-penicillamine used in RA are usually avoided in pregnancy, although the risk of abnormalities is probably low. Cytotoxic drugs, such as cyclophosphamide, methotrexate and chlorambucil, are all highly teratogenic and must be discontinued prior to pregnancy.[3]

Biologic therapies, such as anti-TNF agents (etanercept and infliximab), are used increasingly in inflammatory arthritis. Available data suggest that these agents are safe in pregnancy but that they should ideally be discontinued by 30 weeks gestation [D].[7,8]

## SYSTEMIC LUPUS ERYTHEMATOSUS

This is a relapsing and remitting multisystem connective tissue disorder that predominantly affects women of childbearing age. The diagnostic criteria are shown in Table 6.7.2. It most commonly affects the joints (symmetrical non-erosive peripheral arthritis and arthralgia), the skin (malar rash, photosensitivity, discoid lupus, alopecia, vasculitis, Raynaud's phenomenon), and the kidneys (glomerulonephritis). There may be anaemia, lymphopenia, thrombocytopenia, hypocomplementaemia and a raised ESR. The C-reactive protein (CRP) is not raised.

**Table 6.7.1** Safety in pregnancy of drugs used for autoimmune conditions

| Safe to continue or start in pregnancy | Discontinue or avoid in pregnancy |
| --- | --- |
| Paracetamol | Non-steroidal anti-inflammatory drugs |
| Hydroxychloroquine | Cyclophosphamide |
| Sulfasalazine | Gold |
| Corticosteroids | Penicillamine |
| Azathioprine | Methotrexate |
| | Chlorambucil |
| | Leflunamide |
| | Mycophenolate mofetil |

**Table 6.7.2** American College of Rheumatology criteria for systemic lupus erythematosus (SLE)

| | |
|---|---|
| Malar rash | Renal disorder |
| Discoid rash | Neurological disorder |
| Photosensitivity | Haematological disorder |
| Oral ulcers | Immunological disorder |
| Arthritis | Antinuclear antibody |
| Serositis (e.g. pleurisy, pericarditis) | |

- For a diagnosis of SLE, four of these criteria are required simultaneously or serially.

Systemic lupus erythematosus is associated with ANA and anti-double-stranded DNA (dsDNA) antibodies. There may be antibodies to extractable nuclear antigens (ENA) including Ro and La, or antiphospholipid antibodies (aPL) with or without APS.

## Effect of pregnancy on SLE

Pregnancy is associated with an increased risk of SLE flare, which may occur at any stage of the pregnancy or postpartum. Neither the severity nor the type (e.g. renal or skin) of flare is altered by pregnancy. Flares may be harder to diagnose in pregnancy because many features, such as fatigue, erythema, anaemia and hair fall, are common to both.[9] Pregnancy does not alter the antibody profile but increases the ESR and may exacerbate thrombocytopenia.

## Effect of SLE on pregnancy outcome

In women who have quiescent SLE, have no renal involvement and are Ro/La and aPL negative, there is no adverse effect of their disease on pregnancy.[10] Active disease at conception, renal involvement and APS increase the risks of miscarriage, pre-eclampsia, fetal growth restriction (FGR), preterm delivery and stillbirth.

## Management

This should begin with pre-pregnancy counselling enabling an accurate risk assessment for individual women. Women should be advised to conceive during periods of disease remission. Once pregnancy is confirmed (or pre-pregnancy if there is a delay in conception), NSAIDs are discontinued. Hydroxychloroquine is continued because it is safe, because withdrawal may precipitate flare, and because it has a very long half-life such that the fetus remains exposed for up to three months after the mother discontinues the drug.[9] Prednisolone and azathioprine

are also continued. During pregnancy, SLE flares are treated with new or increased doses of steroids [C].[9,10] Not only are women with renal lupus at increased risk of pre-eclampsia, but also pre-eclampsia may be harder to diagnose in such woman, who already have hypertension and proteinuria. Low platelets, renal impairment, oedema, worsening hypertension and proteinuria may be attributable to either. Pointers to a renal lupus flare include red cells or red cell casts in the urine, hypocomplementaemia (falling levels of C3 and C4), and a rising anti-DNA titre. Pointers to a diagnosis of pre-eclampsia include raised transaminases and hyperuricaemia. Those at high risk of pre-eclampsia and FGR should be offered serial growth scans and tests of fetal well-being as indicated. Regular visits to the joint clinic are important to screen for pre-eclampsia and SLE flare.

## NEONATAL LUPUS SYNDROMES

These are caused by anti-Ro or anti-La antibodies and manifest as cutaneous neonatal lupus, affecting 5 per cent of babies of Ro-positive women, and congenital heart block, affecting 1–2 per cent of babies of Ro-positive women. If the first child is affected, the risk to the second child is 10-fold higher and about 16 per cent, and once two children are affected the risk rises to about 50 per cent. Neonatal cutaneous lupus develops in the first 2 weeks of life and is a geographical skin lesion of the face or scalp. It may be precipitated by exposure to ultraviolet light and usually regresses spontaneously without scarring within six months. Congenital heart block develops *in utero* at 18–30 weeks. There is no treatment, and one in five affected babies die as neonates. About half of those surviving require pacemakers in early infancy and the rest by their teens.[9] Ro-positive women should be offered fetal cardiology screening [C].

## ANTIPHOSPHOLIPID SYNDROME

This describes the association of aPL (either anticardiolipin antibodies or lupus anticoagulant) with the classical clinical features shown in Table 6.7.3.[11]

Additional clinical features include thrombocytopenia, livedo reticularis, epilepsy, migraine, heart valve disease and pulmonary hypertension. Antiphospholipid syndrome may be primary or found in association with SLE, RA or other connective tissue disease. Therefore women with primary APS, even if based on a positive lupus anticoagulant, do not have 'lupus' unless there are features of SLE (see Table 6.7.1).

The pathogenesis of APS involves a co-factor, β2-glycoprotein. Antiphospholipids reduce human chorionic gonadotrophin (hCG) release and inhibit trophoblast invasion *in vitro* – a potential explanation for the association

**Table 6.7.3** Classification criteria for antiphospholipid syndrome

| Clinical criteria | |
|---|---|
| Thrombosis | Venous |
| | Arterial |
| | Small vessel |
| Pregnancy morbidity | Three or more consecutive miscarriages (<10 weeks) |
| | One or more fetal death (>10 weeks) |
| | One or more premature birth (<35 weeks) due to severe pre-eclampsia or placental insufficiency |
| **Laboratory criteria** | |
| Anticardiolipin antibody | IgG or IgM |
| | Medium/high titre |
| | Two or more occasions >12 weeks apart |
| Lupus anticoagulant | Two or more occasions >12 weeks apart |

with miscarriage. However, the 'typical APS' fetal loss occurs in the second trimester and is associated with severe FGR, oligohydramnios and early-onset pre-eclampsia.[12] The common feature is defective or abnormal placentation, possibly related to thrombosis.

Pregnancy in women with APS is associated with an increased risk of thrombosis. This is particularly so for women with previous thrombosis. Antiphospholipd syndrome is a form of acquired thrombophilia. Thrombosis may therefore affect unusual sites such as the axillary or retinal veins. What makes APS particularly dangerous is the fact that thrombosis may also affect arterial and small vessels, causing, for example, stroke or renal disease. In general, those women who have had a previous venous thrombosis are at risk of recurrent venous thromboses, and those with previous arterial thrombosis from recurrent arterial events. Pregnancy also increases the risk of, or may exacerbate, pre-existing thrombocytopenia.

The effect of APS on pregnancy is to increase the risk of early and late miscarriage, stillbirth, placental abruption, FGR and pre-eclampsia.

## Management

Antiphospholipid syndrome should be managed in pregnancy by multidisciplinary teams with expertise of caring for these high-risk pregnancies. Those women with a previous history of arterial or venous thrombosis will usually be on long-term treatment with warfarin. This should be converted to aspirin and high prophylactic doses of low-molecular-weight heparin (LMWH) as soon as pregnancy is confirmed and at least before 6 weeks gestation to avoid warfarin embropathy (see Chapter 8, Medication in pregnancy). LMWH is continued in high prophylactic doses throughout pregnancy and postpartum for 6 weeks or until warfarin is recommenced.

For women without a previous history of thrombosis, there is agreement that low-dose aspirin (75 mg per day) is beneficial, although supportive evidence is mostly from retrospective, non-randomized studies. Indeed, randomized studies do not support a beneficial effect of aspirin, but this is because such studies have included very low risk groups of women, some without any previous history of adverse pregnancy outcome. Low-dose aspirin, is safe and all centres with an interest in APS use aspirin sometimes from pre-conception [D].[12,13] The role of LMWH in addition to aspirin is more controversial.[14] Two prospective studies of women with aPL and recurrent miscarriage demonstrated significantly increased live birth rates in groups allocated to aspirin and LMWH versus those receiving aspirin alone, and current Royal College of Obstetricians and Gynaecologist (RCOG) guidelines advocate the use of LMWH in addition to aspirin for women with recurrent miscarriage and aPL (see Published guidelines at the end of this chapter). However, both these studies had an unusually low live birth rate in the aspirin-alone groups. Two more recent randomized studies failed to show any increased benefit of LMWH over and above aspirin alone in women with APS and recurrent pregnancy loss.[14] That said, in women who have suffered late fetal losses or neonatal deaths attributable to APS, the risks of adverse pregnancy outcomes is higher and it is common to recommend LMWH in these situations [D].[12,13,15]

---

### EBM

- Evidence supports the use of high prophylactic doses of LMWH throughout pregnancy in women with APS who have had previous thromboses.
- Evidence from retrospective and cohort studies supports a role for low-dose aspirin for fetal indications.
- There is growing evidence that the use of LMWH in addition to aspirin for recurrent fetal loss provides no additional benefit.

---

A suggested management plan is given in Table 6.7.4. The risk of pre-eclampsia, abruption, FGR and preterm delivery is less for women with APS diagnosed as a result of recurrent early miscarriage compared to those women with APS diagnosed as a result of later pregnancy adverse outcome.[12,15] Past obstetric history is the best predictor of risk, although success rates for women diagnosed and treated for APS are about 70–80 per cent.[12,14,15] All women require careful and regular monitoring for pre-eclampsia, and serial growth scans and tests of fetal well-being as

**Table 6.7.4** Management recommendations for antiphospholipid syndrome pregnancies

| Antiphospholipid antibodies – no thrombosis or pregnancy loss | Aspirin 75 mg or nothing |
|---|---|
| Previous thrombosis | LMWH and aspirin |
| Previous recurrent (>3) miscarriages (<10 weeks) | Aspirin ± LMWH (? stop LMWH at 13–20 weeks) |
| Fetal loss or severe PET/FGR/NND | Aspirin + LMWH |

- FGR, fetal growth restriction; LMWH, low-molecular-weight heparin; NND, neonatal death; PET, pre-eclampsia.

appropriate [D].[13] Liaison with obstetric anaesthetists is vital prior to delivery in women receiving LMWH for any indication. In those who have had previous thromboses, discontinuation of LMWH peripartum should be minimal, but for those receiving LMWH for purely fetal indications, it may simplify the management of analgesia and anaesthesia for labour and delivery if the LMWH is discontinued prior to delivery.

# SJOGREN'S SYNDROME

This typically causes dry eyes and a dry mouth. The dry eyes may be confirmed objectively with the Schirmer tear test. Similar to APS, Sjogren's syndrome may be primary or associated with SLE, RA or other connective tissue disease. This syndrome is typically associated with positivity for Ro and La, and therefore the risk of neonatal lupus and congenital heart block (see above). Primary Sjogren's is associated with the finding of positive rheumatoid factor and positive ANA, and hypergammaglobulinaemia.

# SCLERODERMA

Scleroderma may occur as a localized cutaneous form, as systemic sclerosis or as part of the CREST syndrome (calcinosis, Raynaud's phenomenon, (o)esophageal involvement, sclerodactyly and telangiectasia). Skin involvement produces characteristic facies with a beaked nose and limited mouth opening, limiting facial expression. Systemic fibrosis involves the oesophagus, the lungs, the heart and the kidneys. There is no effective definitive treatment for scleroderma, although symptoms may be controlled with calcium antagonists, prostacyclin and specific treatments for renal involvement (ACE inhibitors) and pulmonary hypertension (sildenafil, bosentan).

Adverse effects on pregnancy relate to the degree of any renal, lung or cardiac involvement. Women with early diffuse disease are at increased risk in pregnancy and therefore women should be advised to postpone pregnancy until the disease has stabilized.[16] Those with severe pulmonary fibrosis or pulmonary hypertension should be advised against pregnancy [E]. Those with renal involvement and hypertension are at increased risk of pre-eclampsia and FGR. Oesophageal symptoms often increase in pregnancy, but those of Raynaud's may improve secondary to vasodilatation.

## Management

Pre-pregnancy counselling is vital to inform women accurately about the potential risks of pregnancy. Formal lung function and echocardiography to assess the extent of systemic involvement are recommended. During pregnancy, regular multidisciplinary assessment is required, with screens of blood pressure, urinalysis, renal function and maternal symptoms. Scleroderma renal crises are extremely dangerous and ACE inhibitors should not be stopped in pregnancy or withheld [E]. Raynaud's phenomenon may be ameliorated with heated gloves and calcium antagonists. Corticosteroids should be avoided because they may precipitate a renal crisis. Beta-agonists cause vasoconstriction and should also be avoided. Assessment by an obstetric anaesthetist prior to delivery is essential. In women with scleroderma, there are often problems with blood pressure measurement, venous access, capillary oxygen saturation monitoring and difficult airways.

> ## KEY POINTS
>
> - Rheumatoid arthritis usually improves in pregnancy and deteriorates postpartum.
> - SLE is more likely to flare in pregnancy.
> - Adverse pregnancy outcome in SLE is related to the presence of APS, renal involvement, disease activity and the presence of anti-Ro and La antibodies.
> - Ro and La antibodies are associated with Sjogren's syndrome and may cause congenital heart block and neonatal lupus.
> - APS may cause arterial, venous or capillary thrombosis, miscarriage, late fetal loss, early-onset pre-eclampsia and severe FGR.
> - APS is treated in pregnancy with low-dose aspirin and LMWH.
> - Steroids are safe to treat connective tissue disease in pregnancy and are used in preference to NSAIDs.

## Published Guidelines

RCOG guidelines for recurrent miscarriage/APS. Guideline No. 17. London: RCOG.

# Key References

1. Nelson JL, Ostensen M. Pregnancy and rheumatoid arthritis. *Rheum Dis Clin North Am* 1997; **23**: 195–212.

2. Barrett JH, Brennan P, Fiddler M *et al.* Does rheumatoid arthritis remit during pregnancy and relapse postpartum? Results from a Nationwide Study in the United Kingdom performed prospectively from late pregnancy. *Arthritis Rheum* 1999; **42**: 1219–27.

3. Ostensen M, Khamashta M, Lockshin M *et al.* Anti-inflammatory and immunosuppressive drugs and reproduction. *Arthritis Res Ther* 2006; **8**: 209–38.

4. Mendonca LLF, Khamastha MA, Nelson-Piercy C *et al.* Non-steroidal anti-inflammatory drugs as a possible cause for reversible infertility. *Rheumatology* 2000; **39**: 880–25.

5. Carmichael SL, Shaw GM, Ma C *et al*; National Birth Defects Prevention Study. Maternal corticosteroid use and orofacial clefts. *Am J Obstet Gynecol* 2007; **197**: 585: e1–76.

6. Sau A, Clarke S, Bass J *et al.* Azathioprine and breastfeeding: is it safe? *BJOG* 2007; **114**: 498–501.

7. Vinet E, Pineau C, Gordon C *et al.* Biologic therapy and pregnancy outcome in women with rheumatic diseases. *Arthritis Rheum* 2009; **61**: 587–92.

8. Ostensen M, Lockshin M, Doria A *et al.* Update on safety during pregnancy of biological agents and some immunosuppressive anti-rheumatic drugs. *Rheumatology* 2008; **47** (Suppl. 3): iii28–31.

9. McKillop L, Germain S, Nelson-Piercy C. SLE in pregnancy. *BMJ* 2007; **335**: 933–6.

10. Khamashta MA. Systemic lupus erythematosus and pregnancy. *Best Pract Res Clin Rheumatol* 2006; **20**: 685–94

11. Miyakis S, Lockshin MD, Atsumi T *et al.* International consensus statement on an update of the classification criteria for definite antiphospholipid syndrome (APS). *J Thromb Haemost* 2006; **4**: 295–306.

12. Derksen RHWM, Khamashta MA, Ware Branch D. Management of the obstetric antiphospholipid syndrome. *Arthritis Rheum* 2004; **50**: 1028–39.

13. Lakasing L, Bewley SJ, Nelson-Piercy C. Management of antiphospholipid syndrome in pregnancy. In: Khamastha MA (ed). *Hughes syndrome: The Antiphospholipid Syndrome*, 2nd edn. London: Springer, 2006: 555–67.

14. Laskin CA, Spitzer KA, Clark CA *et al.* Low molecular weight heparin and aspirin for recurrent pregnancy loss: results from the randomized controlled HepASA trial. *J Rheumatol* 2009; **36**: 279–87.

15. Bramham K, Hunt BJ, Germain S *et al.* Pregnancy outcome in women with Antiphospholipid syndrome: Management in a tertiary referral centre. *Lupus* 2010; **19**: 58–64.

16. Steen VD. Pregnancy in women with systemic sclerosis. *Obstet Gynecol* 1999; **94**: 15–20.

# 6.8 Liver and gastrointestinal disease

*Catherine Nelson-Piercy*

## MRCOG standards

### Theoretical skills

Understand the epidemiology, aetiology, pathophysiology, clinical characteristics, prognostic features and management of women with liver and gastrointestinal disease.

### Practical skills

Be able to manage independently:

- Crohn's disease and ulcerative colitis,
- irritable bowel syndrome,
- reflux oesophagitis,
- hyperemesis,
- obstetric cholestasis.

Be able to manage under direct supervision pregnant women with:

- acute fatty liver of pregnancy,
- hepatitis.

## INTRODUCTION

Liver disease in pregnancy is encountered relatively rarely, but gastrointestinal problems, including nausea, vomiting, oesophageal reflux and constipation, are almost universal. Liver disease can be dangerous for both the mother and the fetus. This chapter considers the liver conditions specific to pregnancy – obstetric cholestasis and acute fatty liver of pregnancy – and those that predate or coincide with pregnancy – viral hepatitis and chronic liver disease. HELLP syndrome is discussed in Chapter 7.6, Pre-eclampsia and non-proteinuric pregnancy-induced hypertension. Gastrointestinal diseases usually predate the pregnancy; inflammatory bowel disease and irritable bowel syndrome are the most common. Gastrointestinal problems exacerbated or brought on by pregnancy, such as gastro-oesophageal reflux and hyperemesis, are also discussed.

## PHYSIOLOGICAL CHANGES IN PREGNANCY

Pregnancy causes decreased lower oesophageal pressure, decreased gastric peristalsis and delayed gastric emptying. Gastrointestinal motility is reduced, with increased small-bowel and large-bowel transit times. There is a 20–40 per cent fall in serum albumin concentration, partly due to dilution resulting from the increase in total blood volume. Total serum protein concentration also decreases. The alkaline phosphatase concentration more than doubles due to production by the placenta, which increases with gestation. Levels of alanine transaminase (ALT); serum glutamic pyruvic transaminase (SGPT); aspartamine transaminase (AST) and serum glutamic-oxaloacetic transaminase (SGOT) fall and there is a fall in the upper limit of the normal ranges for both enzymes (Table 6.8.1).[1] Thus a mildly abnormal level for transaminases that may be significant in the diagnosis of obstetric cholestasis or in the assessment of pre-eclampsia may be overlooked unless pregnancy-specific ranges are used. The concentrations of other liver enzymes are not substantially altered and there is no significant change in bilirubin concentration during normal pregnancy.

## NAUSEA, VOMITING AND HYPEREMESIS

Nausea and vomiting are common symptoms in early pregnancy, affecting over half of pregnant women. The onset of symptoms is usually early in the first trimester at around 5–6 weeks gestation. Hyperemesis is less common, but causes much morbidity and repeated hospital admissions and can be dangerous if inadequately or inappropriately treated. Nausea and vomiting in pregnancy become hyperemesis if the woman is unable to maintain adequate hydration and nutrition, either because of severity or duration of symptoms. This is associated with marked weight loss, muscle wasting, ketonuria, dehydration and electrolyte disturbance,

**Table 6.8.1** Normal ranges for liver enzymes in non-pregnant and pregnant populations

| Liver enzyme | Non-pregnant | Trimester | | |
|---|---|---|---|---|
| | | 1st | 2nd | 3rd |
| AST (IU/L) | 7–40 | 10–28 | 10–29 | 11–30 |
| ALT (IU/L) | 0–40 | 6–32 | 6–32 | 6–32 |
| Bilirubin (µmol/L) | 0–17 | 4–16 | 3–13 | 3–14 |
| Gamma GT (IU/L) | 11–50 | 5–37 | 5–43 | 3–41 |
| Alkaline phosphatase (IU/L) | 30–130 | 32–100 | 43–135 | 133–418 |

- ALT, alanine transaminase; AST, aspartamine transaminase; GT, glutamyl transpeptidase.

including hypokalaemia and a metabolic hypochloraemic alkalosis. A common associated symptom is ptyalism – the inability to swallow saliva. The risks associated with hyperemesis include fetal growth restriction, maternal hyponatraemia leading to central pontine myelinolysis and thiamine deficiency leading to Wernicke's encephalopathy.[2] Markers of severity include weight loss >10 per cent, abnormal thyroid function tests with raised free thyroxine (T4) and suppressed thyroid-stimulating hormone (TSH) and abnormal liver function tests with raised transaminases.

## Management

Other possible causes of nausea and vomiting should be excluded (Table 6.8.2). These include urinary tract infection (which often coincides with hyperemesis), thyrotoxicosis (where symptoms of weight loss, diarrhoea and tachycardia precede the pregnancy) and cholecystitis. An ultrasound scan of the uterus is important to exclude hydatidiform mole and to diagnose multiple pregnancy, both of which increase the risk of hyperemesis. The most important component of management is to ensure adequate rehydration. This should be with normal saline with added potassium chloride sufficient to correct tachycardia, hypotension and ketonuria and return electrolyte levels to normal. Dextrose-containing fluids are avoided except in women with diabetes. High concentrations of dextrose in particular may precipitate Wernicke's encephalopathy. This is prevented by routine administration of oral or intravenous thiamine. Anti-emetics may be liberally and safely used in pregnancy [A, C].[2–4] Women with severe hyperemesis may require regular parenteral doses of more than one anti-emetic to control their symptoms. Even for women with nausea and vomiting in pregnancy that does not require hospital admission but interferes

**Table 6.8.2** Protocol for the management of hyperemesis

| Investigations | U + E, FBC, LFTs, TFTs<br>MSU<br>US scan uterus |
|---|---|
| Fluid therapy | Normal saline 1 L + 20–40 mmol KCl 8-hourly |
| Vitamin therapy | Thiamine orally 25–50 mg tds *or* thiamine intravenously 100 mg in 100 mL normal saline weekly |
| Anti-emetic therapy | Possible regimens include:<br>Cyclizine 50 mg p.o./i.m./i.v. tds<br>Promethazine 25 mg p.o. nocte<br>Stemetil 5 mg po tds; 12.5 mg i.m./i.v. tds<br>Metoclopramide 10 mg p.o./i.m./i.v. tds<br>Domperidone 10 mg p.o. qds; 30–60 mg p.r. tds<br>Chlorpromazine 10–25 mg p.o.; 25 mg i.m. tds |

- US, ultrasound.

with work and home life, anti-emetics may be appropriate. For women with severe hyperemesis who do not improve despite conventional treatment with intravenous fluids and electrolytes and regular anti-emetics, a trial of corticosteroids may be considered [B].[5,6] Iron supplements may induce nausea and vomiting, and should be withheld until symptoms resolve.

### EBM: Hyperemesis

- There are substantial data from systematic reviews[3] and cohort studies[2] to support the safety of conventional anti-emetics in pregnancy, including the first trimester.
- Several randomized, controlled trials[5] support a beneficial effect of corticosteroids.

## GASTRO-OESOPHAGEAL REFLUX

About two-thirds of women experience heartburn in pregnancy, commonly in the third trimester. This is partly because of increased reflux due to the decreased lower oesophageal pressure, decreased gastric peristalsis and delayed gastric emptying, and partly due to the enlarging uterus. Reflux of acid or alkaline gastric contents into the oesophagus causes inflammation of the oesophageal mucosa, leading to pain, waterbrash and dyspepsia.

## Management

Postural changes, such as sleeping in a semi-recumbent position, may help, especially in late pregnancy. Avoiding food or fluid intake immediately before retiring may also prevent symptoms. Antacids are safe in pregnancy and may be used liberally. Liquid preparations are more effective and should be given to prevent and treat symptoms. Aluminium-containing antacids may cause constipation, and magnesium-containing antacids may cause diarrhoea. Metoclopramide increases lower oesophageal pressure and speeds gastric emptying and may help relieve reflux. Sucralfate and histamine$_2$-receptor blockers (e.g. ranitidine) are both safe throughout pregnancy. Omeprazole, a proton-pump inhibitor and more powerful suppressor of gastric acid secretion, is also safe.[4] It should be reserved for reflux oesophagitis when histamine$_2$-receptor blockers have failed.

## PEPTIC ULCER

Peptic ulceration is rare in pregnancy. Presentation is usually with epigastric pain rather than with complications such as haemorrhage or perforation. Prostaglandins induced by pregnancy have a protective effect on the gastric mucosa, thus explaining the reduced incidence compared to non-pregnant women. Gastrointestinal endoscopy (including the sedation used for the procedure) is safe in pregnancy and should be used to investigate all but minor haematemesis.

## Management

Antacids, sucralfate and histamine$_2$-receptor blockers are all safe in pregnancy. *Helicobacter pylori* has a causal role in peptic ulceration, but eradication therapy is usually deferred until after delivery. Misoprostol, a prostaglandin analogue, protects the gastric mucosa but is contraindicated during pregnancy because of the risk of miscarriage.

## CONSTIPATION

This is another common symptom of normal pregnancy, probably due to reduced colonic motility. Poor dietary intake associated with nausea and vomiting, dehydration, opiate analgesia and iron supplements exacerbate constipation. Management includes advice regarding increased fluid intake and dietary fibre. Temporary cessation of oral iron supplements may help, and laxatives should only be used if the above measures fail. Osmotic laxatives, such as lactulose and magnesium hydrochloride, are safe. Stimulant laxatives, such as glycerol suppositories, and senna (Senokot®) tablets are also safe in pregnancy.

---

**EBM: Gastro-oesophageal reflux, dyspepsia, constipation**

- There are substantial data from systematic reviews[3] to support the safety of antacids, anti-emetics, sucralfate, histamine$_2$-receptor blockers and proton pump inhibitors in pregnancy.
- Misoprostol should be avoided.
- Osmotic and stimulant laxatives are safe to use in pregnancy.

---

## INFLAMMATORY BOWEL DISEASE

Both Crohn's disease and ulcerative colitis tend to present in young adulthood. Ulcerative colitis is more common in women and is encountered more commonly in pregnancy. The course of inflammatory bowel disease (IBD) is not usually affected by pregnancy. The risk of flare in pregnancy is reduced if colitis is quiescent at the time of conception. Most exacerbations occur early in pregnancy and cause abdominal pain, diarrhoea and passage of rectal mucus and blood. Women with Crohn's disease may experience postpartum flare. Pregnancy outcome is usually good in women with IBD, although active disease at the time of conception is associated with an increased risk of miscarriage, and active disease later in pregnancy may adversely affect pregnancy outcome, with an increased rate of preterm delivery.[7,8] Prior surgery, including ileostomy, proctocolectomy and pouch surgery, does not preclude successful pregnancy.

## Management

Women with IBD should be encouraged to conceive during periods of disease remission. Management is not substantially affected by pregnancy. Oral or rectal sulfasalazine (Salazopyrin), mesalazine (Asacol) and other 5-aminosalicylic acid drugs may be safely used throughout pregnancy and breastfeeding, although as sulfasalazine is a dihydrofolate reductase inhibitor, 5 mg daily folic acid should be used pre-conception and in pregnancy to reduce the increased risk of neural tube defects, cardiovascular defects, oral clefts and folate deficiency. Oral and rectal preparations of corticosteroids may be required for acute treatment or maintenance and are safe in pregnancy. Azathioprine may be needed to maintain remission and this should be continued in pregnancy (see Chapter 6.7, Autoimmune conditions).[8] Biologic therapies such as the anti-TNF agents (infliximab and adalimumab) are used increasingly in IBD. Available data suggest that these agents are safe in pregnancy but should ideally be discontinued by 30 weeks gestation [D].[9]

Clinicians must remain alert to the possible dangerous surgical complications of IBD, including intestinal obstruction, haemorrhage, perforation or toxic megacolon. Caesarean section may be indicated in the presence of severe peri-anal Crohn's disease with a deformed, inelastic or scarred rectum and perineum. Active perianal Crohn's may prevent healing of an episiotomy.

## EBM: Inflammatory bowel disease

- Evidence from cohort studies[7] supports an association between conception during periods of active disease and adverse pregnancy outcome.
- Sulfasalazine and related drugs are safe in pregnancy, but folic acid 5 mg/day should be given concomitantly.
- Corticosteroids and azathioprine may safely be used for maintenance or acute management of disease flares.[8]

## ACUTE AND CHRONIC VIRAL HEPATITIS

The course of most viral hepatitis is not altered by pregnancy. Pregnant women may contract acute hepatitis in the same way and with the same clinical features as non-pregnant women (see Chapter 7.4, Infection). Thus fever, malaise, anorexia, jaundice and possible recent exposure should alert the clinician to the diagnosis. The implications of acute hepatitis infection in pregnancy are discussed in Chapter 7.4, Infection. As with acute hepatitis B infections, neonates born to women with chronic hepatitis B virus (HBV) should be given hepatitis B immune globulin and HBV vaccine within 24 hours of birth. Immunization is 85–95 per cent effective at preventing both HBV infection and the chronic carrier state. There is a significant risk (60–80 per cent) of hepatitis C infection progressing to chronic infection, and about 20 per cent of those with chronic infection develop slowly progressive cirrhosis over a period of 10–30 years. Detection of hepatitis C virus (HCV) antibody implies persistent infection rather than immunity. The risk of progressive liver disease with hepatitis C is lower in women and in those aged <40 years who do not abuse alcohol. Women with hepatitis C are at increased risk of obstetric cholestasis (see below).[10]

## CHRONIC LIVER DISEASE

Severe hepatic impairment is associated with infertility. Liver disease may decompensate during pregnancy, and pregnancy should be discouraged in women with severe impairment of hepatic function. Those with portal hypertension and oesophageal varices are at risk from variceal bleeding, especially in the second and third trimesters.

## OBSTETRIC CHOLESTASIS

This is a liver disease specific to pregnancy, characterized by pruritus affecting the whole body but particularly the palms and soles, and abnormal liver function tests. It is more common in women from South America, the Indian subcontinent and Scandinavia. The prevalence in the UK is about 0.7 per cent.[11] The aetiology is unknown, but relates to a genetic predisposition (one-third of patients have a positive family history) to the cholestatic effect of oestrogens.

Obstetric cholestasis most commonly presents in the third trimester at around 30–32 weeks gestation.[11] Women with pruritus but without a rash, other than excoriations, should have liver function tests. These must be interpreted with reference to the normal ranges for pregnancy[1] since often in obstetric cholestasis the hepatic transaminases are only mildly elevated. The most usual abnormality is raised ALT or AST, although a small proportion of women have only a raised gamma GT or raised bile acids.[12] Although raised bile acids are not necessary to confirm the diagnosis, they are useful, especially in those women with typical clinical features but normal standard liver function tests.[12] There may be associated dark urine, pale stools, steatorrhoea and malaise. Obstetric cholestasis is a diagnosis of exclusion, and the differential diagnosis includes extrahepatic obstruction with gallstones, acute or chronic viral hepatitis, primary biliary cirrhosis (PBC) and chronic active hepatitis (CAH). Investigations should therefore include a liver ultrasound, serology for hepatitis A, B and C, Ebstein–Barr virus and cytomegalovirus, and liver autoantibodies (anti-mitochondrial antibodies to exclude PBC and anti-smooth muscle antibodies to exclude CAH).

The risks with obstetric cholestasis include postpartum haemorrhage (related to vitamin K deficiency secondary to malabsorption of fat), preterm labour, meconium-stained liquor, fetal distress (cardiotocograph (CTG) abnormalities) in labour and, rarely, intrauterine death (IUD). The cause of the adverse effects on the fetus is unknown. The risk of IUD increases towards and beyond term but does not correlate with either symptoms or liver function tests. There is a correlation with bile acid levels.[13]

## EBM: Obstetric cholestasis

- Evidence from prospective studies[11,12] supports the need for a high index of clinical suspicion, and therefore serial measurement of liver function tests, in women with onset of pruritus affecting predominantly the palms and soles in the third trimester.
- This evidence also highlights the trade-off between reduced fetal mortality and increased rates of induction, preterm delivery and caesarean section.

## Management

This should involve counselling the woman regarding the above risks. Liver function tests and clotting times should be monitored regularly. Current guidelines suggest that there is insufficient evidence to support the common practice of expediting delivery at 37–38 weeks. Vitamin K should be given to the mother (10 mg orally daily) from the time of diagnosis to reduce the risk of postpartum haemorrhage. No specific method of fetal surveillance can be recommended to predict fetal complications in mothers with obstetric cholestasis. Although such monitoring may serve to reassure the mother and her carers, delivery is rarely indicated earlier than 37 weeks on the basis of such monitoring. Management strategies that involve elective early (by 38 weeks) delivery and fetal surveillance have shown a decreased risk of IUD compared to earlier studies, but also result in increased rates of caesarean section, prematurity and admissions to neonatal intensive care units.[11]

Control of symptoms may be achieved with a combination of antihistamines and emollients or, if these are insufficient, ursodeoxycholic acid (UDCA). This drug usually leads to rapid reduction in liver function tests and pruritus, but there is as yet no evidence for a reduction in fetal risk. A randomized controlled trial is currently in progress to determine the role of UDCA and early elective delivery.

Following delivery, liver function tests return to normal and there is no permanent detrimental effect on maternal liver function. Symptoms may recur with menstruation (cyclical itching) or with oestrogen-containing oral contraceptives, which should therefore be avoided. Recurrence of obstetric cholestasis in subsequent pregnancies exceeds 90 per cent.

---

### KEY POINTS

**Obstetric cholestasis**
- Liver function tests should be requested in any pregnant woman with pruritus without obvious rash.
- Liver function tests should be repeated serially if the itching involves the palms and soles.
- Other causes of pruritus and abnormal liver function tests, including viral hepatitis and gallstones causing extrahepatic obstruction, should be excluded.
- Retrospective studies support active management with elective delivery by 38 weeks.
- Active management increases the risk of caesarean section and prematurity.
- UDCA improves symptoms and liver function tests

The role of UDCA and elective delivery are currently under investigation in a randomized placebo-controlled trial.

---

## ACUTE FATTY LIVER OF PREGNANCY

This is another pregnancy-specific liver disease. It is rare and a recent UK wide study found a prevalence of 5 per 100 000.[14] Acute fatty liver of pregnancy (AFLP) is closely related to and shares many features, and probably pathophysiology, with pre-eclampsia. It usually presents in the third trimester with abdominal pain, nausea, vomiting, anorexia and sometimes jaundice. It is associated with markedly deranged liver function tests, renal impairment, a markedly elevated uric acid, a raised white cell count, hypoglycaemia and coagulopathy.[14] Clinical features of pre-eclampsia may be mild or absent. It is more common in twin pregnancies. It may come to light only after delivery when coagulation is checked because of excessive bleeding. It is also associated with diabetes insipidus and may present with polyuria and polydipsia. Perinatal and maternal mortality and morbidity are increased (10 and 1.8 per cent, respectively).[14]

## Management

This should involve a high-dependency or intensive care unit and a multidisciplinary team. Delivery should be expedited following adequate correction of any hypoglycaemia or coagulopathy with 50 per cent dextrose, intravenous vitamin K and fresh frozen plasma. Management after delivery is conservative, although early referral to a liver unit should be considered if liver function does not improve or if there are any features of hepatic encephalopathy.

## Published Guidelines/Online Resources

RCOG Green top guideline no. 43 Obstetric Cholestasis. Jan 2006 ‹www.rcog.org.uk/files/rcog-corp/uploaded-files/GT43ObstetricCholestasis2006.pdf›

Germain S, Nelson-Piercy C. Liver and Gastrointestinal disease. Maternal Medicine Module. *RCOG Strat-OG* 2nd edn. London: RCOG, 2007.

## Key References

1. Girling JC, Dow E, Smith JH. Liver function tests in pre-eclampsia: importance of comparison with a reference range derived for normal pregnancy. *Br J Obstet Gynaecol* 1997; **104**: 246–50.
2. Nelson-Piercy C. Treatment of nausea and vomiting in pregnancy: when should it be treated and with what? *Drug Saf* 1998; **19**: 155–64.
3. Mazzotta P, Magee LA. A risk–benefit assessment of pharmacological and non-pharmacological treatments for nausea and vomiting of pregnancy. *Drugs* 2000; **59**: 781–800.
4. Kametas N, Nelson-Piercy C. Hyperemesis gravidarum, gastrointestinal and liver disease in pregnancy. *Obstetrics Gynaecol Reprod Med* 2008; **18**: 69–75.

5. Nelson-Piercy C, Fayers P, de Swiet M. Randomized, placebo-controlled trial of corticosteroids for hyperemesis gravidarum. *Br J Obstet Gynaecol* 2001; **108**: 1–7.

6. Moran P, Taylor R. Management of hyperemesis gravidarum: the importance of weight loss as a criterion for steroid therapy. *QJM* 2002; **95**: 153–8.

7. Kornfeld D, Crattingnuis S, Ekbom A. Pregnancy outcomes in women with IBD – a population-based cohort study. *Am J Obstet Gynecol* 1997; **177**: 942–6.

8. Alstead EA, Nelson-Piercy C. Inflammatory bowel disease in pregnancy. *Gut* 2002; **52**: 159–61.

9. Vinet E, Pineau C, Gordon C *et al.* Biologic therapy and pregnancy outcome in women with rheumatic diseases. *Arthritis Rheum* 2009; **61**: 587–92.

10. Locatelli A, Roncaglia N, Arreghini A *et al.* Hepatitis C virus infection is associated with a higher incidence of cholestasis of pregnancy. *Br J Obstet Gynaecol* 1999; **106**: 498–500.

11. Kenyon AP, Nelson-Piercy C, Girling J *et al.* Obstetric cholestasis, outcome with active management: a series of 70 cases. *Br J Obstet Gynaecol* 2002; **109**: 282–8.

12. Kenyon AP, Nelson-Piercy C, Girling J *et al.* Pruritus may precede abnormal liver function tests in pregnant women with obstetric cholestasis: a longitudinal analysis. *Br J Obstet Gynaecol* 2001; **108**: 1190–2.

13. Glantz A, Marschall HU, Mattson LA. Intrahepatic cholestasis of pregnancy: relationship between bile acid levels and fetal complication rates. *Hepatology* 2004; **40**: 467–74.

14. Knight M, Nelson-Piercy C, Kurinczuk JJ *et al.* A prospective national study of acute fatty liver of pregnancy in the UK. *Gut* 2008; **57**: 951–6.

# 6.9 Respiratory conditions

*Louise Kenny*

## PULMONARY DISEASE IN PREGNANCY

The physiological changes occurring within the respiratory system are summarized in Tables 6.9.1 and 6.9.2. Symptomatically, pregnant women may complain of new-onset rhinitis, which may result from oestrogen-induced oedema, hyperaemia and hypersecretion of the upper airways. Although mostly harmless, this contributes to the greater difficulties encountered during intubation of pregnant women. Much more common is the complaint of shortness of breath or 'air hunger'. This dyspnoea is experienced by approximately half of all pregnant women by 20 weeks gestation and by three-quarters by 30 weeks. It rarely occurs at rest and does not significantly impair normal activities. The postulated mechanism is high progesterone levels acting via the hypothalamus to increase respiratory drive.

Anatomically, the lower chest wall circumference increases by 5–7 cm, the diaphragm is elevated 4–5 cm by term and the costal angle widens. These changes occur due to the pressure from the expanding uterus and the relaxation of thoracic ligaments. Diaphragmatic excursion is not reduced, however, the accessory muscles contribute proportionally more than the diaphragm to the increase in tidal volume found in pregnancy.

The metabolic rate becomes elevated in pregnancy, as demonstrated by a rise in resting oxygen uptake ($\dot{V}_{O_2}$) and carbon dioxide output ($\dot{V}_{O_2}$). This extra oxygen turnover is of course necessary for the feto-placental unit and the extra demands made by maternal physiology. Minute ventilation ($\dot{V}_E$) and alveolar ventilation ($\dot{V}_A$) are both increased to meet this demand by an increase in tidal volume ($T_V$) rather than by a change in respiratory rate, which remains constant. This state of relative hyperventilation causes a fall in $PaCO_2$, which results in a chronic respiratory alkalosis. Blood pH is kept within the normal range by a reactionary increase in renal bicarbonate excretion.

Airway function is maintained and peak expiratory flow rate (PEFR) and forced expiratory volume in 1 second ($FEV_1$) measurements are not affected by pregnancy.

## Investigating pulmonary disease in pregnancy

The physiological changes occurring in pregnancy must also be considered when interpreting the results of investigations. The effect on arterial blood gas analysis is clear from Table 6.9.1. The chest x-ray must also be interpreted with caution. The cardiothoracic ratio is elevated, vascular markings may become more prominent, and small pleural effusions are even possible in normal pregnancy. Peak flow and spirometry tests can be interpreted in the usual manner.

Concern is often raised about the safety of various radiological examinations during pregnancy. For a fuller

**Table 6.9.1** Normal arterial blood gas values and the effect of pregnancy

|  | Pre-pregnancy | By term |
|---|---|---|
| $PaO_2$ | 11–13 kPa (83–98 mmHg) | 0.13 kPa (0.98 mmHg) |
| $PaCO_2$ | 4.8–6.0 kPa (36–45 mmHg) | 3.7–4.2 kPa (28–32 mmHg) |
| $HCO_3^-$ | 24–30 mmol/L | 18–21 mmol/L |
| pH | 7.35–7.45 | 7.4–7.45 |

**Table 6.9.2** The effect of pregnancy on lung function

| Lung function | Change by term | Actual volume change |
|---|---|---|
| Total lung capacity | 4% decrease | 200–400 mL |
| Functional residual | 10–20% decrease | 300–500 mL capacity |
| Expiratory reserve | 15–20% decrease | 100–300 mL volume |
| Tidal volume | 30–50% increase | 200 mL |
| Minute ventilation | 30–50% increase | 3 L/min |
| Residual volume | 20–25% decrease | 200–300 mL |
| Respiratory rate | No change |  |
| Vital capacity | No change |  |
| Peak flow | No change |  |
| Metabolic rate | 15% increase |  |
| Oxygen consumption $(V_{O_2})$ | 20–33% increase |  |

description of risks to the fetus, see Chapter 7.3, Malignancy. 5 cGy is often considered the maximum safe exposure for the fetus, although this is gestation dependent [D]. Chest x-ray, venography, pulmonary angiography and ventilation perfusion scanning all expose the fetus to significantly lower levels than this, and the potential benefits of all these investigations are usually thought to outweigh the risks. However, exposure should be minimized where possible. For example:

- Lateral chest x-rays are often unnecessary and carry a greater exposure risk than an AP erect chest film; they can mostly be avoided.
- A mobile chest x-ray carries greater exposure than a departmental film, so the patient should be moved where possible.
- The 'ventilation' component of $\overset{\text{g}}{V}/\overset{\text{g}}{Q}$ scanning can be omitted in women with no previous history of chest disease.
- Pulmonary angiography carries less fetal risk if a brachial route is used in preference to the femoral.

Shielding of the fetus should be used where the situation allows. Computed tomography (CT) scanning utilizes much higher energy levels, and safer alternatives are usually available. However, if the indication is strong enough, even CT has its place. Spiral and non-contiguous axial imaging are techniques that may reduce exposure without compromising diagnostic accuracy. Magnetic resonance imaging (MRI) scanning involves no irradiation and is also considered safe.

## ASTHMA

Asthma is the respiratory illness most likely to be encountered during pregnancy, with a prevalence of between 1 and 4 per cent.

The true effect of pregnancy on asthma severity has been addressed by a number of prospective case-controlled studies which suggest that approximately two-fifths will deteriorate, two-fifths will stay the same and one-fifth will improve.[1] The potential benefits of pregnancy-induced immune system alterations and progesterone-mediated bronchodilatation may be opposed by the reluctance of patients and physicians to treat asthma appropriately for fear of harming the fetus through drug exposure. Women with severe asthma seem more likely to deteriorate, while those showing improvement during pregnancy are more likely to suffer postpartum relapse.[2] Approximately 1 in 10 asthmatics will suffer an acute attack in labour [C].

The precise effect that the asthma has on the pregnancy is unclear. Almost every conceivable obstetric complication has been found to be more common in pregnant asthmatics by one case-control study or another. However, the pattern of antenatal complications varies greatly among studies and this lack of consistency has cast doubt over the findings. Poor controls, varied case mixes and different treatment regimes make resolution of the data very difficult.

**EBM**

Prospective and retrospective studies of women with asthma suggest that pregnancy outcome is usually extremely good.

A prospective case-controlled study by Schatz in 1995 found no increase in the incidence of any obstetric complications among almost 500 asthmatics.[3] These women were managed by an obstetrician and an interested physician and this may explain the normal outcomes. However, only a quarter of the women used steroids of any kind, and the overall mild nature of the condition in this group may have contributed to the favourable outcomes.

It is still accepted that severe and poorly controlled asthma does have a detrimental effect on pregnancy, so closer surveillance for hypertensive disorders, intrauterine growth restriction and preterm rupture of membranes/labour can be justified [E].

# Management of asthma in pregnancy

In the recent Confidential Enquiry into Maternal Deaths (2003–2005), four women died from asthma, all suddenly and unexpectedly. Asthma will usually have been diagnosed prior to pregnancy and treatment already instituted. However, this is not always the case, and the initial presenting signs and symptoms of asthma are the same as those of asthma that is inadequately treated:

- chest tightness and wheeziness;
- cough;
- breathlessness, especially in the early hours of the morning.

The management of asthma in pregnancy is essentially the same as in non-pregnant patients.

Prevention is the key, and known triggers of exacerbations should be eliminated or avoided in the home and at work (Table 6.9.3).

## Pharmacological treatment of asthma

This follows a step-by-step approach, more clearly outlined in the *British National Formulary*.

**Step 1: occasional relief bronchodilators** (up to once per day): short-acting inhaled beta$_2$-agonist, e.g. salbutamol, terbutaline, fenoterol.

**Step 2: regular inhaled preventative**: inhaled short-acting beta$_2$-agonist as required (see above) plus regular inhaled standard dose corticosteroid (beclomethasone, budesonide or fluticasone), cromoglycate or necrodomil.

**Step 3: high-dose inhaled corticosteroid**: inhaled short-acting beta$_2$-agonist as required (see above) plus regular high-dose inhaled corticosteroid.

**Step 4: high-dose inhaled corticosteroids plus regular bronchodilators**: inhaled short-acting beta$_2$-agonist as required (see above) plus regular high-dose inhaled corticosteroid plus one of the following regular long-acting bronchodilators:

long-acting inhaled beta$_2$-agonist;
modified-release oral theophylline;
inhaled ipratropium or oxitropium;
cromoglycate or nedocromil.

**Step 5: regular corticosteroid tablets**: inhaled short-acting beta$_2$-agonist as required (see above) plus regular high-dose inhaled corticosteroid plus one of the regular long-acting bronchodilators (see step 4) plus regular prednisolone tablets.

Short-acting and long-acting beta$_2$-agonists, inhaled steroids and theophylline can all be used with confidence in pregnancy. Neonatal irritability and apnoea have been reported with theophylline; however, this uncommon side effect should not prohibit use of the drug if indication exists. These drugs will suffice for most mild to moderate asthmatics. Limited

**Table 6.9.3** Triggers and provocative stimuli for exacerbations of asthma

| Allergens | Pollen (seasonal) |
| --- | --- |
| | Dust mites, animal danders, moulds (non- seasonal) |
| Occupational | Industrial chemicals, metal salts, wood and vegetable dust |
| Infection | Viral and/or bacterial |
| Environmental pollution | Tobacco smoke, ozone |
| Pharmacological | Aspirin and non-steroidal anti-inflammatory drugs, beta-blockers |
| Emotional stress | |
| Exercise and cold air | |

evidence suggests that leukotriene receptor anatgonists are safe and can be continued in women with more severe asthma who have been stabilized on them prior to pregnancy. It is less likely that pregnant patients will be using antimuscarinic bronchodilators, sodium cromoglycate or nedocromil; however, no adverse effects have been reported in pregnancy. Prednisolone is the oral steroid of choice for pregnancy, as 88 per cent of it is metabolized by the placenta, limiting fetal exposure. Initial worries about an association with isolated cleft lip have been allayed by a recent case-control study which did not support the original animal experimental work [B].[4] However, a subsequent meta-analysis has once again confused the debate with a statistically significant 3-fold increase in oral clefting risk for steroid use in the first trimester [A].[5] Neonatal adrenal suppression has proven to be a theoretical risk rather than a real practical concern. Newer anxieties have arisen about associations with intrauterine growth restriction, neuronal development, long-term hypertension and preterm labour. If real, these complications are likely to occur in the long-term users of higher doses, i.e. those women with more severe asthma. Corticosteroids are usually only prescribed for good medical reasons, and usually outside of the teratogenic period. Most agree that if a need for steroids exists, pregnancy should not be considered a contraindication.

---

**EBM**

The teratogenic risk and possible harmful fetal effects of maternal steroid treatment remain an area of controversy. However, the Committee on Safety of Medicines has concluded that 'there is no convincing evidence that systemic corticosteroids increase the incidence of congenital abnormalities such as cleft lip and palate', but that 'prolonged or repeated doses increase the risk of intrauterine growth restriction'.[6]

---

Specific guidelines also exist for the management of acute asthma attacks and these should also be adhered to in pregnancy.[7] The severity of acute exacerbations is divided into three groups.

1  **Uncontrolled asthma in adults**. Speech must be normal, with a pulse of <110 beats/min and respiratory rate of <25/min. Peak flow should be >50 per cent of predicted or personal best. Treatment involves nebulized salbutamol or terbutaline. Failure to respond should prompt referral to hospital. Otherwise, normal treatment can be stepped up and a course of oral steroids may be prescribed.

2  **Acute severe attack**. These patients will not be able to complete sentences, will have a pulse >110 beats/min, a respiratory rate of >25/min and a peak flow of <50 per cent predicted or personal best. Acute treatment involves oxygen, nebulizers and oral prednisolone. Those not responding well should be transferred to hospital with an aminophylline infusion.

3  **Life-threatening asthma**. This most serious of asthma exacerbations is characterized by a 'silent chest', cyanosis, bradycardia or a peak flow of <33 per cent of predicted or personal best. Immediate hospital treatment is necessary with oxygen, nebulizers, intravenous aminophylline, oral steroids or intravenous hydrocortisone.

It is useful for all clinicians to remember these guidelines. However, there should be a low threshold for the involvement of appropriate physicians in cases of deteriorating asthma in pregnancy. Possible precipitating factors should be addressed with all acute exacerbations. For example, antibiotics are often prescribed for presumed chest infection.

## Managing pregnancy in asthmatic patients

- Well-controlled mild or moderate asthmatics will have a normal outcome with standard antenatal care [B]. For those with poorly controlled or severe asthma, care should be multidisciplinary, preferably through a high-risk antenatal clinic with general medical input [E].
- Baseline investigations, such as peak flow measurements, should be obtained at booking [E].
- Medical treatment should be optimized by following the above protocol, with repeated reassurance about the use of these drugs in pregnancy. A recent study has demonstrated that physicians are still reluctant to prescribe oral steroids during pregnancy.[2]
- In view of the uncertainty over the true impact of severe asthma on pregnancy outcome, the maternity team should remain vigilant for signs of preterm labour and follow fetal growth and well-being with ultrasound [E].
- Induction of labour and caesarean section will mostly be reserved for obstetric indications, although delivery may need to be expedited in the most severe cases [D].
- No form of analgesia is contraindicated, although regional anaesthesia is preferable rather than general for major operative procedures.
- Women taking prednisolone should be screened for glucose intolerance and measures taken to control this

if it is found. Those taking prednisolone at the onset of labour should be given supplementary doses of 100 mg hydrocortisone 6–8-hourly until oral intake is resumed. Advice should also be sought for those women who have had a recent course finishing in the week prior to labour, or for those who have intermittent repeated courses of high-dose steroids [B].

- Ergometrine, prostaglandin $F_{2\alpha}$, aspirin and non-steroidal anti-inflammatory drugs should be avoided where possible, as all have been reported to cause bronchospasm [E].
- The risk of postnatal deterioration should be discussed with the woman.
- Breastfeeding is not contraindicated with any of the medications used, although high-dose oral steroid use (>40 mg/day) carries a risk of neonatal adrenal suppression.

## CYSTIC FIBROSIS

The reporting of pregnancies in women with cystic fibrosis began in the 1960s and the initial outcomes seemed unfavourable. However, with improvements in the care of both individuals with cystic fibrosis and high-risk pregnancies in general, the outlook is more favourable. Although men with cystic fibrosis are usually infertile, this is not the case for women. Menarche is delayed by an average of two years and the incidence of anovulatory cycles and secondary amenorrhoea is indeed higher. Cervical mucus may be more tenacious. However, fertility is the general rule rather than the exception. Average life expectancy for those with cystic fibrosis continues to lengthen and many women are now choosing to start a family and employing specialist assistance where subfertility exists.

The spectrum of disease phenotype and severity is highly varied and only loosely correlated to genotype. Individual counselling, preferably prior to conception, is vital and it must be clearly understood that outcome predictors are imprecise.

### Outcomes

Only one woman with cystic fibrosis features in the most recent Confidential Enquiry into Maternal Deaths. She elected to continue with her pregnancy despite counselling about the very high risk of death in her case. She received excellent multidisciplinary care between the various specialist teams but died a few weeks after an early elective caesarean section. This case illustrates the need wherever possible for adequate pre-conception evaluation in this group of women. Outcomes needing consideration are both the effect of the pregnancy on the cystic fibrosis and, conversely, the effect of the cystic fibrosis on the pregnancy. A number of different markers of disease severity have been proposed as predictors of maternal and fetal outcome (Table 6.9.4).

**Table 6.9.4** Predictors of maternal and fetal outcome in pregnancies complicated by cystic fibrosis

| |
|---|
| Absolute pre-pregnancy pulmonary function |
| Stability of pre-pregnancy pulmonary function |
| Colonization with *Burkholderia cepacia* |
| Presence of pulmonary hypertension |
| Degree of pancreatic insufficiency |
| Glucose intolerance/diabetes (predating pregnancy or gestational) |
| Body mass index |
| Maternal weight gain during pregnancy |
| Presence of liver disease and portal hypertension |

Two recently published series are in general agreement with one another, although the Canadian series from Toronto (*n* = 92 pregnancies in 54 women)[8] includes cases from as long ago as 1961. The patients in this group had slightly milder disease overall than those in Edenborough's UK group (*n* = 22 pregnancies in 20 women)[9] (%FEV$_1$ <50 per cent in 12 and 18 per cent respectively, and pancreatic insufficiency in 60 and 100 per cent, respectively).

## Effect of pregnancy on cystic fibrosis

No women in either of these studies died during or within 6 weeks of pregnancy. However, only 79 per cent of the Canadian women were still alive ten years after the delivery, the earliest death occurring three years after the birth. Only three-quarters were still alive four years after delivery in the UK study, the earliest death occurring only six months postpartum. These mortality rates are, however, no different from those for non-pregnant individuals with cystic fibrosis.

Death is a very crude measure of the effect of pregnancy on cystic fibrosis. Decline in lung function has also been examined. Edenborough found a 13 per cent loss in %FEV$_1$ during pregnancy, although this was mostly regained in the following year, and a net loss of 5 per cent in FEV$_1$ overall at one year following delivery. Gilljam's prediction of 3 per cent is similar; neither deterioration is significantly greater than that expected for the normal cystic fibrosis population [B]. However, caution must be exercised in women with poor pre-pregnancy lung function (<50 per cent predicted %FEV$_1$). There is evidence suggesting that they do suffer a permanent pregnancy-associated decline in lung function,[10] although this, too, is disputed.[8]

The anatomical and physiological changes in cardiorespiratory function during pregnancy might be thought to impair mucus clearance, increase atelectasis and predispose to pulmonary infections. However, serious medical events would appear to be no more common in pregnancy than would be expected from the pre-pregnancy lung function tests.

**EBM**

Retrospective studies suggest that pregnancy only accelerates the loss of respiratory function in 'severe' cases of cystic fibrosis.

## Effect of cystic fibrosis on pregnancy

Studies have not shown an increase in miscarriage or anomaly risk over the general obstetric population,[8–10] although cystic fibrosis was diagnosed in two of the Canadian offspring. In one case, the diagnosis of maternal cystic fibrosis was not made until after the child was born, and in the second, prenatal screening had indicated that there was only a very low risk that the child would be affected (see below). The mean gestation at delivery was >37 weeks in both studies, although one in three babies was born preterm in the UK study. The prematurity rate was no higher than for the general population in the Canadian group (8 per cent). Intrauterine growth restriction was not encountered more frequently than would normally be expected. Only one neonate died, sepsis being the cause following delivery at 31 weeks gestation.

The average maternal weight gain of 10–12 kg during pregnancy demands an extra 300 kcal/day. Pancreatic insufficiency is very common in cystic fibrosis, and enzyme supplements are usually needed to aid digestion. Increasing nutritional intake during pregnancy may be very difficult, especially with confounding factors such as nausea, hyperemesis and indigestion. It is hardly surprising that average maternal weight gain is reduced by approximately half. Furthermore, a compromised pancreas may fail to fulfil its added endocrine responsibilities: gestational diabetes occurred in 8 per cent of those women in the Canadian group who were not pre-existing diabetics.

Caesarean section is normally employed only for obstetric reasons in women with mild to moderate cystic fibrosis. However, one in three women were delivered by preterm section in the UK group, the most common indication being deteriorating lung function. Instrumental delivery rates do not appear to be increased.

The more recent retrospective reviews do suggest a generally good outcome for mother and baby. Problems such as prematurity and maternal death within five years of delivery are mostly confined to cases with poor pre-pregnancy lung function, pancreatic insufficiency (especially glucose intolerance) and lung colonization with *Burkholderia cepacia*. A %FEV$_1$ of <50 per cent is often considered a relative contraindication to pregnancy. Good outcomes with prolonged maternal survival afterwards are nevertheless possible, even with values below this. The presence of pulmonary hypertension causes grave concern.

Serious consideration should be given to termination of the pregnancy to prevent right-sided heart failure.

## Management of cystic fibrosis during pregnancy

### EBM

- A recent and comprehensive guideline has been commissioned by the European Cystic Fibrosis Society; this was based on review of the literature and experience of paediatricians, adult and transplant physicians, and nurses, physiotherapists, dieticians, pharmacists and psychologists experienced in CF and anaesthetists and obstetricians with experience of cystic fibrosis in pregnancy.[11] This document makes broad-based multidisciplinary recommendations for the management of pregnancy in cystic fibrosis, which should be undertaken in specialist centers.

- Ideally, a full discussion should take place prior to conception. Treatment can be optimized and the risks discussed. Patients with poor lung function or pulmonary hypertension may be advised to avoid pregnancy altogether.
- The average age of survival for women with cystic fibrosis in the UK is approximately 28 years. The effect on a child of losing a parent should be considered before conception.
- The issue of prenatal screening should be raised, although this must be done diplomatically, as the condition being screened for is, after all, present in the mother. As cystic fibrosis is an autosomal recessive condition, the offspring will either be all obligate carriers, if the partner is free of mutations, or one in two will be affected if he is a carrier himself. Approximately one in 25 individuals are cystic fibrosis carriers in the UK. DF508 is the most common cystic fibrosis mutation in the UK, accounting for 80 per cent of the total. A 'rare' mutation screen may test for as many as 30 different mutations; however, this will still only detect approximately 90 per cent of all mutations. Hence, even when the partner of the woman with cystic fibrosis has a 'negative' mutation screen, there is still a one in 250 chance he is a carrier (1/25 × 1/10) and therefore a one in 500 chance that the baby will have cystic fibrosis (1/250 × 1/2).
- Vigilance must be maintained for the complications of cystic fibrosis: haemoptysis, pneumothorax, atelectasis, respiratory failure and cor pulmonale.
- There should be no hesitation in performing chest x-rays where these are deemed necessary.
- Chest physiotherapy and bronchial drainage should continue.
- Serial lung function tests, e.g. spirometry and arterial blood gases, should be performed at regular intervals throughout pregnancy.

- Careful surveillance for signs of chest infection becomes even more important due to the complications of pneumonia in pregnancy (see below). *Pseudomonas aeruginosa* is the most common cause of chest infection in cystic fibrosis. Penicillins, cephalosporins and aminoglycosides are the most commonly used antibiotics (intravenously, orally or inhaled). All are considered safe in pregnancy, even gentamicin (the risk of fetal ototoxicity can be minimized by ensuring maternal serum levels do not exceed recommended levels). The risks to the mother and fetus of withholding appropriate antibiotics are greater. Some antibiotic dosing schedules will need to be adjusted due to the larger volume distribution and enhanced renal elimination found in pregnancy.
- Cardiovascular status should be observed during pregnancy, preferably by echocardiography.
- Pancreatic enzymes should be continued and insulin levels adjusted appropriately.
- Termination of pregnancy should be considered by women with very unfavourable features.
- Advice from dieticians will be essential to maintain caloric intake. Rarely, enteral (and even parenteral) feeding is necessary.
- Regular fetal monitoring with growth scans is advisable, especially in more severe cases of lung disease or poor maternal weight gain.
- Ideally, induction of labour and caesarean section are performed only for obstetric reasons. However, deterioration in lung function may prompt intervention. General anaesthesia should be avoided where possible.
- Facial oxygen may be required in labour, and exhaustion should be prevented by instrumental delivery if necessary. Prolonged Valsalva manoeuvres may predispose to pneumothoraces.

## TUBERCULOSIS

Infection with *Mycobacterium tuberculosis* most commonly presents in African and Indian ethnic groups, new immigrant populations, refugees and asylum seekers. Human immunodeficiency virus (HIV) positivity is another well-recognized risk factor and this is one reason cited for the increasing incidence of tuberculosis (TB) since the 1980s. As deaths from tuberculosis appear to be increasing, a prospective national study of tuberculosis in pregnancy was undertaken by the United Kingdom Obstetric Surveillance System (UKOSS) from February 2005 to August 2006.[12] Over this period, there were 52 confirmed cases, representing an incidence rate of 4.6 per 100 000 maternities with a 95 per cent confidence interval from 3.4 to 8.0.

Treatment can be safe and effective in pregnancy and the outcome is normally good. Failure to diagnose the condition and patient non-compliance with medication regimens do put the mother and newborn at increased risk. There were four deaths from tuberculosis in the most recent

Confidential Enquiry into Maternal Deaths (2003–2005), including one late death. In most of these cases, a delayed diagnosis contributed to the poor outcome.

> ## EBM
>
> There is no good evidence to suggest that pregnancy is an independent risk factor for infection with *Mycobacterium tuberculosis* or that the course and outcome of TB are altered by pregnancy.

Primary infection is usually asymptomatic, although fever, cough, conjunctivitis and erythema nodosum may all occur. A cellular immune response can be detected 3–8 weeks later by a positive tuberculin test.

Any further clinical manifestations are known as 'post-primary tuberculosis' and include pulmonary disease (apical lung cavitation, pneumonia, pleural effusion), miliary TB (widespread disseminated TB), pericarditis, peritonitis, meningitis, bone and genitourinary TB. These may occur months or years after the primary infection following a period of 'latency'.

Public health policies towards TB prevention and detection have differed on each side of the Atlantic. In the USA, tuberculin testing (the Mantoux test) is used to screen high-risk groups during pregnancy. A positive result combined with specific risk factors may prompt a screening chest x-ray and sputum testing for mycobacteria. Based on the results of these, the patient is either treated for active TB or given prophylaxis with isoniazid, on the assumption that latent infection is present and could reactivate at any time. In the UK, widespread vaccination of schoolchildren with bacille Calmette Guérin (BCG – said to prevent 70 per cent of infections) reduces the value of routine tuberculin testing, which will be positive in those who have been vaccinated. There is no screening programme for TB in pregnancy in the UK and clinicians must remain hypervigilant for signs and symptoms suggestive of the disease.

Pulmonary manifestations are the most common presenting features of TB, and a chest x-ray may show upper lobe densities and cavitation, fibrosis, pleural effusion, empyema or calcifications. Sputum is examined for acid-fast bacilli using a Ziehl–Nielsen stain and subsequently cultured for antibiotic sensitivity testing. Bronchoscopic washings must be obtained if there is no sputum. Extrapulmonary TB is diagnosed using tissue biopsies in a similar way. Although the Mantoux test is considered safe in pregnancy, it is unable to distinguish active disease from previous disease and BCG vaccination.

Active tuberculosis infections are treated with a combination of antibiotics, determined by the results of the culture sensitivities. Although regimens vary, treatment usually includes therapy with rifampicin, isoniazid, pyrazinamide and sometimes ethambutol. Less well-known drugs may be necessary in cases of multidrug resistance including amikacin, kanamycin and ethionamide.

# The relationship between pregnancy and TB

It is generally agreed that pregnancy has no impact on the course of TB and that TB, if diagnosed and treated expeditiously, has no significant impact on the pregnancy [D]. Delayed or inadequate therapy would appear to be detrimental to both maternal and fetal outcomes, however, increasing the risks of prematurity and intrauterine growth restriction [D].

Presentation and diagnosis are unaffected by pregnancy, although misguided reluctance in performing chest x-rays may lead to further diagnostic delay.

Vertical transmission (congenital TB) is extremely rare and usually only occurs where maternal disease has gone untreated. Fewer than 300 cases have been reported, although placental infection is somewhat more common. Lateral transmission from the mother or other close contacts, occurring after delivery, is a much more likely cause of infant infection. Therefore, strict criteria exist for the diagnosis of congenital TB. One of the following is necessary:

- lesions in the first week of life;
- a primary hepatic complex or caseating granuloma;
- histological evidence of placental or endometrial involvement;
- absence of TB in other carers of the child.

Congenital TB usually presents with fever, lymphadenopathy, hepatosplenomegaly and respiratory distress. It is fatal in one in five cases. In only half of all cases has the diagnosis of maternal TB already been made.

# Treatment of TB during pregnancy

- TB is most likely to be diagnosed by physicians, even during pregnancy, and the specialist advice of a respiratory consultant is essential, along with close involvement by microbiologists [E].
- Isoniazid, rifampicin and ethambutol are used initially. The ethambutol can be stopped when sensitivities show that the other two drugs are adequate. These are then continued for nine months in total. The most significant toxic side effect of isoniazid in animal and human studies is demyelination (causing a peripheral neuropathy). This can be prevented by supplementation with pyridoxine (vitamin B$_6$). Hepatotoxicity may be more common in pregnancy, and liver function tests should be performed monthly [D]. Most studies do not show a significant elevation in the anomaly rate above the background 2–3 per cent in users of rifampicin in pregnancy [B]. Liver enzyme induction, with theoretical vitamin K deficiency, should prompt maternal oral vitamin K supplements in the third trimester to prevent haemorrhagic disease of the newborn. The theoretical risks of fetal ocular toxicity with ethambutol have not been borne out in practice. Although pyrizinamide is usually avoided in pregnancy, there are no data to suggest a harmful effect and it should be used

if needed as a second-line agent. Streptomycin, a previous favourite in TB treatment, has well-recognized fetal oto-toxicity. Safer alternatives are available.

- Non-compliance with drug regimens outside of pregnancy is a major problem. There is no reason to think that it is any less so during pregnancy. Supervision, encouragement and incentive schemes may be necessary to encourage proper use of the prescribed medications.
- All the anti-tuberculous drugs mentioned in this section are compatible with breastfeeding [D].
- There is often concern over the infectious nature of TB in a maternity setting. Provided that the prescribed drugs have been taken properly, an active TB sufferer will become non-infectious within 2 weeks of commencing treatment. If the mother is still sputum positive, specialist infection control nursing will be necessary. The newborn should be immunized with BCG and also given prophylactic antibiotics (usually isoniazid). Separation of the infant from its mother is not necessary unless she is non-compliant or another carer or family member is highly infectious.
- It would seem prudent to send the placenta for microbiological investigation. Evidence of acid-fast bacilli should increase surveillance of the newborn.

# PNEUMONIA

Pneumonia, in otherwise healthy individuals, is no more common in pregnancy than in an age-matched population as a whole, and the maternal outcome, in the main, is no better or worse. The incidence of pneumonia in pregnancy would appear to be on the rise, but this may be accounted for by an increase in the number of pregnancies in women with co-existing problems such as HIV and cystic fibrosis. Four women died in the 2003–2005 Confidential Enquiry into Maternal Deaths. One of these women had presented very late for antenatal care. Generally prompt diagnosis and treatment avoids poor maternal outcomes. In addition, fetal outcome may be affected, and prompt recognition and treatment of pneumonia in pregnancy are essential if this is to be avoided. The main risk would appear to be preterm labour, although growth restriction has also been reported (Table 6.9.5).

**Table 6.9.5** Risk factors for pneumonia

| |
|---|
| History of recent upper respiratory tract infection |
| Chronic respiratory disease (e.g. asthma, cystic fibrosis) |
| Smoking |
| Immunocompromise (HIV, substance abuse, alcoholism, recurrent courses of antenatal steroids) |
| Anaemia |
| Farm workers (*Coxiella burnetii*) |
| General anaesthesia (aspiration pneumonitis) |

- HIV, human immunodeficiency virus.

## Diagnosis of pneumonia in pregnancy

The symptoms and signs of pneumonia are not altered by pregnancy, but may be confused with physiological changes common to pregnancy. Reluctance to perform a chest x-ray may further delay the diagnosis. Obstetricians have a responsibility in educating other physicians that the fetal radiation exposure with appropriate shielding is minimal and that this examination is safe. This message is even more important if risk factors for pneumonia are present.

Sputum should be sent for microbiological examination and culture. Blood can be taken for serological testing for *Mycoplasma* and viral antibodies.

## Treatment of pneumonia in pregnancy

### Common organisms

Frequently, no infectious agent is found and the pneumonia is treated empirically. The most common bacteria causing community-acquired pneumonia are *Streptococcus pneumoniae* and *Haemophilus influenzae*, often occurring after a viral infection. Atypical pneumonias caused by *Mycoplasma* and, less commonly, *Legionella* must also be considered. Penicillins, macrolides and cephalosporins are the treatments of choice and none is contraindicated in pregnancy. Higher doses of amoxycillin should be used to counteract the increased renal clearance found in pregnancy. Erythromycin or clarithromycin should be added if there is suspicion of an atypical pneumonia, and cephalosporins used for penicillin-allergic individuals or hospital-acquired infections. Pneumonias requiring hospitalization are usually treated with a third-generation cephalosporin (e.g. ceftriaxone) with erythromycin.

Common viral causes of pneumonia include the three subtypes of influenza myxovirus. Although amantadine and ribavirin antiviral agents have been used in pregnancy with no obvious harmful effects, their use is not recommended. The generally good outcome of viral pneumonia in pregnancy would support this.

## Less common causes of pneumonia in pregnancy

More unusual pneumonias occur when there are underlying risk factors. *Klebsiella* is said to be typical of alcoholics, often associated with abscess formation. *Coxiella burnetii* is found in the aerosols produced by farm animals. Q fever, the pneumonia caused by this organism, is said to cause miscarriage, intrauterine death and stillbirth. *Staphylococcus aureus* is significantly more likely after influenza infections and may have a sudden and rapid course. Pneumonia following aspiration of stomach contents is rare, but carries a significant mortality, with anaerobic and Gram-negative organisms being the most common infectious agents.

Antenatal complications: maternal

*Streptococcus pneumoniae* and *Pseudomonas aeruginosa* are common causes of pneumonia in HIV-positive individuals. *Pneumocystis carinii* is an acquired immunodeficiency syndrome (AIDS)-defining illness that carries a high mortality rate, whether or not it occurs in pregnancy. The theoretical risks of using Septrin (trimethoprim-sulphamethoxazole) in pregnancy include folate antagonism, and kernicterus or haemolysis in the newborn. The latter is extremely uncommon, and folate supplementation minimizes the risks associated with the trimethoprim. Pentamidine can be used as an alternative in pregnancy. Other unusual organisms to be considered in HIV-positive women, or those with other causes of significant immunocompromise, include atypical *Mycobacteria* and *Cryptococcus*.

The true incidence of pneumonia in adult chickenpox infections is unclear, but mortality from varicella pneumonitis has been quoted as 11 per cent. Whether the depressed cell-mediated immunity of pregnancy truly influences the incidence and mortality of varicella pneumonia in pregnancy is unclear, although many reports suggest it worsens outcome, with mortality rates quoted as being as high as one in three. *Varicella zoster* virus infections in pregnancy are discussed further in Chapter 7.4, Infection and Chapter 13, Fetal infections.

## ACKNOWLEDGEMENT

This chapter has been revised and updated. The author and editors acknowledge the contribution of Alec McEwan to the chapter on this topic in the previous edition of the book.

## Key References

1. Stenius-Aarniala B, Piirila P, Teramo K. Asthma and pregnancy: a prospective study of 198 pregnancies. *Thorax* 1988; **43**: 12–18.

2. Cydulka RK, Emerman CL, Schreiber D *et al.* Acute asthma among pregnant women presenting to the emergency department. *Am J Resp Crit Care Med* 1999; **160**: 887–92.

3. Schatz M, Zeiger RS, Hoffman CP *et al.* Perinatal outcomes in the pregnancies of asthmatic women: a prospective controlled analysis. *Am J Resp Crit Care Med* 1995; **151**: 1170–74.

4. Czeizel AE, Rockenbauer M. Population-based case-control study of teratogenic potential of corticosteroids. *Teratology* 1997; **56**: 335–40.

5. Park-Wyllie L, Mazzotta P, Pastuszak A *et al.* Birth defects after maternal exposure to corticosteroids: prospective cohort study and meta-analysis of epidemiological studies. *Teratology* 2000; **62**: 385–92.

6. Committee on Safety of Medicines/Medicines Control Agency. *Curr Probl Pharmacovig* 1998; **24**: 5–10.

7. British Thoracic Society. The British guidelines on asthma management. *Thorax* 1997; **52** (Suppl.): S1–21.

8. Gilljam MD, Antoniou M, Shin J *et al.* Pregnancy in cystic fibrosis. Fetal and maternal outcome. *Chest* 2000; **118**: 85–91.

9. Edenborough FP, Stableforth DE, Webb AK *et al.* Outcome of pregnancy in women with cystic fibrosis. *Thorax* 1995; **50**: 170–74.

10. Edenborough FP, Mackenzie WE, Conway SP *et al.* The effect of pregnancy on maternal cystic fibrosis vs nulliparous severity matched controls. *Thorax* 1996; **51** (Suppl. 3): A50.

11. Edenborough FP, Borgo G, Knoop C *et al*; European Cystic Fibrosis Society. Guidelines for the management of pregnancy in women with cystic fibrosis. *J Cyst Fibros* 2008; **7** (Suppl 1): S2–32.

12. Knight M, Kurinczuk JJ, Spark P, Brocklehurst P. *United Kingdom Obstetric Surveillance System (UKOSS) Annual Report 2007.* Oxford: National Perinatal Epidemiology Unit; 2007.

# 6.10 Neurological conditions

*Louise Kenny*

---

The focus of this section is mostly on pre-existing medical conditions and how they interact with pregnancy. Neurological disease is fortunately rare. The details of each and every neurological condition are well beyond the bounds of this textbook, and also of the MRCOG. Candidates sitting this examination are not expected to be obstetric physicians. However, competence is demanded in the management of several neurological conditions commonly encountered in the antenatal clinic. Epilepsy is common in women of reproductive age and the use of anticonvulsant drugs in pregnancy represents a model example of how benefits of treatment to the fetus and mother must be weighed against the risks. Multiple sclerosis demonstrates clearly how pregnancy can alter the clinical course of a disease. Myasthenia gravis illustrates how maternal conditions can continue to cause harm, even after delivery, and the 'triplet repeat diseases' highlight the need for specialized pre-pregnancy counselling and prenatal diagnostic services.

Strictly speaking, stroke need not be included here as it tends to feature more as a problem arising during pregnancy. However, in other respects it fits well with this discussion and it is important to recognize those women presenting with risk factors for stroke at booking, when the possibility of prevention exists.

## EPILEPSY

Approximately six in every 1000 pregnancies are complicated by a past or current history of epilepsy, making it the most common pre-existing neurological condition complicating antenatal care. However, on occasion, epilepsy can present for the first time during pregnancy and every obstetrician must have a working differential for the causes of seizure during pregnancy (Table 6.10.1). Familial, cryptogenic and trauma-related epilepsy accounts for the vast majority of cases with an established diagnosis at the onset of pregnancy. A minority of cases are caused by brain tumours, congenital abnormalities and vascular problems and these may require even more specialized care during the pregnancy. Seizure frequency may increase, decrease or stay the same in pregnancy (37, 13 and 50 per cent, respectively),[1] with labour being a particularly high-risk time for convulsions. A recent prospective study in the UK demonstrated no major differences in obstetric outcomes (excluding fetal abnormalities); however, an Icelandic retrospective study found a caesarean section rate almost double that of the control population.[2] A proportion of emergency caesarean sections were performed for seizures occurring during labour.

**Table 6.10.1** A differential diagnosis of seizures during pregnancy and the postpartum period

| Idiopathic epilepsy |
| --- |
| **Epilepsy secondary to a specific cause** |
| Previous trauma |
| Antiphospholipid syndrome |
| Intracranial mass lesions |
| Gestational epilepsy (seizures secondary to pregnancy) |
| **Intracranial infection** |
| Meningitis |
| Encephalitis |
| Brain abscess/subdural empyema |
| Cerebral malaria |
| **Vascular disease** |
| Cerebral infarction |
| Subarachnoid and cerebral haemorrhage |
| Hypertensive encephalopathy |
| Eclampsia |
| Cerebral vein thrombosis |
| Thrombotic thrombocytopenic purpura |
| **Metabolic** |
| Hyponatraemia/hypoglycaemia/hypocalcaemia |
| Liver and renal failure |
| Anoxia |
| Alcohol withdrawal |
| **Drug toxicity** |
| Local anaesthetics, e.g. lignocaine |
| Tricyclic antidepressants |
| Amphetamines |
| Lithium |
| **Pseudoepilepsy (factitious)** |

**Table 6.10.2** Effects of anti-epileptic drugs on the fetus and newborn

| **Teratogenicity** |
| --- |
| Major and minor congenital malformations |
| Characteristic dysmorphic syndrome |
| **Neonatal withdrawal effects** |
| **Vitamin K deficiency with haemorrhagic disease of the newborn** |
| **Developmental delay or behavioural difficulties** |

# Therapeutic aspects

Anti-epileptic drugs (AEDs) may affect the fetus and newborn in a number of ways (Table 6.10.2).

The evidence is confusing and often contradictory. There are no randomized, controlled trials and studies are mostly retrospective with ascertainment bias. This makes patient counselling very difficult. However, a number of points are generally accepted.

- The incidence of congenital anomalies is increased significantly amongst the offspring of epileptic mothers [B].
- AEDs are responsible for most or all of this increase [B].
- The benefits of seizure control during pregnancy outweigh the risks [E].
- Polytherapy with more than one AED carries greater risks to the fetus than monotherapy [B].
- Although certain AEDs are more strongly linked to particular congenital abnormalities, there is significant overlap, and the first-line agents can all cause the fetal anticonvulsant syndrome [B].

Other points are more controversial. No evidence grade is given for these points in view of this uncertainty.

- Women with a history of seizures who are not taking AEDs have a higher risk of congenital anomalies in their offspring than those with no history.
- Women with regular and severe seizure activity during pregnancy carry a higher congenital abnormality risk.
- Lower doses of AED carry a lower risk.
- The use of high-dose folic acid reduces the congenital anomaly risk.
- AED levels should be checked during each trimester as altered pharmacokinetics may disrupt seizure control.

# Congenital abnormalities

The reported incidence of congenital abnormalities among the offspring of epileptic women varies among studies, mainly due to variations in case ascertainment and definition. Major abnormalities (which are less likely to go unreported) are found in 5–10 per cent of women who have taken AEDs [C].[2-4] The incidence of anomalies may actually be determined by a number of different factors:

- an inherent added risk associated with epilepsy, independent of AEDs,
- genetically inherited tendencies,
- the number and severity of seizures during pregnancy,
- the use of AEDs during pregnancy.

Until recently, it was generally agreed that whether treated or not, women with a history of seizures had a higher fetal anomaly rate than those without such a history. A recent prospective study from Newcastle has supported this assertion, finding major abnormality rates among treated epileptics, untreated epileptics and controls to be 4.6, 8 and 2.4 per cent, respectively.[3] However, equivalent figures from the USA published in 2001 have suggested differently (5.7, 0 and 1.8 per cent, respectively),[4] as did a study from Milan, which found severe structural anomalies in 5.3 per cent of AED-exposed pregnancies and none in the 25 pregnancies with a history of seizure but no treatment.[5] There is similar disagreement over the impact that first and

**Table 6.10.3** The fetal anticonvulsant syndrome(s)

| Major abnormalities | Minor abnormalities |
|---|---|
| Microcephaly | Hypertelorism |
| Cleft lip and palate | Distal digital and nail hypoplasia |
| Neural tube defects | Flat nasal bridge |
| Congenital heart defects | Low-set abnormal ears |
| Intrauterine growth restriction | Epicanthic folds |
| Developmental delay | Long philtrum |

second trimester seizure activity has on congenital anomaly rates. These studies found no evidence of increased congenital anomaly rates in the offspring of women with higher level seizure activity.

The medications themselves undoubtedly carry the greatest risk [B]. Non-epileptic women using these drugs for other reasons demonstrate similar anomaly rates.[4] The 'fetal hydantoin syndrome' described by Hanson and Smith in 1975 has been renamed the 'fetal anticonvulsant syndrome' after the realization that AEDs other than phenytoin (carbamazepine, valproate, phenobarbitone, benzodiazepines) could also cause a similar array of abnormalities (Table 6.10.3).

The incidence of this syndrome in AED-exposed pregnancies is two to three times higher than in controls [B]. Behavioural problems, learning difficulties, speech and gross motor delay and features of autism were found in more than 50 per cent of children diagnosed with this syndrome when studied retrospectively [D].[6]

Despite this generic effect seen with most anticonvulsants, certain drugs are more closely associated with particular groups of anomalies. Valproate and, to a lesser extent, carbamazepine are thought to increase the risk of neural tube defects to between 1 and 2 per cent [B]. Doses >1000 mg/day of valproate seem more likely to be associated with this outcome [C]. Valproate may likewise increase the incidence of genitourinary anomalies and, along with phenytoin, cardiac abnormalities also. Prospective studies have estimated a risk as high as one in five of developmental delay with phenytoin and carbamazepine therapy, although this is disputed.

The various studies do agree on one point: polytherapy carries greater risk than treatment with one drug alone [B].[4,5] Holmes and colleagues, for example, found the incidence of major malformations to be 5.7 per cent in the offspring of women using monotherapy, but 8.6 per cent in those using two or more AEDs.[4]

The question is often asked: which anticonvulsant carries least risk of fetal harm? Women presenting already pregnant on AEDs should probably remain on their current regimen, as any teratogenic harm is likely to have occurred already. If a pregnancy is being planned, some have the opinion that valproate should be avoided, as it would appear to carry the greatest teratogenic risk and more recent reports suggest it may also cause developmental delay. Newer drugs, such as lamotrigine, gabapentin and tiagabine, so far have a good record in animal studies, but experience in human pregnancies is still too limited to assess their safety confidently [E].

## Other important drug effects

For reasons that are not entirely clear, carbamazepine, phenytoin, phenobarbitone (and even valproate) cause vitamin K deficiency, perhaps by inducing liver enzymes responsible for its oxidative degradation. Vitamin K is required for the carboxylation of factors II (prothrombin), VII, IX and X, and deficiency in the neonate may cause haemorrhagic disease of the newborn, with catastrophic intracranial and gastrointestinal bleeding occurring in a few. Owing to the extremely low levels of vitamin K in a healthy neonate, deficiency must be measured indirectly by studying 'prothrombin induced by vitamin K absence' (PIVKA) levels. Use of these anticonvulsants has been shown to increase PIVKA levels [B]. This increase can be prevented by maternal therapy with vitamin K supplements in the third trimester [B]. Indeed, some have even postulated that vitamin K deficiency may contribute to some of the structural abnormalities found in the fetal anticonvulsant syndrome, raising the possibility that vitamin K supplements earlier in pregnancy might be warranted.

Neonatal withdrawal effects have been noted with maternal use of phenobarbitone, carbamazepine and valproate, and range from poor feeding to jitteriness and convulsions. Such effects are uncommon now that phenobarbitone is used less frequently.

Phenytoin and carbamazepine may also cause an increase in childhood cancers such as neuroblastoma, although the rarity of these makes statistical certainty difficult [C].

## Drug pharmacokinetics

A number of factors during pregnancy serve to reduce effective serum concentrations of various AEDs:

- the increased volume distribution of pregnancy,
- the increased renal clearance,
- induction of hepatic enzyme metabolism by pregnancy and high folate levels,
- vomiting and delayed malabsorption.

The reduction in serum protein concentration during pregnancy means that a greater proportion of the drug is found in the free (active) state. This is especially true for those AEDs exhibiting strong protein-binding characteristics (Table 6.10.4).

Serum levels of AEDs include both the free and the protein-bound components. Keeping the total level in the low 'normal' range is therefore advised during pregnancy to limit the chances of maternal toxic side effects and fetal complications [E]. In reality, even free levels do not correlate well with seizure control [D] and some authorities disagree with routine testing of serum levels.

Antenatal complications: maternal

**Table 6.10.4** Protein binding of anti-epileptic drugs

| >50% protein bound | <50% protein bound |
| --- | --- |
| Clonazepam | Carbamazepine |
| Gabapentin | Phenytoin |
| Valproate | Lamotrigine |
| | Phenobarbitone |
| | Vigabatrin |

**Table 6.10.5** Enzyme-inducing ability of anti-epileptic drugs

| Enzyme-inducing AEDs | Non-enzyme-inducing AEDs |
| --- | --- |
| Phenobarbitone | Valproate |
| Phenytoin | Lamotrigine |
| Carbamazepine | Gabapentin |
| | Ethosuximide |
| | Clonazepam |

However, testing should be performed in a number of special cases [E]:

- suspected non-compliance (60 per cent of pregnancies in a recent survey),
- increasing seizure activity,
- concerns over toxic side effects,
- polypharmacy with drug interactions.

The enzyme-inducing AEDs may enhance their own metabolism and that of other agents (Table 6.10.5). Valproate may inhibit the enzyme epoxide hydrolase, which metabolizes phenytoin and carbamazepine.

## Managing epilepsy and pregnancy

**EBM**

There are no randomized, controlled trials pertinent to the management of epilepsy in pregnancy. Guidelines such as the one given below are based on evidence of grades C, D and E.[7,8] Retrospective studies highlight how poorly such guidelines are adhered to.

### Pre-pregnancy counselling

As with diabetes, there is much to be gained by planning pregnancy carefully following detailed counselling from a joint team including obstetricians and neurologists [D].

- The diagnosis should be reviewed by a neurologist – this is dubious in a proportion of women using AEDs.
- Consideration should be given to stopping AEDs in those who have been seizure free for more than two years. The risk of relapse is 20–50 per cent, being higher for some

forms of epilepsy (e.g. juvenile myoclonic epilepsy) than others (e.g. absence or tonic-clonic seizures) [C]. Serious health and social consequences may result from a recurrence of seizures (e.g. driving prohibition). If withdrawal is to be attempted, it should occur in small increments over a prolonged period, supervised by a specialist. The patient should not drive during this period.

- Where possible, treatment regimens should be simplified to a single AED and the lowest effective dose used to minimize the risk of congenital abnormalities [E].
- The risks to the mother and the fetus of non-compliance with prescribed medications, especially status epilepticus, must be discussed along with the AED-associated fetal risks [E].
- Folic acid 5 mg should be taken each day periconceptually. This is most important for women taking valproate and carbamazepine, although it is still unclear whether this reduces the risk of neural tube defects in this group [E].
- The risk to the offspring of epilepsy should also be discussed. Few cases of epilepsy exhibit autosomal dominant inheritance. However, having one parent with idiopathic epilepsy confers a 4 per cent risk of epilepsy in the offspring, increasing to 10 per cent when a parent and a sibling are affected, and to 15 per cent when both parents have epilepsy [C].

### Antenatal management

- Care should be carried out by an obstetrician with a special interest in epilepsy, jointly with a neurologist [E].
- All pregnancies occurring in women on anticonvulsant drugs should be notified to the UK Register of Anti-epileptic Drugs in Pregnancy [E].
- Screening for fetal anomalies should be offered to all women with epilepsy, with particular attention paid to those anomalies more commonly found in this group. A fetal cardiac scan may be warranted at 22 weeks gestation [E].
- Drug level monitoring may not need to be carried out as a routine but many clinicians like a 'starting' value and there are other situations that may prompt testing (see above) [E].
- Oral vitamin K supplements should be taken from 36 weeks onwards (10 mg per day) to prevent haemorrhagic disease of the newborn [C].
- If steroids are to be given for the usual obstetric indications, women using enzyme-inducing AEDs should be given 48 mg in total (two doses of 24 mg dexamethasone 24 hours apart) [E].

### Intrapartum care

- Induction of labour and caesarean section are indicated for the usual obstetric indications. Vaginal delivery should otherwise be the aim [E].

- Labour carries a higher risk of seizure due to sleep disruption, reduced intake and absorption of AEDs and hyperventilation, which may alter free levels of AEDs. Every effort must be made to administer anticonvulsants as usual. Intravenous phenytoin can be used if necessary, although it may cause arrhythmias.
- Seizures during labour are best controlled with intravenous benzodiazepines (e.g. clonazepam or diazepam). Rectal diazepam can be used in the absence of intravenous access. Provided the fetal heart rate tracing remains reactive, this is not usually considered an indication for emergency caesarean section. However, status epilepticus or recurrent seizures in labour may warrant abdominal delivery for fetal reasons [E].

## Postpartum care

- The serum levels of AEDs may rise in the postpartum period and monitoring may be necessary to prevent maternal toxic side effects. However, sleep deprivation may lower the normal threshold for seizure activity. If doses have been raised during pregnancy, a reduction in the immediate postpartum period may be necessary [E].
- All anticonvulsants reach breast milk. Neonatal side effects are rare, but sedation and withdrawal effects must be watched for, in particular where phenobarbitone and benzodiazepines have been used. Breastfeeding is to be encouraged [C].
- A single 1 mg intramuscular vitamin K neonatal supplement is advised in order to prevent haemorrhagic disease of the newborn [C].
- Contraceptive advice should be given before discharge home. The enzyme inducers will reduce the contraceptive efficacy of the combined pill, minipill and Depo-Provera injections. A combined oral contraceptive pill containing 50 mg of oestrogen should be used, preferably with a shorter pill-free interval (5–6 days instead of 7). 'Tricycling' will further reduce the chances of ovulation. Depo-Provera should be given every 10 weeks instead of every 12. The Mirena intrauterine system is ideal, as the locally administered progestogen will not be affected by induced liver enzymes [C].
- Special advice should be given to new mothers who also have epilepsy [C].

  - Ask for extra help if you are not getting enough sleep.
  - Ensure that someone else is present when you bath your baby.
  - Surround yourself with cushions and pillows when you are holding your baby.
  - Feed and change your baby on the floor while leaning against a wall to prevent you falling onto the baby in the event of a seizure.

Unfortunately, a recent UK prospective study[3] has shown how poorly such recommendations are being followed. Less than 50 per cent of pregnancies were planned and only one in ten epileptic women took folic acid appropriately. Most did not have pre-pregnancy counselling and one in five were using AEDs despite a fit-free interval of greater than two years prior to the pregnancy. Sixty per cent were looked after solely by general practitioners, and vitamin K was given to only a third of those who should have received supplements in the third trimester.

## Sudden unexpected deaths in epilepsy

Sudden unexpected death in epilepsy (SUDEP) is an uncommon and non-traumatic death that occurs suddenly and unexpectedly in a patient with epilepsy who was otherwise previously healthy. Deaths from SUDEP are usually not witnessed and may or may not occur during a seizure. It is without any obvious clinical or pathological explanations. SUDEP accounts for 10 per cent of all epilepsy-related deaths; 85 per cent of these fatalities occur between the ages of 20 and 50 years. The incidence of SUDEP stands at approximately one in 1000 people with epilepsy per year which is at least ten times of the sudden death rate found in the general population. Eleven women died from epilepsy in the most recent (2003–2005) triennial Confidential Enquiry. Six deaths were classified as SUDEP with a further two late deaths also attributed to this cause. It is not clear whether pregnancy is an independent risk factor for SUDEP; it will, however, be an indirect risk factor since SUPED is known to be more common in patients who do not take prescribed anticonvulsants; many women are reluctant to take anticonvulsants when pregnant or breast-feeding for fear of harming their babies.

# MULTIPLE SCLEROSIS

Multiple sclerosis (MS) is a multifocal autoimmune disease of the central nervous system. Infiltrating lymphocytes and macrophages bring about inflammation, demyelination and axonal damage while further activating inherent central nervous system (CNS) immune cells such as astrocytes and microglia. Optic nerve, brain and spinal cord may all be affected and this may manifest as almost any neurological deficit, symptom or sign. Most cases are characterized by a 'relapsing and remitting' natural history, with slow gradual decline. Less commonly, the MS follows a more rapidly progressive pattern. Diagnoses of MS are either 'probable' or 'definite', depending on whether the clinical features (probable) have been supported by the results of specialized investigations (oligoclonal abnormalities in cerebrospinal fluid, white matter lesions on magnetic resonance imaging (MRI) or prolonged latency of evoked potentials on neurophysiological testing). An inheritable genetic element to the disease does exist, but very rarely is a true Mendelian pattern of autosomal dominance seen. Overall, the risk of the offspring developing MS with one affected parent appears to be approximately 4 per cent. The rate can, however, be as high as 30 per cent if both parents are affected [D]. Viral infection is likely to be a more important aetiological factor and indeed relapses are more common following non-specific viral illness [D].

## Effect of pregnancy on MS

> **EBM**
>
> Various studies, both prospective and retrospective, suggest that pregnancy does not accelerate the course of MS, but relapses are more common in the puerperium. Pregnancy may have a protective effect.

The key part that the immune system plays in MS disease activity is highlighted by the effects of pregnancy on this condition. Pregnancy is characterized by a shift from type 1 (pro-inflammatory) to type 2 (anti-inflammatory) T-cell activity. Although various studies have reached slightly different conclusions, the combined evidence suggests that pregnancy itself is associated with a reduction in the number of relapses [C][9] and that this may even reduce the overall progression of the disease in the long term [D].[10] Also, the incidence of MS may be lower in multiparous women than in women who have never been pregnant [D].[10] As with rheumatoid arthritis, however, relapses in the puerperium are more common [C],[9] although this is not influenced by breastfeeding and one recent study has even reported a possible protective effect.[9] It is important to be aware of potential bias in such studies; women with more active disease are less likely to become pregnant for many reasons. However, the most recent reports have tried to avoid such bias and the above effects remain. Confavreux and colleagues[9] found a relapse rate of 0.2 per woman per year during the third trimester, compared to 0.7 in the year before pregnancy. In the first three months postpartum, this rate increased to 1.2. The overall progression in disability scores was not altered by pregnancy over a three-year time period. The effect of pregnancy on the course of the chronic progressive variant of MS is less clear.

## Management of MS during pregnancy

Multiple sclerosis sufferers experience a wide variety of neurological symptoms and treatment should be tailored to the individual. Non-pharmacological therapy may be sufficient in some cases, but expert help should be requested from a neurologist.

Moderate to severe relapses are traditionally treated with intravenous high-dose methylprednisolone followed by a tapering course of oral steroids. This is not contraindicated in pregnancy. Urinary urgency may be treated with tricyclic antidepressants, such as imipramine, and this is safe to continue. Spasticity and paroxysmal pain may be treated with baclofen (probably safe in pregnancy) and anticonvulsant drugs (see above under Epilepsy). Mood alterations are also common in MS. Depression and hopelessness are just as typical as the frequently mentioned 'euphoria'. Treatment with tricyclic antidepressants is not contraindicated in pregnancy.

Prophylaxis for MS remains an area of controversy. Although cyclophosphamide and azathioprine have been used, they are not as effective as beta-interferon (β-IFN) and glatiramer (a synthetic amino acid polymer). None of these drugs should be continued through pregnancy for prophylactic reasons, although experience to date suggests that β-IFN is not associated with any specific obstetric complications, and the increased miscarriage risk seen in animal studies with high doses has not yet been confirmed in humans. Trials are underway to assess the role of such treatments in the postpartum period. Breastfeeding is not advised whilst using β-IFN, although harmful effects have not been noted.

Induction of labour and caesarean section are mostly reserved for obstetric indications [E], although serious disability may make vaginal delivery impractical and an exacerbation of urinary symptoms and limb spasm may warrant earlier planned delivery. The use of epidural anaesthesia is not contraindicated and does not cause an increased rate of disease progression [C].

## MYASTHENIA GRAVIS

This relatively rare neurological condition nevertheless deserves mention as it is more common in women of child-bearing years and illustrates well how maternal disease can interact with pregnancy in ways not yet covered in this chapter.

Myasthenia gravis (MG) is caused by autoimmune disruption at the nicotinic neuromuscular junction. It may present with double vision, difficulty swallowing, ptosis and respiratory muscle failure. Anti-acetylcholine receptor autoantibodies can be found in 85–90 per cent of patients, and thymic abnormalities (hyperplasia or thymoma) in somewhat fewer. However, these autoantibodies can also be found in women who do not have the disease, and the diagnosis instead is usually made by administration of edrophonium chloride (a short-acting anticholinesterase), which transiently improves symptoms, notably muscle strength, in those with MG (the Tensilon test). Longer acting acetylcholinesterase inhibitors are the mainstay of treatment (neostigmine and pyridostigmine), but immunosuppressive therapy with corticosteroids, azathioprine, cyclosporin A and methotrexate is a second-line option. Plasmapharesis and intravenous immunoglobulin infusions are used for serious exacerbations. Undertreatment and overtreatment both carry their own risks. 'Myasthenic crises' can be precipitated

**Table 6.10.6** Emergencies in myasthenia gravis

| Myasthenic crisis | Cholinergic crisis |
|---|---|
| Nasal regurgitation | Abdominal 'colicky' pain |
| Dysphagia | Diarrhoea |
| Respiratory impairment | Excess salivation and sweating Severe weakness (depolarizing block) Bradycardia |

by infection, aminoglycosides, magnesium sulphate, local anaesthetics, beta-blockers, beta-receptor agonists, narcotics and neuromuscular blockers (Table 6.10.6).

## Interaction between myasthenia and pregnancy

The effect of the pregnancy on MG is unpredictable. A recent retrospective review found deterioration in 19 per cent, improvement in 22 per cent and no change in 59 per cent.[11] Myasthenic symptoms worsened postpartum in approximately a third of the women in this study [D]. The severity of the pre-pregnancy disease did not predict well what would occur during the confinement, although women who have previously undergone thymectomy have been noted in other studies to be less likely to have an exacerbation [D]. Review of further pregnancies in the same women did not show any consistency of effect between pregnancies. Owing to the change in volume distribution of pregnancy, the dose of anticholinesterase inhibitors needed to control symptoms usually increases. Increasing the dosage frequency has been found to be more effective in some cases. Persistent vomiting in the first trimester will necessitate intravenous administration of anticholinesterases. Prolonged labour (associated with delayed gastric emptying and malabsorption) may also be an indication for parenteral drug delivery.

Anticholinesterases are considered safe in pregnancy, although neonatal intestinal tube muscular hypertrophy has been reported following a pregnancy exposed to very high doses. Although there have been concerns regarding the teratogenicity and fetal effects of corticosteroids and azathioprine, their use is not contraindicated [E] and most clinicians will continue using them through pregnancy if an indication exists. Experience with cyclosporin in pregnancy is growing, although there remains an added possible risk of intrauterine growth restriction. Methotrexate should be avoided before and during pregnancy due to its teratogenic effects. The theoretical reduction in serum hormone levels brought about by plasmapharesis has not caused preterm labour in practice. Miscarriage rates and preterm delivery rates are not significantly different from those of a control population [C].

Transplacental passage of the immunoglobulin G auto-antibodies may cause two distinct fetal/neonatal problems.

1 Women with anticholinergic receptor antibodies occasionally deliver infants with arthrogryposis multiplex congenita, a serious congenital syndrome characterized by multiple joint contractures and pulmonary hypoplasia. Although the aetiology of this syndrome is diverse, severely reduced movement *in utero* is thought to be the basic mechanism. Animal experiments have shown that sera from women with anticholinergic receptor antibodies can cause a similar range of anomalies *in vivo*.

2 Neonatal myasthenia gravis (NMG) is a more common manifestation of these antibodies, affecting 10–50 per cent of newborns delivered to women with MG. The onset is usually within 24 hours and most cases are mild, presenting with generalized hypotonia, poor sucking, difficulty in feeding and weak cry. Less commonly, ventilation is required, sometimes for a number of weeks. The newborn is usually treated with anticholinesterases but exchange transfusions, plasma exchange and intravenous immunoglobulins have been used in more resistant cases. The correlation between maternal disease severity, or antibody titres, and the incidence and severity of NMG is not a strong one. However, seronegative mothers may be less likely to have an affected baby, and affected babies themselves are usually seropositive.

Clearly, the pregnancy should be managed in conjunction with a neurologist. Anaesthetic and paediatric colleagues should be informed [E]. Regular fetal surveillance is warranted and polyhydramnios should be excluded. Preterm delivery is only necessary in severe crises and a vaginal delivery should be aimed for [E]. Problems may occur in second stage due to the skeletal muscle fatigue and there should be a low threshold for instrumental delivery. Advice should be taken before any medications are prescribed, as various drugs may precipitate a myasthenic crisis. Magnesium sulphate is contraindicated for the treatment of hypertension or eclampsia. The neonate should be carefully observed for signs of NMG and caution should be exercised with breastfeeding when high doses of anticholinesterases have been used. Drug doses may need to be reduced slowly to pre-pregnancy levels.

## INTRACRANIAL VASCULAR EVENTS: 'STROKE'

'Stroke' is a generic term used to describe a cerebrovascular accident, the causes of which are many and varied. Assigning a diagnosis to 'stroke' is vital for appropriate treatment and prevention of further events.

Stroke can be further classified as shown in Table 6.10.7.

Across all age groups, hypertension, diabetes and cigarette smoking are the most common 'causes' of stroke, working through a common atherosclerotic pathway.

**Table 6.10.7** Stroke classification

| Ischaemic | Arterial |
|---|---|
| | Venous |
| Haemorrhagic | Subarachnoid |
| | Intracerebral |

Various studies have estimated a stroke risk of between five and ten per 100 000 deliveries, although a Canadian retrospective review gave a 6-fold higher risk than this.[12] Most do not find a significant increase in strokes antenatally compared with a female population of the same age distribution, but the increase in the postpartum period is striking. A US study published in 1996 found a relative risk for stroke in pregnancy of 2.4 overall (95 per cent confidence intervals 1.6–3.6); however, when subdivided into antepartum and postpartum periods, the relative risk in the first 6 weeks after delivery was found to be nine for ischaemic stroke (infarcts) and 28 for haemorrhagic [D].[13] Evidence from other studies supports these findings.

**KEY POINTS**

### Causes of pregnancy-associated strokes

Below are the causes of pregnancy-associated strokes found in two recent studies.[12,13]

#### Infarcts
- Pre-eclampsia/eclampsia
- Primary CNS vasculopathy
- Carotid artery dissection
- Cardiac embolic events
- Coagulopathies (e.g. thrombophilias, antiphospholipid syndrome)
- Thrombotic thrombocytopenic purpura (TTP)
- Post-herpetic vasculitis

#### Haemorrhagic
- Pre-eclampsia/eclampsia
- Disseminated intravascular coagulation
- Arteriovenous malformations
- Ruptured aneurysms
- Cocaine abuse
- Primary CNS vasculopathy
- Sarcoid vasculitis

In women under 40 years of age, infarcts are more common than haemorrhagic strokes. However, this predominance of infarcts is less marked in the pregnancy-associated group.

In a significant number of cases, no underlying cause is found. The wide aetiology of stroke in pregnancy presents a diagnostic challenge. The subsequent treatment will depend very much on the diagnosis. Investigations undertaken to determine a cause may include:

- MRI/computed tomography (CT) scanning,
- cerebral angiography,
- echocardiogram,
- thrombophilia screen,
- antiphospholipid testing.

Clearly, treatment and management of the pregnancy will depend on the diagnosis: anticoagulation, for example, may be necessary after a cerebral venous thrombosis. Haemorrhagic strokes caused by bleeding aneurysms or arteriovenous malformations (AVMs) carry a significant risk of rebleeding if left untreated in pregnancy [D].[14] Ideally, such abnormalities would be diagnosed and treated before conception, but some will present for the first time in pregnancy. AVMs, in particular, may enlarge as pregnancy progresses, perhaps in response to hormonal changes. Outside of pregnancy they are a much less common cause of subarachnoid haemorrhage than aneurysms. In the two studies cited above, AVM was found to be the cause of subarachnoid haemorrhage in more cases than was a bleeding aneurysm (eight versus three) [D]. A few will present with recurrent headaches and neurological deficit, but without haemorrhage. Treatment in these cases is the same as in the pre-pregnant state, with surgery (excision of AVM, clipping of aneurysm) or obliteration with neuroradiological techniques. However, some consideration must be given to fetal radiation exposure. Subarachnoid haemorrhage may present with headache, vomiting, reduced consciousness, neck stiffness and focal neurology. In view of the high risk of rebleeding, most advocate early treatment rather than an initial delay. Nimodipine is used to reduce vasospasm, and hypertension must be controlled. Neurosurgery is normally tolerated well by the pregnancy, although decision-making can be complicated by reduced maternal conscious level. Vaginal delivery is encouraged if there is confidence that the source of the bleeding has been treated adequately, although this can be difficult sometimes with AVMs. A longer passive second stage is usually encouraged to reduce the need for the Valsalva manouevre, with early recourse to instrumental delivery [E]. If the aneurysm or AVM has not been treated, or this treatment has occurred recently, an elective caesarean section is advocated, as labour is considered by many to be a high-risk time for a first bleed or a rebleed [E]. Of note, however, is that only one death has occurred from subarachnoid haemorrhage during labour in the last six years in the UK, leading some to believe that this risk has been previously overstated. Poor maternal clinical state (coma, brainstem death) is of course another indication for caesarean section.

Epidurals can be used provided there is no evidence of raised intracranial pressure. Special anaesthetic techniques are used to limit the hypertensive responses found with intubation, which carry the risk of precipitating a rebleed [E].

Investigation and treatment of the pregnant patient with stroke obviously require significant input from neurologists and neurosurgeons. However, all those in maternity care have an important part to play in stroke prevention. For example, women with antiphospholipid syndrome and thrombophilias can be treated, once recognized, with prophylactic anticoagulation [D]. Optimal management of hypertension in pre-eclampsia and eclampsia will also help to reduce the associated stroke risk [D].

# MIGRAINE AND HEADACHE

Tension headaches are more common in pregnancy, and migraines may present for the first time. Clinically, they must be differentiated from much less common but far more serious causes of headache (see below). Making a diagnosis may involve special investigations and the help of a neurologist or radiologist. Treatment will depend on the cause.

A classical migraine attack in a woman with a history of migraines does not normally warrant review by a neurologist. Visual disturbance, aphasia and paraesthesia or numbness usually last no more than an hour or so and are followed by a throbbing unilateral headache with associated nausea, vomiting and photophobia. However, as many as one in ten women with migraine in pregnancy have no previous history [D]. In view of the considerable symptom overlap with other diagnoses, a specialized opinion may be warranted. This applies also to women with migraine who suffer a presumed attack with atypical or prolonged neurological deficits. Hemiplegic migraine, for example, may last for many hours and should raise the possibility of an alternative diagnosis.

---

**KEY POINTS**

**Causes of headache in pregnancy**
- Tension headache
- Migraine
- Pre-eclampsia
- Benign intracranial hypertension
- Cerebral vein thrombosis
- Meningitis
- Subarachnoid haemorrhage (see below)
- Intracranial mass
  Inadvertent dural puncture (spinal headache)

---

Between 60 and 70 per cent of women with migraine will improve, or be symptom free, during pregnancy [C]. Those women who have cycle-related migraines are most likely to note an improvement. No more than 10 per cent seem to deteriorate in pregnancy. Every effort should be made to avoid precipitating factors, such as chocolate and cheese. Non-drug therapies such as relaxation techniques, sleep, massage and ice packs can be tried. Acute attacks in pregnancy are normally treated with paracetamol (rectal may be better than oral administration) and/or codeine-based drugs along with an anti-emetic such as metoclopramide. Occasional use of non-steroidal anti-inflammatory drugs is permitted, but should be avoided after 32–34 weeks [C]. Stronger opiates are sometimes needed. Ergotamine derivatives should be avoided, although studies have failed to show obvious harm. Sumatriptan, a serotonin antagonist, is in common use outside of pregnancy. Initial data collected by the manufacturers of unintended pregnancy exposures have demonstrated no clear problems, but it is still best avoided at present [E].

Prophylaxis against migraine attacks in pregnancy is best provided by low-dose aspirin or amitriptyline (commencing with low doses such as 10 mg per day). Propranolol and atenolol have been used, with the awareness of the associated potential for intrauterine growth restriction. The safety of pizotifen and methysergide in pregnancy is still in question.

# PARAPLEGIA

Pregnancy in a woman with a spinal cord injury (SCI) can present challenges to the patient and her obstetrician. Some problems that occur in able-bodied women are more likely to occur in women with SCI, such as urinary tract infections, anaemia and venous thrombosis. Other problems are specific to women with SCI and include neurogenic bladder, spasticity, decubitus ulcers and autonomic hyperreflexia.

## Antenatal management

- Antenatal management should take into account the level of SCI and the degree of paralysis. A formal assessment of renal, urological or pulmonary status may be appropriate.
- Women with spinal cord lesions at T6 or above are at risk of autonomic hyperreflexia and should be cared for in a setting where invasive monitoring and physicians experienced with autonomic hyperreflexia are available.
- Pre-eclampsia, fetal growth restriction and stillbirth are not more common in this population, and antenatal testing for fetal wellbeing is not indicated in the absence of other obstetric indications.
- Pre-term labour may be slightly more common in this population. In addition, although the majority of patients with SCI are able to perceive labour, the subjective experience may be different to that of able-bodied women and may delay presentation. However, serial cervical assessment (using ultrasound) and home uterine contraction monitoring have not proven useful in detecting women at increased risk of pre-term labour in this population.

Antenatal complications: maternal

## Intrapartum care

- Previous recommendations against performing inductions of labour have been made because of concern of autonomic hyperreflexia. Most studies available do not provide enough detail to suggest that induced labour is more difficult to manage than spontaneous labour with regards to autonomic hyperreflexia and it is therefore reasonable to restrict inductions to obstetric indications.
- The mode of delivery in women with SCI is primarily determined by standard obstetrical indications. However, spasticity and contractures can impair the ability to achieve a vaginal delivery. If the patient has limited abduction and rotation, preventing use of the lithotomy position, she should be assessed for suitability of positioning on her side with flexion of the upper leg at the hip.
- A unique indication for caesarean section in women with SCI is intractable autonomic hyperreflexia unresponsive to pharmacological or anaesthetic manipulation. The surgery will continue to incite the process but can be lifesaving if the time to delivery seems remote.
- Attendant staff need to be aware of the risk of pressure ulcers and traumatic injuries in women with SCI – frequent changes in position are advised.
- Frequent bladder emptying or catheterization will prevent over-distension in patients with neurogenic bladder.
- The level and completeness of the spinal cord lesion determines the patient's perception of labour and the anaesthetic requirements.
  - Pain from the first stage of labour is transmitted by sympathetic fibres that enter the spinal cord at T10–12 and L1.
  - The second stage of labour involves pain from pressure and distension of perineal tissues. These signals travel along the pudendal nerve and enter the spinal cord at S2–4. Therefore, patients with lesions above T10 may not perceive labour at all but those with lesions above T5–6 may benefit from anaesthesia to prevent autonomic hyperreflexia.
- SCI is not a contraindication to regional anaesthesia.

## Post-natal care

- Once again, attendant staff need to be aware of the risk of pressure sores and traumatic injuries in the post-natal period.
- Care should be taken to avoid urinary retention, no matter what the mode of delivery, in order to prevent a deterioration in bladder function and to minimize the risk of urinary infection and autonomic hyperreflexia.
- Breastfeeding should be encouraged; no deficiency in the let down reflex has been observed, even in patients with high cervical lesions.

# PRENATAL DIAGNOSIS OF NEUROLOGICAL DISEASES

Although most severe neurological disorders limit life expectancy, many milder problems do not, and women suffering from these conditions may wish to become pregnant, or may present at the booking clinic. Alternatively, a healthy woman with a previously affected child may come under your care. Such individuals may or may not be interested in recurrence risks in their offspring. Good quality information is needed so that an informed choice can be made. The first step is to seek out the true diagnosis. The term 'cerebral palsy', for example, does not give any indication of aetiology. Although cerebral palsy usually occurs as a result of various environmental factors, genetic factors are responsible for a few cases, raising the recurrence risk. 'Muscular dystrophy' is all too often assumed to be Duchenne's muscular dystrophy (an X-linked recessive condition); in fact, there are many different kinds of muscular dystrophy with different inheritance patterns. A careful family history is vital, but help is likely to be needed from neurologists, paediatricians and clinical geneticists.

Once the maternal diagnosis has been established, empiric recurrence risks can often be quoted. In a few cases, genetic testing offers the possibility of more precise prenatal prediction. This entire process can take many weeks, and plans should be made before the woman actually becomes pregnant, if possible.

The triplet repeat diseases highlight best some of the complexities of prenatal testing. Huntington's chorea, myotonic dystrophy, Friedreich's ataxia and fragile X all share a similar genetic abnormality. A three base pair sequence (the 'triplet') which is repeated a variable number of times in the healthy gene becomes 'expanded', so that many more copies of the triplet are present and gene function becomes disrupted. To a degree, the disease severity may be related to the size of the expansion. Expanded sequences have a tendency to expand further, causing so-called 'anticipation', i.e. the condition becomes more severe in successive generations. Myotonic dystrophy provides the clearest example.

Myotonic dystrophy is the most common muscular dystrophy affecting pregnant women and occurs as a result of the disruption of a gene coding for a protein kinase on chromosome 19. The gene is disrupted by the expansion of a CTG triplet repeat; 5–35 CTG repeats is considered normal. More than 40 is abnormal, and mildly affected individuals will show a degree of expansion beyond this size. Severely affected individuals often have many thousands of repeats. Clinical features include muscle weakness, myotonia of hands and tongue, swallowing and speech disability, cataracts and cardiac arrhythmias, testicular atrophy and peripheral insulin resistance. Mental retardation occurs in those affected severely from a young age.

Myotonic dystrophy is an autosomal dominant condition, affected individuals having one normal and one abnormal allele. Their offspring have a 50 per cent risk of inheriting the mutated allele. Quite how severely affected the child will be is difficult to predict with any degree of accuracy. A woman with moderate to severe disease herself is likely to have a significantly expanded mutation already. If this is inherited by the fetus, further expansion is likely and the neonate will be born with severe congenital myotonic dystrophy. Such a pregnancy may be characterized by polyhydramnios and poor fetal movements. Preterm delivery is more common, and severe hypotonia and respiratory difficulties are evident at birth. Talipes and facial diplegia may be present and survival beyond the neonatal period is followed by significant developmental delay in most cases. A woman with minimal or absent disease (and therefore a shorter expansion) has a risk of approximately one in ten that her child will be severely affected. However, if such a woman has delivered a severely affected newborn in a previous pregnancy, the risk of another badly affected child is higher (approximately 40–80 per cent). This reflects the greater likelihood that she has an inherently unstable mutation.

Inheritance and further expansion of the mutated allele can be detected by molecular testing carried out on placental biopsy material, although precise analysis of expansion size and prediction of outcome can still be difficult.

## ACKNOWLEDGEMENT

This chapter has been revised and updated. The author and editors acknowledge the contribution of Alec McEwan to the chapter on this topic in the previous edition of the book.

## Key References

1. Tomson T, Lindbom U, Ekqvist B, Sundqvist A. Epilepsy and pregnancy: a prospective study of seizure control in relation to free and total plasma concentrations of carbamazepine and phenytoin. *Epilepsia* 1994; **35**: 122–30.

2. Olafsson E, Hallgrimsson JT, Hauser WA *et al.* Pregnancies of women with epilepsy: a population-based study in Iceland. *Epilepsia* 1998; **39**: 887–92.

3. Fairgrieve SD, Jackson M, Jonas P *et al.* Population based, prospective study of the care of women with epilepsy in pregnancy. *BMJ* 2000; **321**: 674–5.

4. Holmes LB, Harvey EA, Coull BA *et al.* The teratogenicity of anticonvulsant drugs. *N Engl J Med* 2001; **344**: 1132–8.

5. Canger R, Battino D, Canevini MP *et al.* Malformations in offspring of women with epilepsy: a prospective study. *Epilepsia* 1999; **40**: 1231–6.

6. Moore SJ, Turnpenny P, Quinn A *et al.* A clinical study of 57 children with fetal anticonvulsant syndromes. *J Med Genet* 2000; **37**: 489–97.

7. Brodie MJ, French J. Management of epilepsy in adolescents and adults. *Lancet* 2000; **356**: 323–9.

8. Scottish Obstetric Guidelines and Audit Project. *The Management of Pregnancy in Women with Epilepsy*. A Clinical Practice Guideline for Professionals Involved in Maternity Care. Aberdeen: SOGAP, 1997.

9. Confavreux C, Hutchinson M, Marie Hours M *et al.* Rate of pregnancy-related relapse in multiple sclerosis. *N Engl J Med* 1998; **339**: 285–91.

10. Rumarker B, Andersen O. Pregnancy is associated with a lower risk of onset and a better prognosis in multiple sclerosis. *Brain* 1995; **118**: 253–61.

11. Batocchi AP, Majolini L, Evoli MD *et al.* Course and treatment of myasthenia gravis during pregnancy. *Neurology* 1999; **52**: 447–52.

12. Jaigobin C, Silver FL. Stroke and pregnancy. *Stroke* 2000; **31**: 2948–51.

13. Kittner SJ, Stern BJ, Feeser BR *et al.* Pregnancy and the risk of stroke. *N Engl J Med* 1996; **335**: 768–74.

14. Stoodley MA, Macdonald RL, Weir BK. Pregnancy and intracranial aneurysms. *Neurosurg Clin North Am* 1998; **9**: 549–56.

# 6.11 Dermatological conditions

*Louise Kenny*

Although this section of the book deals with pre-existing diseases and their interaction with pregnancy, the dermatological conditions of most interest to the obstetrician are the 'dermatoses of pregnancy', i.e. the skin conditions peculiar to pregnancy. These are thus discussed alongside pre-existing conditions.

The skin may be the sole organ affected by a multisystem disease. Skin disorders occurring as part of multisystem disease (connective tissue disease, infections and malignancies) are considered in the appropriate chapters. It is worth remembering, however, that the skin manifestation of these disorders may be the initial presentation of these conditions.

## PHYSIOLOGICAL SKIN CHANGES IN PREGNANCY

Physiological cutaneous skin changes during pregnancy are common and rarely cause major concern. Hyperpigmentation may occur of the nipples and areolae, axillae, linea alba (which becomes the linea nigra), face (melasma or cloasma) and pre-existing pigmented moles and freckles. Oestrogen is probably responsible for cutaneous vascular changes such as an increase in spider naevi, palmar erythema and even the occurrence of head and neck haemangiomas. Oedema is almost universal, and venous varicosities of the legs, vulva and rectum often become more prominent or appear for the first time. Striae gravidarum are pinkish purple linear markings on the lower abdomen and breast, which later fade to white and usually persist after pregnancy is over as depressed, irregular bands. Some women maintain that hair growth and condition improve in pregnancy. Postpartum alopecia, however, is a recognized phenomenon that is usually mild and transient.[1] Sebum secretion increases (see below), but apocrine activity may decline.

## PRE-EXISTING CONDITIONS

Women with pre-existing skin problems are likely to present with a diagnosis already established. As with all pre-existing maternal conditions, one must consider the effect both the disease and its therapies will have on the pregnancy, the labour, the fetus and the neonate. Conversely, the pregnancy may influence the course and nature of the condition itself.

The effect of pregnancy on atopic dermatitis (atopic eczema) and psoriasis is unpredictable.[2] The former often improves in pregnancy but may deteriorate postnatally, due to physical factors such as breastfeeding, environmental agents such as detergents or even immune factors. A generalized pustular psoriasis may occur in pregnancy (see below) and is more common in women with previous psoriasis. Sebum secretion increases in pregnancy and may be responsible for the common deterioration of acne during pregnancy. Apocrine gland activity, on the other hand, declines in pregnancy, meaning that the rare conditions affecting these glands (hidradenitis suppurativa and Fox–Fordyce disease) are likely to improve. The pregnancy-associated suppression of cell-mediated immunity is thought to cause the often marked increase in human papilloma virus warty lesions (condylomata acuminata). In rare cases, these may obstruct the vagina. Only then are they an indication for caesarean section.

Impact of pre-existing skin diseases on the pregnancy itself is usually minimal in the absence of any multisystem involvement (clearly, connective tissue disorders and infections with skin involvement are quite different).

Conditions affecting the abdominal wall may interfere with abdominal delivery and delay wound healing. Vulval problems may similarly affect vaginal delivery and the healing of tears and episiotomies. A rare condition called X-linked ichthyosis is associated with steroid sulphatase deficiency and this in turn is said to delay the onset of labour, increasing the need for induction for prolonged pregnancy.

Certain skin conditions have a genetic component and the offspring may be at risk of the condition themselves. A few examples are cited in Table 6.11.1.

One of the most important factors to consider is the potential impact that dermatological drugs and therapies may have on a pregnancy.[3] A number of such treatments are confirmed teratogens and are absolutely contraindicated in pregnancy (Table 6.11.2). The retinoids are used to treat severe acne and psoriasis. Isotretinoin is especially harmful, causing central nervous system, craniofacial and cardiovascular abnormalities in as many as 50 per cent of exposed pregnancies.

Other drug treatments should only be used with careful consideration in pregnancy, including cyclosporin, hydroxyurea, penicillamine, psoralens and ultraviolet A (PUVA) and rifampicin.

A number of these medications may linger in body tissues for many months after treatment has ended. Great care must be taken that women undergoing such therapies are made aware of the vital role of reliable contraception, which may need to be continued long after the treatment has stopped. The British National Formulary advises the following periods

**Table 6.11.1** Examples of inheritable skin disorders

| Autosomal dominant |
| --- |
| Ichthyosis hystrix and vulgaris |
| Palmoplantar hyperkeratosis (tylosis) |
| Epidermolysis bullosa simplex |
| Ectodermal dysplasia (some forms) |

| X-linked recessive |
| --- |
| X-linked icthyosis |
| Hypohidrotic ectodermal dysplasia |

| Multifactorial |
| --- |
| Atopic eczema (the risk of some allergic problems may reach 50% in the offspring of a couple with one affected person; the risks are higher where both parents are eczema sufferers) |
| Psoriasis (the children of two psoriatic parents have a risk of approximately 50% of being affected themselves) |

**Table 6.11.2** Dermatological treatments to be avoided during pregnancy

| |
| --- |
| Acitretin and tazarotene (retinoids used in psoriasis) |
| Isotretinoin (retinoid used to treat severe acne) |
| Griseofulvin (antifungal treatment) |
| Methotrexate (antimetabolite used to treat psoriasis) |
| Podophyllin (used for genital warts) |
| Tetracycline (used for skin infections/acne) |
| Thalidomide (leprosy treatment) |
| Psoriasis (the children of two psoriatic parents have a risk of approximately 50% of being affected themselves) |

of time during which conception should be avoided after the drugs have been stopped [E]:

- acitretin – two years;
- methotrexate – six months;
- griseofulvin – one month.

It should be noted that these drugs may also carry potential harm through an effect on the male gametes. Men who have used griseofulvin, for example, are advised against fathering offspring within six months of treatment ending.

Emollients, dithranol, coal tar and topical corticosteroids are safe in pregnancy, as is chlorpheniramine.

# DERMATOSES PRECIPITATED BY PREGNANCY

This section covers two groups of conditions:

1  skin conditions in which pregnancy is just one of a number of precipitating factors,
2  skin conditions unique to pregnancy.

Acne, erythema multiforme, erythema nodosum and generalized pustular psoriasis form the first group. Pre-existing acne may deteriorate during pregnancy, but may also present *de novo*. Erythema multiforme and erythema nodosum are both caused by a multitude of other aetiological factors, which must be excluded before it is possible to attribute the onset to pregnancy alone. Generalized pustular psoriasis describes a superficial sterile eruption occurring on the background of widespread erythema, which is associated with fever, systemic upset and hypocalcaemia (with tetany) in the more severe cases. It carries significant perinatal mortality and is more common in those with a history of plaque psoriasis. A clinically identical condition called impetigo herpetiformis was previously thought to be a pregnancy-specific dermatosis, but the two are now considered the same condition. Pregnancy appears to be one of a number of triggers for generalized pustular psoriasis.

This leaves four reasonably well-defined dermatoses found only in pregnancy (see Table 6.11.3).

**Table 6.11.3** Pregnancy-specific dermatoses

| Name | Incidence | Onset | Resolution | Clinical features | Histology | Immunofluorescence | Fetal effects | Recurrence | Management | Associated conditions |
|---|---|---|---|---|---|---|---|---|---|---|
| Polymorphic eruption of pregnancy (pruritic urticarial papules and plaques of pregnancy, toxaemic rash of pregnancy, toxic erythema of pregnancy) | 1 in 250 | 27–40 weeks (usually late third trimester) | Usually within 2 weeks of delivery | Red urticarial papules and plaques. Rarely, vesicles and target lesions. Begins abdominally within striae. Umbilical sparing. May spread to thighs and occasionally limbs | Epidermal/dermal oedema Perivascular infiltration Patchy parakeratosis | Negative | None | Uncomon | Calamine lotion 1% hydrocortisone aqueous cream Antihistamines Systemic steroids | None |
| Pemphigoid gestationis (herpes gestationis) | 1 in 3000–60 000 | 2nd/3rd trimester (occasionally postpartum) | Few weeks postpartum to 1 year | Erythematous urticarial plaques. Vesicles and bullae form at the centre or periphery of plaques. Often begins periumbilically. Spreads to trunk and extremities | Perivascular inflammation Subepidermal blister | Positive | Possible increased risk of IUGR and preterm labour | Common | Moderate/strong topical steroids Systemic steroids Antihistamines | Graves' disease and other autoimmune conditions |
| Prurigo of pregnancy | 1 in 300 | 25–30 weeks | Several months | No urticated lesions. Multiple excoriated papules on abdomen and limbs | See polymorphic eruption of pregnancy | Negative | None | Recorded | Aqueous cream Topical steroids Antihistamines | Atopy |
| Pruritic folliculitis of pregnancy | Uncertain | 2nd/3rd trimester | Within 2 weeks of delivery | Masses of itchy red follicular papules | Non-specific folliculitis | Negative | None | Uncertain | Topical 10% benzoyl peroxide Mild topical steroids Antihistamines | None |

● IUGR, intrauterine growth restriction.

A diagnosis can usually be made on clinical grounds alone; however, pemphigoid gestationis can be confused with polymorphic eruption of pregnancy if there are no vesicles present. The two conditions are easily distinguished by immunofluorescence studies of skin biopsies. Pemphigoid gestationis is characterized by C3 deposition along the epidermal/dermal junction. Immunoglobulin G (IgG) deposition is usually another feature, the target protein being a 180 kDa component of hemidesmosomes. Immunofluorescence studies are negative in polymorphic eruption of pregnancy. Clinical distinction is appropriate as pemphigoid gestationis has been linked to increased rates of stillbirth, intrauterine growth restriction (IUGR) and preterm labour [D]. Although this may represent biased reporting of poor outcomes, extra surveillance would seem warranted in these pregnancies [E].

## ACKNOWLEDGEMENT

This chapter has been revised and updated. The author and editors acknowledge the contribution of Alec McEwan to the chapter on this topic in the previous edition of the book.

## Key References

1. Schiff BL, Kern AB. A study of postpartum alopecia. *Arch Dermatol* 1963; **87**: 609.
2. Winton GB. Skin diseases aggravated by pregnancy. *J Am Acad Dermatol* 1989; **20**: 1–13.
3. Perlman SE, Rudy SJ, Carissa P, Townsend-Akpan C. Caring for women with childbearing potential taking teratogenic dermatologic drugs. *J Reprod Med* 2001; **46** (Suppl. 2): 153–61.

# 6.12 Drug and alcohol misuse

*Louise Kenny*

---

## MRCOG standards

### Relevant standards

Candidates are expected to understand and demonstrate appropriate knowledge, skills and attitudes in relation to pregnant women who misuse alcohol and drugs.

### Theoretical skills

- Awareness of drug and alcohol misuse in pregnancy.
- Knowledge of the pharmacological actions of opioids, cocaine, marijuana, amphetamines, benzodiazepines and alcohol.
- Appreciate the acute and chronic maternal effects and associations of substance abuse to optimize recognition and management during pregnancy.
- Understand the fetal/neonatal effects of *in-utero* exposure to these substances.
- Recognize the association between substance abuse and other health and social problems.

### Practical skills

- Provide preconception counselling to a woman with a history of alcohol or drug misuse.
- Manage a pregnancy complicated by substance abuse.
- Liaise with social and specialist drug services to individualize care.

## INTRODUCTION

The incidence of substance misuse in the UK varies widely by geographical location. Three per cent of the under-35s in the UK are said to have a drug problem, although London, Glasgow, Liverpool and Manchester have traditionally been considered the 'hotspots'. A recent cross-sectional audit of health records in a London specialist perinatal addictions outreach service reported a total of 167 pregnant substance-using women referred between 2002 and 2005. Compared to 1989–1991, there were significantly more

pregnant women presenting at an older age, later gestation, with increased polysubstance use and a higher percentage of women from black or minority ethnic communities. Clearly the problem is increasing, and maternity services must have local guidelines and action plans in place to manage it.

There is a tendency to focus attention on the medical aspects of substance abuse in pregnancy. Although these drugs may involve actual harm to the pregnancy, the associated social and health problems are as important, if not more so. Throughout this chapter it will become clear that separating the two is very difficult, and the contributions made firstly by the drugs themselves and secondly by the socio-economic environment are almost impossible to disentangle. Separating the two is of greater theoretical than practical importance. Substance-exposed pregnancies are 'high risk', and tailored antenatal care must be provided which tackles all the problems, both social and medical.

Substances of abuse are rarely used in isolation. 'Polysubstance' misuse is the norm, and heavy alcohol consumption and tobacco smoking compound the harm done by classified drugs. The following discussion therefore does not tackle each drug independently, but aims to explore their individual contributions to each problem encountered in the pregnancy.

## EBM

Many studies demonstrating harmful effects of substance abuse in pregnancy are retrospective and little or no effort is made to control for confounding factors. Clearly, there are no randomized studies. Better study design is often associated with negative results or a diminution in the harm reported. There is little doubt, however, that drug use during pregnancy is linked to poorer outcomes.

## PHARMACOLOGY

It is valuable to revise the basic pharmacological actions of abused substances, as these actions help to explain both the short-term and long-term effects on the pregnancy outcome.

## Cocaine

Cocaine is a central nervous system (CNS) stimulant. It prevents the reuptake of neurotransmitters (adrenaline, noradrenaline, dopamine) at nerve terminals, causing an exaggerated response to these chemical messengers. Increased motor activity, tremors, convulsions, tachycardia, generalized vasoconstriction, hypertension and hyperpyrexia may result. The sense of euphoria occurs as a result of dopamine accumulation within the mesolimbic system. Chronic cocaine use brings about dopamine depletion. Use of cocaine with alcohol results in a more powerful vasoconstrictor called cocaethylene.

## Opiates

Opiates (heroin, methadone, morphine, buprenorphine) mimic the actions of the endogenous opioid peptides widely distributed throughout the CNS which bind to mu, delta or kappa opioid receptors. These compounds have a wide diversity of physical functions, but are intimately linked with pain perception and mood control. The 'reward circuitry' of the mesolimbic dopaminergic system is influenced by endogenous and exogenous opioids and is responsible for both the pleasurable effects and psychological dependence found with opiate abuse.

## Amphetamines

Amphetamines similarly enhance the dopaminergic neurotransmitter system. *Ecstasy* (3,4-methylenedioxymethamphetamine – MDMA) is a derivative of metamphetamine. It causes accumulation of synaptic serotonin and dopamine, but direct axonal damage and serotonin depletion can occur with prolonged use.

## Alcohol and marijuana

Alcohol and marijuana have fundamental non-specific actions on the neural membrane, in common with the sedative–hypnotic–anaesthetic group of drugs. They differ somewhat in their actions due to differing lipid solubilities, routes of intake, metabolic pathways and different ratios of stimulant and depressant effects. Marijuana, unlike alcohol, has hallucinogenic properties.

## Benzodiazepines

The actions of benzodiazepines (diazepam, temazepam) are mediated through the neuroinhibitory gamma-aminobutyric acid type A (GABA-A) receptor. GABA and benzodiazepines have anxiolytic, sedative and hypnotic effects and also affect cognition. They bring about muscle relaxation and act as anticonvulsants. GABA has trophic effects and this may be important in neurodevelopment. Excessive benzodiazepine use leads to receptor down-regulation and tolerance.

## MATERNAL EFFECTS

The effects of substance abuse on the mother may be acute or chronic and may be specific to the drug used or part of a general pattern of illness found among substance abusers. It is vital for obstetricians to have an understanding of these problems, as they may present in the antenatal clinic or as emergencies on the labour suite. Furthermore, they may be confused with complications of pregnancy.

## Acute maternal effects

Drug abuse is associated with a wide range of health problems, which may present acutely to various different healthcare professionals.

### Overdose

Excess alcohol intake causes ataxia, confusion, stupor and eventually coma. Opiates in excess depress respiratory drive and may also cause coma. Cocaine, amphetamines and ecstasy cause tachycardia, hypertension and hyperthermia and predispose to cardiac arrhythmias, myocardial infarction, seizures and stroke. The potential for diagnostic confusion with fulminating pre-eclampsia and eclampsia is clear. Acute presentations also include aggression, paranoia and psychosis, particularly with the CNS stimulants, such as amphetamines, ecstasy and cannabis.

### Withdrawal

Withdrawal from the physically addictive substances may also present acutely. Alcohol withdrawal may result in blackouts, tremor, hallucinations, delirium and seizures. Opiate withdrawal is characterized by sweating, coryza and lacrimation. Pyrexia, nausea and vomiting, diarrhoea and abdominal pain, tachycardia and hypertension are also common.

### Infections

Drug abuse is often associated with poor diet, poor hygiene and generalized immunosuppression. Pneumonia and tuberculosis (TB) may present acutely. Sexual disinhibition and prostitution increase the risk of sexually transmitted diseases (STDs), including human immunodeficiency virus (HIV). Intravenous substance use predisposes to endocarditis, hepatitis and septicaemia (which may be fungal). Local infections such as cellulitis and osteomyelitis are not uncommon.

### Other acute presentations

Hypoglycaemia, acute or chronic hepatic failure and Wernicke's encephalopathy may result from excessive alcohol consumption. Aspiration pneumonitis, subdural haematomata and rhabdomyolysis with acute renal failure are further examples of acute complications of substance abuse. All types of trauma, including road traffic accidents (RTAs) and grievous bodily harm, are more common among drug users.

## Chronic maternal effects

The effects of HIV infection and chronic hepatitis (whether alcoholic or infectious) are well known. Nutritional deficiencies may cause peripheral neuropathy (vitamin $B_1$ and vitamin $B_{12}$), pellagra (niacin), cerebellar degeneration and Wernicke–Korsakoff syndrome (vitamin $B_1$). Poor venous access is common in intravenous substance users and this may cause difficulty during emergency situations (drug induced or pregnancy related). Femoral nerve neuropathy may result from frequent trauma during injection into the femoral vein. Obstructive and restrictive pulmonary lesions may occur, as can pulmonary hypertension.

## OBSTETRIC PROBLEMS

Substance abuse has been associated with a number of obstetric complications, including:

- miscarriage,
- preterm rupture of membranes,
- preterm labour,
- placenta praevia,
- abruption,
- pre-eclampsia,
- breech presentation,
- chorioamnionitis,
- intrauterine growth restriction (IUGR) and intrauterine death (IUD).

Although plausible biological explanations exist for why substances of abuse might cause these problems, the exact contribution from the drugs themselves is very difficult to isolate from the confounding factors such as smoking, poor nutrition and general health, lack of antenatal care and low socioeconomic status.

## Miscarriage

Studies examining rates of miscarriage in substance-exposed pregnancies are often retrospective and poorly controlled. Confirmation by tissue diagnosis is often missing. Opiates, cocaine and CNS stimulants have all been implicated, but good-quality evidence is mostly lacking.

Most attention has been paid to the effect of alcohol on miscarriage rates, and large quantities have been shown to have abortive properties in animal experiments. There is general agreement that alcoholics have a higher rate of miscarriage, although it is almost impossible to separate

the effect of the alcohol from the confounding effects of ill-health, poor nutrition and low socioeconomic status. Alcohol consumption is closely related to smoking and caffeine use (coffee drinking), both of which have stronger causative relationships with miscarriage. North American studies have linked 'heavy drinking' (more than two drinks per day) with an increase in miscarriage rate, giving relative risk values of between two and three. This association is not, on the whole, confirmed in European and Australian studies, where greater effort has been made to control for confounding factors.[1] Most agree, however, that more than six drinks a day for several days per week is associated with higher miscarriage risk [C].

There is no good evidence to suggest that the other substances discussed in this chapter cause miscarriage.

## Teratogenicity

The only confirmed teratogen amongst this group of substances is alcohol. The fetal alcohol syndrome (FAS) describes a clearly defined group of problems caused by *in-utero* alcohol exposure:

- prenatal or postnatal growth restriction/microcephaly,
- nervous system dysfunction (mental retardation, intellectual impairment, ataxia, attention defects),
- characteristic facial appearance (mid-face hypoplasia, narrow palpebral fissures, underdeveloped philtrum, ptosis, rotated low-set ears).

'Fetal alcohol spectrum' is the term used to describe other alcohol-induced abnormalities which do not qualify for the 'full' diagnosis of FAS.

The relationship between alcohol consumption during early pregnancy and the incidence of FAS is not a simple one. Despite having the highest rates of worldwide alcohol consumption, France has a significantly lower rate of reported FAS than North America, where less alcohol is consumed. A number of reasons have been cited to explain this discrepancy, including a difference in drinking patterns between the two countries and a greater readiness to label newborns with the diagnosis of FAS in the USA. 'Heavy drinking' is defined as more than two drinks per day, or more than 45 per month. This group of women have an approximate incidence of FAS of 4 percent. Alcoholics, or those drinking more than 18 units per day, carry a risk of one in three of their offspring having FAS. These figures are altered by socioeconomic status, general health, smoking and possibly ethnicity, which all act as confounding factors. There is no clear threshold below which alcohol consumption is considered entirely safe; however, the incidence of alcohol-related birth defects (ARBDs) and FAS increases sharply after three units per day [C].[2] 'Binge drinking' of more than five units in one session may be more harmful than taking the same quantity in 'divided doses', although there is no good evidence for this at present. Clearly, this practice should be discouraged during pregnancy [E].

The relationship between benzodiazepine use in the first trimester and congenital anomalies, most notably cleft lip and palate, has been examined many times. A meta-analysis by Dolovich et al.[3] included the 23 most technically robust studies. The cohort studies could not significantly link benzodiazepine use with any fetal abnormalities. The case-control studies, however, gave a 3-fold increase in risk for all major anomalies and an odds ratio of 1.79 (1.13–2.82) for oral clefting. They suggest detailed scanning for those pregnancies exposed in the first trimester.

There are good scientific reasons why ecstasy and cocaine might act as teratogens, although the better controlled studies and meta-analyses have not confirmed the effects found in laboratory animals exposed to high concentrations of these drugs in utero. Neurotransmitters can be found in the fetal brain from very early gestations, and it is likely that they are involved in neuronal migration and establishment of synaptic circuitry. It is simple to imagine how these processes could be disturbed by exposure to such drugs and bring about the microcephaly said to be characteristic of cocaine-exposed neonates.

After maturation of the muscularis layer of fetal cerebral vessels, acute vasoconstriction may lead to infarction followed by the subsequent development of cavitary lesions (e.g. porencephalic cysts). Vascular disruption secondary to cocaine use has also been postulated as a cause for the increase in gut, genitourinary and limb defects reported by some authors. Controlled studies have failed to support these findings.

A recent prospective follow-up study[4] of 136 babies exposed to ecstasy in utero has reported a significant increase in the anomaly rate (15.4 per cent); however, almost half the women used other illegal substances or alcohol and most of the abnormalities were 'minor', raising the possibility of ascertainment bias. To reach statistical significance, the background congenital anomaly rate was quoted as 2–3 per cent; in fact, if minor abnormalities are included, it may be closer to 10 per cent.

Although congenital anomalies will undoubtedly complicate a proportion of pregnancies exposed to marijuana and opiates, no consistent pattern of abnormalities has been found. Most studies show no increase in anomaly risk or are uncontrolled and retrospective.

## Preterm labour and abruption

The obstetric effects of cocaine have perhaps drawn the most attention. Its vasoconstrictive properties are thought to cause abnormal implantation, hypertensive episodes and abruption. Down-regulation of beta-adrenoreceptors in the myometrium may lead to increased uterine irritability and predispose to preterm labour. Amphetamines and ecstasy may have similar effects, although there are much less data. Studies of cocaine use in pregnancy have confirmed the increased risk of preterm labour and abruption; however, these are often lost when confounders (alcohol use and smoking) have been accounted for.[5]

Opiate withdrawal is also thought to cause uterine excitability and result in preterm rupture of membranes and preterm labour [E]. However, smoking is more common among opiate abusers, and minimal antenatal care is the norm. Failure to consider the effect of these confounding factors means the effect of opiates per se is often overestimated.

The effect of prenatal alcohol exposure on the length of gestation remains unclear.

## In-utero growth and development

Intrauterine growth restriction and stillbirth more commonly occur in pregnancies exposed to high alcohol levels, opiates and cocaine. The vasoconstrictive properties of cocaine and ecstasy may cause placental insufficiency and predispose to abruption, uterine irritability and preterm labour. The high metabolic demands of a fetus alternately exposed to opiate 'highs' and withdrawals might also be responsible for IUGR and even stillbirth [E].

Fetal growth restriction is one of the three defining criteria for FAS. Although there are many reasons why growth might be restricted in pregnancies exposed to high levels of alcohol, it is generally held that alcohol per se has a growth-retarding action.

The odds-ratio of producing infants below the tenth centile of weight for gestational age (compared with non-drinkers) for women consuming alcohol, but less than one unit per day, is 1.1. (95% CI 1.00–1.13), one to two units per day 1.62 (1.26–2.09) and three to five units per day 1.96 (1.16–3.31).[6] Among women who continue to drink more than two units per day throughout the third trimester, 45 per cent had an infant with a birth weight below the tenth centile for gestational age, whereas in those who successfully reduced or discontinued their alcohol consumption during the last three months of pregnancy there was no excess of low birth weight, with only 8 per cent falling below the tenth centile. Although low birth weight is a consistent finding in opiate-exposed pregnancies, a causative link between opiate use and IUGR has been difficult to prove due to the action of the following confounding factors:

- 'polydrug' use,
- tobacco smoking and alcohol consumption,
- chaotic and reduced attendance for antenatal care,
- high rates of HIV and other STDs,
- low socioeconomic status,
- poor nutrition.

Substituting methadone for heroin has a beneficial effect on prenatal growth, but this may have more to do with increased levels of antenatal care than the action of the heroin itself (see below).

The vasoconstrictive properties of cocaine suggest it should cause prenatal growth restriction. The Maternal Lifestyles Study (MLS)[7] demonstrated a 450 g reduction in birth weight in cocaine-exposed pregnancies even after the effects of alcohol and tobacco were controlled for [C]. This growth limitation is thought to occur mostly in the third trimester.

## NEONATAL EFFECTS

In the newborn period, substance-exposed infants are more likely to suffer low Apgar scores, infectious complications and CNS disturbance, and opiates may also cause neonatal respiratory depression. Prematurity, low birth weight and IUGR contribute as much to the neonatal problems as do the short-term actions of the drugs themselves.

Finnegan was the first to describe the neonatal abstinence syndrome (NAS). This results from the acute withdrawal of transplacental opioid which occurs at the delivery of a baby born to an opiate-abusing mother. The onset of the syndrome is normally within 24 hours of birth if the opiate used was short acting (e.g. heroin). It consists of:

- irritability, hypertonicity, tremor, exaggerated startle response and occasionally seizures,
- sweating and sneezing,
- abnormal sleep behaviour, high-pitched cry, poor feeding with weak suck and uncoordinated swallowing.

Methadone maintenance does not prevent NAS, but may delay its presentation until the second day of life due to its longer half-life.

Alcohol, cocaine and amphetamines have a less marked effect on neonatal behaviour, if any effect at all. Rare events such as neonatal hypertension, arrhythmias and necrotizing enterocolitis are said to be more common in the offspring of cocaine users, although the confounding effects of prematurity are difficult to separate. Abnormal electroencephalogram (EEG) and brainstem auditory-evoked responses have been demonstrated in these neonates, and the use of neonatal behavioural assessment scales has shown dampened arousal, poor orientation and reduced state control.

Amphetamine-exposed newborns occasionally demonstrate hyperactivity, poor feeding and disrupted sleep patterns. The neonatal effects of marijuana are debated. Greater irritability, tremors and startle responses have been reported, but a well-controlled Jamaican study[8] has suggested that once again the postnatal environment is more important than drug exposure *per se*. In fact, neonatal scores were found to be higher in the offspring of heavy marijuana users. In rural Jamaican society, these women tend to be wealthier and more highly educated. Benzodiazepines may cause neonatal respiratory depression, reduced tone and poor feeding.

## CHILD DEVELOPMENT

Tests of child development are complex and beyond the scope of this chapter. They examine many aspects of behaviour, including language and motor skills, attention and play, cognition and problem-solving and arousal and affective expression. They themselves are open to interpretation and bias.

Mothers willing to participate in longitudinal studies may be more highly motivated, and superior parenting skills in co-operative families may make the effects of the substance abuse appear less significant. Children, as they grow up, may find that society's low expectations of their substance-abusing mothers are reflected onto themselves.

### Alcohol

Impaired development of the CNS is a key criterion of FAS. Although children with FAS have an average IQ of less than 70, the consequences of alcohol consumption that does not result in the full syndrome are less clear. The literature is confusing and does not offer clear guidance, perhaps because of the aetiological difficulties discussed above.

### Opiates

Opiate use in pregnancy is indeed associated with poor developmental outcomes for the offspring; however, it seems that confounding factors are most likely to be responsible, rather than the drug itself. Results of child development tests have been found to be lower at one and two years of age by some researchers. However, a clear harmful effect of opioids themselves on child development is not strongly suggested by the literature.

### Cocaine

Head circumference is inversely related to cocaine exposure during pregnancy. Along with the reported association with serious fetal/neonatal intracranial pathology, it is unsurprising that cocaine itself is thought to be directly damaging to neurodevelopment, with or without confounding social factors. Indeed, neurophysiological testing of such children suggests reduced numbers of oligodendrocytes and impaired myelination.

Closer examination of the data on neurodevelopmental outcome has challenged this view, and the two sides of the debate are difficult to reconcile. The meta-analysis performed by Frank and colleagues[9] selected 36 prospective and blinded studies in which polydrug use was uncommon. After controlling for confounding factors, there was no significant overall association between prenatal cocaine exposure and cognition, language and motor skills, behaviour, attention, affect or neurophysiology, up to six years of age [C].

This controversy is likely to continue. For practical purposes, cocaine use in pregnancy should be considered a marker of 'high risk'. Independent of any direct actions of the drug, pregnancy and neurodevelopmental outcomes are nevertheless poor and will only improve with better access to healthcare and social support.

# SCREENING FOR SUBSTANCE ABUSE IN PREGNANCY

Pregnant women who use drugs may avoid antenatal care for fear of inciting closer scrutiny of their lifestyles, which may often include other criminal activities. They may fear that their child, or children, will be removed from them. Because of this, they may present needing help only at the time of a social, domestic or medical crisis. All those caring for pregnant women should be vigilant for substance abuse and take the opportunity to institute specialized antenatal care whenever presentation occurs. Enquiry about illicit substance use should be routinely made of all pregnant women in a matter-of-fact way. Be prepared to ask more than once. Covert urine testing may confirm substance abuse, but be careful when disclosing this information source, as it may be seen as underhand and untrustworthy and may damage the fragile relationship between the woman and the healthcare services.

Screening for heavy alcohol consumption can be quickly carried out in all pregnant women using the TACE questionnaire. Only four questions are asked:

T (for Tolerance): *how many drinks does it take to make you feel high?* More than two suggests a degree of tolerance and scores two points.

A (for Annoyance): *has anyone annoyed you by criticising your drinking?* Answering 'yes' scores one point.

C (for Cutting down): *have you ever thought you needed to cut down your drinking?* Answering 'yes' scores one point.

E (for 'Eye opener'): *have you ever had a drink first thing in the morning to steady your nerves or to get rid of a hangover?* Answering yes scores one point.

A score of two or more points is considered a positive screen and carries a 70 per cent sensitivity for detection of heavy drinkers. Further questioning and assessment are needed of those who screen positive.

# MANAGEMENT OF PREGNANCY COMPLICATED BY SUBSTANCE ABUSE

A multidisciplinary team approach is necessary to create a confidential, reassuring and non-judgemental environment in which the pregnancy outcome and childbirth experience can be optimized. This team will include social workers, specialist drug services, drug-liaison midwives, general practitioners (GPs), obstetricians and paediatricians.

'Harm minimization' recognizes the futility of simply telling users to stop using. It aims initially to promote a change in the nature of the drug taking, to stabilize lifestyles and reduce criminal behaviour. Stopping drug abuse

altogether is a much longer term aim. Exchanging needles or moving to non-intravenous modes of delivery would be examples of harm reduction. Reducing alcohol and tobacco consumption and establishing methadone maintenance are particularly important aims in pregnancy.

## Antenatal care

Significant improvements in pregnancy outcome are achieved by regular antenatal care, which should be tailored to the individual. Points to consider include:

- carefully targeted history taking,
- counselling about the possible effects of the drug abuse on the pregnancy,
- possible urine testing for illicit substances,
- discussion and delineation of achievable aims to reduce harm,
- ultrasound scanning to accurately date the pregnancy,
- screening for hepatitis B and C, HIV and possibly bacterial vaginosis,
- detailed anomaly scanning,
- serial growth scanning and fetal assessments as necessary,
- reflection on the need for a child protection case conference,
- communication with anaesthetic and paediatric services: cocaine and opiate abusers may pose particular problems for obstetric anaesthetists, and admission to a special care baby unit (SCBU) is very likely, even if only for observation.

---

**Focused history taking from the pregnant drug abuser**
- Type of drug(s) used, when, how often, how much and mode of administration.
- Does her partner use drugs?
- Has the woman particular fears or concerns of her own?
- Are there specific psychological or health problems leading to, or a consequence of, the drug abuse?
- What are the social/financial circumstances?
- Is she in any legal trouble?
- Does she drink alcohol or smoke tobacco?
- Does she practise safe sex?
- Does she share needles?

---

Women using street narcotics should be offered methadone maintenance treatment (MMT). Methadone has a longer half-life than heroin and blood levels remain more stable. Users are provided with a regular but limited supply, which offers the opportunity to remove themselves from the criminal high-risk behaviours often necessary to fund a street habit and which carry such risk to the pregnancy. Having to attend regularly to obtain prescriptions allows close antenatal surveillance and healthcare. The fetus avoids opiate 'highs' and withdrawals and other possible harmful contaminants of street drugs. Compliance with these regimens can reduce neonatal mortality and increase birth weight, although the benefits are lost if MMT is supplemented with street 'top-ups', which many abusers need for the 'highs' not provided by methadone. Negotiating the dose with the user is a difficult task. Low doses (60 mg/day) are associated with higher rates of non-compliance. Twice-daily dosing regimens may minimize the trough levels and reduce relapses.

> ### EBM
>
> Using methadone during pregnancy (as opposed to no opiates at all) is associated with an approximate doubling of neonatal mortality. Use of both methadone *and* heroin carries a 6-fold increase in neonatal mortality risk.

Women established on MMT may consider gradual withdrawal (e.g. a reduction in dose of 2–2.5 mg every 7–10 days). Anecdotal evidence recommends that this should occur in the second trimester, as leaving it until later risks preterm labour [E]. The greater risk of withdrawal during pregnancy is a subsequent relapse of illegal narcotic use. This is considered to carry the greatest risk of fetal harm, and withdrawal during pregnancy should only be attempted in highly motivated women with a stable, supportive and drug-free environment to which they can return.

Unfortunately, there is no such 'replacement' regimen for cocaine users. Harm reduction must involve a reduction in cocaine use. Without an incentive, it may be very difficult to gain the trust and co-operation of pregnant users who fear reprisals for their substance abuse.

Pregnancy is a relative indication for inpatient alcohol detoxification. Most programmes choose to treat the pregnant, alcohol-dependent woman with short-acting barbiturates or benzodiazepines. Chlordiazepoxide and other benzodiazepines, such as diazepam and barbiturates, are valuable for symptomatic treatment during medical withdrawal from alcohol. They are also potentially teratogenic. Some clinicians, therefore, recommend avoiding their use if at all possible. The risks versus the possible benefits of their use need to be assessed.

Disulfiram (Antabuse) is contraindicated during pregnancy. Its use has been associated with clubfoot, VACTERL syndrome and phocomelia of the lower extremities. Women who conceive while taking this drug should receive counselling before deciding to continue the pregnancy.

## Intrapartum care

Labour may be the first time a pregnant substance abuser presents to medical services. It should be managed as normal, with a few additional points to bear in mind.

- Recommend continuous cardiotocography (CTG) monitoring in view of the increased risk of placental insufficiency and fetal compromise.
- Be aware that opiates may influence the CTG and interpretation may be more difficult.
- Avoid, as far as possible, fetal blood sampling, scalp electrodes and episiotomies to reduce the vertical transmission risk of hepatitis and HIV.
- Elective caesarean section before membrane rupture reduces HIV vertical transmission and possibly that of hepatitis C (although this needs confirmation).[10]
- Give normal maintenance doses of methadone to prevent withdrawal. These will not provide analgesia, which should be offered in addition. Epidural analgesia may prove most effective if opioid receptors are already saturated by the illegal opiate.
- Those women who have undergone supervised withdrawal from opiates during the pregnancy should avoid systemic opiates in labour. Nitrous oxide and epidural analgesia are preferable.
- Naloxone should not be given to opiate-dependent mothers or their offspring – severe withdrawal effects may occur.
- In cocaine users, ephedrine may be less effective at reversing hypotension secondary to regional analgesia. Phenylephrine is a useful alternative.

## Postnatal care

Above all, the new mother should be supported in her first few days, as any new parent should be. Indeed, she is likely to have minimal help when she leaves hospital. Ongoing assistance from the specialist midwife is vital.

- If the baby seems well, it should be transferred to the postnatal ward with the mother. NAS usually presents in the first 2 days and the baby must be closely observed for signs of this. Methadone withdrawal may take a little longer, but will usually have begun by 4 days (the minimum time period that women are advised to stay in hospital). If the infant is demonstrating withdrawal symptoms, it will need special care facilities.
- Breastfeeding is encouraged in most women, even those on methadone. Infant weaning should occur gradually; fortunately the quantities of opiates reaching breast milk are small. HIV-positive women, those using large amounts of benzodiazepines and cocaine users are exceptions to this general rule. These women should be advised to bottle-feed. Hepatitis C is not a contraindication to breastfeeding.[10]
- Babies born to hepatitis-B-positive mothers should be immunized.
- Drug misuse by a parent does not necessarily equate with child neglect or abuse, and automatic child abuse registration will only discourage women from seeking antenatal care. Social services should be informed of the delivery and decisions made about the levels of support needed to ensure child safety.
- Appropriate contraceptive advice must be provided before discharge.

# ACKNOWLEDGEMENT

This chapter has been revised and updated. The author and editors acknowledge the contribution of Alec McEwan to the chapter on this topic in the previous edition of the book.

## KEY POINTS

- There is increasing evidence suggesting harm to the fetus from heavy alcohol consumption in pregnancy.
- Binge drinking in early pregnancy may be particularly harmful.
- There is considerable doubt as to whether infrequent low level alcohol consumption conveys any long-term harm.
- Alcohol is the only clear teratogen, although benzodiazepines may predispose to oral clefting.
- Moreover, the effects of alcohol and other drugs on short- and long-term child development are still in question. Potent cellular actions and devastating complications such as intracerebral haemorrhage are well recognized, but have a less striking impact on the results of larger population studies.
- Regardless of the direct harm caused by drug or alcohol abuse during pregnancy, such behaviour is a powerful marker of poor obstetric outcome and should prompt close antenatal surveillance by specialized healthcare workers.
- The aim of antenatal care should be to minimize harm by setting realistic goals.
- All units should have a dedicated team with defined guidelines to optimize outcomes for mother and baby.

## Key References

1. Abel EL. Maternal alcohol consumption and spontaneous abortion. *Alcohol* 1997; **32**: 211–19.
2. Allebeck P, Olsen J. Alcohol and fetal damage. *Alcohol Clin Exp Res* 1998; **22** (Suppl. 7): 329S–325.
3. Dolovich LR, Addis A, Vaillancourt JM *et al.* Benzodiazepine use in pregnancy and major malformations or oral cleft: meta-analysis of cohort and case-control studies. *BMJ* 1998; **317**: 839–43.
4. McElhatton PR, Bateman DN, Evans C *et al.* Congenital anomalies after prenatal ecstasy exposure. *Lancet* 1999; **354**: 1441–2.
5. Sprauve ME, Lindsay MK, Herbert S, Graves W. Adverse perinatal outcome in parturients who use crack cocaine. *Obstet Gynecol* 1997; **89**: 674–8.
6. Mills JL, Graubard BI, Harley EE *et al.* Maternal alcohol consumption and birth weight. *J Am Med Assoc* 1984; **252**: 1875–79.
7. Bada HS, Verter J, Bauer CR *et al.* Maternal Lifestyle Study (MLS): Intrauterine growth of infants exposed to cocaine/opiates *in utero*. *Paediatr Res* 1996; **39**: 256.
8. Dreher MC, Nugent K, Hudgins R. Prenatal marijuana exposure and neonatal outcomes in Jamaica: an ethnographic study. *Pediatrics* 1994; **93**: 254–60.
9. Frank DA, Augustyn M, Knight WG *et al.* Growth, development and behaviour in early childhood following prenatal cocaine exposure. A systematic review. *J Am Med Assoc* 2001; **285**: 1613–26.
10. Gibb DM, Goodall RL, Dunn DT *et al.* Mother-to-child transmission of hepatitis C virus: evidence for preventable peripartum transmission. *Lancet* 2000; **356**: 904–7.

# 6.13 Smoking

*Andrew Shennan*

## INTRODUCTION

Smoking-related morbidity and mortality affect millions of individuals throughout the world. Each year, almost a quarter of all deaths of men can be attributed to a smoking-related cause and although far fewer female deaths are related to smoking, the gap is rapidly closing. More women are becoming smokers in industrialized countries. The cause of this morbidity and mortality is largely related to the effects on cardiovascular disease, although smoking is also a cause of cancer, particularly of the lung.

Although smoking is decreasing in high income countries, there is evidence it is increasing in low and middle income countries, and overall around a quarter of young women smoke. This affects their risks of developing gynaecological cancers such as cancer of the cervix. Other risks, such as that of thromboembolic disease, are increased. Effects on the menopause and miscarriage as well as low birth weight (due to both fetal growth restriction and spontaneous preterm delivery) have been reported. However, in spite of educational programmes to point out these obvious detrimental effects to fetal well-being, it has proved very difficult to introduce preventative strategies as nicotine is highly addictive. Smoking in pregnancy is also strongly linked to poor socioeconomic status, including poor support,

depression and psychological illness. Smoking remains a major preventable cause of low birth weight, preterm delivery and perinatal mortality, as well as neurodevelopmental problems. This section reviews the relationship between smoking and pregnancy outcome, and discusses management strategies to reduce adverse events.

## INCIDENCE IN PREGNANCY

In the developed world, smoking has declined in the last 30 years from around 20–30 per cent of pregnant women, to 10–20 per cent who report smoking.[1,2] As with the non-pregnant population, there is a strong association with socioeconomic background, so that those from lower groups have considerably higher smoking rates, and there is evidence that the decline has been less apparent in the low socioeconomic sector.[2] Generally, actual smoking rates are about 3 per cent higher than reported rates, as evidenced by cotinine levels.[3]

It has been reported that women who continue to smoke, in spite of knowledge of the detrimental effects, are more likely to have problems at work and, in general, are less well supported on a psychosocial basis. Women without partners and who already have children are less likely to stop.

Women are more likely to stop smoking in pregnancy then at other times, and up to 45 per cent spontaneously quit. Women who stop smoking in pregnancy are more likely to smoke less, have non-smoking partners, and have good support and knowledge.[4] However, only a third of quitters remain abstinent after one year. Overall, pregnancy does provide an opportunity to instigate quitting interventions.

## AETIOLOGY AND CLINICAL EFFECTS

### Preterm delivery

There is good epidemiological evidence that smoking is related to the risk of preterm delivery, including early preterm birth. There is also an established relationship with perinatal death [C]. The association is strong and often dose related, which therefore adds considerable evidence that the effect is causative and not related to other associated factors [C].

Women who smoke have approximately double the risk of preterm delivery. This is principally due to spontaneous preterm delivery, but it also can increase the risk of the need for iatrogenic delivery through association with placental abruption and placenta praevia [C]. Smoking is also a risk factor for preterm premature rupture of the fetal membranes.[5]

Lower mean birth weight has been associated with a high mean systolic blood pressure in later life in the children of mothers who smoke. Smoking may therefore be contributing to the possible *in-utero* programming effects with which reduced fetal growth potential is now thought to be associated.

## Intrauterine growth restriction

It is established that low birth weight for gestation is more common in women who smoke.[6] On average, babies will be approximately 200 g lighter as a result of smoking. There is a dose relationship to this effect and it is recognized that women who smoke more than ten cigarettes a day will have lower birth weight than those who smoke less than this number, the effects being greater in male fetuses [C]. Even passive smoking can reduce birth weight.[7]

## Intelligent quotient

Cognitive performance is reduced in the children of the mothers who smoke during pregnancy, even after adjustment for other confounding variables.[8] Longer term effects on the children may include influence on respiratory illness over and above that which may be caused by the children living in a family where smoking continues [C].

## Smoking and pre-eclampsia

There are many studies that demonstrate an association between a reduced risk of pre-eclampsia and smoking [C].[9] However, it is clear that any possible benefit in this reduction is completely superseded by the harmful effects of smoking [D]. Indeed, women who do show the clinical signs of pre-eclampsia have more severe disease. In these women, there are increased rates of perinatal mortality, abruption and intrauterine growth restriction.

## Infertility, ectopics and miscarriage

There is now evidence that both ovarian function and implantation may be affected by smoking, thus reducing the fertility of these women. There is also an increased incidence of ectopic pregnancy that is apparent from recent meta-analyses. The risk of miscarriage is also increased.

# MANAGEMENT: SMOKING CESSATION IN PREGNANCY

Although women are more likely to stop smoking when pregnant than at any other time, only a minority will stop smoking when they become pregnant. These individuals frequently smoke less and have better support from home, including a partner who gives up or is a non-smoker. Programmes that encourage smoking cessation have been associated with some improved outcome, in terms of less low birth weight and premature delivery [C].

A meta-analysis of randomized controlled trials, where smoking cessation was the primary aim of the intervention, included 72 trials, with more than 25 000 women providing data on smoking cessation outcomes in pregnancy. Interventions ranged from advice and counselling (written, electronic or telephone), feedback of fetal health status, provision of pharmacological agents (e.g. nicotine replacement therapy and bupropion), social support and encouragement (including rewards for cessation and hypnosis). Overall, only six women in every 100 stopped smoking. Eight trials that looked at relapse prevention showed that interventions did not work. Overall, smoking cessation programmes were associated with a 17 per cent reduction in low birth weight and a 14 per cent reduction in preterm birth. This represented about a 50 g difference in birth weight.[10] No other perinatal outcomes improved.

Generally, these programmes are highly intensive before they are successful, and standard advice from midwives and other clinicians to stop smoking has had little impact on overall quitting rates during pregnancy [C]. However, a small number of individuals do stop on brief advice and, as this is inexpensive, it is worthwhile [E].

Specialist staff are known to be more effective than others, with more than a doubling of cessation rates [B].[11] Unfortunately, few women are willing, or have the opportunity, to use these counselling services. Self-help material has some benefit in approximately 4 per cent of smokers. There is, however, good evidence that stopping smoking will reduce the adverse effects of smoking in pregnancy; the challenge is to find ways to stop women who do not spontaneously quit.[12]

> **EBM**
>
> Specialist staff trained in counselling women about smoking are more likely to succeed in cessation programmes.

Prevention is better than cure, and overall strategies to stop women commencing smoking pre-pregnancy must be a priority, given the relatively poor uptake following intervention programmes.

Antenatal complications: maternal

## KEY POINTS

- Only a minority of women quit smoking when pregnant.
- Smoking in pregnancy is associated with preterm birth, fetal growth restriction and perinatal death and is the single most preventable cause of these adverse events.
- Most adverse events are dose related and preterm birth and birth weight can be improved with smoking cessation programmes.
- The children of mothers who smoke have lower intelligence quotients.

## Key References

1. Cnattingius S. The epidemiology of smoking during pregnancy: smoking prevalence, maternal characteristics, and pregnancy outcomes. *Nicotine Tob Res* 2004; **6** (S2): S125–S140.

2. US Department of Health and Human Services. *The health consequences of smoking. 2004 Surgeon General's Report*. US Department of Health and Human Services, 2004.

3. Tapen DM, Forward RP, Wilde CJ. Smoking at the end of pregnancy measured by cord blood cotinine assay. *NZ Med J* 1995; **108**: 108–9.

4. McBride CM, Emmons KM, Lipkus IM. Understanding the potential of teachable moments: the case of smoking cessation. *Health Educ Res* 2003; **18**: 156–70.

5. Harger JH, Hsing AW, Tuomala RE *et al.* Risk factors for preterm premature rupture of fetal membranes; a multi-center case control study. *Am J Obstet Gynecol* 1990; **163**: 130–37.

6. Kramer MS. Determinants of low birthweight: methodological assessment and meta analysis. *Bull WHO* 1987; **65**: 663–737.

7. Rubin DH, Krasilnikoff PA, Leventhal JM *et al.* Effect of passive smoking on low birthweight. *Lancet* 1986; **ii**: 415–17.

8. Sexton M, Fox NL, Hebel JR. Prenatal exposure to tobacco: II. Effects on cognitive functioning at age three. *Int J Epidemiol* 1990; **19**: 72–7.

9. Cnattingiuss S, Mills JL, Yuen J *et al.* The paradoxical effect of smoking in pre-eclamptic pregnancies. Smoking reduces the incidence with increases of rates of perinatal mortality, abruptio placentae and intrauterine growth. *Am J Obstet Gynecol* 1997; **177**: 156–61.

10. Lumley J, Chamberlain C, Dowswell T *et al.* Interventions for promoting smoking cessation during pregnancy. *Cochrane Database Syst Rev* 2009; (**3**): CD001055.

11. West R. Helping patients in hospital to quit smoking. Dedicated counselling services are effective – others are not. *BMJ* 2002; **324**: 64.

12. Sexton M, Hebel JR. A clinical trial of change in maternal smoking and its effect on birthweight. *J Am Med Assoc* 1984; **251**: 911–15.

# 7.1 Anaemia

*Tracey A Johnston*

---

## MRCOG standards

### Relevant standard

Candidates are expected to understand the epidemiology, aetiology, pathophysiology, clinical characteristics, prognostic features and management of anaemia.

In addition, we would suggest the following.

### Theoretical skills

* Revise the physiological changes of the blood in pregnancy.

### Practical skills

* Be able to detect and manage antenatally.

---

## INTRODUCTION

Anaemia is the most common medical disorder of pregnancy. Pre-existing bone marrow disorders and inherited haemoglobin (Hb) variants are discussed in Chapter 6.5, Haematological conditions. This chapter aims to revise the physiological changes in pregnancy, and discusses the maternal and fetal risks of anaemia, diagnosis and management.

## PHYSIOLOGICAL CHANGES

* Plasma volume increases by 50 per cent.
* Red cell mass increases by up to 25 per cent.
* There is a consequent fall in Hb concentration, haematocrit and red cell count because of haemodilution.
* Mean cell volume (MCV) increases secondary to erythropoiesis.
* Mean cell Hb concentration (MCHC) remains stable.
* Serum iron and ferritin concentrations decrease secondary to increased utilization.
* Total iron-binding capacity increases.

* Iron requirements increase (due to expanding red cell mass and fetal requirements) from 2.5 mg/day in the first trimester to 6.6 mg/day in the third trimester (700–1400 mg total pregnancy).
* There is a moderate increase in iron absorption.
* Folate requirements increase in pregnancy (due to the fetus, placenta, uterus and expanded maternal red cell mass).
* There is no major effect on $B_{12}$ stores, although levels decrease (preferential active transport to the fetus).

## DEFINITION

*A pathological condition in which the oxygen-carrying capacity of red blood cells is insufficient to meet the body's needs.*

Often the diagnosis is based on blood values, in particular Hb concentration. The World Health Organization (WHO) recommends that the Hb concentration should not fall below 11 g/dL at any time during pregnancy,[1,2] but many clinicians use the figure of 10.5 g/dL as recommended by the Centers for Disease Control of North America.[3]

## INCIDENCE

Around 30–50 per cent of women become anaemic during pregnancy, with iron deficiency being responsible in more than 90 per cent of cases. The incidence of folate deficiency is around 5 per cent (though it is often underdiagnosed) and this is almost always the cause of megaloblastic anaemia in pregnancy, with vitamin $B_{12}$ deficiency being rare.

## CLINICAL FEATURES

Anaemia is very often asymptomatic in pregnancy, with the diagnosis being made on routine screening. Clinical features include tiredness, dizziness, fainting and lethargy. Pallor may be apparent.

## SCREENING

Anaemia is routinely screened for in pregnancy by estimating the Hb concentration by means of a full blood count at the beginning of pregnancy and again later in pregnancy, often at the start of the third trimester, and again at term. This lacks specificity but has the advantage of being cheap and simple to perform. The presence of a low Hb does not reveal the cause of the anaemia.

## IRON DEFICIENCY ANAEMIA

### Aetiology

Iron deficiency anaemia is classically described as a microcytic, hypochromic anaemia because of the reduced MCV and MCHC. This is the most common cause of anaemia in pregnancy, but the diagnosis should still be confirmed. There are significant iron demands during pregnancy, secondary to expanding red cell mass and fetal requirements, which can only be met by a limited increase in iron absorption, and by utilization of iron stores. If iron stores are already depleted because of menstruation, recurrent pregnancies and poor intake, anaemia will develop rapidly. During pregnancy, the total iron-binding capacity (TIBC) increases secondary to the increased plasma volume, and serum iron falls. As iron demands exceed supply during pregnancy, ferritin levels fall. Decreased Hb concentration is a late event in iron deficiency anaemia.

### Consequences

The evidence regarding the consequences of iron deficiency anaemia in pregnancy is conflicting. From the maternal perspective, as well as the clinical features described above, it has been suggested that impaired function of iron-dependent enzymes causes alterations in muscle function, neurotransmitter activity and epithelial changes throughout the body.[4] This has been used as the basis for the explanation for the apparent link between iron deficiency anaemia and preterm delivery, infection, medical intervention during labour and postpartum blood loss. It is clear that women with significant anaemia at the time of delivery will not tolerate blood loss as well, and are more likely to receive blood transfusion postnatally. From the fetal perspective, it is widely accepted that there is an increased risk of preterm delivery and intrauterine growth restriction. However, many of the studies have not controlled for other

factors, such as smoking, that may be important.[5] There is also conflicting evidence regarding the neonatal iron status and cognitive development and behaviour of babies born to iron-deficient mothers.[6]

## Diagnosis

Iron deficiency can be present in the absence of anaemia, and other parameters of the full blood count that usually give a clue to this (reduced MCV, MCH (mean cell haemoglobin) and MCHC) are not as accurate during pregnancy (Table 7.1.1).

The diagnostic test for iron deficiency is a ferritin concentration. This is not affected by pregnancy, and a concentration of <12 mg/L is diagnostic. This could be used as a screening test as iron deficiency is so common in pregnancy, but requires an extra blood test (although many laboratories now have the facilities to estimate the ferritin concentration from the full blood count sample) and adds cost.

## Treatment

### Efficacy of treatment

Although it is clear that iron supplementation improves the haematological indices, there is little robust evidence to prove, especially in cases of mild anaemia in pregnancy with no complications, that such therapy improves clinical outcomes for these mothers or their babies, and consideration should be given to whether benefits outweigh the frequent relatively mild side effects.[7] It has also been demonstrated that intravenous iron is most effective in improving the haematological indices, followed by intramuscular administration, with oral supplementation being least effective.[7] Again this must be balanced against the invasiveness of administration and the possible adverse effects, which are mildest with oral supplementation and most severe with the intravenous route.[7] Having said this, it is standard practice in the UK to treat anaemia in pregnancy.

**Table 7.1.1** Haematological values

|  | Non-pregnant | Pregnant | Iron deficiency |
|---|---|---|---|
| Hb (g/dL) | 12–15 | 11–15 | <10.5 |
| MCV (fL) | 75–99 | More | Less |
| TIBC (mmol/L) | 45–72 | Increases | Decreases by <15% |
| Se Fe (mmol/L) | 13–27 | 13–27 | <12 |
| Fe (mg/L) | 15–300 | 15–300 | <12 |

- Fe, ferritin; Hb, haemoglobin; MCV, mean cell volume; TIBC, total iron-binding capacity; Se Fe, serum ferritin.

## Oral iron

The treatment for iron deficiency is oral iron replacement [B], which is usually effective if there is enough time (maximum increase in Hb is 0.8 g/dL per week). The recommended dose is 120–240 mg of elemental iron per day. Ferrous salts are absorbed better than ferric salts [B] and should be used in preference. There is little to choose between the different ferrous salts in terms of absorption and efficacy, and side effects are related to the amount of elemental iron contained. The choice of preparation should therefore be dictated by cost and patient tolerance, but it should be noted that a reduction in side effects is usually secondary to a reduction in the amount of elemental iron absorbed. Vitamin C taken simultaneously aids absorption [B], hence the common advice to take iron with fresh orange juice. There is, however, little to gain, other than increased cost, by using combination preparations with ascorbic acid included.

There is a 40 per cent risk of side effects with oral iron preparations, mainly gastrointestinal, and this can have a direct effect on tolerance and compliance. Slow-release preparations are often associated with a decrease in the incidence of side effects, but this is mainly secondary to decreased absorption of elemental iron, as most is not released from the preparation until it has passed through the first part of the duodenum, where iron absorption is optimal. For those with proven iron deficiency that cannot be managed with oral therapy because of lack of compliance, severe gastrointestinal side effects, continuing significant blood loss or malabsorption, parenteral preparations exist.

## Intramuscular iron

Iron sorbitol injection has a low molecular weight and thus allows rapid absorption from the injection site, although high levels may be excreted before utilization. It is not suitable for intravenous use. It is administered by deep intramuscular injection and can be associated with pain at the time of injection and tattooing of the skin. The dose is calculated depending on the degree of iron deficiency and patient weight, but requires repeated injections, usually over the course of 2 weeks.

## Intravenous iron

There are various intravenous iron preparations that are now available with significantly fewer side effects compared to iron dextran, which has now been withdrawn from use because of the high incidence of anaphylaxis. These preparations have all been used successfully in pregnancy in selected cases, and are associated with a greater and more rapid rise in Hb concentration with fewer (but more serious) side effects when compared with oral preparations.[7] Depending on the preparation used, this form of therapy can require daily trips to hospital for several days, as well

as an intravenous cannula, and is thus more disruptive and invasive than oral therapy, but is a realistic alternative to blood transfusion when oral therapy has failed. Many units, however, use iron sucrose (Cosmofer™), which is licensed for total dose iron replacement in the second and third trimesters. It is given as a single infusion and takes 4–6 hours to complete.

## Blood transfusion

Towards the end of pregnancy there may not be the time available to increase the Hb with iron therapy, and blood transfusion may be indicated as well as iron therapy. It should be borne in mind that blood transfusion is not without risk,[8] and effective screening programmes should detect anaemia early enough to allow iron therapy to be utilized. However, transfusion is the most rapid way to increase Hb concentration, but is a relatively slow way to increase iron stores.

## Erythropoietin

Recombinant human erythropoietin is mainly used for the anaemia associated with erythropoietin deficiency in chronic renal failure, but can also be used to increase the autologous production of blood in normal individuals. It has been used in cases of severe postpartum anaemia with success, and has been life saving in cases where blood transfusion is declined, for example Jehovah's Witnesses. It has also been used during pregnancy in a small number of renal patients with no adverse maternal or perinatal complications.[7,9]

# Prevention/prophylaxis

Prevention of iron deficiency is usually possible with a good balanced diet in the absence of ongoing blood loss, and identification and treatment of iron deficiency prior to pregnancy are optimal. However, many women enter pregnancy already iron deficient, or become so during pregnancy. Health education by the midwife regarding diet is therefore important.[10]

There has been much work carried out on the role of routine iron supplementation in pregnancy, and this has been the subject of a Cochrane Review.[11] This meta-analysis of 40 trials including 12 706 women concluded that although there is clear evidence of improvement in haematological indices in those women who receive iron supplements during pregnancy, there are not enough data to determine that routine supplementation with iron alone or in combination with folic acid has any substantial benefits or adverse effects on maternal and fetal health and pregnancy outcomes (premature delivery and low birth weight) among populations where anaemia is common. The reviewers felt that there was not enough evidence to suggest a change in current recommended iron and folic acid doses with either modality of supplementation [A].

---

### EBM

- Oral iron therapy with ferrous salts is the treatment of choice for iron deficiency anaemia in pregnancy [B].
- Vitamin C aids absorption but there is no evidence to support the use of combined preparations [B].
- There is no evidence to advise against a policy of routine iron supplementation in pregnancy [A].

---

# FOLATE DEFICIENCY

## Aetiology

There is a significant increase in folate requirements during pregnancy because of the increased cell replication that is taking place in the fetus, uterus and bone marrow (increase in red cell mass). Plasma folate concentrations decrease throughout pregnancy, reaching half the non-pregnant levels by term. The incidence of folate deficiency is higher in multiple pregnancies. Folate deficiency causes a megaloblastic anaemia, the incidence of which in pregnancy is around 5 per cent, although higher rates are found in other parts of the world and are thought to be secondary to poor diet. In the UK, many foods now have folate supplements added, making the recommended daily intake of 800 µg easier to achieve.

## Consequences

There are clear links between periconceptual folate deficiency and neural tube defects,[12] as well as a suggested association with other anomalies,[13] hence the advice that all women planning a pregnancy should take 400 µg/day of folic acid and continue this for the first 12 weeks of pregnancy until the neural tube is closed [A]. From the maternal perspective, the consequences of folate deficiency are not just anaemia, but involvement of tissues with high rates of cell turnover, in particular mucous membranes; the effects of folate deficiency can thus be exacerbated by malabsorption if the gut mucosa is affected.

## Diagnosis

Outside pregnancy, the macrocytosis of folate deficiency anaemia is diagnosed by an increased MCV. However, during pregnancy the MCV is increased, but the macrocytosis may be masked by co-existing iron deficiency leading to a reduced MCV. Red cell indices are therefore not particularly useful for diagnosis. Examining the blood film may be useful, but in pregnancy the diagnosis often entails examination of a bone marrow aspirate.

## Treatment

Severe folate deficiency is extremely rare, but once megaloblastic haematopoiesis is established, treatment is difficult secondary to poor folate absorption from the affected gastrointestinal tract. In this uncommon situation, 5 mg oral pteroylglutamic acid daily or parenteral folate can be used.

## Prevention/prophylaxis

The case for routine prophylaxis with 400 µg/day for the prevention of neural tube defects has already been discussed above. However, there are other situations in which folate prophylaxis is indicated. These include women taking anticonvulsant drugs [E] and those with haemolytic anaemias (see Chapter 8, Medication in pregnancy). In these situations, the recommended prophylactic dose is 5 mg/day throughout pregnancy.

# VITAMIN B₁₂ DEFICIENCY

Vitamin $B_{12}$ deficiency is rare during the reproductive years, and is associated with infertility; therefore, vitamin $B_{12}$ deficiency during pregnancy is very uncommon. Absorption is unchanged by pregnancy, and vitamin $B_{12}$ is actively transported across the placenta to the fetus.

Chronic tropical sprue can give rise to megaloblastic anaemia in pregnancy secondary to both vitamin $B_{12}$ and folate deficiencies.

## Management

In cases of known $B_{12}$ deficiency, treatment should be optimized prior to conception (and may be necessary to allow conception). Women on $B_{12}$ replacement therapy should continue this as normal. Virtually all diets that contain animal products will supply enough $B_{12}$ during pregnancy, although strict vegans may become deficient.

---

### KEY POINTS

- Anaemia is the most common medical disorder of pregnancy, with significant implications for both mother and child.
- Although iron deficiency is the major cause of anaemia in pregnancy, this diagnosis should be established to allow optimal treatment.
- Screening for anaemia in pregnancy is simple, as is treatment of iron deficiency anaemia.
- There is no evidence to support routine iron prophylaxis in the absence of other risk factors.
- The role of periconceptual folate supplementation should be emphasized at pre-conceptual counselling.

## Further Reading

*Why Mothers Die 1997–1999*. Confidential Enquiry into Maternal Deaths in the United Kingdom. Chapter 4, Hall MH. Haemorrhage. London: RCOG Press, 2001.

## Key References

1. World Health Organization. *Nutritional Anaemias*. Technical Report Series. Geneva: WHO, 1972.

2. World Health Organization. Iron deficiency anaemia, assessment, prevention, and control: a guide for programme managers. Available from: www.who.int/reproductive-health/docs/anaemia.pdf

3. Centers for Disease Control. Current Trends: CDC criteria for anaemia in children and child bearing-aged women. *Morb Mortal Wkly Rep* 1989; **38**: 400–4.

4. Finch CA, Cook JD. Iron deficiency. *Am J Clin Nutr* 1984; **39**: 471–7.

5. Scholl TO, Hediger ML. Anemia and iron deficiency anemia: compilation of data on pregnancy outcome. *Am J Clin Nutr* 1994; **59** (Suppl.): 492S–501S.

6. Walter T. Effect of iron-deficiency anaemia on cognitive skills in infancy and childhood. *Baillière's Clin Haematol* 1994; **7**: 815–27.

7. Reveiz L, Gyte GML, Cuervo LG Treatments for iron-deficiency anaemia in pregnancy. *Cochrane Database Syst Rev* 2007; (**2**): CD003094.

8. SHOT Annual Report 2000/2001. London: Serious Hazards of Transfusion Steering Group, 2002.

9. Breymann C, Major A, Richter C *et al.* Recombinant human erythropoietin and parenteral iron in the treatment of pregnancy anemia: a pilot study. *J Perinat Med* 1995; **23**: 89–98.

10. Watson F. Routine iron supplementation – is it necessary? *Modern Midwife* 1997; **7**: 22–6.

11. Pena-Rosasa JP, Viteri FE. Effects of routine oral iron supplementation with or without folic acid for women during pregnancy. *Cochrane Database Syst Rev* 2006; (**3**): CD004736.

12. Lumley J, Watson L, Watson M, Bower C. Periconceptual supplementation with folate and/or multivitamins for preventing neural tube defects. *Cochrane Database Syst Rev* 2001; (**3**): CD001056.

13. Elwood JM. Can vitamins prevent neural tube defects? *Can Med Assoc J* 1983; **129**: 1088–92.

# 7.2 Abdominal pain

*Clare L Tower*

## MRCOG standards

There are no clearly defined knowledge criteria in the core curriculum for the topic of 'abdominal pain'. Instead, specific requirements can be found in the sections relating to individual disorders. However, the diagnosis, investigation and management of acute abdominal pain is a required clinical competence.

A detailed discussion of every cause of abdominal pain in pregnancy is both impractical and cumbersome, and many of the disorders are discussed elsewhere in detail. Thus, this chapter aims to give an overview of the approach to abdominal pain in pregnancy, with a focus on differential diagnoses, and aspects of the approach that are specific to pregnant women.

## INTRODUCTION

Abdominal pain is an extremely common complaint in pregnant women, with the majority of women experiencing it at some point during pregnancy. The vast majority is benign and self limiting. However, an approach to abdominal pain in pregnancy must enable identification of serious pathology to allow successful treatment to be implemented. There are many pitfalls in the assessment of pregnant women with abdominal pain and sadly several are found in the Triennial Maternal Mortality Report.[1] In particular, diagnosis of the 'acute abdomen', often defined as a collection of symptoms and signs of intraperitoneal disease best treated with surgery,[2] is notoriously difficult.

## HISTORY AND EXAMINATION

In the same way as outside pregnancy, a systematic approach to the history and examination of the abdominal pain is required. A detailed outline of this can be found in many undergraduate textbooks. However, the gravid uterus and the physiological changes in pregnancy can mask some of the typical findings seen outside pregnancy. A classic example is the location of the appendix. This becomes displaced upwards as gestation increases. Therefore, whereas the appendix may lie at McBurney's point in the first trimester, by the late third trimester it may become located in the right hypochondrium, or be located behind the pregnant uterus. The enlarging uterus also separates the intra-abdominal organs from the parietal peritoneum with increasing gestation. Therefore, signs of peritonism may be masked as the inflamed abdominal organ no longer irritates the parietal peritoneum. Furthermore, many associated symptoms and signs can also be those common in a normal pregnancy, for example nausea and vomiting. A thorough but focused history and examination will suggest a short list of likely differential diagnoses (Table 7.2.1), thus guiding further investigation. Causes can be considered first as obstetric and non-obstetric, then within a systems review, e.g. gastrointestinal, renal and other. Involvement of other specialists, such as gastroenterologists, urologists or surgeons, may be indicated.

## INVESTIGATIONS AND IMAGING

The list of possible differential diagnoses will guide suitable and targeted investigations (Table 7.2.1). Knowledge of how biochemical and haematological markers differ from the non-pregnant state is imperative in order to understand the significance of the results. White cell counts are typically increased during pregnancy, as is alkaline phosphatase due to placental production. Biochemical markers such as urea and creatinine fall. A summary of the variations seen in the more common investigations performed during pregnancy is given in Table 7.2.2.

There has been much debate about the suitability of varying imaging modalities during pregnancy, largely due to concerns about the effect on the fetus. Ultrasound is considered safe and is widely used, and can be useful in the diagnosis of, for example, appendicitis and renal tract obstruction. Diagnosis of renal tract obstruction

**Table 7.2.1** Differential diagnoses, key finding and investigations

| Disorder | Key clinical features | Specific investigations | Management |
|---|---|---|---|
| **Obstetric – early pregnancy** | | | |
| Miscarriage | Pain and bleeding | USS, HCG and progesterone levels | Expectant, Medical or surgical. See Chapter 57, Problems in early pregnancy |
| Ectopic pregnancy | Pain followed by a small amount of bleeding, peritonism, shoulder tip and rectal pain, may present with diarrhoea | USS, HCG and progesterone levels | Expectant, Medical or surgical. See Chapter 57, Problems in early pregnancy |
| Ruptured corpus luteal cyst | Signs of peritonism | USS | Analgesia ± laparoscopy |
| Adnexal torsion | Twisting pain, peritonism. More common in 1st trimester and postpartum | USS | Analgesia ± laparoscopy |
| **Obstetric – late pregnancy** | | | |
| Round ligament pain | Bilateral, stitch like | None | Analgesia and reassurance |
| Braxton Hicks | Painful/painless tightenings not causing cervical dilatation | Vaginal examination to exclude labour | Reassurance |
| Labour | Painful contractions | Vaginal examination, CTG etc. | Consider tocolysis and steroids if preterm |
| Placental abruption | Constant pain, rigid uterus, sometimes frequent and short-lasting contractions ± bleeding | Fetal assessment, bloods | Resuscitation, delivery |
| Pre-eclampsia | Epigastric, right upper quadrant | All PET investigations | Treat blood pressure, consider delivery |
| Polyhydramnios | Tight, distended abdomen, difficult to feel fetal parts | USS, exclude diabetes, infection (TORCH) | Detailed fetal scan, consider amnio-drainage |
| Adnexal torsion | Twisting pain, peritonism | USS | Analgesia ± laparoscopy |
| Fibroid degeneration | Constant localized pain, over the fibroid | USS to confirm fibroids. Degenerative cystic changes may be present. | Analgesia |
| Uterine rupture | Sudden onset constant pain, haemodynamic collapse, vaginal bleed, haematuria | All bloods, crossmatch, CTG | Resuscitate and surgery |
| Acute fatty liver | Epigastric/right upper quadrant pain, often associated with malaise, nausea and vomiting. May be jaundiced and have ascites | All PET investigations – may have hyperuricaemia, hypoglycaemia, deranged LFTs. USS/CT or MRI liver | Stabilize and deliver |
| Urinary retention (retroverted uterus) | Unable to pass urine, palpable and uncomfortable bladder | Catheter. USS will help exclude other causes | Conservative management. Usually resolves after 12 weeks |
| Physiological obstruction of ureters | Renal angle tenderness | USS to assess renal pelviectasis (2 cm normal) | Usually conservative, if significant, may require nephrostomy |
| Chorioamnionitis | Tender uterus, offensive discharge, systemic signs of sepsis, usually preceded by ruptured membranes | Blood cultures, inflammatory markers, speculum, CTG | Intravenous antibiotics, resuscitate and deliver |

(*Continued*)

Antenatal complications: maternal

| Symphysis pubis dysfunction | Suprapubic tenderness, over bone. Worse on movement and standing on one leg | Full physiotherapy assessment | Physiotherapy, analgesia |
|---|---|---|---|
| Rectus abdominis rupture | Sudden onset pain, usually precipitated by cough or vomit. Rare and usually in multiparous women. May have associated haematoma | Exclude other causes of abdominal pain | Analgesia. Expanding haematoma may require surgical exploration |
| **Non-obstetric** | | | |
| **Renal tract causes** – Urinary tract infection | Dysuria, frequency of micturition | Urine dipstick, urine for culture | Increase oral intake of fluid, antibiotics |
| Pyelonephritis | Loin pain (renal angle tenderness), radiating round to abdomen and into groin, rigors | Blood cultures, urine dipstick and culture, renal ultrasound scan | Antipyretics, i.v. antibiotics, i.v. fluids |
| Renal calculi | Loin pain (renal angle tenderness), radiating round to abdomen and into groin, often colicky in nature | Urine dipstick (microscopic haematuria), urine for culture, renal ultrasound scan | Conservative management with fluids and analgesia, involve urologists |
| **Gastrointestinal tract causes** – Constipation | Constant or colicky abdominal pain, infrequent, hard stools | | Dietary advice, stool softeners |
| Gastritis/peptic ulcer disease | Epigastric pain, often constant or burning. Duodenal ulcers relieved by food, gastric ulcers made worse by food. May be associated with nausea, vomiting, haematemesis | Gastroscopy if severe. Involve gastroenterologists | Antacids and ulcer healing drugs – H2 receptor antagonists/ proton pump inhibitors |
| Appendicitis | Pain, not always localized to right iliac fossa, especially in third trimester. Signs of peritonism. Associated anorexia, nausea, vomiting and pyrexia | Inflammatory markers (white blood cell count, c-reactive protein), ultrasound abdomen. Pyuria may be present | Involve general surgeons, surgical management |
| Bowel obstruction | Colicky abdominal pain, associated with vomiting and nil passed per rectum. High pitched or absent bowel sounds. Usually have risk factors. Perforation will cause signs of peritonism | Abdominal x-ray. Involve general surgeons. Colonoscopy | Conservative management – intravenous fluids, nasogastric tube. May require surgery |
| Cholecystitis/cholelithiasis | Epigastric or right upper quadrant pain (colicky or stabbing). May radiate through to back and be associated with nausea and vomiting. Intolerance of fatty food. Tenderness and guarding | Ultrasound of gallbladder/ liver, liver function tests | Conservative management – analgesia, fluids, antibiotics if infected. Surgery may be indicated (see text) |
| Pancreatitis | Epigastric pain, radiates through to back. Associated with nausea and vomiting | Ultrasound upper abdomen, CT scan liver function tests, amylase and lipase three times normal, calcium low, high blood glucose | Involve surgeons, conservative management. Use of prognostic scoring systems |
| Gastroenteritis | Generalized, usually crampy abdominal pains, associated with diarrhoea and vomiting | Stool sample | Fluids, manage at home if possible |

PART TWO: OBSTETRICS: ANTENATAL

*(Continued)*

| Hepatitis | Right upper quadrant/epigastric pain. May be associated with jaundice | Ultrasound liver, liver function tests, hepatits screen | Involve hepatologist, depends on underlying cause |
|---|---|---|---|
| Strangulated hernia | Peritonism, may be associated with bowel obstruction | Involve surgeons | Involve surgeons, treat bowel obstruction |
| Inflammatory bowel disease | Generalized pain, associated diarrhoea, mucus and rectal bleeding, vomiting, weight loss | Inflammatory markers, sigmoidoscopy, colonoscopy | Involve gastroenterologists, steroids, mesalamine, other immune modulators such as azathrioprine |
| **Other** – abdominal bleeding | Very rare. Ruptured liver capsule, splenic artery aneurysms, aortic aneurysms, cause haemorrhagic shock and abdominal pain | FBC, crossmatch, assess fetal well-being with CTG | Resuscitate, surgical management |
| Pelvic vein thrombosis | Often thrombosis of right/left iliac vein, causing groin tenderness, leg swelling, sometimes pyrexia | Doppler ultrasound, venogram, thrombophilia screen | Anticoagulation using low molecular weight heparin, involve haematologists, may require filter in inferior vena cava |
| Systemic causes, e.g. DKA, increased calcium, sickle cell crisis | Generalized abdominal pain, associated with being systemically unwell | Urea, electrolytes, blood glucose, bone profile | Treatment dependent on cause, involve the general physicians |
| Trauma – remember domestic violence | Associated with bruising. Domestic violence commonly results in abdominal trauma during pregnancy | Assessment of fetal well-being, kleihauer, particularly if rhesus negative. Check for other injuries | Ensure safety, specialist mid-wifery service, social input |
| Pneumonia | Right lower lobe pneumonia may cause right upper quadrant pain. Associated with respiratory symptoms | Chest x-ray, blood gases, inflammatory markers, sputum cultures | Antibiotics, may require oxygen and high dependency support if severe |

**Table 7.2.2** Biochemical and haematological variations in pregnancy

| Investigation | Non-pregnant | Pregnant | Notes |
|---|---|---|---|
| Haemoglobin g/dL | 12–15 | 11–14 | Haemoglobin falls, to lowest at around 32 weeks |
| White cell count $\times 10^9$/L | 4–11 | 6–16 | White cells increase. Further increases in response to steroids when given for lung maturity, and in labour |
| Platelets $\times 10^9$/L | 150–400 | Can fall by around 10% in pregnancy | |
| C reactive protein g/L | Does not vary in pregnancy | | |
| Urea mmol/L | 2.7–7.5 | <4.5 | Falls with increasing gestation |
| Creatinine µmol/L | 65–100 | <75 | |
| Amylase | Generally unchanged in pregnancy | | |
| Uric acid (urate) mmol/L | 0.18–0.35 | Generally considered as $0.1 \times$ no of weeks gestation, e.g. 0.35 at 35 weeks | |
| AST/ALT IU/L | <40 | Both usually lower in pregnancy, with 30 as upper limit of normal | |
| Alkaline phosphatase iu/L | 30–130 | Increases with gestation, up to around 400 | |

**Table 7.2.3** Radiation exposures[4,12,13]

| Procedure | Fetal exposure | Fetal exposure in dose equivalents |
|---|---|---|
| Background radiation exposure | 0.002 cGy/week | 3.1 mSv/year |
| Long haul flight | – | 0.3 mSv |
| Chest/skull x-ray per film | <0.001 cGy | 0.04 mSv |
| Mammogram | 0.0004 cGy | 0.13 mSv |
| Ventilation/perfusion scan with $^{99m}$Tc | <0.2 cGy | 1.5 mSv |
| Abdominal x-ray per film | 0.1 cGy | 1 mSv |
| Intravenous pyelography | >1 cGy depending on number of images | 6 mSv |
| Bone imaging with $^{99m}$Tc | <0.5 cGy | 4.4 mSv |
| Abdominal CT | 2–5 rad | 10 mSv |
| Barium enema | 1.6 cGy | 7 mSv |
| Pelvic CT | 2.5 cGy | 10 mSv |

- Rad is the old non-SI unit of radiation. 1 rad = 0.01 Gray (Gy) = 1 cGy. As different types of radiation have a different impact on the human body, the dose equivalent is used in order to allow meaningful comparisons of damage. This incorporates a modifying factor (energy deposited per unit mass of tissue). The SI unit of this is the Sievert (Sv), and the non-SI is the rem and 1 centi-Sv = 1 rem.

is a common example of difficulties in interpretation of scan findings. Physiological dilatation of the renal collecting system occurs in pregnancy due to a combination of compression and smooth muscle relaxation secondary to progesterone. A physiological dilation of up to 2 cm is considered 'acceptable', and is often greater on the right. Signs helpful in the differentiation of physiological from pathological obstruction have been suggested. In physiological dilatation, the ureter will taper to a normal calibre as is crosses the pelvic brim, but in pathological dilatation, this is lost. Also, ureteric 'jets of urine' entering the bladder can be seen in physiological dilatation, a phenomenon that is also lost in pathological dilatation.[3]

Investigations involving ionizing radiation have often been avoided during pregnancy due to concerns about the radiation effect on the fetus in terms of teratogenesis, pregnancy loss and future malignancy. However, the overall risks are very small. Fetal risks, thought to be maximal with exposure between 8 and 15 weeks, are not increased by exposures less than 5 rad. Risks of subsequent carcinogenesis are also small. It is estimated that a 1–2 rad exposure may increase the risk of leukaemia from 1:3000 to 1:2000.[4]

Table 7.2.3 gives approximate radiation doses of various types of investigation. To put this into context, these are much lower than a long-haul intercontinental flight that provides a 15 mrem dose of radiation, and a short haul flight that provides 6 mrem.[5] Thus, fetal risks are minimal and should not prevent an important investigation in pregnancy.

## DIFFERENTIAL DIAGNOSES

A list of specific differential diagnoses, investigations and management are given in Table 7.2.1. Several are discussed in other sections of the book. Hence, detailed descriptions are given only for significant conditions not discussed elsewhere.

### Appendicitis

Appendicitis is the most common cause of an acute surgical abdomen during pregnancy, with an incidence of 1:500–2000 pregnancies, and it accounts for 25 per cent on surgery for non-obstetric indications. As previously discussed, diagnosis is often hampered due to the physiological effects of pregnancy. Ultrasound is useful, although less so during the third trimester, or if the appendix has perforated. As a result, approximately 40 per cent of pregnant patients who undergo appendicectomy have a normal appendix.[2] Perforation of the appendix is associated with significant fetal and maternal mortality. Fetal loss rates of up to 20–35 per cent have been reported, partly due to the high incidence of preterm labour secondary to peritonitis. Not surprisingly, maternal mortality increases in the third trimester.

Management of appendicitis is surgical, and involving general surgical colleagues early is recommended. Surgery can be open, using an incision over the point of maximal tenderness (may be right paramedian or midline in late pregnancy), or laparoscopic. Laparoscopic surgery is now considered acceptable during pregnancy, even during the third trimester.[6] A 15 mmHg pneumoperitoneum is well tolerated by the fetus. Reports in the literature describe veress needle insertion either in the mid-clavicular line, 2 cm below the inferior costal margin, or the open Hasson technique. The open Hasson entry technique is recommended as it avoids insufflation of the uterus which would be catastrophic to the fetus. In cases in which there is diffuse peritonitis, intravenous antibiotics are recommended pre-operatively. Caesarean section may also need to be considered if the mother is severely unwell, particularly as gestation approaches term.

### Acute cholecystitis

Acute cholecystitis is the second most common surgical cause of an acute abdomen in pregnancy, with an incidence of between 1:1600 and 1:10 000 pregnancies. Over 90 per cent of cases are caused by gallstones, and gallstones are an incidental finding in between 3.5 and 10 per cent of pregnant women.[2] This is likely to increase as women continue to delay pregnancies until they are older. Gallstone formation is more likely in pregnancy as progesterone predisposes to increased bile stasis and high levels of oestrogen increase the lithogenicity of bile. The signs and symptoms are largely the same as those found outside pregnancy and are summarized in Table 7.2.1. Serum levels of direct bilirubin and transaminases may be raised, and amylase may be raised. Alkaline phosphatase is of limited use due to placental production. Ultrasound will detect 95–98 per cent of gallstones, and in acute cholecystits, gallbladder thickening (>3 mm), pericholecystic fluid, sonographic Murphy's sign (focal tenderness under transducer when positioned over gallbladder) and dilatation of the intra- and extrahepatic ducts will be present.

Management can be medical or surgical. Until recently, medical management was more common, with surgery being delayed until after delivery of the baby. However, reports have shown that delaying surgery is associated with a high recurrence rate (44–92 per cent), longer hospital stay, increased risk of gallstone pancreatitis (up to 13 per cent), spontaneous miscarriage and preterm labour.[2] Therefore, surgical management using laparoscopic or open cholecystectomy during pregnancy is growing in popularity. Endoscopic retrograde cholangiopancreatography (ERCP) can also be used during pregnancy, using techniques to reduce the fetal radiation dose.

## Bowel obstruction

The incidence of bowel obstruction in pregnancy is 1:1500–16 000 pregnancies and in most patients is caused by adhesions.[2] Volvulus is a more common cause (approximately 25 per cent) in pregnancy compared with non-pregnancy and is believed to be due to the rapid change in size of the uterus having a physical influence on the surrounding mobile organs such as the caecum. High maternal (6 per cent) and fetal (26 per cent) mortality rates have been reported, particularly in the third trimester.[7] Bowel surgeons should be involved in the management, and series have suggested that nearly a quarter of cases will require surgical resection.[7]

## Pancreatitis

Acute pancreatitis has an incidence of between one in 1000 to one in 3000 pregnancies, and is most common during the second and third trimesters and in the puerperium.[8] As in the non-pregnant state, the two most frequent causes are gallstones and alcohol. Symptoms, signs and management are the same as outside pregnancy. Pancreatitis can range from mild disease through to a severe necrotizing form. Most, around 80 per cent, are mild and self limiting. Serum amylase and lipase are key

in the diagnosis and will typically be three times the upper limit of normal. Lipase is more sensitive and therefore is currently the recommended test.[9] Although these enzymes are useful for diagnosis, they do not aid in assessment of severity or prognosis. Prediction of which patients will progress to severe life-threatening disease is challenging. Therefore, there are several grading systems currently in use: Ranson's criteria, Glasgow score and the APACHE II (Acute Physiology and Chronic Health Evaluation) assessment. Unfortunately, these systems are more complex to use in pregnancy as they do not account for the physiological effects of pregnancy on parameters such as white blood cell count. Therefore, management should involve surgical colleagues and is largely supportive with bowel rest, fluids, monitoring and analgesia. It has been suggested that pethidine and tramadol should be used as analgesia as they do not cause spasm of the sphincter of Oddi.[2] Women who are severely ill may require delivery of the baby.

## Renal stones

Renal stones occur in approximately 1:200–1:2000 pregnancies, and may be associated with preterm labour.[6] Management should involve the urologists, and between 64 and 84 per cent will resolve with conservative management of fluids and analgesia.[10] Ultrasound is the initial investigation, but this may miss a partial blockage. Thus, intravenous urogram (IVU or IVP) may be required. Outside pregnancy, unenhanced helical CT is the gold standard for diagnosis, and reports of use in pregnancy can be found in the literature. However, both these modalities involve a higher radiation dose. The presence of uncontrolled pain, sepsis, single kidney obstruction or preterm labour indicates that further interventions are required. Percututaneous nephrostomy or a ureteric stent can be used to temporarily relieve the obstruction. However, these may require replacing every 6–8 weeks. Ureteroscopy with Holmium laser is an option in pregnancy for stones smaller than 1 cm, and without sepsis.[11]

## KEY POINTS

- Abdominal pain is very common in pregnancy.
- A systematic approach is required to identify serious from non-serious pathology.
- Differential diagnoses should be considered as pregnancy and non-pregnancy related.
- Diagnosis may be hampered by the physiological changes associated with pregnancy.
- Investigations should not be limited by pregnancy, particularly if the well-being of the mother may be adversely influenced.
- Appropriate involvement of other specialties is indicated.

## Key References

1. Lewis G (ed.). *The Confidential Enquiry into Maternal and Child Health (CEMACH). Saving Mothers' Lives: reviewing maternal deaths to make motherhood safer – 2003–2005.* London: CEMACH, 2007.

2. Augustin G, Majerovic M. Non-obstetrical acute abdomen during pregnancy. *Eur J Obstet Gynecol Reprod Biol* 2007; **131**: 4–12.

3. Nair U. Acute abdomen and abdominal pain in pregnancy. *Curr Obstet Gynaecol* 2005; **15**: 359–67.

4. ACOG Committee Opinion. Number 299, September 2004 (replaces No. 158, September 1995). Guidelines for diagnostic imaging during pregnancy. *Obstet Gynecol* 2004; **104**: 647–51.

5. Barish RJ. In-flight radiation exposure during pregnancy. *Obstet Gynecol* 2004; **103**: 1326–30.

6. Kilpatrick CC, Orejuela FJ. Management of the acute abdomen in pregnancy: a review. *Curr Opin Obstet Gynecol* 2008; **20**: 534–9.

7. Perdue PW, Johnson HW Jr, Stafford PW. Intestinal obstruction complicating pregnancy. *Am J Surg* 1992; **164**: 384–8.

8. Ramin KD, Ramin SM, Richey SD, Cunningham FG. Acute pancreatitis in pregnancy. *Am J Obstet Gynecol* 1995; **173**: 187–91.

9. Rickes S, Uhle C. Advances in the diagnosis of acute pancreatitis. *Postgrad Med J* 2009; **85**: 208–12.

10. Srirangam SJ, Hickerton B, Van Cleynenbreugel B. Management of urinary calculi in pregnancy: a review. *J Endourol* 2008; **22**: 867–75.

11. McAleer SJ, Loughlin KR. Nephrolithiasis and pregnancy. *Curr Opin Urol* 2004; **14**: 123–7.

12. Fattibene P, Mazzei F, Nuccetelli C, Risica S. Prenatal exposure to ionising radiation: sources, effects and regulatory aspects. *Acta Paediatr* 1999; **88**: 693–702.

13. Stabin MG. Doses from medical radiation sources. Health Physics Society Articles. Last accessed April 2010. Available from: http://hps.org/hpspublications/articles/dosesfrommedicalradiation.html.

# 7.3 Malignancy

*Louise Kenny*

Pregnancy does not affect the course of cancer *per se*. However, diagnosis is often delayed as the presenting symptoms of malignancy may be confused with the common symptoms of pregnancy. Both the investigation and treatment of a malignancy may carry risks for the fetus, and serious conflict may occur between the desire to treat the mother appropriately while limiting harm to the pregnancy.[1] Future prospects for childbearing may be subsequently limited by surgery, radiotherapy and chemotherapy. Psychological adjustment to a diagnosis of cancer is likely to be more difficult while pregnant.[2]

Managing cancer during pregnancy therefore requires a multidisciplinary approach involving obstetricians, oncologists, paediatricians and counsellors. The role of an individual midwife or oncology nurse should not be underestimated [E].

## EBM

Evidence to support management decisions in pregnancies complicated by cancer is derived mostly from retrospective uncontrolled studies [D]. Few case-control studies have been performed and the paucity of good-quality evidence must be made clear during patient counselling.

## INTRODUCTION

Approximately one in every 1000 pregnancies is complicated by a new diagnosis of cancer. Traditionally, cervical cancer has been reported as the most common malignancy with an incidence of 0.8 per 1000 pregnancies. The incidence in the developed world would appear to have reduced to approximately 0.3 per 1000 with the advent of suitable screening, matching that of breast cancer. In comparison, the incidence of melanoma is variably reported between 0.2:1000 and 2.6:1000, making it potentially the most common malignancy diagnosed during pregnancy. In general, the distribution of cancers occurring in pregnancy mirrors the distribution of cancer in young women. This distribution may change as more women choose to start their families later in life.

## RADIOTHERAPY AND CHEMOTHERAPY DURING PREGNANCY

Fetal exposure to radiation and/or chemotherapeutic agents may potentially have a number of detrimental effects. These include:

- miscarriage and intrauterine fetal death,
- congenital anomalies,
- severe mental retardation (SMR) and microcephaly,
- prenatal and postnatal growth restriction,
- increase in the risk of childhood malignancy,
- infertility in the offspring,
- induction of germline genetic abnormalities.

Counselling couples about the fetal risks associated with cancer treatment is complicated by a lack of high-quality evidence. There have been no randomized trials, and publication and ascertainment bias skew the available data. Studies often involve small numbers and are retrospective and unsystematic in their approach and follow up. Chemotherapy and radiotherapy are often used in combination and the contributory effects of the illness itself on the pregnancy are impossible to isolate from other variables. Data are often out of date and irrelevant to newer management regimes. Experimental data from animal studies can be helpful, but there are marked interspecies differences and caution must be exercised in extrapolating directly to human pregnancies. Remember also that the background fetal anomaly rate is variably quoted as 3–6 per cent. All studies should be interpreted with this in mind.

## Radiation exposure during pregnancy

Radiation dose is measured in Grays and rads.

1 Gray (1 Gy) = 100 rad
1 centiGray (cGy) = 1 rad

Calculating fetal exposure and radiation absorption during radiotherapy and radiological investigations is complicated and often imprecise. Although the primary radiation beam can be accurately directed and quantified, additional exposure occurs from leakage through the head of the linear accelerator, external scatter from beam modifiers and internal scatter within the patient. With appropriate shielding, fetal exposure can be reduced by as much as 50 per cent, although the effects of shielding also can be difficult to quantify. The gestation at which exposure occurs is also important for two reasons. Most importantly, fetal tissues show differential radiosensitivity throughout the course of the pregnancy (see below). Second, a larger fetus is more difficult to shield effectively and may lie closer to the irradiated field.

The effects of prenatal exposure to ionizing radiation are described as either deterministic or stochastic. Deterministic effects are those where loss of function occurs due to cell destruction. The severity of the effect is dose related and a critical threshold exists below which the effect is not seen. Miscarriage, intrauterine death, congenital anomalies and SMR are believed to follow this pattern. Stochastic effects are those where ionizing radiation causes genetic cell modification and loss of cell cycle control, which, after a period of latency, leads to the development of cancer. Stochastic effects also demonstrate a dose–effect relationship, but without a threshold value.[3]

- Very early exposure to radiation during pregnancy (pre-implantation and early organogenesis; 0–2 weeks post-conception) will either result in miscarriage or the pregnancy will continue unaffected.

- Mammalian animal experiments show that congenital abnormalities are more likely when exposure occurs during early organogenesis (3–7 weeks post-conception in a human pregnancy).

- Generalized growth and neurological development continue throughout normal pregnancy. Microcephaly, SMR and permanent growth restriction remain potential risks for the fetus exposed during the remainder of the pregnancy. The 8–15-week period appears to be the time of highest risk and corresponds to a critical stage of cortical formation and organization. There is minimal risk after 25 weeks, unless very high exposures occur.

- An increased predisposition to malignancy later in life appears to be a risk whatever the gestational age at which exposure occurs.

Evidence for the effects of radiation exposure during pregnancy is derived from three sources:

1 animal experiments,[4]
2 accidental human exposures,
3 the Japanese survivors of the atomic bomb.[5,6]

The high rate of fetal loss occurring with exposure during pre-implantation (conception to day 10) has been confirmed by rodent experiments and epidemiological data from Nagasaki and Hiroshima. Miscarriage and intrauterine death occur with a threshold of 10 cGy in these first few weeks; however, this increases steadily towards term, at which time the lower threshold for causing intrauterine death is estimated as >1 Gy.[3]

Animal experiments, mostly involving rodents, have shown that exposure during organogenesis causes a variety of congenital anomalies, notably involving the skeleton, eye and urinary tract. The threshold, extrapolating to humans, is possibly as low as 5 cGy, with a marked dose–response effect. However, human studies have failed to find this effect, with the exception of microcephaly. Teratogenesis should nevertheless remain a concern. It may be that the critically sensitive time in the human fetus is shorter, or that pregnancies with major anomalies abort spontaneously or have gone unrecorded.

Destruction of neural cells or failure of their migration may lead to microcephaly and/or mental retardation. Data from Japan[6] have estimated a lower threshold for microcephaly of 10 rad, with the 8–15-week period being most crucial. The incidence of microcephaly was 40 per cent with exposures of 50 cGy or higher. Severe mental retardation was also found more commonly in the offspring exposed between 8 and 25 weeks, with lower thresholds for SMR of 6 cGy (8–15 weeks) and 28 cGy (16–25 weeks). Studies of intelligence quotient (IQ) reflect these observations.[7]

There are fewer data on the effect of the radiation exposure on developing germ cells. Delayed menarche has been observed in Japanese girls exposed to radiation in utero with a threshold of 25 rad. No increase in the rates of infertility has yet been demonstrated.

A safe exposure limit of 5 cGy during pregnancy has been suggested. However, this does not take account of possible stochastic effects that do not show a lower threshold. An increase in childhood malignancies has been reported in a famous Oxford study of pelvimetry during pregnancy in which exposures were typically 1 cGy (Oxford Survey of Childhood Cancers).[5,8] The background rate of childhood malignancy is one in 1300 before the age of 15. This study gave a relative risk of 1.4 for those offspring exposed *in utero* to pelvimetry. A pelvic computed tomography (CT) scan typically exposes a fetus to approximately 2.5 cGy and this is thought to double the risk of a childhood malignancy. Clearly, setting a 5 cGy 'safe limit' may be considered simplistic, and the debate continues. Table 7.2.3, p. 148, in Chapter 7.2, Abdominal pain, lists the mean fetal dose exposures predicted for various investigations. It is important to realize, however, that the actual dose is dependent on many factors and that the true value may be 5-fold higher.

In practice, if cross-section imaging of the pelvis or abdomen is required during pregnancy, magnetic resonance imaging (MRI) is preferred over the use of CT scanning [E]. It is likely that single exposures to radiation carry greater fetal risk than divided doses, adding further to the difficulties in applying the available human data to real diagnostic and therapeutic scenarios [D].

Radiotherapy to the pelvis is contraindicated in pregnancy due to the effects on the fetus, which cannot be shielded. There are, however, other cancers for which radiotherapy is a viable treatment modality; shielding of the pelvis enables sufficient reduction in exposure to the fetus after the first trimester to allow the use of radiotherapy in the treatment of a number of cancers, e.g. breast cancer and lymphomas.

## KEY POINTS

- The dose required to induce embryonal lethality increases sharply during the first trimester from 0.1 cGy at day 1 to over 1 Gy after the first trimester. The fetal effects of radiation include intrauterine death, congenital malformations, developmental or growth restriction and late malignancy.
- Within the first 2 weeks post-implantation, exposure to radiation is thought to be an all-or-nothing effect (resulting in fetal death if affected). Conversely, anomalies result from exposure (to doses above 0.1 Gy) in the later weeks of the first trimester.
- Radiotherapy to the pelvis is contraindicated in pregnancy due to the effects on the fetus, which cannot be shielded. There are, however, other cancers for which radiotherapy is a viable treatment modality.

## Chemotherapy and pregnancy

Prior to implantation, the blastocyst is immune to the effects of chemotherapy. The period of organogenesis between 5 and 10 weeks is, however, a critically sensitive time. Exposure to chemotherapy during this period may be associated with malformations in 10–20 per cent of cases [D].[9] After 12 weeks gestation, malformations should be less common, although growth and neurological development remain potentially vulnerable throughout pregnancy.

A number of retrospective studies support these generalizations regarding the importance of the timing of chemotherapy during pregnancy. Congenital malformations seem no more likely if chemotherapy is given only during the second and third trimesters [D].[10] First-trimester exposure does indeed seem more hazardous, and this is somewhat dependent on the agents used [D].[9]

Antimetabolites carry the greatest risks to a first-trimester pregnancy. Although miscarriage is the most common outcome, aminopterin may cause neural tube, skeletal and clefting abnormalities. This anti-neoplastic agent has been replaced by methotrexate, which is structurally similar and has the same effects on the early fetus. Both should be avoided in the first trimester and later in the pregnancy where possible. A 14 per cent congenital anomaly risk has been quoted for alkylating agents (e.g. cyclophosphamide) if given in the first trimester. This risk falls to near background levels for administration in the second and third trimester. Antibiotics such as doxorubicin and bleomycin do not have clear teratogenic effects, although they are still to be avoided in the first trimester where possible. Vinca alkaloids, such as vincristine and vinblastine, are harmful in animal pregnancies but this effect is not obvious in the few human pregnancies so far exposed in the first trimester [D]. Information is constantly updated with regard to the use of these drugs during pregnancy and it is wise to consult a drug information bureau before deciding management.

Other effects of fetal exposure to chemotherapy in the second and third trimesters are even less clear. Studies are conflicting with regard to prenatal and postnatal growth restriction, although one review concluded that intrauterine growth restriction occurred in 40 per cent of exposed pregnancies [D].[9]

The longer term effects of fetal exposure to chemotherapy are also unclear. Survivors of cancer who received chemotherapy as children have been followed up closely with the assumption that late complications of treatment in this group might also be expected to occur in individuals exposed *in utero*. Investigators have looked for evidence of impaired intellect, reduced gonadal function (delayed puberty and reduced fertility), visceral damage and mutagenesis within germ cells. However, direct application of findings from individuals treated during childhood to those exposed to chemotherapy *in utero* makes the assumption that fetal cells behave in the same way as those of a child. This may not be the case and fetal germ cells, for example, might be more susceptible to genetic damage than those of an older child. However, there is currently no robust evidence to suggest that future fertility may be affected or to suggest any intellectual impairment or increase in the genetic problems in the next generation.

A more consistent effect of chemotherapy on the fetus is myelosuppression. A third of newborns delivered to women who received treatment for leukaemia during their pregnancy showed evidence of bone marrow suppression in one study [D].[11] Fortunately, this is rarely of clinical importance, and sepsis, serious anaemia and haemorrhage are uncommon in the neonate. However, it is good practice to avoid myelosuppressive agents in the 3 weeks prior to delivery, if possible [E].

Decisions regarding the timing of operative delivery should aim to avoid the increased susceptibility to maternal infection if performed within 2 weeks of a cycle of chemotherapy. Similarly, those prescribing chemotherapy need to be aware of the potentially dramatic dose changes required both during pregnancy and following delivery, due to the attendant physiological changes.

Despite the lack of evidence for major harm from chemotherapy in the second and third trimesters, breastfeeding is usually discouraged if treatment continues into the puerperium [E]. This reflects unresolved uncertainties about the true safety of these agents and the knowledge that significant quantities do reach breast milk.

## SYMPTOM CONTROL IN THE PREGNANT PATIENT WITH CANCER

The symptoms of cancer and of normal pregnancy overlap and can easily be confused. Early satiety, nausea and vomiting, constipation, dyspnoea, fatigue and depression are all common during a normal pregnancy but can also be significant symptoms of malignancy. Every effort should be made to determine symptom aetiology when a known cancer co-exists with pregnancy. Shortness of breath, for example, may simply be the effect of high progesterone levels and expanded tidal volume typical of the third trimester. However, in the cancer patient it may be a sign of pleural effusions, significant anaemia or lung metastases. Similarly, nausea and vomiting may have a more sinister cause, such as hypercalcaemia, electrolyte imbalance, uraemia and even intracranial metastases. Early advice from an oncologist should be sought when new symptoms arise.

Pain should be managed with paracetamol and opiates. Non-steroidal anti-inflammatory drugs are best avoided, especially in the third trimester. Tricyclic antidepressants can be safely used for neuropathic pain, but carbamazepine should not (see Chapter 8, Medication in pregnancy) [B].

Poor appetite may be secondary to depression, pain and nausea and vomiting. Treatments for nausea include metoclopramide, prochlorperazine and cyclizine. Ondansetron and haloperidol can be used if necessary. Prednisone is effective for a number of symptoms, including nausea, anorexia and fatigue. Cannabis seems to be beneficial in a number of ways but is not advised during pregnancy [C]. Constipation is effectively treated with docusate, magnesium hydroxide and senna, all of which are safe in pregnancy.

The psychological adjustment to a diagnosis of cancer is always difficult, seldom more so than during pregnancy. Fears of limited life expectancy deprive couples of future hopes and plans for themselves and their family. Focusing on short-term goals and enjoying the present are so much harder to do during pregnancy. More specifically, there may be anxieties regarding the effect of the disease or its treatment on the fetus. The question of termination of a wanted pregnancy will be extremely distressing. There may be conflict over what is best for the woman herself and what will do least harm to the pregnancy. Concern for other children and anxieties about future fertility add further to the crisis. There is remarkably little research or evidence to guide practice, but the involvement of a mental health team or counselling service should be offered at the very least.

---

## KEY POINTS

- Most cytotoxic chemotherapy molecules are small enough to cross the placenta and affect the fetus.
- The estimated risk of major teratogenicity in the first trimester is approximately 10-20 per cent. Use of combination agents increases the risk.
- Exposure during the second and third trimesters may give rise to growth restriction, prematurity and stillbirth, but is unlikely to be teratogenic.
- Delayed effects of exposure to chemotherapeutic agents appears to be rare. The currently available evidence suggests that there are no significant adverse effects on fertility or intellectual and neurological development in those exposed.
- No published data exist to suggest any increase in the rate of childhood malignancies in those subjected to chemotherapy *in utero*.
- Chemotherapy, where other treatment modalities are considered unsuitable, is therefore considered relatively safe in the second and third trimesters. Patients should be counselled regarding the increased risks of growth restriction (and consequent premature delivery) and stillbirth.
- There is no evidence to support using a reduced dose of chemotherapy in pregnancy [E].

# SPECIFIC EXAMPLES

## Breast cancer

Breast cancer accounts for a quarter of all cancers diagnosed in pregnancy, occurring in approximately one in 3000 pregnancies. Stage for stage, the outcome is no different from that for breast cancers diagnosed outside pregnancy [B].[12] Continuing the pregnancy certainly does not seem to have a deleterious effect on outcome, and termination of pregnancy is not indicated for this reason [D]. However, at diagnosis, pregnancy-associated breast cancer tends to be larger in size, more advanced and more likely to have metastasized to local lymph nodes. This, in part, may be due to the six-month average delay in its diagnosis. This is thought to increase the risk of nodal metastases by at least 10 per cent.

Breast masses are common in pregnancy. Lactational adenomas, galactocoeles, mastitis and infarction of hypertrophied breast tissue are all benign pregnancy-induced breast lumps that may masquerade as malignancy. Breast enlargement, greater vascularity and increased tissue density add to the diagnostic difficulty. Mammography is safe with appropriate shielding but has a lower sensitivity in pregnancy. Fine-needle aspiration or excisional biopsy should be performed if there is any suspicion of malignancy. Once carcinoma has been diagnosed, a chest x-ray may be needed for staging, and once again this is safe with shielding [E]. CT scanning for metastases should be replaced by ultrasound and MRI. If necessary, technetium bone scans can be employed, exposing the pregnancy to 0.5 cGy.

A common surgical option for breast cancer is lumpectomy followed by post-operative chest-wall radiotherapy to reduce local recurrence risks. Radiotherapy for breast cancer might typically be 50 Gy. With appropriate shielding, fetal exposure may be as little as 4 cGy at very early gestations (5 weeks), rising to 14–18 cGy in the second trimester when the uterus is larger. This is above the 'accepted' threshold of safety, and a modified radical mastectomy, which does not necessitate post-operative radiotherapy, should normally be advised during pregnancy instead [E]. The surgery itself carries minimal risk, if any, to the fetus. Conservative breast surgery can sometimes be performed in the third trimester, with adjunctive radiotherapy delayed until the puerperium.

Chemotherapy for breast cancer in the second and third trimesters is not associated with obvious fetal harm.[13] Where possible, the last dose should be given 3 weeks prior to delivery to limit the effects of fetal bone marrow suppression [E]. Tamoxifen use in pregnancy has previously been discouraged. Experiments in rodents have demonstrated anomalies similar to those found with *in-utero* diethylstilbestrol (DES) exposure and an increased intrauterine fetal death rate. Although these effects appear to be species

specific, there are only minimal human data testifying to the safety of tamoxifen in pregnancy and its use is not currently recommended.

Fetal surveillance by regular growth scanning is warranted, although a clear link with prenatal growth restriction has not been established. Placental metastases are found very rarely and there are no reports of breast cancer spreading to the fetus. Some authors suggest delivery at 34 weeks to limit the fetal exposure to chemotherapeutic agents. Others await spontaneous labour if fetal growth is normal. Neonatal blood sampling is necessary to exclude clinically relevant pancytopenia.

## Pregnancy after breast cancer

With the high background incidence of breast cancer and progressive delay in childbearing, it is not uncommon now to be asked for advice on this matter. Four studies are cited which have failed to show any effect on survival if pregnancy occurs after breast cancer [B].[14–17] Although it can be argued that women with a more favourable prognosis are more likely to consider a pregnancy, the survival among node-positive patients was not affected by pregnancy either. It has been suggested that becoming pregnant soon after breast cancer may affect long-term survival and that a delay should be advised. Studies that demonstrate a survival advantage with such a delay may simply be highlighting the improved prognosis for women who remain alive 2–5 years after the diagnosis. For younger women (who have a worse prognosis anyway), a delay of 2–5 years will have minimal impact on fertility. Allowing more time will help to give a more individualized prognosis. Such a delay may be more difficult to justify in women in their late thirties and forties.

The use of tamoxifen during pregnancy is not recommended (see above). Breastfeeding is not contraindicated, but previous surgery and radiotherapy may impair subsequent lactation.

The following points are the recommendations given in the RCOG guideline.

- There is no indication that termination of pregnancy after diagnosis of breast cancer is necessary to improve the prognosis.
- Women planning pregnancy or who become pregnant after breast cancer should consult their clinical oncologist, surgeon and obstetrician.
- There is no evidence that the survival of women who have had breast cancer and subsequently become pregnant is compromised. However, an interval of at least two, and preferably three, years between treatment and conception is recommended.

## Cervical cancer

Cervical cancer is the most common pregnancy-related gynaecological cancer, although the quoted incidence varies from one in 1200 to one in 10 000 pregnancies. It commonly presents with vaginal bleeding, but discharge and pain may also occur. A high proportion of cases are detected by cervical screening and are otherwise asymptomatic.

## Cervical screening in pregnancy

False-positive cervical smears are more likely during pregnancy for a number of reasons:

- eversion of the squamocolumnar junction occurs as a consequence of high oestrogen levels and exposed columnar epithelium undergoes squamous metaplasia;
- cervical infiltration by leukocytes occurs in pregnancy;
- decidualization of the cervix is a frequent finding;
- trophoblasts may be present in the cervical canal;
- relative immunosuppression may allow greater human papilloma virus (HPV) activity.

It is vital that the cytologist reading the smear is aware that it has been taken from a pregnant woman if false positives are to be kept to a minimum. In the UK it is not usual for routine cervical screening to be carried out in pregnancy, and smears are normally deferred until the postnatal appointment. However, if there is clinical concern regarding the cervix, or if it seems unlikely that the individual will return after the pregnancy for a smear to be carried out, there should be no hesitation in performing it while the woman is pregnant.

Most studies show a high degree of concordance between cytology (smears) and colposcopy [B][18] during pregnancy, but the possibility of false-positive or false-negative results must always be considered.

## Management of an abnormal smear in pregnancy

A reluctance to perform cervical smears during pregnancy may also arise from unfounded anxieties over the subsequent management of the abnormal smear. One study of colposcopy during pregnancy found concordance, overestimation and underestimation of the final diagnosis (based on cone histology) in 73, 17 and 10 per cent, respectively, and this did not differ significantly from the non-pregnant control group.[19] Indeed, unsatisfactory colposcopy is less common during pregnancy due to eversion of the squamocolumnar junction. Squamous metaplasia is more common and the cervix will usually look larger and have increased vascularity. Colposcopy during pregnancy therefore requires experience and careful judgement. Hacker and colleagues demonstrated a 99.5 per cent diagnostic accuracy for colposcopy, with only a 0.5 per cent false-negative rate (with no missed invasive lesions) amongst 1064 pregnant women.[20]

If a smear taken in pregnancy has suggested low-grade cervical intraepithelial neoplasia (CIN) and the colposcopic impression agrees, these women can be managed by repeat colposcopy in each trimester, with a further evaluation in the postpartum period. There is no evidence that CIN progresses more rapidly in pregnancy, and indeed regression rates of 25–70 per cent have been documented for high-grade CIN first detected in pregnancy.[21]

If the colposcopic impression is of a higher grade lesion, it is vital that microinvasive and invasive cancers are excluded. Older studies recorded an unacceptably high rate of complications with knife conization during pregnancy, principally a >500 mL blood loss in 7–13 per cent of cases (mostly in the third trimester).[22] Any causative association with miscarriage, preterm rupture of membranes, preterm delivery and chorioamnionitis remains uncertain, but concerns do exist. These concerns have seen a shift away from conization in pregnancy towards the use of directed punch biopsies, which carry less morbidity. Concordance between directed biopsies and the final diagnosis is complete or within one degree of severity in over 95 per cent of cases [B].[19] Missed invasive lesions are extremely uncommon. Treatment of CIN II and III should be delayed to the postpartum period, but colposcopy every 8 weeks antenatally is advised to monitor for progression of the lesion [E].

Despite this discussion, cervical conization may still be warranted during pregnancy. If invasive cancer cannot be excluded by directed punch biopsies, or colposcopy is inadequate, a cone biopsy may be necessary. Also, 'microinvasion' can only be confirmed on a cone specimen. Although diathermy loop conization has been used in pregnancy, the little evidence there is would suggest that cold knife conization gives fewer positive margins and higher quality biopsy specimens.[23]

Postpartum evaluation is extremely important for women who have antenatal colposcopy, even those who have undergone cone biopsy. Lesions may regress, persist or progress, and the diagnosis made during pregnancy may need to be upgraded. High rates of residual intraepithelial neoplasia and cytological abnormalities have been found following conization, which should not necessarily be considered adequate treatment for CIN during pregnancy.[24]

## Management of cervical cancer in pregnancy

Cervical cancer is normally staged clinically by chest x-ray, cystoscopy, pyelogram and CT or MRI scanning. MRI is the investigation of choice for pelvic imaging during pregnancy.

Cervical cancer is usually treated surgically in its early stages. Chemoradiotherapy is reserved for more advanced disease due to the effects this treatment has on ovarian, bladder, bowel and sexual function. Knife conization may be sufficient treatment for Ia1 (microinvasive) cervical cancer outside pregnancy due to the low risk of recurrence or lymph node (LN) metastases. If this diagnosis is made during pregnancy and the cone biopsy margins are clear, the pregnancy should be allowed to continue, with vaginal delivery. However, the significant rate of positive margins and residual disease found with conization in pregnancy make further evaluation in the postpartum period imperative.[24] For women who have completed their families, a postpartum simple hysterectomy with ovarian conservation is recommended [E].

Higher grade lesions (Ib1–IIa) are usually treated by simple or radical hysterectomy with lymph node sampling. Cancers presenting at less than 20 weeks gestation have traditionally been treated immediately [E]. The hysterectomy can usually be performed with the fetus *in situ*, however, a hysterotomy, avoiding the lower part of the uterus, can be employed to remove the pregnancy and improve access if necessary. Delaying treatment until after delivery becomes an increasingly favourable option after 20 weeks gestation for stage I cancers.[25] Nine studies involving 63 patients with stage I cervical cancer have examined the effect of a delay, varying between 1 and 32 weeks. Only one outcome was possibly affected by the delay. However, these studies are clearly non-randomized and the decision to delay should be made with oncologists and neonatologists after careful patient counselling. Steroids should be given to promote fetal lung maturation. Delivery at 32–34 weeks can now be justified with advances in the care of the preterm infant. Caesarean section is normally advised, due to theoretical concerns of haemorrhage from cervical lesions and increased malignant cell dissemination with vaginal delivery [E]. Local recurrence within episiotomy sites is well documented and is associated with a high mortality rate. Radical hysterectomy at the time of caesarean section is associated with greater blood loss, but the rate of other complications is not increased [D].

Consideration should also be given to the use of neoadjuvant chemotherapy in the second and third trimesters. This may limit progression of disease and more confidently allow delay in surgical treatment, although its safety also remains in question.

Radiotherapy is employed with more advanced lesions (stage IIb and above) and usually takes the form of external beam teletherapy and intracavitary brachytherapy. The external beam alone employs 40–50 Gy. Most pregnancies will spontaneously abort after such high doses, usually within 5 weeks [D]. Occasionally, the fetus must be removed surgically. Preterm delivery of the fetus may be necessary at later gestations.

Where a lesion is very advanced, and the maternal prognosis poor, the woman may prefer to compromise her own treatment if this means limiting the risks to the fetus. Careful, sensitive counselling is clearly very important in this situation.

## Ovarian cancer

The incidence of ovarian tumours in pregnancy is quoted as one in 1000 deliveries, although ovarian cancer is much less common (one in 5000–18 000). Adnexal masses are found in approximately one in 100 pregnancies; 50 per cent measure <5 cm, 25 per cent are 5–10 cm and the remaining quarter are >10 cm in size. Table 7.3.1 lists various causes of adnexal mass found in pregnancy, in decreasing order of incidence.

**Table 7.3.1** The most common causes of adnexal mass in pregnancy

| |
|---|
| Functional cyst |
| Mature teratoma (dermoid) |
| Cystadenoma (serous and mucinous) |
| Para-ovarian cyst |
| Endometrioma |
| Leiomyoma |
| Malignancy (3–6 per cent of all cases) |

There are various non-neoplastic ovarian lesions which are unique to pregnancy and which will resolve spontaneously after delivery. These include:

- luteoma of pregnancy,
- follicular cyst of pregnancy,
- hyperreactio luteinalis,
- granulosa cell proliferations,
- hilus cell hyperplasia,
- ectopia deciduo.

With the extensive use of ultrasound for dating and assessing pregnancies, the recognition of adnexal masses in pregnancy has increased. Although most remain asymptomatic, 10–15 per cent will rupture, bleed or cause adnexal torsion [D], and these acute events are thought to increase the risk of miscarriage and preterm labour [D]. Occasionally, an ovarian mass may cause dystocia during labour or virilization. As one in 20–50 ovarian lesions in pregnancy will be malignant[26] and as many as one in six may become symptomatic, a careful management decision has to be made when they are first recognized. Symptomatic adnexal lesions may need to be operated on immediately. Small (<6 cm) unilocular cysts are likely to resolve spontaneously before 16 weeks without causing harm and should be left alone [D].[27] A further ultrasound should be performed at 16 weeks gestation. A persistent complex mass should prompt a laparotomy. Miscarriage is said to be less likely if intervention occurs at this point in the second trimester. Persistent simple cysts that are not associated with ascites and have no solid areas or thick septae within them can be treated conservatively. Dermoid cysts are often confidently diagnosed by ultrasound. These, too, can be left although the risk of a cyst accident must always be considered, as this may increase the risk of miscarriage. MRI may help with diagnosis in selected cases.

Tumour markers, such as Ca125, alpha-fetoprotein (aFP) and human chorionic gonadotrophin (hCG), are helpful for diagnosis and treatment monitoring outside pregnancy. These substances may all be elevated during a normal pregnancy and do not usually feature in the diagnosis or management of the adnexal mass antenatally. Of note, however, an extremely high maternal serum aFP value, performed for fetal anomaly screening, has led to the diagnosis of endodermal sinus tumours on a number of occasions.

Surgery for an adnexal mass in pregnancy usually involves a lower midline incision, which allows adequate access with minimal uterine manipulation. Peritoneal washings should be taken and omental and peritoneal biopsies. Where appropriate, a simple cystectomy with ovarian conservation is attempted. Otherwise, a unilateral salpingoooophorectomy should be performed. Frozen sections of the contralateral ovary can be taken to help intraoperative management, but bilateral oophorectomy should normally be avoided at the initial operation, as even malignant cases are usually early stage, chemosensitive or of low malignant potential. Para-aortic lymph node sampling and debulking should be considered in more complex cases, although it would be unusual for the uterus to need to be removed.

If an ovarian cyst is removed in the first trimester, it may have arisen from the corpus luteum and may have been providing hormonal support to the early pregnancy. It is accepted practice in this situation to provide progesterone supplementation until the second trimester is reached [D].

## Management of ovarian cancer in pregnancy

The histopathological nature of ovarian cancer in pregnancy reflects the younger age of the affected population. Germ cell and epithelial cell cancers each account for 30–40 per cent of cases, but two-thirds of the epithelial group are of 'low malignant potential'. The remainder are mostly sex cord stromal tumours. Dysgerminomas are the most common malignant ovarian tumours found in pregnancy.

Stage I epithelial cancers, tumours of low malignant potential and stage Ia dysgerminomas do not require adjunctive treatment with chemotherapy. Other forms of germ cell tumour and more advanced epithelial cancers would normally be treated with chemotherapy postoperatively. Beyond the first trimester, the use of bleomycin, etoposide, cisplatin and vincristine/vinblastine has not been clearly linked with fetal harm, with a number of successful outcomes having been reported in the literature.[28] However, until more data have been collected, concerns will remain over the use of anti-neoplastic drugs during pregnancy, especially during the first trimester (see above).

## Other malignancies

The principles of managing cancer in pregnancy can be illustrated by further examples.

* Older, uncontrolled studies suggested a poorer outcome stage for stage when melanoma presented during pregnancy. More recent case-controlled studies show no difference in three- and five-year survival rates [B].[29] Although melanoma is the malignancy most likely to metastasize to the placenta and fetus, this nevertheless rarely occurs. However, the placenta should be examined at delivery and sent for histopathology.

* Pregnancy does not alter the course of cancer but may cause a delay in diagnosis.
* Sensitive methods of investigation can be safely employed during pregnancy.
* Safe treatments are available during pregnancy for dealing with all symptoms caused by cancer.
* Chemotherapy in the first trimester is associated with a significantly increased risk of fetal abnormalities. Treatment during the second and third trimesters of pregnancy would seem to be safer, but the data are limited.
* Radiation exposure must be restricted to the very low levels found with investigative x-rays. Radiotherapy for pelvic, abdominal or chest malignancies usually carries excessive fetal risk, even with shielding.
* Management requires a multidisciplinary approach.

The fetus will have metastases in 30 per cent of cases where placental involvement is found. Biopsy of the sentinel or draining node may be useful in predicting spread of malignant melanoma. A blue dye can be used to locate this lymph node, as an alternative to technetium-labelled sulphur colloid, avoiding fetal radiation exposure [D].

* Radiotherapy for head, neck and brain tumours usually carries a fetal dose exposure of <10 cGy due to the distance between the field and the uterus. Abdominal shielding can reduce this to <2 cGy.
* The treatment for Hodgkin's lymphoma and chronic myeloid leukaemia can often be delayed until after the pregnancy. Acute leukaemias and non-Hodgkin's lymphoma must be treated immediately as the risks to the woman and her pregnancy from haemorrhage, anaemia and sepsis outweigh the possible fetal harm from chemotherapy, even in the first trimester [D].

## ACKNOWLEDGEMENT

This chapter has been revised and updated. The author and editors acknowledge the contribution of Alec McEwan to the chapter on this topic in the previous edition of the book.

## Key References

1. Iseminger KA, Lewis MA. Ethical challenges in treating mother and fetus when cancer complicates pregnancy. *Obstet Gynecol Clin North Am* 1998; **25**: 273–85.
2. Schover LR. Psychosocial issues associated with cancer in pregnancy. *Semin Oncol* 2000; **27**: 699–703.

3. Fattibene P, Mazzei F, Nuccetelli C, Risica S. Prenatal exposure to ionising radiation: sources, effects and regulatory aspects. *Acta Paediatr* 1999; **88**: 693–702.

4. Tribukait B, Cekan E. *Developmental Effects of Prenatal Irradiation.* Dose–effect relationship and the significance of fractionated and protracted radiation for the frequency of fetal malformations following X-irradiation of pregnant C3H mice. Stuttgart: Gustave Fischer, 1982: 29–35.

5. Muirhead CR, Kneale GW. Prenatal irradiation and childhood cancer. *J Radiol Prot* 1989; **9**: 209–12.

6. Otake M, Schull W. Radiation-related small head sizes among prenatally exposed A-bomb survivors. *Int J Radiat Oncol Biol Phys* 1992; **63**: 255–70.

7. Mole RH. Irradiation of the embryo and fetus. *Br J Radiol* 1987; **60**: 17–31.

8. Gilman EA, Kneale GW, Knox EG, Stewart AM. Pregnancy x rays and childhood cancers: effects of exposure age and radiation dose. *J Radiol Prot* 1988; **8**: 3–8.

9. Partridge AH, Garber JE. Long-term outcomes of children exposed to anti-neoplastic agents *in utero*. *Semin Oncol* 2000; **27**: 712–26.

10. Doll DC, Ringenberg S, Yarbo JW. Antineoplastic agents and pregnancy. *Semin Oncol* 1989; **16**: 337.

11. Reynosa E, Shepherd F, Messner H *et al.* Acute leukaemia in pregnancy: The Toronto Leukaemia Study Group experience with long-term follow-up of children exposed *in utero* to chemotherapeutic agents. *J Clin Oncol* 1987; **5**: 1098–106.

12. Lethaby AE, O'Neill MA, Mason B *et al.* Overall survival from breast cancer in women pregnant or lactating at or after diagnosis. *Int J Cancer* 1996; **67**: 751–5.

13. Berry DL, Theriault RL, Holmes FA *et al.* Management of breast cancer during pregnancy using a standardised protocol. *J Clin Oncol* 1999; **17**: 855–61.

14. Harvey JC, Rosen PP, Ashikari R *et al.* The effect of pregnancy on the prognosis of carcinoma of the breast following radical mastectomy. *Surg Gynecol Obstet* 1981; **153**: 723–5.

15. Mignot L, Morvan F, Berdah J *et al.* Pregnancy after breast cancer. Results of a case-control study. *Presse Med* 1986; **15**: 1961–4.

16. Ariel I, Kempner R. The prognosis of patients who become pregnant after mastectomy for breast cancer. *Int Surg* 1989; **74**: 185.

17. von Schoultz E, Johansson H, Wilking N, Rutquist LE. Influence of prior and subsequent pregnancy on breast cancer prognosis. *J Clin Oncol* 1995; **13**: 430–4.

18. Guerra B, De Simone P, Gabrielli S *et al.* Combined cytology and colposcopy to screen for cervical cancer in pregnancy. *J Reprod Med* 1998; **43**: 647–53.

19. Baldauf JJ, Dreyfus M, Ritter J, Philippe E. Colposcopy and directed biopsy reliability during pregnancy: a cohort study. *Eur J Obst Gynecol Reprod Biol* 1995; **62**: 31–6.

20. Hacker NF, Berek JS, Lagasse LD *et al.* Carcinoma of the cervix associated with pregnancy. *Obstet Gynecol* 1982; **59**: 735–46.

21. Yost NP, Santoso JT, McIntire DD, Iliya FA. Postpartum regression rates of antepartum cervical intraepithelial neoplasia II and III. *Obstet Gynecol* 1999; **93**: 359–62.

22. Hannigan EV, Whitehouse HH, Atkinson WD, Becker SN. Cone biopsy during pregnancy. *Obstet Gynecol* 1982; **60**: 450–5.

23. Robinson W, Webb S, Tirpack J *et al.* Management of cervical intraepithelial neoplasia during pregnancy with LOOP excision. *Gynecol Oncol* 1997; **64**: 153–5.

24. Connor JP. Noninvasive cervical cancer complicating pregnancy. *Obstet Gynecol Clin North Am* 1998; **25**: 331–42.

25. Duggan B, Muderspach LI, Roman LD *et al.* Cervical cancer in pregnancy: reporting on planned delay in therapy. *Obstet Gynecol* 1993; **82**: 598–602.

26. Creasman WT, Rutledge F, Smith JP. Carcinoma of the ovary associated with pregnancy. *Obstet Gynecol* 1971; **38**: 111–16.

27. Thornton JG, Wells M. Ovarian cysts in pregnancy: does ultrasound make traditional management inappropriate? *Obstet Gynecol* 1987; **69**: 717–21.

28. Boulay R, Podczaski E. Ovarian cancer complicating pregnancy. *Obstet Gynecol Clin North Am* 1998; **25**: 385–99.

29. MacKie RM, Bufalino R, Morabito A. Lack of effect of pregnancy on outcome of melanoma. *Lancet* 1991; **337**: 653–5.

# 7.4 Infection

*Joanna C Gillham*

## INTRODUCTION

The body has a natural resistance to infection, with the ability to 'acquire' resistance to pathogens through natural exposure and vaccines. Immune defences at the body surface are the epithelial barriers of skin and the mucous membranes. Secretory immunoglobulin (Ig) A is found on the mucosa and provides the ability to resist proteolytic enzymes. Chemical factors, for example gastric acid, are active against certain gut pathogens and the low pH maintained in urine and vaginal secretions helps to inhibit their growth. Natural antibodies are present in extracellular fluids. Organisms may be carried by the lymphatics and trapped in lymph nodes where they may become a target for phagocytosis by macrophages. Alternatively, they can enter the circulation where they may be ingested by neutrophils or phagocytic cells in the liver (Kupffer's cells), spleen, bone marrow, pituitary or adrenal gland.

Acquired resistance occurs when the presence of foreign antigens stimulates production of antibodies by plasma cells. The primary response is production of IgM. This is a large molecule that does not cross the placenta. Within 10–14 days, production of IgG begins; this smaller molecule becomes prominent, with the ability to cross the placenta.

Immunity is not always acquired by antibody production. Cell-mediated immunity via T-lymphocytes is important in fungal, viral and some bacterial infections (tuberculosis, syphilis, leprosy, brucellosis). T-lymphocytes possess the ability themselves to be cytotoxic or to produce lymphokines that activate and attract macrophages to the site of infection.

Pregnancy represents a relatively immunocompromised state, with hormonal and immunological changes. Various hormones made by the trophoblast have been shown to interfere with the induction of the immune response. These include progesterone and oestrogen, which inhibit cytotoxic T-cells and natural killer cells. These physiological alterations in immunoregulation may help support the fetoplacental allograph, but may expose the mother to increased susceptibility to various pathogens.

## VIRAL INFECTIONS

### Relevant viral infections

- Herpes viruses: herpes simplex, varicella zoster, cytomegalovirus, Epstein–Barr;
- Parvoviruses: parvovirus B19;

- Togaviruses: rubella;
- Paramyxoviruses: measles;
- Retroviruses: human immunodeficiency virus (HIV);
- Hepatitis viruses: hepatitis A, hepatitis B, hepatitis C, hepatitis D, hepatitis E.

# HERPES VIRUSES

All of the herpes virus group are composed of DNA.

## Herpes simplex virus infection

This virus is classified into types 1 and 2. Type 1 herpes simplex virus (HSV) is classically associated with the orofacial infections and encephalitis, HSV-2 with the genital manifestations. In reality, there is a great amount of overlap with these subtypes.[1]

### Epidemiology and aetiology

The virus is transmitted through close physical contact and sexual intercourse. Herpes simplex virus must contact mucosal surfaces or abraded skin to initiate infection. Herpes simplex virus type 1 is often contracted in childhood, with 80–90 per cent of the adult population having positive serology. Antibodies to both subtypes are thought to offer some cross-protection. The prevalence of type 1 HSV increases with decreasing socioeconomic class. Herpes simplex virus-2 infections are acquired sexually, so their incidence begins to increase in adolescence. Both viruses establish latent infections in sensory neurons. In the orofacial form, the virus can remain latent in the trigeminal nerve; in the genital disease, it remains in the sacral ganglia. There are many reactivation triggers: trauma, febrile illness, stress, menstruation and ultraviolet radiation. Immunocompromised patients can develop severe disseminated HSV infection involving multiple viscera.

### Presentation and diagnosis

Primary infection in the facial area is often asymptomatic. If lesions appear, they can involve the lips, eyes and face. Most characteristic are painful lesions of the oral mucosa. A first attack of genital herpes is usually more severe and symptomatic, presenting with multiple painful genital ulcers after a short incubation period. In 80–90 per cent of cases, primary genital herpes involves the vulva and cervix. All the skin lesions start with erythema, progressing to vesicles, then ulcers and finishing with crusting. These lesions can last up to 2 weeks.

Inguinal lymphadenopathy is associated with most primary cases. Fever, malaise and headaches are present in approximately 30 per cent patients. Retention of urine is a rare symptom. Recurrent infections tend to be less severe. Patients infected with HSV type 2 tend to suffer more frequent episodes. Local tingling and paraesthesiae are often noted 1–2 days before recurrent attack. Some viral carriers may be permanently asymptomatic.

Diagnosis is suggested by clinical history and examination but should be confirmed. Swabs of the affected area for viral culture and isolation of the organism give definitive diagnosis. Subsequent analysis is by viral culture or polymerase chain reaction (PCR) Type-specific HSV serological testing (immunoglobulin G antibodies to HSV-1 and HSV-2) is now widely available.[2]

Full sexually transmitted disease screening by a genitourinary clinic with appropriate contact screening and a cervical smear should be performed.

### Management

This is an unpleasant disease with no cure. It is recurrent, which can lead to relationship and psychosexual problems, making specialist advice and counselling support mandatory. The patients need to be informed that when lesions are noted they are infectious, thus the need to refrain from sexual intercourse.

Treatment involves bathing lesions in warm saline, and simple analgesics. Initial genital or oral HSV infection can be treated with topical, oral or intravenous acyclovir. Topical therapy is less effective. Although intravenous acyclovir is the most effective treatment, oral acyclovir is normally preferable and adequate [C].[1] Secondary bacterial infection is treated with antibiotics. Rarely, hospital admission is needed for stronger analgesia, parenteral acyclovir or catheterization.

#### In relation to pregnancy

##### Antepartum

Data from the USA suggest around 2 per cent of women acquire genital HSV infection in pregnancy, with most cases being asymptomatic or unrecognized.[3] It may be difficult to clinically distinguish from recurrent and primary genital HSV infections. Type-specific HSV antibody testing, which can help differentiate between primary and recurrent infection, should be undertaken if a woman presents with a first episode of genital herpes in the third trimester.[4] The relevant history should be appropriately documented, and the suggested mode of delivery should be discussed. There is no value in performing antepartum maternal viral cultures as they do not predict the infant's risk of exposure to HSV at delivery [C].[5]

Primary HSV infection has been associated with spontaneous abortion, stillbirth, fetal growth restriction (FGR) and preterm labour. Owing to the increased susceptibility of the pregnant immune system, earlier recourse to intravenous acyclovir in suspected primary genital HSV infection is suggested. Management should involve a genitourinary physician. Acyclovir is tolerated in pregnancy and there is no clinical or laboratory evidence of maternal or fetal toxicity.[1] The RCOG green top guidelines[4] state that acyclovir should be used with caution before 20 weeks gestation. Treatment with oral acyclovir is for 5 days at a dose of either 200 mg five times a day or 400 mg three times a day for woman with severe symptoms. Disseminated HSV infection is an indication for intravenous acyclovir.

### Intrapartum

The vulva and cervix should be carefully examined for herpes lesions when women present in labour if they have a previous history of HSV.

Caesarean section is recommended for all women presenting with first-episode genital herpes at the time of delivery or a primary episode within 6 weeks of delivery [C]. If the baby is delivered vaginally in these circumstances, the risk of neonatal herpes is approximately 41 per cent.[4] If the woman opts for a vaginal birth rather than a caesarean section, rupture of membranes should be avoided and invasive procedures not used. Intravenous acyclovir should be given intrapartum to the mother. The neonatologist needs to be informed as acyclovir for the neonate may be necessary [E].[4]

If the first episode is in the first or second trimester and there is no recurrence, a vaginal delivery is permitted.[4] There is insufficient evidence to recommend use of daily suppressive acyclovir from 36 weeks of gestation to reduce the likelihood of HSV lesions at term for women who experience a primary episode of genital herpes earlier in the current pregnancy [E].[4,6]

There is no agreement on the use of caesarean section in the management of patients with a history of recurrent HSV. For women with a history of recurrent genital herpes, who would opt for caesarean delivery if HSV lesions were detected at the onset of labour, daily suppressive acyclovir given from 36 weeks of gestation until delivery may be given to reduce the likelihood of HSV lesions at term [A].[4]

Women presenting with recurrent genital herpes at the onset of labour should be advised that the risk to the baby of neonatal herpes is small, and caesarean section is not routinely recommended for these women [C].[4]

In women with recurrent genital herpes, invasive procedures in labour should be avoided. If confirmed rupture of membranes occurs at term then delivery should be expedited by the appropriate means and the neonatologist informed about these babies.[4]

### Postpartum

If any orofacial lesions are present, parents should be advised to refrain from close contact with the baby in that region. Breastfeeding is recommended unless the mother has lesions around the nipples. Acyclovir is excreted in breast milk but its use is not contraindicated and there are no harmful effects to the infant.

### Fetal infection

The implications to the fetus of HSV infections are discussed in Chapter 13, Fetal infections.

### Co-infection with HIV

These women are at increased risk of more severe and frequent symptomatic recurrent episodes of genital herpes during pregnancy and of asymptomatic shedding of HSV at term. Early liaison with the genito-urinary medicine physicians and paediatricians is vital.

### Neonatal herpes

This can be caused by HSV type 1 and 2. The risks to the neonate are greatest when a woman acquires a new infection (primary genital herpes) in the third trimester, particularly within 6 weeks prior to delivery. This disease can be localized to the skin, eye and/or mouth, local/central nervous disease and or can be disseminated with multiple organ involvement. Disseminated disease carries the worst prognosis; with antiviral treatment, mortality is around 30 per cent and 17 per cent suffer long-term seqeulae.[4]

---

## KEY POINTS

- Management of these patients should be in conjunction with a genitourinary physician.
- Acyclovir is considered appropriate to use in pregnancy.
- There is no value in performing viral cultures in the antenatal period as they do not predict potential neonatal infections.
- There may be a role for treatment with daily suppressive acyclovir in the last 4 weeks of pregnancy in cases of recurrent HSV. This may decrease the need for delivery by caesarean section.
- If the first episode of HSV is within 6 weeks of the due date, delivery by caesarean section should be strongly considered.
- Careful inspection of the vulva and vagina should be performed when a woman presents in labour.
- If a patient has recurrent genital herpes at term, the risk to the baby of neonatal herpes is small and caesarean section is not routinely recommended. However, invasive procedures should be avoided in labour, and labour expedited if there is confirmed rupture of membranes. The neonatologists should be aware of such babies.

---

# Varicella zoster virus

Varicella zoster virus (VZV) has two distinct diseases: varicella (chickenpox) and herpes zoster (shingles).

## Epidemiology and aetiology

The primary infection is chickenpox, which commonly occurs in childhood. The virus enters through the mucosa of the upper respiratory tract and then remains latent in sensory and motor nerve cells. Recurrence tends to occur localized to one dermatome. Patients with both diseases are infective, the virus being spread by direct contact or airborne transmission.

## Presentation and diagnosis

The incubation period for varicella is 14–21 days. Following a prodromal illness of fever and malaise, a florid pruritic rash erupts. Initially a maculopapular rash, this rapidly turns to vesicles and then crusts over. The rash is commonly most extensive on the face and trunk, being minimal on the extremities. Patients are contagious from approximately 2 days before the onset of the rash until the vesicles have crusted over.

Primary varicella infection in adults is associated with more complications: pneumonia, encephalitis and hepatitis are the most common.

Shingles presents with painful and pruritic vesicles along a single sensory or motor nerve. Rarely, there can be systemic involvement with this reactivation, involving multiple visceral inflammation. This tends to be associated with significant immunosuppression.

In both manifestations, the clinical presentation of the disease is classical enough to make a confident diagnosis clinically. Laboratory tests are available to measure IgM and IgG anti-varicella antibodies.

## Management

Although available, VZV vaccination is not routinely used in the UK. However, vaccination pre-pregnancy or postpartum is an option that should be considered for women who are found to be seronegative for VZV IgG before pregnancy or in the postpartum period. Pregnancy should be avoided for three months after the vaccination.[7]

Chickenpox in childhood is usually a self-limiting illness, with both anti-pruritic and anti-pyretic measures being taken to alleviate the symptoms. The non-pregnant adult needs to be more closely monitored, with evidence of any systemic symptoms needing prompt evaluation and treatment by a specialist medical team. Antibiotics may be required for subsequent secondary infection of the vesicles. Routine oral antivirals are not required, but intravenous antiviral agents are utilized with systemic VZV.

### In relation to pregnancy

More than 90 per cent of the antenatal population is seropositive for VZV IgG antibody. Thus potential contact with affected individuals in pregnancy is high, but primary VZV is uncommon – affecting approximately three in 1000 pregnancies.

### Antepartum

A past history of chickenpox should be sought. If there is no positive history, pregnant women should be advised about avoidance of contact with chickenpox or shingles and to contact healthcare personnel immediately if exposure occurs. If a suspected non-immune pregnant woman has contact with VZV, her VZV antibody status should be investigated. This can usually be performed within 24–48 hours on either a current blood sample or serum stored from blood tests performed at the antenatal booking visit.[7]

As pregnancy may confer a mildly immunocompromised state, if the mother is not immune to VZV and she had significant exposure, she should be given VZV immunoglobulin (VZIG) as soon as possible. This is effective up to 10 days after contact, but does not absolutely preclude development of the disease [E].[7] The UK Advisory Group on Chickenpox considers any close contact during the period of infectiousness to be significant. The risk of infection following contact with shingles in a non-exposed area is remote. If shingles is disseminated, in an exposed area or in an immunocompromised individual, then the risk is greater.

Clinicians should be aware of the excess morbidity associated with varicella infection in adults, including pneumonia, hepatitis, encephalitis and occasionally mortality.[7] The UK Advisory Group on Chickenpox[8] recommends that oral acyclovir (800 mg five times a day for 7 days) be prescribed for pregnant women if they present within 24 hours of the onset of the rash and are over 20 weeks gestation [E]. Varicella zoster virus immunoglobulin is of no benefit once chickenpox has developed. Hospital assessment and intravenous acyclovir are required for those patients with varicella pneumonia, those over 36 weeks gestation and patients with clinical deterioration after day 6 of the rash [E].[7]

The obstetrician, the infectious disease team and the virologist should manage pregnant women with chickenpox. A neonatologist is required to be involved should the disease onset coincide with the delivery period.

The risk of developing secondary complications is increased in cigarette smokers and in patients with chronic lung disease, immunosuppression and prolonged courses of steroids.

### Intrapartum

Delivery during the viraemic period can be hazardous to both the mother and baby. Thus treatment with acyclovir is recommended and delivery postponed, if appropriate, until 5–7 days after the onset of maternal rash. Delaying delivery decreases the maternal complications of bleeding, thrombocytopenia and disseminated intravascular coagulation. It also allows time for transfer of protective antibodies from the mother to the fetus, thus decreasing the incidence of varicella of the newborn, which has high associated morbidity and mortality [E].[7]

Maternal shingles at the time of delivery is not a risk to the neonate, as transplacentally acquired antibodies will already be in the fetal system.

### Postnatal

If birth occurs within the 7 days following the onset of the maternal rash, or if the mother develops the chicken pox rash within the 7 day period after birth, the neonate should be given VZIG [E].[7]

### Fetal infection

The risk of miscarriage does not appear to be increased if chickenpox occurs in the first trimester [C,D], but if varicella develops in the first 28 weeks of pregnancy, there is a small risk of fetal varicella infection.[7] The implications to the fetus of VZV infections are discussed in Chapter 13, Fetal infections.

Antenatal complications: maternal

## KEY POINTS

- If a suspected non-immune pregnant woman has contact with VZV, her immunological status should be ascertained.
- If a confirmed non-immune pregnant women has contact with chickenpox or disseminated or exposed shingles, she should be offered VZIG. Similar advice should be preferred to an immunocompromised person exposed to shingles. VZIG is effective up to 10 days after contact.
- If a pregnant woman presents within 24 hours of onset of VZV rash after 20 weeks gestation, oral acyclovir should be administered. Acyclovir should be used cautiously prior to 20 weeks gestation.
- If infection with VZV occurs in pregnancy, management should involve a physician with a specialist interest in infectious diseases.
- Admission to hospital and intravenous acyclovir should be considered if the woman is 36 weeks gestation, has any signs of varicella pneumonia or has any clinical deterioration.
- Delivery in the viraemic period should be avoided if at all possible. Ideally, delivery should be delayed until 7 days after the onset of the maternal illness. This allows transplacental transfer of antibodies.

## Cytomegalovirus

### Epidemiology and aetiology

Transmission can be horizontal via direct human-to-human contact and with sexual activity. Cytomegalovirus (CMV) is excreted in saliva, urine, semen, cervical secretions, stool and tears. It can be transmitted via blood transfusion and organ transplantation. Vertical transmission can occur during pregnancy, delivery and breastfeeding. Viral shedding from the cervix increases as the pregnancy advances in gestation. The lungs, liver, kidney and salivary glands are the most commonly affected organs.

### Presentation and diagnosis

In healthy adults, the presentation is indistinguishable from infectious mononucleosis. Fever and malaise are typical, with lymphadenopathy. The blood picture shows a lymphocytosis, with atypical lymphocytes. Haemolytic anaemia, thrombocytopenia and deranged liver function tests may be present. This disease runs a benign course.

Disseminated, sometimes fatal, infection occurs in the immunocompromised, particularly transplant recipients and patients with acquired immunodeficiency syndrome (AIDS). The varied manifestations include encephalitis, retinitis, pneumonitis and involvement of the gastrointestinal tract. Virology of the urine, saliva, blood, cerebrospinal fluid or nasopharynx secretions is diagnostic. Serological tests can identify past or current infection. Other less utilized tests are detection of monoclonal antibodies to CMV antigens and PCR. However, IgM levels rise with reactivation and cannot therefore be used as a marker for first infection.

### Management

In the normal adult population, infection with CMV will largely go unrecognized. Treatment is directed at alleviation of the symptoms.

#### In relation to pregnancy

There are no implications from a maternal health point of view.

#### Fetal infection

The implications to the fetus of CMV infections are discussed in Chapter 13, Fetal infections.

## Epstein–Barr virus

### Epidemiology and aetiology

This virus causes infectious mononucleosis, commonly referred to as 'glandular fever'. The most common affected age groups are adolescents and young adults. Transmission is via saliva and aerosol droplets. Epstein–Barr virus (EBV) is considered to be the aetiological agent for Burkitt's lymphoma and nasopharyngeal carcinoma.

### Presentation and diagnosis

The predominant symptoms are fever, malaise, sore throat and headache. A petechial rash on the soft palate and a macular rash are common. These rashes typically occur in 90 per cent of patients who have been treated with ampicillin for their sore throat. Characteristic features are cervical lymphadenopathy and splenomegaly. Mild hepatitis is common. Rare complications include meningitis, myocarditis and mesenteric adenitis. In the majority of cases, this is a self-limiting illness, but it can run a protracted course with the patient feeling debilitated for several months.

Peripheral blood film shows atypical mononuclear cells. Serological tests for specific EBV IgM antibodies can demonstrate recent infection. The two classical tests for the virus are the monospot test and the Paul–Bunnell reaction. The latter detects antibodies that agglutinate sheep erythrocytes. False-positive results can occur in hepatitis, Hodgkin's disease and acute leukaemia.

### Management

In the majority of cases no specific treatment is required, although corticosteroid treatment may be necessary if there is neurological involvement.

In relation to pregnancy
There are no special features involving the pregnant woman and no known effects of vertical transmission.

# PARVOVIRUSES

## Human parvovirus B19

The virus is a single-stranded DNA virus. This is a common infection, particularly in infants and younger children, alternatively known as erythema infectiosum or 'Fifth's disease'.

## Epidemiology and aetiology

Aerosol droplets and exchange of bodily fluids transmit this virus. Fifty to 80 per cent of adults are seropositive.

## Presentation and diagnosis

Children typically have a fever and a bright erythematous, photosensitive malar rash – the 'slapped cheek rash'. Most adult infections are asymptomatic. The rash is less prominent but more widespread, involving the face, trunk and extremities. Chronic bone marrow failure can occur in the immunocompromised. Those patients with hereditary blood dyscrasias, for example sickle cell anaemia, are susceptible to aplastic crises.

Serological testing is required for diagnosis as the clinical presentation is similar to that of a number of viral syndromes. The presence of IgG to parvovirus B19 can confirm immunity. If this is not confirmed, paired rising titres 10–14 days after exposure or the presence of specific IgM antibody can indicate those at risk of fetal infection. PCR can detect parvovirus B19 DNA in maternal sera.

## Management

In healthy individuals this is normally a self-limiting illness, with no specific therapy being warranted.

In relation to pregnancy
Spontaneous abortion and intrauterine fetal death have been associated with parvovirus B19 infection. All pregnant women presenting with a non-vesicular rash compatible with a viral infection should be investigated for rubella and parvovirus B19 infection [E]. When serology shows potential for early infection with parvovirus B19, the patient should be referred to a fetal medicine unit capable of fetal blood sampling and intravascular transfusion [E].[9]

### Fetal infection
The implications to the fetus of parvovirus B19 infections are discussed in Chapter 13, Fetal infections.

# TOGAVIRUSES

## Rubella

### Epidemiology and aetiology

This is a fragile, single-stranded RNA virus, easily killed by heat and ultraviolet light. Spread is via respiratory droplets or *in-utero* transmission.

### Presentation and diagnosis

The incubation period varies between 14 and 21 days. Malaise and fever are the common clinical features, with conjunctivitis and lymphadenopathy (particularly postauricular and suboccipital). The classical rash is a pink/red macular type, starting on the forehead and spreading to the trunk and limbs. Rare complications are secondary pulmonary bacterial infection, arthralgia, encephalitis and haemorrhagic manifestations due to thrombocytopenia.

The diagnosis is usually clinical but can be confirmed by culturing the virus from urine, nasopharynx or cerebrospinal fluid. Serological testing for rubella IgG and IgM is available.

### Management

This disease is usually self-limiting and treatment is symptomatic.

In relation to pregnancy
Rubella infection in pregnancy does not confer increased risk to the mother; it is the devastating teratogenic effects of this virus that are of concern (see Chapter 13, Fetal infections). Human Ig can decrease the symptoms of the disease, but does not prevent the teratogenicity.

All children are offered the vaccine in the form of the MMR (measles, mumps and rubella) injection at approximately 15 months of age. All susceptible women who are receiving healthcare should ideally have their serological state tested. Opportunistic testing for this can be performed, for example family planning clinics and infertility investigation. If immunity to rubella is not confirmed, the vaccine should be offered. It is recommended that pregnancy should be avoided for one month after the vaccine is administered.

#### Antepartum
The routine booking bloods taken in the antenatal period include serological testing for the presence of rubella antibodies. If not immune, the patient should be counselled about avoidance of any affected people.

All pregnant women presenting with a non-vesicular rash compatible with a viral infection should be investigated for rubella and parvovirus B19 infection, irrespective of a prior history of rubella vaccination or previous positive rubella antibody tests [E].

### Postpartum

For non-immune individuals, the opportunity should be taken to administer the vaccine in the post-delivery period. With hospital delivery, the vaccine is given on discharge from the hospital.

### Fetal infection

The implications to the fetus of rubella infections are discussed in Chapter 13, Fetal infections.

## PARAMYXOVIRUSES

## Measles

This is a highly contagious virus, mostly occurring in childhood. Immunization in early infancy is with the MMR vaccine. This acute febrile illness is associated with high morbidity and mortality, particularly in developing countries.

### Epidemiology and aetiology

The virus is spread by respiratory droplets.

### Presentation and diagnosis

The incubation period varies from 8 to 14 days. The viraemic phase is prior to the classical measles rash developing. This is characterized by fever, malaise, rhinorrhoea, cough, conjunctivitis and small greyish spots on the buccal mucosa (Koplick's spots). A maculopapular rash then occurs, initially on the face, then spreading to the rest of the body. Complications include otitis media, bacterial pneumonia, myocarditis, hepatitis and encephalomyelitis. Infection in the adult is rare, but is often a more severe illness.

Diagnosis is made on clinical symptoms and signs. Rarely used serological tests include a haemagglutination inhibition antibody that is present by the onset of the rash and remains positive for life.

### Management

Treatment is symptomatic.

#### In relation to pregnancy

As with any acute febrile illness, measles can precipitate spontaneous miscarriage or premature labour. No teratogenic effects of this virus are recognized.

## RETROVIRUSES

## Human immunodeficiency virus

This virus affects the normal immune cells of the body. AIDS occurs when the immune system is so depleted that unusual infections from bacteria and viruses develop. On average, it takes 8–10 years from infection with HIV to the development of AIDS.

### Epidemiology and aetiology

Infection with HIV occurs through sexual contact and contact with infected blood. Women are more likely to be infected through sexual contact than men. Risk factors are frequent unprotected sexual intercourse with different partners and intravenous drug abuse. The presence of other sexually transmitted infections increases shedding of HIV. Among adults newly diagnosed with HIV in the UK, 58 per cent are thought to have acquired their infection through heterosexual exposure. Although the incidence of infections acquired heterosexually in the UK has risen steadily,[10] the majority of cases are of black African ethnicity who were probably infected in sub-Saharan Africa. Perinatal transmission can occur *in utero*, intrapartum or through breastfeeding. In the majority of cord blood samples, HIV is not detected, thus suggesting that the majority of transmission is not in the antenatal period.[11]

#### In relation to pregnancy

##### Antepartum

Voluntary testing for HIV should be an integral part of antenatal care, offered and recommended to all pregnant women, irrespective of their risk factors.[12] Joint care is required from the beginning of pregnancy with a physician expert in HIV.

In HIV-positive women, the initial booking visit should include a thorough history and physical examination. Baseline examination should include fundoscopy, neurological and pelvic examination. The initial visit should include counselling about the perinatal transmission of HIV and the importance of compliance with antiretroviral regimens. Women should be informed that interventions, for example anti-retroviral therapy, caesarean section (in indicated cases) and avoidance of breastfeeding, can reduce the risk of mother to child HIV transmission from 25 to 30 per cent to less than 2 per cent [A].[13] All treatment should be performed in a multidisciplinary setting with involvement of other relevant health professionals. If appropriate, patients should be referred for drug treatment and/or detoxification programmes.

Screening should be undertaken as for all pregnant individuals, with the addition of screening for hepatitis C, tuberculosis, bacterial vaginosis and other sexually transmitted diseases. Baseline antibody titres of *Toxoplasma gondii* and CMV should be obtained. Liver function tests need to be performed. HIV viral load and CD4 lymphocyte count should be measured at the initial visit and repeated each trimester to follow response to therapy or to detect indications for therapy.[13]

The risks of mother-to-child transmission of chorionic villus biopsy or amniocentesis are uncertain. If invasive prenatal diagnosis is contemplated, the advice of a fetal medicine specialist and HIV physician should be sought and prophylaxis with highly active antiretroviral therapy (HAART) considered.[13]

Prophylaxis of opportunistic infections during pregnancy should be based on criteria similar to those for non-pregnant women with HIV. These opportunistic infections are *Pnemocystis carinii* pneumonia, *Mycobacterium avium* infection, toxoplasmosis, tuberculosis and herpes simplex virus.

Approximately 98 per cent of HIV-infected children have acquired the virus from their mothers – during pregnancy, at delivery or through breastfeeding. Thus, prevention of mother-to-child transmission is a major health priority. Varying mother-to-child transmission rates have been quoted, ranging from 13–25 per cent in Europe to 35 per cent in developing countries. Risk factors for transmission are advanced maternal HIV disease, low antenatal CD4 T-lymphocyte counts, high maternal plasma viral loads, mode of delivery, duration of membrane rupture, chorioamnionitis and preterm delivery.[14] Breastfeeding is associated with a two-fold increase in the rate of transmission, from 14 to 28 per cent.[15]

All women who are HIV positive should be advised to take anti-retroviral therapy during pregnancy and at delivery [A]. The optimal regimen should be determined on a case by case basis by an HIV physician. Women with advanced HIV should be treated with a HAART regimen. The start of treatment should be deferred if possible until after the first trimester [A].[13]

The AIDS Clinical Trial Group (ACTG) 076 trial of zidovudine (ZDV) administered this drug to mothers in pregnancy (14–34 weeks gestation) and delivery, and to the newborn for 6 weeks. They showed that transmission could be reduced by as much as two-thirds, reducing to 8.3 per cent [B].

Women who do not require HIV treatment for their own health require anti-retroviral therapy to prevent mother-to-child transmission. Anti-retroviral therapy is usually commenced between 28 and 32 weeks of gestation and should be continued intrapartum [A].[13]

Pregnancy has not been shown to have an adverse affect on the natural history of HIV. No benefit to maternal health from termination of pregnancy has been demonstrated.

HIV is non-teratogenic.

The issue of associated drug abuse is discussed in Chapter 6.12, Drug and alcohol misuse.

### Intrapartum

A meta-analysis of six observational, prospective studies showed a reduction of approximately 30 per cent in transmission with delivery by caesarean section.[16] However, this analysis was based on a crude comparison of transmission rates and was unable to control for potential confounding factors [A]. The European Collaborative Study suggested a reduction of HIV transmission by up to 50 per cent.[17] However, any potential protective benefit of caesarean section has to be balanced against its risks and costs. Morbidity is more common and severe in HIV-infected women. The implications of caesarean section for the health of the mother and child are particularly fraught in developing countries. If there is longer than 4 hours between rupture of the membranes and delivery, the value of caesarean section is decreased.

Women who have a detectable plasma viral load and/or who are not taking HAART should be offered a planned caesarean section as it reduces the risk of mother to child transmission. However, whether elective caesarean section is of benefit in women taking HAART who have an undetectable plasma viral load at the time of delivery is uncertain. There is an increase in the vertical transmission once the membranes have been ruptured for 4 hours. However, if a woman presents with this history, delivery by caesarean section is still recommended.[13]

A zidovudine infusion should be started 4 hours before beginning the caesarean section and should continue until the umbilical cord has been clamped. A maternal sample for plasma viral load should be taken at delivery. The cord should be clamped as early as possible and the baby should be bathed immediately after the birth.[13]

Women who opt for vaginal delivery should have their membranes left intact as long as possible and the use of fetal scalp electrodes and fetal blood sampling should be avoided. Women should continue their HAART regimen throughout labour and if an intravenous zidovudine is required it should be commenced at the onset of labour and continued until the umbilical cord has been clamped [D,E].[13] HIV infection *per se* is not an indication for continuous electronic fetal monitoring.

### Postpartum

In the UK, all women who are HIV positive should be advised not to breastfeed their babies. Anti-retroviral therapy should be discontinued or changed as deemed appropriate by an HIV physician. All infants born to women who are HIV positive should be treated with anti-retroviral therapy from birth.[13]

---

### KEY POINTS

- Testing for HIV in the antenatal period should be offered to all women, irrespective of their supposed risk for the virus.
- If HIV positive, the care of the pregnant woman is managed jointly with a physician with a specialist interest in infectious disease.
- Increased mother-to-child transmission occurs with:
  - a low maternal CD4 count
  - high maternal HIV RNA load
  - invasive procedures during labour – artificial rupture of membranes (ARM), fetal blood sampling (FBS) and fetal scalp electrode (FSE)
  - prolonged interval between rupture of membranes and delivery
  - concurrent ascending bacterial infection
  - vitamin A deficiency.
- Decreased vertical transmission occurs with:
  - undetectable maternal HIV RNA
  - ZDV/nevirapine/HARRT administration
  - all women should be advised to take anti-retroviral therapy during pregnancy and at delivery (even if the woman does

not need it for her own health) as therapy reduces mother-to-child transmission). If given to solely reduce vertical transmission, anti-retroviral therapy is usually commenced between 28 and 32 weeks. Women with advanced HIV should be treated with HART regimen and treatment deferred if possible until after the first trimester
- delivery by elective caesarean section if a detectable plasma viral load and/or who are not taking HAART
- avoidance of breastfeeding.

# HEPATITIS VIRUSES

## Hepatitis A

### Epidemiology and aetiology
The virus is most commonly transmitted by the fecal–oral route by either person-to-person contact or ingestion of contaminated food or water. Hepatitis A is endemic in developing countries due to poor hygiene and sanitation.

### Presentation and diagnosis
Acute hepatitis A infection is clinically indistinguishable from other causes of acute viral hepatitis. Most infected children under the age of six years are asymptomatic. In the older child and adult, clinical manifestations can vary from a mild, non-specific, anicteric infection to fulminant hepatic failure. Symptoms include fever, malaise, anorexia, nausea, vomiting and abdominal discomfort. Jaundice may be present, with dark urine and hepatomegaly. A raised serum alanine transaminase indicates acute hepatic injury. Infection can be diagnosed by the presence of anti-hepatitis A IgM.

### Management
Treatment is supportive, and complete recovery with no long-term illness is the usual outcome. Administration of human serum immunoglobulin protects against hepatitis A by either preventing infection or attenuating symptoms. Protection is short lived, so injections needed to be repeated every 3–6 months. A vaccine is available and provides up to ten years' protection.

#### In relation to pregnancy

**Antepartum**
Advice on travelling to areas where hepatitis A is endemic should be available. The safety of the hepatitis A vaccine in pregnancy has not been determined, although the theoretical risk to the fetus of an inactivated vaccine is low.

**Fetal infection**
There are no long-term fetal consequences of hepatitis A infection.

## Hepatitis B

This is a blood-borne, double-stranded DNA virus. The virus has three major structural antigens: surface antigen (HbsAg), core antigen (HbcAg) and e antigen (HbeAg).

### Epidemiology and aetiology
This is an extremely infectious virus; the UK prevalence may be as high as 1 per cent in inner city areas, with high proportions of immigrant women. Transmission of the virus is by bodily secretions (principally blood) and thus with sexual contact, blood transfusions, intravenous drug abuse and perinatal transmission.

### Clinical presentation and diagnosis
Infection with hepatitis B is often asymptomatic, except in intravenous drug abusers, of whom 30 per cent will develop jaundice. Non-specific symptoms and signs include nausea and vomiting, fatigue and malaise, photophobia and headache, right upper abdominal pain and diarrhoea. Physical examination of patients often shows no abnormality, although hepatomegaly (10 per cent of patients), splenomegaly (5 per cent) and lymphadenopathy (5 per cent) may be present.[18] Hepatitis B virus causes acute and chronic hepatitis and the chances of becoming chronically infected vary with age. Infected neonates and young children are more likely to develop chronic infection.

Acute hepatitis B is usually self-limiting and most patients who contract the virus will clear it completely. Fulminant hepatic failure occurs in about 1 per cent of cases. All cases must be notified and sexual and close household contacts screened and vaccinated.

Non-specific haematological tests commonly show a leukopenia, and may show anaemia and thrombocytopenia. Biochemistry reveals elevated serum aminotransferase.

Diagnosis is by the presence of HbsAg. The presence of HbeAg shows disease is active with viral shedding into the bloodstream. Antibodies to e begin to appear in the serum at the time HbeAg is disappearing. The presence of the e antigen indicates a period of high patient infectivity, as the presence of e antibodies indicates low infectivity. Complete resolution of the disease is indicated by the disappearance of HBsAg and the appearance of surface antibodies. These antibodies provide immunity, whether obtained from resolution of infection or vaccination with HbsAg.

### Management
Patients should be monitored to ensure fulminant liver disease does not develop, and should have serological testing three months after infection to check the virus is cleared from the blood.

About 5–10 per cent of patients will remain positive for HbsAg at three months and a smaller proportion will have ongoing viral replication. These patients require follow up by a hepatologist.[18]

Some individuals with chronic hepatitis B will have clinically insignificant or minimal liver disease and never go on to develop complications. Long-term sequelae can be the development of cirrhosis/hepatocellular carcinoma.

### In relation to pregnancy

**Antepartum**

All women are routinely offered testing for hepatitis B antibodies at their antenatal booking visit. If testing positive for the first time, the infectious state of the patient should be ascertained by serology. Relevant issues include testing of the partner, testing for other sexually transmitted disease including HIV, safe sexual practice, baseline liver function tests and referral to a hepatology physician.

The presence of hepatitis B does not seem to pose additional risk for the pregnancy.

**Intrapartum**

Fetal scalp electrodes and fetal blood sampling should be avoided. The use of forceps rather than ventouse has been suggested as most appropriate for instrumental delivery.

**Postpartum**

Neonates infected at birth have a >90 per cent chance of becoming chronic carriers of hepatitis B virus, with the associated risks of subsequent cirrhosis and hepatocellular carcinoma. Management plans should thus include administration of passive immunoglobulin in the first 24 hours after birth to those neonates with mothers of high infectivity, and administration of the active hepatitis B vaccine to those neonates whose mothers have a low infectivity or those deemed to be going to an 'at-risk' household.

Provided babies are immunized, there is no contraindication to breastfeeding.

---

### EBM

- There is limited research on the most appropriate mode of delivery for hepatitis-B-positive women. Thus, vaginal delivery is considered appropriate.
- Breastfeeding is permitted.

---

### KEY POINTS

- If the patient tests positive for hepatitis B, her infectious state should be ascertained.
- Screen also for hepatitis C, HIV and all other sexually transmitted diseases.
- This disease appears to confer no increased risk on fetal well-being during pregnancy.

---

- Vertical transmission, usually at the time of delivery, is high, reaching 95 per cent in mothers who are both HBsAg-positive and HbeAg-positive.
- In labour, aim to keep the membranes intact for as long as possible. Avoid FBS/FSE use.
- Deliver in a way that confers least trauma to the baby. Forceps delivery is favoured over ventouse by many clinicians, although this is not evidence based.
- Administer hepatitis B immunoglobulin to those neonates born to high-infectivity mothers. Administer hepatitis B vaccine to those neonates born to low-infectivity mothers.

## Hepatitis C

### Epidemiology and aetiology

As with hepatitis B, this virus can be transmitted sexually and perinatally. However, the main group of hepatitis-C-positive individuals is within the intravenous drug culture. A new injection drug user has an 80 per cent chance of becoming positive for hepatitis C antibody within one year.[19]

### Clinical presentation and diagnosis

The clinical features of hepatitis C are non-specific. It is often diagnosed when patients have vague symptoms and are revealed to have abnormal alanine transferase levels. Cirrhosis develops in 20–40 per cent of patients, and in these there is up to 3 per cent annual development of hepatocellular carcinoma.[13]

Early identification and referral of cases of acute hepatitis C infection are important as there is strong evidence to suggest that early treatment with alpha-interferon reduces the risk of chronic infection. The rate of chronicity in untreated patients is approximately 80 per cent.[18] Antibodies to hepatitis C appear relatively late in the course of the infection and if clinical suspicion is high, the patient's serum should be tested for hepatitis C RNA to establish a diagnosis.

### In relation to pregnancy

**Antepartum**

Systematic screening for HCV is not indicated. Screening is indicated in high-risk groups or if a women tests positive for hepatitis B virus or HIV. Antenatal care should involve a physician with a specialist interest in hepatitis C. With a positive hepatitis C virus test, the woman should be counselled about the risk of giving birth to an infected newborn and about the higher infection rate if there is co-existent HIV. Hepatitis C virus RNA determination is useful because, if negative, these patients can be counselled about the lower transmission rate.

**Intrapartum**

This management is the same as for hepatitis B. Further research is required into whether delivery by caesarean section will reduce transmission.

**Postpartum**

There is no contraindication to breastfeeding.

**Fetal infection**

Vertical transmission rates vary greatly in reported studies, although most rates are in the range of 10 to 15 per cent.[18] Increased perinatal transmission occurs in women who

---

**EBM**

- There is limited knowledge about the appropriate mode of delivery in hepatitis C-positive women. Thus vaginal delivery is permitted.
- Breastfeeding does not appear to increase the risk of mother-to-child transmission.

---

have high titres of hepatitis C virus RNA or who are co-infected with HIV.

No immunoprophylaxis is available at this time.

---

**KEY POINTS**

- Screening for hepatitis C is not routinely offered in the antenatal period.
- There is increased mother-to-child transmission with detectable maternal hepatitis C virus RNA and if there is co-existent HIV infection.
- Intrapartum management is the same as for hepatitis B individuals.
- There is no neonatal immunoprophylaxis available.

---

## Hepatitis D

This is a single-stranded RNA virus that requires co-infection with hepatitis B virus. It often increases the severity of the illness. It is usually confined to intravenous drug abusers in the UK.

## Hepatitis E

This virus is transmitted by the fecal–oral route and produces a self-limiting illness similar to hepatitis A. It is common in the developing world. Pregnant women with acute hepatitis E infection have a risk of fulminant liver failure of around 15 per cent, with a mortality of 5 per cent.

# BACTERIAL INFECTIONS

## Gonorrhoea

### Epidemiology and aetiology

The bacterium *Neisseria gonorrhoeae* is a Gram-negative, intracellular diplococcus that can be found in the epithelium

of the genitourinary tract and in the rectum, pharynx and eye. *N. gonorrhoeae* can ascend, causing uterine and tubal infection. It is a sexually transmitted disease. Risk factors include multiple or casual sexual contacts, 20–24 years of age, past or current history of illicit drug use and low socio-economic status.

## Presentation and diagnosis

The incubation period is approximately 10 days. The most common symptom is an increased vaginal discharge, classically a purulent yellow-green. Other symptoms are vaginal itching or burning, bleeding during or after intercourse, urethritis, dysuria and tender Skene's or Bartholin's glands. Between 30 and 60 per cent of infected women will have asymptomatic or subclinical infection.

Infections that are not treated or are treated inadequately may spread from the lower genital tract to the endometrium and Fallopian tubes – pelvic inflammatory disease. Silent episodes of pelvic inflammatory disease can occur, grossly affecting the reproductive capacity of the woman, increasing the risk of tubal infertility/ectopic pregnancy and causing chronic lower abdominal pain.

Disseminated gonoccocal infection is rare, involving fever, arthritis and skin disorders. It is reported to be more common in pregnancy.

The diagnosis is culture of the gonococcal organism from endocervical, urethral, anal or pharyngeal swabs. A quicker, less sensitive method is the demonstration of the Gram-negative diplococci on direct microscopy. PCR can demonstrate gonoccocal DNA, and is an accurate but expensive test.

## Management

Management of the patient should involve a genitourinary physician. Classical treatment of gonorrhoea was by penicillin, but large-scale resistance is occurring by the organism. Concomitant treatment for chlamydia should be given as these infections co-exist in 45 per cent of cases. Classical treatment is a cephalosporin with azithromycin to cover chlamydia.

Management plans should include avoidance of sexual intercourse until treatment is completed, eradication of the organism (confirmed with follow-up cultures), contact tracing with treatment of affected partners, and advice on safe sex practices.

### In relation to pregnancy

#### Antepartum

Acute gonococcal infection is associated with miscarriage, premature labour, pre-labour rupture of membranes, chorioamnionitis and small for gestational age fetus. It has also been associated with stillbirth.

During pregnancy, recommended treatment is with a cephalosporin or spectinomycin. Dilatation and curettage after a miscarriage or for a termination of pregnancy has an increased risk of endometritis if the organism is present. Thus, ideally, vaginal swabs are performed prior to this surgery.

### Intrapartum

*Neisseria gonorrhoeae* can be transmitted from the mother's genital tract to the neonate during labour. The usual manifestation of neonatal infection is gonococcal ophthalmia neonatorum, which has a risk of transmission of 30–50 per cent, which is increased with premature rupture of membranes and premature delivery. It occurs in the first few days of life, presenting as a bilateral, purulent, conjunctivitis. Prompt identification and treatment with antibiotics are necessary as resulting blindness can occur.

### Postpartum

Gonorrhoea can cause endometritis and pelvic sepsis.

---

## KEY POINTS

- Classical symptoms are a purulent vaginal discharge with vaginal itch and urethritis.
- 30–60 per cent of infections are asymptomatic.
- Complications of ascending infection are:
  - pelvic inflammatory disease
  - chronic pelvic pain
  - increased risk of an ectopic pregnancy
  - tubal infertility.
- Management should be within a genitourinary clinic.
- Contact tracing and treatment are vital.
- Treatment of gonorrhoea is with a cephalosporin.
- Concomitant treatment for chlamydia should be administered. These infections co-exist in 45 per cent of cases.

---

## Meningococcal disease

This is any clinical condition caused by the Gram-negative aerobic bacterium *Neisseria meningitidis*. The most prevalent subtypes in Europe are B and C. The conditions include purulent conjunctivitis, septic arthritis, meningitis, and septicaemia with or without meningitis.

### Epidemiology and aetiology

In the UK, the incidence varies from two to eight cases per 100 000 people. Outbreaks may occur among family contacts, school children and students. It is transmitted by close contact, by exchange of upper respiratory tract secretions. The age peaks are under two years and between 15 and 24 years of age. Carriage of meningococcus in the nasopharynx has been reported to be 10–15 per cent.

### Presentation and diagnosis

Meningitis typically presents with headache, fever, neck stiffness, nausea, vomiting and photophobia. Meningococcaemia is characterized by a petechial or purpuric rash. When meningococcus reaches the bloodstream, there is massive production of endotoxin, and shock and disseminated intravascular coagulation are induced. This can lead to hypotension and multi-organ failure. The mortality rate of fulminant meningococcal septicaemia is approximately 30 per cent. Classical diagnosis is culture of the organism, but this has a low sensitivity, especially if antibiotics have been administered prior to the sample. Gram staining or methods detecting polysaccharide antigen can obtain rapid results. Serological testing and PCR can also be utilized.

### Management

Prompt recognition and treatment are essential as the case fatality is 10–20 per cent. Treatment is with penicillin or cephalosporin, for example ceftriaxone. Antibiotics are recommended in people exposed to someone with meningococcal disease – rifampacin, ceftriaxone or ciprofloxacin. There are vaccines available for the serogroups A and C; these are only effective in older children and adults.

#### In relation to pregnancy

The presentation and treatment of the disease are the same in the pregnant woman. As with any acute febrile illness, miscarriage and premature labour are associated complications. There are no teratogenic effects of the pathogen.

## Listeria

*Listeria monocytogenes* is a Gram-positive bacterium. Unusually for a bacterium that does not form spores, it is very resistant to the effects of freezing, drying and heat.

### Epidemiology and aetiology

Up to 10 per cent of humans may carry *Listeria* in their intestinal tract. The infective consequences depend on both the strain of the pathogen and the susceptibility of the victim. Most healthy people are unaware of an infection with *Listeria*. The vulnerable groups are the immunocompromised, pregnant women and the newborn. *Listeria* has been associated with ingestion of various contaminated foods, including raw milk, soft cheese, ice cream, raw meat and vegetables, and is associated with ready-to-eat meals.

### Presentation and diagnosis

The symptoms of listeria can be non-specific with influenza-like symptoms and fever, nausea and vomiting. Complications are septicaemia and meningo-encephalitis.

Diagnosis is by culture of the organism from blood, cerebrospinal fluid or stool or from serological testing.

## Management
Treatment is with penicillin.

### In relation to pregnancy

#### Antepartum
*Listeria* infection predisposes to miscarriage, premature labour and stillbirth, thus advice pertaining to the avoidance of danger foodstuffs during pregnancy should be given.

Meconium presence in liquor at very premature gestation has been associated with *Listeria* infection.

Other bacterial infections are discussed in relevant chapters elsewhere in this book: urinary tract infections/pyelonephritis in Chapter 6.6, Renal disease; bacterial vaginosis in Chapter 21, Preterm labour; and group B *Streptococcus* in Chapter 21, Preterm labour.

# MYCOBACTERIUM INFECTION

## Tuberculosis

The causative organism is *Mycobacterium tuberculosis*. This is a widespread disease, more common in the developing world.

## Epidemiology and aetiology
Upper respiratory tract droplets spread the bacilli. Risk factors for infection are poor living conditions, overcrowding and poor nutrition. People are more susceptible at the extremes of age and if immunocompromised. There is an increased incidence in the immigrant population in the UK.

## Presentation and diagnosis
There are two major patterns of disease with tuberculosis (TB). Primary TB is seen as an initial infection, usually in children. This is a non-specific illness, with a cough and wheeze. The initial focus of infection is a small subpleural granuloma accompanied by hilar lymph node infection. In nearly all cases, these granulomas resolve and there is no further spread of the infection.

Secondary TB, seen mostly in adults, is a reactivation of previous disease, particularly if the health status of the person declines. The granulomatous inflammation is much more florid and widespread. In pulmonary TB, there is typically a gradual onset of symptoms over weeks/months. Malaise, anorexia, weight loss, night sweats and purulent or blood-stained sputum predominate.

Miliary TB is the result of acute diffuse dissemination of tubercle bacilli via the bloodstream.

Sputum is positive for acid-fast bacilli when stained with Ziehl–Nielsen and cultures grown. The tuberculin skin test is based on the type 4 hypersensitivity reaction, i.e. with previous TB infection there will be sensitized lymphocytes that can react to another encounter with antigens from TB organisms. Injection with tuberculin will then produce a wheal and red induration. This test will also be positive if a person has been vaccinated with bacille Calmette Guérin (BCG). A chest x-ray is required.

## Management
Treatment and drug regimens are given by a specialist chest physician. Treatment for TB uses antibiotics to kill the bacteria. The two antibiotics most commonly used are rifampicin and isoniazid. However, instead of the short course of antibiotics typically used to cure other bacterial infections, TB requires much longer periods of treatment (around 6–12 months) to entirely eliminate mycobacteria from the body. Latent TB treatment usually uses a single antibiotic, while active TB disease is best treated with combinations of several antibiotics, to reduce the risk of the bacteria developing antibiotic resistance. Contact tracing is vital. BCG vaccination is traditionally given at approximately 13 years of age. In high-risk populations, the vaccine is given in the neonatal period.

### In relation to pregnancy

#### Antepartum
Tuberculosis discovered during pregnancy should be treated without delay, with immediate involvement of a chest physician. Isoniazid, rifampacin and ethambutol can be used in pregnancy. Pyridoxine is recommended for pregnant women taking isoniazid. No increase in morbidity and mortality from TB has been noted during pregnancy and there does not appear to be an increase in the relapse rate in pregnancy.[20] The one exception is in pregnant women with HIV infection previously infected with TB.

#### Intrapartum
Any patient with active disease should be isolated. Inhalational anaesthesia should be avoided.

#### Postpartum
The small concentration of anti-TB drugs in breast milk does not produce toxicity, so breastfeeding is permitted.[20] The neonate needs to be vaccinated with BCG and may need anti-tuberculous drugs.

#### Fetal infection
Congenital tuberculosis is rare.

# TOXOPLASMOSIS

*Toxoplasma gondii* is an intracellular protozoan parasite.

## Epidemiology and aetiology

The definitive host of this organism is the domestic cat. Transmission may occur transplacentally, by ingestion of raw or undercooked meat containing protozoan cysts, or by exposure to oocysts in soil/cat litter contaminated with cat faeces.

## Presentation and diagnosis

Asymptomatic infections are common, and up to 80 per cent of some populations are infected. The disease mostly has no clinical consequences. Those at risk for severe disease are the developing fetus and the immunocompromised. Serological testing can demonstrate antibodies to *Toxoplasma gondii*, IgM antibody or significant changes in the IgG antibody titre, indicating recent infection.

## Management

Treatment is with spiromycin.

### In relation to pregnancy

#### Antenatal

Routine testing for immunity to toxoplasmosis is not undertaken in the UK. To minimize the risk, pregnant women should not eat undercooked meat or handle cat litter and should wear rubber gloves if gardening. Frequent hand washing is advised.

If testing is performed, present and past infection need to be carefully distinguished. Old toxoplasmosis infection does not pose a fetal risk.

It is not known whether antenatal treatment in women with toxoplasmosis reduces the congenital transmission of *Toxoplasma gondii* [A].

#### Fetal infection

The implications to the fetus of *Toxoplasma* infections are discussed in Chapter 13, Fetal infections.

## CHLAMYDIA

Chlamydia is the most prevalent bacterial sexually transmitted disease. It is an obligatory intracellular bacterium – *Chlamydia trachomatis* – that contains DNA and RNA. There are numerous serotypes, D–K being responsible for the oculogenital and sexually transmitted strains of the disease.[21]

## Epidemiology and aetiology

Risk factors include multiple sexual partners, young age, history of other sexually transmitted diseases and low socioeconomic class.

The cost-effectiveness of the screening and treatment of chlamydia has long been a subject of debate. The greatest rise in chlamydial infection over the past ten years has been in the younger sexually active population – 16–19-year-old females. Although professional awareness of the infection is rising, genitourinary clinics remain the only setting in which nationwide screening of this often symptomatic but devastating disease is undertaken. Screening is recognized to significantly reduce the prevalence of genital tract infections and pelvic inflammatory disease. The prevalence of chlamydia varies considerably in different populations (1–29 per cent); restricted screening would be unlikely to have a great effect on its prevalence as the general population makes limited use of genitourinary clinics.

After identifying demographic and behavioural risk factors, the Chlamydia Advisory Group concluded that, in addition to testing symptomatic patients and those in higher risk groups (people attending genitourinary clinics or those seeking termination of pregnancy), the evidence supported opportunistic screening. Recommendations were that screening should be offered to all sexually active women below the age of 25 years and to those over the age of 25 years with a new sexual partner or who have had two or more partners in the past year. Recommended screening is by the ligase reaction test on a first-catch urine sample, rather than the more invasive endocervical swabs of older, less accurate, tests such as ELISA.

## Presentation and diagnosis

The incubation period is 7–21 days.

Infection with chlamydia can be asymptomatic in up to 75 per cent of cases. Symptoms are increased/unusual vaginal discharge, dyspareunia, intermenstrual bleeding, abdominal pain or dysuria.

The complications of inadequately treated or untreated chlamydia are pelvic inflammatory disease, chronic pelvic pain and salpingitis, thus increasing the risk of future ectopic pregnancies and/or tubal infertility. A perihepatitis can occur, the Fitz–Hugh–Curtis syndrome.

An endocervical swab and/or first void urine are suitable specimens for establishing the diagnosis. Cell culture of the organism is too expensive in non-endemic regions. The most commonly employed diagnostic tests are PCR and ligase chain reaction. These amplification assays possess higher sensitivities than previously used enzyme immunoassay tests.[22]

## Management

These patients should be managed with input from the genitourinary clinic.

Contact tracing and treatment are essential – failure to treat partners is probably the most common cause of 'treatment failure'. First-line agents for treatment outside pregnancy are doxycycline (for 1 week) or a single dose of azithromycin (better compliance but more expensive).

## In relation to pregnancy

### Antepartum

Antibiotic therapy in pregnancy reduces the number of women with positive cultures following treatment by approximately 90 per cent compared with placebo [A].[22]

Classical treatment of chlamydia is with tetracyclines, which are contraindicated in pregnancy. Erythromycin is an acceptable alternative, but can have gastrointestinal side effects and needs a full 7-day course. A recent Cochrane Review cites amoxycillin as an acceptable alternative therapy to erythromycin in pregnancy if the drug is not being tolerated. If amoxycillin/erythromycin are contraindicated or not tolerated, clindamycin or azithromycin (single dose/ fewer side effects compared to erythromycin) may be prescribed [A].[23]

Preterm labour, premature rupture of the membranes and low birth weight have also been associated with chlamydial infection.

### Intrapartum

Perinatally transmitted *Chlamydia trachomatis* can cause conjunctivitis and pneumonitis. In untreated mothers, the incidence of conjunctivitis is 35–50 per cent and of pneumonitis 11–20 per cent. Conjunctivitis occurs earlier, typically between the 5th and 12th postnatal days, with a mucoid discharge that becomes purulent, followed by oedema of the eyelids and conjunctival erythema. Pneumonia occurs later, at 2–3 weeks of age, with symptoms including tachypnoea and cough.

### Postpartum

Chlamydia can cause postpartum endometritis.

---

### EBM

- Antibiotic therapy decreases the number of pregnant women with positive cultures following treatment by 90 per cent.
- Typical treatment of this disease is with tetracyclines. These are contraindicated in pregnancy. Acceptable alternatives are amoxycillin or erythromycin.

---

### KEY POINTS

- Screening for this disease is recommended for all those aged <25 years who are sexually active and all those aged >25 years who have had a new sexual partner in the last year or who have had two or more different partners.
- Screening should be performed on first-catch urine samples and analysed by the ligase chain reaction.
- This disease is asymptomatic in up to 75 per cent of cases.
- Classical symptoms are increased vaginal discharge, intermenstrual bleeding and dyspareunia.

---

- Pelvic complications are the same as for gonorrhoea.
- Management should be in conjunction with a genitourinary clinic.
- Contact tracing and treatment are vital.

---

## SPIROCHAETES

## Syphilis

This disease is caused by the spirochaete *Treponema pallidum* and is usually transmitted by sexual contact. It is a complex systemic disease with multiple clinical manifestations.

### Epidemiology and aetiology

Humans are the natural hosts of *T. pallidum*. The organism usually penetrates abraded or damaged skin or mucous membrane, although intact membrane can be penetrated. Dissemination rapidly occurs. The average incubation period is 28 days.[24] There is an association between syphilis and HIV; it is not known whether syphilis predisposes individuals to HIV acquisition or whether transmission of either disease is potentiated by the presence of the other.

### Presentation and diagnosis

Infection with syphilis is characterized by several stages. Initial disease development is usually denoted by the appearance of a chancre (ulcer). This is the classical primary syphilis lesion at the site of inoculation, which is usually small, firm, round and painless. Most patients then develop secondary syphilis 3 weeks to three months after the primary stage. This is a systemic illness, with fever, malaise, lymphadenopathy, non-pruritic rash and mucosal lesions. Without treatment, these clinical manifestations usually resolve spontaneously. There is then a latent period.[24] In about one-third of untreated patients, latent syphilis develops subsequently into tertiary syphilis, with neurosyphilis, cardiovascular involvement or gummatous disease 3–10 years after the initial stages.

Unlike most bacterial infections, syphilis cannot be cultured quickly or cheaply. Visualization of *T. pallidum* can be made by dark field microscopy, but this is very sensitive to the method of sample collection. Serological testing is the mainstay of screening and diagnosis. There are two main types of test: the non-treponemal and the treponemal tests. Non-treponemal tests detect antibodies to reagin (a cholesterol–lecithin–cardiolipin antigen). The usual tests are the Venereal Disease Research Laboratory (VDRL) and the rapid plasma reagin (RPR), which are positive within about 4–7 days of onset of primary syphilis. However, there is lack of sensitivity in primary syphilis, with 13–41 per cent of affected individuals testing negative. These tests are usually positive in people presenting with secondary syphilis. The tests become negative between 3 and 12 months after treatment.[24] Advantages of non-treponemal tests are that they are inexpensive, easy to perform and sensitive, and therefore good for screening. The disadvantages are consequent upon false-positive results, which may be caused by acute viral infection (such as hepatitis and measles), malaria, TB, advanced malignancy, pregnancy and various autoimmune conditions. The diagnosis of syphilis needs to be confirmed by a treponemal serological test, such as the FTA-ABS (fluorescent-treponemal antibody–absorbed test). These tests remain positive whether or not treatment has been administered.[24]

## Management

Treatment is with a single intramuscular dose of penicillin for patients who have had syphilis for less than a year; greater doses are needed for patients infected for longer. Contact tracing and counselling should be performed through the genitourinary clinic.

### In relation to pregnancy

#### Antepartum

Syphilis is screened for in the routine antenatal booking bloods by the non-treponemal tests. If positive, confirmatory treponemal tests should be performed.

Treatment during pregnancy is with the penicillin regimen appropriate for the stage of syphilis [C]. A complication of treatment is the Jarisch–Herxheimer reaction, a systemic reaction that may occur a few hours after the administration of penicillin, with fever, myalgia and vasodilatation. Women who are treated in the second half of pregnancy need to seek medical help as they are at risk of premature labour or fetal distress. Pregnancy does not affect the course of the disease in the mother.

Syphilis has been associated with spontaneous abortion, stillbirth, non-immune hydrops, intrauterine growth restriction and perinatal death, as well as serious sequelae in liveborn affected children.

#### Fetal infection

The implications to the fetus of syphilis infections are discussed in Chapter 13, Fetal infections.

**KEY POINTS**

- Non-treponemal tests are used for syphilis screening.
- False-positive results on non-treponemal tests can occur with:
  - acute viral infection
  - malaria/tuberculosis
  - advanced malignancy
  - pregnancy
  - autoimmune conditions.
- Treponemal tests are used for the diagnosis of syphilis.
- Management should be in conjunction with the genitourinary clinic.
- Contact tracing and treatment are essential.

# PROTOZOA

## Trichomonas

Trichomoniasis vaginalis is the vaginal infection caused by this flagellated protozoon. It prefers a high vaginal pH (>4.5) and is transmitted by sexual contact.

### Epidemiology and aetiology

Risk factors for trichomoniasis are smoking, Afro-Caribbean/African race, decreased educational level and increased number of sexual partners. There is a high co-infection rate with other sexually transmitted diseases.

### Clinical presentation and diagnosis

Symptoms vary widely, but common presenting complaints are pruritis, frothy copious yellow/green discharge, dyspareunia and vulvovaginal soreness. Signs of the infection are the typical odour of the discharge and erythema of the vulva and cervix. Diagnosis is made on a saline wet preparation and motile flagellated trichomonads can be seen on the periphery of clumps of epithelial cells. More sensitive techniques such as culture, immunofluorescence and enzyme immunoassay are available, although these are more expensive and time consuming.

### Management

Metronidazole is the treatment of choice. Partners must also be treated.

#### In relation to pregnancy

##### Antepartum

Owing to the increased pelvic blood supply in pregnancy, trichomoniasis may result in vaginal bleeding, particularly postcoital.

Trichomoniasis has been associated with preterm birth and other pregnancy complications. Metronidazole treatment provides a parasitological cure but it is not known whether this treatment has any effect on pregnancy outcome; it is only recommended after the first trimester.

# FUNGAL INFECTION

## Candida

Superficial and subcutaneous fungal infections affect the skin, keratinous tissues and mucous membranes. Systemic infection can occur by opportunistic infection in the at-risk host or with more invasive organisms. These systemic infections are associated with a high morbidity and mortality. *Candida albicans* alone is the cause of vaginitis in approximately 85–90 per cent of cases. Other non-albicans species are *Candida glabrata* and *Candida tropicalis*, which are increasing in frequency.

## Epidemiology and aetiology

The normal vaginal flora, lactobacilli, are the most important barrier to candidal infection.

Factors predisposing to an increased colonization by *Candida* are pregnancy, uncontrolled diabetes, oral contraceptives, antibiotic usage, intrauterine contraceptive devices and increased frequency of sexual intercourse.

Most women will suffer from a symptomatic candidial infection ('thrush') at some time, and up to 20 per cent of women in the reproductive age group can be found to have asymptomatic candida. This shows a dramatic decrease after the menopause. It is not a sexually transmitted disease. Approximately 5 per cent of women are inflicted with candida as a chronic condition. Sources of the recurrence can be vaginal inoculation or from a gastrointestinal reservoir.

Recurrent infections are associated with increased candidal virulence, *Candida* non-albicans and host factors such as decreased secretory local immunity or IgE-mediated hypersensitivity reaction.

The incidence of fungal infections is increasing rapidly in relation to the growing number of immunocompromised individuals in the population – on chemotherapy, on immunosuppressive drugs and HIV positive.

## Presentation and diagnosis

Presentation is with itching and pain in the vulval and vaginal area, which may be associated with an increased vaginal discharge and dysuria. Erythema and excoriation can be seen around the vulval area. The vaginal epithelium and cervix may be reddened. There may be a thick, curd-white discharge. A high vaginal swab should be taken to confirm the clinical diagnosis, with microscopy of both the cells and mycelia being stained Gram positive, and subsequent culture of the organisms.

## Management

Self-treatment with anti-mycotics is available in the form of vaginal creams, pessaries and oral tablets. Recurrent self-medicating is not recommended, and microbiological diagnosis of the disease is necessary. Preventative measures, such as avoiding tight synthetic underwear, avoidance of heavily perfumed bath products and perfumes, application of live yoghurt to the affected area and avoiding sweet foods, may decrease the recurrence.

In relation to pregnancy

### Antepartum

Vaginal candida infections are more common in pregnancy. Owing to the higher oestrogen stimulation, there is more glycogen available in the vaginal cells, which provides nutrients promoting candidal multiplication.

Clinical symptoms should have the diagnosis confirmed with a high vaginal swab, and topical treatment is appropriate in pregnancy.

### Fetal infection

There is no risk to the fetus from candidal infection.

## Key References

1. Whitley RJ, Roizman B. Herpes simplex virus infections. *Lancet* 2001; **357**: 1513–18.
2. Ashely, RL. Performance and use of HSV type specific serology test kits. *Herpes* 2002; **9**: 38–45.
3. Brown ZA, Selke S, Zeh, J *et al*. The acquisition of herpes simplex virus during pregnancy. *N Engl J Med* 1997; **337**: 509–15.
4. Low-Beer NM, Kinghorn GR. *Management of genital herpes in pregnancy*. Green top guideline no 30. London: RCOG, September 2007.
5. Arvin AM, Hendsleigh PA, Prober CG *et al*. Failure of antepartum maternal cultures to predict the infant's risk of exposure to herpes simplex virus at delivery. *N Engl J Med* 1986; **315**: 796–800.
6. Scott, LL, Sanchez PJ, Jackson GL *et al*. Acylcovir suppression to prevent caesarean delivery after first episode genital herpes. *Obstet Gynaecol* 1996; **87**: 69–73.
7. Byrne BMP, Crowley PA, Carrington D. *Chickenpox in pregnancy*. Green top guideline no 13. London: RCOG, September 2007.
8. Wallace MR, Bowler WA, Murray NB *et al*. Treatment of adult varicella with oral acyclovir. A randomized placebo controlled trial. *Ann Intern Med* 1992; **117**: 358–63.
9. Brown T, Anand A, Ritchie LD. Intrauterine parvovirus associated with hydrops fetalis. *Lancet* 1984; **2**: 1033–4.
10. Health Protection Agency. HIV and Sexually transmitted infections reviewed on 24 November 2003. Renewing the focus: HIV and other sexually transmitted infections in the United kingdom in 2002. Annual report, November 2003 [www.hpa.org.uk/infections/topics_az/hiv_and_sti/publications/annual2003/anual2003.htm]

11. Giaquinto C, Ruga E, Giacomet O, Rampon R. HIV: mother to child transmission, current knowledge and ongoing studies. *Int J Gynaecol Obstet* 1998; **63** (Suppl. 1): S161–5.

12. Brocklehurst P, Volmink J. Antiretrovirals for reducing the risk of mother to child transmission of HIV infection. *Cochrane Database Syst Rev* 2002; (**1**): CD003510.

13. Low-Beer NM, Smith JR. *Management of HIV in pregnancy.* Green top guideline 39. London: RCOG, April 2004.

14. Risk factors for mother-to-child transmission of HIV12. European Collabarative Study. *Lancet* 1992; **339**: 1007–12.

15. Dunn DT, Newell ML, Ades AE, Peckham CS. Risk of human immunodeficiency virus type 1 transmission through breast feeding. *Lancet* 1992; **340**: 585–8.

16. Villarl P, Spino C, Chalmers TC *et al.* Caesarean section to reduce perinatal transmission of human immunodeficiency virus. A metaanalysis. *Online J Curr Clin Trials* 1993; Doc no 74.

17. The European Collaborative Study. Caesarean section and risk of vertical transmission of HIV-1 infection. *Lancet*; **343**: 464–7.

18. Ryder SD. Acute hepatitis. *BMJ* 2001; **322**: 151–3.

19. Maddrey WC. Update in hepatology. *Ann Intern Med* 2001; **134**: 216–23.

20. Lazarus A, Sanders J. Management of tuberculosis. *Postgrad Med* 2000; **108**: 71–40.

21. Guaschino S, De Seta F. Update on Chlamydia trachomatis. *Ann NY Acad Sci* 2000; **900**: 293–300.

22. Brocklehurst P, Rooney G. Interventions for treating genital chlamydia trachomatis infection in pregnancy. *Cochrane Database Syst Rev* 2000; (**2**): CD000054.

23. Turrentine MA, Newton ER. Amoxycillin or erythromycin the treatment of antenatal chlamydial infection: a meta-analysis. *Obstet Gynecol* 1995; **86**: 1021–5.

24. Walker GJA. Antibiotics for syphilis diagnosed during pregnancy. *Cochrane Database Syst Rev* 2001; (**3**): CD001143.

# 7.5 Gestational diabetes

*Clare L Tower*

## INTRODUCTION

Gestational diabetes (GDM) is defined as impaired carbohydrate tolerance resulting in hyperglycaemia, which first develops or becomes diagnosed during pregnancy. Some of these women will, in fact, have previously undiagnosed diabetes, usually type 2. It is clinically important, both for the management of the pregnancy, but also as it significantly increases an individual's long-term risk of developing type 2 diabetes. Women developing GDM face similar increased risks as diabetic women in terms of macrosomia and its associated complications, neonatal hypoglycaemia and late pregnancy loss. Furthermore, their offspring are at increased risk of obesity and diabetes in the future.

## EPIDEMIOLOGY AND RISK FACTORS

Studies investigating risk factors for development of GDM vary with the definition of the disorder used, which in turn is dependent on the type of testing (see below).

Systematic reviews have suggested the risk factors are obesity, advanced maternal age, family history of diabetes, specific ethnic groups, high weight gain in early adulthood and current smoking [A].[1] The ethnic groups at particularly high risk are women from South Asia (India, Pakistan and Bangladesh have a relative risk of 7.6–11-fold compared to white women) and black Caribbean women (relative risk 3.1). Thus, the overall prevalence of GDM varies with the ethnicity of the population and varies between 1 and 14 per cent.[2,3]

There has been much debate regarding the use of screening strategies to detect GDM, and studies have investigated the use of risk factors to guide screening. A randomized controlled trial comparing risk factor-based screening from the United States found positive predictive values for a first-degree relative with type 1 diabetes (15 per cent), a first-degree relative with type 2 diabetes (6.7 per cent), a previous baby greater than 4.5 kg (12.2 per cent), glycosuria (50 per cent), current suspected macrosomia and polyhydramnios (both 40 per cent).[4] Other traditionally quoted risk factors for which less robust evidence exists include twin pregnancy, polycystic ovarian disease, parity (related to maternal age), previous congenital abnormality and previous stillbirth.

The risks of developing GDM in subsequent pregnancies are high, with recurrence rates between 30 and 84 per cent.[5] A systematic review found that the risk was highest in the ethnic groups at particular risk of an initial presentation of GDM.[6] Furthermore, women who have required insulin treatment for GDM in a previous pregnancy have a recurrence risk of 75 per cent.

The National Institute for Health and Clinical Excellence (NICE) currently recommends that women with the risk factors outlined in Table 7.5.1 be offered testing for GDM in the form of an oral glucose tolerance test (discussed below) [A].[5]

### Pathogenesis

Pregnancy is a state of increased insulin resistance, secondary to the secretion of placental hormones such as progesterone, cortisol, placental lactogen, growth

**Table 7.5.1** Risk factors for gestational diabetes[5]

| Risk factor |
| --- |
| Body mass index >30 kg/m$^2$ |
| Previous macrosomic infant ≥4.5 kg |
| Previous gestational diabetes |
| First-degree relative with diabetes |
| Ethnic origin: |
|    South Asia (India, Pakistan, Bangladesh) |
|    Black Caribbean |
|    Middle Eastern (Saudi Arabia, UAE, Iraq, Jordan, Syria, Oman, Qatar, Kuwait, Lebanon, Egypt) |

**Table 7.5.2** World Health Organization criteria for the 2-hour 75 g oral glucose tolerance test

| | Whole blood venous (mmol/L) | Whole blood capillary (mmol/L) | Plasma venous (mmol/L) | Plasma capillary (mmol/L) |
| --- | --- | --- | --- | --- |
| Fasting | ≥6.1 | ≥6.1 | ≥7.0 | ≥7.0 |
| 2 hours | ≥6.7 | ≥7.8 | ≥7.8 | ≥8.9 |

hormone and prolactin. This insulin resistance, evident by the second trimester, persists throughout the pregnancy and resolves with delivery of the placenta. Normal pregnant women demonstrate an increased pancreatic β cell response and hyperinsulinaemia. This facilitates the supply of glucose to the fetus by altering maternal energy metabolism from carbohydrate to lipids. Women with GDM have an exaggeration of this insulin resistance, possibly due to a limited ability of the pancreatic β cells to increase insulin secretion. This may represent an early marker of deterioration in β cell function. A subset (1–38 per cent) of women with GDM have islet cell autoantibodies, including insulin antibodies and glutamic acid decarboxylase antibodies.[7] These women may be more likely to be of normal weight and are at increased risk of subsequent type 1 diabetes. A minority of women (<5 per cent) have specific glucokinase mutation resulting in β cell dysfunction and inability to compensate for the insulin resistance. During the third trimester, this impaired ability to compensate for the insulin resistance results in an increase in blood glucose levels in response to a glucose load. Although this may not be sufficient to cause symptoms, the excessive glucose load is able to exert an adverse effect on the fetus, through fetal hyperglycaemia and hyperinsulinaemia.

## DIAGNOSIS

The oral glucose tolerance test (OGTT) is used for diagnosis. This involves ingesting a glucose load and testing response to it at varying time intervals. There are at least six different versions of the OGTT performed internationally, varying with glucose load, time of sampling and cut-off criteria for diagnosis. NICE currently recommend the use of the World Health Organization (WHO) 2-hour OGTT which involves ingestion of 75 g of glucose (Table 7.5.2). Outside pregnancy, a plasma venous glucose at 2 hours ≥11.1 mmol/L is diagnostic of diabetes mellitus, and between 7.8 and 11.1 mmol/L indicative of impaired

glucose tolerance. The levels for impaired glucose tolerance are considered to be diagnostic of GDM. The other most commonly used test is the 3-hour 100-g test, as recommended by the American Diabetes Association. NICE guidance is that the WHO 2-hour 75-g test should be used at 24–28 weeks gestation in women with the risk factors in Table 7.5.1. Women with fasting and 2-hour levels above those shown in Table 7.5.2 are diagnosed with GDM, as these criteria are associated with an increased incidence of treatable neonatal and maternal complications [A].[5,8] Using the screening criteria in Table 7.5.1, between 20 and 50 per cent of women will screen positive depending on geographical area.[5]

Women who have had gestational diabetes in a previous pregnancy should be screened much earlier. NICE guidance suggests that they are offered early self-monitoring of blood glucose or a GTT at 16–18 weeks. If normal, this should be repeated at 28 weeks.[5]

## CONGENITAL MALFORMATIONS

As expected from the pathogenesis, there is no excess risk of major congenital malformations in women developing GDM, as blood glucose would be expected to be normal during organogenesis. The exception to this is those women who, on postnatal testing, have previously undiagnosed type 2 diabetes, thus would have had hyperglycaemia during the first trimester. The proportion of these women varies with different populations, but some UK centres have described 12–20 per cent of women with GDM as having persistently impaired glucose tolerance on postnatal testing, thus likely to have type 2 diabetes. Studies have shown that these women are at increased risk of congenital malformations.[9]

## ANTENATAL CARE

For many years, the level of hyperglycaemia at which benefit was to be derived from treatment was unknown. However, in 2005, the Australian Carbohydrate Intolerance Study in Pregnant Women (ACHOIS) trial was published.[8]

This study randomized women with impaired glucose tolerance on the WHO 2-hour test (Table 7.5.2), to routine care or diabetic care (diet, monitoring and insulin, as appropriate). There was a lower rate of serious perinatal complications (defined as death, shoulder dystocia, fractures and nerve injury) in the 490 women in the intervention arm (1 per cent), compared to 4 per cent in the 510 women in the routine care group. More women in the intervention group underwent induction of labour and more babies were admitted to special care, but there was no increase in caesarean section rate and significantly fewer babies had macrosomia. Importantly, the number of women needing treatment to prevent one adverse outcome was 34. Therefore, women with impaired glucose tolerance on the WHO 2-hour GTT should be offered treatment for GDM [A].

The primary goal of treatment is to achieve near-normal glycaemic control, and options include diet, blood glucose monitoring, fetal monitoring, oral hypoglycaemic agents and, for some women, insulin therapy (20 per cent in the ACHOIS). A recent large observational study (23 316 women), the Hyperglycemia and Adverse Pregnancy Outcomes (HAPO) study, attempted to determine a threshold level above which risks were increased.[10] Although no threshold was identified, this study supported the ACHOIS finding that there are increased adverse risks in women with impaired glucose tolerance in pregnancy.

## Blood glucose monitoring

Blood glucose should be monitored in the same way as women with pre-existing diabetes (see Chapter 6.2, Diabetes mellitus). Pre-prandial levels should be 3.5–5.9 mmol/L and 1 hour post-prandial levels should be less than 7.8 mmol/L. In common with pre-existing diabetes, women with GDM are best managed within a specialist service with access to obstetricians, diabetologists, dieticians, specialist nurses and midwives.

## Diet and exercise

As in pre-existing diabetes, post-prandial hyperglycaemia has been associated with poor outcomes in gestational diabetes (see above under Blood glucose monitoring). Initially, lifestyle modifications, such as dietary changes, should be used to reduce these levels. Studies have shown that diets high in low-glycaemic index carbohydrates can improve overall glycaemic control and post-prandial hyperglycaemia [A]. Several small observational studies have suggested that obese pregnant women with gestational diabetes may improve glycaemic control without any risks of ketonuria with a moderate (30 per cent) reduction in calorie intake [C]. Increased exercise may also have beneficial effects, with several small studies showing improved glucose control and reduced need for insulin.

Therefore, NICE guidelines suggest that women with GDM should choose diets containing low-glycaemic index carbohydrates and low-fat proteins. They should also be advised to undertake moderate exercise (30 minutes a day) and restrict calorie intake if the pre-pregnancy body mass index (BMI) is greater than 27 $kg/m^2$.[5]

## Fetal monitoring

Women with GDM are at risk of developing fetal macrosomia. It has been suggested that this can be detected and predicted by the measurement of fetal abdominal circumference on ultrasound. A cohort study of 201 women with GDM reported the sensitivity of abdominal circumference at 30–33 weeks gestation to predict macrosomia as 88 per cent, with a specificity of 83 per cent. The positive predictive value was 56 per cent and the negative predictive value 96 per cent.[11] One randomized controlled trial of 141 women with GDM compared ultrasound at 28 and 32 weeks with 32 weeks alone.[12] Insulin therapy was commenced if the abdominal circumference was greater that the 75th percentile. This study found that there were more macrosomic babies in the group scanned only at 32 weeks. Thus, although there is a lack of robust evidence, NICE suggests that insulin therapy should be considered if the fetal abdominal circumference is greater than the 70th centile at diagnosis [C].[5] There are no studies clearly demonstrating benefits of particular monitoring regimes in terms of frequency of ultrasound scans. However, fetal monitoring should be conducted as for women with pre-existing diabetes (see Chapter 6.2, Diabetic mellitus).

## Pharmacological treatments

Overall, 82–93 per cent of women with GDM will achieve glycaemic control with diet alone.[5] Poor control of blood glucose is associated with similar complications as for women with pre-existing diabetes (macrosomia, birth trauma, neonatal hypoglycaemia, perinatal death, induction of labour and caesarean section). Therefore, NICE guidance suggests that hypoglycaemic therapy should be considered if diet and exercise fail to achieve blood glucose targets over a period of 1–2 weeks.[5] Oral hypoglycaemic agents and insulin have been discussed in detail in Chapter 6.2, Diabetes mellitus. Options for treatment include oral hypoglycaemic agents (metformin or glibenclamide), regular insulin or insulin analogues. The choice is dependent on the particular patient and will depend on glucose control and acceptability. There are several studies demonstrating the clinical and cost effectiveness of glibenclamide and metformin in GDM. However, at the time the NICE guidelines were written, the guideline development group stated that since none of these studies have been conducted in the National Health Service (UK) healthcare setting, insulin would continue to be the treatment of agent of choice.[5] However, a large randomized controlled trial of the use of metformin in GDM was published subsequently.[13] This large Australian study randomized 363 women to receive metformin (46 per cent required supplemental insulin) and 370 to insulin. The primary outcome, a composite of neonatal outcomes including neonatal hypoglycaemia, respiratory complications, birth trauma, phototherapy, low Apgar scores and preterm birth, was the same (32 per cent) in both groups. Interestingly, there was significantly less severe neonatal hypoglycaemia in the metformin group, but also a slightly higher rate of preterm birth less than 37 weeks. There was no difference in birth weight between the two groups, and women in the metformin group demonstrated lower weight gain (although the difference may not be clinically significant). Furthermore, metformin was more acceptable to patients. Although long-term follow-up data for the infants are awaited, it appears that metformin is a safe and acceptable alternative for women with GDM [B].

## Timing and mode of delivery

The majority of studies investigating timing and mode of delivery include women with type 1 and GDM. This is discussed in Chapter 6.2, Diabetes mellitus. Thus, current guidelines do not differentiate between the two, and NICE recommends that pregnant women with diabetes be offered elective birth after 38 completed weeks gestation.[5] However, patient management should be individualized and timing and mode of delivery be considered in the context of glycaemic control and fetal ultrasound findings. A woman with diet-controlled GDM, who has good control and no evidence of macrosomia, may not necessarily require early induction.

## Intrapartum care

Intrapartum maternal hyperglycaemia poses the same risks to the fetus of neonatal hypoglycaemia in GDM as in type 1 and type 2 diabetes. This is discussed in Chapter 6.2, Diabetes mellitus. Thus, blood glucose should be tested every hour and maintained between 4 and 7 mmol/L.[5] A sliding scale of intravenous insulin and dextrose should be instituted if blood glucose falls outside this range. However, this recommendation is based on a single study of 85 women with GDM [C]. Women who have not required treatment with insulin in the antenatal period are less likely to require intravenous insulin and dextrose. Similarly, women undergoing elective caesarean section are unlikely to require intraoperative insulin and dextrose infusions if they have not required antenatal insulin treatment. Women who require steroid treatment for lung maturity should be treated in the same way as women with pre-existing diabetes (see Chapter 6.2,

Diabetes mellitus). In all cases, care of women should be individualized, and a jointly agreed care plan involving the obstetrician and diabetic team should be agreed antenatally and documented in the notes.

## Postnatal care

Women with true GDM are unlikely to require insulin following delivery. However, in order to detect women with previously undiagnosed type 1 or type 2 diabetes, it is recommended that blood glucose monitoring be conducted in the early postnatal period.[5] NICE do not recommend a particular regime for postnatal testing, but pre-meal and bedtime testing until blood glucose levels return to normal (4–6 mmol/L), then once daily while an inpatient would be appropriate. Contraception should also be discussed prior to discharge.

## FUTURE RISK OF DEVELOPING DIABETES

Women who have developed GDM are at increased risks of subsequent type 2 diabetes. A recent comprehensive systematic review and meta-analysis estimated this increased risk to be 7.43-fold overall.[14] The duration of follow-up varied from 6 weeks to 28 years. Another systematic review reported an incidence of between 3 and 70 per cent.[15] It is therefore recommended that women undergo testing for diabetes at the 6 weeks postnatal check and annually thereafter [A].[5]

Women should be advised of the symptoms of hyperglycaemia and advised that lifestyle modifications may reduce the likelihood of developing type 2 diabetes.[5] However, this advice is based on studies conducted on a different population to women who have had GDM. A systematic review and meta-analysis concluded that lifestyle interventions reduced the progression of impaired glucose tolerance to type 2 diabetes with a hazard ratio of 0.51 [A].[16] However, the studies included men and were conducted on older populations than women who have been recently pregnant. There are no published studies addressing the risks and impact of treatments in women who have had GDM. Until publication of the recent NICE guidelines, the recommended test was the 75-g oral glucose tolerance test at 6 weeks postpartum and annually thereafter.[17] However, the recent NICE guidelines considered evidence suggesting that a postnatal fasting plasma glucose of 6.0 mmol/L or more could be used to select women who should undergo a full glucose tolerance test.[18] In this study of 122 women tested 6 weeks postnatally, the fasting plasma glucose had a sensitivity of 100 per cent and a specificity of 94 per cent for identifying diabetes compared to a glucose tolerance test [D]. Thus, NICE suggested that changing from a

## KEY POINTS

- Gestational diabetes (GDM) is impaired carbohydrate tolerance which first develops during pregnancy.
- GDM is associated with increased risks of macrosomia and its associated complications, neonatal hypoglycaemia and late pregnancy loss.
- There are many well-defined risk factors, the main ones being ethnic origin, obesity and GDM in a previous pregnancy.
- Women at risk should be tested using the 2-hour 75-g oral glucose tolerance test at 24–28 weeks gestation.
- Women who have had GDM in a previous pregnancy should be offered early self-monitoring of blood glucose or a glucose tolerance test at 16–18 weeks gestation.
- Treating GDM reduces the incidence of complications.
- Most (82–93 per cent) women will achieve control of blood glucose with lifestyle modifications alone.
- Treatment can be with oral hypoglycaemic agents or insulin.
- Pregnant women with diabetes should be managed in a joint obstetric/diabetic clinic involving the input of obstetricians, diabetologists, dieticians, specialist nurses and midwives.
- Pre-prandial blood glucose should be 3.5–5.9 mmol/L.
- Post-prandial levels should be less than 7.8 mmol/L.
- Post-prandial blood glucose levels, rather than levels of $HbA_{1c}$, should be used to monitor glycaemic control in the second and third trimesters as these associate better with outcome.
- Diabetic women should be offered monitoring of fetal growth and well-being, although there is no good evidence that these monitoring strategies reduce the risks of stillbirth and macrosomia.
- Diabetic women should be offered delivery after 38–39 weeks, as there is evidence that this reduces risk shoulder dystocia and caesarean section. Care should be individualized and will depend on glycaemic control and development of macrosomia.
- Women with macrosomia should have the risks and benefits of different modes of delivery discussed with them.
- Maternal blood glucose should be monitored hourly during labour and be kept between 4 and 7 mmol/L during labour and delivery. Women who are diet controlled are unlikely to need any specific treatment during labour.
- Women with true GDM are unlikely to require insulin postnatally.
- Women should undergo early postnatal glucose monitoring to ensure their blood glucose is in the normal range.
- Women who have had GDM are at high risk of developing type 2 diabetes in the future. This risk can probably be reduced by lifestyle modifications.
- Women should be screened for diabetes at the 6-week postnatal check and annually thereafter.
- All women should receive postnatal advice regarding contraception and planning their next pregnancy.

glucose tolerance test to fasting plasma glucose could represent a cost saving to the NHS.[5]

# Key References

1. Scott DA, Loveman E, McIntyre L, Waugh N. Screening for gestational diabetes: a systematic review and economic evaluation. *Health Technol Assess* 2002; **6**: 1–161.
2. Report of the Expert Committee on the Diagnosis and Classification of Diabetes Mellitus. *Diabetes Care* 2003; **26** (Suppl. 1): S5–20.
3. American Diabetes Association. Gestational diabetes mellitus. *Diabetes Care* 2004; **27** (Suppl. 1): S88–90.
4. Griffin ME, Coffey M, Johnson H et al. Universal vs. risk factor-based screening for gestational diabetes mellitus: detection rates, gestation at diagnosis and outcome. *Diabet Med* 2000; **17**: 26–32.
5. National Institute for Health and Clinical Excellence. Diabetes in pregnancy. Management of diabetes and its complications from pre-conception to the postnatal period. London: NICE, 2008.
6. Kim C, Berger DK, Chamany S. Recurrence of gestational diabetes mellitus: a systematic review. *Diabetes Care* 2007; **30**: 1314–19.
7. Mauricio D, Balsells M, Morales J et al. Islet cell autoimmunity in women with gestational diabetes and risk of progression to insulin-dependent diabetes mellitus. *Diabetes Metab Rev* 1996; **12**: 275–85.
8. Crowther CA, Hiller JE, Moss JR et al. Effect of treatment of gestational diabetes mellitus on pregnancy outcomes. *N Engl J Med* 2005; **352**: 2477–86.
9. Fraser R, Heller S. Gestational diabetes: aetiology and management. *Obstet Gynaecol Rep Med* 2007; **17**: 345–8.
10. Metzger BE, Lowe LP, Dyer AR et al. Hyperglycemia and adverse pregnancy outcomes. *N Engl J Med* 2008; **358**: 1991–2002.
11. Bochner CJ, Medearis AL, Williams J 3rd et al. Early third-trimester ultrasound screening in gestational diabetes to determine the risk of macrosomia and labor dystocia at term. *Am J Obstet Gynecol* 1987; **157**: 703–8.
12. Rossi G, Somigliana E, Moschetta M et al. Adequate timing of fetal ultrasound to guide metabolic therapy in mild gestational diabetes mellitus. Results from a randomized study. *Acta Obstet Gynecol Scand* 2000; **79**: 649–54.
13. Rowan JA, Hague WM, Gao W et al. Metformin versus insulin for the treatment of gestational diabetes. *N Engl J Med* 2008; **358**: 2003–15.
14. Bellamy L, Casas JP, Hingorani AD, Williams D. Type 2 diabetes mellitus after gestational diabetes: a systematic review and meta-analysis. *Lancet* 2009; **373**: 1773–9.

15. Kim C, Newton KM, Knopp RH. Gestational diabetes and the incidence of type 2 diabetes: a systematic review. *Diabetes Care* 2002; **25**: 1862–8.

16. Gillies CL, Abrams KR, Lambert PC *et al.* Pharmacological and lifestyle interventions to prevent or delay type 2 diabetes in people with impaired glucose tolerance: systematic review and meta-analysis. *BMJ* 2007; **334**: 299.

17. Department of Health. National Service Framework for Diabetes: Standards. London: Department of Health, 2002.

18. Holt RI, Goddard JR, Clarke P, Coleman MA. A postnatal fasting plasma glucose is useful in determining which women with gestational diabetes should undergo a postnatal oral glucose tolerance test. *Diabet Med* 2003; **20**: 594–8.

# 7.6 Pre-eclampsia and non-proteinuric pregnancy-induced hypertension

*Andrew Shennan*

## MRCOG standards

- Conduct pre-pregnancy counselling to a level expected in independent primary care.
- Manage severe pre-eclampsia/eclampsia.

In addition, we would suggest the following:

### Theoretical skills

- Distinguish between the different causes of hypertension in pregnancy.
- Understand the principles underlying the pathophysiology of pre-eclampsia.
- Describe and quantify the risk factors for pre-eclampsia.
- Know the principles of management of the woman who presents with pre-eclampsia.
- Advise a woman with a previous history of pre-eclampsia.

### Practical skills

- Know how to manage the woman with severe pre-eclampsia; this will involve detailed knowledge of fluid management, hypertension control, anticonvulsant prophylaxis and anaesthetic issues.
- Be able to treat eclampsia.

## INTRODUCTION

Women who are hypertensive and pregnant must be subdivided into those with:

- chronic hypertension (see Chapter 6.1),
- pregnancy-induced or gestational hypertension (PIH).

Women with PIH are subdivided further: the majority have non-proteinuric PIH, a condition associated with less maternal or perinatal mortality/morbidity, whereas a minority have the major pregnancy complication of pre-eclampsia.[1]

It is imperative that every effort is made to accurately classify women with hypertension in pregnancy as having chronic hypertension, non-proteinuric PIH or pre-eclampsia. The aetiology and management of the three conditions are very disparate, as are implications for future pregnancies. The aetiology and management of chronic hypertension in pregnancy are discussed in Chapter 6.1. Women with non-proteinuric pregnancy-induced hypertension (PIH) need to be monitored to ensure that proteinuria does not develop and pre-eclampsia become apparent; non-proteinuric PIH is not an indication for admission,[2] but induction of labour or antihypertensive treatment may be considered depending on gestation and blood pressure. This chapter focuses on pre-eclampsia.

Even in developed countries, women still die from pre-eclampsia and eclampsia.[3] In the United Kingdom, fewer than ten women die each year. Eclampsia is now rarely associated with mortality, although severe hypertension and cerebral vascular accidents still occur.[4] Prevalence of maternal death is not falling; between 2003 and 2005 there were 18 direct deaths attributed to pre-eclampsia and eclampsia, with a mortality rate of 0.85 per 100 000 pregnancies. This was greater than the previous triennia (0.70 per 100 000 pregnancies). Eclampsia has an estimated incidence in the UK of 26.8 cases per 100 000 maternities.[4] There were no maternal deaths in any eclamptic women, possibly attributed to the more judicious use of magnesium sulphate. Worldwide, however, maternal mortality from hypertensive disease accounts for approximately 60 000 deaths per year.

Because of concerns about the potential adverse effects of pre-eclampsia, many women who have a normal outcome require intensive surveillance; up to a quarter of antenatal admissions are as a direct result of monitoring and managing women with hypertension. Antenatal care is directed towards identifying women with hypertension and proteinuria. Day units reduce the need for inpatient management, but current methods for screening women at risk are poor and the onset and progression of the disease are unpredictable.

Perinatal mortality is also increased with pre-eclampsia. Pre-eclampsia is associated with intrauterine growth restriction (IUGR), particularly when early in onset. Placental involvement also explains the association with placental abruptions. As delivery is the only cure, the hypertensive diseases of pregnancy have become the most common cause of iatrogenic preterm birth. They account for 15 per cent of all preterm births, but up to a quarter of very low birth weight infants. There is strong evidence linking size at birth to health in adulthood, i.e. that there are fetal origins of adult disease.[5] Thus, the small babies resulting from pregnancies affected by pre-eclampsia have health implications in adult life, including an increased risk of hypertension, heart disease and diabetes when they become adults. Additional and significant longer-term health service resource implications result from subsequent learning disabilities and low intelligence quotient (IQ). Maternal disease severity and fetal involvement do not always correlate; for example, the babies of women who have eclampsia at term often have normal birth weight.[4]

## CLASSIFICATION AND DEFINITION

The term pregnancy-induced hypertension usually implies hypertension caused by, but unrelated to other pathology associated with the pregnancy, a diagnosis that is difficult to make until after the pregnancy has ended.

Blood pressure and proteinuria define pre-eclampsia, but they are not fundamental to the aetiology and are more indicative of end-organ damage. In clinical practice, the threshold of abnormality is set low to identify at-risk cases, but this results in many women being identified with hypertension and/or proteinuria who are not at increased risk.

The International Society for the Study of Hypertension in Pregnancy (ISSHP), based on the recommendation of Davey and MacGillivray,[6] uses the term 'gestational hypertension' to include all women with PIH whether proteinuric or not, as long as they had been previously normotensive and not proteinuric. Once proteinuria has developed, this is assumed to be pre-eclampsia (Table 7.6.1).

If any organ system known to have the potential to be affected by pre-eclampsia is involved, the possibility of the disease must be suspected; hypertension and proteinuria cannot be relied upon to define the disease. However, for pragmatic reasons, these signs must remain hallmarks for definition. Tests for liver, kidney, blood and placental involvement should always be sought if pre-eclampsia is suspected (see below).

**Table 7.6.1** The International Society for the Study of Hypertension in Pregnancy (ISSHP) classification (modified and abbreviated)

| |
|---|
| **A. Gestational hypertension and/or proteinuria developing during pregnancy, labour or the puerperium in a previously normotensive non-proteinuric woman** |
| 1. Gestational hypertension (without proteinuria) |
| 2. Gestational proteinuria (without hypertension) |
| 3. Gestational proteinuric hypertension (pre-eclampsia) |
| **B. Chronic hypertension (before the 20th week of pregnancy) and chronic renal disease (proteinuria before the 20th week of pregnancy)** |
| 1. Chronic hypertension (without proteinuria) |
| 2. Chronic renal disease (proteinuria with or without hypertension) |
| 3. Chronic hypertension with superimposed pre-eclampsia (new-onset proteinuria) |
| **C. Unclassified hypertension and/or proteinuria** |
| **D. Eclampsia** |

- Definitions
  Hypertension in pregnancy:
  - Diastolic BP >110 mmHg on any one occasion or
  - Diastolic BP >90 mmHg on two or more consecutive occasions >4 hours apart
  Proteinuria in pregnancy:
  - One 24-hour collection with total protein excretion >300 mg/24 hours *or*
  - Two 'clean-catch-midstream' or catheter specimens of urine collected >4 hours apart with ≥2+ on reagent strip

## INCIDENCE

The prevalence of pre-eclampsia varies with the definition used and the population studied; however, pre-eclampsia occurs in less than 5 per cent of an average antenatal population. In some recent prospective studies, the incidence has been as low as 2.2 per cent, even in a primigravid population, in which the condition is known to have the highest prevalence.[7] The incidence of non-proteinuric PIH is approximately three times greater. In the United States, the incidence of pre-eclampsia has been reported to be slightly higher, possibly because of the high-risk status of the populations studied (usually primiparous women at large teaching centres). The incidence of pre-eclampsia in women with a single risk factor is approximately 15 per cent.

# AETIOLOGY

Although the primary events leading to pre-eclampsia are still unclear, it is now widely believed that a cascade of events leads to the clinical syndrome (summarized in Figure 7.6.1). Although the inheritance of pre-eclampsia has yet to be characterized, there is a strong familial predisposition: a family history in either mother or sister increases the risk of pre-eclampsia four- to eight-fold. This genetic predisposition leads to a faulty interplay between the invading extravillous trophoblast cells (of fetal origin) and the maternal immunologically active decidual cells.

The faulty interplay results in a failure of trophoblast invasion into the myometrium and the maternal spiral arteries do not undergo their physiological vasodilatation.[8] Only the most superficial decidual portion of the spiral artery is invaded by the trophoblast. This inadequate trophoblast invasion is also seen in pregnancies complicated by fetal growth restriction (without pre-eclampsia), demonstrating that the maternal syndrome of pre-eclampsia must be related to additional factors.

The diminished dilatation of the spiral arteries, associated increased resistance in the uteroplacental circulation and an impaired intervillous blood flow probably result in an inadequately perfused placenta. Ischaemia or ischaemia/reperfusion in the second half of gestation produces reactive oxygen species and oxidative stress in the placenta.

The placental hypoperfusion is also postulated to result in the secretion of a factor(s) into the maternal circulation that causes 'activation' of vascular endothelium.[9]

Endothelial cell activation explains the widespread manifestations of the disease, as the vascular endothelium supplies all organ systems involved. Many markers of endothelial damage are raised. Pre-eclampsia is associated with lipid changes (there is a two-fold increase in triglycerides and free fatty acids), and an increase in lipid peroxidation, both in the placenta and systemically, suggests that oxidative stress (an imbalance between free radical synthesis and antioxidant defence) may be involved in the endothelial cell changes.

# MANAGEMENT

## Screening for pre-eclampsia

### History

More than a third of pre-eclampsia occurs in women with risk factors; a careful history will allow the clinician to assess risk.

A family history in a first-degree relative increases the risk of pre-eclampsia four- to eight-fold, illustrating the strong genetic influence [D]. A woman has double the risk of pre-eclampsia if pregnant by a partner who had previously fathered an affected pregnancy [D].

An immunological element to the disease process is evidenced by the effect of exposure to the paternal antigen, via either the fetus or the partner. Pre-eclampsia occurs more commonly in first pregnancies; miscarriages or terminations of pregnancy provide some reduction in risk in subsequent pregnancies [D]. However, in women with chronic hypertension, a prior miscarriage is a risk factor for progression to pre-eclampsia. A new partner increases risk, whereas non-barrier methods of contraception and increased duration of sexual cohabitation reduce risk [D]. Exposure to a partner's 'foreign' antigens is common to these phenomena. Teenage mothers and pregnancies conceived by donor insemination have increased risk of pre-eclampsia, presumably due to the lack of exposure to such antigens [D].

Underlying medical disorders, particularly those involving vascular disease – such as chronic hypertension – increase the risk of pre-eclampsia (to over 20 per cent); this highlights the importance of the maternal susceptibility, as well as the placental aetiology in the disease process. All forms of glucose intolerance, including gestational diabetes, are associated with an increased risk [D]. This may be related to obesity, which is an independent risk factor. Women with antiphospholipid syndrome and multiple pregnancies are at increased risk. Risk may be related to the size of the placenta; molar pregnancies have been associated with pre-eclampsia, as have pregnancies complicated by hydrops fetalis (mirror syndrome) or trisomy chromosomal complement.

Women with a history of pre-eclampsia, particularly those requiring delivery before 37 weeks, all have about a 20 per cent chance of developing pre-eclampsia again [D].

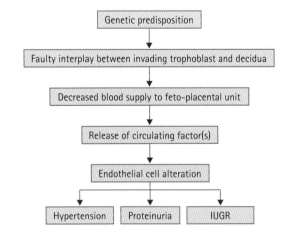

**Figure 7.6.1** Aetiology of pre-eclampsia. IUGR, intrauterine growth restriction

## Biophysical tests

The detection of raised blood pressure in early gestation is related to the subsequent risk of pre-eclampsia, even within the normal blood pressure range (i.e. the lower the blood pressure, the lower the risk). Automated blood pressure monitoring removes many of the errors of standard sphygmomanometry, but is only a weak indicator of risk, and these monitors may underread in pre-eclampsia [D].[7] Two other biophysical tests have been investigated, but are not useful: isometric exercise testing and the roll-over test. Problems with reproducibility and poor predictor values mean that these have not been introduced into clinical practice. The angiotensin II sensitivity test, involving assessing the blood pressure response to infusion of the vasoconstrictor angiotensin II, has also shown poor predictor values in larger studies and is invasive, time-consuming and costly [B].

In contrast, Doppler analysis of the uterine artery waveform has reasonable sensitivity and specificity, and is relatively quick, non-invasive and relatively inexpensive if performed at the same time as other ultrasound scans. Poor placental perfusion is a characteristic feature of pregnancies destined to develop pre-eclampsia and therefore it would seem logical to identify those women who have increased resistance in this circulation. In pregnancies at increased risk of pre-eclampsia, there is persistence of a relatively high resistance circulation with a notch. The later this test is performed, the better the predictive values [D]. At 20 weeks gestation in a low-risk population, approximately one in five women will develop pre-eclampsia,[10] if they have an abnormal waveform; the prediction value is considerably greater at 24 weeks [D]. This screening test does allow women to be targeted for increased surveillance and possible prophylactic therapies. The importance of screening tests will escalate if an adequate treatment to prevent pre-eclampsia is established.

## Biochemical tests

The simple measurements of plasma volume, haemoglobin concentration and haematocrit all have a weak association with the development of pre-eclampsia, but poor prediction values [D]. Uric acid and platelets are sometimes measured in women with chronic hypertension to predict superimposed pre-eclampsia, but are lacking in sensitivity and specificity. The measurement of second trimester human chorionic gonadotrophin and maternal serum alpha-fetoprotein is associated with a two-fold increase in pre-eclampsia, and is likely to reflect the disease process that occurs at the uteroplacental interface [D]. This may also explain why low pregnancy associated plasma protein A (PAPP-A) is associated with higher risks in later pregnancy. These increases in risk are not sufficient to alter clinical practice significantly. Many markers of endothelial activation have been shown to be increased in pre-eclampsia. Some will rise before the clinical manifestations of the disease, but there is invariably overlap between the women who are subsequently normal and those who develop pre-eclampsia, again limiting clinical usefulness. Urinary excretion of calcium, microalbuminuria and prostacyclin metabolites have been investigated, as well as urinary kallikrein:creatinine ratios, and further work may eventually establish a combination of tests that could be clinically useful, perhaps by combining endothelial and placental markers of the disease. More recently, soluble fms-like tyrosine kinase-1 (sFLT) and placental growth factors (PLGF) have been used as a ratio to enhance prediction with better prediction then previous tests, but these have not been adopted into clinical practice.

## Role of prophylaxis

Surveillance and timely delivery are the essence of current antenatal management in order to prevent the consequences of pre-eclampsia. Preventing the manifestation of the disease would be highly preferred. There are a number of potential therapies that have been investigated in an effort to prevent the occurrence of pre-eclampsia. Aspirin, calcium and fish oils have gained the most focus in this regard, although other substances, such as magnesium, zinc and even rhubarb, have been investigated. Aspirin, a cyclo-oxygenase enzyme inhibitor, reverses the imbalance between the vasoconstrictor thromboxane $A_2$ and the vasodilator prostacyclin that is known to occur in pre-eclampsia. In a meta-analysis of individual patient data (31 randomized trials and 32 217 women), the use of anti-platelet agents (particularly low-dose aspirin) resulted in a significant 10 per cent reduction in the relative risk of both pre-eclampsia and serious adverse outcome.[11] The number needed to treat in order to prevent pre-eclampsia was 114 and to prevent one serious adverse outcome was 51. Aspirin should be seriously considered in the management of very high-risk women and is likely to be safe. The dose, timing and the populations to be targeted are still being thoroughly investigated.

In a review of 12 randomized controlled trials in 15 206 women, calcium supplementation resulted in a significant reduction (52 per cent) in the relative risk of pre-eclampsia with a higher effect in those at high risk (78 per cent) and with low calcium intake (64 per cent). Calcium supplementation may reduce parathyroid release and intracellular calcium leading to a reduction in smooth muscle contractility in women at risk of developing pre-eclampsia.[12] Calcium supplementation warrants further research.

Fish oils containing n-3 fatty acids are thought to inhibit platelet thromboxane $A_2$. However, the four trials that have investigated their use have not shown any reduction in pre-eclampsia [A].

The potential role of oxidative stress in the aetiology of the maternal syndrome of pre-eclampsia has resulted in a number of studies of the antioxidants vitamin C and E supplementation. However, none of these have shown benefit.

## Maternal and fetal assessment

Before any management decisions are made, the first task is to confirm the diagnosis of pre-eclampsia (see above under Screening for pre-eclampsia), in order to ensure that iatrogenic morbidity does not ensue [E].

When women present with hypertension, both the gestational age and the previous pregnancy history are important factors in establishing risk of progression to pre-eclampsia: late-onset hypertension after 37 weeks gestation rarely results in serious morbidity to mother or baby [D]. However, hypertension that presents early, particularly before 28 weeks, will result in pre-eclampsia developing in almost half of women.

Care in assessing blood pressure will prevent misdiagnosis; blood pressure measurement is poorly performed in clinical practice, for example digit preference (the practice of rounding the final digit of the blood pressure to 0) occurs in more than 80 per cent of antenatal measurements. The antenatal population within the UK has a significant proportion of obese women. The standard bladder used in sphygmomanometer cuffs ($23 \times 12$ cm) undercuffs about a quarter of the antenatal population, resulting in the overdiagnosis of hypertension, usually by more than 10 mmHg. Overcuffing underestimates measurements, but usually by less than 5 mmHg, and is preferable in cases of doubt. Keeping the rate of deflation during measurement to 2–3 mm/s will prevent overdiagnosing diastolic hypertension. A similar effect is achieved by using Korotkoff 5; fewer women will be diagnosed as hypertensive than when Korotkoff 4 is used. Korotkoff 4 is also less reproducible [C], and randomized, controlled clinical trials have confirmed that all healthcare providers should be using Korotkoff 5 when measuring blood pressure in pregnancy [B]. Repeating the blood pressure, or obtaining a series of readings in the day unit, will limit the overdiagnosis of hypertension [E].

Errors in the interpretation of proteinuria are also common with dipstick urine analysis, and 24-hour collections of urine are necessary to confirm the diagnosis [E]. More than 300 mg in 24 hours is considered abnormal. Newer automated devices that can be used by the bedside relate the proteinuria to creatinine, and closely equate to 24-hour collections. The point-of-care test for albumin/creatinine ratio has an overall sensitivity of 97 per cent, a specificity of 98 per cent, a positive predictive value of 92 per cent and a negative predictive value of 99 per cent, which is equally effective regardless of the time of testing.

Every effort should be made to identify women at risk of life-threatening complications. Most women who present with eclampsia will not have had a recent blood pressure or urine analysis that was sufficiently abnormal to have identified them as at risk. Only just over half of women who presented with eclampsia had had prior hypertension and proteinuria diagnosed together. Blood pressure and proteinuria cannot be relied upon alone. The syndrome of pre-eclampsia is multisystemic and it is the ease of measurements of hypertension and proteinuria that has led to their adoption in the diagnosis of pre-eclampsia. Other organ involvement must be considered, such as fetal involvement, or other signs, such as epigastric tenderness. For pragmatic reasons, other signs have not been introduced to define the disease, but they are equally important.

## Management remote from term

Early-onset pre-eclampsia is frequently associated with placental insufficiency, which can result in IUGR, abruption of the placenta and fetal death [C]. Fetal well-being must be carefully considered in all cases. A symphyseal–fundal height should be carefully measured in all women who present with pre-eclampsia, in addition to an enquiry as to fetal movements [E]. At early gestations, or in pregnancies with suspected IUGR, it is usual to confirm fetal growth with ultrasound, and to assess the amniotic fluid volume and umbilical artery Doppler waveform [E]. Suspected fetal compromise is a frequent cause for delivery in pre-eclampsia.

Involvement of other organ systems in the affected women must be sought.

- *Platelets* are consumed due to the endothelial activation. A platelet count $>50 \times 10^9$/L is likely to support normal haemostasis [E]; however, a falling platelet count, particularly to $<100 \times 10^9$/L, may indicate a need to consider delivery [E].
- Hypovolaemia results in an increased *haematocrit* and the *haemoglobin* may also be raised.
- If delivery or induction of labour is likely to be imminent, or if the platelet count is low, it is also sensible to screen for *clotting abnormalities* [E]. Pre-eclampsia can cause disseminated intravascular coagulation, and clotting must be adequate for regional anaesthesia.
- *Uric acid*, a measure of fine renal tubular function, is used to assess the disease severity, although severe disease can still occur with a normal uric acid level. Spuriously high levels of uric acid are associated with acute fatty liver of pregnancy.
- Raised *urea* and *creatinine* are associated with late renal involvement, but are not useful as an early indicator of disease severity (serial measurements may identify renal disease progression) [E].
- Pre-eclampsia can cause subcapsular haematoma, liver rupture and hepatic infarction, and liver *transaminases*

should be measured. Aspartate aminotransferase (AST) and other transaminases indicate hepatocellular damage, and elevated levels may again indicate a need to consider delivery. It should be remembered that the normal range for transaminases is approximately 20 per cent lower than the non-pregnant range [C].

When liver involvement is associated with haemolysis and low platelets, this is known as HELLP syndrome, which is a severe variant of pre-eclampsia. If proteinuria excretion is high (usually >3 g/24 hours), circulating albumin may fall, increasing the risk of pulmonary oedema. A raised AST can be associated with either haemolysis or liver involvement; lactate dehydrogenase levels are also elevated in the presence of haemolysis.

Corticosteroids should be given to enhance fetal lung maturity and are safe in pre-eclampsia [D]. Steroid therapy may assist in the recovery from HELLP syndrome and has been used in the postpartum period. It is not unusual to see a slight improvement in biochemical parameters in the antenatal period associated with corticosteroid use [D].

The treatment of moderate hypertension may be detrimental to fetal growth [D].[13] However, severe hypertension should be avoided, and blood pressures >170/110 mmHg require urgent therapy (see below) [E].[13]

In women with an established diagnosis of pre-eclampsia, delivery should be considered once fetal lung maturity is likely (approximately 32 weeks gestation), particularly if either maternal multi-organ involvement or fetal compromise is apparent. However, women with pre-eclampsiapresenting between 28 and 32 weeks can often be managed conservatively without substantial risk to the mother, as long as close inpatient supervision is maintained (E). In such cases, conservative management reduces neonatal morbiditywithout significantly increasing maternal morbidity.

Maternal indications for delivery include an inability to control hypertension, deteriorating liver or renal function, progressive fall in platelets or neurological complications. A non-reactive cardiotograph (CTG) with decelerations or a fetal condition that is clearly deteriorating often warrants delivery.

# Labour ward management of pre-eclampsia

A set protocol should be followed when a women has severe pre-eclampsia [E]. All staff working on the labour ward must be familiar with the protocol in use. Typical entry criteria for such a protocol would be:[14]

- eclampsia, or
- severe hypertension (>170/110 mmHg) with + or >1 g/24 hours proteinuria, or
- hypertension (>140/90 mmHg) with ++ or >3 g/24 hours proteinuria with an additional complication such

as headache, visual disturbance, epigastric pain, clonus (more than three beats) or a platelet count $<100 \times 10^9$/L or AST >50 IU/L.

The two main reasons why women die, as demonstrated by the Confidential Enquiry, are cerebral haemorrhage and adult or acute respiratory distress syndrome,[3] and the two most important aetiological factors for these are severe hypertension and excess fluid intake. Control of blood pressure and fluid balance is therefore crucial.

## Intrapartum blood pressure control

Blood pressure should be measured frequently (every 15 minutes) [E]. To facilitate this, automated sphygmomanometers may be used, but these oscillometric devices underread the blood pressure in pre-eclampsia. Large changes in blood pressure should therefore be confirmed with a mercury sphygmomanometer [E].

Intracerebral haemorrhage complicated 7/15 deaths in the last Confidential Enquiries into Maternal Deaths (CEMD).[3] Mean arterial pressures (MAPs) are used to guide management, and most protocols recommend the instigation of intravenous anti-hypertensive therapy at MAP >125 mmHg [E]. Labatolol or hydralazine is the usual first-line treatment [C]. Regimens vary (although there is an increasing trend towards regional protocols), for example:

- Labetolol: bolus of 20 mg i.v. if the MAP remains >125 mmHg, followed at 10-minute intervals by 40-, 80-, 80-mg boluses, up to a cumulative dose of 220 mg. Once the MAP is <125 mmHg, an infusion of 40 mg/hour is commenced, doubling (if necessary) at 30-minute intervals, until a satisfactory response or a dose of 160 mg/hour is attained.
- Hydralazine: bolus of 5 mg i.v. if the MAP remains >125 mmHg, followed by further boluses of 5 mg up to a cumulative dose of 15 mg. Once the MAP is <125 mmHg, an infusion of 10 mg/hour is commenced, doubling (if necessary) at 30-minute intervals, until a satisfactory response or a dose of 40 mg/hour is attained. Colloid should be infused prior to treatment if the baby is undelivered, to protect the uteroplacental circulation and prevent hypotension and fetal distress [E].

If one agent is ineffective, or if side effects occur (e.g. tachycardia with hydralazine), the other agent can be used. Third-line agents include sodium nitroprusside and nifedipine.

## Fluid management

As women with pre-eclampsia can have a reduced intravascular volume, leaky capillary membranes and low albumin levels, they are prone to pulmonary oedema. Renal failure is a rare complication of pre-eclampsia that usually follows acute blood loss, when there has been inadequate transfusion, or as a result of profound hypotension. Oliguria without a rising serum urea or creatinine is a manifestation of severe pre-eclampsia and not of incipient renal failure. Administration of intravenous fluid in response to oliguria must be performed with caution [E].

Most protocols limit fluid intake (in the form of intravenous crystalloid) to approximately 1 mL/kg per hour [E]. A Foley catheter should be inserted and fluid balance recorded.

In a well-perfused women, oliguria (<400 mL/24 hours) requires no treatment per se. A low threshold for central venous pressure (CVP) assessment is recommended; in the absence of invasive monitoring, repetitive fluid challenges are to be avoided. If the CVP is high (>8 mmHg) with persistent oliguria, a dopamine infusion can be considered (1 µg/kg per minute) [E]. If the creatinine or potassium rises, haemodialysis or haemofiltration may be necessary, and the advice of a renal physician should be sought. The administration of diuretics temporarily improves urine output, but further decreases the circulating volume and exacerbates electrolyte disturbances; frusemide should only be given if there are signs of pulmonary oedema [E]. In particularly difficult cases, pulmonary artery catheterization should be considered.

## Anticonvulsant therapy

Magnesium sulphate can be used to control an eclamptic fit (up to 8 g). Alternatively, diazepam (10 mg) can be used [E]. An eclamptic fit is usually self-limiting, and prolonged fitting warrants a brain scan to rule out other pathology, such as an intracerebral bleed [E].

If an eclamptic fit occurs, magnesium sulphate is the prophylaxis of choice, as demonstrated by the Eclampsia Trial [B].[15] In addition to reducing the incidence of further fits, the benefits of magnesium sulphate over both diazepam and phenytoin include a significantly lower need for maternal ventilation, less pneumonia and fewer intensive care admissions. Magnesium sulphate acts as a membrane stabilizer and vasodilator and reduces intracerebral ischaemia. It is usually given as a 2 g intravenous loading dose and a maintenance infusion at 1–2 g/hour. In cases of oliguria, care must be taken, as magnesium sulphate is renally excreted. Toxicity is detected by the absence of patellar reflexes, but ultimately respiratory arrest and muscle paralysis or cardiac arrest will occur. The antidote is 10 mL of 10 per cent calcium gluconate.

Even with severe pre-eclampsia, eclamptic fits are rare (<1 per cent). However, the Magpie Trial evaluated magnesium sulphate versus placebo in women with pre-eclampsia and demonstrated a clear benefit of prophylactic therapy [A]. Magnesium sulphate halved the risk of eclampsia and probably reduced the risk of maternal death. There did not appear to be any substantive harmful short-term effects to either the mother or baby.[15,16]

## Anaesthesia

A general anaesthetic can be dangerous, as endotracheal intubation can cause severe hypertension. Regional blockade is the preferred method of analgesia for labour and of anaesthesia for operative deliveries [E], but a coagulopathy must be excluded. Platelet levels of $<80 \times 10^9/L$ should ensure haemostasis, and most obstetric anaesthetists will insert a regional block under these circumstances. Care must be taken to avoid arterial hypotension (particularly following postpartum haemorrhage) in view of the vasoconstriction and reduced intravascular volume. A low threshold for central invasive monitoring is necessary in women who require a caesarean section [E].

## Postpartum care

As a third of eclamptic fits occur postpartum, intensive monitoring is required, usually for 48 hours after delivery. Although eclampsia has been reported beyond this time, it is unlikely to be associated with serious morbidity. Blood pressure is frequently at its highest 3–4 days after delivery. Anti-hypertensive therapy may therefore need to be continued after discharge home; in the absence of fetal considerations, the most effective therapy can be used – and drugs such as methyldopa discontinued.

All women who have suffered severe pre-eclampsia should be reviewed at a hospital postnatal clinic 6–12 weeks after delivery [E]. In addition to blood pressure and urine testing, tests of renal and liver function should be instigated; residual disease may merit referral to a physician. Underlying predispositions to pre-eclampsia, such as an inherited thrombophilia or antiphospholipid syndrome, should be excluded (multiparous women are more likely to have an underlying cause). The postnatal visit is also an excellent opportunity to discuss complications of the pregnancy and the planned management of any future pregnancy.

## FUTURE CARDIOVASCULAR RISK

Women with pre-eclampsia have a four-fold increased risk of developing hypertension and nearly a two-fold increased risk of ischaemic heart disease, stroke and venous thromboembolism, even up to 14 years after the index pregnancy. Women having early pre-eclampsia are at highest risk.[17] This reflects a possible common aetiology or a long-term effect on disease development and highlights the possible need for earlier cardiovascular risk assessment and the commencement of preventative therapies at an earlier age. It is plausible that active assessment of cardiovascular risk up to six months postpartum may lead to earlier identification of cardiovascular risk and the potential for lifestyle modification.[18]

## KEY POINTS

- Pre-eclampsia is a multisystem disorder involving the placenta, liver, kidneys, blood, and neurological and cardiovascular systems; hypertension and proteinuria are diagnostic signs.
- Both maternal and fetal morbidity and mortality are more likely to occur with early-onset disease.
- Despite the many tests being investigated, pre-eclampsia cannot be accurately predicted. An abnormal uterine artery Doppler at 20 weeks will increase risk approximately six-fold in both high- and low-risk women.
- Cerebral haemorrhage and adult respiratory distress are common causes of death in pre-eclampsia; therefore acute management focuses on controlling blood pressure and restricting fluid intake.
- The use of anti-hypertensive therapy in moderately hypertensive women demonstrates a significant reduction in severe hypertension only; there are no other proven additional benefits.
- Low-dose aspirin in pregnancy results in a small (10 per cent), but significant reduction in pre-eclampsia; there is an associated reduction in preterm delivery.
- Magnesium sulphate is the anticonvulsant of choice following an eclamptic fit, resulting in fewer fits and less maternal morbidity compared to diazepam and phenytoin. There is also a clear benefit to prophylactic magnesium sulphate therapy – the risk of eclampsia is halved.

## Key References

1. Hayman R, Baker PN. *Hypertension in Pregnancy: Definition, Diagnosis and Investigation. A CME Self-assessment Test.* London: RCOG Press, 1997.

2. Hayman R, Baker PN. *Hypertension in Pregnancy: Management. A CME Self-assessment Test.* London: RCOG Press, 1997.

3. Lewis G (ed.). The Confidential Enquiry into Maternal and Child health (CEMACH). Saving Mothers' Lives: reviewing maternal deaths to make motherhood safer – 2003–2005. The Seventh Report on Confidential Enquiries into Maternal Deaths in the United Kingdom. London: CEMACH, 2007.

4. Knight M. Eclampsia in the United Kingdom 2005. *Br J Obstet Gynaecol* 2007; **114**: 1072–8.

5. Barker DJP, Bull AR, Osmond C. Fetal and placental size and risk of hypertension in adult life. *BMJ* 1990; **301**: 259–61.

6. Davey DA, MacGillivray I. The classification and definition of the hypertensive disorders of pregnancy. *Am J Obstet Gynecol* 1988; **158**: 892–8.

7. Higgins JR, Walshe JJ, Halligan A *et al.* Can 24-hour ambulatory blood pressure measurement predict the development of hypertension in primigravidae? *Br J Obstet Gynaecol* 1997; **104**: 356–62.

8. Brosens IA. Morphological changes in the utero–placental bed in pregnancy hypertension. *Clin Obstet Gynecol* 1977; **77**: 573–93.

9. Roberts JM, Taylor RN, Musci TJ *et al.* Pre-eclampsia: an endothelial cell disorder. *Am J Obstet Gynecol* 1989; **161**: 1200–4.

10. Mires GJ, Williams FL, Leslie J, Howie PW. Assessment of uterine arterial notching as a screening test for adverse pregnancy outcome. *Am J Obstet Gynecol* 1998; **179**: 1317–23.

11. Askie LM, Duley L, Henderson-Smart D *et al.* Antiplatelet agents for prevention of pre-eclampsia: a meta-analysis of individual patient data. *Lancet* 2007; **369**: 1791–8.

12. Hofmeyr GJ, Duley L, Atallah A. Dietary calcium supplementation for prevention of pre-eclampsia and related problems: a systematic review and commentary. *Br J Obstet Gynaecol* 2007; **114**: 933–43.

13. Von Dadelszen P, Ornstein MP, Bull SB *et al.* Fall in mean arterial pressure and fetal growth restriction in pregnancy hypertension: a meta-analysis. *Lancet* 2000; **355**: 87–92.

14. North West Pre-eclampsia Care Group. Regional guidelines for the management of severe pre-eclampsia. In: Baker PN, Kingdom J (eds). *Pre-eclampsia: Aetiology and Management.* London: Parthenon, 2004.

15. Which anticonvulsant for women with eclampsia? Evidence from the Collaborative Eclampsia Trial. *Lancet* 1995; **345**:1455–63.

16. The Magpie Collaborative Group. Do women with pre-eclampsia, and their babies, benefit from magnesium sulphate? The Magpie Trial: a randomised placebo-controlled trial. *Lancet* 2002; **359**: 1877–90.

17. Bellamy L, Casas JP, Hingorami AD, Williams DJ. Pre-eclampsia and risk of cardiovascular disease and cancer in later life: systematic review and meta-analysis. *BMJ* 2007; **335**: 974.

18. Magee L, von Dadelszen P. Pre-eclampsia and increased cardiovascular risk. *BMJ* 2007; **335**: 945–6.

# Medication in pregnancy

*Clare L Tower*

## INTRODUCTION

Pregnant women conceive taking a wide variety of both prescription and over-the-counter medications. Many pregnant women require medication for specific pregnancy and non-pregnancy related conditions. Therefore, a broad understanding of the impact of pregnancy on drug pharmacokinetics (drug handling) and pharmacodynamics (drug actions) is required. Furthermore, the large majority of drugs cross the placenta, and some drugs have significant fetal effects. For this reason, most drugs are not licensed for use in pregnancy, thus prescribing in pregnancy often lies outside licensed indications. A detailed discussion of all drugs is beyond the scope of this book. Therefore, this chapter will review the general principles and provide examples. A detailed discussion of prescribing for particular disorders during pregnancy can be found in the relevant sections of this book.

## PRE-CONCEPTION COUNSELLING

Encountering women of reproductive age with significant medical problems, for which they are taking prescribed medications, is becoming increasingly common. It is beneficial for many of these women to be seen pre-conceptually for several reasons. First, it allows optimization of therapy such that pregnancy can be commenced with the lowest achievable risks. Typical examples of this include optimization of glycaemic control in diabetic women and the

prescription of high-dose folic acid groups at particular risk. Second, it allows drugs with potentially terotogenic effects to be changed to a safer alternative. Furthermore, it allows the opportunity to discuss particular risks and concerns, of both the medical problem itself and the medications that will be prescribed during pregnancy. Pregnant women often have many concerns about the effects of medications on an unborn baby, and it is usual for them to put the unborn baby's needs above their own. Thus, women may suddenly stop drugs in early pregnancy that may have a significant impact on their own health. Discussions in the pre-conception period will prevent such non-compliance in early pregnancy of important medications, such as anti-epileptics or immunosuppressants.

## EFFECTS OF PREGNANCY ON PHARMACOKINETICS AND PHARMACODYNAMICS

### Absorption

Pregnancy is associated with a reduction in gastric motility and an increase in gastric pH, both of which could be expected to affect drug absorption. However, studies have demonstrated that pregnancy has no measurable affect on drug bioavailability via these mechanisms.[1]

### Distribution

The volume of distribution is defined as the volume in which an amount of drug would need to be distributed to produce a particular blood concentration. Therefore, for drugs which are highly bound in the tissues, such as basic drugs like amphetamine, the volume of distribution is large, but the plasma concentration is low. For acidic drugs, such as warfarin, which are highly protein bound, the volume of distribution is relatively low, but the plasma concentration high. Therefore, the volume of distribution is dependent upon plasma volume, tissue volume, the amount of binding of a drug in the tissues and to plasma proteins. Pregnancy causes an increase in plasma volume that reaches a peak at around 32 weeks gestation. In addition, the concentrations of the two main drug-binding proteins, albumin and $\alpha_1$-acid glycoprotein fall during to around 70–80 per cent of pre-pregnancy levels by term. Therefore, pregnancy results in an increase in volume of distribution (due to increased plasma volume) and an increase in the fraction of a drug that is unbound, or active, in the plasma (due to a fall in plasma proteins). Thus, measurements of total drug concentration, which are used for medications such as phenytoin and sodium valproate, underestimate the corresponding unbound or active concentrations. This may result in prescribing higher doses than necessary, which is particularly important as the teratogenicity of both these drugs is reported in registries to be dose dependent [D]. Thus, measurement of unbound concentrations should be used wherever possible. This is of particular relevance to drugs with a narrow therapeutic window.

## Metabolism

Following oral ingestion, drugs are absorbed by the gut and undergo first pass metabolism in the liver by numerous enzymes. Although the liver smooth endoplasmic reticulum is the main site of enzymatic metabolism, virtually all cells have the ability to metabolize drugs to some degree, with other main sites being the epithelial cells of the gut, kidney, lung and skin. There are many enzymes involved and their activity is modified by pregnancy. Furthermore, there may be an increase in hepatic blood flow in pregnancy.[2]

The cytochrome P450 (CYP) system is a major enzymatic system involved in drug metabolism, of which there are now 57 human genes and 59 pseudogenes described, divided into 18 classes. Not only does pregnancy alter the activity of these enzymes, but it also varies with gestation, drug interactions (for examples, enzyme inducers) and genotype. Different genotypes at CYP loci result in an individual being a poor metabolizer or an extensive metabolizer for a particular enzyme. The uridine 5′-diphosphate glucuronosyltransferase (UGT) is a further enzyme system demonstrating modification during pregnancy. Changes in drug metabolism can have a significant effect on active drug levels. Enzymes demonstrating increased activity will result in reduced plasma levels of a drug, requiring an increase in dose and vice versa. Thus, variation of drug metabolism with pregnancy is complex, and although the majority of enzymes increase in activity, some decrease. The overall effect is further compounded by genetic variation and the effect of plasma volume and plasma proteins described above. Table 8.1 illustrates this with examples of drugs in which variation in metabolism is observed. This should be considered when prescribing in pregnancy, and since there are so many unknown factors, clinicians must be guided by the overall clinical effect of a drug.

**Table 8.1** Examples of modification of enzyme activity with pregnancy.[2]

| Enzyme | Change | Drug | Effect |
|--------|--------|------|--------|
| CYP1A2 | ↓ | Caffeine, clozapine, olanzapine | Increased half-life, increased unbound and active drug |
| CYP2A6 | ↑ | Nicotine | Lower levels |
| CYP2C9 | ↑ | Phenytoin, losartan, NSAIDs | Reduced levels |
| CYP2C19 | ↓ | Proguanil, PPIs | Higher plasma levels |
| CYP2D6 | ↑ | >40 drugs, e.g. beta-blockers, SSRIs anti-arrhythmics | Reduced levels |
| CYP3A4 | Variable | >50% drugs, e.g. nifedipine | Variable effects |
| UGT | ↑↑ | Lamotrigine, zidovudine, morphine | Increased clearance, thus reduced levels |

- PPIs, proton pump inhibitors, such as omeprazole; SSRIs, selective serotonin reuptake inhibitors, such as fluoxetine.

## Renal clearance

Pregnancy causes an increase in renal blood flow and glomerular filtration rate of more than 50 per cent, which can have a significant effect on drugs that are predominantly excreted by the kidneys. Thus, the clearance of beta-lactam antibiotics, such as penicillins and cephalosporins, is increased during pregnancy [C]. Although there may be lower plasma levels as a result, levels in urine may be higher, which may be a desired effect for treating urinary tract infections. Low molecular weight heparins, such as dalteparin and enoxaparin, also demonstrate increased renal clearance during pregnancy, which may require dose adjustments [C].[3] Thus, a 20–65 per cent increase in dose for drugs that are renally excreted may be needed to maintain therapeutic levels [E].[2]

## Drug transfer across the placenta

The majority of drugs are able to cross the placenta to the fetus to some degree, and there are very few that demonstrate no placental transfer. Transfer of drugs across the placenta can occur by passive transfer, active transport, facilitated diffusion, phagocytosis and pinocytosis.[2] By far the most common method is passive diffusion, or movement of a molecule down a concentration gradient, and this is determined by the lipid solubility, polarity and molecular weight of the drug. Therefore, small, un-ionized lipid-soluble drugs are able to cross at the fastest rate. This can be influenced by the degree of plasma protein binding and by placental metabolism. Drugs with a molecular weight <500 Da, which is the large majority, are able to cross the placenta by passive diffusion. Heparin (both unfractionated and low molecular weight) is the most well-known drug that is unable to cross the placenta due to its high molecular weight of between 3000 and 5000 Da, depending on the preparation.

While it is generally considered that facilitated diffusion, phagocytosis and pinocytosis play little significant role in drug transfer, there is growing interest in placental active transport, utilizing energy-requiring drug transporters. Energy is usually derived from ATP, or from electrochemical gradients. All these transporters work against a concentration gradient, and several have now been described within the placenta. These include P-glycoprotein (multidrug-resistant gene MDR1 product) that is able to transport digoxin and dexamethasone, multidrug resistance proteins 1–3, able to transport methotrexate and ampicillin and the monocarboxylate and sodium/multivitamin transporters, able to transport valproate and carbemezepine.[4]

## Placental drug metabolism

There is growing evidence that the placenta expresses many of the enzymes able to metabolize drugs. These include many of the CYP enzymes, UGT, glutathione S-transferase and sulphotransferases. The study of the clinical effects of many of these enzymes is in its infancy. However, it is known that, for some enzymes it varies with gestation, and the activity of many is altered by alcohol and cigarette smoking. Drugs that undergo metabolism in the placenta include steroids, such as dexamethasone, and alcohol.[5]

A better understanding of placental transfer and metabolism of individual drugs may help in the development of fetal therapy. For example, transplacental passage of anti-arrhythmic drugs has been used to treat fetal supraventricular tachycardias since the first report in 1980.[6] The success rate of monotherapy is in the order of 50 per cent.[7] Transfer of digoxin across the placenta is complex, involving both passive diffusion and active transport via the P-glycoprotein. Co-administration of other anti-arrhythmic drugs has been suggested to improve success by modifying P-glycoprotein transport of digoxin.[5]

## Teratogenicity

A teratogen is an agent that is able to permanently alter the development, growth, structure or function of a developing embryo or fetus. The effect of drugs in the pre-implantation period (fertilization to implantation) is often considered to be an 'all or nothing' phenomenon.[8] In other words, a drug will result in injury to a large number of cells, resulting in complete loss, or only a few cells are affected and the remaining cells can compensate at this early stage, resulting in no malformation. The period of organogenesis (embryonic phase, weeks 2–8 post-conception) is the most critical. Within this period, each structure has a period of maximal vulnerability, and usually, the earlier the insult the more severe the resulting malformation. However, some structures that have initially formed during embryogenesis are still vulnerable to effects in the fetal period of development (9 weeks to term). For example, failure of neural tube closure arises during the day 17–30 day post-fertilization to cause anencephaly and neural tube defects. However, encephalocoeles have been described post-closure during the fetal period.[8] Unfortunately, teratogenicity of most drugs is only established after initial drug licensing, as pregnant women are excluded from human trials of new drugs. The classic and most famous example of this is thalidomide, which was introduced as an anti-emetic in the 1950s and was subsequently withdrawn when it was found to cause phocomelia.

## Lactation

The principles of drug transfer from the maternal circulation into breast milk are the same as those across any membrane, and thus will depend on the lipophilic properties, degree of ionization and plasma protein binding of the drug. The amount of drug that the infant is exposed to will be dependent upon volume of milk ingested, maternal plasma levels and infant excretion (which probably varies with age and is less with increasing immaturity). Plasma protein binding has been shown to have a significant impact on levels in breast milk. Drugs which are highly protein bound result in less infant exposure via breast milk. Measurable infant levels were only found for drugs with less than 70 per cent plasma protein binding.[2] Unfortunately, there are very few good data available on the drug exposure to infants via breast milk for the large majority of drugs, thus a risk–benefit analysis must be conducted on an individual basis. However, there are very few drugs for which breastfeeding is contraindicated.[8] In general terms, the lowest effective dose should be used, and if there are concerns (or if there are no data about a drug), timing breast feeds to avoid times of peak maternal plasma levels should be recommended [E].

## Specific drug considerations in pregnancy

Prescribing during pregnancy requires careful consideration of the risks and benefits, in discussion with the woman herself. In general, use of the lowest number of drugs (monotherapy where possible) and the lowest effective dose is recommended, remembering the effects of pregnancy on plasma levels of a drug [E]. Table 8.2 shows examples of the key considerations, applying the above principles, for particular drug classes during pregnancy and lactation. For obvious reasons, this is in no way exhaustive and more detailed discussions can be found in the literature referenced at the end of this chapter, or in the relevant sections of this book.

**Table 8.2** Examples of drug prescribing considerations during pregnancy

| Drug | Pre-conception | Effects of pregnancy | Fetal considerations | Lactation |
|---|---|---|---|---|
| **Cardiovascular system** | | | | |
| ACE inhibitors, ARBs | Should be changed to alternative if possible | Avoid – only use if no alternative with fetal monitoring of growth and liquor volume. Stop if oligohydramnios [D,E] | Teratogenic in first trimester. Renal and cardiac problems in late gestation [D,E] | Considered compatible |
| Anti-hypertensives | Optimize blood pressure control | Nifedipine may demonstrate increased clearance in third trimester [D] | Beta-blockers associated with fetal growth restriction (less so with labetalol). Intravenous doses should be given with fetal monitoring | Present in breast milk (except nifedipine, which is >90% protein bound). Infants reported normotensive, so considered safe |
| Statins | – | – | Usually stop as may adversely effect placental development. Studies ongoing | Considered compatible |
| **Antibiotics** | | | | |
| Penicillins/ cephalosporins | – | Increased renal excretion, lower plasma levels | Cross placenta, considered safe | Small amounts in breast milk, safe |
| Tetracyclines | – | – | Increased risk NTD, cleft palate and cardiovascular effects (not doxycycline). Tooth discolouration [D,E] | Found in breast milk. Concerns about effects on teeth |
| Ciprofloxacin | – | – | Only small amounts cross placenta, but has been associated with bone/cartilage problems. However, few data | Concentrated in breast milk. Neonatal *Clostridium difficile* has been reported [D] |
| **Analgesics** | | | | |
| Paracetamol | – | – | Safe | Safe |
| NSAIDS | – | – | Premature closure of ductus and kidney dysfunction >32 weeks [A] | Considered safe |
| Opiates | – | – | No major effects known, fetal dependence and withdrawal [D] | May improve fetal withdrawal symptoms [D] |
| **Immunosuppressants** | | | | |
| Steroids | – | Usual maternal side effects. Risk–benefit analysis to continuing treatment | Weak association with cleft lip. Placenta metabolizes 90% of prednisolone. Association with reduced fetal weight [C] | Unknown levels in breast milk, but usually considered safe |
| Azathioprine | Counsel safe [D,E] | Considered safe [D,E] | Fetal liver lacks enzyme to convert to active metabolite (6-mercaptopurine) | Low concentrations of metabolites in breast milk. However, theoretical of immunosuppression, thus usually not recommended for breastfeeding [E] |
| Cyclosporin | Counsel safe [D,E] | Counsel safe [D,E] | Increased risks of fetal growth restriction [D,E] | As above |

*(Continued)*

Antenatal complications: maternal

| Drug | Pre-conception | Effects of pregnancy | Fetal considerations | Lactation |
|---|---|---|---|---|
| **Psychiatric drugs** | | | | |
| SSRIs | Consider changing to ones with lowest association with abnormalities (i.e. change from paroxetine). Discuss risks and benefits | May require increased dose [D,E] | Paroxetine and sertraline associated with teratogenicity, such as cardiac defects, omphalocoele (risk low approximately 2/1000). Fluoxetine crosses placenta, but not considered teratogen [D,E] | Present in breast milk. Avoid feeding at times of peak plasma levels [E] |
| Lithium | Risk–benefit analysis involving psychiatrist | Risk–benefit analysis involving psychiatrist. Some suggest reducing/stopping just prior to delivery [D,E] | Cardiovascular malformations, floppy infant, neonatal arrhythmias, hypoglycaemia, thyroid dysfunction [D] | Found in breast milk. Breastfeeding generally avoided as neonatal clearance slower than adult [E] |
| **Anti-epileptics** | | | | |
| Sodium valproate | Optimize treatment on lowest dose, avoid if possible | Total concentrations fall, but more so than the unbound concentrations. As teratogenicity is dose dependent, need to measure unbound levels [D,E] | Teratogen that is rapidly transported to fetus. Associated with 'Valproate syndrome', developmental delay [D,E] | Enters breast milk. Neonatal serum levels <10% of maternal levels [D,E] |
| Carbamezepine | Obtain control on lowest dose possible | – | Associated with facial dysmorphism, developmental delay, NTD, phalanx and nail hypoplasia [D,E] | Probably safe in breastfeeding [D,E] |
| Phenytoin | Obtain control on lowest dose possible | Total concentrations fall, but more so than the unbound concentrations. As teratogenicity is dose dependent, need to measure unbound levels [D,E] | Associated with congenital heart defects and cleft palate [D,E] | Low transfer in breast milk. Considered safe [D,E] |
| Lamotrigine | Obtain control on lowest dose possible | Increased clearance due to increased UGT activity [D,E] | Crosses placenta, limited data as newer drug [D,E] | Low transfer in breast milk, therefore considered safe [D,E] |
| **Anti-coagulants** | | | | |
| Warfarin | Discuss risks, and make plan for pregnancy. Depends on indication for anti-coagulation | Depends on reason for use. In general, avoid use at period of greatest teratogenicity and after 36 weeks. May be safe to use heparin as alternative throughout pregnancy, but for women with metal valves this may not provide sufficient anti-coagulation [E] | Teratogen. Exposure between 6 and 10 weeks associated with embryopathy. Higher dose (>5 mg/day) associated with higher fetal risk [D,E] | Does not enter breast milk as highly protein bound [D] |
| Heparin | Reassure safe in pregnancy | Safe in pregnancy. Increased renal clearance, may require increased dose. Monitoring of Xa levels if therapeutic (rather than prophylaxis is required) [D,E] | Does not cross placenta due to molecular size | Safe in breastfeeding |

• ACE, angiotensin converting enzyme; ARB, angiotensin type 1 receptor blocker; SSRIs, selective serotonin reuptake inhibitors.

## KEY POINTS

- Pre-conception counselling offers an opportunity to optimize drug therapy, change medications with teratogenic potential and discuss compliance of important medications.
- Absorption of drugs is not significantly altered by pregnancy.
- Pregnancy is associated with increased plasma volume and reduced levels of albumin and $\alpha_1$-acid glycoprotein (plasma binding proteins), which results in an increased unbound, or active, drug concentration.
- Pregnancy alters the activity of many of the enzymes involved in drug metabolism. Effects vary with enzyme, gestation, genotype and other prescribed drugs, thus are often difficult to predict.
- Renal clearance of drugs increases during pregnancy, resulting in lower plasma levels of drugs that are predominantly excreted via this route.
- Drugs cross the placenta predominantly by passive diffusion and there is growing interest in the active transporters. Thus, small lipid soluble, non-ionized drugs cross at the highest rate.
- The embryonic period of human gestation (weeks 2–8 post-fertilization) is the period of greatest vulnerability to the teratogenic effect of drugs.
- Transfer of drugs into breast milk is determined by lipophilic properties of a drug, molecular size and polarity. Highly plasma bound drugs (probably greater than 70 per cent) do not cross into breast milk.
- In general, drugs in pregnancy and breastfeeding should be used at the lowest effective dose, using the lowest number of drugs (monotherapy where possible).

## Key References

1. Loebstein R, Lalkin A, Koren G. Pharmacokinetic changes during pregnancy and their clinical relevance. *Clin Pharmacokinet* 1997; **33**: 328–43.
2. Anderson GD. Using pharmacokinetics to predict the effects of pregnancy and maternal-infant transfer of drugs during lactation. *Exp Opin Drug Metab Toxicol* 2006; **2**: 947–60.
3. Ensom MH, Stephenson MD. Pharmacokinetics of low molecular weight heparin and unfractionated heparin in pregnancy. *J Soc Gynecol Invest* 2004; **11**: 377–83.
4. Ganapathy V, Prasad PD, Ganapathy ME, Leibach FH. Placental transporters relevant to drug distribution across the maternal-fetal interface. *J Pharmacol Exp Ther* 2000; **294**: 413–20.
5. Syme MR, Paxton JW, Keelan JA. Drug transfer and metabolism by the human placenta. *Clin Pharmacokinet* 2004; **43**: 487–514.
6. Kerenyi T, Gleicher N, Meller J. Transplacental cardioversion of intrauterine supraventricular tachycardia with digitalis. *Lancet* 1980; **2**: 393–4.
7. Ito S. Transplacental treatment of fetal tachycardia: implications of drug transporting proteins in the placenta. *Semin Perinatol* 2001; **25**: 196–201.
8. Buhimschi CS, Weiner CP. Medications in pregnancy and lactation. Part 1, Teratology. *Obstet Gynecol* 2009; **113**: 166–88.

# Maternal mortality

*James Drife*

## MRCOG standards

### Theoretical skills

- Candidates should be familiar with the most recent report of the Confidential Enquiry into Maternal Deaths in the UK. (These reports are published every three years with new findings and recommendations, so candidates should not rely on out-of-date reports.)
- Candidates from overseas should know the leading causes of maternal death in the countries in which they work.

### Practical skills

Preventing maternal deaths requires a wide range of skills.

- Clinical skills are required to treat conditions such as postpartum haemorrhage and severe hypertension.
- Administrative skills are required to implement preventive measures such as routine thromboprophylaxis.
- Organizational skills on a wider scale may be needed to ensure that care is available to at-risk women.

## INTRODUCTION

Maternal death is still common in many parts of the world, but has become rare in developed countries. In the United Kingdom, its infrequency means that when a maternal death does occur it can be a shattering experience for everyone involved. Lessons for prevention are best learned by aggregating cases nationally, and the Confidential Enquiry into Maternal Deaths has now been running continuously in England and Wales for over 50 years. Its methods are now being emulated in many countries across the world.

## INCIDENCE

### Worldwide

The World Health Organization (WHO) estimates that in 2005 there were 536 000 maternal deaths – equivalent to one every minute of every day – and that the global maternal mortality rate (MMR) is now 400/100 000 live births.[1] Over 99 per cent of the deaths are in developing countries. In Africa, the overall estimated MMR is 820/100 000, and when this is combined with high fertility rates, the result is disastrous. For example, in Ethiopia a young woman enters the reproductive phase of her life with a one in ten chance that she will die as a result of pregnancy or delivery (Figure 9.1).

### United Kingdom

In the United Kingdom, maternal death occurs in around 1 in 10 000 pregnancies. The MMR, however, has risen from 9.9/100 000 pregnancies in 1985–87 to 13.9/100 000 in 2003–05, partly (but not entirely) due to more complete reporting of indirect deaths, which now outnumber direct deaths (see Table 9.1).[2]

Incomplete reporting of maternal deaths occurs in all countries. Death certificate data are inadequate and if the UK relied only on these, the MMR would be 7.05/100 000 – around half the true rate. Instead, the UK makes strenuous efforts to ascertain as many of the deaths as possible. In 1994–96, a computer program was introduced linking birth and death registration, and in 2003 the establishment of the Confidential Enquiry into Maternal and Child Health (CEMACH) provided dedicated staff in each region, helping to identify deaths that might previously have been missed. The high ascertainment in the UK makes comparisons with other countries potentially misleading.

### Confidential enquiries into maternal deaths

Since 1952, every maternal death in England and Wales has been the subject of a detailed enquiry, conducted by clinicians – doctors and, nowadays, midwives. Any death during pregnancy or within a year after delivery

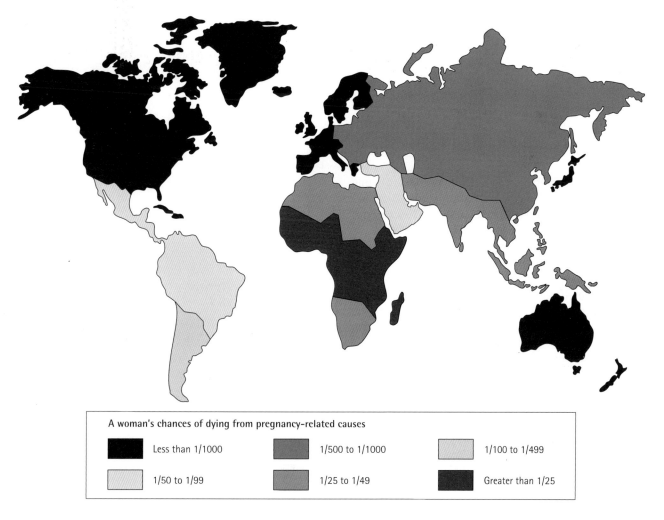

**Figure 9.1** World map of maternal mortality

**Table 9.1** Number of maternal deaths in the United Kingdom

|  | 1994–96 | 1997–99 | 2000–2002 | 2003–2005 |
|---|---|---|---|---|
| Direct | 134 | 106 | 106 | 132 |
| Indirect | 134 | 136 | 155 | 163 |
| Coincidental | 36 | 29 | 36 | 55 |
| Late direct | 4 | 7 | 4 | 11 |
| Late indirect | 32 | 39 | 45 | 71[a] |
| Total | 340 | 317 | 346 | 432 |

[a]This increase in late indirect deaths was due to improved ascertainment.

is reported to CEMACH, which in 2009 became the Centre for Maternal and Child Enquiries (CMACE). A form requesting all relevant details is sent to all staff involved, including the general practitioner (GP), midwife, obstetrician, anaesthetist and other specialists. The completed form is sent to regional assessors and then to the Department of Health, where it is anonymized before being seen by national assessors in obstetrics, pathology, midwifery and other specialties such as anaesthetics, general medicine or psychiatry, as appropriate.

Anonymity allows those involved to comment frankly and make their own suggestions for improvements. No blame is attached to individuals, and the forms are destroyed as soon as the national report is produced. Similar systems exist in Scotland and Northern Ireland and the final reports are UK-wide, making the identification of individual cases more difficult. The reports, which are published every three years, list the causes of death, draw attention to substandard care and make recommendations for improving practice.[2]

## DEFINITIONS

The definitions given here are those used by the Confidential Enquiries.

- *Maternal death.* Death of a woman while pregnant or within 42 days of termination of pregnancy, from any cause related to or aggravated by the pregnancy or its management, but not from accidental or incidental causes.
- *Direct death.* Death resulting from obstetric complications of the pregnant state (pregnancy, labour and puerperium), from interventions, omissions, incorrect treatment or from a chain of events resulting from any of the above.
- *Indirect death.* Death resulting from previous existing disease or disease that developed during pregnancy and was not due to direct obstetric causes, but was aggravated by the physiological effects of pregnancy.
- *Late death.* Death occurring between 42 days and one year after abortion, miscarriage or delivery, due to 'direct' or 'indirect' maternal causes.
- *Coincidental death.* Death from an unrelated cause which happens to occur in pregnancy or the puerperium. The word 'coincidental' has replaced the term 'fortuitous'.
- *Maternal mortality rate.* This is expressed in the UK as the number of deaths per 100 000 maternities. A 'maternity' is a clinical pregnancy ending in live birth, stillbirth, miscarriage or abortion.
- The WHO, however, defines the maternal mortality rate as 'the number of maternal deaths per 100 000 women of reproductive age', and the maternal mortality ratio as 'the number of maternal deaths per 100 000 live births'. Close attention needs to be paid to definitions and denominators.

## AETIOLOGY

The causes of maternal mortality are similar all over the world, although overall rates and the relative contribution of each cause vary from country to country.

### Worldwide

Estimates published by WHO (see Table 9.2) show the numbers of women dying of direct causes which are largely treatable. The underlying causes in many developing countries include lack of access to contraception, unsafe abortion, lack of primary care or transport facilities, and inadequate equipment and staffing in district hospitals. Only 55 per cent of deliveries within the developing world are attended by a trained attendant and only 37 per cent of deliveries occur within health facilities.

Education of women is important. In India, the states with high rates of female literacy also have high rates of contraceptive use and low maternal mortality rates. In all countries, safer care could be provided to illiterate women if there were the political will to do so.

**Table 9.2** Causes of maternal mortality worldwide

| Causes of maternal death | Estimated No. of deaths in 2002 | Projected No. for 2008 |
|---|---|---|
| Total | 510 262 | 424 000 |
| Haemorrhage | 141 767 | 112 000 |
| Sepsis | 75 827 | 50 000 |
| Hypertensive diseases | 71 503 | 49 000 |
| Obstructed labour | 43 113 | 27 000 |
| Abortion | 65 969 | 55 000 |
| Other maternal conditions | 112 082 | |

- Data from the World Health Organization.

**Table 9.3** Causes of maternal deaths in the UK 2003–2005[2]

| Cause | Total | Major substandard care |
|---|---|---|
| **Direct** | | |
| Thromboembolism | | |
|    Pulmonary embolism | 33 | 18 |
|    Cerebral thrombosis | 8 | 1 |
| Pre-eclampsia/eclampsia | 18 | 9 |
| Haemorrhage | 17 | 10 |
| Amniotic fluid embolism | 17 | 6 |
| Early pregnancy deaths | 14 | 10 |
| Genital tract sepsis | 18 | 12 |
| Anaesthetic | 6 | 6 |
| Total direct deaths | 132 | 72 |
| **Indirect** | | |
| Cardiac | 48 | 15 |
| Psychiatric | 19 | 3 |
| Cancer | 10 | 2 |
| **Other indirect** | **86** | **25** |
| Total indirect deaths | 163 | 45 |

### United Kingdom

The specific causes of maternal death in the UK are shown in Table 9.3. The number of direct deaths has changed little in the last 12 years, but the number of indirect deaths has steadily increased.

### Direct deaths

The causes of direct death have also changed very little.

## Thromboembolism

This has been the leading direct cause of maternal death in the United Kingdom since 1985. The 33 deaths from pulmonary embolism in 2003–05 (there were also eight deaths from cerebral embolism) were almost equally divided between antepartum and postpartum deaths. Eleven occurred before 12 weeks of pregnancy.

## Hypertensive disease

When the Enquiry began in 1952–54, there were 246 deaths from hypertensive disease in England and Wales. In 2003–05 in the UK, the total was 18. The condition is no less common, but care is now better. Of the 18 deaths in 2003–05, ten were from intracranial haemorrhage.

## Haemorrhage

Haemorrhage is treated well in the UK. Out of over 2 million pregnancies in the triennium 2003–05, there were only 17 deaths from this cause. Three were from placenta praevia and two from abruption. Postpartum haemorrhage (PPH) caused nine deaths, though there must have been over 7000 cases of life-threatening PPH, as studies of severe maternal morbidity show that it occurs in around 1 in 300 deliveries.[2] Three of the deaths were from obstetric trauma. Until 2003–05, a separate chapter was devoted to genital tract trauma, but the reduction in deaths from this cause made this unnecessary.

## Amniotic fluid embolism

Formerly, amniotic fluid embolism (AFE) was diagnosed only when the pathologist confirmed fetal squames in the lungs. From 1991–93, clinically obvious cases have also been included, but only after assiduous assessment to rule out misclassification. There were six clinically diagnosed cases in 2003–05 – four in which autopsy was inadequate and two in which death occurred many weeks after initial collapse. The number of histologically confirmed cases has remained around 8–10 per triennium for 20 years.

## Early pregnancy deaths

This category covers deaths before 24 weeks gestation (formerly the upper limit was 20 weeks). In 2003–05, ten were from ectopic pregnancy (out of an estimated 32 000 cases), and one was from miscarriage. There were two deaths from termination, one of which was due to criminal abortion – the first maternal death from this cause in the UK since 1982. Before the Abortion Act of 1967, there were around 30 deaths every year from criminal abortion. The recent case was of a woman who had not long been in the UK and there may have been cultural issues or coercion. When she presented to the Emergency Department with rigors and severe lower abdominal pain, the cause and severity of her condition were not recognized.

## Sepsis

Until 1935, streptococcal puerperal sepsis was the leading cause of maternal death in the UK, causing hundreds of deaths each year. Within 50 years, this cause was eliminated and in the 1982–84 report a modest sentence – 'No deaths could be directly attributed to puerperal sepsis' – marked one of the great medical achievements of the twentieth century. Since 1985, however, there has been a small but steady rise in the number of deaths from sepsis to 18 in 2003–05, with three of these being due to puerperal sepsis. As with septic abortion, the seriousness of puerperal sepsis in its early stages is now difficult to recognize because it is so rarely seen.

## Anaesthesia

Despite the rising caesarean section rate, the number of maternal deaths from anaesthesia fell steadily from 37 in 1970–72 to only one in 1994–96. Since then the number has risen to six in 2003–05. This illustrates the need to maintain vigilance – then as now, the main lesson is that trainees must know the limits of their competence.

# Indirect deaths

The 163 indirect deaths in 2003–05 were divided into 48 cardiac and 18 psychiatric cases, ten cases of malignancy possibly affected by pregnancy, and 87 'others'.

## Cardiac disease

The total of 48 deaths made this the leading cause of maternal death in 2003–05. Formerly, the major cardiac problem was rheumatic heart disease, as it still is in many developing countries, but now in the UK the main causes of death are myocardial infarction and (when late deaths are included) cardiomyopathy (Table 9.4). These conditions are linked with increasing obesity, increasing age at child bearing and the continuing high rate of smoking among women in the UK.

## Psychiatric

In 2003–05, 12 women committed suicide (usually by violent means) within 6 weeks of delivery and another 21

**Table 9.4** Deaths from cardiac disease in the UK, 2003-2005[2]

| Cardiac disease | Indirect | Late |
| --- | --- | --- |
| Aortic dissection | 9 | 0 |
| Myocardial infarction | 12 | 4 |
| Ischaemic heart disease | 4 | 0 |
| Sudden adult death syndrome (SADS) | 3 | 9 |
| Cardiomyopathy (including peripartum) | 1 | 16 |
| Myocarditis or myocardial fibrosis | 5 | 0 |
| Mitral stenosis or valve disease | 3 | 0 |
| Infectious endocarditis | 2 | 2 |
| Ventricular hypertrophy/heart failure | 2 | 1 |
| Congenital heart disease | 6 | 2 |
| Total | 47 | 34 |

Antenatal complications: maternal

suicides were late indirect deaths. There were a further 65 cases in which psychiatric disorder caused or contributed to the death. In the past, not all psychiatric deaths were reported, but after the enquiry highlighted the problem in the 1990s, case ascertainment improved. Suicide was the leading cause of death in 2000–02, but the rate decreased in 2003–05, possibly because of recommendations in previous reports that women at risk should be identified and management plans developed.

### Cancer

In most countries, death from cancer during pregnancy is classed as 'coincidental' but in the UK, deaths from cancer are classed as indirect if it appears that the pregnancy may have masked the disease or affected the diagnosis or outcome. Central nervous system (CNS) tumours, in particular, fall into this category.

### Other indirect deaths

There were 87 'other indirect' deaths in 2003–05. The main causes were diseases of the central nervous system (37 deaths) and infectious diseases (16 deaths). Among the CNS diseases, 22 deaths were due to subarachnoid or intracerebral haemorrhage and 11 were due to epilepsy. Among the infectious diseases, five of the 16 deaths were due to human immunodeficiency virus.

## Coincidental deaths

Formerly called 'fortuitous' deaths, the 52 coincidental deaths included 14 cases of neoplasia unaffected by the presence of pregnancy, 24 road traffic accidents and ten cases of homicide – in each case by the woman's partner or close relative. When late deaths were included, the total number of murders was 19, all but two committed by a partner or family member who had a known history of domestic abuse. Domestic violence is now a major concern to the maternity services and a chapter in the 2003–05 report is devoted to this problem. Of the 361 women whose deaths were reported to the Enquiry, 70 (19 per cent) had features of domestic abuse, including four with genital mutilation/cutting.

## PREVENTION

### Worldwide

Almost 200 countries have signed up to the Millennium Development Goals (MDGs) agreed at the United Nations Millennium Summit in 2000. MDG 5 is a 75 per cent reduction in the global MMR from its 1990 level by the year 2015. Table 9.2 illustrates how slow the progress is towards this goal, though many agencies, including WHO and the World Bank, are promoting initiatives and some countries are achieving success. Several countries – such as South Africa and Malaysia – have set up confidential enquiries similar to the UK model. Enquiries can identify the major problems, but implementing their recommendations requires commitment from politicians, doctors, other healthcare workers and the population as a whole.

Postpartum haemorrhage can be reduced by routine oxytocics at delivery, and unsafe abortion by contraceptive services and legal termination of pregnancy. Otherwise, the main need is less for prevention than for prompt treatment of pregnancy complications. This requires transport, trained healthcare workers, drugs and equipment. The importance of medical care in pregnancy and childbirth was underlined by a comparative study in the United States, which showed that a religious group that had good general health, but refused all modern medical care, had a maternal mortality rate similar to those in developing countries.[3]

## Past experience in the United Kingdom

Until 1935, the UK's maternal mortality rate was around 400/100 000 (one death in 250 births), but it fell steadily between 1936 and 1985 (Figure 9.2). Other indicators of public health, such as infant mortality, fell slowly and steadily during the twentieth century, but maternal mortality, by contrast, fell rapidly during and after the Second World War, when social conditions could hardly be said to be improving. This strongly suggests that the fall was due to specific factors, such as:

- antibiotics: sulphonamides were introduced in 1937 and penicillin in 1944; death rates from puerperal sepsis quickly fell;
- blood transfusion became safe during the 1940s;
- ergometrine, for the treatment and prevention of postpartum haemorrhage, was introduced in the 1940s;
- better training of midwives and obstetricians: Midwives Acts were passed in 1902 and 1936, and the Royal College of Obstetricians and Gynaecologists was founded in 1929;
- reduced parity: the average family size began to fall long before the pill was introduced in 1961;
- legalization of abortion in 1967 was followed by elimination of criminal abortion as a cause of maternal death (Figure 9.3).

## The current picture in the United Kingdom

Preventing maternal deaths involves targeting the women most at risk. Using denominator data collected by the Office of National Statistics, general risk factors can be identified.

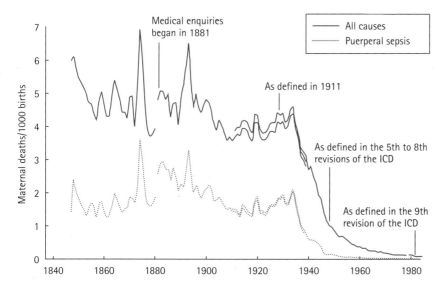

**Figure 9.2** Maternal mortality rate in England and Wales, 1847–1984 (reproduced from *Report on Confidential Enquiries into Maternal Deaths in England and Wales 1982–84*, published by HMSO, 1989)

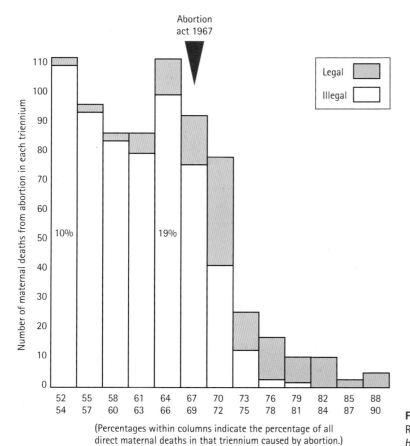

(Percentages within columns indicate the percentage of all direct maternal deaths in that triennium caused by abortion.)

**Figure 9.3** Maternal deaths from abortion, 1952–90. Reproduced with permission from *Maternal and Child Health 1994; 19*: 348

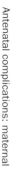

## General risk factors

- *Age.* The 'grande multipara' has long been recognized as a high-risk case, and in 1997–99 the MMR was 6.2 among primigravidae and 35 among women of parity 4 or more. However, age and parity go together and as high parity is now uncommon, the importance of maternal age has become clearer. In 2003–05, the MMR was 9.8 in the 20–24 age group and 29.4 among women aged over 40.

- *Ethnicity.* A higher risk among black women has been found in many countries including the United States,

France and Holland, and was documented in the UK for the first time in 1994–96. Since then, there has been no improvement. The effect of ethnicity in 2003–05 is shown in Table 9.5. Black African women in the UK are almost six times more likely to die than white women. Of the Black African women who died, only four were UK citizens, most of the others being recently arrived immigrants, refugees or asylum seekers. Black Caribbean women are much less likely to have language difficulties, but are still almost four times more likely to die than white women. The cause of these differences remains unclear: suggested reasons – cultural factors and social circumstances – may in reality mean poor communication between maternity services and the woman and her family, problems with the organization of services, failure of the woman or her family to access services, or failure of the services to appreciate the seriousness of symptoms when they occur.

- *Social class*. The huge effect of social class was shockingly illustrated in the 1997–99 report, which showed that the MMR among the lowest social class in Britain was 135/100 000 – similar to that in a developing country – and that 97 of the 242 maternal deaths occurred in social class 9. This group includes itinerant people (travellers), who tend to turn up at the wrong time or day at the antenatal clinic or fail to keep appointments. It is all too easy to overlook such people's needs in a service that caters mainly to the wishes of more articulate and better organized women. Such detailed data are no longer available, but the 2003–2005 report shows that women with unemployed partners are seven times more likely to die than women with employed partners.
- *Obesity*. In 27 per cent of cases in 2003–05 the woman's body mass index (BMI) was not reported but among the remainder, over 50 per cent were overweight or obese, with the figure rising to 65 per cent among deaths from thromboembolism and 73 per cent among deaths from sepsis. Morbid obesity (BMI 40 or over) was present in 8 per cent of cases. CEMACH is conducting a study of obesity in pregnancy which is due to be completed in 2011.
- *Assisted conception*. Twelve of the women who died in 2003–05 were known to have undergone *in vitro* fertilization (IVF), and four of these deaths were due to ovarian hyperstimulation syndrome. In addition, multiple pregnancy is associated with a doubling of the risk of maternal death.

## Substandard care

The Confidential Enquiries also identify substandard care. Standards are rising all the time and the proportion of cases in which care falls below current standards has not changed over the years. Substandard care may involve only a minor aspect of the treatment and does not necessarily mean that the death could have been avoided.

**Table 9.5** Ethnicity and maternal mortality in the UK, 2003-2005[2]

| Ethnic group | Direct and indirect deaths | MMR/ 100 000 maternities | Relative risk[a] |
|---|---|---|---|
| White | 162 | 11.1 | 1.0 |
| Mixed | 1 | 5.2 | 0.5 |
| Black African | 30 | 62.4 | 5.6 |
| Black Caribbean | 9 | 41.1 | 3.7 |
| Indian | 9 | 20.3 | 1.9 |
| Pakistani | 6 | 9.2 | 0.8 |
| Bangladeshi | 6 | 23.6 | 2.1 |
| Chinese/ other Asian | 1 | 14.0 | 1.3 |
| Middle East | 7 | 32.0 | 2.9 |
| Other | 2 | 28.0 | 2.5 |
| Total | 233 | 13.5 | |

[a] Compared with white.
- MMR, maternal mortality rate.

Nevertheless, major substandard care was identified in almost 40 per cent of cases in 2003–05, and examining these cases helps to indicate how deaths may be avoided. There is an increasing emphasis on guidelines and protocols, but these can only save lives if they are understood and implemented.

## Direct deaths

### Thromboembolism

Most women who died from thromboembolism had obvious risk factors which were disregarded. Obesity, a personal or family history of thromboembolism, and age over 35 years can be identified early in pregnancy. Women should be routinely weighed at booking to identify those with a BMI >30 kg/m². During pregnancy, new risk factors may appear, such as immobilization or long-haul air travel.

An important factor is caesarean section. In 1995, the RCOG produced recommendations[4] on thromboprophylaxis after caesarean section and in the next triennium deaths from thromboembolism after caesarean section fell dramatically (Table 9.6). Deaths after vaginal delivery did not change, however, and in 2004 the RCOG produced a guideline[5] for pregnancy and vaginal delivery, indicating which women require prophylaxis with low molecular weight heparin in addition to standard measures, such as early mobilization and compression stockings.

The other way in which substandard care occurs is when symptoms are ignored. Most deaths from thromboembolism are preceded by chest pain, cough or leg pain, the

**Table 9.6** Puerperal deaths from thromboembolism

| Mode of delivery | 1994-96 | 1997-99 |
|---|---|---|
| Vaginal delivery | 10 | 10 |
| Caesarean section | 15 | 4 |
| Total | 25 | 14 |

significance of which becomes only too clear in retrospect. Classic symptoms require recognition and investigation, especially in high-risk women.

### Hypertensive disease

Eight of the 20 deaths from pre-eclampsia in 1994–96 were due to pulmonary oedema caused by fluid overload during treatment. Fluid balance protocols have been improved and there were no deaths from this cause in 2003–05. Nevertheless, there were 12 deaths from intracranial haemorrhage due to inadequate anti-hypertensive therapy. It became clear that systolic blood pressure was often being ignored as attention was focussed on the diastolic. The 2003–05 report introduced a set of Top Ten key recommendations, one of which is: 'All pregnant women with a systolic blood pressure of 160 mmHg or more require antihypertensive treatment'. The report also recommended that syntometrine should be avoided in the third stage in these cases and drew attention to repeated failures to carry out routine urine testing for proteinuria.

### Haemorrhage

One of the manifestations of substandard care in 2003–05 was failure to recognize signs of intra-abdominal bleeding, and another of the Top Ten key recommendations is wider use of early warning scores, as used in critical care units. Management of uterine atony was often inadequate, and the report recommended regular training for all staff on the identification and management of maternal collapse. A third major concern was placenta accreta. The rising caesarean section rate has led to more cases of placenta praevia implanted over a uterine scar. The key recommendations include the need to warn women about the future risks of caesarean section, and the need for placental localization in women with a previous caesarean section. The reports have repeatedly stated that caesarean section for placenta praevia must be carried out by an experienced surgeon. The current report stresses the importance of multi-disciplinary planning when problems are anticipated and recommends calling a second consultant when severe haemorrhage occurs.

Prompt blood transfusion is life-saving, but deaths continue to occur among women who refuse transfusion for religious or other reasons. Guidelines have been produced for the management of such cases and should be discussed with all staff. Maternal death in these circumstances is particularly distressing.

### Amniotic fluid embolism

Amniotic fluid embolism (AFE) is often thought of as having a hopeless prognosis, but care was still judged to be substandard in seven of the 19 deaths in 2003–05. In most cases, this was due to delay in instituting resuscitation. Premonitory symptoms including breathlessness, chest pain and panic were recorded in 11 of the cases, with the interval between onset of symptoms and delivery varying from almost immediately to over 4 hours. Reasons for delayed resuscitation included failure to recognize the severity of the illness, unnecessary investigations, lack of relevant drugs and equipment, and inability of the cardiac arrest team to gain access to the labour ward. One woman collapsed after a 7–8 hour second stage of labour, and in three cases emergency caesarean section was delayed. The UK Obstetric Surveillance System (UKOSS) is continuing to register all cases of AFE, whatever the outcome, and the incidence in the UK is now estimated at 1.8 cases per 100 000 maternities.

### Early pregnancy deaths

Diagnosing pregnancy is now easy, but only if someone thinks of the possibility and arranges a test. Ectopic pregnancy is notoriously deceptive, and GPs and casualty officers should perform a urinary pregnancy test on any woman of reproductive age with unexplained abdominal pain. Gastrointestinal symptoms may mask the diagnosis. Protocols for medical management of ectopic pregnancy must be strictly adhered to. Death from ovarian hyperstimulation syndrome (OHSS) is an emerging concern and it is now recommended that women admitted with OHSS must receive thromboprophylaxis.

### Sepsis

Streptococci can still produce overwhelming sepsis in a relatively short time, even after a woman has gone home after a short post-natal stay. Now that puerperal sepsis has become rare, doctors and midwives have little experience of recognizing the early signs of serious disease. Maternal tachycardia is an important sign that must not be overlooked. Others are constant abdominal pain and tenderness. Immediate treatment may be life-saving and high-dose broad-spectrum intravenous antibiotic treatment must be started immediately without waiting for microbiology results. An unusual feature of the 2003–05 report was that eight of the 22 deaths from sepsis were from genital tract infection present before delivery.

### Genital tract trauma

As mentioned above, death from genital tract trauma is now rare, partly because difficult forceps deliveries are rarely attempted. In 2003–05, trauma caused three deaths, including one from uterine rupture after induction of labour with a standard regimen of prostaglandin in a parous woman. The classic picture of ruptured uterus – precipitate labour, fetal bradycardia and maternal shock – was not recognized until too late.

Antenatal complications: maternal

## Anaesthesia

Increased use of regional anaesthesia, and ensuring that only appropriately trained staff give anaesthetics in the labour ward, have achieved a gratifying fall in maternal deaths from anaesthesia despite a rising caesarean section rate. Nevertheless, problems are still being identified, for example in the recovery area after early-pregnancy surgery. In the labour ward, morbidly obese women pose a particular problem and direct supervision is essential in these cases. It is still necessary for the report to point out that trainee anaesthetists must be able to obtain prompt advice from a designated consultant at all times.

## Indirect deaths

Although the proportion of cases with substandard care is lower among indirect deaths than among direct deaths (Table 9.3), there is nevertheless potential for improvement.

### Cardiac disease

The spectrum of cardiac disease has changed over the years. Rheumatic heart disease is still seen among immigrant women, who require a complete medical examination, including cardiovascular examination, by an appropriately trained doctor at booking. Specialist referral is essential if rheumatic heart disease is identified. In all pregnant women, symptoms of breathlessness and tachycardia require investigation, particularly when there are risk factors such as obesity, a family history of heart disease, existing hypertension, smoking or age over 35 years. All the deaths from ischaemic heart disease in 2003–05 were in women who had risk factors. Four had a BMI over 40. It is concerning that in the 2003–05 report, midwives and doctors failed to recognize classic symptoms of myocardial infarction, such as crushing chest pain radiating to the jaw. It was also necessary for the report to point out that if a clinician is not competent to interpret an ECG, he/she should consult someone who is.

### Psychiatric disease

A new recommendation in the 2003–05 report is that women who have been referred to child protection services are at particular risk, and communication between agencies is essential. Also at risk are women who have requested termination, but have had to continue with the pregnancy. Other recommendations from previous reports remain important. All women should be routinely asked in early pregnancy about current and previous mental health problems. Questioning should be sensitive, but explicit. Women with a past history of severe mental illness complicating pregnancy have a 33–55 per cent chance of recurrence. Each unit should have a protocol for the management of women at high risk. An emerging problem is inadequate communication between midwives who are looking after women in pregnancy and GPs who have the information about women's previous history. There

is a need for assessment and management of psychiatric illness by a specialist perinatal mental health team, and every region should have a mother and baby unit to which women may be admitted.[6]

### Other indirect deaths

Among the many lessons from the indirect deaths is one repeated several times in the 2003–05 report – the need for modified early warning scoring systems to reduce delay in the recognition of serious illness. When a serious medical condition is identified in pregnancy, rapid specialist referral is essential and normal referral pathways may need to be bypassed. Sudden death in epilepsy (SUDEP) continues to be a problem: the risk may not be greater in pregnancy than in the non-pregnant state, but epilepsy may be more difficult to control in pregnancy, and women should have specialist care in pregnancy from a consultant obstetrician and a neurologist or specialist physician with an interest in epilepsy and pregnancy.

## Coincidental deaths

### Road traffic accidents

Pregnancy is not a contraindication to the use of seat belts, and women should be advised that the belt is placed 'over and under the bump'.

### Domestic violence

Domestic violence may begin or worsen during pregnancy and may be the reason for late booking or poor attendance, or conversely for repeated attendance with minor injuries or non-existent complaints. Other warning signs include drug or alcohol abuse, or the constant presence of a partner at examinations. Staff need sensitivity and ingenuity to help an affected woman to communicate with them. There should be routine enquiries about violence when a social history is taken, and local strategies for referral, and every woman should be seen on her own at least once during the pregnancy. Staff must adopt a non-judgemental and supportive attitude[7] and should remember that health professionals, too, may be victims of abuse.

## THE FUTURE

As maternal mortality has fallen in the UK, attention has turned to 'near misses' – incidents that might have resulted in a maternal death but for prompt and effective treatment. In the 1990s, criteria were developed for the definition of near misses.[8] The most recent CEMD report included a summary of the Scottish Confidential Audit of Severe Maternal Morbidity, which collected national data during 2003–05 and showed that the annual rate of severe morbidity varied from 4.6 to 6.1 per 1000 maternities. By far the most common cause was major obstetric haemorrhage, defined as an estimated blood loss of 2.5 litres or more. Of the 329 cases of severe morbidity in 2005, 235 were of severe haemorrhage. Similar findings were reported in a survey of the three Dublin maternity hospitals in 2004–2005, where the prevalence of severe maternal morbidity was found to be 3.2/1000 maternities.[9] Of the 158 cases identified, 74 were of hypovolaemia requiring transfusion of more than five units of red cells.

These emerging data from severe morbidity surveys underline the message that the risks of pregnancy have not gone away and that the low rates of maternal mortality in developed countries are due to effective intervention when problems occur. The rates of severe morbidity reported in current studies (3–4/1000) are similar to the rates of mortality in the UK before 1935, and to the global MMR today.[1] Vigilance is still essential, and new lessons continue to emerge from national surveillance by the confidential enquiry.

## SUMMARY

The worldwide total of over 500 000 maternal deaths every year is a largely preventable tragedy. We know how to treat the conditions that cause these deaths. Ensuring that treatment reaches the women who need it, however, is a matter of political will, and obstetricians have a duty to act as advocates for the women at risk.

In the United Kingdom, the maternity services have been successful in making pregnancy safe for most women, but substandard care still occurs. It is very concerning that the number of maternal deaths is now rising. Women from ethnic minorities are at increased risk, as are the most deprived sections of the community. The confidential enquiry has led the way in revealing these disturbing facts, and others such as the risks associated with psychiatric disease, domestic violence and now obesity. The purpose of the enquiry is to save lives, and its recommendations are always firmly based on its findings. The importance of this process is increasingly recognized in the UK and worldwide.

### KEY POINTS

- Maternal death is the death of a woman while pregnant or within 42 days after the end of pregnancy. Direct deaths result from obstetric complications and indirect deaths from disease aggravated by, but not directly due to, pregnancy.
- Across the world, the average MMR is 400 per 100 000. Of the estimated global total of 536 000 maternal deaths every year, 99 per cent are in developing regions.

- In developed countries, the MMR is around ten per 100 000 maternities. In Britain between 1936 and 1985, the MMR fell steadily due to antibiotics, blood transfusion, ergometrine, better training of midwives and obstetricians and the 1967 Abortion Act.
- Direct deaths in the UK have not fallen during the last decade. The leading cause of direct death is thromboembolism.
- Indirect deaths in the UK are increasing and now outnumber direct deaths. The leading causes are cardiac disease and (when late deaths are included) psychiatric disease.
- Risk factors for maternal death include age, obesity, low social class and belonging to an ethnic minority.
- Most of the deaths worldwide, and many in the UK, are preventable.

## Key References

1. World Health Organization. Maternal Mortality in 2005. Estimates developed by WHO, UNICEF, UNFPA and The World Bank. Geneva: WHO, 2007.
2. Lewis G (ed.). The Confidential Enquiry into Maternal and Child Health (CEMACH). *Saving Mothers' Lives: reviewing maternal deaths to make motherhood safer – 2003–2005*. The Seventh Report on Confidential Enquiries into Maternal Deaths in the United Kingdom. London: CEMACH, 2007.
3. Kaunitz AM, Spence C, Danielson TS et al. Perinatal and maternal mortality in a religious group avoiding obstetric care. *Am J Obstet Gynecol* 1994; **150**: 826–31.
4. RCOG Working Party. *Thromboprophylaxis in Obstetrics and Gynaecology*. Report of a Working Group. London: RCOG Press, 1995.
5. RCOG Guidelines and Audit Committee. Thromboprophylaxis during pregnancy, labour and after vaginal delivery. Guideline No. 37. London: RCOG, 2004.
6. Royal College of Psychiatrists. *Perinatal Mental Health Services*. Council Report CR88. London: Royal College of Psychiatrists, 2000.
7. Aston G, Bewley S. Abortion and domestic violence. *Obstet Gynaecol* 2009; **11**: 163–8.
8. Mantel GD, Buchmann E, Rees H, Pattinson RC. Severe acute maternal morbidity: a pilot study for a definition of a near-miss. *Br J Obstet Gynaecol* 1998; **105**: 985–90.
9. Murphy CM, Murad K, Deane R et al. Severe maternal morbidity for 2004–2005 in the three Dublin maternity hospitals. *Eur J Obstet Gynecol Reprod Biol* 2009; **143**: 34–7.

# SECTION B
Antenatal complications:
fetal conditions

# 10.1 Biochemical screening

*Michele P Mohajer*

**MRCOG standards**

**Theoretical skills**

- Understand the biochemical components used in maternal serum screening and how they relate to the specific malformations.
- Understand the limitations of maternal serum screening and the situations in which screening may be unreliable.

**Practical skills**

- Be able to counsel a woman about the screening tests available to her.
- Be able to explain about detection rates and limitations of screening.
- Be able to counsel parents who have had a screen-positive result.

## INTRODUCTION

Over the last 50 years, many biochemical substances produced by the feto-placental unit have been identified in maternal serum. A number of these have been found to be associated with certain fetal conditions and have been incorporated into national screening programmes. This section aims to describe those programmes, along with their advantages and disadvantages.

In 1956, the first biochemical marker identified in maternal serum was alpha-fetoprotein (AFP); the association between a raised serum AFP and open spina bifida was not demonstrated until 1974.[1]

## BIOCHEMICAL SCREENING FOR NEURAL TUBE DEFECTS

Alpha-fetoprotein is produced by the fetal liver. It crosses into the maternal serum from the amniotic fluid or via the placenta.

Maternal serum AFP (MSAFP) rises throughout most of pregnancy (from 12 to 32 weeks), hence accurate determination of gestational age is mandatory. To allow for the increase in concentration in the second trimester, it is convenient to express all AFP values as a multiple of the normal median (MoM) at the relevant gestational age. The separation between the distribution of MSAFP levels in pregnancies with open fetal defects and normal pregnancies is greatest at 16–18 weeks gestation, and therefore screening is optimum at this stage.

Alpha-fetoprotein screening was intended for the detection of open spina bifida, and not closed spina bifida. Using a cut-off level of 2.5 MoM, 79 per cent open spina bifida and 88 per cent anencephaly can be detected [C]. If all neural tube defects (NTDs) are considered, the detection rate is 72 per cent, with a false-positive rate of 0.001 per cent.[2]

Raised MSAFP is also associated with other fetal malformations or conditions, including:

- multiple pregnancy,
- abdominal wall defects (gastroschisis, exomphalos, bladder extrophy),
- congenital nephrosis,
- spontaneous fetal loss.

There is also some degree of association between a raised MSAFP and the following conditions:

- pre-eclampsia,
- preterm delivery,
- low birth weight,
- underestimated gestation,
- low maternal weight,
- Afro-Caribbean ethnic origin,
- male fetus,
- raised MSAFP in a previous pregnancy,
- smoking.

Levels of MSAFP may be lowered in association with other conditions, including:

- Down's syndrome (trisomy 21),
- Edward's syndrome (trisomy 18),
- insulin-dependent diabetes,
- overestimated gestation,
- high maternal weight.

Alpha-fetoprotein screening now has a relatively minor role in the detection of fetal defects due to the widespread use of sophisticated ultrasound techniques. Using ultrasound to demonstrate the characteristic cranial signs of spina bifida (the 'lemon and banana' sign), the detection rate of all NTDs is 81per cent [C] with a false-positive rate of 0.0003 per cent (see Chapter 10.2, Ultrasound screening).[3] This detection rate exceeds that of AFP screening programmes. However, AFP screening is still used in areas of high NTD prevalence, or where high-resolution ultrasound is not routinely available.

## The role of amniocentesis in MSAFP screening

Prior to high-resolution ultrasound, amniocentesis was routinely performed to detect increased levels of AFP and acetylcholinesterase (AChE) in the amniotic fluid in an attempt to diagnose open fetal defects. The risk of fetal loss may be eight times higher when amniocentesis is performed in these circumstances [A], and it therefore should not be performed as an initial investigation.[4]

Many more biochemical substances have been identified that are produced during pregnancy. Many of these have been investigated for their usefulness in detecting pregnancy complications. Two notable hormones, human placental lactogen (hPL) and oestriol (E3), were used widely to assess placental function. These have now been abandoned due to the development of better biophysical methods.

## BIOCHEMICAL SCREENING FOR DOWN'S SYNDROME

The main area of development of other biochemical markers in pregnancy has been in screening for Down's syndrome (trisomy 21).

Down's syndrome is still the most common cause of severe mental retardation. The natural birth prevalence increases with maternal age, from one in 1500 under the age of 25, to one in 1000 at age 30, and to one in 100 at age 40. The overall incidence of the condition has increased due to women having their babies at an older age.

In the early 1980s, antenatal screening relied on identifying women above a specified age (e.g. 35 years) and offering them amniocentesis. In 1984, low MSAFP levels in the mid-trimester were found to be associated with Down's syndrome.[5] Later, human chorionic gonadotrophin (hCG) was found to be raised in Down's syndrome, and unconjugated oestriol (uE3) was found to be reduced. Division of hCG into its free subunits (alpha-hCG and beta-hCG) provided additional value in screening. More recently, a fourth biochemical marker,

inhibin-A, has been found to be raised in Down's syndrome pregnancies.[6]

Subsequently, measurement of biochemical substances in the first trimester of pregnancy has also demonstrated an association with Down's syndrome. The two markers used are free beta-hCG and pregnancy-associated plasma protein A (PAPP-A).

Accurate gestational age assessment is vital to the utility of these biochemical markers. Screening is only applicable to singleton pregnancies, so ultrasonic assessment is again mandatory. All markers vary with gestation, and so MoMs are used to determine abnormal values.

## Second trimester screening

Second trimester screening is carried out between 15 and 22 weeks of pregnancy. Serum screening programmes incorporate:

- two components (MSAFP and total hCG or free beta-hCG): the double test;
- three components (MSAFP, hCG and uE3): the triple test; or
- four components (MSAFP, hCG, uE3 and inhibin): the quadruple test.

The screening performance of these markers improves with the addition of markers, such that for a false-positive rate of 5 per cent, the detection rates for the double, triple and quadruple tests are 59, 69 and 76 per cent, respectively.[7] However, the extra cost of using additional serum markers must be considered.

Certain factors can influence serum markers.

- Insulin-dependent diabetes and increased maternal weight lower all markers.
- Twin gestation produces approximately twice the level of all serum markers.
- Minor variations occur with ethnic differences and in smokers.
- Other conditions in which serum screening may be unreliable include maternal renal failure and severe dehydration (e.g. severe hyperemesis gravidarum).

The aim of screening is to maximize the detection rate with a low false-positive rate, in order that invasive testing is minimized. It is likely that even combinations of serum analytes measured in the second trimester will not have adequate detection rates or, perhaps most importantly, intervention rates to be used for population screening for Down's syndrome (see National recommendations below).

## First trimester screening

Two biochemical markers, namely free beta-hCG and PAPP-A, when measured between 8 and 14 weeks in combination with maternal age, can detect 62 per cent of Down's syndrome pregnancies, with a 5 per cent false-positive rate.[8]

Data suggest that this method of screening is as effective as those serum markers in established use at 15–20 weeks [B]. These serum markers, when combined with maternal age and nuchal translucency (NT) measurement (see Chapter 10.2, Ultrasound screening), comprise the triple test or combined test, which has an estimated detection rate of 85 per cent for a 5 per cent false-positive rate.[9] This test is usually performed in a single visit, which reduces the anxiety of waiting for a result.

First trimester screening provides the opportunity to establish a diagnosis in early pregnancy (if chorionic villus sampling is utilized). To introduce this method of screening on a nationwide basis would require enormous financial support for the training and education of health professionals, the provision of information and counselling services, and the expansion of expertise in diagnostic ultrasound and invasive tests, such as chorionic villus sampling [C].

## Integrated/hybrid screening

Simultaneously using markers from both trimesters yields a better screening performance than using markers in either trimester alone. Thus, if the first trimester triple test is combined with the second trimester quadruple test, the detection rate for Down's syndrome has been estimated at 94 per cent for a 5 per cent false-positive rate.[10] If the false-positive rate is fixed at 1 per cent, the detection rate will be 85 per cent. This approach therefore yields a higher detection rate than any other screening test at a given false-positive rate. The SURUSS report showed that if the risk cut off level is fixed at 1:200, the detection rate is 89 per cent for a 2.4 per cent false positive rate.[11] The FASTER trial showed comparable results.[12] However, the logistics of introducing such a screening system need to be considered. The result of the first trimester screen would need to be concealed from the woman, and thus would negate the advantage of early prenatal diagnosis. If ultrasound facilities are not sufficiently developed to perform reliable NT measurement, the full, integrated test cannot be provided. In the absence of NT, the detection rate for the integrated test is 85 per cent for a 5.5 per cent false-positive rate.[10] In addition, the infrastructure necessary for the organization and counselling of integrated/hybrid screening far exceeds that required for the present screening programmes. Nevertheless, the enormous financial and emotional advantage of a test with a 1 per cent false-positive rate cannot be denied.

## National recommendation for Down's screening

Current recommendations state that all pregnant women should be offered first trimester screening (by 13 weeks and 6 days), but that provision should be made to allow for later screening (as late as 20 weeks 0 days).[13] Ideally, the combined test (NT + beta HCG + PAPPA) should be offered between 11 weeks 0 days and 13 weeks 6 days. For women who book later in pregnancy, the most clinically effective serum screening (triple or quadruple test) should be offered between 15 weeks 0 days and 20 weeks 0 days.

## BIOCHEMICAL SCREENING FOR OTHER ABNORMALITIES

A number of other chromosomal abnormalities have been shown to be associated with biochemical markers.

- *Trisomy 18.* Trisomy 18 (Edward's syndrome) is the second most common aneuploidy surviving to birth. In the second trimester, MSAFP, hCG and uE3 levels are all low. Risk assessment for trisomy 18 has been incorporated into some screening programmes.
- *Triploidy.* This chromosomal abnormality is inconsistent with survival. Affected pregnancies may be identified in the mid-trimester, as there are very high or very low levels of AFP and hCG, and low levels of E3.
- *Turner's syndrome (45, X).* In Turner's syndrome associated with hydrops, the serum markers show a pattern similar to that of Down's syndrome pregnancies. In those without hydrops, the hCG level is low.
- *Smith–Lemlie–Opitz syndrome.* This is an autosomal recessive condition associated with moderate to severe mental retardation. In these pregnancies, uE3 is very low or undetectable, and MSAFP and hCG tend to be low. The risk of a pregnancy affected with this condition can thus be calculated, and the diagnosis is confirmed by measuring 7-dehydrocholesterol (7-DHCO) in the amniotic fluid.

## HEALTH ECONOMICS OF SCREENING

A major challenge in the delivery of Down's screening services is the need to set up an adequate organizational structure. This not only means dedicated laboratory facilities with computer-assisted test interpretation and expertise to provide invasive prenatal testing, but also a team of experienced co-ordinators to undertake the enormous workload of counselling. This counselling is essential, both prior to undertaking the test and in the event of a screen-positive result when invasive testing is contemplated. It is this last service provision that has poor structure in many screening programmes, and fiscal implications are generally underestimated. In the ideal structure, each unit should have a clear screening policy agreed centrally. A screening co-ordinator is responsible for reporting results to women and co-ordinating the local screening service. A local director of screening, of consultant status, guides and supports the service and is attentive to advances in screening and their controlled introduction into practice.

## EBM

- High-resolution ultrasound has a better detection rate for open fetal defects than a high MSAFP [C].
- With accurate ultrasound dating, second trimester biochemical screening using four markers can detect 76 per cent of Down's syndrome pregnancies [B].
- First trimester serum screening is as effective as mid-trimester serum screening [B].

## KEY POINTS

- A raised MSAFP has good sensitivity but poor specificity for open fetal defects, but is still used in areas of high NTD prevalence.
- Mid-trimester serum screening for Down's syndrome is widely available in the UK.
- Detection rates vary depending on the number of markers used.
- A dating scan must be performed prior to Down's syndrome screening.
- Combined (first trimester) screening is recommended but may be difficult to implement due to cost and limited expertise.
- Counselling before and after testing accounts for the bulk of the workload.

## Published Guidelines

Grudzinskas JG, Ward RHT (eds). Screening for Down's Syndrome in the First Trimester. Recommendations arising from the Study Group. London: RCOG Press, 1997.

*Antenatal screening for Down's Syndrome.* London: RCOG Press, July 2003.

NICE Clinical Care Guideline 62- Antenatal Care, 2008.

## Key References

1. Wald NJ, Brock DJH, Bonnar J. Prenatal diagnosis of spina bifida and anencephaly by maternal serum alpha-fetoprotein measurement. A controlled study. *Lancet* 1974; **1**: 765–7.

2. Report of UK Collaborative Study on Alpha-fetoprotein in Relation to Neural Tube Defects. Maternal serum alpha-fetoprotein measurement in antenatal screening for anencephaly and spina bifida in early pregnancy. *Lancet* 1977; **1**: 1323–32.

3. Papp Z, Toth-Pal E, Papp CS, Torok O. Impact of prenatal mid-trimester screening on the prevalence of fetal structure anomalies: a prospective epidemiological study. *Ultrasound Obstet Gynecol* 1995; **6**: 320–6.

4. Morrow RJ, McNay MB, Whittle MJ. Ultrasound detection of neural tube defects in patients with elevated maternal serum AFP levels. *Obstet Gynecol* 1991; **78**: 1055–7.

5. Cuckle HS, Wald NJ, Lindenbaum RH. Maternal serum alpha-fetoprotein measurement. A screening test for Down's syndrome. *Lancet* 1984; **1**: 926–9.

6. Wald NJ, Densem JW, George L *et al*. Prenatal screening for Down's syndrome using Inhibin-A as a serum marker. *Prenat Diagn* 1996; **16**: 143–53.

7. Wald NJ, Densem JW, Smith D, Klee GG. Four marker serum screening for Down's syndrome. *Prenat Diagn* 1994; **14**: 707–16.

8. Wald NJ, George L, Smith D *et al*. Serum screening for Down's syndrome between 8 and 14 weeks of pregnancy. *Br J Obstet Gynaecol* 1996; **103**: 407–12.

9. Wald NJ, Hackshaw AK. Combining ultrasound and biochemistry in first trimester screening for Down's syndrome. *Prenat Diagn* 1997; **17**: 821–9.

10. Wald NJ, Watt HC, Hackshaw AK. Integrated screening for Down's syndrome based on tests performed during the first and second trimesters. *N Engl J Med* 1999; **341**: 461–7.

11. Wald NJ, Rodeck C, Hackshaw AK *et al*. First and second trimester screening for Down's syndrome: the results of the serum, urine and ultrasound screening study (SURUSS). *J Med Screen* 2003; **10**: 56–104.

12. Malone FD, Canick JA, Ball RH *et al*. First trimester screening or second trimester screening, or both, for Down's syndrome. *N Engl J Med* 2005; **353**: 2001–11.

13. NICE clinical care guideline No. 62-Antenatal Care 2008.

# 10.2 Ultrasound screening

*Michele P Mohajer*

## INTRODUCTION

The incidence of major structural fetal abnormality is 2–3 per cent, and far exceeds all chromosomal abnormalities or single gene defects. As a result of the technological development in high-resolution ultrasound equipment, the prenatal diagnosis of most major structural malformations is possible. As a consequence, there has been a significant fall in perinatal mortality rates due to the termination of affected fetuses. In addition to this role, ultrasound scanning is vital in determining gestation, viability and number of fetuses. The advent of such technological development has provided the foundation for the subspecialty of fetal medicine.

## WHAT IS SCREENING?

The purpose of screening for fetal malformation is not simply to terminate the fetus prior to viability in order to reduce perinatal mortality rates. Although screening does reduce perinatal mortality rates, the identification of fetal malformation allows parents to make informed choices regarding their pregnancy. This facilitates physical and psychological preparation for the delivery of an infant with a birth defect, which may even take place in another centre. In addition, identification of certain abnormalities may allow parents to avail themselves of *in-utero* treatments that can improve the infant's condition prior to birth. Ultrasound screening can also be used to identify some fetuses with chromosomal disease in which case invasive diagnostic procedures can be performed.

## WHO SHOULD BE SCREENED?

Certain conditions increase a woman's chance of having a malformed fetus. So-called 'high-risk' groups can be identified, such as women with insulin-dependent diabetes, maternal drug ingestion (e.g. anticonvulsants, warfarin), or a positive family history. However, 95 per cent of abnormalities occur in fetuses born to mothers who have no risk factors at all.[1] Therefore, routine ultrasound scanning of all pregnancies has been suggested as the preferred method to identify structural malformations [A]. Evidence to support this recommendation is unsatisfactory. Vast differences exist in detection rates, ranging from 16 to 85 per cent.[2–4]

The reasons for these differences are unclear. The skill and training of the operator are important, but perhaps an important variable is the gestational age at which the scan is done. The optimum time for the identification of structural fetal anomalies is 18–21 weeks [B].[5,6]

Prior to performing the ultrasound scan, it is vital that the parents understand the objectives, the limitations and also the detection rates for the major malformations.[6] This is ideally done by the provision of information leaflets [C].

## TIMING OF SCREENING

### The detailed fetal anomaly scan at 18–21 weeks

The scan initially checks viability and number of fetuses, as well as placental site and amniotic fluid volume. Standard views of the fetus are then taken. These are:

1 transverse section through the fetal head, assessing head shape and internal structures;
2 fetal spine: sagittal, coronal and transverse views;
3 fetal abdomen: longitudinal and transverse; identifying intra-abdominal organs: stomach, kidneys, bladder and ventral wall integrity and cord insertion;
4 transverse section through fetal thorax to examine four-chamber view of the heart and outflow tracts;
5 limbs: identify three long bones in each limb.

Inability to obtain the standard images may occur due to fetal position or maternal size.

# MAJOR STRUCTURAL MALFORMATIONS

## Central nervous system malformations

Many major structural defects of the central nervous system (CNS) may be identified at the 20-week scan, and certain malformations can be identified at earlier gestations.

### Neural tube defects

These malformations occur when there is a failure of dorsal fusion in early embryological life, such that neural tissue is exposed. Neural tube defects (anencephaly, cephaloceles and spina bifida) are the most common CNS malformations in the UK, and much energy has been applied to the screening and prevention of these anomalies. Anencephaly is characterized by the absence of the cerebral hemispheres and cranial vault, and can be identified from as early as 11–12 weeks. The prognosis is uniformly fatal within the first hours or days of life. Cephalocele is a protrusion of the intracranial contents through a bony defect of the skull. These contents may include only meninges (cranial meningocele) or brain tissue (encephalocele). Ultrasound examination can identify a solid or cystic paracranial mass. The prognosis depends on the presence of brain tissue within the sac and other associated intracranial features. Spina bifida, in which the defect exists in the vertebral fusion, is the most common CNS malformation. Demonstration of the lesion itself by ultrasound may be difficult. However, the intracranial signs associated with spina bifida, the Arnold–Chiari malformation (herniation of the cerebellum and brainstem through the foramen magnum), are more easily identifiable.[7] This demonstration of the 'lemon and banana' sign has displaced maternal serum alpha-fetoprotein (MSAFP) as the main screening test for spina bifida in many units. The detection rate for open spina bifida on ultrasound screening is 81 per cent, with a false-positive rate of 0.0003 per cent.[8]

### Hydrocephalus

This condition arises when there is an abnormal accumulation of cerebrospinal fluid (CSF), resulting in enlargement of the ventricular system. In itself, it is not a diagnosis based upon aetiology but is commonly associated with other intracranial and extracranial abnormalities. Diagnosis on ultrasound examination is achieved by demonstration of enlarged lateral ventricles and anterior displacement of the choroid plexus. The three major forms are aqueduct stenosis, communicating hydrocephalus and Dandy–Walker syndrome. This last syndrome is characterized by the addition of a cyst in the posterior fossa and defect in the cerebellar vermis, both of which are detectable on ultrasound. The prognosis is variable, again depending on the severity of the hydrocephalus and presence of additional malformations.

Other less common CNS malformations may be identified on ultrasound. These include holoprosencephaly, iniencephaly, arachnoid cysts, porencephalic cysts, agenesis of the corpus callosum, hydrancephaly, microcephaly, intracranial tumours and aneurysm of the vein of Galen.

## Cardiac malformations

Systematic examination of the fetal heart has enabled the prenatal diagnosis of many congenital heart defects. Since the fetal heart is almost horizontal, a transverse section through the fetal chest will demonstrate a four-chamber view. This standard view provides information about the position and size of the fetal heart, the cardiac chambers and the atrioventricular connections. Congenital heart abnormalities associated with an abnormal four-chamber view include:

- hypoplastic left heart
- hypoplastic right heart
- atrioventricular canal defect
- large ventricular septal defect
- large atrial septal defect
- single ventricle
- valve stenosis or atresia
- Ebstein's anomaly
- cardiac tumour
- cardiac situs abnormalities.

However, there is a wide variation in the ability of ultrasound screening for cardiac abnormalities, with detection rates varying from 6 to 77 per cent.[1,4] These differences may be related to the gestational age at which the scan is performed, the type of congenital heart abnormality, as well as the experience of the operator. Several cardiac defects are associated with a normal standard four-chamber view. These include:

- tetralogy of Fallot
- transposition of the great arteries
- small atrial and ventricular septal defects
- mild pulmonary or aortic valve stenosis
- mild coarctation of the aorta.

With the improvements in paediatric cardiac surgery, prenatal diagnosis of cardiac conditions has become much more important. Parents can make informed choices, if given the realistic expectations of the problem.

## Thoracic malformations

By obtaining transverse and longitudinal views of the fetal chest, space-occupying lesions, solid or cystic, may be diagnosed. The fetal lungs are uniformly echogenic. Fluid within the pleural cavity (pleural effusions) may be identified as a result of certain fetal conditions. Chylothorax, a relatively common cause of pleural effusion in neonatal life, is an accumulation of chyle in the pleural cavity. Bronchogenic cysts may appear as sonolucent areas within the fetal chest.

Congenital cystic adenomatous malformation of the lung (CCAML) is a condition whereby there is overgrowth of terminal bronchioles at the expense of saccular spaces. The ultrasound appearance varies according to the type: either macrocystic, with large cystic structures within the chest, or microcystic, where there is increased echogenicity of the lung tissue. Lung sequestrations may also appear as an echogenic mass. Cystic structures within the chest may also be demonstrated in the fetus with congenital diaphragmatic hernia. When there is a defect, the stomach or other abdominal contents may be demonstrated above the level of the diaphragm.

## Gastrointestinal and abdominal wall malformations

Demonstration of the integrity of the abdominal wall is made on transverse and longitudinal views. Ventral wall defects, gastroschisis and exomphalos may be identified.

Gastroschisis is a para-umbilical defect, and can be diagnosed by the presence of herniated organs floating freely within the amniotic cavity. An exomphalos is a central defect surrounded by a membrane on which the umbilical cord is inserted. These defects may also be associated with an elevated MSAFP. In isolation, the prognosis for both of these malformations is good with surgical correction, but karyotyping should be considered in the case of exomphalos, as an association with aneuploidy exists. Rarer defects in the abdominal wall may be diagnosed, known as bladder and cloacal extrophy.

Intra-abdominal pathology may be diagnosed on ultrasound such as:

- fetal ascites
- small and large bowel obstruction
- meconium peritonitis
- mesenteric, omental and retroperitoneal cysts.

Many of the obstructive malformations may be associated with polyhydramnios.

## Urogenital malformations

The fetal kidneys and bladder are relatively easily identified structures in the mid-trimester. Many fetal renal problems are associated with a disturbance in amniotic fluid volume. By 16 weeks, the majority of the amniotic fluid is produced by the fetal kidneys. If oligohydramnios is diagnosed in the mid-trimester, in the absence of a history of ruptured membranes, fetal renal malformation must be suspected.

Renal agenesis may be bilateral or unilateral. If bilateral, there is associated an hydramnios and the condition is fatal. Visualization of the fetal kidneys in this situation is difficult due to loss of the acoustic window and may be facilitated by an amnio-infusion.

Infantile polycystic kidney disease is an autosomal recessive disease. Ultrasound diagnosis is made by the demonstration of bilateral enlarged hyperechogenic fetal kidneys, absent fetal bladder and associated oligohydramnios. The prognosis is poor.

Obstructive uropathy may occur due to an obstruction at the urethra or ureter. Urethral obstruction, due either to urethral atresia or posterior urethral valves, may be demonstrated by the presence of a distended fetal bladder, hydroureter and hydronephrosis. Ureteric obstruction, which may be unilateral or bilateral, can be diagnosed by ultrasound by the demonstration of hydronephrosis.

In multicystic dysplastic kidney disease (MDKD), ultrasound examination of the fetal kidneys shows the presence of multiple cysts, and increased echogenicity of the surrounding parenchyma. The kidneys are enlarged and where there is bilateral disease, the prognosis is fatal.

Tumours of the kidney and adrenal gland, if present in fetal life, can also be diagnosed on ultrasound scans.

## Skeletal malformations

Diagnosis of skeletal abnormalities requires a full examination of the fetus, with a skeletal survey. This involves both morphological and biometric examination of the skull, vertebrae, ribs, long bones and digits of the hands and feet. Measurement of the femur length at a dating scan may be the first clue to a skeletal problem.

Skeletal malformations may affect the whole skeleton and may be lethal, such as:

- achondrogenesis
- thanatophoric dysplasia
- short-rib polydactyly syndromes
- fibrochondrogenesis
- homozygous achondroplasia
- osteogenesis imperfecta (perinatal type)
- hypophosphatasia (perinatal type).

Lethality is usually dependent on thoracic cage involvement and subsequent development of pulmonary hypoplasia.

Other skeletal problems, such as radial anomalies, talipes equinovarus, femoral hypoplasia, facial clefts and digital anomalies, may be identified and may form part of another syndrome, including chromosome anomalies.

The prognosis depends on the involvement of other, non-skeletal, malformations.

The overall detection rate of skeletal problems is 90 per cent.[9]

## Hydrops fetalis and cystic hygroma

This is a condition in which fluid accumulates within the body cavities and soft tissues of the fetus. The aetiologies of this condition are numerous (see Chapter 17, Fetal hydrops).[10] Visualization of fluid within the fetus is relatively easy, and the most common area of fluid accumulation is at the fetal neck, the cystic hygroma. This is usually due to lymphatic obstruction, and is recognized as a cystic structure adjacent to the fetal neck. Cystic hygromas are frequently associated with chromosomal abnormalities. Smaller degrees of fluid in this area are referred to as nuchal oedema or nuchal translucency. As detailed below, it is this latter anomaly that has been identified at earlier gestations (11–14 weeks), and has now been incorporated into screening programmes for aneuploidy.

## Screening for chromosomal disease

Many structural malformations identified on scan may be associated with chromosomal disease, such as:

- cystic hygroma
- cardiac defects
- exomphalos
- holoprosencephaly
- microcephaly
- diaphragmatic hernia
- oesophageal/duodenal atresia
- renal anomalies
- radial aplasia
- micrognathia
- clinodactyly of the fifth finger
- polydactyly
- talipes.

At the time of the 20-week scan, minor ultrasound abnormalities may be seen that may also be associated with aneuploidy. These are known as 'soft markers'. They may not constitute a structural defect, but when seen along with another risk factor for chromosomal disease, karyotyping may be considered. Soft markers include:

- nuchal oedema
- mild renal pyelectasis
- hyperechogenic bowel
- echogenic intracardiac foci
- strawberry-shaped skull
- mild ventriculomegaly
- shortened long bones
- choroid plexus cysts

- clenched fists
- rocker bottom feet
- sandal gap
- single umbilical artery.

These soft markers have been included in some screening programmes for Down's syndrome. However, apart from nuchal oedema, there is no strong evidence at present that the other soft markers are helpful in identifying Down's syndrome [A].[11]

A recent NHS fetal anomaly screening programme[12] has refined recommendations such that only the follow markers should be referred for further management:

- nuchal oedema (>6 mm)
- ventriculomgaly (atrium 10 mm or greater)
- echogenic bowel
- renal pelvic dilatation (greater than 7 mm AP)
- small measurements compared to the dating scan (<3rd centile)
- facial clefting.

Choroid plexus cysts, head shape, cysterna magna (in the absence of brain abnormality), echogenic foci and two vessel cord should not be recorded or referred and should be considered as 'normal variants'.[13]

## FIRST TRIMESTER SCREENING

Ultrasound scanning in the first trimester was primarily introduced for viability and accurate dating. However, from 2010, the national Screening Committee in the UK have recommended the introduction of the $11-13^{+6}$ week scan in screening for Down's syndrome. With improved resolution of ultrasound and examination of the fetus in the first trimester, an increasing number of anomalies will be detected at this earlier gestation. A number of fetal defects may also be seen, such as:

- anencephaly
- holoprosencephaly
- encephalocele
- Dandy–Walker syndrome
- cardiac anomalies
- gastroschisis
- exomphalos
- megacystis
- diaphragmatic hernia
- multidysplastic kidney
- some skeletal dysplasias.

Using a combination of transabdominal and transvaginal ultrasound, up to 59 per cent of major structural defects may be diagnosed at the 11–14-week scan.[14,15]

An important component of the first trimester scan is the NT measurement, which is the maximum thickness of the subcutaneous translucency between the skin and the soft tissue overlying the cervical spine. It has not only been shown to be an effective screening test for aneuploidy, but also may identify a fetus at risk of cardiac defects, skeletal dysplasias and genetic syndromes.[16] There are sufficient data to show that NT screening for Down's syndrome at 10–14 weeks is superior to serum screening with multiple markers at 15–20 weeks gestation [A]. Assessment of the fetal nasal bone during the first trimester may improve the detection of Down's syndrome. However, studies of general population screening have not been able to support this.[15] Although proven to be useful, the availability of nuchal screening in the UK is still limited. The counselling, expertise and training required to successfully implement such a national screening test may be difficult to achieve.

## HAZARDS OF ULTRASOUND SCAN

Many epidemiological and laboratory studies have been performed to search for evidence of possible biological effects of diagnostic ultrasound. Childhood cancer, dyslexia, non-right handedness, delayed speech development and reduced birth weight have all been implicated, but as yet there is no good evidence to establish a firm link between ultrasound and these endpoints.[1]

Although a sophisticated investigation, there are limitations to ultrasound. Adequate visualization of the fetal anatomy may not be possible due to the fetal position or maternal habitus. In situations of gross maternal obesity, confirmation of fetal viability may be extremely difficult.

Visual confirmation of fetal normality appears to promote a positive attitude towards the pregnancy, with improved compliance on healthcare issues such as smoking and alcohol.[17] However, the detection of fetal defects and, in particular, soft ultrasound markers may generate immense anxiety and rejection, even if the subsequent invasive testing proves the fetus is healthy. Hence, for the successful maintenance of ultrasound screening programmes, a framework of skilled midwives, sonographers and counsellors is necessary. This is not only to deal with parents in whom a fetal abnormality has been diagnosed, but also to ensure that prior to the ultrasound scan, women have a clear idea about what the test is likely to achieve and its reliability in doing so.

---

**EBM**

- Screening the whole population rather than selective scanning is the most reliable way to identify fetal abnormality [A].
- A scan undertaken between 18 and 21 weeks is the most effective method to identify a wide range of fetal abnormality [B].
- Screening for fetal abnormality reduces the perinatal mortality rates through identification and termination of affected pregnancies [A].

---

**KEY POINTS**

- Detailed ultrasound at 18-21 weeks is an important screening examination in which most life-threatening malformations can be diagnosed.
- Pregnant women should receive clear information regarding the objectives of the ultrasound examination and the likelihood of finding an abnormality.
- Success of the ultrasound examination depends on the operator, the ultrasound equipment, the fetal position and the maternal habitus.
- When an abnormality is detected on ultrasound, the parents should have ready access to skilled counsellors who are able to provide them with full information, options and support in order to allow them to make an informed choice.

## Published Guidelines

Grudzinskas JG, Ward RHT (eds). *Recommendations Arising from the Study Group on Screening for Down's Syndrome in the First Trimester*. London: RCOG Press, 1997.

Fetal Anomaly Ultrasound Screening Programme. UK National Screening Committee, 2006.

Clinical Care Guideline No 62. *Antenatal Care. Routine Care for the Healthy Pregnant woman*. NICE, March 2008.

## Key References

1. Whittle M. *Ultrasound Screening for Fetal Abnormalities*. Report of the RCOG Working Party. London: RCOG Press, 1997.
2. Crane JP, LeFevre ML, Winborn RC *et al*. and the RADIUS Study Group. A randomized trial of prenatal ultrasonographic screening: impact on the detection, management and outcome of anomalous fetuses. *Am J Obstet Gynecol* 1994; **171**: 392–9.
3. Luck C. Value of routine ultrasound scanning at 19 weeks: a four year study of 8849 deliveries. *BMJ* 1992; **304**: 1474–8.
4. Carvalho JS, Mavrides E, Shinebourne EA *et al*. Improving the effectiveness of routine prenatal screening for major congenital heart defects. *Heart* 2002; **88**: 387–91.
5. Drife JO, Donnai D (eds). *Antenatal Diagnosis of Fetal Abnormalities*. London: RCOG Press, 1991: 354–5.
6. Clinical Care Guideline No 62; *Antenatal Care. Routine Care for the Healthy Pregnant Woman*. NICE March 2008.
7. Nicolaides KH, Campbell S, Gabbe SG, Guidetti R. Ultrasound screening for spina bifida: cranial and cerebellar signs. *Lancet* 1986; **ii**: 72–4.

8. Papp Z, Toth-Pal E, Papp CS, Torok O. Impact of prenatal mid-trimester screening on the prevalence of fetal structure anomalies: a prospective epidemiological study. *Ultrasound Obstet Gynecol* 1995; **6**: 320–26.

9. Whittle MJ. *Routine Ultrasound Screening in Pregnancy.* Report of the RCOG Working Party. London: RCOG Press, 2000: 7–12.

10. James D. Fetal hydrops. In: *The Yearbook of Obstetrics and Gynaecology*, vol. 9. London: RCOG Press, 2001: 277–87.

11. Smith-Bindman R, Hosmer W, Feldstein VA *et al.* Second-trimester ultrasound to detect fetuses with Down's syndrome. A meta-analysis. *J Am Med Assoc* 2001; **285**: 1044–55.

12. UK National Screening Committee. Fetal Anomaly Ultrasound screening Programme. Soft Marker screening policy, 2009.

13. Reading AE, Campbell S, Cox DN, Sledmere CM. Health beliefs and health care behaviour in pregnancy. *Psychol Med* 1982; **12**: 379–83.

14. Whitlow BJ, Chatzipapas IK, Lazanakis ML *et al.* The value of sonography in early pregnancy for the detection of fetal abnormalities in an unselected population. *Br J Obstet Gynaecol* 1999; **106**: 929–36.

15. Malone FD, Ball RH, Nyberg DA *et al.* First trimester nasal bone evaluation for aneuploidy in the general population. *Obstet Gynecol* 2004; **104**: 1222–28.

16. Nicolaides KH, Heath V, Liao AW. The 11–14 week scan. *Clin Obstet Gynaecol* 2000; **14**: 581–94.

17. Souka AP, Pilalis A, Kavalakis I *et al.* Screening for major structural abnormalites at the 11–14 week ultrasound scan. *Am J Obstet Gynecol* 2006; **194**: 393–6.

# 10.3 Invasive prenatal diagnosis

*Michele P Mohajer*

## INTRODUCTION

High-resolution ultrasound imaging has enabled direct access to the different constituents of the gestational sac from the middle of the first trimester of pregnancy. An ever-increasing range of invasive techniques is being developed to facilitate the diagnosis of chromosomal and single gene defects, metabolic disorders, intrauterine infection, fetal anaemia, thrombocytopenia and some structural problems.

All invasive procedures carry a small risk of fetal loss. Early prenatal testing provides the opportunity for surgical termination of the pregnancy if required, but the earlier invasive testing tends to increase the fetal loss rate. Non-invasive techniques for identifying fetal cells in maternal blood and cervical mucus have been the focus of much research.[1] Developments in techniques employing multiplex PCR have enabled reliable prenatal diagnosis of fetal blood groups[2] and fetal aneuploidy.[3]

The routinely used invasive procedures are amniocentesis, chorionic villus sampling (CVS) and fetal blood sampling (FBS).

## AMNIOCENTESIS

Amniocentesis involves the aspiration of amniotic fluid from the amniotic sac via a needle inserted through the maternal abdomen. It is the most common prenatal diagnostic procedure in the UK. It was first introduced in 1966 for the diagnosis of genetic disease[4] and subsequently used to confirm open neural tube defects the presence of a raised maternal serum alpha-fetoprotein (see Chapter 10.1, Biochemical screening).[5] It is usually performed between 15 and 16 weeks gestation.

## Method

Using an aseptic technique, a 22-gauge needle is inserted through the maternal abdomen under direct real-time ultrasound control with continuous needle-tip visualization. This method is more successful than blind techniques [B]. Fifteen to 20 mL of fluid containing fetal cells is aspirated into a syringe. The cells are then cultured for 2–3 weeks before further testing can be performed.

## Indications for amniocentesis

The main indication for amniocentesis is for fetal karyotyping. In view of the risk of miscarriage, the procedure is offered when there is an increased risk of aneuploidy, such as for:

- women with positive screening for Down's syndrome;
- women of advanced maternal age (traditionally >35 years);
- ultrasound detection of an abnormality or soft markers;
- parental balanced translocation;
- a previous history of chromosomal abnormality.

One of the major disadvantages for the woman has been the long wait for the result, which may take from 2 to 4 weeks. Molecular genetics has developed two techniques which have permitted the rapid diagnosis of many major chromosomal abnormalities. These two tests, fluorescence *in-situ* hybridization (FISH) and quantitative fluorescence polymerase chain reaction (QF-PCR), can provide results in 24–48 hours.[6] FISH relies on the unique ability of a portion of single-stranded DNA (known as a probe) to hybridize with its complementary target DNA sequence. By attaching a fluorescent label to the appropriate probe, diagnosis of autosomal trisomies for chromosomes 13, 18, 21 and X and Y chromosomes can be made in 6–8 hours by direct fluorescent microscopy. QF-PCR uses highly polymorphic small tandem repeat markers, which allow distinction between normal and trisomic DNA samples. Diagnosis of the major chromosomal abnormalities (trisomies 13, 18, 21 and sex chromosome copy number abnormalities) can be performed in 24–48 hours. Both techniques share the same diagnostic dilemma in that conventional chromosomal analysis is required to detect other chromosomal disorders. However, as a result of its reliability, rapidity and relatively low cost, QF-PCR has been introduced in most laboratories as an adjunct to long-term culture.[7]

Amniocentesis is also used for the diagnosis of single gene disorders. However, culture of the cells and extraction of the DNA often means a significant delay in receiving the result.

Using PCR techniques, amniocentesis can also be used to facilitate the diagnosis of certain congenital infections (see Chapter 13, Fetal infections), such as cytomegalovirus and toxoplasmosis.

Amniocentesis has a role to play in isoimmunized pregnancies. PCR techniques can be used to identify the blood group of the fetus and, later on, the optical density difference at the wavelength 450 nm (AOD450) provides an indirect measurement of the bilirubin. However, in view of the increased likelihood of further sensitization, other non-invasive methods for estimating the degree of fetal anaemia are now in routine use (fetal middle cerebral artery Doppler peak systolic velocity).[8]

Amniocentesis is no longer routinely used to estimate the alpha-fetoprotein and acetylcholinesterase for the diagnosis of neural tube defects. Amniocentesis performed in the presence of raised maternal serum alpha-fetoprotein is associated with a significant increase in fetal loss [A].

## Complications

The fetal loss rate from the procedure varies, but the only randomized, controlled trial of low-risk women reports a rate of 1 per cent [A].[9] Many units report their own miscarriage rate based on their own individual audit data. Operator experience has been shown to be important [B]. Adequate levels of training (>30 procedures per year) are necessary to maintain success and reduce complications. Cell culture may fail in 0.5 per cent of amniocenteses, necessitating a further invasive test.

## Early amniocentesis

Owing to the relative ease of the procedure, amniocentesis at earlier gestations was performed in order to provide women with the advantages of early prenatal diagnosis. Early amniocentesis can be performed from 10 weeks gestation, but the technique has been largely abandoned due to the increased fetal loss rates, fetal talipes and reduced amniocyte culture rate [A].[10] It is therefore recommended that this procedure is not performed.

## CHORIONIC VILLUS SAMPLING AND PLACENTAL BIOPSY

These procedures refer to the sampling of placental tissue. 'Placental biopsy' is the term used when the procedure is performed after the first trimester. Placental tissue can be obtained by catheter, needle aspiration or biopsy forceps. Transabdominal and transcervical methods are both used. The procedure can be performed from 10 weeks gestation. Early diagnosis allows the woman the option of termination before 13 weeks gestation.

### Transabdominal CVS

Using aseptic techniques, an 18–20-gauge needle is inserted through the maternal abdomen to the placental site under direct ultrasound guidance. Placental tissue is aspirated into a syringe attached to the needle. Similarly, a fine biopsy forceps can be used through an outer guide needle. If the placenta is completely posterior and low lying, access via the transabdominal route may not be possible.

### Transcervical CVS

This method is ideal for the posterior low-lying placenta. The cervix and vagina are visualized through a speculum and cleaned with sterile solution. Transabdominal ultrasound is performed to visualize the cervical canal. The needle, catheter or biopsy forceps is then introduced through the cervix towards the placenta under ultrasound guidance, and a sample is taken.

The choice of a transabdominal or transcervical approach should be dependent on operator experience, the placental site and the axis of the uterus. Transcervical CVS is associated with less discomfort than the transabdominal approach, but the potential risk of infection and then procedure-related loss is higher with the transcervical route.

### Indications for CVS

Chorionic villus sampling has the advantage of yielding a large amount of tissue and is therefore the method of choice when large amounts of DNA are required in the diagnosis of monogenic disorders. With the increasing use of early screening tests for Down's syndrome, and with high-resolution ultrasound detecting abnormalities in the first trimester, CVS is more frequently requested.

Although direct chromosome preparations and other rapid cell culture techniques have allowed rapid karyotyping, QF-PCR is now widely used for rapid test reporting.[7] This is advantageous to parents who do not wish to wait for results and who wish to avail themselves of early termination if an affected fetus is found.

## Complications

Fetal loss rate has always been considered to be higher with CVS than with amniocentesis. Second trimester amniocentesis is safer than early amniocentesis or transcervical CVS, and is the procedure of choice in the second trimester [A]. Transabdominal CVS should be regarded the procedure of choice when testing is required before 15 weeks gestation. The procedure-related loss above the individual background risk is considered to be 1 per cent.[11]

Confined placental mosaicisms can occur in about 2 per cent of cases. This presents counselling difficulties and necessitates further invasive testing to obtain fetal cells.

There has been concern regarding the association of CVS and limb defects. This complication appears to be related to the procedure being performed at earlier gestations. Subsequent studies have shown no association when the procedure is performed after 10 weeks.[12]

## FETAL BLOOD SAMPLING

Sampling of blood from the fetal circulation has now been used for a variety of diagnostic purposes. It requires expertise and should be performed by clinicians with extensive experience in all other ultrasound-guided procedures.

## Method

The procedure can be performed from 16 to 18 weeks gestation, onwards. However, before 20 weeks it carries increased risk of cord accidents. A 20-gauge needle is introduced through the maternal abdomen under direct ultrasound control. Fetal blood can be aspirated from either the placental insertion or fetal insertion of the umbilical cord. Cardiac puncture or intrahepatic vessels may also be sampled.

## Indications for fetal blood sampling

Rapid high-quality karyotyping can be obtained with this method within 48–72 hours. This is particularly useful when an abnormality is detected late in the pregnancy.

Fetal blood sampling is also vital in the diagnosis of fetal haematological problems, such as anaemia and thrombocytopenia. It has also been used to assess the acid-base status of the fetus in growth restriction, but non-invasive biophysical methods and Doppler studies are more routinely used.

## Complications

Bleeding at the site of the needle and fetal bradycardia may occur as a result of the procedure, especially in association with the umbilical artery site. The overall procedure-related fetal loss is 1–2 per cent. Introduction of infection may occur and, more importantly, if the mother is carrying human immunodeficiency virus (HIV) or other viruses, transmission to the fetus may occur.[13]

## FETOSCOPY

With improvement in fibreoptic technology, direct *in-utero* visualization of the fetus can now be achieved. This may be useful for identifying small structural abnormalities and facilitating direct organ biopsy, such as skin and muscle biopsy. Organ biopsy can also be performed under ultrasound control. This is only used in specialist centres and >80% of indications is for the treatment of severe twin-to-twin transfusion syndrome.

## COUNSELLING

The decision as to which invasive test is required must be tailored to the individual mother. It is imperative that she is given full details of the range of tests available, the procedures, advantages and disadvantages, and risk of fetal loss or damage. This information should be given well before the procedure is attempted, allowing her to make her decision, and should be non-directive. The discussion should be followed up with written information.[14]

## CONCLUSIONS

These invasive procedures allow the diagnosis and assessment of a large number of abnormalities, so that parents can make choices about the continuation or otherwise of their pregnancies. Early diagnostic procedures provide the advantage of early termination, if sought, but must be balanced against the increased fetal loss, or the possibility of terminating a fetus that may have miscarried spontaneously. Rapid molecular tests have improved the waiting time for results but have limitations. Further developments in the identification of fetal cells in maternal tissues may reduce the necessity of invasive diagnostic tests.

## EBM

- The rate of miscarriage following amniocentesis is approximately 1 per cent [A].
- Early amniocentesis has a higher complication rate than CVS and mid-trimester amniocentesis [A].
- Amniocentesis performed under direct ultrasound visualization is associated with higher rates of success [B].

## KEY POINTS

- Amniocentesis is the most commonly performed prenatal diagnostic procedure.
- Chronic villus sampling should not be performed at less than 10 weeks gestation because of the association of limb defects.
- Most invasive tests other than amniocentesis are generally performed in a tertiary referral centre.
- The specific invasive test should be tailored to the individual woman's circumstances and wishes.
- A team of specialist counsellors should be available for the parents both before and after invasive techniques are performed.

## Published Guidelines

Amniocentesis Consent Advice RCOG: setting Standards to improve women's health. London: RCOG Press, 2006.

Whittle MJ. *Amniocentesis and chorion villus sampling.* RCOG 'Green Top' Guideline No. 8, January. London: RCOG Press, 2009.

## Key References

1. Lamvu G, Kuller JA. Prenatal diagnosis using fetal cells from the maternal circulation. *Obstet Gynaecol Surv* 1997; **52**: 433–7.
2. Daniels G, Finning K, Martin P, Massey E. Non invasive prenatal diagnosis of fetal blood group phenotypes: current practice and future prospects. *Prenatal Diagn* 2009; **29**: 101–7.
3. Lo YM. Noninvasive prenatal detection of fetal chromosome aneuploidies by maternal plasma nucleic acid analysis: a review of the current state of the art. *BJOG* 2009; **116**: 152–7.
4. Steele MW, Breg WR. Chromosome analysis of human amniotic fluid cells. *Lancet* 1966; **1**: 383–5.
5. Bennet MJ. Fetal loss after second trimester amniocentesis in women with raised serum alpha-fetoprotein. *Lancet* 1978; **2**: 987.
6. Thein AT, Abdel-Fattah SA, Kyle PM, Soothhill PW. An assessment of the use of interphase FISH with chromosome specific probes as an alternative to cytogenetics in prenatal diagnosis. *Prenat Diagn* 2000; **4**: 275–80.
7. Cirigliano V, Voglno G, Marongiu A *et al.* Rapid prenatal diagnosis by QF-PCR: evaluation of 30,000 consecutive clinical samples and future applications. *Ann NY Acad Sci* 2006; **1075**: 288–98
8. Oepkes D, Seward PG, Vandenbussche FP *et al.* Doppler ultrasonography versus amniocentesis to predict fetal anaemia. *N Eng J Med* 2006; **355**: 156–64.
9. Tabor A, Philip J, Madsen M *et al.* Randomised controlled trial of genetic amniocentesis in 4606 low-risk women. *Lancet* 1986; **1**: 1287–93.
10. Nicolaides K, Brizot M de L, Patel F, Snijders R. Comparison of chorionic villus sampling and amniocentesis for fetal karyotyping at 10–13 weeks gestation. *Lancet* 1994; **344**: 435–9.
11. Alfirevic Z, Mujezinovic F, Sundberg K. Amniocentesis and chorion villus sampling for prenatal diagnosis. *Cochrane Database Syst Rev* 2009.
12. Froster UG, Jackson L. Limb defects and chorion-villus sampling: results from an international registry, 1992–94. *Lancet* 1996; **347**: 489–94.
13. Workman MR, Philpott-Howard J. Risk of fetal infection from invasive procedures. *J Hosp Infect* 1997; **35**: 169–74.
14. Amniocentesis and Chorion Villus sampling. Policy, standards and protocols. May 2008. NHS Fetal Anomaly Screening Programme.

# 10.4 Management of fetal anomalies

*Michele P Mohajer*

---

## MRCOG standards

### Theoretical skills

- Familiarize yourself with the more common diagnosable fetal anomalies and their prognoses.
- Understand the advantages and disadvantages of surgical and medical termination of pregnancy.
- Understand the pattern of inheritance of the more common genetic disorders.

### Practical skills

- Be able to perform a first trimester termination of pregnancy under indirect supervision.
- Be able to manage early and late (medical) termination of pregnancy.
- Have taken part or observed bereavement counselling with parents who have suffered fetal loss.

## INTRODUCTION

The management of the pregnancy in which an abnormal fetus is identified involves a whole multidisciplinary team of specialists. This team comprises the sonographer, fetal medicine specialist, geneticist, neonatologist and paediatric surgeon, along with the nurse specialists within each specialty. When the diagnosis is made, clear information should be made available to the parents regarding the condition, prognosis and level of disability, should the baby be born alive. This may be very difficult to achieve. Many conditions have such a wide variation in outcome (e.g. Down's syndrome and spina bifida) that accurate prediction may not be possible. When given an adverse prenatal diagnosis, parents are deeply shocked and experience acute grief. They may not be able to take in the information given to them. Written information, contact numbers and support groups are important, but parents may have great difficulty reaching a decision, especially one that results in the termination of the pregnancy. Therefore, management includes not only the practical aspect of the specific disorder, but also the psychological support for the parents and family involved in the pregnancy.

## PRACTICAL MANAGEMENT

### Termination of pregnancy

When parents are told of a fetal abnormality, they must make decisions, the most important being whether to continue or terminate the pregnancy. The response to diagnosis will be tempered by the options available to the parents, including *in-utero* treatment, postnatal treatment or termination. If the condition is lethal, the decision to terminate may be easier, but more often than not, the condition carries a risk of physical or mental impairment, which is difficult to quantify. Once a serious abnormality has been diagnosed, evidence shows that the parents will terminate the pregnancy in 80–90 per cent of cases.[1]

Conditions that are considered lethal include:

- anencephaly
- bilateral renal agenesis
- lethal skeletal dysplasias
- some severe complex cardiac defects
- triploidy
- trisomy 18, 13, 15.

Other conditions which are not lethal, but are well documented as being associated with long-term handicap, include:

- spina bifida
- trisomy 21 and other chromosomal abnormalities
- cardiovascular abnormalities
- muscular dystrophies
- phocomelia.

If the decision to terminate is reached, the methods available and associated risks must be discussed with the parents.

# METHODS OF TERMINATION

## Surgical termination

Surgical termination may be performed by vacuum aspiration or dilatation and evacuation. Vacuum aspiration or suction curettage is the method used until the end of the first trimester. Dilatation of the cervix prior to surgery is achieved by passing graduated metal dilatators or inserting vaginal prostaglandin preparations. Abortion is then performed by the use of a Perspex suction tube connected to vacuum apparatus. The inherent risk associated with abortion relates to the use of general anaesthesia and the invasive nature of the procedure – with complications of haemorrhage, uterine perforation and infection. The incidence of haemorrhage is 1.5/1000, the incidence of uterine perforation is 1–4/1000 and of cervical trauma <1 per cent. Post-abortion infection occurs in up to 10 per cent of cases and is significantly reduced if prophylactic antibiotics are given [B]. Suction curettage has been shown to produce lower risks of these complications than sharp curettage.[2] Complications are lessened the earlier the gestation. Couples should also be informed of the risk of failed abortion, which occurs in 2.3/1000 surgical terminations.

Dilatation and evacuation is performed in some areas up until 20 weeks gestation. Mechanical dilatation of the cervix to 14 mm is performed, and fetal parts are extracted with the use of appropriate instruments. This may be carried out under ultrasound control. Cervical dilatation may be complicated by cervical tears, uterine perforation and the creation of false passages. The use of cervical priming agents such as mifepristone, misoprostol and gemeprost has improved the safety of the procedure [B].[3] It is a very distressing procedure, but safe and effective when undertaken by specialist practitioners with a sufficiently large caseload [A]. However, it is not widely available. It also prevents a full post-mortem examination of the fetus being carried out in order to confirm any ultrasound diagnosis. Consideration should be given to karyotyping the fetus by sending placental tissue for cytogenetic analysis (with informed consent).

## Medical termination

Medical termination of pregnancy has been revolutionized by the introduction of prostaglandins and the antiprogesterone mifepristone.

Gestations of 9 weeks (63 days) or less can be successfully terminated with mifepristone 600 mg, followed 48 hours later by a prostaglandin (gemeprost or misoprostol). Less than 0.5 per cent will fail to respond to this regimen,[4] which should be the method of choice at these gestations [A]. However, the diagnosis of fetal abnormality is extremely rare by 9 weeks gestation and so medical termination is usually performed in the second trimester. Medical termination has the additional advantage of allowing the opportunity for a post-mortem examination. Pre-treatment with mifepristone (200 mg) sensitizes the myometrium to prostaglandin agents and so reduces the induction–abortion interval [B]. Misoprostol is the prostaglandin of choice as it requires specific conditions for storage and transfer. The risk of failure to terminate the pregnancy is 6/1000. The standard regimen is: mifepristone 200 mg orally, followed 36–48 hours later by misoprostol 800 µg vaginally, then misoprostol 400 µg orally to a maximum of four oral doses. Consideration should be given to karyotyping the fetus by sending placental tissue for cytogenetic analysis (with informed consent).

## Third trimester termination and intrauterine fetocide

Since 1990, termination of pregnancy after 24 weeks has become legal if there is a lethal abnormality or sufficient evidence that the infant will be born with serious mental or physical disability.[5] This is an extremely distressing situation to all involved, including the parents, obstetricians and midwives. The safety of medical termination has made late termination much safer, but the law states that the fetus must not be born alive. This requires intrauterine fetocide – which is achieved by fetal intracardiac injection of potassium chloride (KCl) via a 20-gauge trans-abdominal needle under ultrasound control. This procedure should be performed by an operator experienced in invasive fetal procedures. Fetal sedation may be necessary prior to the fetocide. This is achieved by the administration of diazepam or pethidine into the fetal circulation. An ultrasound should be performed 1 hour after the injection of KCl to ensure cessation of fetal heart pulsation.

The assessment of the level of disability is an extremely difficult area. Although the outcome of some abnormalities is well documented, an accurate prognosis of many prenatally detected anomalies is not possible. Advice from genetic specialists, counsellors and support groups may be sought, but ultimately the decision to terminate the pregnancy will rest with the parents. Consideration should be given to karyotyping the fetus by sending a fetal blood sample (and banking DNA) for cytogenetic analysis (with informed consent).

## The post-mortem examination

Parents may find the prospect of a post-mortem examination of their baby very distressing, but it is a vital part of the management. Although high-quality ultrasound provides an accurate diagnosis of major fetal pathology, post-mortem provides more detail, identifies abnormalities that permit a more specific diagnosis and modifies genetic counselling. Important diagnostic refinements are identified in up to 40 per cent of cases.[6]

The issue of post-mortem has become further complicated by the legal requirement of consent. Consent is now required for the post-mortem examination of fetuses at all gestations and, additionally, if tissues or organs are retained for later study or research. If parents do not consent to a post-mortem, it is important to request photographs, x-rays and a sample of tissue (skin or placenta) for cytogenetic studies, which may provide additional information.

## THE CONTINUING PREGNANCY

The pregnancy may continue for many reasons. For example, the condition may be amenable to postnatal treatment. This particularly applies to structural malformations that can be surgically corrected, such as:

- gastroschisis
- exomphalos
- diaphragmatic hernia
- duodenal atresia
- some cardiac defects (Fallot's tetralogy, atrial septal defect, ventricular septal defect, transposition of the great vessels)
- posterior urethral valves
- cleft lip.

It is important that parents receive full information regarding the treatment and long-term outcome of the condition; this is preferably provided by the surgeon performing the procedure. Certain conditions, such as gastroschisis, will require continued fetal surveillance throughout pregnancy as there may be growth problems or loops of bowel may become obstructed. Most pregnancies will also require continued surveillance for psychological support. Even though parents have been given optimistic expectations of the outcome, they will be anxious throughout, and need constant reassurance from all members of the team. If paediatric surgical teams are not within the hospital, parents may have to travel to a main centre to receive both prenatal counselling and delivery if their neonatal unit is unable to cope with their situation.

Certain fetal conditions are amenable to intrauterine therapy.

Hydrops fetalis is discussed in Chapter 17, Fetal hydrops. Cases secondary to fetal anaemia may respond to intrauterine fetal blood transfusion. Fetal tachydysrhythmias may also result in fetal hydrops. Maternal administration of antidysrhythmic drugs (digoxin, flecainide, amiodarone) is effective in converting the fetal rate to sinus rhythm and also reversing the hydrops.[7]

If fluid is in a particular cavity, for example a pleural effusion, its presence may compromise normal lung development. Pleural drainage may be performed, as both a diagnostic and a therapeutic procedure. If the fluid accumulates, a pleuro-amniotic shunt can be inserted. This shunt procedure can be applied to other conditions. In the case of posterior urethral valves, outflow obstruction can be so severe as to cause bilateral hydronephrosis and irreversible renal damage. A vesico-amniotic shunt can be inserted into the fetal bladder and so bypass the urethral obstruction.

Sophisticated techniques to perform intrauterine surgery have been developed. If a diaphragmatic hernia is present early in pregnancy, the presence of a mass in the fetal chest compromises fetal lung development such that the infants often die of pulmonary hypoplasia. *In-utero* repair of the diaphragmatic defect has been performed with some success, but only in extremely specialized units, and not without significant maternal morbidity.[8]

Parents may elect to proceed with the pregnancy because there is not enough certainty or evidence that the malformation will result in a significant degree of mental or physical disability. This decision will vary among individuals and depending on their own particular circumstances, for example an infertile couple with a long-awaited pregnancy may accept the risk of potential handicap more than a multigravid mother for whom the risk of a handicapped child may compromise the well-being of her existing family.

Examples of such abnormalities include:

- Dandy–Walker malformation
- agenesis of the corpus callosum
- distal limb abnormalities
- some cardiac defects.

Finally, parents may not want termination, even if the condition has 100 per cent mortality, because of religious or moral beliefs. These wishes must be respected.

The management of these continuing pregnancies requires skilled, personalized care. There are few published data that consider the psychological impact of continuing the pregnancy with a prenatally diagnosed abnormality. There are reasons to hypothesize that women who elect to continue a pregnancy may experience a better psychological outcome than women who terminate: such women are thought to be spared the guilt associated with decision-making. However, some reports suggest that these women would seek early prenatal diagnosis in a subsequent pregnancy. Management of continuing pregnancies includes communication between hospital and community health workers, continuity of care with the same personnel, adequate time and repeated counselling (outside routine clinic hours), written information and contacts with support groups.[9] Serial ultrasound scans may be requested to provide reassurance that the baby is still alive and growing.

The management of the pregnancy with a malformation requires additional considerations as well as emotional support. Parents need to be prepared for:

- how, where and when their baby will be delivered,
- what their baby will look like,
- what will happen to their baby after delivery.

There may also be practical difficulties if delivery is to take place in a tertiary centre. The costs of transport, childcare and subsistence must be considered.

Discussion needs to occur with other healthcare professions as to the timing and appropriate place of delivery of the fetus.

## PLAN FOR THE FUTURE

Once the pregnancy is over, carefully planned follow up is an essential part of the management. In the case of termination or death of the infant, time for grieving must be allowed. Grief reactions will vary among individuals depending on different circumstances. Some couples want intensive counselling and contact with the medical team, whereas others want time away from what has become an emotionally painful environment. Post-mortem results may provide additional information as to the precise diagnosis. This could influence the management of a subsequent pregnancy and the choice of a prenatal test.

Referral to a genetic specialist may be required in order to assess the risk of recurrence and possibly to investigate other family members. Follow up with the paediatric or neonatal team involved is an important part of the bereavement counselling.

Parents will require information on the availability of early, reliable prenatal diagnosis if another pregnancy is contemplated.

Couples may require more than one bereavement counselling session, either because the results are incomplete or because they wish it. Sensitivity to the individual's needs is essential in this situation.

Finally, a letter summarizing the discussion should be sent to the parents. This provides documentation and also allows the information to be assimilated at a later date, away from the hospital environment.

### EBM

- Termination of pregnancy is more likely if the diagnosis is made earlier in gestation [C].
- The risks of termination of pregnancy are reduced if abortion is performed at earlier gestations [B].
- Psychological stress is high after termination, with 40 per cent of women showing symptoms of psychiatric morbidity [B].

### KEY POINTS

- Parents must have as much access to information as possible before making a choice.
- Referral to a tertiary centre may be necessary for further investigation or treatment.
- Psychological morbidity is high following termination for fetal abnormality using either surgical or medical methods.
- Whether or not they continue the pregnancy, the parents will need long-term support from both hospital specialists and the community.

## Published Guidelines

Fetal vesico-amniotic shunt for lower urinary tract outflow obstruction. NICE interventional procedure guidance 202. December 2006.

Penney G. *The Care of Women Requesting Induced Abortion.* Evidence-Based Clinical Guidelines No. 7. London: RCOG Press, 2004.

## Key References

1. Royal College of Obstetricians and Gynaecologists. *Ultrasound Screening for Fetal Abnormalities.* Report of the RCOG Working Party. London: RCOG Press, 1997: 2–3.
2. Edelman DA, Brener WE, Berger GS. The effectiveness and complications of abortion by dilatation and vacuum aspiration versus dilatation and rigid metal curettage. *Am J Obstet Gynecol* 1974; **119**: 473–80.
3. Schulz KF, Grimes DA, Cates W. Measures to prevent cervical injury during suction curettage abortion. *Lancet* 1983; **i**: 1182–4.
4. UK Multicentre Trial. The efficacy and tolerance of mifepristone and prostaglandin in first trimester termination of pregnancy. *Br J Obstet Gynaecol* 1990; **97**: 480–6.
5. Gevers S. Third trimester abortion for fetal abnormality. *Bioethics* 1999; **13**: 306–13.
6. Clayton-Smith J, Farndon PA, McKeown C, Donnai D. Examination of fetuses after induced abortion for fetal abnormality. *BMJ* 1990; **300**: 295–7.
7. van Engelen AD, Weijtens O, Brenner J *et al.* Management outcome and follow-up of fetal tachycardia. *J Am Coll Cardiol* 1994; **24**: 1371–5.
8. Flake AW. Fetal surgery for congenital diaphragmatic hernia. *Semin Paediatr Surg* 1996; **5**: 266–74.
9. Chitty LS, Barnes CA, Berry C. Continuing with pregnancy after a diagnosis of lethal abnormality: experience of five couples and recommendations for management. *BMJ* 1996; **313**: 478–80.

# Previous history of fetal loss

*Arri Coomarasamy*

---

## INTRODUCTION

Some 3.2 million stillbirths occur worldwide every year, with 98 per cent of these in the developing world.[1] The stillbirth rate is approximately 5 per 1000 deliveries in the developed world, and 25/1000 in the developing world, rising to 32/1000 in Sub-Saharan Africa and South Asia.[1] Qualitative studies show that women who have experienced a previous pregnancy loss have omnipresent worry during a subsequent pregnancy.[2] Their pregnancies are characterized by a see-saw course of varying emotions, vigilance, seeking reassurance and physical symptoms, such as headaches. Moreover, many women with a history of pregnancy loss have increased risks for future pregnancy loss and other obstetric complications. Therefore, expert support is often required and this should be provided by staff who have the right attitude, experience, knowledge and skills.

## DEFINITIONS

A fetal loss up to 24 completed weeks of gestation is defined as a miscarriage. A late fetal loss is defined as *in utero* death delivering between $22^{+0}$ to $23^{+6}$.[3] A stillbirth is defined as a baby delivering with no signs of life after 24 completed weeks of pregnancy. For the purposes of this chapter, we have grouped late fetal losses and stillbirths. It is noteworthy (particularly when international comparisons are being made) that the World Health Organization (WHO) and Canada use 22 weeks gestation, and Australia uses 20 weeks gestation as thresholds for defining stillbirths.

Stillbirth rate is the number of stillbirths per 1000 total births, which incorporates live births and still births. In the United Kingdom, the stillbirth rate was 5.2 per 1000 total births in 2007.[3] This represents a marginal improvement compared to the previous years.

## CAUSES AND ASSOCIATIONS

There are several factors associated with fetal loss (Table 11.1). Some of these have a clear causal link (for example, an abruption or a cord event), while others may contribute indirectly to fetal loss (for example, obesity). Some losses may be associated with multiple aetiologies; for example, a fetal loss could be directly linked to an abruption, but the woman may have risk factors, such as anti-phospholipid positivity and pre-eclampsia. Thus even when there appears to be an obvious cause for a fetal loss, it is important to investigate comprehensively, guided by protocols or guidelines. The importance of comprehensive investigations lies in the fact that they are needed to provide an accurate risk prediction and plan risk modification. Many of the risk factors may be modifiable or treatable, for example, maternal obesity, smoking, anti-phospholipid syndrome and pre-eclampsia. Knowledge of these risk factors will, therefore, help tailor the management pre-conceptually and during pregnancy.

In an effort to classify the causes and risk factors for stillbirths, numerous classification systems have emerged. Six of the contemporary internationally accepted systems (Amended Aberdeen, Extended Wigglesworth; PSANZ-PDC, ReCoDe, Tulip and CODAC) were recently evaluated for interobserver agreement and proportion of unexplained stillbirths.[4] Aberdeen and Wigglesworth showed poor agreement with kappas of 0.35 and 0.25, respectively, with Tulip performing the best with a kappa of 0.74. Wigglesworth and Aberdeen also resulted in a high proportion of unexplained stillbirths, with CODAC and Tulip giving the lowest. Given these findings,

**Table 11.1** Risk factors for stillbirth: management principles

| Risk factor | Prevalence | Estimated rate of stillbirth | Risks | Specific management approaches |
|---|---|---|---|---|
| Unselected population | – | 5.2/1000 | – | – |
| **Maternal age** | | | | |
| <20 years | 6.5% | 5.6/1000 | Preterm birth<br>Fetal growth restriction<br>Pre-eclampsia | Support |
| >40 years | 3.6% | 7.7/1000 | Diabetes<br>Chromosomal abnormalities<br>Preterm birth<br>Pre-eclampsia<br>Growth restriction<br>Multiple pregnancies | Consider CVS or amniocentesis |
| **Hypertensive disorder** | | | | |
| Chronic hypertension | 6–10% | 6–25/1000 | | Aspirin (75 mg/day) from 12 to 36 weeks; Antihypertensives (see Chapter 6.1) |
| Mild pregnancy-induced hypertension | 5.8–7.7% | 9–51/1000 | | Surveillance |
| Severe pregnancy-induced hypertension | 1.3–3.3% | 12–29/1000 | | Antihypertensives (see Chapter 7.6) |
| **Diabetes** | | | | |
| Treated with diet | 2.5–5% | 6–10/1000 | Pre-eclampsia<br>Thromboembolic disease<br>Macrosomia<br>Fetal growth restriction | Good glycaemic control (see Chapter 6.2) |
| Treated with insulin | 2.4% | 6–35/1000 | | |
| SLE | <1% | 40–150/1000 | Superimposed PET<br>Abruption<br>FGR<br>Renal dysfunction<br>Thromboembolic events<br>(Risks increase if lupus positive) | Surveillance<br>Tight control of SLE<br>Consider heparin and aspirin<br>See Chapter 6.7 |
| Renal disease | <1% | 15–200/1000 | PET<br>FGR | See Chapter 6.6 |
| Thyroid disorders | 0.2–2% | 12–20/1000 | Preterm birth<br>Neurodevelopmental problems in offspring of hypothyroid mothers | See Chapter 6.4 |
| Thrombophilia | 1–5% | 18–40/1000 | Thromboembolic disease<br>PET<br>Abruption | Consider aspirin ± heparin (see Chapter 6.7) |
| Cholestasis of pregnancy | <0.1% | 12–30/1000 | Sudden unexpected fetal deaths | |
| Smoking >10 cigarettes | 20–30% | 10–15/1000 | Preterm birth<br>Fetal growth restriction<br>Cognitive impairment in offspring | Smoking cessation programmes (see Chapter 6.13) |

*(continued)*

**Table 11.1** (continued)

| Risk factor | Prevalence | Estimated rate of stillbirth | Risks | Specific management approaches |
|---|---|---|---|---|
| **Obesity (pre-pregnancy)** | | | | |
| BMI 25–29.9 kg/m² | 21% | 12–15/1000 | | |
| BMI >30 | 20% | 20/1000 | Diabetes<br>Pre-eclampsia<br>Thromboembolic disease<br>Macrosomia<br>Fetal growth restriction | Weight reduction strategies |
| Previous growth-restricted infant | 5–10% | 12–30/1000 | FGR<br>PET | See Chapter 15 |
| Previous stillbirth | 0.5–1.0% | 9–20/1000 | | Consider induction of labour at 38–39 weeks |
| **Multiple gestation** | | | | |
| Twins | 3% | 12/1000 | Preterm birth<br>Fetal growth restriction<br>Ante-partum haemorrhage<br>Congenital abnormalities<br>Twin to twin infusion (if mono-chorionic twins)<br>Cerebral palsy | See Chapter 12 |
| Triplets | 0.1% | 15–50/1000 | | Consider fetal reduction |
| **Ethnicity (UK HES data)** | | | | |
| White | 80% | 3.9/1000 | | |
| Black | 5.3% | 10.7/1000 | Pre-eclampsia<br>Diabetes<br>Sickle cell disease | Improve access to healthcare |
| Asian | 10.1% | 7.8/1000 | Diabetes | |
| Chinese | 0.6% | 5.1/1000 | | |
| **Deprivation status** | | | | |
| Least deprived quintile | 16% | 3.6/1000 | | |
| Most deprived quintile | 28% | 6.5/1000 | | Improve access to healthcare |
| True umbilical knots | 1% | 27/1000 | | |

- Data from Fretts et al.[5] and CEMACH 2009,[3] ONS and HES.

there is a need to reconsider the continued use of the well-established Wigglesworth and Aberdeen classification systems in the UK. In January 2008, a new perinatal death notification (PND) form, including a new classification of cause of death, was introduced by CEMACH.[3] However, it would be several years before the utility of this tool becomes fully apparent.

In the most recent CEMACH report (June 2009, reporting on perinatal deaths in 2007[3]), 76 per cent of stillbirths were categorized as 'unexplained' using the Wigglesworth classification system (Figure 11.1). Aberdeen obstetric classification was then applied to these 'unexplained' stillbirths, but 74 per cent of the original 76 per cent remained still unexplained. The most common identifiable cause of stillbirths was congenital malformations (8.2 per cent), followed by death from intrapartum events (6.4 per cent).

In the recent CEMACH report, the main factors associated with stillbirths and neonatal deaths are extremes of maternal age, obesity, social deprivation and ethnicity.[3] Mothers aged less than 20 and above 40 years had the highest rates of stillbirth, neonatal and perinatal deaths. Previous CEMACH reports showed a BMI over 30 was associated with stillbirths and neonatal deaths. The stillbirth rate of women in the most deprived quintile was 1.8 times higher than in the least deprived quintile. In comparison to women of White ethnicity, women of Black ethnicity and Asian ethnicity had approximately twice the rate of stillbirths and neonatal deaths.

Antenatal complications: fetal

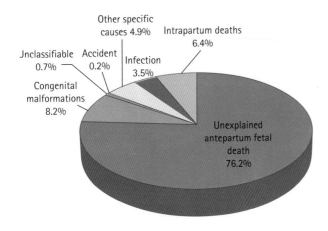

Other specific
causes 4.9%    Intrapartum deaths
6.4%

Unclassifiable   Accident
0.7%             0.2%    Infection
                         3.5%

Congenital
malformations
8.2%

Unexplained
antepartum fetal
death
76.2%

**Figure 11.1** Causes of stillbirths in the United Kingdom in 2007. *Source*: CEMACH, Perinatal Mortality 2007.[3]

One important contributory factor to stillbirths is fetal growth restriction – 38 per cent of unexplained stillbirths have a birth weight below the tenth centile for gestation, and a quarter of them below the third centile.[3]

The risk factors for stillbirth, with their prevalence,[3,5] estimated risk of stillbirth,[3,5] appropriate investigations, and possible approaches to risk modifications or treatment are given in Table 11.1. It is important to identify and focus on specific risk factors or causes of stillbirth, as evidence shows that the greatest reductions in stillbirth in the past have occurred with targeted strategies; for example, since the introduction of Rhesus (Rh) immune prophylaxis, there has been a 95 per cent reduction in stillbirths from Rh isoimmunization.

# MANAGEMENT

The timing of pregnancy and the likelihood of recurrence of pregnancy loss are the primary concerns for couples who plan to have another pregnancy. They may yearn for a baby, but fear the pain of a pregnancy loss. Studies suggest fathers often want to have a baby as soon as possible, but mothers wish to wait longer until they feel physically or emotionally ready.[6,7]

SANDS Guidelines for Professionals[8] suggest the following approach in helping couples planning to have a baby after a previous pregnancy loss:

- Offer parents time to discuss their ideas, concerns, expectations and feelings, together as a couple and individually, to help reach a decision about timing of pregnancy.
- Offer parents the opportunity to discuss the specific individualized risks for the mother and baby in a future pregnancy.
- Reassure parents that there is no specific right time for them to try for a baby.
- Encourage the parents to look after and look out for each other physically and emotionally, particularly focusing on ways of reducing their anxiety (e.g. with the use of relaxation techniques).

- Offer preconception advice to reduce or manage risks, e.g. cessation of smoking and weight reduction.
- Offer and organize referral to other specialists as appropriate, e.g. geneticists and counsellors.
- Acknowledge that a future pregnancy is likely to be stressful, but emphasize that there will be support to ensure the couple's and baby's health.

## Investigations and risk assessment

The risk assessment will entail careful review of the history, previous notes and investigation results, as well as arranging of any necessary additional investigations. It may be necessary to write to another hospital to obtain records; if so, it is worth asking for a copy of the notes and actual investigation reports rather than a summary letter. Many of the following investigations would generally have been performed after a stillbirth:

- Post-mortem (full or limited); if not, x-ray or magnetic resonance imaging (MRI) of the stillborn baby. Post-mortem should have ideally been performed by a pathologist with expertise in perinatal pathology.
- Chromosomal analysis of the stillborn baby.
- Infection screening: syphilis (VDRL), human parvovirus B19, listeria, cytomegalovirus (CMV), toxoplasmosis, rubella and vaginal swab (for GBS). Malaria testing if the woman is from a malaria risk area. Although GBS, *Ureoplasma urealyticum* and *Mycoplasma hominis* have been associated with stillbirth,[9] colonization with these pathogens is so common that a definite association with stillbirth has not been firmly established.
- Testing for maternal diabetes.
- Testing for thrombophilias:
  - acquired: Lupus anticoagulant and anticardiolipin antibodies (IgG and IgM).
  - congenital: Factor V Leiden (activated protein C resistance), antithrombin III, protein C and protein S.
- HbA1C and random blood glucose.
- Full blood count, blood group and antibody screen, Kleihauer.
- Liver function tests and bile acids.
- Thyroid function tests and antithyroid antibodies: The presence of antithyroid antibodies (particularly thyroid peroxidase antibodies), regardless of TSH or free T4 levels, is associated with miscarriages and preterm births.

Once a cause and/or associated risk factors have been established, the care provider should attempt to estimate the risk of adverse obstetric outcomes, particularly stillbirth, for the specific woman. Given all the various factors that influence outcomes, this is easier said than done; interactive prediction software that takes into account the interdependence of various risk factors may be helpful in the future. For now, the information in Table 11.1 can be used in estimating the stillbirth risk for a specific woman.

For many couples with a previous pregnancy loss, risk identification, future risk estimation, and indeed future pregnancy management plans may have been worked out in the follow-up consultation(s) after their previous loss. Generally, such plans should be adhered to, unless there are clear reasons to deviate. If changes are necessary, it is important to explain to the couple the need for the changes.

## SPECIFIC MANAGEMENT APPROACHES

The last column of Table 11.1 provides specific measures that can be taken if risk factors are identified. Box 11.1

### Box 11.1   Summary of evidence for interventions to prevent still births

| Behavioural and nutritional interventions before and during pregnancy | Prevention and treatment of medical disorders and infections during pregnancy | Screening and monitoring during pregnancy and labour | Intrapartum care interventions |
|---|---|---|---|
| Prevention of female genital mutilation (FGM) and care for woman with FGM | Calcium supplementation to prevent pregnancy-induced hypertension | Pregnancy risk screening | Instrumental delivery (vacuum vs. forceps) |
| Promotion of birth spacing | Anti-hypertensives in pregnancy | Fetal movement counting for high-risk pregnancies | Emergency obstetric care packages, including caesarean section** |
| Reduction of exposure to indoor air pollution | Anti-platelet agents in high-risk pregnancies | Ultrasound scanning | Elective induction of labour for post-term pregnancies |
| Smoking cessation during pregnancy** | Anti-oxidants in pregnancy | Umbilical artery Doppler velocimetry for high-risk pregnancies | Drugs for cervical ripening and induction of labour |
| Reduction of exposure to smokeless tobacco | Heparin for certain maternal conditions including clotting disorders | Pelvimetry | Planned caesarean section for breech deliveries*/** |
| Antenatal care (ANC) packages | Management of intrahepatic cholestasis during pregnancy | Detection and management of maternal diabetes mellitus during pregnancy | Maternal hyperoxygenation |
| Peri-conceptional folic acid supplementation** | Plasma exchange during high risk pregnancies | Antepartum fetal heart rate monitoring with cardiotocography (non-stress test and contraction stress test) | Amnioinfusion during labour |
| Routine iron (iron-folate) supplementation** | Cervical cerclage for high-risk pregnancy | Fetal biophysical profile scoring during pregnancy | Magnesium sulphate for pre-eclampsia/ eclampsia and preterm labour |
| Vitamin A/β-carotene supplementation during pregnancy | Anti-helminthic treatment** | Vibroacoustic stimulation | |
| Multiple micronutrient supplementation during pregnancy | Syphilis screening and treatment** | Amniotic fluid volume assessment | |
| Antenatal magnesium supplementation in deficient populations | Antibiotics for maternal reproductive tract and bladder infections | Home vs. hospital bed rest and monitoring for high-risk pregnancies | |
| Balanced protein-energy supplementation during pregnancy | Antibiotics for PROM/PPROM | In-hospital fetal surveillance units | |
| | Antimalarials in malaria-endemic areas** | Partograph use | |
| | Insecticide treated bed nets (ITNs) during pregnancy** | Intrapartum cardiotocography with or without pulse oximetry | |
| | PMTCT for HIV** | | |
| | Periodontal care during pregnancy | | |

☐ Uncertain evidence of impact: further research required before including in programmes

▨ Some evidence of impact: can include in programmes but further research recommended

▮ Interventions of benefit recommended for inclusion and scaling up in programmes

*Recommended only where access to referral-level care is good.

**Clear benefit for maternal and/or neonatal health.

● Reproduced with permission from Ref. 10.

● PMTCT: Preventing mother-to-child transmission.

Antenatal complications: fetal

provides a comprehensive list of interventions[10] that have been studied for stillbirth prevention, taking a developing world perspective, where 98 per cent of stillbirths occur.

Timely diagnosis and management of growth restriction is an important aspect of care in those with previous fetal losses. Ultrasound should be considered in these patients. A customized growth chart is likely to be more accurate in identifying a truly growth restricted fetus, as opposed to a constitutionally small fetus.

By 38–39 weeks, many couples will be extremely anxious, and would often want labour induced. The risk of respiratory distress syndrome (albeit small) and risks of induction (e.g. abnormal CTG, uterine hyperstimulation and instrumental deliveries) will need to be balanced against continuation of pregnancy which carries a small risk of stillbirth and possible adverse effect on the couple's psychological well-being. Many practitioners and parents would consider induction of labour at 38–39 weeks a reasonable course of action.

---

- – planned caesarean section for breech [A]
- – fetal movement monitoring in high risk pregnancies [B]
- – intrapartum cardiotocography [C]
- – appropriate management of obstetric cholestasis [D]
- – anti-helminthic [A] and anti-malarial treatment [A]
- – insecticide-treated bednets (ITNs) during pregnancy to reduce risk of malaria. [A]
- Induction of labour at 38–39 weeks is preferred by many couples with a past history of stillbirth, and is endorsed by most obstetricians. [E]

---

## KEY POINTS

- Stillbirth rate in the United Kingdom is 5.2/1000.
- Ninety-eight per cent of all stillbirths occur in the developing world.
- Most stillbirths remain unexplained, by the commonly used Wigglesworth or Aberdeen classifications. The most common identifiable cause of stillbirths is congenital malformation.
- Risk factors for stillbirths include: extremes of maternal age, obesity, social depravation, non-White ethnicity, smoking, growth restriction, hypertensive disorders, diabetes, systemic lupus erythematosus (SLE), renal disease, thrombophilia and multiple pregnancies.
- Timing of pregnancy and likelihood of another pregnancy loss are major issues to couples with previous fetal loss; follow SANDS guidelines to counsel such couples. [E]
- Risk evaluation should include a careful review of past history, notes and investigation results, and assessment for current risk factors (e.g. smoking and BMI). [E]
- In future pregnancies, fetal growth evaluation, ideally using a customized growth chart reference, is essential. [C]
- A systematic review has shown the following interventions to have some or clear evidence of benefit in reducing stillbirths:
  - – antiplatelet agents in high-risk pregnancies [A]
  - – heparin for antiphospholipid antibodies [A]
  - – umbilical artery Doppler in high risk pregnancies [A]

## Key References

1. Stanton C, Lawn JE, Rahman H *et al.* Stillbirth rates: delivering estimates in 190 countries. *Lancet* 2006; **367**: 1487–94.
2. Cote-Arsenault D, Donato KL, Earl SS. Watching and worrying: early pregnancy after loss experiences. *MCN Am J Matern Child Nurs* 2006; **31**: 356–63.
3. Confidential Enquiry into Maternal and Child Health (CEMACH). *Perinatal Mortality 2007: United Kingdom.* London: CEMACH, 2009.
4. Flenady V, Froen JF, Pinar H *et al.* An evaluation of classification systems for stillbirth. *BMC Pregnancy Childbirth* 2009; **9**: 24.
5. Fretts RC. Etiology and prevention of stillbirth. *Am J Obstet Gynecol* 2005; **193**: 1923–35.
6. Turton P, Badenhorst W, Hughes P *et al.* Psychological impact of stillbirth on fathers in the subsequent pregnancy and puerperium. *Br J Psychiatry* 2006; **188**: 165–72.
7. Swanson KM, Karmali ZA, Powell SH, Pulvermakher F. Miscarriage effects on couples' interpersonal and sexual relationships during the first year after loss: women's perceptions. *Psychosom Med* 2003; **65**: 902–10.
8. Schott J, Henley A, Kohner N. *Pregnancy Loss and the Death of a Baby: Guidelines for Professionals*, 3rd edn. Shepperton: Bosun Press, 2007 (SANDS: Stillbirth and neonatal death charity).
9. Gibbs RS. The origins of stillbirth: infectious diseases. *Semin Perinatol* 2002; **26**: 75–8.
10. Bhutta ZA, Darmstadt GL, Haws RA *et al.* Delivering interventions to reduce the global burden of stillbirths: improving service supply and community demand. *BMC Pregnancy Childbirth* 2009; **9** (Suppl. 1): S7.

# Multiple pregnancy

*Bill Martin*

## MRCOG standards

### Theoretical skills

- Understand the different types of twins and their risks.
- Understand the potential problems of multiple pregnancies and the general principles of management.

### Practical skills

- Be able to discuss with a patient the differences between monochorionic and dichorionic placentation.
- Be able to discuss the general complications of multiple pregnancies.
- Be able to discuss the increased perinatal risk of multiple pregnancies.

## INTRODUCTION

Dizygous pregnancy rates vary with maternal age, race, nutrition and geography. The highest rates are reported in sub-Saharan Africa (Nigeria) and the lowest in the Far East (Japan). Monozygous twinning rates are, however, fairly constant, at 3–5/1000 births, although there is some anecdotal evidence that the incidence is also increasing. Multiple pregnancies have increased in the UK from 11.1/1000 maternities in 1988 to 15.3/1000 maternities in 2007, with triplets and higher order multiples increasing almost three-fold.[1] This increase is largely due to assisted conception techniques, which result in multiple rates of up to 30 per cent. Though predominantly dizygotic, pregnancies which result from assisted conception techniques are at greater risk of monozygotic division than those spontaneously conceived. Both the British Fertility Society and the Human Fertilisation and Embryology Authority suggest transferring a maximum of two embryos in each treatment cycle, without compromising pregnancy success.

## MATERNAL RISKS

The mother is at increased risk for several pregnancy complications, including miscarriage, hyperemesis gravidarum, premature labour and delivery, anaemia, pre-eclampsia, antepartum and postpartum haemorrhage, polyhydramnios, operative delivery and increased stay in hospital. Women who have twins are also at increased risk of having problems with breastfeeding and developing postnatal depression.

## FETAL RISKS

Multiple pregnancies are associated with an increase in fetal and neonatal mortality compared with singleton pregnancies. The perinatal morbidity and mortality increases with increasing order of multiple pregnancy. The majority of perinatal deaths are associated with preterm birth and intrauterine growth restriction (discussed further below). Perinatal mortality rates are 27.2 and 81.8 per 1000 total births for twins, triplets and higher order multiple births respectively.[2] Monochorionic (MC) twins have an increased loss rate (14.2 per cent) compared with dichorionic (DC) twins (2.6 per cent), mainly due to losses before 24 weeks. The differential loss rate is mainly the result of twin–twin transfusion syndrome (TTTS).[3]

### Preterm labour

Twins are five times more likely to be born preterm compared with singletons, and delivery before 32 weeks is approximately twice as common in monochorionic compared with dichorionic twins.[4] Over 25 per cent of triplets deliver prior to 32 weeks.

### Intrauterine growth restriction

Growth restriction of one or more of the fetuses in a multiple pregnancy is very common. The aetiology is not well understood, but occurs in 9.1 per cent of all twins and 9.9 per cent of MC twins.[5] The incidence is similar for MC and DC twins when twin–twin transfusion syndrome is excluded. Twin birth weight discordance has been demonstrated to be a risk factor for preterm birth and adverse perinatal outcome. This effect was found particularly with discordances >40 per cent before 32 weeks gestation and was usually attributable to fetal growth restriction, most often in the second twin.[6] The presence of discordant growth in twins presents difficulties in management more so in MC compared with DC due to the presence of vascular anastomoses in the former.

## Single fetal death

This may occur either early in gestation or later as the pregnancy progresses. Fetal death after 24 weeks gestation is relatively uncommon, occurring in 1.1 and 3.6 per cent of dichorionic diamniotic (DC/DA) and monochorionic diamniotic (MC/DA) twin pregnancies respectively.[7] Morbidity to the surviving fetus depends very much on the chorionicity of the pregnancy. When one monochorionic twin dies *in utero*, there is a 12 per cent risk of death and an 18 per cent risk of neurological damage. The same figures for DC twins are 4 and 1 per cent. These complications are usually as a consequence of severe hypotension occurring during the death of the other twin.

The risk of cerebral palsy is increased in the surviving twin after a co-twin death, and same-sex twins are at greater risk than unlike-sex twins. The likely cause, in addition to the consequences of prematurity, is twin–twin transfusion problems associated with monochorionicity.

## Twin–twin transfusion syndrome

Twin–twin transfusion syndrome is a condition that complicates up to 15 per cent of monochorionic twin pregnancies. It is characterized by haemodynamic imbalances caused by unidirectional deep arteriovenous vessels and a relative lack of superficial vascular anastomoses (arterio-arterial anastomatoses (AAA) and veno-venous anastomatoses (VVA)) which have bidirectional potential and can, if present, protect against those imbalances. Twin–twin transfusion syndrome can occur in MC/MA twins but is rarer, possibly because of the presence of protective AAA.[3] In 5 per cent of cases TTTS can reverse with the donor becoming the recipient and vice versa. This can occur after treatment with amnioreduction or laser.[3]

The diagnosis requires the ultrasound demonstration of polyhydramnios around one twin (the recipient) and oligohydramnios around the other twin (the donor), with the separating membrane completely covering this fetus (stuck twin). The recipient twin is usually appropriately grown for gestational age, has a large distended bladder and may, if severely compromised, be hydropic (see Chapter 17, Fetal hydrops). Recipient fetuses may also develop cardiac dysfunction and neonatal hypertension. The donor twin, on the other hand, is frequently severely growth restricted, with abnormal umbilical artery Doppler waveforms. If untreated, the perinatal mortality of TTTS is extremely high (>90 per cent). Although twin–twin transfusion is usually a gradual process, it can happen suddenly with the death of one twin, usually the recipient.

## Twin reversed arterial perfusion sequence

This complication occurs in approximately 1 per cent of MC pregnancies. It is characterized by an acardiac twin, which receives its blood supply via a large arterio-arterial anastomosis from a normal co-twin (known as the 'pump' twin). This results in absent or rudimentary development of the upper body structures as the acardiac twin is supplied with deoxygenated blood. The perinatal mortality of the pump twin is considerable, with death usually occurring through complications of high output cardiac failure leading to hydrops fetalis or polyhydramnios-induced preterm delivery.

## Congenital anomalies

There is an excess of malformations in twins compared with singleton pregnancies.[8] These include malformations arising from the process of development and are often midline structural anomalies (e.g. neural tube defects, cardiac and cleft lip anomalies). An extreme example is the development of conjoined twins. Other malformations occur through disruption in a previously normally formed fetus. Disruptions are more common in monochorionic pregnancies and consist of predominantly vascular-type lesions (e.g. hydrancephaly, porencephaly, small bowel atresia). A further mechanism leading to maldevelopment is the constraint of sharing the uterine cavity (e.g. talipes, congenital dislocation of the hip).

## Other fetal risks

There are complications that usually arise in the third trimester and in particular in the intrapartum period. These include intrapartum hypoxaemia through entanglement (interlocking twins); umbilical cord accidents such as cord prolapse which are more likely in multiple pregnancy due to an increased frequency of malposition; or cord entanglement in monoamniotic twins.[3]

---

**KEY POINTS**

- Preterm labour and delivery are the biggest cause of adverse perinatal outcome in multiple pregnancy [B].
- Maternal risks relate mainly to increased uterine distension and the development of pre-eclampsia [B].
- An excess of congenital malformations means that examination of multiple pregnancies by detailed ultrasound scanning is mandatory [B].

# MANAGEMENT

## Diagnosis and determination of chorionicity

Dizygous twins are always DCDA. The chorionicity of monozygotic twins depends on the timing of embryo splitting after fertilization. They may be:

- dichorionic diamniotic (DCDA, if <3 days)
- monochorionic diamniotic (MCDA, 4–7 days).
- monochorionic monoamniotic (MCMA, 8+ days).

The early establishment of chorionicity is crucial to management of twins. Complications are greater in MC compared with DC twins. Twenty per cent of twins are monochorionic, but such pregnancies are associated with an almost 26 per cent risk of perinatal mortality.

In the first trimester, chorionicity may be determined with nearly 100 per cent accuracy. In contrast, mid-trimester assessment is only 80–90 per cent accurate. If two placentae are visualized or if the fetuses are discordant for gender, the pregnancy must be dichorionic. Visualization of the twin-peak or lambda sign is also useful in the diagnosis of dichorionicity; however, the absence of this sign is not as reliable in the confirmation of monochorionicity. Membrane thickness has also been used to assign chorionicity. In difficult cases, zygosity studies may need to be performed, but there is no evidence that this approach improves overall outcome in monochorionic twins.

## Screening for aneuploidy and prenatal diagnosis

Serum screening in multiple pregnancies is not as reliable as in singletons. Therefore the screening method of choice is nuchal translucency, which can be performed in the first trimester and allows calculation of an individual risk for each fetus. It may also be predictive for the development of TTTS if monochorionic pregnancies are discordant for nuchal thickness and crown rump length. The efficacy of nuchal translucency measurement screening in twins might be improved when combined with first trimester maternal serum screening, but this is not widely available currently.

Before any invasive procedure is undertaken for karyotyping, careful ultrasound mapping of the different placentae and gestational sacs is mandatory to assist in subsequent management when the karyotype results are available. The pregnancy loss rates for genetic amniocentesis in twins are considered similar to those seen in singletons. No data exist on loss rates with amniocentesis for higher order multiples. Chorionic villus sampling (CVS) is also possible in multiple pregnancies. Although CVS carries a higher loss rate, it has the advantage of being performed earlier (see Chapter 17, Fetal hydrops), but may be less reliable than amniocentesis as up to 4 per cent of CVS samples show evidence of co-twin contamination.

## Monitoring of fetal growth

Serial growth scans should be performed to evaluate fetal growth velocity and to detect any abnormalities in umbilical/artery Doppler waveform analysis and amniotic fluid volume. A sensible policy to monitor twins is 4-weekly scans from 24 weeks in dichorionic pregnancies to try and identify growth restriction, with more frequent scans if growth appears suboptimal. Monochorionic pregnancies should be monitored fortnightly from 16 weeks.[3]

The management of growth restriction in twin pregnancies needs to consider the risks to both the fetuses. Severe growth restriction in one fetus in a DC pregnancy might warrant a conservative approach (even allowing the growth restricted fetus to succumb *in utero*), thus sparing the healthy fetus the risks of iatrogenic prematurity. This situation is more complicated in MC pregnancy due to the presence of vascular anastamoses which could lead to damage/demise of the co-twin under these circumstances (see below).

## Multi-fetal pregnancy reduction

In higher multiple pregnancies, multi-fetal pregnancy reduction (MFPR) may substantially reduce the risk of perinatal morbidity and mortality. With increasing experience, post-procedure miscarriage rates are now <10 per cent, such that reductions from triplets to twins and from quadruplets to twins carry outcomes as good as those of unreduced twin gestations, and the chance of taking home a live baby increases from 80 to 90 per cent. The evidence is less clearly in favour of improved outcome with triplets reduced to twins but becomes more compelling in quadruplets and higher.

When offering MFPR, women should be carefully counselled about preterm delivery rates with expectant management (i.e. non-reduction) of 17 and 28 per cent at less than 29 weeks for triplets and quadruplets, respectively.[9] In addition, triplets and quadruplets have higher rates of other adverse outcomes including increased perinatal death, major anomalies, need for neonatal intensive care, respiratory distress syndrome, intrauterine growth restriction and serious neurological morbidity, which should also be discussed.

## Preterm labour

Prediction of preterm labour in twin pregnancies is as difficult as in singleton pregnancies. Cervical assessment has been suggested as one method to evaluate the risk of preterm labour. However, the frequency of monitoring/assessment of the cervix is unclear. In singleton pregnancy, a cervical length of 15 mm is predictive of preterm labour. In twin pregnancies, the mean cervical length is similar to that of singletons (38 mm), but a cervical length of 25 mm at 23 weeks gestation predicts about 80 per cent of women who deliver spontaneously at <30 weeks, with a false-positive rate of approximately 11 per cent.[10]

Home uterine monitoring, fetal fibronectin estimation, prophylactic cervical cerclage, progesterone supplementation and beta-mimetic therapy have not been shown to reduce the incidence of preterm labour in twin pregnancies and have largely been abandoned.

There is currently not enough evidence to support a policy of routine hospitalization for bed rest in multiple pregnancies. No reduction in the risk of preterm birth or perinatal death is evident, although there is a suggestion that fetal growth is improved. Indeed, in uncomplicated twin pregnancies, there is a suggestion that bed rest may be harmful in that the risk of very preterm birth is increased.

## Antenatal steroids

The efficacy of antenatal steroids in twin pregnancies is uncertain, however some benefit is apparent. There is concern that a larger dose of steroids may be beneficial in multiple pregnancies due to altered pharmacodynamics, although recent evidence suggests this is not an issue.[11]

## Treatment of twin–twin transfusion syndrome and twin reversed arterial perfusion

Treatment options have included serial amnioreduction, septostomy, selective feticide and laser ablation of the communicating anastomoses. Recent evidence has shown an improved outcome using laser ablation with survivals of 80–85 per cent for one twin reported. The major advance appears to be a reduced risk of neurologic damage in the event of a single twin demise to around 5 per cent.[12] The recent RCOG Green Top Guidelines Management of MC twins (no. 51)[3] concludes that TTTS before 26 weeks should be treated at regional fetal medicine centres by laser ablation. Selective feticide allows the survival of one twin with an 85 per cent success rate. Current management therefore favours amnioreduction or expectant management for stage 1; laser ablation for stages 2–4; selective reduction if imminent fetal demise of one twin threatens the co-twin.

In cases of twin reversed arterial perfusion (TRAP), disruption of the acardiac twin's cord or intrafetal vessel ablation with laser or diathermy are the available treatments with survival reported in >70 per cent of pump twins.[13]

## Treatment of co-twin death

In dichorionic pregnancies, expectant management is indicated. Regular assessment of the pregnant woman's coagulation status is necessary in order to detect changes in the coagulation system that may occur. In monochorionic pregnancies, if one twin dies there is a 12 per cent risk of death of the co-twin and an 18 per cent risk of neurological

damage. This is six and four times greater, respectively, than for DC twins.[14] Management depends upon the gestation and on the elapsed time since the fetal death. When death has occurred within 24–36 hours at an early gestation, fetal blood sampling with rescue transfusion may be considered if the surviving fetus is anaemic as indicated by middle cerebral artery Doppler.[3] At later gestations, delivery may more appropriate if there are significant concerns regarding the well-being of the survivor. However, caution must be exercised as any damage is likely to have occurred and delivery may only add risks of prematurity and not improve outcome.

If a co-twin death has occurred some time previously, consideration should be given to appropriate imaging of the surviving fetus's brain with either ultrasound or magnetic resonance imaging to detect cystic changes. If these changes do evolve and are apparent, offering termination of the pregnancy is an option.

## Labour and delivery

Timing of delivery in uncomplicated monochorionic twins is controversial. There is no conclusive evidence as to when delivery should be undertaken. Management in the UK is as diverse as caesarean section at 34 weeks to induction of labour at 38 weeks and all variations in between. If there is evidence of TTTS or other complications, timing of delivery must be individualized. In dichorionic twins, most obstetricians would recommend delivery by 38 weeks.

The mode of delivery is decided on standard principles based on the presentation of the first twin. Vaginal delivery is preferred in vertex–vertex presentations. The optimal mode of birth for the second twin presenting as non-vertex is unknown with retrospective reviews in the literature providing support for both caesarean birth and vaginal birth for the second non-vertex twin.

For the very low birth weight infant (1500 g), opinion is divided as to the optimal mode of delivery. Whereas some advocate caesarean delivery in all cases, there is little evidence that caesarean section improves perinatal outcome.

For MCMA twins, delivery should be around 32 weeks by caesarean section [C].[3] Although some authors suggest that triplets and higher order multiples may be safely delivered vaginally despite the obvious difficulties in monitoring, caesarean section is the more usual mode of delivery.

## CONCLUSIONS

The management of a multiple pregnancy is a major challenge for obstetricians. These pregnancies are at increased risk of maternal and fetal complications that require specialized management. There is an increasing vogue to manage these patients in specialized multiple pregnancy clinics, with access to a fetal medicine specialist with a special interest in multiple pregnancy.

## KEY POINTS

- Determination of chorionicity is important to allocate pregnancy risk [B].
- Nuchal translucency is the method of choice for aneuploidy screening [B].
- Prenatal diagnosis using amniocentesis or CVS is suitable in multiple pregnancy [B].
- Ultrasound assessment should be carried out every 4 weeks from 20 weeks in DC twins and every 2 weeks from 16 weeks in MC twins.[15]
- The management of TTTS and TRAP necessitates referral to an appropriate fetal medicine unit [B,D]. Such conditions carry high perinatal mortality, even with treatment.
- Optimal treatment of TTTS is laser ablation (A).
- Cervical length measurement may be useful in predicting preterm birth in multiple pregnancy [B].
- Uncomplicated MC twins aim to deliver vaginally by 36-37 weeks.[15]
- Uncomplicated DC twins aim to deliver vaginally by 37-38 weeks.[15]

## ACKNOWLEDGEMENTS

This chapter has been revised and updated. The author and editors acknowledge the contribution of Sailesh Kumar to the chapter on this topic in the previous edition of the book.

## Key References

1. ONS (2008) Birth statistics 2007 series FMI no. 36.
2. Confidential Enquiry into Maternal and Child Health (CEMACH) Perinatal Mortality 2006: England, Wales and Northern Ireland. CEMACH: London, 2008.
3. RCOG Guideline No. 51 *Management of Monochorionic Twin Pregnancy*. London: RCOG, 2009.
4. Sebire NJ, Snijders RJ, Hughes K *et al*. The hidden mortality of monochorionic twin pregnancies. *Br J Obstet Gynaecol* 1997; **104**: 1203–7.
5. Russell Z, Quintero RA, Kontopoulos EV. Intrauterine growth restriction in monochorionic twins. *Semin Fet Neon Med* 2007; **12**: 439–49.
6. Cooperstock MS, Tummaru R, Bakewell J, Schramm W. Twin birth weight discordance and risk of preterm birth. *Am J Obstet Gynecol* 2000; **183**: 63–7.
7. Lee YM, Wylie BJ, Simpson LL, D'Alton ME. Twin chorionicity and the risk of stillbirth. *Obstet Gynecol* 2008; **111**: 301–8.
8. Rustico MA, Baietti MG, Coviello D *et al*. Managing twins discordant for fetal anomaly. *Prenat Diagn* 2005; **25**: 766–71.
9. Luke B, Brown MB. Maternal morbidity and infant death in twin vs triplet and quadruplet pregnancies. *Am J Obstet Gynecol* 2008; **198**: 401.e1–10.
10. Souka AP, Heath V, Flint S *et al*. Cervical length at 23 weeks in twins in predicting spontaneous preterm delivery. *Obstet Gynecol* 1999; **94**: 450–54.
11. Battista L, Winovitch KC, Rumney PJ *et al*. A case-control comparison of the effectiveness of betamethasone to prevent neonatal morbidity and mortality in preterm twin and singleton pregnancies. *Am J Perinatol* 2008; **25**: 449–53.
12. Roberts D, Neilson JP, Kilby MD, Gates S. Intervention for the treatment of twin-twin transfusion syndrome. *Cochrane Database Syst Rev* 2008; (**1**): CD002073.
13. Rossi AC, D'Addario V. Umbilical cord occlusion for selective feticide in complicated monochorionic twins: a systematic review of literature. *Am J Obstet Gynecol* 2009; **200**: 123–9.
14. Ong SSC, Zamora J, Khan K, Kilby MD Prognosis for the co-twin following single twin death: A systematic review. *BJOG* 2006; **113**: 992–8.
15. Kilby M, Baker P, Critchley H, Field D (eds). *Consensus views arising from the 50th Study Group: Multiples Pregnancy*. London: RCOG Press, 2006: 283–6.

# Fetal infections

*Sailesh Kumar*

---

## MRCOG standards

### Theoretical skills

- Know the different infectious agents that can cause a range of serious fetal morbidity and mortality.
- Understand the relevant and specific maternal and fetal diagnostic tests to confirm the *in-utero* infection.
- Appreciate the potential perinatal complications of fetal infections.
- Understand that prevention of maternal infection through vaccination and appropriate health education are important measures in preventing fetal infection and morbidity.

### Practical skills

- Be able to counsel and refer appropriately a patient with a fetal viral infection.

---

## INTRODUCTION

Congenital infections may cause significant morbidity and mortality through various different mechanisms. Some infectious agents cause a self-limiting maternal illness with minimal or no adverse fetal consequences, whereas others cause major sequelae in the form of malformations, neurodevelopmental delay and even long-term childhood consequences.

Infectious agents may affect the fetus by vertical transmission, which can be either blood borne or at the time of delivery (e.g. varicella, rubella, cytomegalovirus (CMV) infection, toxoplasmosis and listeriosis). Pre-pregnancy or routine antenatal screening for the presence of some of these infections and appropriate management can prevent adverse fetal or perinatal outcomes. If an infection is suspected because of a positive antenatal test result, confirmatory tests for maternal and, if indicated, fetal infection are essential before intervention is considered. In addition, screening for past infection and immunization to increase herd immunity are also an important public health measure.

The diagnosis of fetal infection is important in order to counsel the mother about the likely sequelae. In some cases the risk of congenital malformations may be so high that an offer of termination of pregnancy may be appropriate (i.e. congenital rubella syndrome). There are numerous infectious agents, and many have either a direct or indirect affect on pregnancy. It is beyond the scope of this chapter to discuss all infectious agents; however, the following are discussed in specific detail: rubella virus, varicella zoster virus (VZV), CMV, toxoplasma, parvovirus B19 and *Treponema pallidum*.

## RUBELLA

Rubella (German measles) is a self-limiting, mild viral illness that poses little danger to children or adults (see also Chapter 7.4, Infection). For the developing fetus, however, infection with rubella virus is a grave threat, capable of inducing severe anomalies and permanent disability. In general terms, the earlier the gestational age at which infection occurs, the greater the risk of fetal morbidity. Despite widespread vaccination programmes, populations of susceptible individuals persist, among them women of childbearing age, whose pregnancies remain vulnerable to congenital rubella syndrome. Natural infections of rubella occur only in humans and are generally mild.

The primary public health concern of rubella infection is its teratogenicity. Infection during the first trimester of pregnancy can induce a spectrum of congenital defects in the newborn, known as congenital rubella syndrome (CRS). The mechanism of infection leading to teratogenesis is not clear, but analysis of infected fetal tissues suggests hypoxia, necrosis and/or apoptosis, as well as inhibition of cell division of critical precursor cells involved in organogenesis. Although malformations can occur in almost all organ systems, the eyes, heart and ears seem to be preferentially affected. Cataracts, retinopathy, microphthalmia, glaucoma, patent ductus arteriosus, pulmonary valve lesions and sensorineural deafness are common abnormalities seen in early fetal infection.[1] The risk of fetal infection and congenital abnormalities is in excess of 80 per cent if infection occurs in the first trimester,[2] and decreases to approximately 25 per cent in early second trimester [C].[1] The risk of congenital abnormalities continues to decrease as pregnancy progresses.

There is emerging evidence indicating that *in-utero* exposure to rubella infection may have more long-term consequences, with such individuals being at higher risk of schizophrenia. It is hypothesized that prenatal infection increases the liability to schizophrenia in adulthood by adversely affecting the maturation of critical brain structural and functional components implicated in the aetiology of this disorder.[3]

Although national immunization programmes in many countries have made this disease increasingly rare because of herd immunity, immigrants to the UK may be susceptible and therefore a high index of suspicion is needed for this infection in recent immigrants from countries with no immunization programme. Mothers born abroad, particularly in Sub-Saharan Africa and South Asia, are more likely to be seronegative than UK-born mothers, with adjusted odds ratios of 4.2 (95 per cent CI 3.1–5.6) and 5.0 (3.8–6.5), respectively.[4] Targeted immunization for such groups should be considered [D]. Recognition of rubella susceptibility prior to pregnancy is an important preventative strategy as it allows immunization of these seronegative women. The need for re-screening of previously seropositive women is controversial. As with many other viruses, re-infection does result in a secondary immune response and evidence of viral replication prior immunity usually prevents viraemia. Congenital rubella syndrome can only occur if viraemia is present. Although postpartum re-immunization of women with low antibody titres could potentially prevent the risk of congenital infection, there is insufficient evidence to support rescreening of previously seropositive women and no data to support or refute the value of offering rubella vaccine to women who have low titres.

## Diagnosis

The clinical diagnosis of rubella is difficult as it is frequently subclinical and the rash is similar to that of other viral infections; therefore serology remains the mainstay of diagnosis.[5] In the mother, acute infection may be diagnosed by isolation of the virus from throat swabs, but it is more common for an acute rubella-specific immunoglobulin (IgM) response to be detected [C] in an individual previously noted to be non-immune using fluorescent immunoassay techniques. Rubella-specific IgG indicates previous infection or immunization. Immunity is usually life-long.

## Management

Vaccination of children remains the cornerstone of the preventative strategy for this devastating fetal disease. Primary

rubella vaccine failure is rare with many studies showing a 100 per cent seroconversion rate. Rubella vaccination has been shown to be cost effective in both developing and developed countries if coverage rates of more than 80 per cent are achieved. Pre-pregnancy counselling should include evidence of immunity and vaccination should be offered to susceptible individuals [C].

If infection is confirmed in the first trimester, termination of pregnancy should be offered as the sequelae of congenital infection are devastating. Later in pregnancy, evidence for fetal infection may be sought. Fetal blood sampling to measure levels of rubella-specific IgM5 may be performed and rubella-specific RNA identified using reverse transcriptase–polymerase chain reaction (RT-PCR) [C,D].[6] There is no prenatal treatment once the fetus is affected. The rubella vaccine is a live attenuated virus and therefore theoretically should be avoided in pregnancy. However, the Centers for Disease Control in the USA have monitored cases of inadvertent rubella vaccination during pregnancy (1971–89) and no adverse sequelae have been documented [C].[7]

> ## KEY POINTS
>
> - Early pregnancy infection results in an extremely high fetal transmission rate [C].
> - Termination of pregnancy should be discussed with patients if maternal infection occurs in the first trimester because of the very high risk of congenital malformation [C].

# CYTOMEGALOVIRUS

Cytomegalovirus, a member of the herpes virus family, is the most common cause of congenital infection in humans (see also Chapter 7.4, Infection). Maternal CMV is a systemic infection that can be transmitted transplacentally to the fetus. An estimated 0.6–0.7 per cent of infants are born with congenital CMV infection, which is diagnosed by the presence of the virus in urine or saliva shortly after birth. The virus has a high prevalence in the general population, is unpredictable in its transmission, and causes an asymptomatic disease in otherwise healthy women. Intrauterine infection with CMV remains the most common congenital virus infection in many regions of the world. Approximately 11 per cent of infected infants are symptomatic at birth. The birth prevalence of congenital CMV infection is estimated to be around 1 per cent, although there is some geographical variation.[8] Primary maternal CMV infection occurs in 0.7–4.1 per cent of pregnancies, is transmitted to the fetus in about one-third of cases[8] and is much more likely to cause fetal damage. Of all such infected newborns, 0.5 per cent die and about 17–20 per cent will have permanent disabilities.[9] The majority of infected babies are born to women whose pregnancies are uncomplicated and who were unaware of the infection during pregnancy. Although most CMV-infected newborns lack signs of infection, approximately 10 per cent have low birth weight, jaundice, hepatosplenomegaly, skin rash, microcephaly and chorioretinitis. Other fetal consequences of CMV infection include haemolytic anaemia, ventriculomegaly, cerebral atrophy and intracranial calcification. The sequelae of fetal infection are gestation dependent: early fetal infection causes brain anomalies, whereas symptomatic late fetal infection results in hepatitis and thrombocytopenia. Neonates with signs of CMV infection at birth have high rates of audiologic and neurodevelopmental sequelae. Congenital CMV infection is the leading infectious cause of deafness, learning disabilities and mental retardation in children (rubella, measles and mumps have become rare due to vaccination).

## Diagnosis

Recent advances in the screening of pregnant women with CMV IgM, CMV IgG and CMV IgG avidity serological tests have led to more accurate diagnosis of CMV infection. When serological screening is performed early in gestation, it is possible to identify those women at risk of intrauterine transmission of the virus (women with a primary CMV infection). The diagnosis of congenital infection in the fetus can sometimes be made using either fetal blood or amniotic fluid. Quantitative PCR on amniotic fluid from pregnant women at 21–22 weeks of gestation is an effective prenatal diagnostic tool [B]. Quantitative PCR on peripheral blood leukocytes from CMV-infected newborns can be used to monitor viral load.[10]

Once structural abnormalities are detected on antenatal ultrasound, the prognosis for the fetus worsens considerably. Abnormalities that may be evident include hydrops, ventriculomegaly, periventricular calcifications, hepatomegaly, intrabdominal calcifications, microcephaly and fetal growth restriction.

## Management

There is no effective fetal therapy. Although postnatal therapy with ganciclovir transiently reduces virus shedding and may lessen the audiological consequences of CMV in some infected infants [C,D], additional strategies are needed to prevent congenital CMV disease.

Some cases of intrauterine infections can be prevented in susceptible women by avoiding contact with the urine or saliva of young children who may be shedding CMV. Vaccines against CMV remain in the experimental stages of development. Termination of pregnancy can be offered to women whose infants have evidence of intrauterine CMV infection and sonographic signs of central nervous system (CNS) damage. Infants who survive symptomatic intrauterine infections have high rates of neurodevelopmental sequelae and require comprehensive evaluation and therapy through centre-based and home-based early intervention programmes.

Women who work in high-risk professions should be given pre-pregnancy advice. If maternal infection is confirmed, consideration should be given to performing an invasive procedure to obtain fetal samples for analysis. Tests can be performed on chorionic villus samples, amniotic fluid or fetal blood [C].[11]

CMV glycoprotein b vaccine has the potential to decrease incident cases of maternal and congenital CMV infection, with a recent publication[12] suggesting a 50 per cent vaccine efficacy rate. However, phase 3 trials have yet to be conducted.

## KEY POINTS

- Pre-pregnancy immunity to CMV infection is socio-economically dependent, ranging from 55 to 85 per cent.
- The rate of primary CMV infection is 1–4 per cent and it carries a 40 per cent risk of fetal transmission [C].
- There is no gestation-dependent alteration of fetal risk from primary perinatal infection with gestation.
- The incidence of congenital infection varies between 0.3 and 3 per cent [C].
- Of these, 5 per cent will be symptomatic at birth, with a 30 per cent neonatal mortality and long-term morbidity in the majority of survivors. This includes neurodevelopmental delay in up to 90 per cent and hearing loss in 60 per cent [C].

## TOXOPLASMA

*Toxoplasma gondii* is a unicellular protozoon (see also Chapter 7.4, Infection). The cat is the definitive host and produces oocysts and sporozoites. Ingestion leads to the formation of tachyzoites, which cause parasitaemia and further dissemination, and subsequent bradyzoites, which lead to latent infection with the formation of tissue cysts in skeletal muscle, heart muscle and CNS tissue. Disease progression is influenced by many factors including parasite, host and environmental elements. There appears to be wide consensus among experts that acquiring toxoplasmosis is often associated with unsafe eating habits. Many demographic indicators (gender, age, race, urban/rural residence, occupation) suggest an increase in the number of people, particularly pregnant women, at high risk of contracting toxoplasmosis through the consumption of raw contaminated meat.

Toxoplasmosis can be transmitted to humans by:

- ingestion of tissue cysts in raw or inadequately cooked infected meat or in uncooked foods that have come in contact with contaminated meat;
- inadvertent ingestion of oocysts and sporozoites in cat faeces; or
- transplacentally.

Immunocompetent adults and adolescents with primary infection are generally asymptomatic, but symptoms may include mild malaise, lethargy and lymphadenopathy. Specific treatment for non-pregnant adults and adolescents is not required. In severely immunocompromised, chronically infected pregnant women (patients with HIV/AIDS and those receiving high-dose immunosuppressive therapy, including organ transplant recipients and patients with malignancies), reactivation of latent *T. gondii* infection can result in congenital transmission of the parasite to the fetus. Immunosuppressed patients may experience more severe manifestations, including splenomegaly, chorioretinitis, pneumonitis, encephalitis and multisystem organ failure. These patients are also prone to reactivation of latent infection involving the CNS.

Congenital toxoplasmosis is marked by the classic triad of chorioretinitis, intracranial calcifications and hydrocephalus. If congenital infection occurs in the first trimester, spontaneous miscarriage is common. The risk of fetal infection rises throughout gestation, with approximately 65 per cent of fetuses affected in the third trimester. Early first trimester maternal infections are less likely to result in congenital infection, but the sequelae are more severe. Transplacental passage is more common when maternal infection occurs in the latter half of pregnancy, but fetal injury is usually much less severe. The majority of infants are born without any obvious problems. There is no accurate logarithm to predict the severity of fetal infection, although high maternal antibody levels may be weakly correlative.[13]

## Diagnosis

For serological diagnosis, IgG, IgM, IgA, IgE antibodies, IgG avidity and the differential agglutination (AC/HS) tests can be used in an attempt to distinguish the acute versus the chronic stage of the infection.[14] Except for measurement of IgG and IgM antibodies, most of these tests are performed only in reference laboratories. All positive screening tests in pregnant women must be confirmed at a toxoplasma reference laboratory using a specific and sensitive ELISA testing [C]. Paired serological titres are important in confirming acute maternal infection. Recent studies have shown that PCR testing of amniotic fluid is useful for identification or exclusion of fetal *T. gondii* infection [C].[15] In addition to the gestational age, the parasite load in amniotic fluid is an independent risk factor for severity of fetal infection. Maternal infections acquired before 20 weeks of gestation with a parasite load 1100 parasites/mL of amniotic fluid is associated with the highest risk of severe outcome in the fetus. Ultrasound evidence of intracranial infections can be used as an adjunct to serological screening, but cannot itself definitively diagnose disease because of the relatively low sensitivity and specificity of diagnosis. Once structural anomalies are present, the prognosis for the fetus worsens

and the option of termination of pregnancy should be discussed with the parents.

## Management

Prevention of primary maternal infection is critical in this regard. This is best achieved by adequate public education through health campaigns to ensure that non-immune pregnant women handle and cook meat appropriately, use gloves when handling cat litter and avoid contact with objects that are potentially contaminated with cat faeces.

If maternal infection is confirmed, spiramycin should be commenced to reduce the likelihood of fetal infection; this treatment reduces the risk of transmission by almost 60 per cent [C].[15] Spiramycin should be started as soon as maternal infection has been confirmed, as the longer the delay the greater the risk of fetal damage [C]. The drug is administered until delivery even in those patients with negative results of amniotic fluid PCR, because of the theoretical possibility that fetal infection can occur later in pregnancy from a placenta that was infected earlier in gestation. If fetal infection is confirmed by a positive result of PCR of amniotic fluid at 18 weeks of gestation or later, treatment with pyrimethamine, sulfadiazine, and folinic acid is recommended (if the patient is already receiving spiramycin, the recommendation is to switch to this combination) (see review by Montoya and Remington[16]). Pyrimethamine is potentially teratogenic and should not be used in the first trimester of pregnancy.

A recent study failed to detect a beneficial effect of early or more potent prenatal anti-toxoplasma treatment (pyrimethamine-sulfadiazine) on the risks of intracranial or ocular lesions in children with congenital toxoplasmosis [C].[17]

Termination of pregnancy is also an option if infection occurs early in gestation or if there is ultrasound evidence of congenital infection.

### KEY POINTS

- In the UK, the risk of congenital toxoplasmosis infection is deemed to be relatively low. Health-economic evaluation has indicated that routine screening of pregnant women would not be cost effective [C].
- Both prenatal and antenatal health education of women with regard to the food that may cause vertical transmission is important.
- In women who have been investigated and are positive for an acute toxoplasmosis infection, investigation and management in a fetal medicine centre is advisable, with maternal treatment to reduce transplacental transmission and minimize acute fetal infection [C].
- If infection occurs in the first or second trimester, the risk of severe congenital disease approaches 25 per cent.

# VARICELLA

Varicella zoster virus (VZV) (chickenpox) is a highly contagious DNA virus of the herpes family that is usually transmitted by respiratory droplets and by direct personal contact with vesicle fluid (see also Chapter 7.4, Infection). The primary infection is characterized by fever, malaise and a pruritic rash that becomes maculopapular and vesicular and finally crusts over before healing. The incubation period is 10–21 days and the disease is infectious 48 hours before the rash appears and until the vesicles crust over. Primary VZV infection is worse in adults, especially pregnant women, than in children. Only about 2 per cent of all cases occur in adults, but these cases account for 25 per cent of all VZV-related deaths. VZV pneumonitis is 25 times more common in adults and occurs in up to 20 per cent of VZV-infected pregnant women. More than 90 per cent of pregnant women are seropositive for varicella zoster IgG (VZIG).

Spontaneous miscarriage does not appear to be increased if chickenpox occurs in the first trimester.[18] Maternal infection before 20 weeks may result in fetal varicella syndrome. However, only 1–2 per cent of maternal varicella infections that occur before 20 weeks gestation result in the fetal varicella syndrome.[18] Typical fetal and neonatal manifestations include skin scarring in a dermatomal distribution, eye defects (microphthalmia, chorioretinitis, cataracts), hypoplasia of the limbs and neurological abnormalities (microcephaly, cortical atrophy, mental retardation and dysfunction of bowel and bladder sphincters). Maternal infection after 20 weeks and up to 36 weeks does not appear to be associated with adverse fetal effects.

## Diagnosis

Prenatal diagnosis is possible using detailed assessment ultrasound, when findings such as limb deformity, microcephaly, hydrocephalus, soft tissue calcification and intrauterine growth restriction may be detected some weeks after the initial infection.[18] VZV DNA can be detected by PCR in amniotic fluid or fetal blood, but its presence does not necessarily indicate development of the fetal varicella syndrome [D]. Passive immunization may reduce the risk of fetal infection, but there is no evidence that it prevents fetal viraemia [D]. There are also no controlled studies concerning the role of antiviral chemotherapy in preventing the fetal syndrome. The varicella vaccine is a live attenuated vaccine and is contraindicated in pregnancy. It is recommended that pregnancy be avoided for 1–3 months after vaccination because the effect of the vaccine on the developing fetus is unknown. Although the numbers of exposures are not sufficient to rule out a very low risk, data collected in the pregnancy registry to date do not support a relationship between the occurrence of congenital varicella syndrome or other birth defects and varicella vaccine exposure during pregnancy.[19]

## Management

The management of women who have either been exposed to or develop chickenpox is discussed in Chapter 7.4, Infection. There is no evidence that VZIG given within 24 hours of contact prevents intrauterine infection [C].

# PARVOVIRUS B19

Parvovirus B19 (erythema infectiosum, Fifth disease) is a small, single-stranded DNA virus that can cause fetal infection (see also Chapter 7.4, Infection). Approximately 50 per cent of adults will be seropositive, indicating past infection and immunity. Among non-immune individuals, approximately one in five carries a risk of acute infection if exposed to erythema infectiosum. There is no evidence that the infection is teratogenic [D], but in the fetus the virus has a predilection for erythropoietic cells, causing a transient but severe pancytopenia.[20] Parvovirus may cause unexpected stillbirths at term and late miscarriages; however, the main concern with fetal infection is the potential to develop hydrops secondary to fetal anaemia or cardiac dysfunction from acute myocarditis [C,D].[20]

## Diagnosis

The diagnosis of human parvovirus B19 in a hydropic fetus requires the isolation of the virus (by PCR) and/or parvovirus-specific IgM from paired maternal and fetal blood [C].[20] Hydrops may occur 2–4 weeks after acute fetal infection (see Chapter 17, Fetal hydrops) [C].[20]

## Management

The anaemic hydropic fetus may be salvaged by aggressive in-utero transfusions of red cells [C]. Infantile red cell aplasia has been reported following in-utero transfusions, and hence these babies should be followed up to detect this potential complication.

## KEY POINTS

- In non-immune pregnant individuals (50 per cent of the population), the presence of an acute infection carries at least a one in five risk of transplacental transmission [C].
- Overall, the fetal death rate associated with acute human parvovirus B19 infection is 9 per cent [C].
- After acute exposure, the interval between maternal infection and fetal consequences is 4–5 weeks.
- The fetal consequences of human parvovirus B19 infection are potentially self-limiting and/or treatable. Investigation and management should take place in a regional fetal medicine centre [C,E].

# SYPHILIS

Syphilis is caused by the spirochaete *Treponema pallidum* (see also Chapter 7.4, Infection). Pregnancy has no known effect on the clinical course of syphilis. The mother can transmit the infection to the fetus either transplacentally or by contact of the newborn with a genital lesion. *Treponema pallidum* can infect the fetus from as early as 9–10 weeks.[21,22]

Untreated syphilis during pregnancy can profoundly affect pregnancy outcome, resulting in spontaneous abortion, stillbirth, non-immune hydrops, growth restriction, preterm delivery, neonatal death, and infant disorders such as deafness, neurological impairment and bone deformities.

Traditionally, congenital syphilis has been divided into two clinical syndromes: early and late congenital syphilis. Early disease refers to clinical manifestations that appear within the first two years of life. Late syphilis occurs after two years, usually around puberty.

## Diagnosis

In routine clinical practice, serological tests on maternal blood such as the VDRL, RPR, FTA-Abs, MHA-TP or TPI assay are used to make the diagnosis (see Chapter 17, Fetal hydrops).

Prenatal laboratory diagnosis of fetal infection is possible. As maternal IgM does not cross the placenta, detection of fetal IgM is indicative of transplacental infection. Fetal blood can be obtained either by cordocentesis or from the intrahepatic vein. *Treponema pallidum* DNA can also be detected using PCR techniques with amniotic fluid, and this method has been shown to be sensitive and specific [C].[23] Ultrasound can also be used to detect some of the manifestations of syphilis in the fetus. Hydrops, hepatosplenomegaly, placentomegaly and small bowel dilatation have all been demonstrated.[24–26] Hepatomegaly seems to be the most sensitive ultrasound marker of fetal infection [D].

## Management

Treatment of syphilis during pregnancy should be with the penicillin regimen appropriate for the mother's stage of syphilis [C]. Monthly follow up of serological titres is recommended for the evaluation of the adequacy of treatment. Despite administration of the recommended penicillin regimen to pregnant women, as many as 14 per cent will have a fetal death or deliver infants with clinical evidence of congenital syphilis [C].[27–29] Any infant at risk for congenital syphilis should also undergo full evaluation and testing for HIV infection. The major factor accounting for the failure to prevent congenital infection is the lack of adequate antenatal care. This is particularly relevant in underdeveloped countries and among the socially deprived in industrialized communities. Routine prenatal screening remains the major line of defence against congenital syphilis [C].

## KEY POINTS

- Congenital syphilis is still a major cause of perinatal morbidity and mortality worldwide.
- The risk of perinatal transmission is greatest within the first year of untreated disease.
- If untreated, 30 per cent of infected fetuses will die *in utero*, 30 per cent will die in the early neonatal period and the remainder will develop late symptomatic syphilis.
- It is a common cause of poor *in-utero* growth worldwide.

## Key References

1. Miller E, Cradock-Watson JE, Pollock TM. Consequences of confirmed maternal rubella at successive stages of pregnancy. *Lancet* 1982; **2**: 781–4.
2. Mellinger AK, Cragan JD, Atkinson WL *et al.* High incidence of congenital rubella syndrome after a rubella outbreak. *Pediatr Infect Dis J* 1995; **14**: 573–8.
3. Brown AS, Susser ES. *In utero* infection and adult schizophrenia. *Ment Retard Dev Disabil Res Rev* 2002; **8**: 51–7.
4. Hardelid P, Cortina-Borja M, Williams D *et al.* Rubella seroprevalence in pregnant women in North Thames: estimates based on newborn screening samples. *J Med Screen* 2009; **16**: 1–6.
5. Daffos F, Forestier F, Grangeot-Keros L *et al.* Prenatal diagnosis of congenital rubella. *Lancet* 1984; **2**: 1–3.
6. Bosma TJ, Corbett KM, O'Shea S *et al.* PCR for detection of rubella virus RNA in clinical samples. *J Clin Microbiol* 1995; **33**: 1075–9.
7. Centers for Disease Control. Rubella vaccination during pregnancy – United States, 1971–1988. *MMWR Morb Mortal Wkly Rep* 1989; **38**: 289–91.
8. Kenneson A, Cannon MJ. Review and meta-analysis of the epidemiology of congenital cytomegalovirus (CMV) infection. *Rev Med Virol* 2007; **17**: 253–76.
9. Dollard SC, Grosse SD, Ross DS. New estimates of the prevalence of neurological and sensory sequelae and mortality associated with congenital cytomegalovirus infection. *Rev Med Virol* 2007; **17**: 355–63.
10. Maine GT, Lazzarotto T, Landini MP. New developments in the diagnosis of maternal and congenital CMV infection. *Expert Rev Mol Diagn* 2001; **1**: 19–29.
11. Enders G, Bader U, Lindemann L *et al.* Prenatal diagnosis of congenital cytomegalovirus infection in 189 pregnancies with known outcome. *Prenat Diagn* 2001; **21**: 362–77.
12. Pass RF, Zhang C, Evans A *et al.* Vaccine prevention of maternal cytomegalovirus infection. *N Engl J Med* 2009; **360**: 1191–9.
13. Sever JL, Ellenberg JH, Ley AC *et al.* Toxoplasmosis: maternal and pediatric findings in 23,000 pregnancies. *Pediatrics* 1988; **82**: 181–92.
14. Montoya JG. Laboratory diagnosis of *Toxoplasma gondii* infection and toxoplasmosis. *J Infect Dis* 2002; **185** (Suppl. 1): S73–82.

15. Hohlfeld P, Daffos F, Costa JM *et al.* Prenatal diagnosis of congenital toxoplasmosis with a polymerase-chain-reaction test on amniotic fluid. *N Engl J Med* 1994; **331**: 695–9.

16. Montoya JG, Remington JS. Clinical practice: Management of *Toxoplasma gondii* infection during pregnancy. *Clin Infect Dis* 2008; **47**: 554–66.

17. Gras L, Gilbert RE, Ades AE, Dunn DT. Effect of prenatal treatment on the risk of intracranial and ocular lesions in children with congenital toxoplasmosis. *Int J Epidemiol* 2001; **30**: 1309–13.

18. Pastuszak AL, Levy M, Schick B *et al.* Outcome after maternal varicella infection in the first 20 weeks of pregnancy. *N Engl J Med* 1994; **330**: 901–5.

19. Wilson E, Goss MA, Martin M *et al.* Varicella vaccine exposure during pregnancy: data from 10 years of the pregnancy registry. *J Infect Dis* 2008; **197** (Suppl. 2): S178–84.

20. Ismail K, Kilby MD. Human parvovirus B19 and pregnancy. *Obstet Gynecol* 2003; **5**: 4–9.

21. Harter C, Benirschke K. Fetal syphilis in the first trimester. *Am J Obstet Gynecol* 1976; **124**: 705–11.

22. Nathan L, Bohman VR, Sanchez PJ *et al. In utero* infection with *Treponema pallidum* in early pregnancy. *Prenat Diagn* 1997; **17**: 119–23.

23. Zoechling N, Schluepen EM, Soyer HP *et al.* Molecular detection of *Treponema pallidum* in secondary and tertiary syphilis. *Br J Dermatol* 1997; **136**: 683–6.

24. Hill LM, Maloney JB. An unusual constellation of sonographic findings associated with congenital syphilis. *Obstet Gynecol* 1991; **78**: 895–7.

25. Satin AJ, Twickler DM, Wendel GD Jr. Congenital syphilis associated with dilation of fetal small bowel. A case report. *J Ultrasound Med* 1992; **11**: 49–2.

26. Nathan L, Twickler DM, Peters MT *et al.* Fetal syphilis: correlation of sonographic findings and rabbit infectivity testing of amniotic fluid. *J Ultrasound Med* 1993; **12**: 97–101.

27. McFarlin BL, Bottoms SF, Dock BS, Isada NB. Epidemic syphilis: maternal factors associated with congenital infection. *Am J Obstet Gynecol* 1994; **170**: 535–40.

28. Mascola L, Pelosi R, Alexander CE. Inadequate treatment of syphilis in pregnancy. *Am J Obstet Gynecol* 1984; **150**: 945–7.

29. Conover CS, Rend CA, Miller GB Jr, Schmid GP. Congenital syphilis after treatment of maternal syphilis with a penicillin regimen exceeding CDC guidelines. *Infect Dis Obstet Gynecol* 1998; **6**: 134–7.

# Tests of fetal well-being

*Linda Watkins and Murray Luckas*

---

## INTRODUCTION

Assessing fetal well-being should reduce perinatal mortality and morbidity; however, the outcome of pregnancy in the developed world is usually good, with adverse perinatal outcomes being relatively rare. It therefore follows that the majority of fetuses subjected to tests designed to assess fetal well-being will be healthy. Those tests should not only be sensitive in their ability to detect a compromised fetus, but also specific in that they do not give an abnormal result when the fetus is well; poor specificity may lead to unnecessary parental anxiety and rates of intervention.

A major problem in the evaluation of tests of fetal well-being is the absence of useful outcome criteria. Perinatal mortality is now too rare an occurrence and too late an outcome measure to be useful. The condition of the neonate at birth is of little help, because it is difficult to separate the effects of parturition from factors present antenatally. Long-term neurodevelopment can be assessed, but such an assessment is subject to many influences and is probably best done some five years after birth.

The ideal test will be quick and easy to perform and will yield readily interpreted results that are reproducible. It should clearly identify the compromised fetus at a stage at which intervention will improve the outcome, but in turn it should not give an abnormal result for a healthy fetus. Unfortunately, this ideal test does not yet exist!

## DEFINITIONS

For the purposes of this chapter, we regard fetal compromise as 'a fetus that is at risk of damage from hypoxia'. Energy, in the form of adenosine triphosphate (ATP) and its sister molecules, is vital for the metabolism of cells. In the absence of sufficient quantities of this energy, cells will no longer be able to function and will eventually die. The production of ATP via oxidative phosphorylation from polysaccharides (glucose), fats and proteins requires oxygen – so-called oxidative metabolism. Where oxygen levels are insufficient to support oxidative phosphorylation, anaerobic metabolism occurs. This is an inefficient process, resulting in reduced production of ATP per molecule of glucose compared to aerobic metabolism (2 versus 24 molecules of ATP). Ultimately, the hypoxic fetus will no longer be able to maintain cellular metabolism, with resultant cell damage and death. The developing brain, myocardium and kidneys are the organs most sensitive to this damage, although fetal demise will eventually occur.

In addition, hypoxia leads to build up of byproducts such as lactic acid, resulting in metabolic acidaemia, which in itself may exacerbate the effects of hypoxia on cellular metabolism. This is a more chronic process than respiratory acidosis, which occurs because of an inability of the feto-placental unit to rid the fetus of carbon dioxide.

## AETIOLOGY

An exhaustive list of the causes of fetal hypoxia is beyond the remit of this chapter. However, the causes include:

- reduced maternal oxygenation such as chronic disease states,
- utero-placental damage (see Chapter 15, Fetal growth restriction),

- impaired fetal blood supply to the placenta, as in cord accidents,
- intrinsic fetal conditions resulting in poor tissue oxygenation, such as fetal anaemia.

## PHYSIOLOGY

The human fetus demonstrates complex patterns of activity from early pregnancy. These include fetal breathing movements, gross body movements and fine motor movements. The linkage of gross body movements to other behavioural patterns has led to the description of fetal behavioural states.[1] Fetal body movements are frequent during state 2F (periods of activity analogous to rapid eye movement (REM) sleep), whereas in 1F, the fetus is quiescent (analogous to non-REM sleep). A third state, 4F, occurs when the fetus displays frequent and vigorous gross body movements; this appears to represent fetal wakefulness.

Human fetal breathing movements occur 30 per cent of the time and gross body movements 10 per cent of the time during the last 10 weeks of pregnancy.[2,3] Cycling between activity and quiescence occurs over a time span of approximately 60 minutes at term. In most fetuses, activity is highest in late evening. Fetal heart rate variation increases during fetal activity, and accelerations are associated with fetal body movements.[4]

As outlined above, a fetus exposed to hypoxia will become progressively more acidotic and will eventually suffer irreversible damage, leading ultimately to death. During this process, the fetus will demonstrate several adaptations designed to conserve energy and reduce oxygen.

One of the first responses of the fetus is to reduce movements, although the human fetus may well adapt to hypoxia in the absence of acidaemia, with breathing movements, in particular, reverting to normal.[5] It would appear that reduced fetal heart rate reactivity and absence of fetal breathing movements are earlier manifestations of fetal hypoxia. With more severe hypoxia, fetal body movements and tone become abnormal. Blood is distributed preferentially to the brain, myocardium and adrenals at the expense of organs such as the kidney. This renal hypoperfusion results in a reduced glomerular filtration rate, oliguria and hence reduced liquor volume. As fetal growth accounts for a substantial fraction of the total substrate consumption, it is reduced – leading to fetal growth restriction (FGR). The majority of the currently available tests of fetal well-being are designed to detect these adaptive changes.

## TESTS OF FETAL WELL-BEING

### Fetal movement counting

Maternal perception of fetal movements occurs from the second trimester. It is well recognized that, on an individual basis, reduced maternal perception of movements may be the harbinger of a sick fetus. However, all too often the mother will present too late, with her fetus already dead. Alternatively, the fetus may well be demonstrating normal activity with the mother failing to recognize those movements.

Structured fetal movement counting (FMC) has been advocated in an attempt to reduce these confounding effects. In the largest study to date, Grant et al.[6] reported a randomized controlled trial (RCT) evaluating the effects of FMC involving 68 000 women. The authors concluded that routine daily counting by women, followed by appropriate action when movements are reduced, seemed to offer no advantage over informal inquiry about movements during standard antenatal care and selective use of formal counting in high-risk cases [B]. Although the study did not rule out a beneficial effect of FMC, the policy would have to be used by 1250 women to prevent one perinatal death, and an adverse effect of FMC was just as likely. Based on this study the NICE guidance on antenatal care recommends that evidence to provide formal 'fetal movement' counting does not exist and therefore should not be routinely provided.[7]

The effect of FMC in high-risk pregnancies is not known; however, it would seem prudent to advise women deemed at high risk of fetal compromise to pay careful attention to their fetal movements. It is recommended that women who report a reduction or an alteration in the movements of their fetus should be offered some form of assessment of fetal well-being [E].

## Fetal heart rate recording

### Cardiotocography

Fetal heart rate recording by non-stress test (NST) cardiotocography (CTG) is perhaps the most commonly performed antenatal test of fetal well-being. Although it is quick and simple to perform, interpretation can be difficult; indeed, over 20 studies have demonstrated poor agreement between experts in assessing the various components of the CTG. This reduces the reliability and the predictive value of the CTG. A normal NST would be regarded as a CTG demonstrating two accelerations (15 beats per minute increase lasting for 15 seconds) within a 30-minute trace.[8]

As outlined above, fetal heart rate accelerations are linked closely with fetal movements and are thought to be due to increased sympathetic output. They are strongly indicative of fetal well-being. The long-term variability of the heart rate is produced by a balance between sympathetic and parasympathetic tone, whereas short-term variability (baseline or bandwidth variability) reflects parasympathetic (vagal) tone. Heart rate variability is usually reduced in the compromised fetus and is virtually always absent prior to fetal death. Despite these observations, the predictive value for an abnormal NST for perinatal morbidity and mortality is less than 40 per cent.[8]

Analysis of 13 trials of NST has failed to demonstrate any significant effect on perinatal outcome. Indeed, in a systematic review of four RCTs, NST was associated with a trend towards increased perinatal mortality.[9] It is therefore apparent that NST should not be relied upon as the sole means of establishing fetal well-being [A].

In an effort to improve the predictive ability of antenatal CTG, fetal stress testing has been tried. The basis of this test is to invoke uterine contractions, thereby reducing placental perfusion and unmasking fetal compromise. This can be performed by inducing natural oxytocin release (nipple stimulation) or by maternal oxytocin administration, with the appearance of late fetal heart rate decelerations indicating fetal compromise. The role of this technique has yet to be established and it has been associated with reports of fetal death in cases of unrecognized severe fetal compromise [E].

Stimulation of the fetus by shaking, vibration or even by sound profoundly alters fetal behaviour and heart rate. When used in conjunction with antenatal CTG, vibroacoustic stimulation of the fetus has been found to reduce the number of unreactive traces due to fetal sleep states; however, the effect on the predictive ability of the CTG remains obscure.[10]

## Computerized cardiotocography

In an attempt to improve the objectivity of antenatal CTG, computer programs have been developed to analyse the fetal heart rate recoding. The most advanced and widely used is that developed by the Oxford Group utilizing the Dawes Redman Criteria (Table 14.1).[11] This system places major emphasis on the fetal heart rate variability and, unlike conventional CTG, allows the measurement of short-term variability (STV – defined as the variation measured in 3.75 s epochs). Fetal heart rate variability has been found to be a better predictor of fetal compromise than the presence or absence of fetal heart rate acceleration or decelerations.[12] Indeed, the likelihood of metabolic acidaemia or intrauterine death can be calculated according to the STV.[13]

In addition to the promising evidence of observational studies, one RCT comparing conventional and computerized NST concluded that computerized NST is associated with fewer additional fetal surveillance examinations and less time spent in testing. However, the study was not large enough to demonstrate any effect on severe perinatal morbidity or mortality rates [B].[14] Results from larger RCTs are awaited.

## Biophysical activity

Assessment of fetal activity has been used as a predictor of fetal compromise, with perhaps the best known system being described by Manning in the 1980s.[15] This biophysical profile (BPP) depends on the ultrasonic assessment over 30 minutes of liquor, fetal tone, body and breathing movements and finally NST. Each component is scored discretely as normal (2) or abnormal (0), with a maximum of 10 and scores under 8 being regarded as abnormal (Table 14.2). Observational data based on over 80 000 high-risk pregnancies show that BPP has a negative predictive value of 99.946

**Table 14.1** The Dawes Redman criteria for a normal antenatal computerized cardiotocogram[9]

| |
|---|
| There must be an episode of high variation that is above the first centile for gestational age, high variation being defined as a section of trace where the 1 minute peak-to peak variation is above a predefined threshold for 5 out of 6 consecutive minutes. These episodes of high variation must be greater than the first centile for gestation (11 beats/minute at 38 weeks). |
| There must be no large decelerations (>20 lost beats) |
| The basal heart rate must be between 116 and 160 beats per minute. A slightly lower or higher rate may be acceptable after 30 minutes if all else is normal |
| At least one fetal movement or three accelerations |
| There should be no evidence of a sinusoidal FHR rhythm |
| The short-term variation should be 3 ms or greater |
| Either an acceleration or variability in high episodes the tenth centile and fetal movements >20 |
| There should be no errors or decelerations at the end of the record |

- FHR, fetal heart rate.

**Table 14.2** Parameters of biophysical profile scoring[15]

| |
|---|
| **Fetal breathing movements** – More than one episode of 30 seconds duration or more within a 30 minute period |
| **Gross body/limb movements** – Four or more discrete body movements (including fine motor movements, including thumb sucking, etc.) |
| **Fetal tone and posture** – Active extension and return to flexion opening and closing of mouth and hands, etc. |
| **Fetal heart rate reactivity** – Normal non-stress test over 20 minutes |
| **Amniotic fluid volume evaluation** – One pocket >3 cm and subjectively normal |

per cent and a positive predictive value of 35 per cent for perinatal morbidity including low Apgar scores, acidaemia at birth, fetal distress and fetal growth restriction.[15]

It must be remembered, however, that adverse outcomes are rare, and therefore the false-negative rates of BPP will inevitably be low (1.9/1000 in the series reported by Harman's group[15] giving a false-negative rate of a placebo test of 99.81 per cent). In addition, although there does appear to be a direct relationship between an abnormal BPP and adverse perinatal outcomes, even a borderline score (6) is associated with a 6-fold increase in perinatal mortality rates, indicating that the test may not give sufficient warning to allow effective intervention.

The BPP is a difficult and time-consuming test to perform. In addition, cessation of movements can occur for up to 40–60 minutes due to cycling in fetal behavioural states. Systematic review of five RCTs has failed to demonstrate any significant benefit of BPP on pregnancy outcome when compared to conventional assessment (NST). However, these trials have included fewer than 3000 women and therefore the review concluded that the current evidence is insufficient to reach any definite conclusions about the benefit or otherwise of the BPP [A].[16] Of concern is the observation in one small RCT that use of the BPP was associated with an increase in obstetric interventions without any benefit in perinatal outcomes when compared with assessment by NST and liquor measurement alone.[17] Indeed, the false-positive rate of BPP is in the order of 70 per cent,[15] and this may well lead to increased rates of unnecessary intervention. The most powerful components of the BPP would seem to be liquor volume assessment and NST and therefore assessment of fetal well-being using these two tools alone may well be as effective as formal BPP [B].[17]

### Biophysical profile in pregnancies complicated by pre-labour rupture of the membranes

The observation that fetal activity (in particular fetal breathing movements) is reduced in the presence of chorioamnionitis has led to the suggestion that BPP is of benefit in monitoring women with pre-labour amniorrhexis. However, the sensitivity for abnormal BPP in the presence of chorioamnionitis appears to be no greater than 25 per cent [B].[18] The value of BPP in this context is thus limited; indeed, absence of fetal breathing movements may correlate more to the onset of labour with intrauterine infection than the infection itself.[5]

### Placental grading

Placental grading according to senescent changes seen on ultrasound examination – the Grannum classification – has been demonstrated to reduce perinatal mortality in one RCT.[19] However, this study was small and needs repeating.

This technique has been incorporated in the BPP to give an overall score out of 12 rather than 10.

## Fetal biometry and Doppler ultrasonography

These are covered in Chapter 15, Fetal growth restriction.

## SUMMARY

There is a distinct lack of reliable evidence on which to base protocols for assessing fetal well-being. It is likely that those protocols should incorporate some form of CTG, but this must not form the sole basis for the assessment of the fetus. Computerized CTG may well be more effective than standard CTG. Formal assessment of the BPP does not appear to hold any advantage over assessment of liquor volume alone. Where fetal growth restriction is suspected, fetal biometry and assessment of umbilical artery waveforms by Doppler ultrasonography should be incorporated.

### KEY POINTS

- Systematic review of 20 trials has failed to demonstrate any beneficial effect of CTG alone on perinatal outcomes.
- Observational data from 12 studies and one small RCT have demonstrated that computerized CTG is more efficient than standard CTG.
- Systematic review of seven trials demonstrates that vibro-acoustic stimulation may well reduce the number of false-positive NST CTGs.
- Although observational data based on 80 000 pregnancies show that formal BPP is effective in monitoring the 'at-risk' fetus, systematic review of four RCTs has failed to demonstrate any advantage over simple methods of fetal assessment.
- One RCT has demonstrated that simple monitoring by CTG and liquor assessment is associated with reduced levels of intervention, with similar perinatal outcome compared to BPP.
- Placental grading has been found to be associated with a reduction in perinatal mortality in one small RCT.
- Systematic review of 11 RCTs indicates that the use of umbilical artery Doppler waveform analysis is of benefit in monitoring high-risk pregnancies.

### Key References

1. Nijhuis JG, Prechtl HF, Martin CB Jr, Bots RS. Are there behavioural states in the human fetus? *Early Hum Dev* 1982; **6**: 177–95.
2. Patrick J, Campbell K, Carmichael L *et al.* Patterns of human fetal breathing during the last 10 weeks of pregnancy. *Obstet Gynecol* 1980; **56**: 24–30.

3. Patrick J, Campbell K, Carmichael L *et al*. Patterns of gross fetal body movements over 24-hour observation intervals during the last 10 weeks of pregnancy. *Am J Obstet Gynecol* 1982; **142**: 363–71.

4. Timor-Tritsch IE, Dierker LJ, Zador I *et al*. Fetal movements associated with fetal heart rate accelerations and decelerations. *Am J Obstet Gynecol* 1978; **131**: 276–80.

5. Richardson B. Biophysical activity. In: Rodeck CH, Whittle MJ (eds). *Fetal Medicine: Basic Science and Clinical Practice*. London: Churchill Livingstone, 1999: 919–37.

6. Grant A, Elbourne D, Valentin L, Alexander S. Routine formal fetal movement counting and risk of antepartum late death in normally formed singletons. *Lancet* 1989; **2**: 345–9.

7. National Institute for Health and Clinical Excellence. NICE clinical guideline 62 Antenatal care: routine care for the healthy pregnant woman. London: NICE, 2008.

8. Devoe LD, Castillo RA, Sherline DM. The nonstress test as a diagnostic test: a critical reappraisal. *Am J Obstet Gynecol* 1985; **152**: 1047–53.

9. Pattison N, McCowan L. Cardiotocography for antepartum fetal assessment. *Cochrane Database Syst Rev* 1999; (**2**): CD001068.

10. Tan KH, Smyth R. Fetal vibroacoustic stimulation for facilitation of tests of fetal wellbeing. *Cochrane Database Syst Rev* 2001; (**1**): CD002963.

11. Dawes GS, Moulden M, Redman CW. Improvements in computerized fetal heart rate analysis antepartum. *J Perinat Med* 1996; **24**: 25–36.

12. Dawes GS, Moulden M, Redman CW. The advantages of computerized fetal heart rate analysis. *J Perinat Med* 1991; **19**: 39–45.

13. Dawes GS, Moulden M, Redman CW. Short-term fetal heart rate variation, decelerations, and umbilical flow velocity waveforms before labor. *Obstet Gynecol* 1992; **80**: 673–8.

14. Bracero LA, Morgan S, Byrne DW. Comparison of visual and computerized interpretation of nonstress test results in a randomized controlled trial. *Am J Obstet Gynecol* 1999; **181**: 1254–8.

15. Dayal AK, Manning FA, Berck DJ *et al*. Fetal death after normal biophysical profile score: An eighteen-year experience. *Am J Obstet Gynecol* 1999; **181**: 1231–6.

16. Lalor JG, Fawole B, Alfirevic Z, Devane D. Biophysical profile for fetal assessment in high risk pregnancies. *Cochrane Database of Syst Rev* 2008; (**1**): CD000038.

17. Alfirevic Z, Walkinshaw SA. A randomised controlled trial of simple compared with complex antenatal fetal monitoring after 42 weeks of gestation. *Br J Obstet Gynaecol* 1995; **102**: 638–43.

18. Lewis DF, Adair CD, Weeks JW *et al*. A randomized clinical trial of daily nonstress testing versus biophysical profile in the management of preterm premature rupture of membranes. *Am J Obstet Gynecol* 1999; **181**: 1495–9.

19. Proud J, Grant AM. Third trimester placental grading by ultrasound as a test of fetal wellbeing. *BMJ* 1987; **294**: 1641–4.

# Fetal growth restriction

*Linda Watkins and Murray Luckas*

## INTRODUCTION

One of the most challenging areas currently facing obstetricians is the detection and management of pregnancies in which the growth of the fetus is poor. There is little doubt that these fetuses experience not only increased rates of perinatal morbidity and mortality, but also higher levels of morbidity extending into adult life.

As many as 40 per cent of so-called unexplained stillbirths are small for gestational age (SGA), leading to the suggestion that early detection and timely delivery may well prevent many fetal deaths. Some 30 per cent of sudden infant death syndrome (SIDS) cases were SGA at birth, and the overall infant mortality of infants suffering from fetal growth restriction (FGR) is as much as 8-fold greater than that for appropriately grown infants. These infants are also at high risk of perinatal hypoxia and acidaemia, operative delivery and neonatal encephalopathy. Neonatal problems include hypoglycaemia, hypothermia, hypocalcaemia and polycythaemia. Paradoxically, these infants have a slightly reduced incidence of respiratory distress syndrome, presumably because of the intrauterine stress resulting in increased surfactant production.

It is possible that babies who suffer with FGR are at increased risk of early cognitive and neurological impairment and cerebral palsy. Long-term data from the 1970 British Birth Cohort indicate that adults who were born SGA had significant differences in academic achievement and professional attainment compared with adults who were of normal birth weight. It would also appear that the uterine environment to which the fetus is exposed can lead to 'programming', resulting in consequences in adulthood – the so-called Barker hypothesis. SGA is associated with an increased risk of hypertension, glucose intolerance and atheromatous vascular disease in later life.[1]

## DEFINITIONS

Traditionally, FGR has been synonymous with SGA based on fetal biometry or birth weight, the latter being one of the few unambiguous measurements made in obstetrics. Being SGA is merely a statistical observation, and the incidence of SGA infants will depend on which cut-off is used. The World Health Organization (WHO) suggests that the cut-off should be made at the tenth centile, thus labelling 10 per cent of all infants as SGA.

This approach would appear to be overly simplistic. Chard *et al.*[2] argue that there is no evidence of a distinct subpopulation of low birth weight babies among the whole population of babies at term, and that the majority of SGA babies are in fact 'healthy but small'. Instead, they suggest that the diagnosis of FGR should be reserved for infants that have failed to reach their genetic growth potential. This definition does not adequately categorize abnormalities such as Edward's syndrome (trisomy 18), which commonly have FGR as a feature of their genetic make up. A better definition would be fetuses whose growth velocity slows down or stops completely because of inadequate oxygen and nutritional supply or utilization. It is this group of fetuses with FGR that is most at risk of the sequelae associated with poor growth.

It is self-evident that not all infants suffering from FGR will be SGA and that not all infants who are SGA will suffer from FGR. Indeed, as few as 15 per cent of SGA fetuses may be small as a result of FGR. Although FGR can afflict larger infants – indeed, theoretically, some 70 per cent of fetuses suffering from reduced growth velocity will have a birth weight considered appropriate for gestational age – it does not seem to affect neonatal outcomes unless the fetus is also small, with an abdominal circumference under the fifth centile.[3] It is therefore logical to concentrate on the SGA fetus that is suffering from FGR.

Thus, in summary, using the model espoused by Bobrow and Soothill,[3] SGA fetuses can be categorized according to aetiology into:

1   normal SGA: no structural anomalies, with normal liquor, normal umbilical artery Doppler waveforms (UADWs) and normal growth velocity;
2   abnormal SGA: those with structural or genetic abnormalities;
3   FGR: those with impaired placental function identified by abnormal UADWs and reduced growth velocity.

Biometrical measurement of the fetus allows a further categorization of SGA into symmetrical and asymmetrical. Where the fetus is symmetrically small, both the head and the abdomen are equally affected. This pattern is seen where the fetal insult occurs in early pregnancy, such as with fetal infection, or where the fetus is abnormal. Asymmetrical SGA is seen where the abdomen is small but the head is relatively spared. This pattern is typical of FGR, although it should be remembered that early-onset placental dysfunction can lead to symmetrical SGA.

# AETIOLOGY

The determinants of fetal size are multifactorial. Maternal size is of greater importance in determining fetal size than paternal build. In addition, ethnic and socioeconomic factors play a role, male fetuses being on average some 200 g heavier than their female counterparts at term. The aetiology of SGA can be divided up into maternal factors, fetal factors and, lastly, placental factors.

## Maternal factors

### Nutrition
Population studies such as those performed during the Dutch Hunger Winter in 1944 have demonstrated that significant effects were only seen at the extremes of starvation. Even then, the fetus is relatively protected during the first and second trimesters. Anorexic mothers have twice the risk of having a SGA baby, with a similar level of risk being seen in women whose booking body mass index (BMI) is <19.

### Smoking
There is extensive evidence implicating a link between maternal smoking and SGA, infants of women who smoke being some 460 g lighter than the offspring of non-smokers.

Of concern is the observation that infants delivered by women exposed to passive smoking are 190 g lighter than babies born to women not exposed to tobacco smoke. The causal mechanism of this effect is not clear, but is probably related to increased levels of fetal carboxyhaemoglobin.

## Alcohol and drugs of abuse
The infants of alcoholic women have a 12-fold increase in their risk of SGA. Consumption of more than 15 units (120 g) of alcohol has been associated with a small reduction (66 g) in birth weight, leading the Royal College of Obstetricians and Gynaecologists to recommend that pregnant women keep their alcohol consumption below this threshold [C]. It is unclear whether marijuana and cocaine are independent risk factors for SGA, but heroin does appear to cause a reduction in fetal size (see Chapter 6.12, Drug and alcohol misuse).

## Maternal therapeutic drug administration
Maternal ingestion of beta-blockers, particularly Atenolol, in the second trimester has been linked to SGA infants, as have anticonvulsants, particularly the hydantoins such as phenytoin.

## Maternal disease
Many severe maternal debilitating conditions can lead to a reduction in fetal growth. Severe cardiorespiratory compromise resulting in a failure of adaptation to pregnancy and maternal hypoxaemia can result in reduced fetal growth. Maternal conditions such as sickle cell disease, collagen vascular diseases and the antiphospholipid antibody syndrome, which result in reduced placental bed perfusion, can also result in reduced fetal growth. Meta-analysis shows that women with intrauterine growth restriction had a higher prevalence of heterozygous G20210A prothrombin gene mutation, homozygous MTHFR C677T gene mutation and protein S deficiency than controls [A].[4] Although maternal diabetes is usually associated with fetal overgrowth, where it is complicated by microvascular disease (retinopathy or nephropathy) it can result in poor placental bed perfusion. Lastly, maternal chronic hypertension, particularly if associated with renal impairment, is often associated with reduced fetal growth.

## Fetal factors

### Fetal abnormality
In the second trimester, 20 per cent of SGA fetuses have chromosomal abnormalities, although this rate falls to 1–2 per cent by mid third trimester.[5] Triploidy is the most common finding under 26 weeks, trisomy 18 being the most common abnormality after this time. Growth restriction

is not usually a feature of trisomy 21. Low birth weight is often a feature of non-chromosomal structural anomalies. Major cardiac defects can affect fetal blood flow to the placenta. Gastroschisis is commonly associated with FGR.

## Infection

Reduced fetal growth is frequently seen in intrauterine fetal infection. Examples include varicella, cytomegalovirus, rubella, syphilis and toxoplasmosis. Worldwide, the malaria parasites are a common cause of SGA.

## Placental factors

Placental mosaicism, often associated with chromosomes 16 and 22, is a frequent finding at chorionic villus sampling. This can be associated with reduced placental bulk and placental dysfunction, resulting in severe FGR.

The adequacy of blood supply to the placenta requires invasions and remodelling of the maternal spiral arteries by fetal extravillous trophoblast cells. The end result is destruction of the smooth muscle in the spiral arteries, converting them from high-resistance vessels to low-resistance circulation, thereby promoting an increase in maternal blood supply to the placental bed.

In pregnancies affected by pre-eclampsia and FGR, there is a failure in the second wave of trophoblast invasion, resulting in reduced maternal blood supply to the placental bed (see Chapter 7.6, Pre-eclampsia and non-proteinuric pregnancy-induced hypertension). This does not appear to result in hypoxia in the intervillous spaces but in a reduction in oxygen transfer to the fetus.

On the fetal side of the placenta, this reduced oxygen transfer leads to high impedance of the fetal blood supply to the intervillous space. This may be due to obliteration or defective angiogenesis leading to a reduction in the tertiary villi. It is this high-resistance fetal circulation in the placenta which leads to reduced end-diastolic flow (EDF) velocities detected by UADW analysis (Figure 15.1).

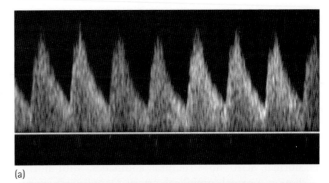

(a)

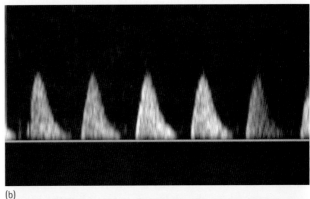

(b)

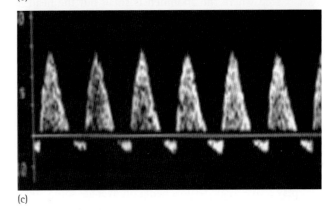

(c)

**Figure 15.1** (a) Umbilical artery Doppler waveforms (UADW) with normal end diastolic flow. (b) Umbilical artery Doppler waveforms (UADW) with absent end diastolic flow. (c) Umbilical artery Doppler waveforms (UADW) with reversed end diastolic flow

## PREDICTION

Accurate prediction of those pregnancies destined to be complicated by FGR would allow increased vigilance and fetal monitoring, which in theory would enable intervention to improve outcomes. Currently, such interventions are limited to avoiding certain risk factors, such as smoking, and timely delivery, thereby avoiding the worst sequelae of FGR.

## History/examination

As outlined above, several risk factors can be identified at booking, such as a BMI <19 and maternal smoking, which place a pregnancy at high risk of FGR. In addition,

a past history of having an SGA baby increases the risk of recurrence in subsequent pregnancies. Congenital uterine anomalies have been associated with a reduction in fetal growth, as have large maternal fibroids. Babies born to older mothers are significantly smaller than the offspring of younger women, although this effect seems to be largely confined to nulliparous women over the age of 40.

Pregnancy-specific complications are also associated with FGR. Pre-eclampsia is perhaps the best known, and many of the placental abnormalities are common to both conditions. Retroplacental haemorrhage in the second and third trimesters can impair placental function sufficiently to reduce fetal growth.

## Maternal serum screening

Several biochemical markers measured in the maternal serum in the second trimester are associated with reduced growth in later pregnancy. These include alpha-fetoprotein (AFP) oestriol (E3), human placental lactogen (HPL) and human chorionic gonadotrophin (hCG). Of these, the most robust is AFP: if the level is 2.5 or more multiples of the median for gestation in the absence of fetal anomaly, there is a 5–10-fold increase in the risk of FGR.

## Ultrasound markers

The best known ultrasonic predictor of subsequent FGR is abnormal uterine artery Doppler velocimetry; this reflects high impedance levels in the maternal arterial blood supply to the placental unit resulting from deficient trophoblast invasion of the maternal spiral arteries. The abnormalities are apparent as either reduced EDF or so-called notching of the waveform. Systematic review of 27 studies involving 12 994 women has shown that abnormal uterine artery Doppler flow velocity is associated with a roughly 3-fold increase in the risk of FGR, although the diagnostic accuracy of the technique is limited [A].[6] It would appear that the combination of unexplained elevated maternal AFP and uterine artery Doppler velocimetry is a much more power predictor of adverse perinatal outcomes (particularly FGR).

Bright or echogenic fetal bowel in the second trimester is associated with an elevated risk of subsequent FGR. Again, a combination of elevated maternal serum AFP (MSAFP) and this ultrasonic marker provides a more precise estimate of the risk of FGR than either predictor alone.

## Scoring systems

Several different scoring systems utilizing various risk factors for reduced fetal growth have been devised to better predict women at particular risk of having an FGR baby. All suffer from poor specificity and sensitivity and are therefore of limited clinical use.

## SCREENING AND DETECTION

Currently, the mainstay of detection of FGR remains the identification of high-risk groups for increased obstetric vigilance, which in most instances includes serial ultrasound examination of the fetus to measure size and growth velocity. Detection of FGR in low-risk women depends upon the identification of SGA fetuses by clinical assessment. Despite the best efforts of providers of obstetric care, it is recognized that only one-quarter of SGA infants in low-risk pregnancies will be recognized in the antenatal period.

## Clinical assessment

Although maternal weight gain in pregnancy has been traditionally recorded, its effectiveness in detecting FGR has never been tested by randomized studies, and observational data give little evidence that it is of benefit. Palpation of the gravid uterus is the standard technique of clinically assessing fetal size; however, it should be remembered that parous women have proven to be more accurate in the estimate of the size of their fetuses than either care providers or one-off fetal measurement by ultrasound. Fundal height measurement (FHM) was introduced as a more objective assessment of the size of the fetus. However, both palpation and FHM to assess the size of the fetus are subject to various factors that reduce their accuracy, such as maternal shape, fetal lie and liquor. A systematic review could only include one controlled study of 1639 women and concluded that there was too little evidence to show whether FHM measurement held advantage over palpation alone [C].[7] Interestingly, Gardosi and Francis[8] have demonstrated in a controlled trial that a policy of serial FHM using a standard technique with plotting on customized antenatal growth charts (adjusted for variables such as maternal height, weight and ethnic group) significantly increased the detection rate of SGA babies, as compared to standard clinical assessment (48 versus 29 per cent) [C]. Although more work is needed, this technique holds promise for increasing the detection rate of SGA babies in low-risk women.

## Ultrasound assessment

Ultrasound examination of the fetus allows biometric measurements; the fetal abdominal circumference is the most accurate predictor of the fetal weight. An estimate of the fetal weight can be made using this measurement, the head circumference, biparietal diameter and the femur length. All these measurements can be plotted on centile charts and should allow the identification of the SGA infant. In addition, comparison of the head and abdominal circumferences will indicate whether the small fetus is symmetrically or asymmetrically small. However, a single set of measurements will not differentiate the normal SGA fetus from the SGA fetus suffering from FGR;[3] this requires serial measurements over time.

Despite the theoretical advantages of screening for FGR by ultrasound, systematic review of seven trials involving some 25 000 low-risk women, comparing a policy of routine ultrasound examination after 24 weeks gestation with scanning based on standard clinical indications, found no advantage of routine ultrasound examination. Routine scanning did not increase the pick-up rate of SGA babies, nor did it significantly affect the perinatal mortality rate [A].[9]

The most effective way of detecting FGR would appear to be by measuring fetal growth over time with serial ultrasound examinations. Serial growth scans are indicated in the woman who is identified as high risk for FGR and/or whose baby is SGA. Although this policy has been universally adopted, it has not been shown to be of benefit in clinical trials [E]. This method of screening for FGR has a high false-positive rate. Mongelli and Gardosi[10] have demonstrated that the use of customized fetal growth charts (again adjusted for variables, such as weight of previous children, maternal height, weight and ethnic group) may reduce this [C]. A 4-week measurement interval was shown to be superior to a 2-week interval, in terms of reducing the false-positive rate.[11] Fortnightly scans should be undertaken where linear growth velocity is not maintained or where the abdominal circumference is below the third centile [E].

The main problem with this approach of serial fetal measurement is one of practicality: clinical imperatives may demand that a diagnosis of FGR is made within a matter of days rather than weeks. Additional indicators of fetal condition may be given by liquor volume, Doppler analysis of the umbilical artery waveform, a careful history of the maternal perception of movements and cardiotocography (CTG).

## Liquor volume

Reduced liquor volumes are a common finding in association with FGR. Progressive fetal hypoxaemia results in blood flow redistribution, with blood being preferentially directed to the brain, with resultant diminished renal perfusion and fetal urine output. The degree of reduction in liquor volume appears to correlate well with the degree of fetal hypoxaemia as reflected by fetal blood $PO_2$ measured at cordocentesis.

## Umbilical artery Doppler velocity studies

Doppler assessment of the umbilical artery waveform demonstrates that, in normal pregnancy, there is forward flow from the fetus to the placenta throughout the cardiac cycle. In the placentae of fetuses suffering from FGR, there is increased vascular resistance, which leads to reduced flow in the diastolic component of the fetal cardiac cycle in the umbilical artery. This reduced flow, together with absent end-diastolic flow (AEDF) or, at the most extreme, reversed end-diastolic flow (REDF), reflects progressive degrees of placental pathology. The degree of abnormality in the UADW correlates well with the risk of fetal hypoxia. In high-risk pregnancies with AEDF, 80 per cent of fetuses will be hypoxic and 46 per cent acidaemic, with the relative risk of perinatal mortality rate being 1.0 where EDF is present, 4.0 with AEDF and 10.6 with REDF.[12]

In a systematic review of 11 randomized, controlled trials conducted in high-risk pregnancies, particularly those complicated by FGR, Neilson and Alfirevic[13] concluded that the use of UADW analysis significantly improved several pregnancy outcomes, including fewer inductions of labour and hospital admissions. In addition, it was associated with

a strong trend towards reducing perinatal mortality (odds ratio 0.71, 95 per cent CI 0.5–1.01). It would thus appear that UADW studies are a valuable tool in the assessment of the SGA infant [A]. In contrast, the use of UADW studies in low-risk pregnancies seems to hold no advantage [A].[14]

Bobrow and Soothill[3] proposed that UADW studies were pivotal in the assessment of the SGA fetus, and allowed the separation of the normal SGA from FGR. This approach has been challenged by an observational study which concluded that abnormal umbilical artery Doppler studies reflect earlier onset and more severe FGR; however, 'normal' SGA fetuses still had high levels of malnutrition at birth and were not all just normal small babies [C].[15] Therefore vigilance is still important for SGA fetuses with normal UADW studies.

Thus, in summary, once a SGA fetus is detected, it is important to consider the causation. A careful history must be obtained from the mother and detailed fetal anatomical assessment, exclusion of fetal infection and karyotyping should be considered. The distinction between normal SGA and FGR can only be made by observing the fetal growth velocity over time. Markers, such as reduced liquor volume and UADW assessment, can aid the distinction.

## MANAGEMENT

## Prophylaxis and treatment

Several prophylactic and therapeutic interventions have been evaluated, perhaps the best known of which is low-dose aspirin administration. Despite promise from early trials, the Collaborative Low-dose Aspirin Study in Pregnancy (CLASP) trial concluded that the prophylactic or therapeutic administration of low-dose aspirin was of no benefit in women deemed as high risk [B].[16] Since then, interventional studies with aspirin have focused on women deemed at high risk not on the basis of history alone but by abnormal maternal uterine artery waveforms. Analysis of these studies indicates that this approach is not justified.[17] The only measures which do seem to be of benefit are smoking cessation, anti-malarial treatment (in high-risk areas) and protein/energy supplementation in poorly nourished women [B].[18] Maternal nutrient supplementation in an attempt to increase fetal weight gain in established cases of FGR may well increase adverse outcomes, and this certainly appears to be true of vitamin C and vitamin E supplementation.

## Monitoring the normal SGA fetus

For the normal SGA fetus, conservative management by fetal surveillance is appropriate. Intervention by delivery is only appropriate if there is evidence of fetal compromise. Umbilical artery Doppler waveform analysis has proved superior to biophysical profile score and computerized CTG analysis in predicting perinatal morbidity in this group,[19] and its inclusion in monitoring policies for these pregnancies is warranted [A].[13]

It must be remembered that AEDF or REDF is unusual in the late third trimester, because the size of the placenta at this stage of pregnancy protects against changes in placental resistance. Fetal compromise is thus possible at this late stage in pregnancy with a normal UADW.

The most important aspect of the biophysical profile would appear to be liquor assessment, and it should also be monitored closely (see Chapter 14, Antenatal tests of fetal well-being). A reduction in the growth velocity of the abdominal circumference often mirrors UADW abnormalities, and continued monitoring of the growth velocity of these fetuses should be performed to detect superimposed FGR [E].

The optimal frequency for fetal assessment in normal SGA is unclear; however, a recent pilot randomized, controlled trial found twice-weekly surveillance held no advantage when compared to fortnightly review.[20] In the absence of other signs of fetal compromise, it is thus appropriate to monitor normal SGA fetuses on a fortnightly basis [B]. The fetal assessment should include biometry, UADW analysis and liquor assessment. Although computerized CTG assessment is superior to conventional CTG assessment, the role of CTGs in the assessment of normal SGA is unclear.

## Monitoring the growth-restricted fetus

Once growth restriction is diagnosed, management options are limited to timely delivery, balancing the risks of continuing with the pregnancy against the risks of prematurity. This policy is based on the assumption that timely delivery will improve the outcome; however, this has never been tested (nor is it ever likely to be) by an interventional trial. The Growth Restriction Intervention Trial (GRIT) randomized women to delivery or conservative management where the clinician was uncertain. This trial found no significant difference in deaths before discharge between immediate delivery and delayed delivery.[21] The overall rate of death or severe disability at two years was 55 (19 per cent) of 290 immediate births, and 44 (16 per cent) of 283 delayed births. With adjustment for gestational age and umbilical-artery Doppler category, the odds ratio (95 per cent CI) was 1.1 (0.7–1.8). Most of the observed difference was in disability in babies younger than 31 weeks of gestation at randomization: 14 (13 per cent) immediate versus five (5 per cent) delayed deliveries. No important differences in the median Griffiths developmental quotient in survivors were seen [B].[22]

If a diagnosis of FGR in a SGA fetus (on the basis of reduced growth velocity, severely reduced liquor volume or abnormal uterine artery waveform) is made after 34 weeks gestation, delivery is indicated [E].

Under 34 weeks gestation, steroids should be administered prior to delivery if possible; there is no clear evidence to guide management. Between 28 and 34 weeks gestation, the presence of REDF should prompt delivery [E]. The

management of AEDF under 34 weeks gestation and indeed REDF under 28 weeks gestation is more controversial.

It is apparent that the interval between the loss of EDF and fetal demise may vary from days to weeks and that the onset of CTG abnormalities is very late in the process – at which stage fetal damage may well be irreversible. Thus, particularly at the extremes of viability, much interest has been paid to methods of fetal surveillance that would allow pregnancy to be prolonged in cases of FGR with AEDF. In these fetuses, so-called brain sparing can be detected by changes in Doppler waveform indices of the middle cerebral artery (MCA), which represent increased flow. Long-term follow up of fetuses demonstrating increased MCA flow indicate that it is a benign adaptive mechanism. Although this increase in cerebral blood flow occurs sequentially after reduced growth velocity and loss of umbilical artery EDF, reversal of this adaptation is sudden and is associated with a poor prognosis. Thus, serial assessment of the MCA waveform does not give suitable forewarning of deterioration for it to be used in monitoring fetuses with AEDF. Many other arterial waveforms, including those from the fetal aorta and renal arteries, have been assessed, although none seems to be able to predict decompensation in FGR with AEDF. One area of interest is the examination of fetal venous systems. Increased pulsatility in the umbilical veins and vena cava and reversed flow during atrial contraction in the ductus venous do seem to give adequate warning of fetal decompensation, with the latter being particularly promising.[23] This may be an area addressed by a new Cochrane review protocol; fetal and umbilical ultrasound in high risk pregnancy.[24] The management of pregnancies complicated by FGR and AEDF in the umbilical artery should be in units capable of providing intensive neonatal care and should be provided by clinicians with a special interest in fetal medicine [E].

## Labour and delivery

Growth-restricted fetuses are at high risk of intrapartum hypoxia and acidaemia. At gestations under 37 weeks, delivery by caesarean section is usually the best option [E]. It would appear that fetuses with normal UADW tolerate labour well, making induction of labour a possibility at more advanced gestations. It is imperative that adequate plans are made for the management of labour, and these must be clearly documented in the notes. Continual electronic fetal monitoring with early recourse to fetal scalp sampling is strongly advisable. Because of the risk of uterine hypertonicity, prostaglandins and oxytocin must be used with great care [E].

## SUMMARY

The prediction and detection of SGA must be a priority of obstetric care. However, the SGA fetus is not necessarily sick, and efforts should be made to discover why the fetus

Antenatal complications: fetal

is small. If FGR is detected, close monitoring and early intervention for suspected fetal compromise are warranted. If the fetus is normal SGA, providing adequate fetal surveillance is undertaken, a conservative approach is appropriate.

## KEY POINTS

- Observational data indicate that only one-quarter of SGA fetuses are detected antenatally.
- One controlled trial has demonstrated that the detection rate is increased using systematic FHM and customized charts.
- Systematic review of seven RCTs shows no benefit of the routine use of ultrasound in late pregnancy in detecting FGR.
- Systematic review of 11 RCTs indicates that the use of UADW analysis is of benefit.
- Observational data support the use of liquor volume assessment in FGR. There is no clear evidence that formal biophysical profiling is warranted.
- Limited evidence is available to demonstrate an improvement in outcome with timely compared to conservative management for FGR.
- Expert opinion advocates delivery for FGR where the fetus is viable and shows signs of significant compromise.
- One observational study concluded that caesarean section is advisable in the presence of significant abnormalities of the UADW.

## Published Guidelines

Royal College of Obstetricians and Gynaecologists. *Investigation and management of the small-for-gestational-age fetus.* Green top guideline No. 31. London: RCOG, 2002.

## Key References

1. Barker DJ. The long-term outcome of retarded fetal growth. *Clin Obstet Gynecol* 1997; **40**: 853–63.
2. Chard T, Yoong A, Macintosh M. The myth of fetal growth retardation at term. *Br J Obstet Gynaecol* 1993; **100**: 1076–81.
3. Bobrow CS, Soothill PW. Fetal growth velocity: a cautionary tale. *Lancet* 1999; **353**: 1460.
4. Alfirevic Z, Roberts D, Martlew V. How strong is the association between maternal thrombophilia and adverse pregnancy outcome? A systematic review. *Eur J Obstet Gynecol Reprod Biol* 2002; **101**: 6–14.
5. Snijders RJ, Sherrod C, Gosden CM, Nicolaides KH. Fetal growth retardation: associated malformations and chromosomal abnormalities. *Am J Obstet Gynecol* 1993; **168**: 547–55.
6. Chien PF, Arnott N, Gordon A *et al.* How useful is uterine artery Doppler flow velocimetry in the prediction of pre-eclampsia, intrauterine growth retardation and perinatal death? An overview. *Br J Obstet Gynaecol* 2000; **107**: 196–208.
7. Neilson JP. Symphysis–fundal height measurement in pregnancy. *Cochrane Database Syst Rev* 2000; (**2**): CD000944.
8. Gardosi J, Francis A. Controlled trial of fundal height measurement plotted on customised antenatal growth charts. *Br J Obstet Gynaecol* 1999; **106**: 309–17.
9. Bricker L, Neilson JP, Dowswell T. Routine ultrasound in late pregnancy (after 24 weeks gestation). *Cochrane Database Syst Rev* 2008; (**4**): CD001451.
10. Mongelli M, Gardosi J. Reduction of false-positive diagnosis of fetal growth restriction by application of customized fetal growth standards. *Obstet Gynecol* 1996; **88**: 844–8.
11. Owen P, Maharaj S, Khan KS, Howie PW. Interval between fetal measurements in predicting growth restriction. *Obstet Gynecol* 2001; **97**: 499–504.
12. Karsdorp VH, van Vugt JM, van Geijn HP *et al.* Clinical significance of absent or reversed end diastolic velocity waveforms in umbilical artery. *Lancet* 1994; **344**: 1664–8.
13. Neilson JP, Alfirevic Z. Doppler ultrasound for fetal assessment in high risk pregnancies. *Cochrane Database Syst Rev* 2000; (**2**): CD000073.
14. Bricker L, Neilson JP. Routine Doppler ultrasound in pregnancy. *Cochrane Database Syst Rev* 2000; (**2**): CD001450.
15. McCowan LM, Harding JE, Stewart AW. Umbilical artery Doppler studies in small for gestational age babies reflect disease severity. *Br J Obstet Gynaecol* 2000; **107**: 916–25.
16. CLASP: a randomised trial of low-dose aspirin for the prevention and treatment of pre-eclampsia among 9364 pregnant women. CLASP (Collaborative Low-dose Aspirin Study in Pregnancy) Collaborative Group. *Lancet* 1994; **343**: 619–29.
17. Goffinet F, Aboulker D, Paris-Llado J *et al.* Screening with a uterine Doppler in low risk pregnant women followed by low dose aspirin in women with abnormal results: a multicentre randomised controlled trial. *Br J Obstet Gynaecol* 2001; **108**: 510–18.
18. Gulmezoglu M, de Onis M, Villar J. Effectiveness of interventions to prevent or treat impaired fetal growth. *Obstet Gynecol Surg* 1997; **52**: 139–49.
19. Soothill PW, Ajayi RA, Campbell S, Nicolaides KH. Prediction of morbidity in small and normally grown fetuses by fetal heart rate variability, biophysical profile score and umbilical artery Doppler studies. *Br J Obstet Gynaecol* 1993; **100**: 742–5.
20. McCowan LM, Harding JE, Roberts AB *et al.* A pilot randomized controlled trial of two regimens of fetal surveillance for small-for-gestational-age fetuses with normal results of umbilical artery Doppler velocimetry. *Am J Obstet Gynecol* 2000; **182**: 81–6.

21. GRIT Study Group. A randomised trial of timed delivery for the compromised preterm fetus: short term outcomes and Bayesian interpretation. *BJOG* 2003; **110**: 27–32.

22. GRIT study group. Infant wellbeing at 2 years of age in the Growth Restriction Intervention Trial (GRIT): multicentred randomised controlled trial. *Lancet* 2004; **364**: 513-20.

23. Baschat AA, Cosmi E, Bilardo CM *et al.* Predictors of neonatal outcome in early-onset placental dysfunction. *Obstet Gynecol* 2007; **109**: 253–61.

24. Alfirevic Z, Stampalija T, Gyte GML, Neilson JP. Fetal and umbilical Doppler ultrasound in high-risk pregnancies (Protocol). *Cochrane Database Syst Rev* 2010; (**1**): CD007529.

# Aberrant liquor volume

*Sailesh Kumar*

## MRCOG standards

- Know the physiology of amniotic fluid production throughout gestation.
- Understand the various stages of development of the fetal lung.
- Know the common causes of amniotic fluid volume abnormalities.
- Appreciation of a logical plan of investigation and management.

## INTRODUCTION

Amniotic fluid surrounds the fetus in intrauterine life, providing protected, low-resistance space suitable for growth and development. The total amniotic fluid volume (AFV) arises from secondary partitioning of body water within the fetoplacental extracellular space and reflects fetal fluid balance, which is in a homeostatic state of constant flux.

There is a wide variation in amniotic fluid volume throughout gestation, with a gradual increase as pregnancy progresses before decreasing after 36 weeks gestation. Amniotic fluid volume is the net result between inflow and outflow of fluid into the amniotic cavity. In early gestation the most likely source of amniotic fluid is active transport of solute by the amnion into the amniotic space with water moving passively along. Later in pregnancy, fetal urine, secretions from the respiratory tract, transfer of fluid across the chorionic plate and umbilical cord (intramembranous flow) and movement of fluid directly between the amniotic cavity and maternal blood across the wall of the uterus (transmembranous flow) all contribute to amniotic fluid volume. Fetal urine is present in the amniotic space as early as 8–11 weeks gestation, but is the major contributor of amniotic fluid only later in pregnancy. At term, fetal urine flow may be as much as 1000–1200 mL/day. Any condition that prevents either the formation of urine (renal agenesis, renal dysplasia) or its egress into the amniotic sac (bladder outlet obstruction, fetal growth restriction) will cause

oligohydramnios. Any condition that causes increased fetal urine production (maternal diabetes) may cause polyhydramnios.

After approximately 20 weeks, when the fetal skin keratinizes, there are several potential mechanisms that allow fluid to either enter or leave the amniotic space. The excretion of fetal urine and swallowing of amniotic fluid by the fetus represent one of the main pathways for the formation and clearance of amniotic fluid. The fetal lungs also contribute significantly to amniotic fluid by secreting large volumes of fluid every day. Other potential mechanisms include fluid transfer across the placenta and secretions from the fetal oro-nasal cavities. Fetal swallowing plays an important role in maintaining amniotic fluid volume during the latter half of the pregnancy. Obstruction to the upper gastrointestinal tract (esophageal atresia, duodenal atresia) or any condition that impairs fetal swallowing will result in polyhydramnios. Table 16.1 shows the various contributions to the inflow and outflow of amniotic fluid in the human fetus.

In the first trimester, amniotic fluid has an electrolyte composition and osmolality similar to that of fetal and maternal blood. As fetal urine begins to enter the amniotic cavity, amniotic fluid osmolality decreases compared with fetal blood. Near term, the amniotic fluid osmolality is lowest (250–260 mOsm/kg water) compared with fetal blood osmolality of 280 mOsm/kg water. This low osmolality is a result of extremely hypotonic fetal urine (60–140 mOsm/kg water) in combination with a lesser volume of isotonic lung fluid.

Clinical assessment of AFV is unreliable, and objective definitions of abnormalities in AVF depend essentially on non-invasive methods such as ultrasound. These include the deepest vertical pool (DVP) or the amniotic fluid index (AFI), which is the total of the DVPs in each of the four quadrants and a more sensitive indicator of AFV throughout gestation.[1,2] In general terms, the DVP is easier to perform and has been demonstrated to be a sensitive ultrasound measure of fetal well-being.[3,4] There is some evidence that AFI is a more sensitive measure of fetal well-being [C]. A recent Cochrane review[5] demonstrated that using the amniotic fluid index increased the number of pregnant

**Table 16.1** Daily amniotic fluid dynamics in the human fetus

| Inflow | Outflow |
|---|---|
| Urine flow (1000–1200 mL) | Swallowing (500–1000 mL) |
| Lung fluid (340 mL) (50 per cent swallowed) | Intramembranous (200–500 mL) |
| Pharyngeal fluid (10 mL) | Transmembranous (10 mL) |

women who were diagnosed with oligohydramnios and induced for an abnormal fluid volume when compared with the deepest vertical pocket measure. These women also had a higher rate of caesarean section for so-called fetal distress. Yet the rate of admission to neonatal intensive care units and the occurrence of neonatal acidosis, an objective assessment of fetal well-being, were similar between the two groups. Other authors suggest that because the AFI excessively identifies pregnancies at risk, leading to greater intervention without any improvement in perinatal outcome, its use should be abandoned in favour of the DVP.[6]

# OLIGOHYDRAMNIOS

Oligohydramnios defined by a DVP of less than 2 cm complicates approximately 3.9 per cent of pregnancies.[3] When oligohydramnios occurs later in pregnancy, the perinatal outcome is poor, with perinatal mortality rates approaching 90 per cent.[4,7,8] This increased perinatal mortality is mainly related to the underlying aetiology and gestation from which oligohydramnios occurs. The common causes of oligohydramnios are shown in Table 16.2.

Perhaps the most common cause of oligohydramnios is preterm premature rupture of membranes (PPROM), which occurs in approximately 3–17 per cent of all pregnancies. Although clinical evidence for membrane rupture is obvious in the majority of cases, ultrasonic evidence of decreased liquor is present in only 5–44 per cent.[9,10]

Oligohydramnios may be associated with intrauterine growth restriction, when it is often associated with a fetal abdominal circumference (AC) measurement (using ultrasound) below the 10th centile for gestation, poor fetal growth velocity (DAC of >1 S.D. over 14 days) and abnormal

**Table 16.2** Causes of oligohydramnios

| |
|---|
| Preterm premature rupture of membranes |
| Placental insufficiency (intrauterine growth restriction) |
| Congenital fetal anomalies |
|     Renal agenesis |
|     Urethral obstruction (atresia or posterior urethral valves) |
|     Renal dysplasia |

umbilical artery waveform velocimetry. Such findings are associated with increased perinatal risk, as is oligohydramnios in isolation.[11] In cases of early-onset intrauterine growth restriction (<24 weeks), there is a strong association with abnormal maternal uterine artery Doppler waveforms (indicating malplacentation), but if these waveform velocities are normal, the association with aneuploidy and structural anomalies is as high as 25 per cent.

Renal anomalies account for up to 57 per cent[12] of cases, with severe oligohydramnios presenting in the mid-second trimester of pregnancy. Such anomalies are severe and include bilateral renal agenesis, multicystic or dysplastic kidneys or bladder outlet obstruction, resulting in impaired urine production that is primary or secondary to urinary tract obstruction.

## Fetal and maternal risks

The main fetal risks relate primarily to pulmonary hypoplasia, chorioamnionitis subsequent to PPROM, and prematurity. Perinatal mortality is increased largely due to prematurity and the association with congenital malformations. Approximately 7 per cent of pregnancies complicated by oligohydramnios are associated with congenital malformations. This incidence rises to almost 35 per cent when amniorrhexis occurs in the second trimester.[12,13] The sequelae of oligohydramnios, flattened facies, postural deformities and pulmonary hypoplasia, are referred to as the Potter syndrome, first reported in association with bilateral renal agenesis. The main risk associated with severe oligohydramnios is pulmonary hypoplasia, which depends critically on the gestation at which it occurs and, to a slightly lesser extent, on its duration and severity. At gestations less than 22 weeks, the perinatal mortality is extremely high. The true incidence of pulmonary hypoplasia is probably underestimated at between 9 and 11/10 000 live births. PPROM before 25 weeks where the DVP is <1 cm has a predicted mortality rate of more than 90 per cent.[14,15]

There are very few maternal risks, unless fetal therapy is considered (i.e. the placement of a vesicoamniotic shunt or amniodrainage). These procedures carry the risk of abruptio placentae and chorioamnionitis.

## Management

The main management objective is to confirm the aetiology of the oligohydramnios and therefore to define prognosis. PPROM is often apparent from the history and clinical examination (the diagnosis and management of PPROM are discussed in Chapter 22, Premature rupture of membranes). The earlier the amniorrhexis occurs, the higher the incidence of subsequent pulmonary hypoplasia [C].[14]

An AFI <5 cm after preterm premature rupture of the membranes between 24 and 32 weeks gestation is associated with an increased risk of perinatal infection and a shorter latency preceding delivery.[16]

In general terms, there is a strong association with severe oligohydramnios/anhydramnios and perinatal mortality associated with pulmonary hypoplasia [C]. Small series of treatment with amnioinfusion have been attempted in the past, but with no reduction in perinatal mortality [D]. Consequently, severe oligohydramnios prior to 24 weeks carries a poor prognosis.[14]

Clinical examination may reveal the presence of chronic hypertension or pre-eclampsia and/or a symphysiofundal height that is small for gestation. Subsequent ultrasound biometry may reveal intrauterine growth restriction[11] or the presence of structural anomalies. A combination of biophysical studies and Doppler waveform analyses (of both uterine and umbilical circulations) may be used to assess fetal well-being and as indirect measures of placental function [A].[17]

The exclusion of congenital anomalies in combination with aneuploidy or isolated is mandatory. Renal agenesis may be difficult to confirm because of the large size of the fetal adrenal glands. However, the inability to visualize a fetal bladder on serial ultrasound examinations and bilateral absence of renal arteries using colour/power Doppler increase the sensitivity of this diagnosis. In cases of urinary outflow tract obstruction, vesicoamniotic shunting in selected cases may significantly increase fetal survival [A].[18] However, long-term renal function may still be significantly impaired, with many children developing end-stage renal failure, need for dialysis and finally renal transplantation.

---

### EBM

- The aetiology of oligohydramnios has a large impact on subsequent perinatal mortality [C]. This group is heterogenous in terms of fetal survival.
- There is a strong association between early-onset oligohydramnios and perinatal mortality, because of an association with preterm labour in amniorrhexis and developmental pulmonary hypoplasia [C].

---

## POLYHYDRAMNIOS

Polyhydramnios is usually defined as a DVP >8 cm or an AFI above the 95th centile for the gestational age. It complicates between 1 and 3.5 per cent of all pregnancies,[4,19,20] and has been shown to be an independent risk factor for perinatal mortality and intrapartum complications among preterm births.[20] In general, polyhydramnios may be caused by increased production of urine from the renal system or by impaired swallowing and intestinal

**Table 16.3** Causes of polyhydramnios

| |
|---|
| Idiopathic |
| Diabetes mellitus |
| Intestinal obstruction (oesophageal or duodenal atresia) |
| Impaired fetal swallowing (anencephaly, aneuploidy, muscular dystrophy) |
| Fetal polyuria (twin-twin transfusion syndrome, Barter syndrome) |
| Cardiac failure secondary to significantly lowered fetal vascular resistance (i.e. sacrococcygeal teratoma, vein of Galen aneurysm) or fetal anaemia (i.e. maternal alloimmunization or parvovirus B19 infection) |
| Fetal infections |

reabsorption of amniotic fluid. The mechanism of polyhydramnios in maternal diabetes mellitus is thought to be secondary to osmotic diuresis in the fetus. However, a large proportion of cases are idiopathic as no obvious cause can be ascertained. The common causes of polyhydramnios are summarized in Table 16.3.

## Fetal and maternal risks

Maternal complications of polyhydramnios mainly relate to distension of the uterus and include preterm labour, abdominal discomfort and uterine atony postpartum. Unstable lie, placental abruption and an increased incidence of caesarean section also result from severe polyhydramnios.

Perinatal mortality in cases of polyhydramnios is increased 10–30 per cent[17,21] and is secondary to the presence of congenital malformations and preterm delivery. Fetal malformations associated with polyhydramnios include pharyngeal/oesophageal obstruction, upper small bowel obstruction (duodenal or jejunal atresia), open neural tube defects, neuromuscular disorders (myotonic dystrophy), cardiac abnormalities, tumours, vascular malformations (Vein of Galen aneurysm), infections, skeletal dysplasias, etc. Aneuploidy is present in up to 10 per cent of fetuses with malformations and in 1 per cent when the polyhydramnios is isolated. In persistent polyhydramnios, the risk of aneuploidy is increased (10–20 per cent) compared with polyhydramnios that resolves.

## Management

It is important to evaluate each case thoroughly in a systematic manner. A careful history, with attention to maternal symptoms, diseases such as diabetes mellitus or red cell alloimmunization or recent viral infections, is important.

High-resolution ultrasound should be performed to assess the degree of polyhydramnios, identify multiple pregnancies, and target assessment of fetal anomalies. Fetal assessment should include examination of the fetal thorax, central nervous system and gastrointestinal and renal systems. Karyotyping should be offered, particularly in association with structural anomalies. If a viral infection is suspected, appropriate fetal and maternal samples should be obtained (see Chapter 7.4, Infection and Chapter 13, Fetal infections). If the excess liquor is associated with anaemia, the fetus is almost always hydropic. Assessing the fetal middle cerebral peak systolic velocity helps identify anaemic fetuses with 100 per cent sensitivity. Correction of the underlying condition with serial *in-utero* fetal transfusions frequently results in amelioration of the polyhydramnios [C].

A major management aim is to reduce maternal discomfort and prolong the pregnancy. Treatment is only indicated when there is severe polyhydramnios (AFI >40 cm; DVP >12 cm), as this is associated with increases in intra-amniotic pressure [C].[22]

Treatment options include pharmacological management with cyclo-oxygenase inhibitors (i.e. indomethacin and sulindac). Prostaglandin synthase inhibitors and, more recently, selective cyclo-oxygenase-2 (COX-2) inhibitors may also be used to decrease fetal urine output and hence reduce the polyhydramnios. Prostaglandin synthase inhibitors, such as indomethacin, are associated with renal failure in neonates and premature closure of the ductus arteriosus, resulting in perinatal mortality [E]. There are also reports of necrotizing enterocolitis and intracranial haemorrhage in infants treated with indomethacin *in utero* [E]. Serial amnioreduction in singleton pregnancies has been advocated but carries the risk of precipitating preterm labour and leads to rapid re-accumulation of liquor.

Polyhydramnios associated with twin–twin transfusion syndrome (stage 1 or 2) is often treated with serial amnioreduction. In more advanced disease (stage 3 or 4), fetoscopic ablation of placental vascular anastomoses is the treatment of choice and is associated with not only resolution of the polyhydramnios in the recipient twin's sac, but also survival rates of greater than 75 per cent (see Chapter 12, Multiple pregnancy).[23]

Termination of pregnancy should be offered for aneuploidy, lethal anomalies and major malformations. Counselling by a paediatric surgeon is helpful if a surgical cause is felt likely. The patient should be counselled about risks of preterm membrane rupture (preterm labour, malpresentation, cord prolapse, chorioamnionitis). If the polyhydramnios persists, elective delivery by 38 weeks is reasonable in view of the increased risk of unexplained stillbirth. There is 2–5 times increased risk of perinatal mortality. Vaginal delivery is possible if the fetal head is reasonably fixed in the pelvis. Labour needs to be monitored carefully as there is an increased incidence of cord prolapse and fetal distress.

## KEY POINTS

- Polyhydramnios is associated with increased perinatal morbidity and mortality [C].
- A careful search for the underlying cause is mandatory.
- In cases in which no secondary cause is identifiable, the gestational age of delivery may be prolonged by the use of cyclo-oxygenase inhibitors [D]. However, this form of pharmacotherapy is not without risk.

## Key References

1. Moore TR, Cayle JE. The amniotic fluid index in normal human pregnancy. *Am J Obstet Gynecol* 1990; **162**: 1168–73.

2. Moore TR. Superiority of the four-quadrant sum over the single-deepest-pocket technique in ultrasonographic identification of abnormal amniotic fluid volumes. *Am J Obstet Gynecol* 1990; **163**: 762–7.

3. Philipson EH, Sokol RJ, Williams T. Oligohydramnios: clinical associations and predictive value for intrauterine growth retardation. *Am J Obstet Gynecol* 1983; **146**: 271–8.

4. Chamberlain PF, Manning FA, Morrison I *et al.* Ultrasound evaluation of amniotic fluid volume. II. The relationship of increased amniotic fluid volume to perinatal outcome. *Am J Obstet Gynecol* 1984; **150**: 250–4.

5. Nabhan AF, Abdelmoula YA. Amniotic fluid index versus single deepest vertical pocket as a screening test for preventing adverse pregnancy outcome. *Cochrane Database Syst Rev* 2008; (**3**): CD006593.

6. Magann EF, Chauhan SP, Doherty DA *et al.* The evidence for abandoning the amniotic fluid index in favor of the single deepest pocket. *Am J Perinatol* 2007; **24**: 549–55.

7. Barss VA, Benacerraf BR, Frigoletto FD Jr. Second trimester oligohydramnios, a predictor of poor fetal outcome. *Obstet Gynecol* 1984; **64**: 608–10.

8. Mercer LJ, Brown LG. Fetal outcome with oligohydramnios in the second trimester. *Obstet Gynecol* 1986; **67**: 840–2.

9. Gonik B, Bottoms SF, Cotton DB. Amniotic fluid volume as a risk factor in preterm premature rupture of the membranes. *Obstet Gynecol* 1985; **65**: 456–9.

10. Robson MS, Turner MJ, Stronge JM, O'Herlihy C. Is amniotic fluid quantitation of value in the diagnosis and conservative management of prelabour membrane rupture at term? *Br J Obstet Gynaecol* 1990; **97**: 324–8.

11. Chang TC, Robson SC, Boys RJ, Spencer JA. Prediction of the small for gestational age infant: which ultrasonic measurement is best? *Obstet Gynecol* 1992; **80**: 1030–8.

12. Moore TR, Longo J, Leopold GR *et al.* The reliability and predictive value of an amniotic fluid scoring

system in severe second-trimester oligohydramnios. *Obstet Gynecol* 1989; **73**: 739–42.

13. Mercer LJ, Brown LG, Petres RE, Messer RH. A survey of pregnancies complicated by decreased amniotic fluid. *Am J Obstet Gynecol* 1984; **149**: 355–61.

14. Kilbride HW, Yeast J, Thibeault DW. Defining limits of survival: lethal pulmonary hypoplasia after midtrimester premature rupture of membranes. *Am J Obstet Gynecol* 1996; **175**: 675–81.

15. Kilbride HW, Thibeault DW. Neonatal complications of preterm premature rupture of membranes. Pathophysiology and management. *Clin Perinatol* 2001; **28**: 761–85.

16. Vermillion ST, Kooba AM, Soper DE. Amniotic fluid indexes after preterm rupture of the membranes and subsequent perinatal infection. *Am J Obstet Gynecol* 2000; **183**: 271–6.

17. Alfirevic Z, Neilson JP. Doppler ultrasonography in high-risk pregnancies: systematic review with meta-analysis. *Am J Obstet Gynecol* 1995; **172**: 1379–87.

18. Clark TJ, Martin WL, Divakaran TG *et al.* Prenatal bladder drainage in the management of the fetal lower urinary tract obstruction: a systematic review and meta-analysis. *Obstet Gynecol* 2003; **102**: 367–82.

19. Hill LM, Breckle R, Thomas ML, Fries JK. Polyhydramnios: ultrasonically detected prevalence and neonatal outcome. *Obstet Gynecol* 1987; **69**: 21–5.

20. Mazor M, Ghezzi F, Maymon E *et al.* Polyhydramnios is an independent risk factor for perinatal mortality and intrapartum morbidity in preterm delivery. *Eur J Obstet Gynecol Reprod Biol* 1996; **70**: 41–7.

21. Carlson DE, Platt LD, Medearis AL, Horenstein J. Quantifiable polyhydramnios: diagnosis and management. *Obstet Gynecol* 1990; **75**: 989–93.

22. Fisk NM, Tannirandorn Y, Nicolini U *et al.* Amniotic pressure in disorders of amniotic fluid volume. *Obstet Gynecol* 1990; **76**: 210–14.

23. Fox C, Kilby MD, Khan KS. Contemporary treatments for twin-twin transfusion syndrome. *Obstet Gynecol* 2005; **105**: 1469–77.

# Chapter 17

# Fetal hydrops

*Sailesh Kumar*

---

## MRCOG standards

- Know the pathophysiology of fetal hydrops.
- Understand the various causes of fetal hydrops (particularly non-immune hydrops).
- Appreciate the non-Rh causes of immune fetal hydrops.
- Know the relevant maternal and fetal investigations.

## INTRODUCTION

Hydrops is defined as the accumulation of fluid in the interstitial tissue (skin) and two serous cavities.[1,2] It is further subdivided into 'immune' (IH) or 'non-immune' (NIH), a distinction made on the presence of maternal alloimmunization (i.e. blood group incompatibility). Table 17.1 indicates the distribution of aetiologies of hydrops fetalis in a contemporary published series. Hydrops is an end-stage process for a number of fetal diseases resulting in tissue oedema and/or fluid collection (ascites, pleural effusion, pericardial effusion) in various sites. Its aetiology may be either immune or non-immune, depending on the presence or absence of red cell alloimmunization. Non-immune causes now account for 90 per cent of all cases of hydrops. The most common causes associated with hydrops are congenital heart abnormalities, abnormalities in heart rate, twin-to-twin transfusion syndrome, congenital anomalies, aneuploidy, infections, congenital anemia and congenital chylothorax. In general terms, it carries a high perinatal mortality (in some series up to 80 per cent) but the variability of outcome is reflected in its many possible underlying aetiologies.[1,2]

## INCIDENCE

Historically, Rhesus (Rh) alloimmunization accounted for the majority of cases of fetal hydrops. However, with the advent of large-scale antenatal anti-D prophylaxis, NIH

**Table 17.1** Number of cases of hydrops by aetiology ($n = 63$)[2]

| Aetiology | Number | Percentage |
|---|---|---|
| **A – Immune hydrops** | 8/63 | 12.7 |
| Anti-D antibodies[a] | 5/8 | 62.5 |
| Anti-Kell antibodies | 2/8 | 25 |
| Anti-c | 1/8 | 12.5 |
| **B – Non-immune hydrops** | 55/63 | 87.3 |
| HPVB19 | 8/55 | 14.5 |
| Thoracic/pulmonary causes | 6/55 | 10.9 |
| Chylothorax | 4/6 | 66.7 |
| Cystic adenomatoid malformation | 1/6 | 16.7 |
| Diaphragmatic hernia | 1/6 | 16.7 |
| Chromosomal abnormality | 14/55 | 25.5 |
| Trisomy 21 | 6/14 | 42.9 |
| Trisomy 13 | 1/14 | 7.1 |
| Turner's syndrome | 5/14 | 35.7 |
| Others[b] | 2/14 | 14.2 |
| Feto-maternal haemorrhage | 1/55 | 1.8 |
| Cardiac causes | 5/55 | 9.1 |
| SVT | 3/5 | 60 |
| CCHB | 1/5 | 20 |
| Congenital heart defects | 1/5 | 20 |
| Cystic hygroma | 6/55 | 10.9 |
| Fetal akinesia | 1/55 | 1.8 |
| Congenital myotonic dystrophy | 1/55 | 1.8 |
| TTTs | 2/55 | 3.6 |
| Idiopathic | 8/55 | 14.5 |
| Unclassified | 3/55 | 5.5 |

[a] Anti-C antibodies were found in the maternal serum of four patients, and anti-E 1 Fya antibodies in the fifth.

[b] The karyotypes were 46XY add10, q24 (*de novo*) and 46XX, t(1;4) (q42;q32) (*de novo*).

- HPVB19, human parvovirus B19; SVT, supraventricular tachycardia; CCHB, complete congenital heart block; TTTs, twin-to-twin transfusion syndrome.

- Reproduced from reference 2 with permission from Parthenon Publishing.

now represents the major challenge facing obstetricians and most contemporaneous studies indicate that NIH is more common.[1,2] The true incidence of NIH is population variable and probably also subject to seasonal variation. For example, homozygous alpha-thalassaemia is the most common cause of fetal hydrops in South East Asia and arguably the leading cause of NIH worldwide. However, this is an uncommon cause of the condition in the UK; aneuploidy, structural anomalies and human parvovirus are more commonly noted associations.[2,3]

## DIAGNOSIS

The diagnosis of fetal hydrops is made most commonly on ultrasound examination of the fetus, although it can be made pathologically. The condition is characterized by skin oedema and serous effusion in two or more body cavities (pleural or pericardial effusions and ascites).[3] There is some evidence that the distribution of serous effusion relates to the underlying aetiologies (Figure 17.1) [C]. The umbilical cord and placenta are frequently affected and are often oedematous. Polyhydramnios is also a common association (see Chapter 16, Aberrant liquor volume).

## PATHOPHYSIOLOGY OF FETAL HYDROPS

The exact pathophysiological process is not defined, but the microvascular fluid exchange system is defined by Starling's law controlling intravascular–interstitial fluid exchange. This is believed to be associated with changes in the movement of fluid across transmembranous pathways associated with a combination of reduced lymphatic drainage, raised intravascular hydrostatic pressure, decreased intravascular oncotic pressure or raised interstitial oncotic pressure [E]. A disturbance of one or a combination of such factors may lead to the development of fetal hydrops.

Extravascular accumulation of fluid may occur as a result of decreased intravascular osmotic pressure, increased intravascular hydrostatic pressure, or aberrations in lymphatic flow. Hypoalbuminaemia may cause low intravascular oncotic pressure. Hypoxic mediated endothelial damage may result in leaking of albumin into the interstitial space. Fetal liver dysfunction (in chronically anaemic fetuses with increased extramedullary erythropoiesis or portal hypertension) can also result in decreased hepatic production of proteins that result in reduced intravascular oncotic pressure. Fetal cardiac dysfunction or increased intrathoracic pressure (because of lung masses or effusions) can lead to increased central venous pressure and delayed lymphatic drainage which results in the development of hydrops. In most cases, the cause of hydrops is multifactorial.[4]

## COMMON CONDITIONS CAUSING FETAL HYDROPS

### Cardiac abnormalities

Cardiac malformations account for the majority of cases of hydrops. These include hypoplastic left or right heart syndrome, atrioventricular canal abnormalities and valvular lesions. The likely mechanism leading to fetal hydrops is raised central venous pressure secondary to increased right heart pressure or juxtaposition of systemic arterial pressure onto the right heart causing myocardial failure (see Table 17.2 for common conditions causing fetal hydrops[2,3]).

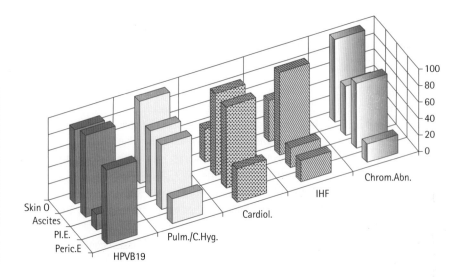

**Figure 17.1** The alterations in fluid distribution by body cavity for different aetiologies.[2] Cardiol., cardiac anomaly; Chrom. Abn., chromosomal abnormalities; HPVB 19, human parvovirus B19; IHF, immune hydrops fetalis; Pulm./C. Hyg., pulmonary anomaly and cystic hygoma; Peric. E., pericardial effusion; Pl. E., pleural effusions; Skin O., skin oedema. Reproduced from reference 2 with permission from Parthenon Publishing

**Table 17.2** Conditions associated with non-immune hydrops

**Cardiovascular**
  Hypoplastic left heart
  Hypoplastic right heart
  A-V canal defects
  Premature closure of foramen ovale
  Transposition of the great vessels
  Ebstein's anomaly
  Atrial flutter
  Supraventricular tachycardia
  Complete heart block
  Placental chorioangioma
  Sacrococcygeal teratoma
  Umbilical cord haemangioma
  Cardiomyopathy

**Chromosomal**
  45X
  Trisomy 13, 18, 21
  Triploidy

**Thoracic**
  Congenital cystic adenomatoid malformation of the lung
  Diaphragmatic hernia
  Pulmonary sequestration
  Primary hydrothorax
  Bronchogenic cyst
  Intrathoracic mass

**Haematologic**
  Alpha-thalassaemia
  Feto-maternal haemorrhage
  Red cell enzyme deficiencies

**Infections**
  Parvovirus B19
  Cytomegalovirus
  Syphilis
  Herpes
  Rubella

**Genetic syndromes**
  Arthrogryposis
  Lethal multiple pterygium syndrome
  Pena–Shokeir syndrome
  Myotonic dystrophy

**Metabolic disorders**
  Gangliosidosis
  Galactosialidosis
  Gaucher's disease

**Twin pregnancy**
  Twin–twin transfusion syndrome
  Acardiac twin

Cardiac dysrhythmia is associated with fetal hydrops, with both tachyarrhythmia and bradyarrhythmia being implicated. Atrial flutter, supraventricular tachycardia (SVT) and complete heart block can all cause hydrops secondary to abnormalities of diastole and direct hypoxia upon myocardial function. As a result, the central venous pressure may rise, causing transudation of fluid into the interstitial space and a consequent inability of the lymphatic system to return the excess fluid into the vascular compartment.

Sacrococcygeal teratomas, placental chorioangioma and vein of Galen aneurysms can all cause hydrops by acting as a large peripheral arteriovenous shunt (decreasing peripheral vascular resistance and afterload). Finally, 'high output' heart failure occurs *in utero*.

## Aneuploidy

Chromosome abnormalities are commonly associated with fetal hydrops in association with or independent of congenital structural anomalies. Turner's syndrome and trisomy 21 together account for the majority of cases and are commonly associated with septate or non-septated cystic hygromata.[2,3] Karyotyping is therefore always indicated as one of the primary investigations in these fetuses.

## Thoracic anomalies

Diaphragmatic hernia, congenital cystic adenomatoid malformation of the lung and pulmonary sequestration cause hydrops by significantly raising intrathoracic pressure and impairing venous return. Compression of the oesophagus may also obstruct fetal swallowing and cause polyhydramnios. Longstanding compression of the fetal lung, either by effusions or by herniated abdominal contents, can cause pulmonary hypoplasia, with accordingly increased perinatal mortality.

## Fetal infections

Parvovirus B19 (erythema infectiosum, Fifth disease) is a significant cause of fetal hydrops; the infection commonly results in an erythematous rash and has high infectivity amongst young children.[5] The transplacental infection rate is approximately 33 per cent, with 9 per cent fetal loss rate. This virus has also been implicated in unexpected stillbirths at term and late miscarriages.[5,6] Parvovirus causes anaemia by destroying cells of the erythroid series, although neutrophils and platelets may also decrease.[6,7] Parvovirus can also directly infect cardiomyocytes and cause myocarditis and cardiac dysfunction, thereby further aggravating the hydrops.[7] The diagnosis of human parvovirus B19 in a hydropic fetus is difficult and requires the isolation of either the viral DNA using polymerase chain reaction (PCR) or parvovirus-specific immunoglobulin M (IgM) from fetal samples.[8] Hydrops tends to occur 2–4 weeks after fetal infection and, as this virus is not known to be associated with congenital malformations or long-term sequelae, fetal therapy in the form of intrauterine, intravascular transfusion(s) may be of benefit. Typically, transfusion of red cells can be of considerable benefit in salvaging some anaemic hydropic fetuses [E].[9,10] However, there has been a report of congenital red cell aplasia in infants who underwent *in-utero* transfusions following parvovirus infection, and hence fetuses treated antenatally should be followed up to detect this potential complication.

A multitude of other viruses (cytomegalovirus, rubella, herpes simplex, coxsackie), bacteria (streptococci), spirochaete (syphilis) and parasites (*Toxoplasma*) can cause fetal infection and occasionally hydrops (see Chapter 13, Fetal infections). However, the effects are variable and no organism consistently or predictably results in either congenital infection or fetal hydrops. Although it is believed that the most common mechanism for the development of hydrops is anaemia, myocarditis and/or hepatitis, other pathways that have yet to be identified may also be responsible. These other viral agents are often associated with high perinatal morbidity and mortality.

## Other causes of fetal hydrops

Structural anomalies of the urinary tract (i.e. urethral atresia) may cause isolated ascites but rarely true hydrops. Urinary ascites occurs when there is rupture of the bladder or renal pelvis secondary to over-distension in lower urinary tract obstruction (posterior urethral valves or urethral atresia). In such cases, both renal dysplasia and severe oligohydramnios are usually present.

Genetic conditions, metabolic disorders and skeletal dysplasias can all cause hydrops by different means. The diagnosis should be considered when a pregnant woman has a positive family history. It is important to try to make as accurate a diagnosis as possible as many of these conditions carry significant recurrence risks, and these patients should receive genetic counselling. In the absence of a family history or definitive diagnosis, most genetic disorders will be undiagnosed and the cause of the hydrops will remain speculative and unexplained. In twin–twin transfusion syndrome complicating monochorionic twins (stage IV or above), the recipient fetus may show signs of hydrops associated with high-output cardiac failure (see Chapter 12, Multiple pregnancy).

## Maternal risks and complications

The maternal 'mirror' syndrome can be associated with fetal hydrops. This is characterized by an unusual type of pre-eclampsia, which has an extremely rapid onset and deterioration. This appears to occur when the placenta is severely oedematous. An increased risk of postpartum haemorrhage and amniotic fluid embolism has also been reported [D].[2]

### KEY POINTS

- There are no EBM guidelines for the treatment of non-immune fetal hydrops; most evidence is in the form of small series from specialist centres [C].
- It is extremely important to exclude aneuploidy and structural malformations using ultrasound.
- Anaemia caused by parvovirus infection is potentially the most treatable condition [E].
- Management should be in a tertiary referral fetal medicine centre [E].

## IMMUNE HYDROPS

The Rh blood group system consists of five major antigens, D, C, c, E and e, all of which can produce erythrocyte alloimmunization.[11] The erythrocyte D antigen is strongly immunogenic and therefore both more important and more common than the other Rh antigens.[11] In classical Rh disease, the mother is RhD negative and the fetus RhD positive. Fetal red cells can enter the maternal circulation at any time during pregnancy through occult fetomaternal haemorrhage. The risk of fetomaternal haemorrhage antenatally increases with gestation from 3 per cent in the first trimester to approximately 65 per cent in the last.

Once maternal sensitization occurs, IgG crosses the placenta and may have very serious effects on the fetus.[11] The concentration of antibody appears to be the most important factor in determining the severity of the disease. The fetus may develop anaemia due to anti-D antibody binding to fetal RhD-positive red blood cells, which are then sequestered in the fetal spleen and undergo haemolysis. Erythropoiesis is stimulated in the fetal liver, which enlarges but is eventually unable to meet the increased demand. Large numbers of erythroblasts are found in the fetal circulation (hence the historical term 'erythroblastosis fetalis'). Severe anaemia develops with cardiac failure, skin oedema, hepatosplenomegaly, ascites and pericardial and pleural effusions. Untreated, these fetuses die or are delivered with hydrops. Less severely anaemic fetuses may be delivered before hydrops occurs but will experience increasingly severe hyperbilirubinaemia (icterus gravis neonatorum), which may proceed to kernicterus due to deposition of unconjugated bilirubin in the grey matter nuclei of the central nervous system.

The frequency and pattern of this condition has changed considerably over the last half century following the introduction of effective prophylaxis using anti-D immunoglobulin administered to the mother after delivery or after any sensitizing events that occur antenatally. Deaths attributable to RhD alloimmunization fell from 46/100 000 births in 1969 to 1.6/100 000 in 1990 in the UK. Similar decreases in prevalence have also been seen worldwide.

The list of antigens other than the Rh system that may cause haemolytic disease is extensive. In practice, atypical antibodies most likely to cause problems include anti-c, anti-kell and anti-E. Haemolytic disease of the ABO system is frequently mild, tends to occur in the first pregnancy and rarely causes severe anaemia or hydrops, causing neonatal jaundice. In contrast to Rh disease, antibodies produced in maternal Kell alloimmunization may cause unpredictably severe and early-onset fetal anaemia [C]. This is secondary to both reticulo-endothelial erythrocyte destruction and suppression of erythropoiesis.[11] The severity and outcome of this form of alloimmunization appear equally unpredictable, whether caused by fetomaternal haemorrhage or exogenous antigen presentation (i.e. transfusion). From 1996, many regions in the UK use Kell-type packed red cells for transfusion in women of reproductive age.

## KEY POINTS

The incidence of Rh disease has decreased dramatically due to the implementation of effective anti-D prophylaxis programmes [A]. Management of Rhesus disease should be based on:

- the maternal antibody titres,
- the paternal genotype,
- the past obstetric history,
- specific screening tests of fetal anaemia.

These factors are designed to detect fetal anaemia prior to the onset of hydrops [C].

- Kell alloimmunization may produce severe early-onset fetal anaemia out of proportion to the antibody titres [C].
- Management should be co-ordinated in fetal medicine centres [E].

# MANAGEMENT OF THE FETUS WITH HYDROPS

Patients whose fetuses are affected with hydrops should be referred to a fetal medicine centre where the necessary expertise and experience are available [E]. A detailed ultrasound scan, including Doppler insonation of the fetal cerebral vasculature and liquor volume, is mandatory [C]. The ultrasound scan must also include careful evaluation of the fetal anatomy and, particularly if skeletal dysplasia is suspected, all the long bones, hands, feet, skull shape and thoracic circumference must be examined.[3]

Karyotyping is mandatory in all cases. Amniocentesis is the method of choice unless anaemia is suspected. Samples should be sent for cytogenetics and infection screen. The placenta and umbilical cord should be carefully examined to exclude a chorioangioma or other vascular abnormalities. This

should also include fetal echocardiography, excluding cardiac malformations and noting normal atrial and ventricular rate and rhythm. Some indication of the cause of hydrops may be obtained from the sites of fluid collection. More recently, the finding that fetal anaemia can be predicted with up to 100 per cent sensitivity using the peak systolic velocity in the middle cerebral artery[12] has significantly improved the assessment of these fetuses. Invasive fetal assessment in hydrops almost always involves fetal blood sampling [C]. This enables fetal blood to be obtained for a variety of investigations (full blood count, karyotype, virology, enzyme studies, liver function tests, acid–base status and protein concentrations). The volume of blood required for these tests is small and should not compromise the fetus. Some of the investigations, such as karyotype or viral studies, can also be carried out on amniotic fluid or chorionic villi; however, fetal blood is preferable for complete haematological, biochemical and metabolic information. The risks of fetal blood sampling in a hydropic fetus are significantly greater than in the non-hydropic state. However, when balanced against the high mortality in such situations, the risk becomes more acceptable [E].

Maternal blood should also be checked for atypical antibodies (indirect Coombs test), full blood count and haemoglobin electrophoresis, viral serology (TORCH titres) and, in selected cases, G6PD and pyruvate kinase carrier status. A Kleihauer–Betke test should be performed to exclude a fetomaternal haemorrhage.[13] Other tests, such as for the presence of anti-Ro and anti-La antibodies, should be performed if the hydropic fetus is severely bradycardic. Many of the tests are selected depending on the clinical picture and family history. If more evidence emerges of unusual viral infections causing hydrops, specific tests to detect these agents may be necessary.

## TREATMENT

Fetal anaemia is treated by *in-utero* intravascular transfusions in hydrops.[13,14] This is the treatment of choice for fetuses affected by red cell alloimmunization, and in experienced hands carries a risk of perinatal death of <10 per cent, with perinatal loss in the hydropic cohort being higher, at 12–15 per cent [C]. Arrhythmias of the fetal heart can be treated either indirectly by administering specific cardiotrophic drugs to the mother or directly to the fetus [C,E]. Although the transfer of drugs through an oedematous placenta is believed to be impaired, cardioversion is certainly possible in many instances.[15] Hydrops secondary to fetal brady-arrhythmias are frequently associated with structural heart abnormalities. The mortality in this group of fetuses is significantly worse.[16]

Pleural effusions can be treated by pleuroamniotic shunting [C],[17,18] and large fetal tumours can be treated either *in utero* or occasionally by open surgery [C,E]. Hydrops in the recipient fetus in twin–twin transfusion syndrome may be treated by either serial amnioreduction or direct fetoscopic laser ablation of communicating placental vessels (see Chapter 12, Multiple pregnancy) [C]. In severe cases where the recipient fetus is hydropic and pre-terminal, selective fetocide using cord occlusion may be the only option if its co-twin is to survive [C].

## OUTCOME

Overall, perinatal mortality in cases of NIH is high (>85 per cent)[2,19,20] despite improvements in diagnosis and management. Early development of hydrops has a particularly poor prognosis. The mortality rate is highest among neonates with congenital anomalies (60 per cent) and lowest among neonates with congenital chylothorax (6 per cent). Mortality is higher in premature infants and those delivered in poor condition (lower 5-minute Apgar scores, higher levels of inspired oxygen support, and more often treated with high-frequency ventilation during the first day after birth). Once the diagnosis is made, urgent referral to a fetal medicine unit is essential.

The outcome in cases of IH treated by serial intrauterine transfusions is much better (85–88 per cent survival).[21] In severe twin–twin transfusion syndrome, the outcome is poor, especially in stage IV disease when the recipient is hydropic.[22]

### KEY POINTS

- Non-immune causes account for the majority of cases of hydrops.
- Karyotyping is essential as part of the diagnostic work up.
- Intrauterine transfusion for foetal anaemia has a high success rate (C).
- Should be managed in a tertiary foetal medicine centre.

## CONCLUSION

Although the aetiology in many cases of NIH is now clearer; fetal NIH remains a difficult clinical problem. Recent advances in fetal therapy have increased the number of treatable conditions, but the overall perinatal morbidity and mortality rates remain high.

## Key References

1. Warsof SL, Nicolaides KH, Rodeck C. Immune and non-immune hydrops. *Clin Obstet Gynecol* 1986; **29**: 533–42.
2. Ismail KMK, Martin WL, Ghosh S *et al.* Etiology and outcome of hydrops fetalis. *J Maternal–Fetal Med* 2001; **10**: 1–7.
3. Saltzman DH, Frigoletto FD, Harlow BL *et al.* Sonographic evaluation of hydrops fetalis. *Obstet Gynecol* 1989; **74**: 106–11.
4. Poeschmann RP, Verheijen RH, Van Dongen PW. Differential diagnosis and causes of nonimmunological hydrops fetalis: a review. *Obstet Gynecol Surv* 1991; **46**: 223–31.
5. Tolfvenstam T, Papadogiannakis N, Norbeck O *et al.* Frequency of human parvovirus B19 infection in intrauterine fetal death. *Lancet* 2001; **357**: 1494–7.
6. Potter CG, Potter AC, Hatton CS *et al.* Variation of erythroid and myeloid precursors in the marrow and peripheral blood of volunteer subjects infected with human parvovirus (B19). *J Clin Invest* 1987; **79**: 1486–92.
7. Naides SJ, Weiner CP. Antenatal diagnosis and palliative treatment of non-immune hydrops fetalis secondary to fetal parvovirus B19 infection. *Prenat Diagn* 1989; **9**: 105–14.
8. Smoleniec JS, Pillai M. Management of fetal hydrops associated with parvovirus B19 infection. *Br J Obstet Gynaecol* 1994; **101**: 1079–81.
9. Brown KE, Green SW, Antunez de Mayolo J *et al.* Congenital anaemia after transplacental B19 parvovirus infection. *Lancet* 1994; **343**: 895–6.
10. Ismail KMK, Kilby MD. Human parvovirus B19 infection and pregnancy. *Obstet Gynecol* 2003; **5**: 4–9.
11. Moise KJ, Schumacher B. Anaemia. In: Fisk NM, Moise KJ (eds). *Fetal Therapy: Invasive and Transplacental.* Cambridge: Cambridge University Press, 1995: 141–63.
12. Mari G, Deter RL, Carpenter RL *et al.* Noninvasive diagnosis by Doppler ultrasonography of fetal anaemia due to maternal red-cell alloimmunization. Collaborative Group for Doppler Assessment of the Blood Velocity in Anemic Fetuses. *N Engl J Med* 2000; **342**: 9–14.
13. Montgomery LD, Belfort MA, Adam K. Massive fetomaternal hemorrhage treated with serial combined intravascular and intraperitoneal fetal transfusions. *Am J Obstet Gynecol* 1995; **173**: 234–5.
14. Fairley CK, Smoleniec JS, Caul OE, Miller E. Observational study of effect of intrauterine transfusions on outcome of fetal hydrops after parvovirus B19 infection. *Lancet* 1995; **346**: 1335–7.
15. van Engelen AD, Weijtens O, Brenner JI *et al.* Management outcome and follow-up of fetal tachycardia. *J Am Coll Cardiol* 1994; **24**: 1371–5.
16. Lopes LM, Tavares GM, Damiano AP *et al.* Perinatal outcome of fetal atrioventricular block: one-hundred-sixteen cases from a single institution. *Circulation* 2008; **118**: 1268–75.
17. Rodeck CH, Fisk NM, Fraser DI, Nicolini U. Long-term *in utero* drainage of fetal hydrothorax. *N Engl J Med* 1988; **319**: 1135–8.
18. Chan V, Greenough A, Nicolaides KN. Antenatal and postnatal treatment of pleural effusion and extra-lobar

pulmonary sequestration. *J Perinat Med* 1996; **24**: 335–8.

19. McCoy MC, Katz VL, Gould N, Kuller JA. Non-immune hydrops after 20 weeks gestation: review of 10 years' experience with suggestions for management. *Obstet Gynecol* 1995; **85**: 578–82.

20. Iskaros J, Jauniaux E, Rodeck C. Outcome of nonimmune hydrops fetalis diagnosed during the first half of pregnancy. *Obstet Gynecol* 1997; **90**: 321–5.

21. Harman CR, Bowman JM, Manning FA, Menticoglou SM. Intrauterine transfusion–intraperitoneal versus intravascular approach: a case-control comparison. *Am J Obstet Gynecol* 1990; **162**: 1053–9.

22. Mari G, Roberts A, Detti L *et al*. Perinatal morbidity and mortality rates in severe twin–twin transfusion syndrome: results of the International Amnioreduction Registry. *Am J Obstet Gynecol* 2001; **185**: 708–15.

# Malpresentation

*Ellen Knox*

## INTRODUCTION

Presentation refers to the part of the fetus that is lowermost within the maternal pelvis.

A malpresentation is any presentation other than the vertex and therefore includes brow and face presentations. This is not to be confused with malposition of the occiput. Malpresentations are associated with maternal and fetal morbidity.

Maternal morbidity is related to the surgical and anaesthetic risks related to operative delivery. In the absence of prompt medical care, most notably in the developing world, malpresentations can also result in obstructed labour with its risks of tissue necrosis and subsequent fistula formation or uterine rupture, sepsis and death.

The presence of fetal abnormality and prematurity are associated with a higher incidence of malpresentation and vice versa. In addition, intrapartum fetal risks of malpresentations include hypoxia from prolonged labour or cord prolapse.

## BREECH PRESENTATION

### Incidence and aetiology

Breech presentation is more common preterm – 28 per cent at 20 weeks, 15 per cent at 28 weeks, falling to 3 per cent at term.[1]

### Maternal abnormalities associated with breech presentation

- Uterine abnormality, e.g. bicornuate uterus.
- Pelvic abnormality.
- Pelvic mass (cervical fibromyomata, ovarian cyst).
- Drug and alcohol abuse.
- Anticonvulsant therapy.

### Fetal abnormalities associated with breech presentation

- Intrauterine growth restriction.
- Abnormality, especially central nervous system (CNS):
  - hydrocephalus;
  - myelomeningocele;
  - Prader–Willi syndrome;
  - aneuploidy/trisomy.

### Feto-maternal abnormalities associated with breech presentation

- Gestational prematurity.
- Placenta praevia.
- Previous pregnancy complicated by a breech presentation at term.
- Multiple pregnancy.
- Oligohydramnios or polyhydramnios.

### Clinical findings

The mother may complain of subcostal discomfort related to the fetal head position. Abdominal palpation reveals a 'ballotable head' at the uterine fundus, although this may be difficult to confirm clinically especially if maternal body mass index is raised. Ultrasound examination should be used to confirm a malpresentation and can also be useful to determine the type of breech and the presence of any associated fetal anomalies, as described above, placental site and liquor volume. It is less useful at term to determine uterine anomalies.

Breech presentation may be extended, or frank, with hips flexed and knees extending; flexed, or complete, with hips and knees flexed; or footling, or incomplete, with hips and knees flexed and feet presenting. Vaginal examination in the cases of extended or flexed breech reveals a soft presenting part, the only bony landmarks being the ischial tuberosities. The anus and genitalia may also be palpable, depending upon the cervical dilatation.

## Evidence from clinical trials

### Mode of delivery at term

The most recent Cochrane systematic review of randomized trials comparing planned breech delivery versus elective caesarean section at term includes three trials with 2369 patients.[2] The majority of data comes from the Term Breech trial, a multicentre randomized controlled trial, published in 2000 [B].[3] Perinatal or neonatal death or short term neonatal morbidity was reduced with planned caesarean section (RR 0.33, 95 per cent CI 0.19–0.56). The combined risk of perinatal mortality, neonatal mortality or serious perinatal morbidity was reduced in the planned cesarean section group compared to the planned vaginal birth group (RR 0.49, 95 per cent CI 0.26–0.91), even after excluding those deliveries that followed a prolonged labour, cases that were induced or augmented with oxytocin or prostaglandins, cases where there was a footling or uncertain type of breech presentation at delivery and cases where delivery took place without a skilled or experienced clinician present.[3] Another subgroup analysis showed a significant reduction in adverse outcome due to complications of both labour (RR 0.14, 95 per cent CI 0.04–0.45) and delivery (RR 0.37, 95 per cent CI 0.16–0.87) for those in the planned cesarean group compared to the planned vaginal birth.[4] In a secondary analysis of the Term Breech trial (not according to group allocation), adverse perinatal outcome was lowest with prelabour cesarean section and increased with cesarean section in early labour, in active labour and vaginal birth.[5] For further discussion – see Chapter 35, Breech presentation.

### Mode of delivery preterm

The Royal College of Obstetricians and Gynaecologists (RCOG) Greentop guidelines do not advise routine caesarean section for the delivery of preterm breech presentation.[6] Evidence from the Term Breech trial cannot be directly extrapolated to preterm breech delivery, which remains an area of clinical controversy, and there is insufficient evidence to support routine caesarean section for preterm breech delivery [D]. One randomized trial of planned caesarean section for preterm breech was stopped prior to completion because of inadequate enrolment.[7] The added difficulty at this gestation is determining when labour is established, as it may either progress quickly, preventing time for operative delivery, or subside with the risk of iatrogenic prematurity if caesarean delivery is undertaken too soon. There is retrospective cohort study evidence that suggests caesarean section confers a better outcome, although the authors caution against concluding causality [D].[8] Conversely, studies exist that suggest mortality is not related to delivery mode.[9] It is likely that prematurity *per se* impacts considerably on outcome. A management algorithm is shown in Figure 18.1. See Chapter 35, Breech presentation, for further discussion.

## External cephalic version

External cephalic version has been demonstrated to reduce the incidence of non-cephalic presentation at delivery (RR 0.38, 95 per cent CI 0.18–0.80) and also the caesarean section rate by lowering the incidence of breech presentation (RR 0.55, 95 per cent CI 0.33–0.91) without any increased risk to the baby.[10] The Royal College of Obstericians and Gynaecologists recommend offering external cephalic version (ECV) to all women with an uncomplicated breech presentation from 36 weeks in a nulliparous woman and from 37 weeks in a multiparous woman.[11] This does not apply to those women who would otherwise be delivering by caesarean section for additional indications. External cephalic version should not be offered routinely before term, as it has not been shown to improve outcomes; a Cochrane review of preterm ECV did not show a reduction in the incidence of caesarean section or non-cephalic presentation at term.[12] Successful ECV has been reported as late as 42 weeks gestation.

## Management

It is current best practice that all women with an uncomplicated breech pregnancy at term (37–42 weeks) should be offered ECV [A].

Although several studies have reported significant benefits from routine tocolysis in facilitating the procedure of EVC, with success rates ranging from 3 to 40 per cent in these trials, there remains insufficient evidence upon which to base the routine use of tocolysis. Because of the recognized adverse effects of beta-sympathomimetics, there is considerable interest in the evaluation of the benefits and risks of alternative agents.

Despite this, ECV has been successfully introduced into routine practice in many units in the UK. Although the success rates (conversion to cephalic presentation) are less than those quoted in some countries (e.g. 40 per cent in the UK, >80 per cent in Africa), a more comprehensive nationwide implementation would result in a significant reduction in the numbers of caesarean sections performed for breech presentation. It is possible to achieve higher success rates with case selection, and it is undoubtedly the

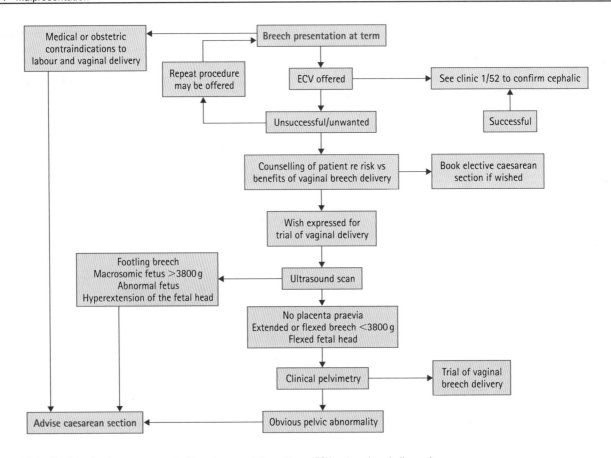

**Figure 18.1** Algorithm for the management of breech presentation at term. ECV, external cephalic version

case that operators improve with experience. Patients can be informed that, following successful ECV, 97.5 per cent of fetuses remain cephalic.

A number of factors have been found to increase the likelihood of successful ECV. These include:

- multiparity;
- adequate liquor volume;
- breech above the pelvic brim;
- fetal head easy to feel – placenta not anterior.

Although various interventions for improving the success rate of ECV have been suggested, neither vibroacoustic stimulation nor amnio-infusion has been proven to be effective in controlled trials and each requires further evaluation.

A few small randomized, controlled studies have shown that regional epidural anaesthesia improves version success without any increase in fetal or maternal morbidity. However, a more recent study of spinal anaesthesia has been published that does not support improved outcome with regional anaesthesia. Once again, no adverse effects on the mother or fetus were reported. In addition, an economic analysis has suggested that with epidural use in institutions where caesarean sections are systematically performed for breech presentations, substantial cost savings are possible. However, no studies have reported any outcomes related to maternal satisfaction or quality of life. Further research in this area is recommended.

Following ECV, whether successful or not, anti-D should be administered to all women who are Rhesus negative.

## Benefits to the fetus of external cephalic version

External cephalic version reduces the incidence of breech presentation at term. However, it should be noted that the rate of delivery by caesarean section may be higher than average for those babies successfully turned when compared to 'genuine' cephalic presentations.[13] It should also be remembered that even when ECV has been successful, these now cephalic-presenting fetuses, when subject to the stress of labour, are more likely to display signs of fetal compromise, and thus should still be regarded as a high-risk group requiring continuous monitoring in labour. Consequently, women requesting an ECV to enable then to experience a home birth should understand the higher risk of fetal compromise and be counselled accordingly.

## Risks to the fetus of external cephalic version

Transient bradycardia occurs in up to 8 per cent of cases. Abruption or direct effects on the placenta or cord (prolapse or direct trauma) occur far less frequently. Feto-maternal haemorrhage has an occurrence rate of between 5 and

28 per cent, although this is often minor and of little clinical significance as long as anti-D is administered appropriately. It is important that such risks are always compared with those incurred during vaginal *or* abdominal breech delivery, procedures that are not risk free themselves. Randomized controlled trials have shown no increase in neonatal mortality and morbidity, although the numbers involved are too small to power for this.

## Benefits to the mother of external cephalic version

Implementing the practice of ECV has been shown to result in a decrease in the number of vaginal breech deliveries and deliveries by caesarean section. Such practice invariably reduces maternal morbidity and mortality (both of which are increased by caesarean section and vaginal breech delivery). As detailed above, there is a higher rate of obstetric intervention (caesarean delivery and instrumental delivery) for those women who have successful ECVs in comparison to those women whose babies were not breech at term.[13]

## Risks to the mother of external cephalic version

An immediate caesarean delivery rate of approximately 0.5 per cent has been suggested in large series.

## Procedure of external cephalic version

Such procedures are best managed by following an agreed protocol (Figure 18.2).

### Indications for external cephalic version

- Any breech presentation after 37 completed weeks in an otherwise uncomplicated pregnancy.
- Maternal request.

### Relative contraindications

- Previous lower segment caesarean section (LSCS).
- Maternal disease, e.g. hypertension, diabetes.
- Fetal growth restriction or oligohydramnios.
- Maternal obesity: if the maternal body mass index (BMI) is >20 per cent of ideal, the procedure is less likely to succeed.

### Absolute contraindications for external cephalic version

- Multiple pregnancy.
- Antepartum haemorrhage (within the last 7 days).
- Need for caesarean section regardless of presentation (e.g. placenta praevia).
- Ruptured membranes.
- Fetal abnormality.
- Need for urgent delivery to ensure fetal well-being – any suspected fetal compromise.
- Declined consent.

Although there is no evidence that reduced fetal growth makes ECV any more difficult to perform, it may be a marker for the existence of some fetal compromise already.

Before attending for ECV, women should be asked to drink plenty of fluid, as this has been shown to optimize liquor volume [A]. There should be no need to starve women before the procedure, as the chance of emergency caesarean section being required is very small.

Ultrasound should be performed before the procedure to confirm the presentation, but is also useful to:

- confirm the presence of a normal fetus;
- ensure an adequate liquor volume;
- confirm the placental position;
- observe for the presence of a nuchal cord;
- detail the fetal attitude and position of the fetal legs. It should be routine practice to:
- perform a cardiotocogram (CTG) to confirm a normal reactive pattern. A cardiotocograph should be performed prior to and after the procedure. There may be CTG abnormalities following ECV which are usually transient and have been described in one small series in approximately 10 per cent of cases;[14]
- obtain informed consent, specifically detailing the risks (failure, caesarean delivery, need for anti-D if Rhesus negative);
- ensure that facilities for delivery by immediate caesarean section are present.

External cephalic version should be performed in a facility with rapid access for operative delivery if required. Once the prerequisites have been completed, the woman is positioned supine with slight lateral tilt. Tocolysis may be given (e.g. 250 mg terbutaline i.v./s.c.) and a short time allowed for the drug to exert its effect.

The operator should perform the ECV in one manoeuvre and uterine manipulation should be limited to a total of 10 minutes' duration (the vast majority will turn within 5 minutes). A variety of techniques may be employed, but essentially:

- the breech is manipulated out of the pelvis by steady and continuous abdominal pressure (the patient having a full bladder may aid this manoeuvre, although this often increases the abdominal discomfort experienced);
- a forward or backward roll/somersault of the fetus can then be performed; pressure should be maximally aimed at moving the breech upward; one hand can be used to maintain the head in flexion – a rocking manoeuvre is sometimes helpful;
- if this sequence should prove unsuccessful, rotation in the opposite direction may be tried; a fetus will often rotate easily one way but not the other; it is not always easy to predict which way will be more successful.

If successful, the attitude of the fetus should be maintained manually for a couple of minutes, during which time fetal

Date ..................................

Identification label

Exclude the following (tick)

☐    Multiple pregnancy

☐    Previous Caesarean section

☐    Antepartum haemorrhage after 20 weeks

☐    Need for caesarean section regardless of presentation

☐    Ruptured membranes

☐    IUGR/oligohydramnios

☐    Fetal abnormality

Parity ☐          Gestation by scan ☐

Explain the procedure and the following risks

•    Need for immediate caesarean section if signs of fetal distress on CTG following procedure

•    Small risk of feto-maternal haemorrhage therefore anti-D needed if rh negative.

•    Need to return for check of presentation next week.

•    Very small risk that the baby can turn back (no documented cases in our experience to date)

**Procedure**

Ultrasound scan
Presentation          Breech extended ☐      Flexed ☐      Footling ☐      Cephalic ☐

Nuchal cord          No ☐

Liquor volume        Normal ☐              Increased ☐

Placental site       Anterior ☐            Posterior ☐

Pre ECV CTG satisfactory          Yes ☐

Fetal head easy to feel           Yes ☐      No ☐

Breech deep in pelvis             Yes ☐      No ☐

Ritodrine dose .................................................................. (see protocol)

Procedure

Signed ..................................

Successful                        Yes ☐      No ☐

Post ECV CTG satisfactory         Yes ☐      No ☐

Blood group ....................... Kleihauer ........................... Anti-D given ........................ date

Outcome          Home (without ECV) ☐          Home after ECV ☐

                 Immediate delivery ☐

**Figure 18.2** Proforma, external cephalic version

monitoring can be commenced. Fetal monitoring should also be commenced if the procedure is unsuccessful. The CTG should be continued until a normal and reassuring pattern can be observed and, once this has been obtained, the patient should be allowed home with an appointment after a few days to confirm the persistence of the cephalic presentation.

Mothers should be told that:

- the procedure does not normally precipitate labour;
- only 2 per cent of babies will revert to a breech;
- the fetus should continue to be active and that a reduction in fetal movements must be reported;
- any vaginal loss (blood or fluid) must be reported.

If reversion to breech occurs, a repeat ECV may be attempted or delivery by caesarean section may be offered. If the ECV is unsuccessful, a full discussion should take place regarding delivery. It should be remembered that ECV can be offered in early labour if the membranes are intact.

As mentioned previously, if the patient is Rhesus negative, anti-D may be administered prophylactically once maternal blood has been obtained for Kleihauer estimation of feto-maternal transfusion.

External cephalic version: summary
- Tocolysis is effective, both when used routinely and when used selectively.
- ECV should be carried out near to facilities for emergency delivery.
- CTG is necessary before and after ECV.
- Ultrasound is an essential adjunct to the management.

If ECV is declined or unsuccessful, women should be informed that elective caesarean section carries a reduced perinatal mortality and early morbidity for babies with a breech presentation at term compared with a vaginal delivery [A]. However, there is no difference in long-term health. All risks and benefits should be explained to the mother. This should include risks of immediate surgical complications and long-term risks such as scar dehiscence in future pregnancy, placenta accrete and increased risk of repeat caesarean section, all of which are difficult to quantify. Elective delivery should occur at 39 weeks gestation to aim to minimize risk of transient tachypnoea of the newborn, which is more prevalent at earlier gestations or the increased risk of emergency delivery if the date is delayed. Ultrasound examination should occur immediately prior to surgery because of the small chance of spontaneous version.

If caesarean section is declined, careful fetal assessment prior to counselling should have ensured that there are no contraindications to vaginal delivery, such as placenta praevia. In addition, hyperextension of the fetal neck increases the risk of head entrapment and cord presentation or footling breech increase the risk of cord prolapse. Although ultrasound estimation of fetal weight is associated with error, estimated weights >3.8 or <2 kg carry an increased

risk to the fetus and the woman should be advised of this. A clinically inadequate pelvis may also reduce the chance of a successful delivery but x-ray pelvimetry does not aid clinical evaluation of likely success in labour [C].[15] In the presence of adverse clinical features, women should be counselled regarding the increased risk to them and their babies by attempting vaginal breech birth.

These factors should be revisited once a woman is admitted in labour. Likewise, they can be assessed if a woman with a previously undiagnosed breech presents in labour.

The Term Breech trial analysis suggested that the absence of an experienced senior practitioner was also associated with an increase in adverse outcomes.[3] Although the relative rarity of vaginal breech delivery means this experience is more difficult to obtain, clinicians should be prepared for this eventuality. In the Term Breech trial, 10 per cent of women allocated to elective cesarean section delivered vaginally; delivery may be too quick for surgical intervention. Regular 'skills drills' can aid development and maintenance of the skills required for vaginal breech delivery, both for the individual clinician and for the whole team. The management in labour, consequent on a decision to aim for a vaginal breech delivery, is discussed in detail in Chapter 35, Breech presentation.

## MANAGEMENT IN PARTICULAR CIRCUMSTANCES

### Preterm labour

As discussed above, there is no evidence to support elective preterm delivery by caesarean section and decisions should be made on an individual basis.

### Twin breech

Currently, a large trial of elective caesarean versus vaginal delivery is underway for twin pregnancies (The Twin Birth Study). In the meantime:

#### First twin breech
The theoretical risk for first twin breech is that of interlocked twins. This is thought to be rare with one study reporting rates of 1/817 twin pregnancies when the first twin was breech and second cephalic.[16] However, it presents a very difficult delivery challenge and most UK obstetricians would recommend elective caesarean section in this case. The RCOG guidelines suggest that in the absence of trial data it would be reasonable to use data from singleton breech presentation to aid decision making. As with a singleton breech, women should be advised of the short-term morbidity risks of caesarean section and risk to future pregnancies, balanced against the benefits of perinatal mortality.

## Second twin breech

Neither RCOG guidelines or the Cochrane review recommend elective caesarean delivery for breech second twin [E]. Evidence from one small randomized trial showed no difference in neonatal morbidity between the two groups, but the study was insufficiently powered to do so [B].[17] Observational studies have shown similar findings, although numbers were again small.

The second twin's position may change following delivery of the first twin in 20 per cent of cases.

Results from the ongoing randomized controlled trial may, however, dictate mode of delivery for all twins.

### KEY POINTS

- ECV after 37 weeks gestation is effective at reducing the incidence of non-cephalic births and caesarean sections [A].
- Elective caesarean section for persistent breech at term reduces perinatal morbidity and mortality [A].
- There is no evidence to support a policy of elective caesarean section for breech presentation in preterm labour [C].

## FACE PRESENTATION

### Incidence and aetiology

The incidence of face presentation is quoted at 1/500. However, this is a historical figure and includes cases of undiagnosed anencephaly which is now unlikely to occur.

Face presentation is also associated with prematurity, fetal goiters, uterine anomalies, polyhydramnios and placenta praevia.

### Clinical findings

Abdominal palpation reveals a deep depression between the anterior shoulder and the fetal head in which no fetal part can be felt. However, the diagnosis is usually made as labour advances on vaginal examination. The landmarks are the mandible, mouth, nose, malar and orbital ridges. Care should be taken to avoid damage to the eyes on examination. Facial oedema can make the distinction between a face and breech presentation difficult and ultrasound should be used if there is any doubt.

Delay in the first or second stage of labour can also occur.

### Evidence from clinical trials

There are no clinical trials involving face presentation and management is therefore based on expert opinion [E].

## Management

- Ultrasound examination should be performed to exclude fetal or pelvic abnormality that may preclude vaginal delivery.
- Vaginal delivery is possible with the mento-anterior position, but not mento-posterior. However, mento-posterior position may rotate during the second stage to mento-anterior. The risks to the fetus are that of facial soft tissue trauma which may persist for several days and can cause feeding difficulties. The maternal risks are perineal injury, sphincter damage and second stage caesarean section.
- Following diagnosis in the first stage of labour, the mother should be fully informed of all the possible risks. At the time of diagnosis, facial oedema and bruising may have already occurred. The diagnosis may occur at the time of diagnosis of failure to progress [E].
- Although augmentation has been used, it is generally not advised and lack of progress should usually prompt delivery by caesarean section [E].
- In the second stage of labour, given a mento-anterior position, the fetal head may be born by flexion, assisted if required by forceps.
- The vacuum delivery is contraindicated [E].

### KEY POINTS

- Face presentation may precede vaginal delivery if the position is mento-anterior.
- Caesarean section may avoid maternal perineal trauma and reduce fetal facial oedema and bruising.

## BROW PRESENTATION

### Incidence and aetiology

The incidence of brow presentation is quoted at 1/1000 deliveries. It is due to a deflexed head and is associated with prematurity. Other rare associations are fetal neck tumours (including goitre) which cause obstruction to head flexion.

### Clinical findings

In labour, failure to progress in the first or second stage may be noted. Care must be taken in assessment of such women, especially in the presence of multiparity when labour progress is less likely to halt secondary to ineffective uterine action. On vaginal examination, the forehead is the leading part felt through the cervix. The anteroposterior diameter of the head is therefore 'mento-vertical' and is about 13 cm at term. In contrast, the average anteroposterior and lateral diameters of the female mid-pelvis are

12 × 12 cm and therefore the 13 cm brow will not usually be able to pass the mid pelvis.

## Evidence from clinical trials

There are no clinical trials involving brow presentation and therefore management is based on expert opinion [E].

## Management

- Diagnosis in the early first stage may warrant expectant management for a short time (2–3 hours) as the brow may flex into a vertex or deflex to a face presentation and thus become amenable to vaginal delivery [E].
- Diagnosis is often made in the late first or second stage of labour when caesarean delivery is advised.
- If associated with failure to progress, caesarean delivery is advised [E].
- Augmentation with syntocinon has been described but is not advised as this could result in uterine rupture [E].
- The mento-vertical dimensions may be smaller in a preterm fetus, thus allowing vaginal delivery. However, caesarean should still be considered, especially in the context of failure to progress because of the risk of cervical cord or intracranial damage.

---

### KEY POINTS

- Brow presentation in early labour can convert to a vertex or a face presentation.
- If the brow persists and the head remains high, delivery by caesarean section is required.

---

# UNSTABLE LIE/TRANSVERSE LIE/ OBLIQUE LIE

## Incidence and aetiology

An incidence of 1/320 is recorded in historical studies. There is an association with progressive multiparity which is likely to be related to progressive laxity of the uterine musculature with each pregnancy.

The presence of polyhydramnios gives greater freedom of fetal movement and can predispose to these malpresentations. Placenta praevia may act as a physical obstruction to fetal engagement, as may any pelvic tumour, significant uterine anomaly or, more rarely, a contracted maternal pelvis.

Hydrocephalus and fetal tumours of the neck or sacrum may prevent engagement of the fetal head in the pelvis. Fetal neuromuscular dysfunction may impede engagement secondary to reduced fetal movement.

## Clinical findings

The absence of a fetal pole in the pelvis on abdominal or vaginal examination, either antenatally or in labour, should raise the likelihood of an unstable/non-longitudinal lie.

## Evidence from clinical trials

There are no randomized trials on which to base the management of these problems, which is therefore based on expert opinion [E].

## Management

- Clinical findings should be confirmed by ultrasound examination [E]. This should also look for fetal-anomaly, measure liquor volume and check placental site. The presence of pelvic tumours or congenital uterine anomalies may be difficult to identify in late pregnancy. Following exclusion of placenta praevia, vaginal examination is usually sufficient to exclude significant pelvic deformity or space-occupying lesion. X-ray pelvimetry does not add additional useful information to aid management.
- In the presence of obstructive fetal or uterine pathology that precludes vaginal delivery: caesarean section should be planned at the appropriate gestation [E]. This may need to be a classical caesarean depending on the extent of the anomaly, and the woman should be counselled regarding that possibility. The risk of cord prolapse in the event of contractions or rupture of membranes should also be discussed and women advised to attend hospital promptly if these occur.
- Even in the absence of an obstructive cause, inpatient management should be recommended from 37 weeks because of the risk of cord prolapse, to enable rapid intervention if required [E]. In the majority of cases, spontaneous version to longitudinal lie will occur prior to membrane rupture or labour onset. Conservative management involves daily review and discharge home prior to the lie stabilizing longitudinally for 48 hours. Active management involves attempting an ECV, with discharge home if the lie remains longitudinal. However, recent RCOG guidelines suggest that ECV for unstable lie should only be done with immediate induction 'stabilizing induction'.[11] Stabilizing induction requires a favorable cervix and immediate facilities for caesarean section in the event of a cord prolapse.
- Should the fetal lie remain non-longitudinal post term, an elective caesarean section should be offered.
- Should the patient present in early labour, ECV can be attempted but with immediate recourse to caesarean section if unsuccessful. ECV should not be attempted with ruptured membranes. Internal podalic version

should not be attempted except on occasion for the second twin.

- Caesarean delivery can be complicated by lack of liquor and difficulty in manoeuvring the fetus into a longitudinal lie. A vertical uterine incision (classical caesarean) may be required.

### KEY POINTS

- The majority of unstable lies will resolve spontaneously.
- Inpatient management is advised from 37 weeks until the lie stabilizes or delivery occurs, because of the risk of cord prolapse.
- Delivery by caesarean section may be difficult especially in the presence of ruptured membranes.

# SHOULDER PRESENTATION/ COMPOUND PRESENTATION/CORD PRESENTATION

## Incidence and aetiology

Cord presentation describes the cord below the presenting part of the fetus, with the membranes intact.

Cord prolapse describes the cord descending through the cervix into the vagina in the presence of ruptured membranes.

Compound presentation refers to more than one fetal part presenting simultaneously.

All are associated with prematurity and prior intrauterine death. All can complicate an unstable lie in labour or at the time of prelabour rupture of membranes. Cord prolapse or presentation can also complicate a 'high' fetal head or breech, or footling breech presentation. They may also be procedure related, following artificial rupture of membranes, fetal scalp electrode placement, stabilizing induction of labour, external cephalic version or internal podalic version. Historically, the incidence of cord presentation/cord prolapse is 1/200–300 deliveries. More recent studies suggest rates of 0.1–0.6 per cent of all births and just above 1 per cent for breech presentations.

## Clinical findings

The presence of a 'high' presenting part (head or breech) in early labour should prompt ultrasound, which may detect the presence of a cord presentation. In advanced labour, the findings are self-explanatory. The cord may be felt pulsating.

Abnormal cardiotocography, such as persistent fetal bradycardia or recurrent decelerations, should raise the possibility of cord prolapse and a vaginal examination should take place to investigate this as a cause.

## Evidence from clinical trials

There are no clinical trials on which to base management, which is therefore based on expert opinion [E].

## Management

- Cord prolapse is an emergency and delivery should be prompt. Fetal hypoxia occurs secondary to pressure of the presenting part and bony pelvis on the cord occluding fetal placental circulation. In addition, prolapse of the cord beyond the introitus causes arterial spasm. The cord should be replaced in the vaginal with minimal handling and the presenting part elevated to avoid compression of the cord. This may involve simultaneous manual displacement of the presenting part, head down tilt or maternal knee to chest position. Immediate plans for delivery should occur in the presence of a viable fetus.
- Continuous fetal monitoring should be in place while delivery is expedited. Ultrasound assessment of the fetal heart may be necessary as audible heart tones and cord pulsations may cease prior to delivery even though the fetus remains viable.
- Terbutaline (0.25 mg subcutaneously) should also be considered as a tocolytic to minimize cord compression from uterine activity [E].[18]
- The use of an indwelling catheter has also been described to fill the maternal bladder and again elevate the fetal presenting part from the cord. This can provide valuable time if delivery is unavoidably detained. A 16-gauge Foley catheter is placed in the bladder and filled with 500–700 mL physiological saline before being clamped. Just before delivery, the clamp is released.
- In the presence of full dilatation, if delivery can be expedited by instrumental delivery, this is may be appropriate.
- Cord presentation necessitates urgent caesarean delivery as rupture of membranes may precipitate cord prolapsed [E].
- Compound presentation of a limb beside the fetal head may be managed expectantly if progress is satisfactory and there is no fetal distress.
- Shoulder presentation and other compound presentations necessitate immediate caesarean delivery to avoid uterine rupture [E].
- Caesarean delivery may be difficult and consideration should be given to vertical uterine incision (classical caesarean) [E].

## KEY POINTS

- Cord prolapse is an emergency which is managed by replacing the cord in the vagina, elevating the presenting part and immediate delivery (usually by caesarean section).
- Compound presentation involving a limb alongside the vertex often resolves and may lead to vaginal delivery if progress is satisfactory.
- All other compound presentations/shoulder presentations require delivery by caesarean section if the fetus is still alive.
- Caesarean delivery may be difficult.

## CONCLUSIONS

- Malpresentations are associated with risk of maternal and fetal morbidity and mortality.
- In labour, suspicions may be raised in the presence of delayed progress.
- Ultrasound can be invaluable to aid diagnosis and management.
- Senior skilled clinicians should be involved in management.
- Regular 'skills drills' can help clinicians to maintain their skills, particularly when clinical situations occur relatively infrequently.
- Many malpresentations require caesarean delivery and these operations can be difficult.
- Following the Term Breech trial, RCOG guidelines recommend offering ECV for breech presentation from 37 weeks and caesarean delivery if this is unsuccessful.

## Key References

1. Hickok DE, Gordon DC, Milberg JA *et al*. The frequency of breech presentation by gestational age at birth: a large population-based study. *Am J Obstet Gynecol* 1992; **166**: 851–2.
2. Hofmeyr GJ, Hannah ME. Planned caesarean section for term breech delivery. *Cochrane Database Syst Rev* 2003 (**2**): CD000166.
3. Hannah ME, Hannah WJ, Hewson SA *et al*. Planned caesarean section versus planned vaginal birth for breech presentation at term: a randomized multicentre trial. *Lancet* 2000; **356**: 1375–83.
4. Su M, Hannah WJ, Willan A *et al*. Term Breech trial Collaborative Group. Planned casarean section decreases the risk of adverse perinatal outcome due to both labour and delivery complications in the Term Breech trial. *BJOG* 2004; **111**: 1065–74.
5. Su M, McLeod L, Ross S *et al*. Factors associated with adverse perinatal outcome in the Term Breech trial. *Am J Obstet Gynecol* 2003; **189**: 740–45.
6. RCOG. The management of Breech presentation RCOG guideline No 20b. London: RCOG Press, 2006.
7. Penn ZJ, Steer PJ, Grant A. A multicentre randomized controlled trial comparing elective and selective caesarean section for the delivery of the preterm infant. *BJOG* 1996; **103**: 684–9.
8. Muhuri PK, Macdorman MF, Menacker F. Method of delivery and neonatal mortality among very low birth weight infants in the United States. *Matern Child Health J* 2006; **10**: 47–53.
9. Kayem G, Baumann R, Goffinet F *et al*. Early preterm breech delivery: is a policy of planned vaginal delivery associated with increased risk of neonatal death? *Am J Obstet Gynecol* 2008; **198**: e1–6.
10. Hofmeyr GJ, Kulier R. External cephalic version for breech presentation at term. *Cochrane Database Syst Rev* 2000; (**2**): CD000083.
11. RCOG External cephalic version and reducing the incidence of breech presentation RCOG Guideline No 20a. London: RCOG Press, 2006.
12. Hutton EK, Hofmeyr GJ. External cephalic version for breech presentation before term. *Cochrane Database Syst Rev* 2006; (**1**): CD000084.
13. Vezina Y, Bujold E, Varin J *et al*. Cesarean delivery after successful external cephalic version of breech presentation at term: a comparative study. *Am J Obstet Gynecol* 2004; **190**: 763–8.
14. Hofmeyr GJ, Sonnendecker EW. Cardiotocographic changes after external cephalic version. *Br J Obstet Gynaecol* 1983; **90**: 914–18.
15. Broche DE, Riethmuller D, Vidal C *et al*. Obstetric and perinatal outcomes of a disreputable presentation: the nonfrank breech. *J Obstet Biol Reprod* 2005; **34**: 781–8.
16. Cohen M, Kohl SG, Roisenthal AH. Fetal interlocking complicating twin gestation. *Am J Obstet Gynecol* 1965; **91**: 407.
17. Rabinovici J, Barkai G, Reichmen B *et al*. Randomised management of the second nonvertex twin: vaginal delivery or cesarean section. *Am J Obstet Gynecol* 1987; **156**: 52–6.
18. Katz Z, Shaoham Z, Lancet M *et al*. Management of labour with umbilical cord prolapse: a 5 year study. *Obstet Gynecol* 1994; **94**: 278–81.

# Prolonged pregnancy

*Devender Roberts*

## INTRODUCTION

Prolonged pregnancy can be a cause of anxiety for both women and obstetricians. It is a common situation and is perceived as being associated with increased risk to the fetus. In addition, many women find the physical burden of pregnancy at or near term to be intolerable. There has been debate over the best method of management of post-term pregnancy with regards to whether a policy of routine induction of labour at a set gestation is more likely to avoid the risks than an expectant approach.

## DEFINITION

The standard international definition accepted by both the World Health Organization (WHO) and the International Federation of Gynaecology and Obstetrics (FIGO) is 42 completed weeks (294 days) or more, the gestational age having been established by ultrasound prior to 16 weeks.

## INCIDENCE

Using the definition of 294 days, the incidence of post-term pregnancy lies between 5 and 10 per cent.[3] It has been recognized that women who attend late for antenatal care may be of uncertain gestation and may have been over-represented in populations of post-term pregnancies. Dating by the last menstrual period (LMP) alone has a tendency to overestimate the gestational age. Gardosi *et al.*[4] argued that most pregnancies that are induced for post-term are not, in fact, post-term when assessed by ultrasound dates. The use of early ultrasound alone to calculate the rate of post-term pregnancy in women who laboured spontaneously significantly reduced the post-term rate from 9.5 to 1.5 per cent.

Meta-analysis of four randomized controlled trials (RCTs) included in a Cochrane review has demonstrated that the routine use of early ultrasound to calculate gestational age significantly reduces the incidence of post-term pregnancy.[5] The NICE guideline on induction of labour recommends that the gestational age should be established by ultrasound before 16 weeks gestation [A].[2]

## AETIOLOGY

The cause of prolonged pregnancy is not clear and it may represent simple biological variation. Post-term pregnancy is more common in primigravid women, and those with a single previous post-term pregnancy have a 30 per cent chance of recurrence.

Infants who suffer fetal distress at term have elevated cortisol levels, whereas those with fetal distress post-term have reduced cortisol levels. A relative adrenocortical insufficiency may contribute to a delay in the onset of labour and an increased risk of intrapartum hypoxia or even death in post-term pregnancy. Further support for the theory that some infants born post-term may have an inherent biological defect comes from the fact that infants delivered following a post-term pregnancy are at increased risk of demise up to two years of age. Sudden infant death syndrome is also more common in infants born after 41 completed weeks of gestation. However, the hypothesis that post-term fetuses are fundamentally different from term fetuses remains unproven.

Amniotic fluid volumes fall in otherwise normal post-term pregnancies.[6] However, there appears to be no deterioration in cardiac output in post-term fetuses in otherwise uncomplicated pregnancies, compared to term fetuses. Doppler velocimetry in uterine, umbilical, middle cerebral, thoracic descending aorta and renal arteries in uncomplicated post-term pregnancies is no different from that in term pregnancies. Long-term pulse interval measured by computerized evaluation of the fetal heart rate correlates with fetal oxygenation and seems to fall progressively from 41 weeks [C,D].[7]

## Fetal and neonatal risks of post-term pregnancies

Post-term pregnancy *per se* is not a pathological condition and should not be confused with the post-maturity syndrome described by Clifford in 1954. This syndrome closely resembles intrauterine growth restriction, with associations with meconium-stained amniotic fluid, oligohydramnios and fetal distress and evidence of loss of subcutaneous fat and dry, cracked skin reflecting placental insufficiency. It is apparent that not every post-term pregnancy is complicated by the post-maturity syndrome, but it is likely that the majority of morbidity and mortality associated with post-term pregnancies arises because of post-maturity.

It has long been recognized that a pregnancy which goes beyond 40 weeks is associated with increased perinatal mortality and morbidity [D].[8,9] A retrospective analysis of 171 527 notified births in the UK revealed a rate of 2.3 stillbirths/1000 total births at term (37–41 weeks) and 1.9/1000 post-term. Calculated per 1000 ongoing pregnancies however, the rate of stillbirth increased from 0.86/1000 at 40 weeks to 2.12/1000 at 43 weeks – almost a 3-fold increase. The same study demonstrated that the neonatal and post-neonatal mortality rates double from 1.57/1000 at 40 weeks to 3.71/1000 at 43 weeks.[8]

A systematic review of 19 RCTs suggests that although the relative risk increases, the overall risks of perinatal death associated with prolonged pregnancy is small 2–3/1000.[2,10]

When lethal congenital abnormalities are excluded, intrapartum fetal death is four times more common and neonatal death three times more common in infants born after 42 weeks gestation. In addition, meconium staining of the amniotic fluid and the need for intrapartum fetal blood sampling were much more common in post-term pregnancies compared to those delivered at 40 weeks.[1,10,11]

Prolonged pregnancy is thus associated with an increased risk not only of meconium staining of the liquor, but also of intrapartum fetal hypoxia, which may result in fetal acidosis, neonatal seizures and perinatal death. Post-term pregnancy is also a risk factor for birth trauma and shoulder dystocia.

## Maternal risks of post-term pregnancy

The risk for both mother and fetus increases as the pregnancy advances beyond 40 weeks.[1] Maternal risks of post-term pregnancies include increased operative delivery, haemorrhage and infection. In addition, post-term pregnancies are associated with considerable psychological morbidity. The pregnancy is perceived by many women as becoming high risk once the estimated date of confinement is passed.

## MANAGEMENT

The data from 21 RCTs comparing elective induction of labour were analysed in a systematic review, which has governed policy for many units in the UK over the past decade.[5] The conclusions of the analysis favoured a policy of induction of labour at 41 completed weeks and beyond, to reduce perinatal mortality, decrease meconium staining of the amniotic fluid and cause a small decrease in caesarean section, compared to conservative management [A]. This systematic review has been updated recently with the addition of six new trials.[10] Eight trials from the original review were removed due to methodological reasons. The current review found that a policy of induction of labour at 41+0 weeks and beyond is associated with fewer deaths when compared to expectant management (1/2986 versus 9/2953; RR 0.30, CI 0.09–0.99, 19 trials). There were no deaths in the induction of labour group and seven in the expectant management group. The causes for perinatal death in the expectant management groups were meconium aspiration (four), intrauterine death at 292 days (one), stillbirth with abnormal maternal GTT (one) and neonatal pneumonia (one). The review did not find a significant difference in the incidence of caesarean section (559/2883 versus 630/2872; RR 0.92, CI 0.76–1.12 at 41 weeks; 110/407 versus 111/403; RR 0.97, CI 0.72–1.31). There were fewer babies with meconium aspiration syndrome in the groups induced at 41 and 42 weeks. The implications for practice from this review were that induction at 41 completed weeks should be offered to low risk women as such a policy is associated with fewer deaths, the risk of assisted vaginal or abdominal delivery is not increased. The largest RCT in this review, by Hannah *et al.*[12] showed a lower caesarean section rate in the induction group as compared with the monitoring group (21.2 versus 24.5 per cent, *p* = 0.03).

An RCT from Sweden[13] which was published after the Cochrane review compared women offered induction of labour at 41+2 weeks gestation with those monitored every third day until spontaneous labour occurred or labour was induced at 300 days for operative births. The study showed no significant difference in operative delivery, haemorrhage >500 mL, perineal trauma, meconium-stained liquor, NICU admission, intrauterine death (no deaths in either group) or neonatal death (0 versus one due to asphyxia from true knot in cord) [B].

The recommendations of the Society of Obstetricians and Gynaecologists of Canada for management of pregnancy[14] at 41–42 weeks are broadly in agreement with these findings. Induction of labour is recommended and monitoring should be instituted in those pregnancies where expectant management is planned.

The American College of Obstetricians and Gynaecologists recommendations on management of post-term pregnancy also support a policy of induction of labour.[15]

Sweeping the membranes at or beyond 40 weeks appears not only to significantly reduce the incidence of post-term pregnancy but also the frequency of using other methods for induction [A].[1] A systematic review evaluating interventions aimed at prevention or improvement of outcomes of delivery beyond term showed that the risk reduction of a formal induction of labour was 21.3 versus 36.3 per cent (RR 0.59, CI 0.50–0.70; NNT 7). The risk of operative delivery is not changed by the intervention.[5] There was no difference in other measures of effectiveness or adverse maternal outcomes. Sweeping the membranes in women at term reduced the delay between randomization and spontaneous onset of labour, or between randomization and birth, by a mean of 3 days. It increased the likelihood of both spontaneous labour within 48 hours (63.8 versus 83.0 per cent; RR 0.77, 95 per cent CI 0.70–0.84; NNT 5) and of birth within 1 week (48.0 versus 66.0 per cent; RR 0.73, 95 per cent CI 0.66–0.80; NNT 5). Sweeping the membranes performed as a general policy from 38 to 40 weeks onwards decreased the frequency of prolonged pregnancy: more than 42 weeks: 3.4 versus 12.9 per cent; RR 0.27, 95 per cent CI 0.15–0.49; NNT: 11; more than 41 weeks: 18.6 versus 29.87 per cent, RR 0.62, 95 per cent CI 0.49–0.79; NNT: 8.579.

Other interventions designed to reduce the incidence of post-term pregnancy include nipple stimulation, but have not been shown to be of benefit [A].[5]

## MONITORING POST-TERM PREGNANCY

The NICE antenatal guideline recommends increased antenatal monitoring consisting of at least twice-weekly cardiotocography and ultrasound estimation of maximum amniotic pool depth in women who decline induction of labour (see Chapter 14, Tests of fetal well-being)[E]. These recommendations are supported by both the American College of Obstetricians and Gynaecologists and the Society of Obstetricians and Gynaecologists of Canada, despite lack of evidence that it improves perinatal mortality. This recommendation is based on the evidence that perinatal morbidity and mortality increase as gestational age advances.

It has been suggested that amniotic fluid index (AFI) is preferable to maximum pool depth (MPD) liquor volume assessment in these pregnancies. However, there is still debate about what constitutes the best cut-off values for both measurements, as liquor volumes fall after term. An RCT comparing the two methodologies showed that use of AFI did not improve perinatal outcomes but was associated with an increase in the intervention rate. Thus, MPD is probably the tool of choice for assessing liquor in these post-term pregnancies [B].[11] More complex fetal monitoring with a formal biophysical scoring system has been suggested, but an RCT showed that it holds no advantage over simple monitoring with non-stress test (NST) cardiotocography (CTG) and liquor assessment [B].[16]

CTG monitoring is usually applied on the basis of observational data, although it is of no proven benefit [D]. It has been suggested that computerized CTG may be superior to conventional CTG, but this has yet to be tested in clinical trials. The use of Doppler analysis of various fetal arterial systems has also been advocated in the assessment of post-term pregnancies, but again this has not been evaluated by

### EBM

- Current guidance for the management of prolonged pregnancy in the UK is based on NICE guideline on induction of labour and antenatal care.[1] Although, systematic review data have not shown induction of labour reduces the risk of caesarean section for the mother, the guideline recommends that on the basis of epidemiological data, trial data and health economic analysis, induction of labour should be offered from 41+0 week onwards. The guideline detailed that induction of labour became more acceptable to women as gestation advanced (45 per cent wanted expectant management at 37 weeks versus 31 per cent at 41 weeks, *p* <0.05).

RCT. In addition, complex arterial Doppler assessment is not suitable as a screening tool in standard practice. The use of umbilical artery Doppler is claimed to be of benefit; however, the alterations in the waveforms are subtle.[17]

In the largest study to date, only 31 per cent of women at 41 weeks gestation opted for conservative management despite this being the unit's policy.[18] Despite this, many women will see induction as interference with a natural process, and loss of maternal choice is a major determinant of maternal dissatisfaction with the management of pregnancy and labour. It is therefore vital that each woman is treated on an individual basis and counselled regarding the risks of post-term pregnancy, to allow her to make her own decision about induction.

---

## EBM

- Systematic review of four RCTs indicates that the use of early ultrasound dating reduces the incidence of post-term pregnancy.
- Systematic review of 19 RCTs indicates that induction of labour after 41+ weeks reduces perinatal mortality rates without increasing caesarean section rates.
- Systematic review of one RCT demonstrates that sweeping the membranes significantly reduces the incidence of post-term pregnancy and the need for other methods of induction.
- No clear evidence exists to support the hypothesis that fetal monitoring can reduce the perinatal mortality in post-term pregnancy, but it is suggested as good practice by the NICE antenatal guideline.
- Uncontrolled studies support the use of NST CTG and liquor assessment in monitoring post-term pregnancy.
- MPD is the tool of choice for monitoring liquor in post-term pregnancy.

---

## ACKNOWLEDGEMENT

This chapter has been revised and updated. The author and editors acknowledge the contribution of Murray Luckas to the chapter on this topic in the previous edition of the book.

---

## KEY POINTS

- Post-term pregnancy is a condition associated with increased perinatal risk albeit small (overall risk 2-3/1000).
- The risk of stillbirth should be calculated in terms of ongoing pregnancies at a particular gestation, to avoid

---

- underestimation. This gives a 6-fold increase in risk from 37 to 43 weeks gestation.
- Induction of labour at 41 completed weeks and beyond significantly reduces the perinatal mortality rate. Nevertheless, some women will opt for conservative management with fetal surveillance.
- Monitoring of post-term pregnancy beyond 42 completed weeks should at the minimum consist of twice weekly CTG and ultrasound measurement of the maximum amniotic pool depth.

## Key References

1. NICE guideline 62. *Antenatal care – routine care for the healthy pregnant woman*. National Collaborating Centre for Women's and Children's Health, RCOG Press, March 2008.
2. NICE guideline 70. *Induction of labour*. National Collaborating Centre for Women's and Children's Health, RCOG Press, June 2008.
3. Shea KM, Wilcox AJ, Little RE. Post term delivery: a challenge for epidemiologic research. *Epidemiology* 1998; **9**: 199–204.
4. Gardosi J, Vanner T, Francis A. Gestational age and induction of labour for prolonged pregnancy. *Br J Obstet Gynaecol* 1997; **104**: 792–7.
5. Crowley P. Interventions for preventing or improving the outcome of delivery at or beyond term. *Cochrane Database Syst Rev* 2000; (**2**): CD000170.
6. Nwosu EC, Welch CR, Manasse PR, Walkinshaw SA. Longitudinal assessment of amniotic-fluid index. *Br J Obstet Gynaecol* 1993; **100**: 816–19.
7. Mandruzzato G, Meir YJ, Dottavio G *et al*. Computerised evaluation of fetal heart rate in post-term fetuses: long term variation. *Br J Obstet Gynaecol* 1998; **105**: 356–9.
8. Hilder L, Costeloe K, Thilaganathan B. Prolonged pregnancy: evaluating gestation-specific risks of fetal and infant mortality. *Br J Obstet Gynaecol* 1998; **105**: 169–73.
9. Smith GC. Life-table analysis of the risk of perinatal death at term and post term in singleton pregnancies. *Am J Obstet Gynecol* 2001; **184**: 489–96.
10. Gülmezoglu AM, Crowther CA, Middleton P. Induction of labour for improving birth outcomes for women at or beyond term. *Cochrane Database Syst Rev* 2006; (**4**): CD004945.
11. Alfirevic Z, Luckas M, Walkinshaw SA *et al*. A randomised comparison between amniotic fluid index and maximum pool depth in the monitoring of post-term pregnancy. *Br J Obstet Gynaecol* 1997; **104**: 207–11.
12. Hannah ME, Hannah WJ, Hellmann J *et al*. Induction of labor as compared with serial antenatal monitoring in post-term pregnancy. A randomized controlled trial.

The Canadian Multicenter Post-term Pregnancy Trial Group. *N Engl J Med.* 1992; **326**: 1587–92.

13. Heimstad R, Skogvoll E, Mattsson LA *et al.* Induction of labor or serial antenatal fetal monitoring in post-term pregnancy. A randomized controlled trial. *Obstet Gynecol* 2007; **109**: 609–17.

14. SOGC Clinical Practice Guideline. *Guidelines for the Management of Pregnancy at 41+0 to 42+0 Weeks.* No. 214, September 2008.

15. American College of Obstetricians and Gynecologists (ACOG). *Management of postterm pregnancy.* Washington (DC): ACOG practice bulletin; no. 55, 2004 Sep. 8.

16. Alfirevic Z, Walkinshaw SA. A randomised controlled trial of simple compared with complex antenatal fetal monitoring after 42 weeks of gestation. *Br J Obstet Gynaecol* 1995; **102**: 638–43.

17. Fischer RL, Kuhlman KA, Depp R, Wapner RJ. Doppler evaluation of umbilical and uterine-arcuate arteries in the postdates pregnancy. *Obstet Gynecol* 1991; **78**: 363–8.

18. Roberts LJ, Young KR. The management of prolonged pregnancy – an analysis of women's attitudes before and after term. *Br J Obstet Gynaecol* 1991; **98**: 1102–6.

# Routine intrapartum care: an overview

*Harold Gee*

## INTRODUCTION

Labour is a physiological process. Superficially, it appears simple but this belies a complexity that produces paradoxes and unexpected consequences. Furthermore, our interventions may not always produce the desired effects and can be counterproductive. When it becomes aberrant, there can be serious sequelae for both mother and fetus. It is also a process that is highly charged, emotionally. Thus, it should not be surprising to find that managing labour and delivery is, perhaps, the most demanding discipline but can be the most rewarding.

Our current concepts of labour management evolved during the 1960s and 1970s. The association between prolonged labour and increased morbidity and mortality was recognized and accepted. It was assumed that correction of delay would avoid the sequelae. Friedman's documentation and graphical representation of progress offered the prospect of early detection of aberrance. Clinicians were optimistic that effective interventions could be had. The availability of synthetic oxytocin and improved methods of administering it gave it the appearance of a panacea. Only the powers were considered open to manipulation. The other two variables, the passages and the passenger, could only be influenced indirectly via the powers. A pragmatic step was taken to use intravenous oxytocin on a 'try and see' basis to augment the powers, correct delay and avoid the problems of prolonged labour.[1] The enthusiasm for the perceived benefits overtook scientific evaluation. Poor progress remained and still does. Not until the 1990s was practice questioned. Since that time, randomized, controlled clinical trials and meta-analyses have shown that although rule-of-thumb interventions such as oxytocin augmentation[2,3] and routine amniotomy[4,5] may speed up labour, they do not, necessarily, improve clinical outcomes [A]. This is not to say that management strategies that include these have no merit, but other components such as the correct diagnosis of labour, psychological support for the woman in labour and one-to-one midwifery care[6] have been shown to be at least as important [A], but continue to be under-valued.

## THE ONSET OF LABOUR

Despite the apparent simplicity of the uterus, its physiology remains poorly understood. The myometrium changes from relative quiescence in pregnancy to rhythmic, forceful activity in labour while, simultaneously, the cervix loses its rigidity to become compliant. There are common mediators for these changes, for example oestrogens and prostaglandins, but they have different effects on the myometrium and cervix. Furthermore, and this makes investigation more difficult, these agents are often paracrine in their activity, i.e. they have their effects over short distances. For example, the decidua and membranes, which produce prostaglandins, are in direct contact with the myometrium and cervix on which they act.

Progesterone inhibits labour. Oestrogens and prostaglandins are facilitatory, and oxytocin maintains labour once the process has begun. Though there are changes in the balance of these hormones, no single 'trigger' for labour has been defined in the human. Evidence indicates that the fetus has a part to play (Figure 20.1). Placental corticotrophin-releasing hormone (PCRH) acts on the fetal pituitary to stimulate adrenal corticosteroid production via adrenocorticotrophic hormone (ACTH). Progesterone downregulates the PCRH gene, while adrenal steroids (cortisol in particular) upregulate it. The sensitivity of the gene is much greater to cortisol than to progesterone. During most of pregnancy progesterone is dominant, but small increments in cortisol will upregulate the gene and at some point over-ride or 'switch' it over to a large output of PCRH. This process constitutes a positive feedback loop in the fetus.

Dehydroepiandrostenedione from the fetal adrenal is metabolized by the placenta, producing a rise in maternal oestriol. This has many effects. It changes smooth muscle cell membrane potentials towards their firing threshold, thereby increasing spontaneous activity. It induces prostaglandin synthesis in the decidua and promotes cervical ripening.

No sudden fall in peripheral serum progesterone has been demonstrated in the human, although it has in other mammals. However, there is a relative reduction in its effect as oestrogen levels rise. Furthermore, as the uterus grows, the placental implantation site, relative to the total internal uterine surface, decreases. Thus, more of the myometrium escapes the paracrine suppressive effect of progesterone from the placenta. Uterine distension itself increases spontaneous activity of the myometrium.

Oxytocin levels do not change markedly at the onset of labour but prostaglandins from the decidua potentiate oxytocin, that is to say the activity produced by the action of oxytocin plus prostaglandin is more than the sum of their individual effects. Oxytocin binds to specific

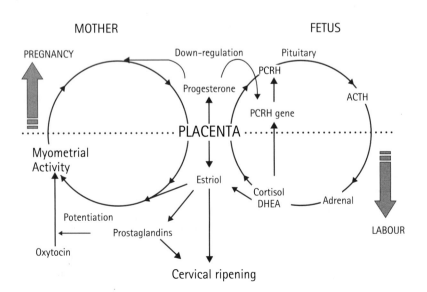

**Figure 20.1** Maternal and fetal positive feedback systems in the initiation of labour. ACTH, adrenocorticotrophic hormone; DHEA, dehydroepiandrostenedione; PCRH, placental corticotrophin-releasing hormone

receptors, opening calcium-activated channels and depolarizing the cell membrane. This depolarization, in turn, opens voltage-dependent calcium channels, resulting in an influx of calcium ions, development of action potentials and contractions. Thus, spontaneous smooth muscle activity increases. However, propagation across the myometrium is slowed by oxytocin, ensuring more muscle fibres are active from any single source. This source can be anywhere in the myometrium – not, as was once thought, only in the cornua. The result is a more rhythmic, co-ordinated myometrium. Release of prostaglandins with contractions further stimulates this positive feedback system in the mother.

Thus, it is likely that labour is initiated and maintained by the interaction of at least two positive feedback systems. Positive feedback loops carry potential dangers. They have no built-in safety mechanism, as do negative feedbacks. Care has to be exercised when stimulating these systems, for example when augmenting uterine activity in an attempt to correct delay.

## UTERINE PHYSIOLOGY IN LABOUR

### Myometrium

Smooth muscle cells are spontaneously active. Contractions occur in the myometrium throughout pregnancy. However, uterine activity in pregnancy is decremental, i.e. activity arising in one cell is unlikely to activate many of its neighbours. During the preparation for labour, oestrogens and prostaglandins develop specialized gap junctions between muscle cells that preferentially conduct electrical potentials. These facilitate propagated activity for labour to become established.

In the first stage of labour, contractions are virtually isometric, i.e. tension is developed without significant change in length. This results in a rise in intrauterine pressure (IUP). IUP can be measured with catheters and intrauterine transducers, but because repetition frequency, amplitude and duration are physiologically linked, albeit non-linearly, semi-objective assessment by timing repetition frequency and duration is adequate for clinical needs [B].[7]

In the second stage, contractions transform from isometric to isotonic, i.e. there is shortening of the muscle fibres as the uterine contents are expelled, with little change in tension. Permanent shortening is known as retraction. Retraction of the fibres compresses blood vessels as they traverse the myometrium to the placenta, and at the same time a shrinking placental implantation site shears off the placenta. Separation of the placenta and control of blood supply to the placenta are crucial to the prevention of haemorrhage in the third stage, although the process begins during the second stage. These physiological changes may account for some of the fetal heart rate irregularities seen at full dilatation and into the second stage.

## The cervix and cervical ripening

The cervix consists primarily of connective tissue in which collagen fibres are embedded in ground substance. Collagen is inelastic and highly tensile (strong). Ground substance is a gel. Its physical properties can be changed rapidly according to its chemical composition and its degree of hydration. Gelatin is a familiar example of a ground substance. In its concentrated form, it is hard and rubbery, but when treated with water and/or heated, it softens and liquefies.

During cervical ripening, structural glycoproteins (dermatin sulphate and chondroitin sulphate) that bind collagen are reduced in concentration, while 'packing' glycoproteins without such affinity (heparan sulphate) increase. Furthermore, hydration is increased by rising levels of hyaluronic acid, a glycoprotein that carries water. These changes in the ground substance allow the collagen fibres to become more loosely packed and able to move relative to each other.

Thus, the cervix changes from its pregnancy state – a rigid, tubular structure, whose canal is held closed by tightly wound, circumferential, collagen fibres bonded together by a firm ground substance – to one in which the ground substance becomes fluid, permitting change in the whole form of the cervix, with the effect that its resistance to delivery is reduced. Tissue redistribution from the cervix to the lower segment is recognized as 'effacement' and the reduction in resistance it produces facilitates subsequent dilatation. The formation of the lower segment is familiar to every obstetrician but the precise processes and anatomical changes have yet to be defined.

## EFFECTS OF LABOUR ON THE FETUS

Contractions affect placental blood flow. Observations *in vivo* suggest that significant impairment of placental perfusion takes place when the intrauterine pressure rises above 35 mmHg (about half to two-thirds maximum IUP), even during physiological contractions. During these periods, the fetus may experience transient hypoxaemia. The response of a healthy fetus to this may be bradycardia. However, bradycardia may also be caused by the response of baroreceptors in the circulatory system to external IUP and from raised intracranial pressure from head compression. Thus, decelerations on cardiotocography may arise from physiological changes in the fetal environment, none of which is going to harm the fetus providing there is adequate recovery time between contractions. Hyperstimulation and poor uteroplacental function impair recovery. Growth-restricted fetuses may not have the energy reserves to maintain anaerobic metabolism during periods of hypoxia. In these instances, physiological labour may pose a threat to the fetus.

## CLINICAL DIAGNOSIS OF LABOUR

This is perhaps the single most crucial point in labour management.

Labour is recognized by the combination of two features:

1 regular, purposeful uterine activity (contractions),
2 cervical change,

but there are many vagaries here.

Friedman defined labour as regular painful contractions. Most women would identify with this but often, particularly in nulliparous women, such features are present long before cervical dilatation begins. Others would say that labour is established only when there is progressive cervical dilatation and anything prior to this is 'pre-labour'. This may appear merely to be a matter of semantics, but when applying limits to progress it is essential that they are applied only to that part of labour for which they were designed. In practice, cervicograms only describe cervical dilatation in the active phase of labour. Thus, for practical purposes, it is better to diagnose 'labour' only when there is evidence of progressive cervical dilatation to indicate entry into the active phase. NICE guidance advises this limit be set at 4 cm [E].[8] There is another reason for this. Oxytocin augmentation for poor progress (slow cervical dilatation) is ineffective in the latent phase. Thus, when women present in early labour (<4 cm), particularly if they are nulliparous, check that all is well with mother and baby, explain sympathetically to the mother that preparation is under way for progressive labour, be patient and buy time. Once there is evidence of progressive cervical change beyond 4 cm, active labour is established and cervicogram monitoring can commence.

## PROGRESS IN LABOUR

Normally, the head engages in the pelvis in an attitude of flexion with the occiput lateral (left or right). In first labours, engagement will normally have taken place in the later weeks of pregnancy but in women who have delivered before, engagement may not take place until labour becomes established. Cervical dilatation is the prime feature of the first stage of labour and is the parameter used to define progress. In the second stage, after full dilatation, rotation and descent of the presenting part takes place. Rotation takes place in the mid-cavity of the pelvis with the occiput moving from lateral to anterior. The head has to be in an antero-posterior position to negotiate the outlet to the pelvis – ideally occipito-anterior. A flexed, occipito-anterior position allows for the head to deflex as it follows the curve of the birth canal through the pelvis. Malposition, for example persistence of an occipito-posterior position, leads to deflexion, relative increase in the presenting dimensions, delay in progress and possible frank obstruction.

Classically, progress is defined in terms of:

- powers
- passages
- passenger.

### Powers

Efficient contractions impart tension to the cervix and produce dilatation in the first stage and, coupled with maternal effort, rotation and descent in the second. Flexion and rotation of the presenting part depend on good expulsive forces. There is no doubt that efficient powers are at the centre of efficient labour. In any labour showing poor progress, poor uterine activity should be suspected first and treated if confirmed.

Assessment of contractions by an experienced attendant has been found to be adequate for clinical practice, with no advantage from invasive monitoring.[7] IUP measurement is used mainly as a research tool but may be indicated when contractions are difficult to palpate, for example in obese patients.

### Paradoxes

There are everyday paradoxes that indicate force and progress are not always in a simple, direct relationship.

- Multiparous women have faster labours than nulliparous women and expend less uterine activity per centimetre of dilatation. Thus, progress is not a simple function of force.
- Precipitate spontaneous labour may be associated with low levels of uterine activity. Any reported morbidity associated with such deliveries usually results from delivery in unprepared settings rather than from the labour itself.
- Many premature deliveries take place with minimal uterine activity.

These paradoxes can be explained if resistance, or lack of it, from the cervix is taken into account. Reduction of resistance may prove more logical than increasing force, especially if uterine activity already appears to be adequate. Unfortunately, the clinical means to manipulate resistance safely have not been developed.

### Passages

These have customarily been considered in terms of the bony pelvis. However, frank contracture of the pelvis is rare in developed societies, today. Pelvic pathology can result from metabolic disorders, congenital deformity of the spine or lower limbs and trauma.

The soft tissues have taken second place, perhaps wrongly. As noted above, the cervix offers resistance in the first stage and the perineum can delay delivery in the later part of the second stage. Poor ripening and abnormal glycoprotein balance in the cervix have been associated with poor progress.

## Passenger

There is statistical evidence for slight increases in birth weight over time, but these are unlikely to have been clinically significant. However, growing concerns over maternal obesity, which in turn influences birthweight, means that further surveillance is required. Fetal macrosomia results in a tendency to shoulder dystocia rather than cephalo-pelvic disproportion. Unlike cephalo-pelvic disproportion, shoulder dystocia does not necessarily give warning of its likelihood by aberrance in cervimetric progress. Furthermore, while increasing birthweight is associated with increased operative delivery rates, other variables such as flexion and rotation are as important in determining outcome.

## GRAPHIC REPRESENTATION OF PROGRESS

### First stage

The first stage of labour was subdivided by Friedman into two main phases: latent and active. The latent phase is very variable, not least because its onset is not precise. Friedman's data show that the latent phase in nulliparous women can last up to 20 hours (mean 8.6 hours), and 14 hours (mean 5.3 hours) in multiparae. During the latent phase, there is relatively little dilatation, but effacement is taking place. Effacement and dilatation tend to be more discrete in first labours than in subsequent ones (see Figure 20.2 for a graphic representation of progress).

The active phase of dilatation is characterized by rapid, progressive dilatation of the cervix. Friedman divided the active phase further into three parts: phases of 'acceleration' and 'deceleration' on either side of the most important part, that of 'maximum slope'. The phases of acceleration and deceleration have been questioned. A more recent and better statistical analysis of labour shows a progressively accelerating rate of cervical dilatation as the active phase progresses.[9]

Friedman selected 200 primigravidae, retrospectively, from a larger heterogeneous group of patients[10] (a second paper follows similar practice for multigravidae[11]) to identify 'ideal' labour, i.e. no iatrogenic interventions (apart from 'prophylactic low forceps'), vaginal deliveries and average-sized, healthy neonates. These patients' labour curves were analysed to identify statistical limits. Means and standard deviations were calculated. From these data, the lower limit of maximum slope dilatation of 1 cm/hour was produced. This value has now become almost universally accepted for clinical practice, but it may be an overestimate for the following two reasons.

1    The data are not normally distributed, with a skew towards higher rates of dilatation.
2    Most clinicians use an average minimum of 1 cm/hour for the whole of the active phase, including the slower phases of acceleration and deceleration and not just the phase of maximum slope.

### Second stage

Progress in the second stage of labour is judged by descent and rotation of the presenting part. This can be done in two ways: by the amount of the presenting part palpable per abdomen or by the station of the presenting part on vaginal examination. The former is practical only with cephalic presentations. The latter can be performed with malpresentations and allows determination of position as well. Partograms for the second stage have been produced,[12] but have not found widespread use.

Arbitary limits have been placed on the duration of the second stage: 3 hours for first deliveries and 2 hours for second and subsequent ones with alert to delay to be had at 2 hours and 1 hour, respectively [E].[8]

In normal labour, full dilatation and entry to the second stage is usually recognized by the mother feeling the urge to push. Epidural analgesia may dull this response so that the second stage may not be diagnosed for some time after full dilatation. This has resulted in a recognition that the length of the second stage may vary considerably. However, once the mother starts to push – the active second stage – and descent takes place, changes in the acid-base status of the fetus occurs. While the passive part of the second stage, i.e. that part before pushing, can be variable without detriment to mother or fetus, there is good reason to limit the duration of pushing, assuming pushing is effective. Good quality evidence on limits is not available but from a practical

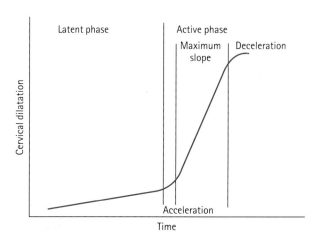

**Figure 20.2** Friedman's division of labour

standpoint 45 minutes for first deliveries and 30 minutes for second and subsequent ones is suggested. When instrumental delivery is required, additional time is required to prepare. These limits, though apparently stringent, allow for this.

## MONITORING

### Partogram

The partogram (Figure 20.3) is a composite, graphical record of key data entered against time as labour progresses. Both maternal and fetal data are represented.

#### Maternal

- Vital signs (blood pressure, temperature 4-hourly recording and pulse rate hourly)
- Uterine activity (every 30 mins)
- Cervimetric progress
- Drugs given
- Analgesia
- Fluid balance (frequency of bladder emptying, urinalysis).

#### Fetal

- Heart rate (immediately after contractions for 1 minute, minimum, every 15 minutes in first stage and 5 minutes in second stage).
- Descent/station
- Presentation
- Position
- Liquor – membranes intact or not and presence of meconium.

A large, prospective, observational study on the use of partograms with strict definition of established labour and agreed policies for intervention has showed an association with reduced use of oxytocin and, possibly, small but significant benefits in outcome [C].[13] However, these benefits have been called into question by randomized trials and meta-analysis [A].[14]

### Cervicogram

An essential part of the partogram is the cervicogram. Vaginal examination to assess cervical dilatation may be performed 2-, 3- or 4-hourly. The interval does not affect clinical outcome. Therefore, the lowest frequency should be adopted routinely with shorter intervals of assessment only when indicated.

Delay can be recognized in active labour when cervical dilatation rate falls below 2 cm in 4 hours or a slowing in rate in women in second or subsequent deliveries [E].[8]

It is common practice to adopt a rate of progress of 1 cm/hour for active phase dilatation, as noted above. A line set on the partogram at this rate of progress may be termed an alert line, that is to say progress slower than this alerts attendants to deviation from low to increased risk. Action lines have been set at varying intervals after the alert line. A randomized trial[15] has shown that an action line set 4 hours after the alert line reduces intervention and gives similar clinical outcomes to a line set at 2 hours. Thus, an action line 4 hours behind the alert line should be adopted [B].[8]

Cervicograms should be aids to the management of labour. Aberrant progress and patterns thereof do not constitute diagnoses in themselves. They are signs for which underlying diagnoses should be sought, though this may not always be successful.

### Uterine activity

Contractions are most commonly assessed by palpation and recorded as frequency per 10 minutes. Amplitude is assessed subjectively and duration may also be timed. External guard-ring tocodynamometers, designed to be part of continuous electronic fetal heart rate monitoring, give no indication of amplitude and do not necessarily record the true duration because positioning on the abdomen affects sensitivity.

Uterine activity normally increases as the first stage progresses towards full dilatation. There is no fixed frequency or level of uterine activity for spontaneous, progressing labour. When augmentation is performed, a maximum of five contractions per 10 minutes has been recommended [E].[8]

### Fetal monitoring

Fetal monitoring is performed in all labours. Low-risk labours should be monitored by intermittent auscultation by ear or by using hand-held Doppler devices every 15 minutes with observation immediately after contractions for a minimum of 1 minute. High-risk labours and any associated with mecomium-stained liquor, bleeding and maternal pyrexia should employ continuous electronic fetal heart rate monitoring [B].[8] Either way, the rate is recorded on the partogram.

### Posture

It has become customary in western society for women to labour on beds in a recumbent position, although there is no clear rationale for this. Pregnant women should not lie supine, as this can produce vena caval compression and compromise the placental circulation. Conventional epidural analgesia limits mobility and may contribute to current trends. If all is well, the labouring woman can adopt whatever position she finds most comfortable. Kneeling on all fours is commonly chosen. Maternal position has not been shown to affect fetal position or the mechanics of labour.

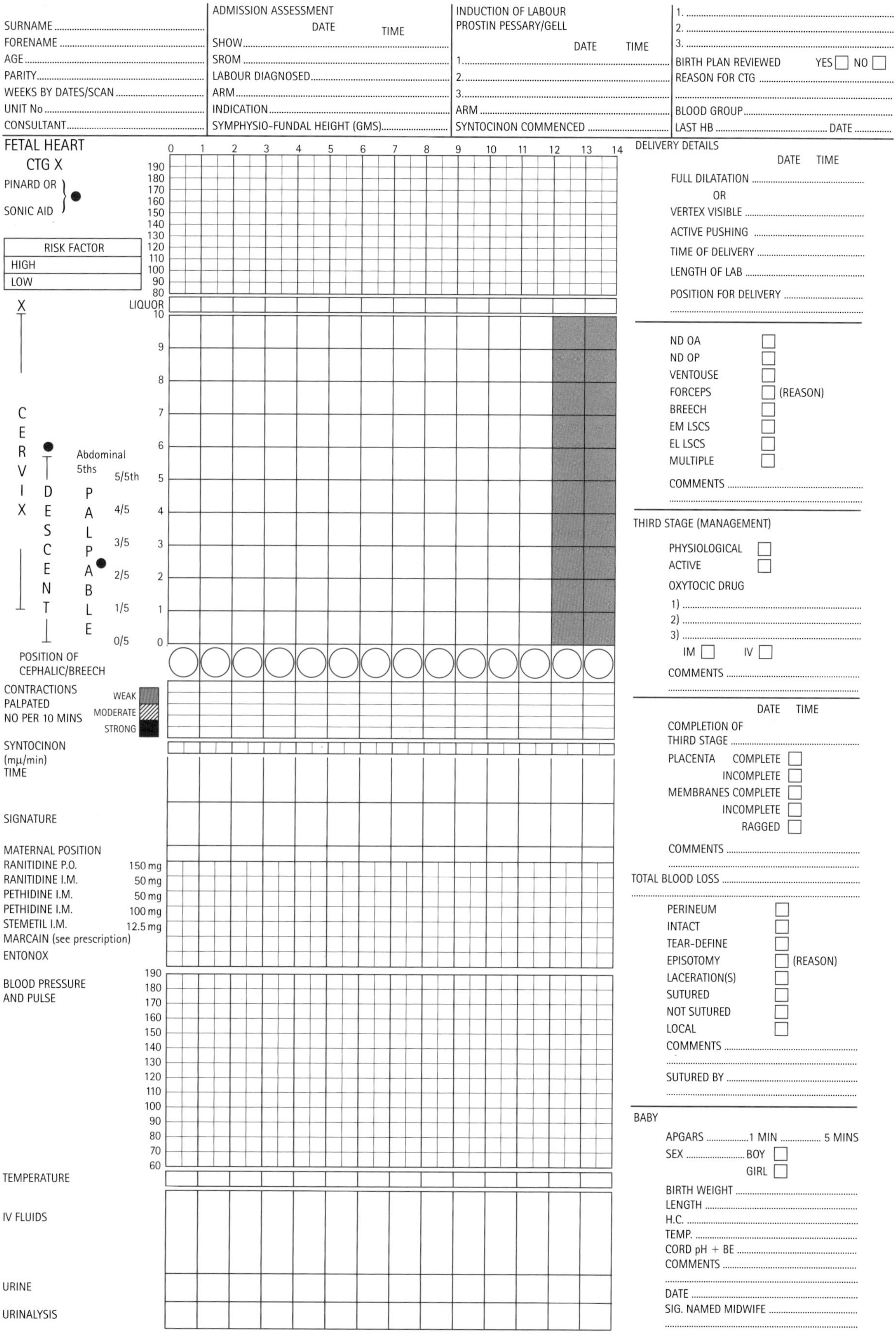

SURNAME .................................
FORENAME .................................
AGE .................................
PARITY .................................
WEEKS BY DATES/SCAN .................................
UNIT No .................................
CONSULTANT .................................

ADMISSION ASSESSMENT
                    DATE        TIME
SHOW .................................
SROM .................................
LABOUR DIAGNOSED .................................
ARM .................................
INDICATION .................................
SYMPHYSIO-FUNDAL HEIGHT (GMS) .................................

INDUCTION OF LABOUR
PROSTIN PESSARY/GELL
                              DATE      TIME
1. .................................
2. .................................
3. .................................
ARM .................................
SYNTOCINON COMMENCED .................................

1. .................................
2. .................................
3. .................................
BIRTH PLAN REVIEWED        YES ☐   NO ☐
REASON FOR CTG .................................
BLOOD GROUP .................................
LAST HB .................................   DATE .................................

FETAL HEART
CTG X
PINARD OR ⎱
            } ●
SONIC AID ⎰

| RISK FACTOR |
| --- |
| HIGH |
| LOW |

X

C
E
R
V
I
X

D
E
S
C
E
N
T

Abdominal
5ths

P
A
L
P
A
B
L
E

5/5th
4/5
3/5
2/5
1/5
0/5

190 180 170 160 150 140 130 120 110 100 90 80

LIQUOR
10

0  1  2  3  4  5  6  7  8  9  10  11  12  13  14

9
8
7
6
5/5th  5
4/5    4
3/5    3
2/5    2
1/5    1
0/5    0

POSITION OF
CEPHALIC/BREECH

CONTRACTIONS
PALPATED
NO PER 10 MINS

WEAK
MODERATE
STRONG

SYNTOCINON
(mμ/min)
TIME

SIGNATURE

MATERNAL POSITION
RANITIDINE P.O.      150 mg
RANITIDINE I.M.       50 mg
PETHIDINE I.M.        50 mg
PETHIDINE I.M.       100 mg
STEMETIL I.M.        12.5 mg
MARCAIN (see prescription)
ENTONOX

BLOOD PRESSURE
AND PULSE

190 180 170 160 150 140 130 120 110 100 90 80 70 60

TEMPERATURE

IV FLUIDS

URINE

URINALYSIS

DELIVERY DETAILS
                                    DATE    TIME
FULL DILATATION .................................
            OR
VERTEX VISIBLE .................................
ACTIVE PUSHING .................................
TIME OF DELIVERY .................................
LENGTH OF LAB .................................
POSITION FOR DELIVERY .................................
.................................

ND OA          ☐
ND OP          ☐
VENTOUSE       ☐
FORCEPS        ☐  (REASON)
BREECH         ☐
EM LSCS        ☐
EL LSCS        ☐
MULTIPLE       ☐

COMMENTS .................................
.................................

THIRD STAGE (MANAGEMENT)

PHYSIOLOGICAL   ☐
ACTIVE          ☐
OXYTOCIC DRUG
1) .................................
2) .................................
3) .................................
IM ☐    IV ☐
COMMENTS .................................
.................................

                                    DATE    TIME
COMPLETION OF
THIRD STAGE .................................
PLACENTA    COMPLETE    ☐
            INCOMPLETE  ☐
MEMBRANES COMPLETE      ☐
            INCOMPLETE  ☐
            RAGGED      ☐

COMMENTS .................................

TOTAL BLOOD LOSS .................................

PERINEUM       ☐
INTACT         ☐
TEAR-DEFINE    ☐
EPISOTOMY      ☐  (REASON)
LACERATION(S)  ☐
SUTURED        ☐
NOT SUTURED    ☐
LOCAL          ☐
COMMENTS .................................
.................................
SUTURED BY .................................

BABY
APGARS .............1 MIN .............5 MINS
SEX .............BOY ☐
            GIRL ☐
BIRTH WEIGHT .................................
LENGTH .................................
H.C. .................................
TEMP. .................................
CORD pH + BE .................................
COMMENTS .................................
.................................
DATE .................................
SIG. NAMED MIDWIFE .................................
.................................

**Figure 20.3** A typical partogram

An upright posture for the second stage has been shown to increase spontaneous vaginal delivery,[16] but perineal trauma and blood loss may be greater [A], although there are few good-quality clinical trials.

Water births, providing immersion in warm water plus buoyancy, offer a soothing environment, which may relax the mother and reduce her requirement for analgesia. Delivery of the baby into water is more controversial and there are risks associated with the water temperature, infection and clearing the baby's oropharynx. Providing adequate guidelines are followed, these risks can be managed [E].

## Episiotomy

Routine episiotomy should not be performed but the procedure may be indicated on a case to case basis. When performed, right medio-lateral episiotomy is recommended.[8]

## Nutrition and fluid balance

Dehydration and ketosis can contribute to poor uterine activity and withholding oral intake has been advocated by some because of the worry over the risk of aspiration, should general anaesthesia be required in an emergency. Data from a randomized controlled trial show that the risks of aspiration are minimal with modern techniques of regional anaesthesia and that there is no particular benefit of light diet over adequate fluid intake.[17] Thus, it seems reasonable to maintain hydration, orally, and be guided by the woman's wishes regarding dietary intake [B].

## PROFESSIONAL ROLES

In the UK, the role of the midwife has been highly developed. The midwife is the expert in normal childbirth and will be in contact with the woman more than any other professional. (S)he should prepare the mother-to-be for labour, give her confidence and offer support, advice and encouragement during labour [A]. This is crucial. Even if continuity of carer is not possible, there should be one-to-one midwifery care in labour. Midwives are independent practitioners and can thus offer total care to low-risk cases.

When complications are found, the midwife should liaise with the medical team to ensure continuity. The roles of midwife and obstetrician are complementary. Even with medical need, the midwife will continue to collect and record data and support the woman through the rest of labour and delivery.

## PSYCHOLOGICAL SUPPORT

Childbirth is a highly emotive event that engenders anxiety and apprehension for all concerned, not least the mother.

Such feelings can be ameliorated by surroundings familiar to the mother and by supportive companions, whether professional or otherwise. These are reasons why some women opt for home delivery. There has been, and still is, a long-running debate about the safety of home delivery. With careful selection and proper attention to contingencies, home delivery can be rewarding.

If the woman understands what is happening and is well prepared, she feels more in control. All too often the delivery environment has focused on perceived medical need, and economies have eaten away at professional input to the preparation for labour. Management decisions may not be explained, thereby disempowering the woman. The result is apprehension and anxiety. These feelings may adversely affect the labour in a number of ways, for example reduced pain threshold, need for more analgesia, increased stress hormones and muscular tension.

These 'soft' issues were once ignored but preparation and support of the woman have significant strongest impact on clinical outcome [A].[6] Doulas (non-professional patient supporters) have been shown to be highly effective and may have advantages over midwives in that they are not distracted from their prime purpose – supporting the labouring woman – by routine monitoring duties.

> ## KEY POINTS
>
> For good labour management:
> - Understand the physiology.
> - Do not diagnose 'labour' until clearly established – evidence of progressive cervical dilatation (>4 cm dilatation).
> - Understand the monitoring and what it tells us.
> - When there is aberrance, try to identify a diagnosis (although this may not always be possible).
> - Understand interventions and identify what you want from them.
> - Establish guidelines and practice on best available evidence.
> - Agree guidelines across professional groups so that practice is consistent.
> - Audit against these standards.
> - Prepare women for their labour and support and encourage them during it.

## Key References

1. O'Driscoll K, Jackson JA, Gallagher JT. Prevention of prolonged labour. *BMJ* 1969; **2**: 447–80.
2. Cardozo L, Pearce JM. Oxytocin in active-phase abnormalities of labour: A randomised study. *Obstet Gynecol* 1991; **75**: 152–7.
3. Hinshaw K, Simpson S, Cummings S *et al.* A randomised controlled trial of early versus delayed oxytocin augmentation to treat primary dysfunctional labour in nulliparous women. *BJOG* 2008; **115**: 1289–95.

4. Group UA. A multicentre randomised trial of amniotomy in spontaneous first labour at term. *BJOG* 1994; **101**: 307–9.

5. Smyth R, Alldred S, Markham C. Amniotomy for shortening spontaneous labour. *Cochrane Database Syst Rev* 2007; (**4**): CD006167.

6. Hodnett ED, Gates S, Hofmeyr GJ, Sakala C. Continuous support for women during childbirth. *Cochrane Database Syst Rev* 2007; (**3**): CD003766.

7. Chua S, Kurup A, Arulkumaran S, Ratnam SS. Augmentation of labour: Does internal tocography result in better obstetric outcome. *Obstet Gynaecol* 1990; (**76**): 164–7.

8. NICE. *Intra-partum care (Guideline 55)*. London: National Institute for Health and Clinical Excellence, 2007: 51.

9. Zhang J, Troendle JF, Yancey MK. Reassessing the labor curve in nulliparous women. *Am J Obstet Gynecol* 2002; **187**: 824–8.

10. Friedman EA. Primigravid labor. *Obstet Gynecol* 1955; **6**: 567–89.

11. Friedman EA. Labor in multiparas. *Obstet Gynecol* 1956; **8**: 691–703.

12. Sizer AR, Evans J, Bailey SM, Wiener J. A second-stage partogram. *Obstet Gynecol* 2000; **96**: 678–83.

13. WHO, World Health Organisation partograph in the management of labor. World Health Organization Maternal Health and Safe Motherhood Programme. *Lancet* 1994; **343**: 1399–404.

14. Lavender T, Hart A, Smyth RM. Effect of partogram use on outcomes for women in spontaneous labour at term. *Cochrane Database Syst Rev* 2008; (**4**): CD005461.

15. Lavender T, Alfirevic Z, Walkinshaw S. Effect of different partogram action lines on birth outcomes: a randomized controlled trial. *Obstet Gynecol* 2006; **108**: 295–302.

16. Gupta JK, Hofmeyer GJ, Smyth R. Position in the second stage of labour for women without epidural anaesthesia. *Cochrane Database Syst Rev* 2004; (**1**): CD002006.

17. O'Sullivan G, Liu B, Hart D *et al.* Effect of food intake during labour on obstetric outcome: randomised controlled trial. *BMJ* 2009; **338**: 784.

Antenatal complications: fetal

# SECTION C
## Late pregnancy/ intrapartum events

# Chapter 21

# Preterm labour

*Myles Taylor*

## MRCOG standards

Candidates are expected to:
- be conversant with the appropriate use of tocolysis and steroids in preterm labour;
- be able to manage preterm labour and *in-utero* transfer of the mother;
- be able to recognize and manage intrauterine infection.

In addition, we would suggest the following:

### Theoretical skills
- Understand the contribution of spontaneous preterm delivery to overall perinatal morbidity and mortality.
- Have access to and utilize mortality and morbidity figures, stratified by gestation.
- Be aware of the aetiologies behind spontaneous preterm labour and how they vary with gestation.
- Recognize major and minor risk factors for spontaneous preterm birth.
- Be aware of specialized screening tests for predicting preterm delivery.

### Practical skills
- Formulate a plan for the antenatal management of asymptomatic women recognized to be at increased risk of spontaneous preterm birth.
- Be able to manage women in threatened preterm labour with regard to obstetric interventions and counselling regarding neonatal prognosis.
- Perform an ultrasound scan to confirm presentation and gestation.
- Be able to use tocolytic agents safely, with regard to dosage, route of administration, side effects and contraindications.
- Be able to undertake a preterm delivery, including delivery by caesarean section.

## INTRODUCTION

There are two major clinical subtypes of preterm births. Indicated preterm deliveries, undertaken for maternal or fetal reasons, make up approximately one-third of all such births. The remaining two-thirds are classified as spontaneous preterm births and have two subdivisions: spontaneous preterm labour and preterm pre-labour rupture of the membranes (PPROM).

## DEFINITION

In the United Kingdom, preterm birth includes all deliveries between $24^{+0}$ and $36^{+6}$ weeks. Many developed countries now officially register all deliveries with a birth weight above 500 g.

In 1994–95, 6.6 per cent of all UK births were preterm, amounting to approximately 40 000 per annum. For reasons related to aetiology, outcome and recurrence risk, preterm deliveries should be divided into three gestational periods: mildly preterm births at $32^{+0}$ to $36^{+6}$ weeks (incidence 5.5 per cent), moderately preterm births at $28^{+0}$ to $31^{+6}$ weeks (incidence 0.7 per cent) and extremely preterm births at $24^{+0}$ to $27^{+6}$ weeks (incidence 0.4 per cent).

Significantly higher rates of preterm birth of up to 12 per cent are reported from the United States. Conversely, many Nordic countries quote rates below 5 per cent. This must reflect differing aetiological, socioeconomic and cultural factors.

## NEONATAL OUTCOMES

### Survival

When counselling parents, doctors must use perinatal statistics that are up to date and, where possible, reflect local outcomes. Figures from a total population within a UK Health Region have been published (Figure 21.1).[1,2]

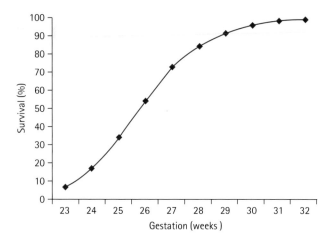

**Figure 21.1** Percentage predicted survival for European infants known to be alive at the onset of labour

Predicted survival can be modified by accurate estimates of fetal weight or antenatal assessments of fetal well-being.

## Morbidity

The risks of later neurodevelopmental impairment, disability and handicap are especially significant within the 24–26-week gestational window. The UK-based EPIcure Study reported that 50 per cent of the survivors at 23–25 weeks gestation were impaired, half with severe disability.[3] In another study, up to 40 per cent of survivors born before 26 weeks gestation were found to have a head circumference below the third centile at two years of age, after which little 'catch-up' growth is possible.[4] Follow up of very low birth weight children to school age has also shown later educational difficulties. Additional concerns relate to social behaviour and criminality, as well as subsequent influences on adult health.

## AETIOLOGY

## Infection

Subclinical infection of the choriodecidual space and amniotic fluid is the most widely studied aetiological factor underlying spontaneous prematurity. Many indirect lines of evidence support the role of subclinical infection in human preterm labour, including the following:

- Vaginal colonization with a variety of microorganisms has been associated with an increased risk of spontaneous prematurity. However, it is plausible that the presence of such pathogens may simply be markers for other socio-economic, sexual or behavioural factors that ultimately lead to preterm labour.

- If an amniocentesis is performed in preterm labour with intact membranes, 10–15 per cent of amniotic fluid samples result in positive cultures.
- Histological chorioamnionitis is much more common after spontaneous preterm birth. Of note, most cases are subclinical, with only 10 per cent of histologically proven cases of chorioamnionitis having overt clinical signs of infection.

## Vascular

Spontaneous prematurity has been associated with an increase in membrane haemosiderin deposits, thought to reflect decidual haemorrhages. The link between placental abruption and either uterine activity or PPROM is well recognized.

## Uterine overdistension

### Multiple pregnancy

In 1999, 1.44 per cent of all maternities in the UK involved multiple pregnancies, mostly twin pregnancies. The median gestation at delivery for twins is approximately 35 weeks and for triplets 33 weeks. Presently, assisted reproduction techniques are responsible for 35 per cent of twin pregnancies and 77 per cent of triplets, leading to an increasing burden of preterm births. Multi-fetal reduction has been shown to reduce risk in higher order pregnancies and should always be considered.

### Polyhydramnios

Fetal anomalies, such as atresias of the gastrointestinal tract, are the most common cause of polyhydramnios leading to preterm delivery.

## Cervical weakness

This remains a notoriously difficult diagnosis to make either within or outside of pregnancy. Even a careful review of the clinical events leading up to preterm labour and delivery does not necessarily show correlation with the aetiology.

## Intercurrent illness

Serious infective illnesses such as pyelonephritis, appendicitis and pneumonia are associated with preterm labour. This association is presumed to be due either to direct blood-borne spread of infection to the uterine cavity or indirectly to chemical triggers, such as endotoxins or cytokines. Many other medical complications, such as cholestasis of pregnancy, and any surgical procedures are associated with preterm labour, although the mechanisms remain obscure.

## Relationship between gestation and aetiology

Studies involving the use of amniocentesis in threatened preterm labour found most positive amniotic fluid cultures to be from pregnancies presenting before 30 weeks gestation. The incidence and severity of histological chorioamnionitis also show an inverse relationship with gestational age. Thus, the earliest births carry the highest risk of an infectious aetiology.

Intrauterine infection has also been associated with an increased risk of various neonatal morbidities, independent of gestation at birth. These include:

- periventricular leukomalacia,
- cerebral palsy,
- bronchopulmonary dysplasia.

These pathologies are presumed to be secondary to high circulating levels of inflammatory cytokines. This leads to the paradox of prematurity, namely, those fetuses who stand to gain most by delaying delivery also carry the greatest risk from prolonged exposure in a potentially hostile uterine environment.

## RISK GROUPS

Owing to limited resources and a paucity of beneficial interventions in low-risk women, most aspects of prematurity prevention should be targeted at women with major risk factors for preterm birth. These major risk factors include the following:

- *Previous preterm birth.* After one preterm birth, the risk in the next pregnancy is approximately 20 per cent. After two preterm deliveries, this risk increases to 35–40 per cent. Where the most recent birth was at term, but the penultimate delivery was preterm, recurrence risks are intermediate. As well as a tendency for preterm births to recur in the same gestational age group, the earliest births have the highest recurrence risks.[5] This presumably reflects differing aetiologies predominating at different gestations.
- *Uterine overdistension.* Multiple pregnancies or pregnancies known to be at risk of polyhydramnios require careful monitoring.
- *Uterine abnormalities.* Cervical surgery, such as cone biopsy, remains a classic risk factor and recent meta-analysis has also implicated large loop excision of the transformation zone.[6] Also, epidemiological evidence casts doubt on the benign nature of surgical cervical dilatation, the risk of subsequent preterm delivery increasing with the number of previous cervical dilatations.
- Although there is little evidence upon which to estimate either individual risk or the total contribution to

preterm births, the malformed uterus has long been associated with spontaneous prematurity. This may be mediated by cervical weakness, although recent evidence suggests that abnormalities of uterine vascularity may also play a role.

- Maternal diethylstilbestrol (DES) exposure in the 1960s led to a cohort of female offspring with congenital uterine and cervical anomalies. The women in this cohort are now approaching the end of their reproductive years. The role of fibroids in preterm delivery remains controversial; considering their frequency, their influence is probably minimal in the absence of cervical involvement.
- *Factors in current pregnancy.* Examples include:
  - intercurrent illness,
  - surgery,
  - recurrent vaginal bleeding.

There is also a variety of minor risk factors for spontaneous preterm birth that carry importance in epidemiological terms. The relative risk attributable to each factor is small. Attempts have been made to develop scoring systems (such as the Creasy score), but these have not proved helpful.

Some minor risk factors carry importance because they are potentially modifiable. These include:

- smoking,
- low body mass index (BMI),
- interpregnancy interval of less than one year.

Other risk factors that are not amenable to influence include:

- maternal age (teenage multiparae),
- parity (nulliparous or grandmultiparous),
- ethnicity (black women),
- socioeconomic deprivation,
- unemployment,
- low levels of education.

## MANAGEMENT OF ASYMPTOMATIC HIGH-RISK WOMEN

A careful analysis of events surrounding the previous birth should be undertaken. The risk of recurrence may be adjusted if there were non-recurring phenomena, such as fetal anomaly or intercurrent illness.

### Investigation and treatment outside of pregnancy

Ideally, women should be seen postnatally and the events leading to their preterm birth reviewed. Following this, a clear management plan for any subsequent pregnancy should be made [E]. The importance of smoking cessation should be stressed [C] and the potential benefit of leaving

12 months between pregnancies should be discussed [C]. Dietician referral may be appropriate for women with a low BMI.

## Investigation and treatment during pregnancy

### Early dating scan

A first trimester dating scan is essential to time subsequent investigations. It also ensures precise gestational age assessment should preterm labour recur near the limits of neonatal viability [E].

### Bacterial vaginosis

Bacterial vaginosis (BV) has been associated with an increased risk of preterm birth in many observational studies. The detection of BV does not involve conventional culture techniques. A vaginal swab is rolled on to a glass slide in a similar fashion to a cervical smear test. Gram staining and microscopy are then used to diagnose BV, using the Nugent scoring system. Randomized studies, such as that of Hauth et al.,[7] have demonstrated that oral metronidazole significantly lowers the risk of preterm birth, by 60 per cent in high-risk women positive for BV [A].

As there is concern that BV may reflect chronic intra-uterine infection, 5–7 days of oral therapy at standard doses seems appropriate. A large trial using briefer therapy has not shown benefit. Several randomized, placebo-controlled studies have suggested an increase in moderately preterm birth (32–34 weeks) in BV-positive women randomized to vaginal clindamycin cream. One hypothesis is that topical therapy adequately treats vaginosis, but fails to affect pre-existing intrauterine infection.

### Asymptomatic bacteriuria

This carries an increased risk of preterm birth. Although it may simply be a marker for heavy vaginal microbial colonization, a meta-analysis of many trials confirms that risk is reduced by appropriate antibiotic treatment [A]. An alternative explanation for the association with preterm birth may be an increased risk of pyelonephritis in women presenting with asymptomatic bacteriuria.

### Group B streptococcal colonization

Group B streptococcal (GBS) colonization has been linked to prematurity. Preterm infants are certainly more susceptible to early-onset GBS infection, acquired during passage through the birth canal. However, evidence that it is one of the major causal organisms behind spontaneous prematurity remains weak. In women known to be at increased risk of preterm delivery, testing for GBS antenatally allows appropriate intrapartum prophylaxis to be planned. Optimal screening involves the use of a combined low vaginal/rectal swab. As maternal carriage can change during pregnancy, later repeat screening should be considered. Only intrapartum treatment should be given [A], as antenatal antibiotics have not been shown to lower perinatal transmission.

It is, of course, very common for women who know they are colonized to request antenatal treatment. Women should be advised that several studies from North America have reported that overaggressive prophylactic treatment of GBS has led to an increase in neonatal infections with penicillin-resistant Escherichia coli. In pregnancy, as elsewhere, antibiotics have the potential for harm.

### Other organisms

Organisms such as Chlamydia trachomatis, Neisseria gonococcus and Trichomonas vaginalis have been associated with preterm delivery, but again, a causal link has not been established. Antenatal treatment of chlamydia has not been shown to lower prematurity rates, although it may prevent perinatal transmission. Treatment of chlamydia and gonococcus must always include contact tracing and treatment of the partner. These are best accomplished in conjunction with the department of genitourinary medicine. A test of cure should always be performed.

### Cervical ultrasound

Cervical length can be accurately and repeatedly measured by ultrasound. The risk of prematurity is inversely related to cervical length [C].[8] These measurements should only be made by transvaginal scanning, as the full bladder necessary for visualization transabdominally leads to false lengthening and can obliterate gross funnelling. Transvaginal ultrasound has been shown to be more accurate than digital measurements for assessing cervical length. The test has predictive ability in all groups of women (low risk, high risk, twins, symptomatic, etc.).

In asymptomatic women with a short cervix, the risk of moderately preterm delivery rises only slightly, to 4 per cent with lengths of 11–20 mm. At 10 mm, the risk is 15 per cent and it increases dramatically as length decreases further. The technique is certainly able to identify a group of women at risk of cervical weakness.

### Cervical cerclage

After documentation of a shortened cervix on ultrasound, randomized trials of cerclage versus observation have shown contradictory results. Perhaps more importantly, cervical ultrasound is able to exclude weakness – if the cervix is long, surgical intervention can be avoided. The Medical Research Council Randomised Trial of Cervical Cerclage highlighted overintervention based on simple clinical assessment, suggesting benefit in only 4 per cent of cases.[9] In a more detailed analysis, cerclage led to improved outcomes only after three or more previous very early deliveries [B]. The relative merits of McDonald versus Shirodkar cerclage have long been debated and remain unresolved. Certainly, a Shirodkar cerclage is located much closer to the internal os. Whether this translates into a better outcome is unknown.

Some authors have advocated transabdominal sutures. These are placed at the level of the internal os via a Pfannenstiel incision or performed laparoscopically. They are permanent and necessitate caesarean section for delivery. Their use has not been subjected to rigorous testing. They have a number of theoretical disadvantages, including the need for abdominal delivery if preterm labour occurs regardless of gestation, and they are associated with the operative morbidity of any abdominal procedure. They are probably only rarely required and their use should be restricted to clinical trials.

## Progesterone supplementation

There is increasing evidence suggesting that progesterone supplementation can reduce the incidence of preterm delivery, particularly in high risk groups. Progesterone is available in two forms – natural, usually administered vaginally, and synthetic, 17-alpha-hydroxyprogesterone administered intramuscularly. In singleton pregnancies with a history of previous preterm delivery, two randomized controlled trials[10,11] showed a reduction in the risk of delivering <37 weeks approaching 50 per cent. Subsequent meta-analyses have confirmed these findings. However, it has not been demonstrated that this observed prolongation of at risk pregnancies is associated with an improvement in perinatal outcomes. Intriguingly, progesterone supplementation does not appear to prevent preterm birth in multiple pregnancies. Further studies are required to define the optimum preparation, dose, timing, route of administration and indications for progesterone supplementation. Currently, the American College of Obstetricans and Gynaecologists recommend progesterone supplementation be restricted to women with a singleton pregnancy and a previous history of spontaneous preterm birth.[12]

## Cervico-vaginal fibronectin testing

This is undertaken after 23 weeks, as levels are often high prior to this gestation. Fetal fibronectin (fFN) is a 'glue-like' protein binding the choriodecidual membranes. It is rarely present in vaginal secretions between 23 and 34 weeks. Any disruption at the choriodecidual interface results in fFN release and possible detection in the cervico-vaginal secretions. A bedside test is available that gives a positive/negative result.

Technique is important in performing the bedside test. Digital examination of the cervix should not have been performed prior to fFN testing and no lubricating jelly used.

In addition:

- Only the swab supplied with the testing kit should be used.
- The swab should be rotated in the posterior fornix for 15–20 seconds to ensure the tip is saturated.
- Endocervical swabbing should not be undertaken.
- The test result should be read within 15 minutes, if using the bedside kit.
  False-positive results can occur if:
- There has been sexual intercourse within 24 hours.
- There is vaginal bleeding.

For high-risk asymptomatic women with a positive fFN test at 24 weeks gestation, 46 per cent will deliver before 30 weeks gestation.[13] Conversely, the risk of preterm delivery is <1 per cent with a negative test.

There is no proven treatment for a positive fFN test, although several groups are studying the potential role of antibiotics. Presently, clinicians can use the high negative predictive value to either withhold treatments or optimize their timing.

## Salivary oestriol

A salivary oestriol surge has been reported up to 3 weeks before onset of labour. Its usefulness in predicting preterm birth has not been proven.

## Home uterine activity monitors

An increase in painless uterine activity may precede the onset of labour. However, the early detection of this increased activity has not been found to reduce the incidence of prematurity. This is not surprising, as no effective prophylactic treatment has yet been found that suppresses contractions. Many studies, meta-analyses and reviews have shown no evidence of benefit from oral ritodrine. At present, the conclusions for other maintenance tocolytics, such as nifedipine or glyceryl trinitrate (GTN) patches, must be similar, given the paucity of well-controlled studies supporting their use.

## Lifestyle modification

Women at high risk should be counselled about smoking [C].

Work from France suggested that increased social and economic support for women believed to be at risk of preterm delivery led to a reduction in early births. Such results have not been replicated elsewhere. Randomized trials of social support in the UK failed to improve pregnancy outcomes [B]. In some situations, hospitalization for bed rest led to an increase in preterm births [A]. The roles of sexual abstinence and/or psychological support are no clearer and should not be recommended as a universal or general measure in high-risk women.

# MANAGEMENT OF SYMPTOMATIC WOMEN

## History

The diagnosis of preterm labour remains notoriously difficult in the absence of advanced dilatation or ruptured membranes. Pre-assessment odds of spontaneous preterm delivery based on historical risk factors are a useful starting point, analogous to the diagnostic approach for thromboembolism or screening for Down's syndrome.

A detailed review of current symptoms is necessary. Symptoms such as low backache or cramping are often cyclical. Vague complaints, such as pelvic pressure or increased discharge, are usually common. The coexistence of vaginal bleeding should always be taken seriously. In a women presenting with contractions, the risk of delivery within 7 days if she has vaginal bleeding and a closed cervix is actually greater than if she presented with no bleeding, but 2 cm of cervical dilatation.

## Examination

Abdominal examination may reveal the presence of uterine tenderness, suggesting abruption or chorioamnionitis. A careful speculum examination by an experienced clinician can yield valuable information. Pooling of amniotic fluid, blood and/or abnormal discharge should all be commented on. A visual assessment of cervical dilatation is usually possible and has been shown to be as accurate as digital examination findings. Medical staff should try to limit digital examinations to cases in which speculum assessment is inconclusive, as they are known to stimulate prostaglandin production and may introduce organisms into the cervical canal. When undertaken in cases of PPROM, digital examinations are associated with a significant reduction in the latent interval before labour.

## Further investigation

### Repeat vaginal examination

Repeat vaginal examination in 1–4 hours should be considered essential in the absence of secondary tests. The interval between assessments should be guided by the severity of the symptoms.

### Post-assessment risk

This should be based on the complete picture. A realistic end-point should be the chance of delivery within the next 7 days. If this risk is judged to be low, serial observation and review are appropriate. If the risk is high, treatment strategies to optimize perinatal outcome should be implemented.

## Bedside fibronectin testing

This offers a rapid assessment of risk in symptomatic women who do not have advanced dilatation. If done correctly, these tests have a greater predictive value than digital examination. In one study, 30 per cent of women with a positive fibronectin test delivered within 7 days, compared with only 10 per cent of women who were 2–3 cm dilated.[14]

## Cervical length measurement

Cervical length measurement by transvaginal ultrasound in symptomatic women has also been shown to improve diagnostic accuracy. Although measurements can be repeated frequently and with little expense, skilled ultrasonographers and suitable machines with transvaginal probes are required.

In symptomatic women, a positive fibronectin test carries a risk of delivery within 28 days of up to 70 per cent, regardless of initial cervical length. Combination testing refines the prediction of deliveries in the next 7 days. In the group with a positive fibronectin test but a normal cervical length, only 5 per cent will deliver within 1 week.[15] However, if the cervix is also short when tested, the risk of delivery within 7 days climbs to 50 per cent. This is particularly useful, as many interventions (tocolytics, steroids and in-utero transfer) should be based on this end-point.

# THERAPY

## Transplacental therapy

### Steroids

Current evidence shows that a single course of maternal steroids given between 26 and 34 weeks gestation and received within 7 days of delivery results in markedly improved neonatal outcomes [A], with a significant reduction in rates of:

- respiratory distress syndrome,
- neonatal death,
- intraventricular haemorrhage.

Maximum benefit from the injection is seen after 24 hours. In the most recent Cochrane review (2006) of this subject, treatment over a wide gestational range (26–34[+6] weeks) resulted in clinical benefit. On the other hand, courses received less than 24 hours and more than 7 days before delivery did not produce a significant reduction in respiratory distress syndrome.

In general, no convincing difference is seen between betamethasone and dexamethasone, although a recent study hinted at improved neurological outcomes with betamethasone.

There is considerable reassuring evidence about the long-term safety of single courses of maternal steroids from paediatric follow up into the teenage years. However, clinicians should only cautiously employ repeat courses, as there is growing concern about adverse consequences and little evidence of improved outcome.[16,17]

Published examples of potentially harmful effects of repeated doses include:

- increased sepsis in PPROM,
- restricted fetal body and brain growth,
- adrenal suppression.

Most worrying is the increased risk of neonatal death seen when three or more courses of antenatal steroids were given in the American Thyrotropin Releasing Hormone (TRH) Study.[18]

Any extensions to the accepted gestational window should also be made cautiously. There may be a limited steroid responsiveness in fetuses at or below 25 weeks gestation. As there is little proof that steroids are beneficial, their use may lead to overoptimism. Although the Royal College of Obstetricians and Gynaecologists Greentop guideline *Antenatal Corticosteroids to Prevent Respiratory Distress Syndrome* (2004) recommends steroids from 24 weeks gestation, this recommendation is not based on evidence from randomized trials. More worryingly, using steroids when inappropriate may hinder later use, particularly when clinicians are wary of multiple courses. The upper gestation at which steroids should be used is also controversial. In comparison to PPROM and pretem labour (PTL), elective non-labour deliveries after 33 weeks are at increased risk of respiratory difficulties and may benefit from prophylactic steroids.

Although there is a paucity of proof that steroids are beneficial in multiple pregnancy, most expert opinion supports their use. Even more caution should be used before embarking on repeat courses in this situation.

Corticosteroids can cause significant glycaemic disruption in diabetic women. They should be used in conjunction with increased glucose monitoring and adjusted insulin doses. The effects can last up to 24 hours after the second dose of steroids.

## Thyrotropin-releasing hormone, vitamin K or phenobarbitone

The use of thyrotropin-releasing hormone (TRH), vitamin K and phenobarbitone to improve neonatal outcome has been studied in randomized trials, but has not been shown to be beneficial [B].

## Tocolytics

The Canadian trial remains the most influential tocolytic trial to date.[19] This trial concluded that ritodrine had no significant benefit on perinatal mortality or the prolongation of pregnancy to term, although it was able to reduce the number of women delivering within 48 hours by 40 per cent [A]. This window of opportunity is the sole rationale for using tocolytics. The use of tocolytics is usually inappropriate if steroids have been given and intensive care cots are available.

### Beta-agonists

These drugs have significant maternal side effects, including hypotension, tachycardia, anxiety and palpitations. Maternal deaths from acute cardiopulmonary compromise are described, with greatest risks:

- if beta-agonists are given in large fluid volumes,
- in multiple pregnancy,
- in women with cardiac disease.

In women with diabetes, significant extra glycaemic disruption additional to that caused by steroids occurs with beta-agonists.

### Oxytocin antagonist

The oxytocin antagonist, atosiban, is now widely used in the UK mainly because of the significantly reduced frequency of side effects compared to beta-agonists. However, its clinical effectiveness is no greater than that of the beta-agonists and costs are higher [B].

### Other agents

Other smooth muscle relaxants used to treat preterm labour include magnesium sulphate, nifedipine and GTN. There is little evidence to suggest increased efficacy or improved outcomes [B] and none has a license for use in pregnancy.

As prostaglandins appear to be one of the pivotal chemicals involved in parturition, non-steroidal anti-inflammatory drugs (NSAIDs), such as indomethacin, have attracted considerable interest as tocolytics. There are potential fetal side effects, but these can be limited by restricting their use to less than 72 hours and only below 30 weeks gestation.

## Antibiotics

The UK Oracle II Study found no evidence of benefit for the use of antibiotics in uncomplicated preterm labour [A][20] and seven-year follow up showed a significant increase in the incidence of cerebral palsy.[21] On the other hand, significant advantages are obtained when antibiotics are prescribed to women with preterm prelabour rupture of membranes without an associated increase in cerebral palsy in the long term.[22]

## Emergency cervical cerclage

Occasionally, women present in the mid-trimester with relatively minor symptoms (pelvic pressure, watery discharge, etc.) and, when examined, are found to have membranes bulging into the upper vagina. If considering emergency cerclage, clinicians need to be aware that there is no randomized evidence for guidance and few reports of the outcome after expectant management. Two clinical issues must be considered.

First, is this a reflection of marked cervical weakness or is the cervix responding to uterine activity? A history of significant cervical surgery may be helpful. If symptomatic contractions are present, the answer is clear. Otherwise, all clinicians can do is reassess the cervical dilatation after several hours. This can be precisely and repeatedly measured non-invasively using transperineal ultrasound.

Second, is there any evidence of intrauterine infection? Only 10 per cent of cases of chorioamnionitis are clinically obvious but, if present, cerclage is doomed to fail. A suggested way to assess this is by amniocentesis, but this is rarely performed in practice.

### *In-utero* transfer

*In-utero* transfer to a unit with adequate neonatal facilities is recommended where these are not available in the admitting unit [D]. It would seem logical that this will improve outcome for babies. It should certainly be considered where neonatal stabilization would be difficult or impossible. It may also help to keep mother and baby together where transfer of the mother after delivery is likely to be difficult. All units should have guidelines for referral and communication.

## FETAL ASSESSMENT

Maternal steroid therapy can suppress both fetal activity and heart rate variability. Umbilical artery Doppler studies can also be influenced. In fetuses with absent/reversed end-diastolic flow (EDF), a short-term return of end diastolic flow is commonly observed.

When labour has started or is thought to be imminent:

- whenever possible, the presentation in preterm labour should be confirmed by ultrasound, as clinical palpation is notoriously unreliable;
- an accurate estimated fetal weight, particularly below 28 weeks, can aid parental counselling.

There are considerable difficulties surrounding the interpretation of the fetal heart rate in preterm infants, particularly at extremely early gestations. Simply applying the criteria used at term is inappropriate. Some work has suggested that the baseline rate is more important than either decelerations or variability. Of note, randomized, controlled trials have failed to show any benefit from continuous as opposed to intermittent monitoring in moderately preterm births [B].[23] Decisions regarding monitoring in labour at very preterm gestations must be discussed with parents. Intervention on the basis of fetal heart rate monitoring may not be justifiable near the limits of viability.

## MODE OF DELIVERY

Many clinicians feel that fetal morbidity and mortality, the difficulty in diagnosing intrapartum hypoxia/acidosis and the maternal risk do not justify caesarean section for fetal indications below 26 weeks. At this early gestation, intrapartum caesarean section has not been shown to improve neonatal outcomes.

As gestation advances, both neonatal outcomes and the ability to diagnose fetal compromise improve, and intervention for fetal reasons becomes universally appropriate. The safety of breech vaginal delivery is often questioned, based on observational data suggesting an increased mortality and morbidity to the preterm breech born vaginally (see Chapter 35, Breech presentation). However, there are recent similar studies that conclude the opposite.[24] Although the obstetric community agreed on the need for a well-conducted randomized trial to answer this question, this was not translated into recruitment when trials were attempted. A careful attempt at vaginal breech delivery, preferably under epidural analgesia, is not absolutely contraindicated [C].

### Type of caesarean section

At the earliest gestations, the lower segment is poorly formed, often leading to vertical uterine incisions. A classical uterine incision carries up to a 12 per cent risk of uterine rupture in subsequent pregnancies, some of which will occur antenatally. The modified DeLee vertical lower segment incision does not appear to carry any greater risk than a conventional transverse incision and should be used in preference [D]. Alternatively, it is often possible to perform an en-caul delivery through a transverse incision if the membranes are left intact.

## ANALGESIA

In terms of intrapartum analgesia, the use of epidural anaesthesia is frequently advocated. There has been little research on the subject. Postulated benefits include avoiding expulsive efforts before full dilatation or a precipitous delivery, a relaxed pelvic floor and perineum, and the ability to proceed quickly to abdominal delivery. Concerns are often expressed about the prolonged effects of narcotic analgesia on a preterm infant with limited metabolic capacity.

## COMMUNICATION

There are two vital areas of communication in the management of women with threatened preterm labour:

(1) communication with the woman and her family and (2) communication with the neonatal paediatricians.

Where possible, a clear management plan should be discussed with the parents. This should include monitoring in labour, potential interventions, and what will happen to the baby afterwards. Involvement of the neonatal paediatricians is helpful, especially where there are difficult issues to cover, such as the management of an extremely preterm infant. Even when resuscitation would not be appropriate, parents often appreciate the opportunity to have discussed the care of their baby with the paediatricians.

When labour does occur, it is vital to alert the neonatologists. Outcomes in very preterm infants have been shown to be improved if there is a senior paediatrician present at delivery. This can usually only be accomplished with some advanced warning.

## SUMMARY

- Oral metronidazole significantly lowers the risk of preterm birth, by 60 per cent in high-risk women positive for bacterial vaginosis.
- Asymptomatic bacteriuria carries an increased risk of preterm birth; the risk is reduced by appropriate antibiotic treatment.
- Mothers at risk of preterm delivery should be screened for GBS colonization. If positive, intrapartum antibiotics should be offered.
- When based on historical factors alone, cervical cerclage improves outcomes only in women with three or more previous very early deliveries.
- Hospitalization for bed rest leads to an increase in preterm births.
- Tocolytics have no significant benefit on perinatal mortality or the prolongation of pregnancy to term, but do reduce the number of women delivering within 48 hours by 40 per cent.
- A single course of maternal steroids given between 28 and 34 weeks gestation and received within 7 days of delivery results in markedly improved neonatal outcomes.
- There is no evidence of benefit and some evidence of harm associated with the use of antibiotics in uncomplicated preterm labour with intact membranes.

## ACKNOWLEDGEMENT

This chapter has been revised and updated. The author and editors acknowledge the contribution of Griff Jones to the chapter on this topic in the previous edition of the book.

## KEY POINTS

- Beneficial antenatal treatments for high-risk women include metronidazole for bacterial vaginosis, antibiotics for asymptomatic bacteriuria, cerclage for three or more second trimester losses or very preterm births and progesterone supplementation.
- In symptomatic women, the following factors are associated with a high risk of delivery within 7 days: cervical dilatation >3 cm, ruptured membranes or any vaginal bleeding.
- A single course of corticosteroids should be given when delivery before 34 weeks is likely within the next 7 days. In general, repeat courses should be avoided, as they may carry risk without conferring benefit.
- After the diagnosis of preterm labour is confirmed, consideration should be given to the issues of neonatology consultation, fetal monitoring, mode of delivery and intrapartum antibiotics if a known GBS carrier.

## Published Guidelines

American College of Obstetricians and Gynaecologists Practice Bulletin. Assessment of risk factors for preterm birth. *Obstet Gynecol* 2001; **98**: 709–16.

Australian National Health and Medical Research Council Clinical Practice Guideline. *Care around Preterm Birth.* ‹www.health.gov.au/hfs/nhmrc›.

Joint Statement of the Fetus and Newborn Committee, Canadian Paediatric Society and Maternal–Fetal Medicine Committee, Society of Obstetricians and Gynaecologists of Canada. *Management of the Woman with Threatened Birth of an Infant of Extremely Low Gestational Age.* ‹www.cps.ca/english/statements›.

Royal College of Obstetricians and Gynaecologists. Clinical guideline. *Tocolytic Drugs for Women in Preterm Labour.* London: RCOG Press, October 2002. ‹www.rcog.org.uk›.

Royal College of Obstetricians and Gynaecologists. Clinical guideline. *Antenatal Corticosteroids to Prevent Respiratory Distress Syndrome.* London: RCOG Press, February 2004. ‹www.rcog.org.uk›.

Royal College of Obstetricians and Gynaecologists. Clinical guideline. *Antenatal Corticosteroids to Prevent Respiratory Distress Syndrome.* London: RCOG Press, February 2004. ‹www.rcog.org.uk›.

## Key References

1. Draper ES, Manktelow B, Field DJ, James D. Prediction of survival for preterm births by weight and gestational age: retrospective population based study. *BMJ* 1999; **319**: 1093–7.
2. Draper ES, Manktelow B, Field DJ, James D. Tables for predicting survival for preterm births are updated. *BMJ* 2003; **327**: 872.

Late pregnancy/intrapartum events

3. Wood NS, Marlow N, Costeloe K *et al.* Neurologic and developmental disability after extremely preterm birth. EPICure Study Group. *N Engl J Med* 2000; **343**: 378–84.

4. Bohin S, Draper ES, Field DJ. Health status of a population of infants born before 26 weeks gestation derived from routine data collected between 21 and 27 months post-delivery. *Early Hum Dev* 1999; **55**: 9–18.

5. Mercer BM, Goldenberg RL, Moawad AH *et al.* The preterm prediction study: effect of gestational age and cause of preterm birth on subsequent obstetric outcome. National Institute of Child Health and Human Development Maternal-Fetal Medicine Units Network. *Am J Obstet Gynecol* 1999; **181**: 1216–21.

6. Kyrgiou M, Koliopoulos G, Martin-Hirsch P *et al.* Obstetric outcomes after conservative treatment for intraepithelial or early invasive cervical lesions: systematic review and meta-analysis. *Lancet* 2006; **367**: 489–98.

7. Hauth JC, Goldenberg RL, Andrews WW *et al.* Reduced incidence of preterm delivery with metronidazole and erythromycin in women with bacterial vaginosis. *N Engl J Med* 1995; **333**: 1732–6.

8. Heath VC, Southall TR, Souka AP *et al.* Cervical length at 23 weeks of gestation: prediction of spontaneous preterm delivery. *Ultrasound Obstet Gynecol* 1998; **12**: 312–17.

9. Medical Research Council/Royal College of Obstetricians and Gynaecologists. Final report of the Medical Research Council/Royal College of Obstetricians and Gynaecologists multicentre randomised trial of cervical cerclage. MRC/RCOG Working Party on Cervical Cerclage. *Br J Obstet Gynaecol* 1993; **100**: 516–23.

10. Meis PJ, Klebanoff M, Thom E *et al.* Prevention of recurrent preterm delivery by 17 alpha-hydroxy-progesterone caproate. *N Engl J Med* 2003; **348**: 2379–85.

11. da Fonseca EB, Bittar RE, Carvalho MH, Zugaib M. Prophylactic administration of progesterone by vaginal suppository to reduce the incidence of spontaneous preterm birth in women at increased risk: a randomized placebo-controlled double-blind study. *Am J Obstet Gynecol* 2003; **188**: 419–24.

12. ACOG Committee Opinion No. 419 October 2008 (replaces No. 291, November 2003). Use of progesterone to reduce preterm birth. *Obstet Gynecol* 2008; **112**: 963–5.

13. Goldenberg RL, Iams JD, Mercer BM *et al.* The preterm prediction study: the value of new vs standard risk factors in predicting early and all spontaneous preterm births. NICHD MFMU Network. *Am J Public Health* 1998; **88**: 233–8.

14. Iams JD, Casal D, McGregor JA *et al.* Fetal fibronectin improves the accuracy of diagnosis of preterm labor. *Am J Obstet Gynecol* 1995; **173**: 141–5.

15. Rizzo G, Capponi A, Arduini D *et al.* The value of fetal fibronectin in cervical and vaginal secretions and of ultrasonographic examination of the uterine cervix in predicting premature delivery for patients with preterm labor and intact membranes. *Am J Obstet Gynecol* 1996; **175**: 1146–51.

16. Wapner RJ, Sorokin Y, Mele L *et al.* Long-term outcomes after repeat doses of antenatal corticosteroids. *N Engl J Med* 2007; **357**: 1190–8.

17. Murphy KE, Hannah ME, Willan AR *et al.* Multiple courses of antenatal corticosteroids for preterm birth (MACS): a randomised controlled trial. *Lancet* 2008; **372**: 2143–51.

18. Banks BA, Cnaan A, Morgan MA *et al.* Multiple courses of antenatal corticosteroids and outcome of premature neonates. North American Thyrotropin-Releasing Hormone Study Group. *Am J Obstet Gynecol* 1999; **181**: 709–17.

19. The Canadian Preterm Labor Investigators Group. Treatment of preterm labor with the beta-adrenergic agonist ritodrine. *N Engl J Med* 1992; **327**: 308–12.

20. Kenyon SL, Taylor DJ, Tarnow-Mordi W. Broad-spectrum antibiotics for spontaneous preterm labour: the ORACLE II randomised trial. ORACLE Collaborative Group. *Lancet* 2001; **357**: 989–94.

21. Kenyon S, Pike K, Jones DR *et al.* Childhood outcomes after prescription of antibiotics to pregnant women with spontaneous preterm labour: 7-year follow-up of the ORACLE II trial. *Lancet* 2008; **372**: 1319–27.

22. Kenyon S, Pike K, Jones DR *et al.* Childhood outcomes after prescription of antibiotics to pregnant women with preterm rupture of the membranes: 7-year follow-up of the ORACLE I trial. *Lancet* 2008; **372**: 1310–18.

23. Shy KK, Luthy DA, Bennett FC *et al.* Effects of electronic fetal-heart-rate monitoring, as compared with periodic auscultation, on the neurologic development of premature infants. *N Engl J Med* 1990; **322**: 588–93.

24. Wolf H, Schaap AH, Bruinse HW *et al.* Vaginal delivery compared with caesarean section in early preterm breech delivery: a comparison of long term outcome. *Br J Obstet Gynaecol* 1999; **106**: 486–91.

# Pre-labour rupture of the membranes

*Myles Taylor*

## INTRODUCTION

Pre-labour rupture of the membranes is a common clinical problem, and the assessment of women with possible membrane rupture is a management issue faced in everyday practice. When PROM occurs, the fetus loses the relative isolation and protection afforded within the amniotic cavity.

## DEFINITION

In general, PROM refers to rupture of the membranes with leakage of amniotic fluid in the absence of uterine activity. Pre-term PROM (PPROM) occurs when rupture of membranes occurs before 37 weeks gestation.

At term, approximately 75 per cent of women will labour within 24 hours of membrane rupture. The latency period tends to be longer with decreasing gestational age: at 26 weeks, only half of women are in labour within 1 week; at 32 weeks, half will labour within 24–48 hours.

## INCIDENCE

Pre-labour rupture of the membranes occurs in approximately 8 per cent of term pregnancies and complicates 2–3 per cent of pregnancies that have not reached 37 weeks gestation. Preterm PROM is associated with approximately one-third of all deliveries before 37 weeks gestation. It is important to make a distinction between term PROM and preterm PROM, as the conditions have different aetiologies, risks and recommended management plans.

## AETIOLOGY

The pathophysiology of PROM is not understood but probably includes a variety of mechanical, infective and constitutional mechanisms.[1] The main risk factors for PPROM include a history of PPROM in a previous pregnancy, genital tract infection, antepartum bleeding and smoking.[2]

### Term PROM

Rupture of the membranes at term usually reflects physiological (as opposed to pathophysiological) processes. Apoptosis (programmed cell death) refers to the natural deterioration and breakdown of cells and cellular structure over time. The role of apoptosis in PROM has attracted considerable research interest.

As term approaches, uterine activity is known to increase and Braxton–Hicks contractions are prominent. Such repetitive stretching of the membranes may lead to weakening via several mechanisms. First, it induces focal thinning of the membranes. Second, it leads to strain hardening, a biomechanical phenomenon associated with materials becoming less elastic and less able to withstand stress. Such stretch-induced weakening will be most likely at the internal cervical os, where physiological ripening of the cervix will allow a degree of membrane prolapse.

## Preterm PROM

In contrast to the 'natural' phenomenon occurring at term, PPROM usually has pathological origins. Ascending infection appears to be one of the major causes and, indeed, appears to be a more frequent aetiology than in preterm labour with intact membranes. That chorioamnionitis can be associated with membrane weakening is easily understood. As with preterm labour, the majority of these infections are subclinical and give few signs or symptoms until fluid loss has occurred.

Another factor strongly linked with PPROM is antepartum haemorrhage, particularly when it occurs recurrently. A weak cervix can also predispose to early membrane rupture. It will fail as a barrier to ascending infection and, by allowing membrane prolapse, will allow localized biomechanical weakening, as described for term PROM.

There is a strong epidemiological link between maternal smoking and PPROM, which is dose dependent. As smoking is a modifiable behaviour and a reduction in smoking has been shown to reduce risk, this should be pointed out to women, particularly those with a history of PPROM in a previous pregnancy.

## CLINICAL ASSESSMENT

The correct diagnosis of PROM, either preterm or at term, is crucial – many interventions will be based upon the diagnosis. If undertaken unnecessarily, these interventions will undoubtedly increase maternal and fetal morbidity.

## History

A history from the mother of 'a gush of fluid' followed by recurrent dampness will correctly identify over 90 per cent of cases of pre-labour membrane rupture.[3]

## Examination

Pre-labour rupture of membranes should be confirmed by a sterile speculum examination, performed after the mother has rested supine for 20–30 minutes. Amniotic fluid can be seen pooling in the posterior fornix, either spontaneously or after fundal pressure. The presence of meconium should be noted. At preterm gestations, meconium is suggestive but not diagnostic of intra-amniotic infection; at term, it is a relative contraindication to expectant management. The absence of any pooling is an equally important finding. The cervix can usually also be seen, allowing assessment of length and dilatation.

A digital examination must be avoided unless the patient is thought to be in established labour, as it is known to increase the incidence of:

- chorioamnionitis
- postpartum endometritis
- neonatal infection.

A digital examination also decreases the length of the latent period before the onset of labour, with the greatest decreases seen at the earliest gestations.[4]

## Basic bedside tests

Concern about the consequences of misdiagnosing true PROM has led investigators to seek secondary tests that can be used at presentation. The two most common tests use either nitrazine sticks (relying on the higher alkaline pH of amniotic fluid) or the ferning pattern seen when amniotic fluid is dried onto a glass slide and then viewed under a microscope. Importantly, neither of these tests has been shown to be more reliable than a basic history and examination.[3] Both have appreciable false-positive and false-negative rates, which appear to be further increased in women with prior negative speculum examinations. Repeated dry pads argue against the diagnosis while the use of pads which change colour when in contact with fluids with a pH >5.2 are now available.[5]

## Misdiagnosed PROM

Ladfors et al.[6] have studied the outcome of women presenting with possible PROM after 34 weeks gestation in whom amniotic fluid could not be seen on speculum examination. Vaginal samples were taken and blindly analysed later for diamine oxidase, an enzyme that is absent from urine or vaginal secretions but present in large amounts in amniotic fluid. Of the women with negative speculum examinations, 12 per cent tested positive for diamine oxidase. Nearly 90 per cent of these diamine oxidase-positive women went into labour within 48 hours, compared to only 45 per cent of the diamine oxidase-negative women. Crucially, no difference in maternal or neonatal outcome was seen between the two groups. This suggests that a delay in the diagnosis of PROM in women with an initially negative speculum examination is of no clinical consequence [C].

## Specialized tests

### Vaginal swabs

Many more technologically advanced and expensive tests have been proposed to confirm or refute the diagnosis of PROM in women with negative speculum examinations. Substances which are present in high concentrations in amniotic fluid and are therefore contenders for a diagnostic test include fetal fibronectin, insulin-like growth factor binding protein 1 (IGFBP1), beta-human chorionic gonadotrophin (β-hCG) and alpha microglobulin-1 protein. All have commercially available rapid bedside tests. These tests have reported sensitivities of 94 and 75 per cent and specificities of 97 per cent, respectively. Fetal fibronectin testing has been shown to become negative in some women after membranes have been ruptured for more than 12 hours if liquor is not seen on speculum examination.

### Ultrasound

Amniotic fluid volume can be assessed by ultrasound. Even at term, the normal variation in directly measured amniotic fluid volume is considerable, ranging from 250 to 1200 mL. This limits the usefulness of ultrasound as a primary diagnostic tool. However, ultrasound may be a useful additional investigation in those women with a strong history of PROM but a negative speculum examination, particularly if their symptoms persist for 48 hours or more. As the variation in amniotic fluid volume can be much greater in preterm gestations, the diagnostic role of ultrasound in PPROM is very limited. Despite this, the ultrasound assessment of amniotic fluid volume has been reported to correlate with latency in PPROM and with neonatal mortality and morbidity in mid-trimester PROM.

## CLINICAL MANAGEMENT

### Term PROM

The predominant risk to the fetus after PROM at term is ascending infection. The risks to the mother are of uterine infection, via either chorioamnionitis or postpartum endometritis. The risks of a policy of induction of labour must also be considered. These include intrapartum complications, operative delivery and postnatal morbidity.

The Canadian TERMPROM Study[7] and subsequent secondary analyses[8–12] have provided considerable evidence to share with prospective parents. The trial compared four management policies, namely immediate induction with intravenous oxytocin, immediate induction with vaginal prostaglandins, expectant management for up to 4 days followed by induction with oxytocin, or expectant management followed by induction with vaginal prostaglandins. As the absolute risks associated with any policy were found to be small, personal preference should be allowed considerable influence [B]. Table 22.1 outlines the differences in labour outcome among the four management policies. None reached statistical significance. In Table 22.2, the risks of maternal and neonatal infection are reviewed. Although clear trends are obvious in these tables, readers are referred to the original publication for tests of significance.

Four points from the original trial are worthy of separate mention.

1   The use of prostaglandins did not reduce the subsequent need for oxytocin; this was no different between the two groups randomized to prostaglandins and the expectantly managed group randomized to induction with oxytocin.
2   Only a minority of women (approximately 18 per cent) randomized to expectant management waited 4 days before induction.

**Table 22.1** Delivery outcomes after membrane rupture at term, TERMPROM Study[7]

|  | Immediate induction | | Expectant management | |
| --- | --- | --- | --- | --- |
|  | Oxytocin (%) | Prostaglandin (%) | Oxytocin (%) | Prostaglandin (%) |
| C-sect (overall) | 10.1 | 9.6 | 9.7 | 10.9 |
| C-sect (multiparous) | 4.3 | 3.5 | 3.9 | 4.6 |
| C-sect (nulliparous) | 14.1 | 13.7 | 13.7 | 15.2 |
| C-sect (nulliparous, unfavourable cervix) | 14.8 | 14.1 | 15.0 | 14.9 |
| SVD, nulliparous | 60.8 | 60.8 | 58.0 | 58.9 |
| Use of oxytocin | 91.9 | 43.1 | 49.9 | 43.8 |
| PROM–delivery interval | 17.2 hours | 23.0 hours | 33.3 hours | 32.6 hours |

- C-sect, caesarean section; PROM, pre-labour rupture of membranes; SVD, spontaneous vaginal delivery.

**Table 22.2** Perinatal infectious morbidity after membrane rupture at term, TERMPROM Study[7]

| | Immediate induction | | Expectant management | |
|---|---|---|---|---|
| | Oxytocin (%) | Prostaglandin (%) | Oxytocin (%) | Prostaglandin (%) |
| Fever before or during labour | 3.8 | 5.8 | 8.7 | 6.7 |
| Antibiotics before or during labour | 7.5 | 9.0 | 11.9 | 11.6 |
| Postpartum fever | 1.9 | 3.1 | 3.6 | 3.0 |
| Neonatal infection | 2.0 | 3.0 | 2.8 | 2.7 |
| Neonatal antibiotics | 7.5 | 10.9 | 13.7 | 12.2 |
| NICU stay >24 hours | 6.6 | 9.2 | 11.6 | 10.2 |

● NICU, neonatal intensive care unit.

3　The four babies that unexpectedly died in the trial were all in the expectant management arms. Two were antepartum stillbirths and two were related to fetal distress in advanced labour, both of which started spontaneously.

4　The views of the women participating in the trial showed a preference for immediate induction, as opposed to expectant management.

Later publications from the same investigators showed that the least expensive policy was immediate induction of labour using oxytocin.[12] In terms of where to undertake expectant management, the evidence suggested an increased risk of infection and caesarean section when women were allowed home. If this was translated into clinical practice, and women needed to remain in hospital, it would clearly increase the cost of expectant management further. In contrast, maternal satisfaction, particularly among multiparous women, was greater with management at home.[10]

Regardless of whether a policy of immediate induction or expectant management is pursued, factors linked with perinatal infection include an increasing number of vaginal examinations after membrane rupture, an increasing interval between membrane rupture and labour onset, and an increasing duration of active labour.[8,9] There is also clear evidence that immediate induction of labour using oxytocin should be recommended for women known to be colonized with group B *Streptococcus* [B].[11] Expectant management in this situation was associated with a 3–4-fold increase in risk of neonatal infection, and even immediate induction with prostaglandins failed to lower this.

In general, the evidence suggests that immediate induction is associated with less maternal and neonatal infection and a shorter interval from membrane rupture to delivery [A]. There is no evidence that mode of delivery is influenced. When oxytocin is used initially, healthcare costs are lower and the interval to delivery is shortest. However, meta-analysis has suggested that the use of epidural analgesia is increased [A]. When prostaglandins are used initially,

infection risks may be marginally greater, the interval to delivery slightly increased, and oxytocin required subsequently in nearly half of the women [A].

A considerable body of work has investigated the use of misoprostol in this situation. The cost of misoprostol is dramatically lower than that of the other agents, and the ability to use it orally may lower the risk of infection. With further studies, it is expected that a role for oral, vaginal or buccal misoprostol will become established.

## Preterm PROM

The major risks in preterm PROM are:

● chorioamnionitis
● abruption
● preterm delivery.

Other risks include cord prolapse and operative delivery. Many tests have been used to predict chorioamnionitis, which is usually subclinical. Serum markers, such as white cell count and C-reactive protein, have a poor predictive ability and should principally be used to support a clinical diagnosis. Oligohydramnios, as assessed by ultrasound, can select a group at higher risk of infection and/or earlier delivery, but again is not diagnostic. Amniocentesis can give valuable information but remains technically difficult when little amniotic fluid remains and is not recommended practice in the UK. In contrast to preterm labour with intact membranes, transvaginal ultrasound measurements of cervical length are not predictive of early delivery. As well as PPROM being a common sequela of antepartum haemorrhage, early membrane rupture carries a 5 per cent risk of subsequent abruption. However, this risk varies inversely with gestational age and is reportedly as high as 50 per cent below 24 weeks.[13]

Although neonates born after PPROM are reported to have lower incidences of respiratory distress syndrome when compared to preterm labour, maternal steroids still appear to reduce the risk further [A]. There does not appear to be any significant increase in maternal sepsis after single steroid courses. Tocolytics are relatively contraindicated in this situation and are known to be less effective.

The UK ORACLE I trial demonstrated a role for oral erythromycin in PPROM regimens.[14] In this study, women with PPROM were randomized to one of four oral regimes:

1  erythromycin (250 mg qds)
2  co-amoxiclav (325 mg qds)
3  both erythromycin (250 mg qds) and co-amoxiclav (325 mg qds)
4  placebo.

The antibiotics were taken for 10 days. In singleton pregnancies, erythromycin alone was associated with a significant reduction (from 14.4 to 11.2 per cent) in the composite primary outcome, a measure of neonatal mortality and major morbidity [B]. The reductions with either co-amoxiclav or both antibiotics failed to reach significance. Unfortunately, the 10-day course of co-amoxiclav led to a significant increase in proven neonatal necrotizing enterocolitis, from 0.5 to 1.9 per cent. Once again, antibiotics have been demonstrated to have the potential for harm. In contrast to those in preterm labour with intact membranes (see Chapter 21, Preterm labour), seven-year follow-up of those children prescribed antibiotics for PPROM in the Oracle I trial did not show any functional impairment. Thus, the prophylactic use of erthryomycin is currently recommended when PPROM is diagnosed (RCOG guideline number 44).

Chorioamnionitis remains a notoriously difficult diagnosis. For research purposes, it requires:

- a maternal pyrexia (>38°C)

and at least two of either:

- maternal tachycardia >100 bpm
- fetal tachycardia >160 bpm
- uterine tenderness
- raised C-reactive protein
- offensive vaginal discharge.

When clinically suspected, delivery is almost always appropriate, as antibiotic therapy is rarely curative. Based on the culture results after amniocentesis in PPROM, anaerobes are the most common isolate, followed by group B *Streptococcus* and then other streptococci.

Novel management strategies have included serial transabdominal amnio-infusion, which has been suggested to increase latency and reduce perinatal mortality. When PPROM occurs in the presence of cervical cerclage, suture removal should be considered [E]. The care of women known to be group B *Streptococcus* carriers has been simplified by the ORACLE trial, as the organism is usually sensitive to erythromycin. After completion of a 10-day course, further antibiotics should probably be withheld until labour starts.

There are two gestational age epochs that require special consideration.

## Pre-viable PROM below 23–24 weeks gestation

Lung development has reached a critical stage and appears to be at least partly reliant on normal amniotic fluid volumes. There are significant risks of lethal pulmonary hypoplasia, a condition that cannot be reliably predicted on prenatal ultrasound. These risks are highest early in the mid-trimester and when severe oligohydramnios is found on serial ultrasound monitoring.

As there are additional risks of:

- chronic pulmonary morbidity,
- fetal limb contractures,
- extremely preterm birth with consequent co-existent morbidity and mortality,

many parents will opt for termination of pregnancy. Researchers have investigated the role of minimally invasive surgery and membrane sealants in this situation, as the prognosis is otherwise very poor, but results have proved disappointing.

## PPROM at 34–37 weeks gestation

This is another controversial area. Randomized trials have suggested that a policy of induction, as opposed to expectant management, may lead to less hospitalization, less perinatal infection and less neonatal morbidity [B].[13,14]

## In-patient versus outpatient care

For some women who rupture membranes early without immediately ensuing labour, the dilemma of best place of management must be considered. There are no good trials to inform practice. As it is recognized that 48–72 hours is a critical time during which many women will labour or develop clinical chorioamnionitis, it is recommended that all women with PPROM are managed as in-patients during this time. After this, a decision to change to outpatient management must be taken at consultant level. Women must know the potential risks and be educated in measurement of their temperature and signs and symptoms of developing chorioamnionitis. It is suggested that women measure their temperature twice daily (RCOG guideline 44).

Neither umbilical artery Doppler analysis nor biophysical testing has proven effective at early identification of the infected fetus. However, given that PPROM is associated with growth restriction monitoring of fetal growth by ultrasound seems reasonable.

## ACKNOWLEDGEMENT

This chapter has been revised and updated. The author and editors acknowledge the contribution of Griff Jones to the chapter on this topic in the previous edition of the book.

## KEY POINTS

- At term, the outcomes for women with PROM are as good in women induced immediately as in those managed conservatively. Where possible, women should be offered the choice.
- At term, women known to be colonized with group B *Streptococcus* should be encouraged to allow immediate induction of labour using oxytocin after PROM.
- Immediate induction is associated with increased use of epidural analgesia.
- Maternal steroid use in PPROM reduces the risk of respiratory distress syndrome.
- Erythromycin used for 10 days after PPROM is associated with a significant reduction (from 14.4 to 11.2 per cent) in neonatal mortality and major morbidity.
- Co-amoxiclav when used for PPROM leads to a significant increase in proven neonatal necrotizing enterocolitis, from 0.5 to 1.9 per cent.
- Term PROM is usually a reflection of normal physiology, whereas pathological processes, such as infection and antepartum haemorrhage, often underlie PPROM.
- Accurate diagnosis of membrane rupture is essential and can usually be achieved by simple history and speculum examination alone.
- A digital vaginal examination should always be avoided after PPROM unless advanced labour is suspected.
- At term, early induction using oxytocin appears to reduce perinatal infection and shorten hospital stay without increasing operative intervention. It should be strongly recommended to women known to be group B *Streptococcus* positive.
- After PPROM, optimal management includes maternal steroids and oral erythromycin.

## Published Guidelines

National Institute for Health and Clinical Excellence. *Induction of Labour.* London: RCOG, July 2008.

Royal College of Obstetricians and Gynaecologists Evidence-based Clinical Guideline Number 44. *Preterm prelabour rupture of membranes.* London: RCOG, November 2006.

## Key References

1. French JI, McGregor JA. The pathobiology of premature rupture of membranes. *Semin Perinatol* 1996; **20**: 344-68.
2. Harger JH, Hsing AW, Tuomala RE *et al.* Risk factors for preterm premature rupture of fetal membranes: a multicenter case-control study. *Am J Obstet Gynecol* 1990; **163**: 130–37.
3. Friedman ML, McElin TW. Diagnosis of ruptured fetal membranes. Clinical study and review of the literature. *Am J Obstet Gynecol* 1969; **104**: 544–50.
4. Lewis DF, Major CA, Towers CV *et al.* Effects of digital vaginal examinations on latency period in preterm premature rupture of membranes. *Obstet Gynecol* 1992; **80**: 630-34.
5. Mulhair L, Carter J, Poston L *et al.* Prospective cohort study investigating the reliability of the AmnioSense method for detection of spontaneous rupture of membranes. *BJOG* 2009; **116**: 313–18.
6. Ladfors L, Mattsson LA, Eriksson M, Fall O. Is a speculum examination sufficient for excluding the diagnosis of ruptured fetal membranes? *Acta Obstet Gynecol Scand* 1997; **76**: 739-42.
7. Hannah ME, Ohlsson A, Farine D *et al.* Induction of labor compared with expectant management for prelabor rupture of the membranes at term. TERMPROM Study Group. *N Engl J Med* 1996; **334**: 1005–10.
8. Seaward PG, Hannah ME, Myhr TL *et al.* International Multicentre Term Prelabor Rupture of Membranes Study: evaluation of predictors of clinical chorioamnionitis and postpartum fever in patients with prelabor rupture of membranes at term. *Am J Obstet Gynecol* 1997; **177**: 1024–9.
9. Seaward PG, Hannah ME, Myhr TL *et al.* International multicenter term PROM study: evaluation of predictors of neonatal infection in infants born to patients with premature rupture of membranes at term. Premature Rupture of the Membranes. *Am J Obstet Gynecol* 1998; **179**: 635–9.
10. Hannah ME, Hodnett ED, Willan A *et al.* Prelabor rupture of the membranes at term: expectant management at home or in hospital? The TermPROM Study Group. *Obstet Gynecol* 2000; **96**: 533–8.
11. Hannah ME, Ohlsson A, Wang EE *et al.* Maternal colonization with group B Streptococcus and prelabor rupture of membranes at term: the role of induction of labor. TermPROM Study Group. *Am J Obstet Gynecol* 1997; **177**: 780–85.
12. Gafni A, Goeree R, Myhr TL *et al.* Induction of labour versus expectant management for prelabour rupture of the membranes at term: an economic evaluation. TERMPROM Study Group. Term Prelabour Rupture of the Membranes. *CMAJ* 1997; **157**: 1519–25.
13. Holmgren PA, Olofsson JI. Preterm premature rupture of membranes and the associated risk for placental abruption. Inverse correlation to gestational length. *Acta Obstet Gynecol Scand* 1997; **76**: 743–7.
14. Kenyon SL, Taylor DJ, Tarnow-Mordi W. Broad-spectrum antibiotics for preterm, prelabour rupture of fetal membranes: the ORACLE I randomised trial. ORACLE Collaborative Group. *Lancet* 2001; **357**: 979–88.
15. Kenyon S, Pike K, Jones DR *et al.* Childhood outcomes after prescription of antibiotics to pregnant women with preterm rupture of the membranes: 7-year follow-up of the ORACLE I trial. *Lancet* 2008; **372**: 1310–18.

# Antepartum haemorrhage

*Lucy Kean*

---

## INTRODUCTION

### Definitions

Antepartum haemorrhage (APH) is variously described as bleeding from the genital tract in pregnancy before the onset of labour at gestations from 20 to 24 weeks. For the purposes of this chapter, the threshold of 20 weeks will be used, as this is often the gestation at which women will be admitted to the labour suite rather than the gynaecology ward.

Antepartum haemorrhage is one of the most common reasons for admission in pregnancy. It affects approximately 4 per cent of all pregnancies and is associated with increased rates of fetal and maternal morbidity and mortality.

### Aetiology

The causes of APH can be divided into three main groups:

1 placenta praevia
2 placental abruption
3 others:
   a. marginal placental bleeding
   b. show
   c. friable cervical ectropion/cervical trauma
   d. local infection of the cervix/vagina
   e. genital tract tumours
   f. varicosities
   g. ruptured vasa praevia.

Placenta praevia and abruption together account for 50 per cent of bleeding and represent the greatest threat to the fetus and mother. Despite the other causes appearing to be more minor (vasa praevia when a fetal vessel ruptures being the exception), these carry an increased perinatal mortality of at least 3 per cent, and must therefore represent a group of pathological conditions. Thus, all APH must be fully investigated and evaluated.

## PLACENTA PRAEVIA

The incidence of placenta praevia is variable depending on the population and background caesarean section rate, with rates reported from 0.4 to 0.8 per cent.

### Definitions

Placenta praevia is defined as a placenta partially or wholly situated in the lower uterine segment. It is graded in two ways, as either grades 1–4 or minor/major.

- Grade 1: the placental edge is in the lower segment, but does not reach the internal os.
- Grade 2: the placental edge reaches but does not cover the internal os.

These grades represent a minor degree of placenta praevia.

- Grade 3: the placenta covers the internal os and is asymmetrically situated.
- Grade 4: the placenta covers the internal os and is centrally situated.

These grades represent a major placenta praevia.

## Aetiology and associations

### Uterine surgery

Placenta praevia is strongly associated with previous uterine surgery. Its incidence increases with the number of procedures performed (Table 23.1) [C].[1]

Women with two or more previous abortions have a 2.1 (95 per cent CI 1.2–3.5) times increased risk of subsequently developing placenta praevia. Other procedures, such as curettage and myomectomy, also increase the risks of praevia.

### Maternal age

Placenta praevia increases dramatically with advancing maternal age, with women older than 40 years having a nearly nine-fold greater risk than women under the age of 20, after adjustment for potential confounders, including parity [C].[1]

### Smoking

The relationship between smoking and placenta praevia is not clear, but there does appear to be a small but significant increase in risk in smokers.

### Associations

- Fetal abnormality: the rate of fetal abnormality is approximately doubled in women with placenta praevia [C].[1]
- Intrauterine growth restriction is common in women with multiple bleeds from a placenta praevia. The overall rate is 15 per cent [C].
- Ten per cent of women with a bleeding placenta praevia will have a coexistent abruption [C].

**Table 23.1** The relationship between placenta praevia and caesarean section

| No. previous caesarean sections | Incidence of placenta praevia (%) | Incidence of placenta accreta in those with placenta praevia (%) | Overall risk of placenta accreta (%) |
|---|---|---|---|
| 0 | 0.26 | 5 | 0.01 |
| 1 | 0.65 | 24 | 0.16 |
| 2 | 1.8 | 47 | 0.85 |
| 3 | 3 | 40 | 1.2 |
| 4 | 10 | 67 | 6.7 |

## Diagnosis

- Placenta praevia usually presents with painless bleeding (although 10 per cent will have concurrent abruption).
- Often a small bleed or number of small bleeds will precede a much larger one (although this is not always the case).
- The presenting part is usually high, being prevented from engaging by the placenta lying in the lower segment.
- The fetal condition generally remains good until the maternal blood loss causes compromise, or an abruption coexists.

It is difficult to diagnose a placenta praevia until the lower segment begins to form at about 28 weeks; however, a low-lying placenta can cause bleeding from the second trimester onwards.

Many cases are now detected on routine ultrasound at 18–23 weeks. Five per cent of women have ultrasound evidence of a low placenta at 16–18 weeks, but only 0.5 per cent have a placenta praevia at delivery. Transabdominal ultrasound is usually the test performed first, although it can be very difficult to determine the placental edge with a posterior placenta. Transvaginal imaging is better and the woman does not need a full bladder, thus avoiding maternal discomfort. Also there is less distortion of the anatomy of the lower uterine segment and cervix. Transvaginal ultrasound does not appear to provoke vaginal bleeding [B].[2]

Magnetic resonance imaging has also been used to identify placenta praevia, though it is expensive and not superior to TV scanning performed by an experienced person.

The following factors on second trimester ultrasound are associated with the persistence of a placenta praevia in the third trimester:

- The placenta covers the internal os with an overlap of greater than 2.5 cm [C].[3]
- The leading edge of the placenta is thick [C].[4]
- The placenta is posterior.
- There is a uterine scar.

## Morbidly adherent placenta

Morbidly adherent placentae occur in approximately 1 in 200–400 deliveries in the United States and 1 in 800 deliveries in the United Kingdom. The major risk factor is uterine scarring, and thus the incidence is increasing with the increasing caesarean section rate. However, prior manual removal or uterine curettage may also cause scarring and an increase in risk. A short caesarean section to conception interval has also been causally related.

Three degrees of adherence have been described, accreta, increta and percreta, where the placenta adheres to or invades into or through the uterine wall because of abnormal development of the decidua basalis.

Accreta is the most common, comprising 80 per cent. Postpartum haemorrhage will occur in most cases, particularly if the accreta is partial, where non-contracted portions of myometrium are adjacent to adherent placenta. Diagnosis in an increasing number of cases is made antenatally,[5] but still many are only diagnosed in the third stage. Antenatal diagnosis using colour flow or power Doppler ultrasound and magnetic resonance imaging has been described. A full discussion of the identification of a morbidly adherent placenta can be found in Chapter 26, Management of previous caesarean section. It is worthwhile trying to determine whether an accreta is present in women at most risk (repeated caesarean sections with an anterior placenta praevia), as it can be helpful in forward planning and discussion of options with the woman.

# MANAGEMENT OF PLACENTA PRAEVIA

## Management of the woman who does not bleed or in whom bleeding is minor and settled

### Maternal risks

#### Bleeding
Antepartum haemorrhage is the cardinal sign of placenta praevia and it is unusual for a woman to reach the late third trimester without vaginal bleeding. Bleeding becomes more likely as the frequency and strength of contractions increase, causing shearing of the placenta at the level of the internal os. The bleeding is said to be painless, though a considerable number (10 per cent) of women who bleed from a placenta praevia will have a coexistent abruption. It is also reported that most women experience a minor bleed before any major bleeding. While this is true for many women, some will have a significant haemorrhage as their first event.

#### Hospitalization
There are few data on which to base the management of placenta praevia. The only randomized study examined hospital versus home care for symptomatic women, i.e. women who had already experienced bleeding.[6] This study included only 47 women and concluded that there was no advantage in hospitalizing women with symptomatic praevia. However, one of the women with sufficient haemorrhage to require immediate delivery was in the home care arm.

Management decisions regarding women who have not bled are difficult and must be made individually. Important factors may include:

- whether the placenta praevia is major or minor;
- where the woman lives in relationship to the hospital and whether she has an adult with her at home;
- the gestation;
- other factors that may make a placenta praevia more difficult to manage, such as a scarred uterus.

Because there have been no trials on this aspect of management, the decision to manage as an outpatient must be made at a senior level and fully discussed with the woman and her partner. It is important to remember that long-term hospitalization carries significant financial and psychological implications for women and their families and may not be justified for women who have never bled.

For women who have had bleeding, most obstetricians would recommend inpatient management from 32–34 weeks. However, there may be exceptions, such as a placenta that migrates enough for vaginal delivery to become an option, or women with very early bleeding only and a minor degree of placenta praevia. Women who are managed as inpatients show a trend towards later delivery. The Royal College of Obstetricians and Gynaecologists recommends inpatient management for women with a major praevia who have bled from 34 weeks [E].[7]

### Surveillance
The rate of fetal abnormality is approximately double the background rate in women with placenta praevia. When a diagnosis of placenta praevia is made, a careful reassessment of the fetal anatomy must be undertaken.

There is a considerable false-positive rate of diagnosis of low-lying placenta at 18–20 weeks using transabdominal (TA) scanning. A repeat transvaginal (TV) scan at 20–24 weeks will reduce the number of women who require follow up and minimize anxiety for these women. Where the placenta appears to cover the internal os, a rescan at 32 weeks is recommended as these women have a lower chance of placental migration, and require more careful management in the third trimester.[7] In women with a minor praevia, a full assessment should take place at approximately 36 weeks. If the placenta is anterior, a vaginal delivery is usually achieved if the distance from the os is >2 cm. If the placenta is posterior, 3 cm seems to be critical distance. The thickness of the placental edge is also important; a thin leading edge is a more favourable finding for vaginal delivery. If the placenta is still low, a further scan in a week or two may show some changes.

### Tocolysis
Tocolysis for the treatment of uterine activity has been used to good effect in some studies [C].[7,8] It appears to be safe to use, gaining on average 13 days when compared to women in whom it was not used. It must be used judiciously to settle uterine activity that is causing bleeding. It must never be considered in women who show signs of cardiovascular instability or where there is evidence of fetal compromise. Studies have mainly used beta-sympathomimetics, which have a theoretical disadvantage. Where tocolysis is considered, agents other than beta-agonists should be considered first. Given the lack of cardiovascular side effects, an oxytocic antagonist would probably be the first choice.

## Planning for delivery

In the woman who has not bled or in whom bleeding has been minor, there are a number of factors that need to be taken into account. These include:

- making a final decision about how to deliver for women with minor praevia;
- timing in relationship to the gestation of the pregnancy;
- ensuring a fully experienced and prepared team is assembled for delivery.

## Deciding when to attempt a vaginal delivery

There has been much debate about when a vaginal delivery can be expected and when it is unlikely to occur. The Royal College of Obstetricians and Gynaecologists guideline suggests that the decision regarding mode of delivery should be made on clinical grounds, supplemented by sonographic assessment.[7]

One large observational study has shown that if the placenta is within 2 cm of the internal os, the vast majority of women will require caesarean section [C].[9] This is therefore accepted as a reasonable cut-off for expecting to need to perform a caesarean section. However, where the leading edge of the placenta is thick, the placenta may still have an impact at this distance.[4] Once the placenta is more than 4.5 cm from the internal os, it is unlikely to be problematic. The grey area of 2–4.5 cm must be managed clinically and will depend on features such as the station of the fetal head and the position of the placenta (anterior or posterior, anterior being slightly less problematic as the anterior lower segment tends to retract more in labour).

Ideally, all women will have had a planned third trimester with repeat scanning, admission where necessary and plans made for delivery if this occurs earlier than anticipated. However, very occasionally an examination in theatre may be required to determine the true relationship between the placental edge and cervix. This may be needed when:

- labour occurs without a definitive ultrasound assessment being performed;
- facilities are not available for ultrasound assessment and delivery needs to be considered;
- despite ultrasound assessment, a clear diagnosis cannot be reached;
- there is a suspicion of a low accessory lobe where the main body of the placenta is normally sited;
- the placenta is said to be a minor praevia, the clinical picture suggests a vaginal delivery may be feasible, and bleeding or labour requires a decision regarding delivery to be made.

## Procedure for examination in theatre

This should only be undertaken when a decision has been made that delivery should be expedited and that a vaginal delivery is considered a safe and valid option if feasible (i.e. the mother and fetus are well and a major placenta praevia is not suspected).

The team should be assembled so that if a placenta praevia is confirmed, a caesarean section can be performed.

A full assessment is much easier with some form of anaesthesia. Given that regional anaesthesia is now becoming more widespread (see below) for delivery in the presence of a praevia, an epidural or combined spinal/epidural is probably appropriate. This can then provide analgesia for labour if required.

Blood must be cross-matched in advance.

The woman should be placed in the lithotomy position and draped. The bladder should be empty to allow full descent of the head. Initially, a vaginal examination is performed to palpate in each fornix. The placenta can be felt as sponginess between the fetal head and the fornix. The whole 360° of the cervix should be palpated against the fetal head. If, on working round the cervix, no placenta is felt, an index finger should be passed through the cervix and a gentle examination performed to feel for the edge of the placenta. This is the most difficult part in practice, but if the placenta is felt it usually precipitates bleeding, making the diagnosis. If the fetal head is felt with no apparent placenta and no bleeding, the membranes should be ruptured and Syntocinon started if the labour has not already begun.

If the cervix is so unfavourable as not to allow a rupture of the membranes, delivery by caesarean section is probably the safest option.

# PLANNED CAESAREAN SECTION FOR PLACENTA PRAEVIA

## Timing of caesarean section

Pre-labour caesarean section carries an increased risk of respiratory complications in the newborn. Occasionally, these are severe enough to require intensive intervention. Table 23.2 shows the incidence of respiratory morbidity for each week of gestation in babies delivered prior to labour from 37 to 41 weeks [D].[10]

**Table 23.2** Respiratory morbidity amongst infants delivered by elective caesarean section

| Gestation | Respiratory morbidity/1000 (95% CI) | Odds ratio compared to vaginal delivery at term (95% CI) |
|---|---|---|
| 37 + 0-37 + 6 | 73.8 (49.1-106.1) | 14.3 (8.9-23.1) |
| 38 + 0-38 + 6 | 42.3 (31.1-56.2) | 8.2 (5.5-12.3) |
| 39 + 0-39 + 6 | 17.8 ( 8.0-33.5) | 3.5 (1.7-7.1) |

It has also been noted that the incidence of respiratory distress syndrome is higher among infants born to mothers delivered by elective caesarean section for placenta praevia that relates to lower cortisol levels in these infants [C].[11] This suggests that the maturing processes in these infants are not accelerated. These data suggest that when bleeding has not occurred, caesarean section should be planned no earlier than 38 weeks, and if a planned caesarean section is to be performed before this time for placenta praevia, it may be worthwhile administering corticosteroids 48 hours prior to delivery.

When bleeding is occurring, the risks and benefits of delivery versus conservative management can only be assessed on an individual basis. However, there is often pressure to deliver earlier because of hospital inpatient management. If there are no compelling medical reasons for delivery before 38 weeks, the risks to the fetus must be fully discussed with the mother before delivery.

## Planning the caesarean section

The degree of technical difficulty of caesarean section for placenta praevia will be related to:

- gestation,
- degree of praevia,
- whether the praevia is anterior,
- presence of other risk factors making a morbidly adherent placenta more likely,
- the sonographic or MRI appearances of the placenta,
- multiple previous abdominal procedures, which may make the access to the uterus more difficult,
- morbid obesity.

It is useful to have as much idea as possible prior to the procedure about the likelihood of placenta accreta. This will enable the mobilization of appropriate personnel and resources.

Autologous blood transfusion is not recommended in the management of placenta praevia, as when blood is needed it is often required in very large amounts.[7] Haemoglobin should be optimized before delivery. Cell saving should be considered.

Radiological assessment with a view to catheterization of the internal iliac or uterine vessels should be considered where there is a high level of suspicion of an accreta.

A planned caesarean section must enlist the help of all those thought to be necessary. This will include at the very least:

- senior obstetrician,
- senior anaesthetist,
- experienced midwives, anaesthetic assistants and theatre staff.

Where a morbidly adherent placenta is a strong possibility, discussion with a surgical/urological team may be necessary as bladder involvement is not uncommon. Because of the risk of ureteric injury when a hysterectomy is required

for an accreta, ureteric stent placement has been suggested prior to caesarean section, as this reduces the risk of ureteric damage.[5]

When a caesarean section is likely to involve significant haemorrhage, the haematology staff (medical and laboratory) should be alerted. The appropriate amount of blood should be cross-matched in advance. The laboratory should be warned if there is likely to be a need for more blood or blood products.

## Consent

It is important that the potential outcomes are discussed with the mother before delivery. This must include a discussion of management in the presence of continued or heavy bleeding and the possibility of the need for hysterectomy or other techniques.

## Type of anaesthetic

The type of anaesthesia used is the ultimate responsibility of the anaesthetist. The final decision can only be made when the anaesthetist has all the facts at his or her disposal. Good communication before the delivery is vital.

There is increasing evidence that blood loss at caesarean section for placenta praevia is less when regional anaesthesia is used and that this does not compromise mothers [C].[12] (Elective delivery is different from delivery of the cardiovascularly unstable woman with acute bleeding, as discussed below.) When procedures are likely to take slightly longer, a combined spinal–epidural approach may be undertaken.

## Surgery

The surgery must be performed or supervised by an experienced obstetrician. The Confidential Enquiry into Maternal Deaths in the United Kingdom 1994–96 recommended that a consultant be present during surgery for a placenta praevia. The main reason for this recommendation is that a decision to proceed to life-saving hysterectomy is likely to be made earlier by a senior person. Despite this recommendation, there were three deaths due to placenta praevia in the last enquiry, even though a consultant obstetrician was present in all three cases.

The surgeon must avail him/herself of all the available information before commencing the caesarean section. It is prudent to try to plan how the uterine incision will relate to the placenta before starting. Careful ultrasound mapping of the placental site prior to operation may help the surgeon to know in which direction the nearest edge of a placenta-overlying uterine incision will be located. The use of radiological embolization should be considered where an accreta is likely.

It is also the responsibility of the surgeon to ensure that appropriate consent has been gained, that all the team members are aware the procedure is about to commence, and that the blood is available in theatre. These vital steps should not be delegated to anyone else in an elective situation.

## Technique

### Uterine incision

Caesarean section is usually performed through a transverse skin incision and through the lower segment of the uterus, but if there is an anterior placenta praevia, the vessels may cover the entire anterior lower segment and the placenta will be encountered underneath the uterine incision. Some authors have recommended a classical caesarean section in this situation, but this may make any repeat caesarean section even more hazardous, and lower segment bleeding can be difficult to see and secure in this case. In cases of a centrally implanted praevia with the potential for an accreta, an upper segment incision, avoiding the placenta entirely with the aim of leaving the placenta *in utero* or performing a planned hysterectomy can be considered [D].[5,7]

### Delivery

The baby may be delivered by the obstetrician passing a hand round the margins of the placenta, or by incising the placenta. It is often easier to bring down one of the baby's feet and perform breech extraction than to try to deliver a very high head past the placenta that occupies the uterine incision. Prolonged delay in delivery can lead to fetal exsanguination if the placenta has been cut. Some authors have recommended clamping the cord as soon as the uterine incision is made, to prevent fetal bleeding if the placenta is cut. However, in many cases this is not easy and can add unnecessary delay.

### Third stage

Oxytocics should be administered (5 units Syntocinon i.v.) as soon as the baby is delivered. An oxytocin infusion may then be commenced to continue uterine contraction. The uterine angles should be secured with Green–Armytage clamps before delivery of the placenta, and any large bleeding venous sinuses in the incision can also be secured.

The placenta should be delivered by controlled cord traction. If at this point a placenta accreta is diagnosed (and it is usually obvious, as no plane of cleavage can be found where the placenta adheres to the old scar), a decision to proceed to hysterectomy should be made, or iliac artery balloon embolization used (if catheters are *in situ*).

Once the placenta is delivered, the lower segment can be examined. Delivery of the uterus may improve visualization. Bleeding with a placenta praevia at this stage is most troublesome from the lower segment as this contracts poorly. Various strategies have been employed to improve haemostasis. These include:

- over-sewing individual bleeding sinuses;
- packing the uterine cavity;
- siting a balloon device, which can be inflated to provide uterine compression and removed later *per vaginum*;

- extra oxytocics, including prostaglandin $F_{2a}$, intramyometrial vasopressin, misoprostol;
- radiographic embolization techniques;
- uterine or internal iliac artery ligation.

What is most important is that if haemorrhage is continuing and excessive, early recourse to hysterectomy is the safest strategy and the abdomen should not be closed until haemostasis is assured.

## Post-delivery monitoring

Women delivered with a major placenta praevia or who have had significant intraoperative haemorrhage must be carefully monitored in a high-dependency setting until continuing loss has been excluded.

The management of major post-partum haemorrhage is discussed in Chapter 42, Postpartum haemorrhage. Again it is vital that if haemorrhage is continuing, early recourse to hysterectomy is undertaken.

## Post-natal counselling

When haemorrhage has been severe, women will need the opportunity to go through events with the senior member of the team. The anaesthetist may wish to be involved. It is important that women understand what implications there may be for future deliveries, especially where there has been particularly difficult surgery.

The management of women with severe antepartum bleeding with placenta praevia utilizes the steps above. Further management of the woman with severe bleeding is discussed below.

## PLACENTAL ABRUPTION

### Definition

Abruption is defined as bleeding following premature separation of a normally sited placenta.

It occurs in as many as 5 per cent of pregnancies, although the majority of these is small and only visible on placental examination after delivery. It can most easily be graded as follows.

0    An asymptomatic retroplacental clot seen after placental delivery.
1    Vaginal bleeding and uterine tenderness; visible retroplacental clot after delivery.
2    Revealed bleeding may or may not be present, but placental separation is significant enough to produce evidence of fetal compromise and retroplacental clot visible after delivery.

3 Revealed bleeding may or may not be seen, but there are significant maternal signs (uterine tetany, hypovolaemia, abdominal pain), with late stage fetal compromise or fetal death. Thirty per cent of these women will develop disseminated intravascular coagulopathy (DIC).

Abruption has historically been associated with very poor fetal and maternal outcomes. Perinatal mortality rates vary widely as the diagnostic criteria are generally clinical and broad. The minimal perinatal mortality rate is at least 4 per 1000. In the last Confidential Enquiry into Maternal Deaths, two deaths were due to abruption, though these were not thought to have been preventable.

## Aetiology and associations

The aetiology of placental abruption is unclear, but there are a number of recognized associations.

The risk factors for abruption include:

- previous abruption/family history of abruption,
- fetal abnormality,
- rapid uterine decompression (rupture of membranes with polyhydramnios),
- trauma,
- chronic chorioamnionitis,
- smoking,
- abnormal placentation (circumvallate placenta, etc.),
- pre-eclampsia,
- underlying thrombophilias.

It is clear that abnormal placentation in its widest context predisposes to abruption. This probably encompasses the last four associations, all of which may represent disturbances in placentation. Abruption is increased in the majority of thrombophilias, including factor V Leiden and prothrombin gene heterozygotes and homozygotes, protein C and S deficiency and antiphospholipid syndromes [C].[13] What is as yet unproven is whether there are any effective interventions to prevent abruption in women with underlying thrombophilias. Women who have previously had an abruption are approximately six times more likely to do so again than women who have never abrupted. Women who have a sister who has had a significant abruption are at increased risk themselves (odds ratio 2).[14]

Given that placental abruption is associated with disturbed placentation, any factor also seen in these cases will be associated with an increased risk of abruption. These include growth restriction, oligohydramnios, fetal abnormality (especially aneuploidy) and abnormal umbilical artery Doppler velocities.

## Diagnosis

The diagnosis of placental abruption is primarily a clinical one. There may or may not be revealed bleeding. The woman may have had pain preceding or during the bleed and the uterus may be irritable; alternatively, if a large abruption is present, the uterus may be hard and tender.

In grades 2 and 3, the clinical picture is usually clear and the management will be dictated by the fetal and maternal condition. Grades 0 and 1 may be much more difficult to diagnose. There will be much overlap between women with marginal bleeding and bleeding due to other causes. This is largely irrelevant clinically, as all women with APH represent a high-risk group for whom surveillance in pregnancy needs to be increased.

Ultrasonography is not a good method of diagnosing placental abruption. Small areas are difficult to visualize and, in the acute phase, large abruptions can be isoechoic and look like placenta. When an abruption is clinically suspected, it is prudent to manage with that as the diagnosis. Ultrasound should be used to:

- confirm fetal viability,
- assess fetal growth,
- measure liquor volume,
- perform umbilical artery Doppler velocities,
- confirm fetal normality as far as possible,
- exclude placenta praevia.

Kleihauer testing should be performed in women who are rhesus negative. This will ensure that an appropriate dose of anti-D is given should a large fetomaternal haemorrhage be detected. Kleihauer testing as a diagnostic tool has not been shown to be of clinical value in determining whether pain or bleeding is secondary to abruption.[15]

## Management specific to abruption

### When to deliver

The main management decision to be made with abruption is whether to deliver the fetus. This will, of course, depend on the clinical picture and the gestation.

Approximately 50 per cent of women who abrupt will present in labour, and the decision then must be how to deliver the fetus.

When fetal compromise is confirmed at viable gestations, the aim should be to deliver the fetus. Studies comparing neonatal outcomes at gestations of viability suggest that caesarean section is a better choice for the fetus; however, even when caesarean section is performed, perinatal mortality rates of 15–20 per cent are reported in this group. At very low gestations, a vaginal delivery should be the aim. Labour is often quick and although prostaglandins can be used, they are rarely needed.

It is important when performing a caesarean section to alert the haematology laboratory and to arrange to have blood cross-matched as soon as possible (see below). Whether there is time to delay to await the results of clotting screens and cross-matching will depend on the degree of maternal bleeding and the condition of the fetus.

It is important to:

- remember that there may already be considerable unrevealed bleeding which may increase the blood loss well above that which has been revealed;

- be as prepared as possible;
- seek senior help if this is thought likely to be necessary;
- expect heavy postpartum bleeding.

If the fetus is already dead, a vaginal delivery should be the expectation. At least 30 per cent of women will develop DIC and delivery should be expedited. The management is discussed further below.

The time taken to achieve delivery will depend entirely on the rate of bleeding, the rate of change in the clotting studies and the clinical condition of the mother. Fortunately, delivery is usually rapid and after delivery the DIC will usually begin to resolve.

If the abruption is small, the fetus uncompromised and the mother well, a conservative approach may be utilized. There can only be gains for the mother and fetus if there are benefits in terms of maturity and the option to give steroids. If abruption is thought to be the diagnosis and the fetus is mature, delivery in a controlled manner is probably the best management plan. After 38 weeks, in most cases of suspected abruption, delivery should be considered. Between 34 and 38 weeks, cases must be managed on an individual basis. When a conservative approach is undertaken, increased surveillance is essential. In the acute phase, a period of inpatient management with twice-daily cardiotocography until stability is confirmed is warranted. Fetal growth must be serially assessed, and umbilical artery Doppler waveform analysis is also helpful.[16]

## Bleeding of other causes

The group of other causes comprises a wide range of conditions. As a group, these causes carry an increased risk of perinatal mortality of approximately five-fold and therefore warrant careful consideration.

Management will depend on the individual cause, but there are some general principles.

- It is preferable to err on the side of caution, and safer to increase surveillance rather than to assume that the cause must be benign.
- There is no evidence to support a policy of delivery at term in the well fetus, but steps to ensure fetal well-being must be continued if a conservative approach is adopted.

## MANAGEMENT OF THE WOMAN PRESENTING WITH ANTEPARTUM HAEMORRHAGE

### Management at initial presentation

A rapid assessment of the condition of both the mother and the fetus is a vital first step.

A clinical history can be quickly taken in an acute situation. A more detailed history can be taken once the immediate clinical picture is established. When taking the initial history, questions should be asked regarding:

- dates by previous scan,
- amount of bleeding,
- associated or initiating factors,
- abdominal pain,
- coitus,
- trauma,
- leakage of fluid,
- previous episodes of bleeding,
- previous uterine surgery (including induced abortions and surgically managed miscarriages),
- smoking and use of illegal drugs (especially cocaine),
- fetal movements,
- blood group,
- position of the placenta, if known from a previous scan.

Smoking increases the risk of placenta praevia, placental abruption and marginal bleeding. This is a dose-dependent effect. Fetal growth restriction is associated with both marginal placental bleeding and placental abruption. The mother may have noticed a reduction in fetal movements. The use of cocaine and crack cocaine is strongly associated with placental abruption.

### Maternal assessment

In the initial stages, maternal assessment should include:

- pulse,
- blood pressure,
- uterine palpation for size, tenderness, presenting part.

A vaginal examination must not be performed until a placenta praevia has been excluded.

### Fetal assessment

It should be established whether a fetal heart can be heard, making sure it is fetal not maternal (the mother may be very tachycardic). If a fetal heart is heard and the gestation is estimated to be 26 weeks or more, fetal heart rate monitoring should be commenced.

These initial steps take very little time. Following this initial assessment, women will fall into one of two categories.

1  The bleeding is minor or settling, and neither the mother nor fetus is compromised.
2  The bleeding is heavy and continuing and the mother or fetus is or soon will be compromised.

### Group 1: bleeding is minor or settling and neither the mother nor fetus is compromised

This is the most common group. It is usually clearly apparent that neither mother nor fetus is in danger on admission.

Time can then be taken to conduct a full and thorough history and examination.

Once it is clear that the placenta is not low, a vaginal examination can be undertaken with the following aims:

- to assess the degree of bleeding;
- to ascertain cervical changes, which may be indicative of labour;
- to assess local causes of bleeding (trauma, polyps, cervical lesions, etc.);
- to take bacteriological samples if infection is suspected (high vaginal and endocervical swabs, urine polymerase chain reaction (PCR) or endocervical swabs for chlamydia, plus viral swabs if herpes is suspected).

After a careful history and examination, is should be possible to use selected investigations to help establish a diagnosis.

## Further investigations

- Full blood count.
- Kleihauer testing in women known to be Rhesus negative or in women with unknown blood group.
- Grouping and saving of serum, with blood cross-matched if there is continuing or severe bleeding.
- Clotting screen in cases of suspected abruption or heavy bleeding.

Ultrasound is useful for:

- measurement of fetal size,
- assessment of liquor volume,
- location of the placenta in relation to the internal cervical os,
- establishment of fetal well-being:
  - biophysical profile (see Chapter 14, Tests of fetal well-being),
  - umbilical artery Doppler velocimetry.

Ultrasound is not generally helpful in diagnosing abruption. Acute abruptions can be difficult to see as they may have the same echogenicity as placenta. It should be made clear that the ultrasound examination is primarily to assess the position of the placenta and the well-being of the fetus. Women are often disappointed if they have been led to believe the ultrasound will identify the cause of the bleeding.

If the source of bleeding is fetal, the fetus is usually quickly compromised. This may present with a fetal tachycardia progressing rapidly to a sinusoidal cardiotocography and finally a terminal bradycardia. Very rarely, an Apt's test (which relies on the resistance of fetal haemoglobin to denaturization by acid) can help if fetal blood loss is suspected.

A Kleihauer test is mandatory for all Rhesus-negative women. All RhD-negative women will require 500 IU anti-D (unless they are already sensitized). The Kleihauer test must be done to determine whether there has been a large fetomaternal haemorrhage, in which case more anti-D will be needed.

The Kleihauer is not a useful test to differentiate small abruptions from bleeding of other causes [C].[14] Fetal cells may appear in the maternal circulation in as many as 15 per cent of women at some time in pregnancy, and a lack of fetal cells in the maternal circulation does not preclude an abruption.

When any pregnant woman complains of episodes of vaginal bleeding in pregnancy, other than confirmed causes of haemorrhage, cervical cancer must be excluded by direct observation of the cervix and a cervical smear taken. This should be undertaken irrespective of her past medical history or reports of normal past cervical smears [E].

## Surveillance after a limited antepartum haemorrhage

Although some units admit women who have had APH for 24 hours, there is no evidence to suggest that this improves outcome once fetal and maternal well-being has been established [D]. Management must be individualized, taking into account the suspected cause of bleeding, gestation, fetal assessment and continuing maternal risk factors.

The following must be borne in mind:

- No bleeding, however light, should be dismissed without full investigation.
- Once APH has occurred, the pregnancy becomes high risk, and a management plan for ongoing fetal surveillance must be formulated and discussed with the mother.
- Women must be advised to watch for warning signs, such as a decrease in the frequency of fetal movements, further bleeding or pain, and should be assessed again should any of these occur.

## Planning for the rest of pregnancy

If bleeding settles and the mother is discharged, a clear plan for the remainder of the pregnancy should be made. Even if the cause is thought to be minor, extra fetal surveillance is needed as a higher fetal mortality rate is seen compared with background. Fetal surveillance for growth and well-being should be instituted, as guided by the clinical picture. If all remains well, induction of labour at term is not needed, but the degree of surveillance after the due date may need to be increased.

## Group 2: severe ongoing bleeding, compromised mother and/or fetus

Delivery must be expedited if the mother is compromised. If the fetus is compromised, the decision to deliver will be based on the gestational age. In most cases, delivery will be indicated.

The method of delivery will be determined by the cause and severity of the bleeding, the fetal gestation and status.

Women with major haemorrhage from a placenta praevia will need delivery by caesarean section.

Placental abruption causing maternal or fetal compromise necessitates delivery. If the fetus is already dead, vaginal delivery after stabilization of the mother is usually the safest option. However, if the bleeding continues, and the mother's condition cannot be stabilized, delivery should be achieved by the quickest method, which may be caesarean section. Coagulopathy will only begin to resolve once the placenta is delivered, and may be severe enough to warrant replacement with fresh frozen plasma (FFP), cryoprecipitate and platelets. These women usually labour very quickly. Epidural or spinal anaesthesia must not be used if the clotting studies are abnormal or not available. Central venous pressure (CVP) lines can be useful, but should be sited through an antecubital long line, and not sited or removed until clotting is normal.

It can be difficult to measure obstetric blood loss accurately, as the loss may be concealed (placental abruption) or diluted by amniotic fluid.

Major haemorrhage can be defined by blood loss and/or vital signs:

- blood loss >1000 mL,
- disturbance of conscious state,
- systolic pressure <100 mmHg,
- blood pulse >120 beats per minute (bpm),
- reduced peripheral perfusion.

Disturbances of coagulation due to loss or consumption of platelets and clotting factors may occur during haemorrhage. DIC is the coagulation problem most often encountered in obstetric patients. This and the other complications – fetal or maternal death, adult respiratory distress syndrome, renal and hepatic failure – are more likely to occur if adequate replacement of blood volume is not instigated rapidly.

## Aims of treatment of major haemorrhage

- Rapid restoration of the circulation blood volume and oxygen-carrying capacity.
- Cessation of further blood loss.
- Restoration/maintenance of normal blood coagulation.
- Delivery of the live fetus (where appropriate).

Resuscitation should aim to keep the haemoglobin concentration above 8 g/dL, the pulse rate below 100 bpm, and the systolic blood pressure above 100 mmHg. Four units of cross-matched blood should be available at all times. The British Committee for Standards in Haematology recommend aiming to keep the platelet count above $75 \times 10^9$, the prothrombin and activated prothrombin times <1.5 × mean control, fibrinogen >1 g/L [E].[17]

The success of treatment is dependent on careful organization as well as prompt treatment and the use of appropriate blood products and non-blood volume expanders.

The patient, her partner and relatives must be kept fully informed.

## When major haemorrhage is identified

1   Call for help. The immediate team will consist of:
    a.  the obstetric specialist registrar
    b.  the obstetric senior house officer
    c.  the anaesthetic registrar
    d.  the senior midwife.

The consultant obstetrician and anaesthetist should be informed. A member of staff should be nominated to run samples and record events. The haematology laboratory must be informed that there is a major obstetric haemorrhage.

2   Start facial oxygen 10–15 L/min (hypoxia will reduce uterine contractions).
3   Insert two intravenous cannulae (14-gauge brown/orange), one into each antecubital fossa.
4   Take 30 mL of blood for:
    a.  full blood count (FBC);
    b.  clotting screen (including fibrinogen and fibrin – degradation products or d-dimers if DIC is suspected);
    c.  cross-match 6 units;
    d.  urea and electrolytes, liver function.
5   Commence the following infusions:
    a.  up to 2 L normal saline/Hartmann's solution;
    b.  colloid (up to 1.5 L);
    c.  uncross-matched Rh-negative blood or group-specific blood (if clinical condition is critical);
    d.  cross-matched blood as soon as available.

Cross-matched blood is the ideal, but crystalloid first and colloid second should be used until blood is available. Group O RhD-negative blood should only be used as a last resort, but can be life saving when haemorrhage is severe. Group O RhD-negative blood must not be given to patients known to have anti-c antibodies from their antenatal records [E].

Fluids should be warmed, as cold injury exacerbates DIC.

6   Site an indwelling catheter to monitor urine output and aim to keep output above 30 mL/h.
7   One member of staff should be assigned to record the following:
    a.  pulse,
    b.  blood pressure,
    c.  CVP (half-hourly) if a line is present (see below),
    d.  continuous fetal heart rate (where appropriate),
    e.  fundal height (abruption/post-partum haemorrhage),
    f.  urine output,
    g.  fluid input (type, volume and i.v. site),
    h.  any drug administration (time, type, dose),
    i.  measured blood loss.
8   The senior obstetrician present should co-ordinate and manage the clinical situation, i.e. prompt treatment of the cause of haemorrhage, adequate fluid replacement and regular checking of FBC and clotting status in order to prevent and treat DIC.

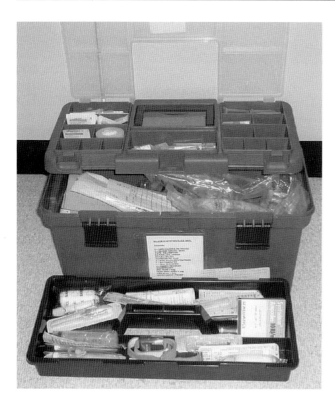

**Figure 23.1** A major haemorrhage box

A major haemorrhage box is an asset on any acute unit. It should contain everything needed for the initial resuscitation (fluids, cannulae, tourniquet, blood bottles and forms, oxytocics, etc.) (Figure 23.1).

## BLOOD TRANSFUSION CONSIDERATIONS

Packed cells and stored blood lack platelets and clotting factors. Fresh whole blood is not available because of potential hazards of viral transmission. FFP and sometimes cryoprecipitate are usually necessary to compensate after transfusion of 4–6 units. Stored blood also is a source of thromboplastins and can lead to or exacerbate DIC when large amounts are transfused. In most units, up to 4 units of FFP may be issued before the coagulation screen result is known for a patient in critical condition (usually 6 units already transfused and blood loss continuing), provided that coagulation studies are being processed.

Thrombocytopenia can also occur during massive transfusion, but in DIC a platelet transfusion is rarely required unless the platelet count falls below $50 \times 10^9$ and there is continued blood loss.

Blood should be administered through blood-warming equipment and rapid administration of warmed fluid should be achieved by the use of a compression cuff on the infusion bag. The use of a blood filter is not necessary. Cold injury increases the risk of DIC.

Extra blood and products should be ordered early – the amount of each will depend on the clinical situation and FBC and coagulation screen results. In established DIC, extra FFP or cryoprecipitate and platelets may be needed, according to instructions from the haematologist.

Recombinant factor VIIa (NovoSeven) has been used in cases of severe continuing haemorrhage. It does not work where there is hypofibrinogenaemia or thrombocytopaenia (fibrinogen <1 g/L, platelets less than $20 \times 10^9$) so should be given after cryoprecipitate and platelets if needed in cases where continued bleeding is thought to be secondary to thrombostatic failure [C].[17] The prothrombotic properties of recombinant factor VIIa neccesitate careful postnatal precautions for thromboembolism deterrence. In the immediate post-haemorrhage period, good hydration and compression devices should be used, with heparin added when clinically safe.

Once bleeding has been stopped, the patient should be managed in an obstetric high-dependency setting or adult intensive therapy unit.

## Central venous pressure monitoring

Central venous pressure (CVP) monitoring can be helpful where there has been massive haemorrhage, concealed blood loss or when blood loss is continuing.

A long line should be used if there are concerns regarding clotting.

A pressure between 3 and 7 cm $H_2O$, using the angle of Louis as the reference zero, should be established.

- Ensure that the rate of transfusion at least equals the rate of continuing blood loss and is, in addition, adequate to replace the loss already measured.
- Do not over-transfuse the patient with cell-free colloid, as this will result in a severely anaemic patient, with a high CVP, preventing further blood transfusion.
- Do not exceed a CVP of 7 cm $H_2O$ (this leads to a high risk of pulmonary oedema due to low colloid oncotic pressure).
- Do not use or rely on increasing the CVP excessively to correct oliguria.
- Consider using a fluid challenge test if you are unsure of the adequacy of fluid replacement:

Infuse 250 mL Hartmann's or normal saline rapidly (2 minutes). Observe the CVP changes over the following 5–10 minutes.

- *Hypovolaemia*: rapid rise and fall back to previous CVP level.
- *Isovolaemia*: rise and fall back to slightly higher CVP level.
- *Hypervolaemia*: rise to higher CVP level sustained for more than 10 minutes.

# MAJOR HAEMORRHAGE AND SPECIFIC ANTEPARTUM CONDITIONS

## Placenta praevia

It is unusual for the placental site to be unknown, as most women have a detailed fetal anomaly scan. Bleeding significant enough to cause maternal hypotension requires delivery.

If the placenta is known to be praevia, delivery by caesarean section is needed. If the placental site is unknown, the following strategy is helpful.

- Is the presenting part engaged? If so, a placenta praevia is less likely.
- Ultrasound scan can be performed to confirm the leading edge of the placenta, but only if the practitioner is trained to do so.
- If the presenting part is high and delivery is needed, an examination in theatre should be considered if the diagnosis is still unclear.
- The consultant must be informed prior to delivery and should be present for delivery or as soon as possible.

# MAJOR ABRUPTION

Large abruptions can lead on to DIC in 30 per cent of women. Management must be directed at ensuring the safety of the mother and fetus. Abruption is associated with a high risk for post-partum haemorrhage.

- Usually presents with pain and vaginal bleeding with a woody, hard, tender uterus.
- If fetal heart is present, continuous monitoring is needed.
- Vaginal examination should be performed with due caution.
- Follow the guidelines for massive obstetric haemorrhage above.
- Prevent post-partum haemorrhage and monitor for renal failure.
- Discuss with consultant haematologist.
- If no fetal heart is detected, ultrasound confirmation should be performed, membranes should be ruptured and Syntocinon commenced to empty the uterus.
- FBC and clotting must be monitored at least 4-hourly as these can deteriorate quickly.

# DISSEMINATED INTRAVASCULAR COAGULATION

This is defined as inappropriate activation of the clotting cascade, leading to widespread coagulation, increased fibrinolysis and end organ failure.

The obstetric causes can be divided into three areas:

1  Injury to vascular endothelium:
  a. pre-eclampsia,
  b. hypovolaemic shock,
  c. septicaemia,
  d. cold injury (large amounts of cold fluid).
2  Release of thrombogenic tissue factors:
  a. placental abruption,
  b. amniotic fluid embolism,
  c. prolonged intrauterine fetal death.
3  Production of procoagulant phospholipids:
  a. incompatible blood transfusion,
  b. septicaemia.

Disseminated intravascular coagulation represents a cascade of events which can vary in severity, and range from a compensated state with only laboratory evidence of increased coagulation and fibrinolytic factor turnover, through to massive uncontrollable haemorrhage with very low concentrations of plasma fibrinogen, raised fibrin degradation products (FDPs) and thrombocytopenia. The evolution of events leading to DIC is shown in Figure 23.2. End organ damage is caused by hypotension, fibrin–platelet clump deposition in small vessels, and persisting endothelial damage leading to increased vascular permeability.

The following organs are most susceptible to damage:

- Kidneys:
  – acute tubular necrosis,
  – glomerular damage.
- Lungs:
  – pulmonary oedema,
  – adult respiratory distress syndrome/systemic inflammatory response syndrome.
- Central nervous system:
  – infarcts,
  – cerebral oedema.

The principles of management are:

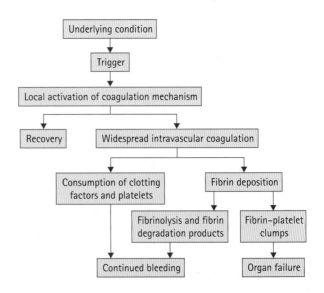

**Figure 23.2** Evolution of disseminated intravascular coagulation

- maternal resuscitation,
- treatment of the cause,
- replacement of blood and clotting factors,
- intensive monitoring until resolution.

Prompt and aggressive fluid replacement will limit damage to the endothelium and allow rapid clearance of fibrin–platelet clumps.

A full coagulation screen should be obtained for any patient at risk of DIC (this should include FPDs or D-dimers and fibrinogen; a thrombin time is useful if fibrinogen testing cannot be done). In DIC, all aspects of the routine clotting study are deranged (activated partial thromboplastin time, partial thromboplastin time and thrombin time). In pregnancy, the normal range for fibrinogen is increased, with the lower limit of normal being 4 g/L. In any woman in whom the fibrinogen falls to 1 g/L, a cryoprecipitate infusion (which is rich in fibrinogen) should be considered. Measurement of fibrin degradation products can be useful; D-dimers that are more specific may also be measured when other indices of coagulation are abnormal.

## Management of disseminated intravascular coagulation

Senior haematological advice should always be sought if DIC is suspected. The mainstay of the management of massive haemorrhage treatment is to stop further loss of blood and resuscitate with appropriate blood products. Mild DIC may be controlled by adequate transfusion with stored blood and FFP. More FFP will be required in severe cases. FFP provides factors V and VIII, other labile coagulation factors and some antithrombin IIIa and fibrinogen. Cryoprecipitate (with a higher concentration of fibrinogen) and platelets may also be needed. After initial resuscitation, management will be dependent on repeated checks of the haemoglobin, platelet count and coagulation status.

- Remember that stored blood contains thromboplastins and can exacerbate DIC once 6 units have been given.
- Remember fibrinogen reference range in pregnancy is >4 g/L. Any woman with a fibrinogen of <1 g/L requires cryoprecipitate if there is active bleeding.

## Treatment of the cause

Disseminated intravascular coagulation will not settle until the cause resolves. The urgency of treatment will be determined by the severity of the DIC and other factors such as maternal and fetal condition.

In general, following abruption and intrauterine fetal death, vaginal delivery should be the aim. Usually, this will be accomplished within 4–6 hours. If DIC becomes uncontrollable during this time, more rapid delivery will be needed. Although it is considered that transfusion of replacement clotting factors may add fuel to the fire of DIC, it is recommended that replacement is aggressively pursued, while delivery is being accomplished.

After delivery, steps to avoid post-partum haemorrhage should be instituted.

## Post-delivery surveillance

The aims are to:

- ensure adequate blood and clotting factor replacement,
- prevent further bleeding,
- monitor renal function and urine output until resolution,
- be vigilant for signs of impending lung involvement.

Fortunately, most women make a rapid recovery following delivery. It is important to ensure that the patient and her partner have the opportunity for a full debriefing.

## SUMMARY

Antepartum haemorrhage increases the risk of perinatal death, regardless of the cause. All women with APH therefore warrant careful fetal and maternal evaluation. In many cases a cause cannot be found, but the increase in perinatal mortality requires careful fetal surveillance for the remainder of all such pregnancies. Abruption carries the largest fetal and maternal risk. Women with underlying placental disease carry the highest risk for abruption.

Placenta praevia is becoming increasingly prevalent. As repeated caesarean sections are performed, the risk of a placenta praevia with a morbidly adherent placenta increases. A multidisciplinary approach is needed to ensure good maternal outcomes in the most difficult cases.

- Transvaginal ultrasound provides the most information and is safe in the diagnosis of placenta praevia.
- The risk of placenta praevia and accreta increases with each subsequent caesarean section.
- Regional anaesthesia for elective caesarean section for placenta praevia is safe and is associated with less maternal bleeding than general anaesthesia.

### KEY POINTS

- The major causes of APH are abruption, placenta praevia and a mixed category of other causes.
- APH of any cause carries an increase in the risk of perinatal death for that pregnancy.
- Maternal deaths related to abruption and placenta praevia continue to be reported. Senior involvement is needed in the delivery of women with placenta praevia.
- Placenta praevia and accreta are likely to become more common as the caesarean section rate rises.
- Increased surveillance is required for all ongoing pregnancies complicated by APH.
- Large abruptions carry a high risk of DIC and require a multidisciplinary approach to optimize care.

# Key References

1. Sheiner E, Shoham-Vardi I, Hallak M *et al.* Placenta previa: obstetric risk factors and pregnancy outcome. *J Matern Fetal Med* 2001; **10**: 414–19.

2. Sherman SJ, Carlson DE, Platt LD, Mediaris AL. Transvaginal ultrasound: does it help in the diagnosis of placenta praevia? *Ultrasound Obstet Gynecol* 1992; **2**: 256–60.

3. Becker RH, Vonk R, Mende BC *et al.* The relevance of placental location at 20–23 gestational weeks for prediction of placenta previa at delivery: evaluation of 8650 cases. *Ultrasound Obstet Gynecol* 2001; **17**: 496–501.

4. Ghourab S. Third-trimester transvaginal ultrasonography in placenta previa: does the shape of the lower placental edge predict clinical outcome? *Ultrasound Obstet Gynecol* 2001; **18**: 103–8.

5. Eller AG, Porter TF, Soisson P, Silver RM. Optimal management strategies for placenta accreta. *BJOG* 2009; **116**: 648–54.

6. Wing DA, Paul RH, Millar LK. Management of the symptomatic placenta praevia: a randomized, controlled trial of inpatient versus outpatient expectant management. *Am J Obstet Gynecol* 1996; **175**: 806–11.

7. Royal College of Obstetricians and Gynaecologists. *Placenta Praevia and Placenta Accreta: Diagnosis and Management*. Green Top Guideline No. 27. London: RCOG, 2005.

8. Besinger RE, Moniak CW, Paskiewicz LS *et al.* The effect of tocolytic use in the management of symptomatic placenta praevia. *Am J Obstet Gynecol* 1995; **172**: 1770–8.

9. Oppemheimer LW, Farine D, Knox Ritchie JW *et al.* What is a low-lying placenta? *Am J Obstet Gynecol* 1991; **165**: 1036–8.

10. Morrison JJ, Rennie JM, Milton PJ. Neonatal respiratory morbidity and mode of delivery at term: influence of timing of elective caesarean section. *Br J Obstet Gynaecol* 1995; **102**: 101–6.

11. Bekku S, Mitsuda N, Ogita K *et al.* High incidence of respiratory distress syndrome (RDS) in infants born to mothers with placenta previa. *J Matern Fetal Med* 2000; **9**: 110–13.

12. Parekh N, Husaini SWU, Russell IF. Caesarean section for placenta praevia: a retrospective study of anaesthetic management. *Br J Anaesth* 2000; **84**: 725–30.

13. Alfirevic Z, Roberts D, Martlew V. How strong is the association between maternal thrombophilia and adverse pregnancy outcome? A systematic review. *Eur J Obstet Gynecol Reprod Biol* 2002; **101**: 6–14.

14. Rasmussen S, Irgens LM. Occurrence of placental abruption in relatives. *BJOG* 2009; **116**: 693–9.

15. Emery CL, Morway LF, Chung-Park M *et al.* The Kleihauer–Betke test. Clinical utility, indication, and correlation in patients with placental abruption and cocaine use. *Arch Pathol Lab Med* 1995; **119**: 1032–7.

16. Neilson JP, Alfirevic Z. Doppler ultrasound for fetal assessment in high risk pregnancies. *Cochrane Database Syst Rev* 2000; (**2**): CD000073.

17. Royal College of Obstetricians and Gynaecologists. *Postpartum Haemorrhage: Prevention and Management*. Green Top Guideline No. 52. London: RCOG, 2009.

# Chapter 24

# Intrauterine fetal death

*Lucy Kean*

---

## MRCOG standards

### Theoretical skills

- To be able to manage intrauterine fetal death in a labour ward setting.
- To have attended a course or training session on counselling after fetal loss.
- Candidates are encouraged to attend post-mortem examinations in cases they have personally managed.

### Practical skills

- Be able to confirm fetal death using ultrasound.

## INTRODUCTION

Intrauterine fetal death (IUFD) or stillbirth is variously defined in different countries, by gestation or birth weight. In England and Wales, stillbirth is defined as a baby delivered with no signs of life known to have died at 24 completed weeks of pregnancy onwards. This definition allows fetuses known to have died before this time, but not expelled from the uterus until after 24 weeks, to be categorized as miscarriages. Therefore parents are not required to notify the registrar of births and deaths of these earlier losses. Most of these are co-twin deaths, which remain *in utero*.[1]

The variety of definitions used across the world makes comparisons of stillbirth rates difficult. In the United States, data are collected from 20 weeks. The rate of early stillbirth (20–27 weeks) is 3.2/1000 births and 3.1/1000 births for ≥28 weeks. These rates are very similar to those seen in the UK.

In the United Kingdom, there was a significant fall in the stillbirth rate from 5.7 per 1000 births in 2002–2004 to 5.2 per 1000 births in 2007.[2] A small decline in the rates of stillbirth among singleton pregnancies was recorded, while the decline in deaths among multiple pregnancies was significantly greater. In singletons, the largest reductions occurred in intrapartum-related deaths, and deaths due to congenital anomalies, antepartum haemorrhage and pre-eclampsia. There was little change in the rate of unexplained antepartum death occurring at term (RR 0.97, 95 per cent CI 0.84–1.11) or preterm (RR 0.94, 95 per cent CI 0.82–1.07); these account for about half of all late fetal deaths.

For the purposes of this chapter, fetal death after 20 weeks gestation is taken as the focus, as these women are generally managed on the labour ward.

## AETIOLOGY

The ability to determine the cause of a IUFD will be related to the rate of uptake of post-mortem examination, the quality of the examination and the experience of the examiner.

From 2007, the Confidential Enquiry into Maternal and Child Health (CEMACH) used the extended Wigglesworth and Obstetric (Aberdeen) classification of cause of death to categorize stillbirths. Using the Wigglesworth categorization, the majority (76.1 per cent) were classified as unexplained. For the unexplained stillbirths, the Obstetric (Aberdeen) classification showed the additional factors identified that may have been associated with deaths. After analysis of the obstetric factors, 74.4 per cent of the original 76.1 per cent were still unexplained. Of these, 37.9 per cent were small for gestational age (birth weight less than 10th centile for gestation).[2] It is hoped that the recognition of the need for specialized paediatric pathology services will reduce the number of IUFDs categorized as unexplained. In large studies, the percentage of fetal deaths designated unexplained has reduced to 10 per cent from previously quoted rates of 40 per cent.[3] CEMACH has now developed a new classification system which aims to reduce the proportion of deaths with an unexplained or non-specific cause.[2]

Clearly, among the group of unexplained IUFD, there are a large proportion of fetuses for which poor growth is suspected if maternal characteristics are included when calculating birth-weight centiles.[3] The implication of this finding is that fetal undergrowth is associated with many unexplained losses, although the pathological mechanism remains unclear [C].

**Table 24.1** Causes of intrauterine fetal death

| Fetal |
|---|
| Cord accidents |
| Feto-fetal transfusion |
| Feto-maternal haemorrhage |
| Chromosomal and genetic disease |
| Structural abnormality |
| Infection |
| Anaemias of fetal origin, e.g. alpha-thalassaemia |
| **Direct maternal effects** |
| Obstetric cholestasis |
| Metabolic disturbance, e.g. diabetic ketoacidosis |
| Reduced oxygen states, e.g. cystic fibrosis, obstructive sleep apnoea |
| Uterine abnormalities, e.g. Ashermann's syndrome |
| Antibody production, e.g. Rhesus disease, platelet alloimmunization, congenital heart block |
| **Maternal placental effects** |
| Pre-eclampsia |
| Renal disease |
| Antiphospholipid syndromes |
| Thrombophilia |
| Smoking |
| Drug abuse, e.g. cocaine |

The causes of fetal death are many (Table 24.1). An understanding of the aetiology and associations can better direct investigations.

## ASSOCIATIONS

It is recognized that IUFD is more common among certain groups, though the exact aetiology for the increase in risk is uncertain. Advanced maternal age, obesity, advanced gestation and social deprivation are all associated with increased risk. Non-white ethnic origin and booking after 12 weeks are also associated with higher risk [C]. Multiple pregnancies have an increased risk, as do women with diabetes and hypertension.[2]

The contribution of each of the above factors to fetal death may be variable. Many of these diseases or conditions are common and yet fetal death is uncommon. It is vitally important not to ascribe causation to associations without investigation, as this may lead to important further information being missed. Although abruption may lead to fetal demise, it may not be the whole story, as abruption is more common in fetal abnormality, thrombophilias, growth restriction, smoking and drug use. Equally, thrombophilias

are common (affecting more than 5 per cent of the population), and while they have been shown to contribute to fetal death in some women, they may also be an incidental finding after a fetal death of another cause. There is still much controversy regarding the role of thrombophilia in stillbirth. Large randomized trials have not been performed and thrombophilia is not a single entity. Association is strongest among women who deliver a very growth restricted baby.

Diabetes is associated with stillbirth as gestation increases. Current guidance advises delivery at 38 weeks in women with diabetes.[4]

Obstetric cholestasis is discussed further in Chapter 6.8, Liver and gastrointestinal disease. It is strongly associated with fetal death as gestation increases. It is an important diagnosis to make, as it may recur in up to 80 per cent of subsequent pregnancies. It is a difficult diagnosis to make at post-mortem as the features are very non-specific in the fetus (generally just an anoxic mode of death). Direct questioning about itching may point to the diagnosis, which can be confirmed by measurement of maternal bile acids.[5]

Cord accidents are often attributed as the cause of death, as the finding of a cord knot or tight nuchal cord is easily seen at delivery and is often seen as a clear demonstration of the cause of death which parents can understand. However, it is rare for knots or cord entanglement to cause antepartum stillbirth. These findings are seen as often in pregnancies resulting in live births. Only if pathological confirmation is obtained should these be deemed causal. Many parents decline post-mortem because causation is erroneously ascribed to a cord accident.

## DIAGNOSIS OF THE DEATH

Intrauterine fetal death presents with decreased fetal movement in as many as 50 per cent of cases. Others present with an unexpected finding at a routine ultrasound or antenatal visit or with signs of an acute event such as abruption, ruptured membranes or the onset of labour. When an IUFD is suspected, it is vitally important to establish the diagnosis as soon as possible. It is natural for parents to cling on to every shred of hope for as long as possible, and delay in diagnosis can lead to a false elevation of hope.

Fetal death must be diagnosed by ultrasound. Cardiotocography can be very misleading as the heart rate tracing of an anxious mother is usually identical to that of a fetus. Even heart rate tracings achieved by scalp electrode can record the maternal heart rate when the fetus is dead.

The ultrasound must be performed by someone trained to do it. Colour-flow mapping can be very useful, especially in the obese woman. It is sometimes, but not always, helpful to the parents to be shown the still fetal heart.

Ultrasound can also confirm features that may be helpful in further investigation. There may be:

- Spalding's sign (overlapping of the fetal skull bones when the fetus has been dead for some time),
- oligohydramnios,
- signs of fetal hydrops.

Once the ultrasound has confirmed fetal death, it is very important that the news is given to the parents in an unambiguous and sensitive way. Phases such as 'I cannot see a fetal heart beat' can be taken by parents to mean that the operator cannot be sure or is not sufficiently trained. It is much better to explain that the baby has died and to express your sorrow.

The initial reaction of parents will vary according to their prior suspicions, and many parents will initially feel anger. It is helpful for parents to be able to express their distress freely and without interruption. Do not try to challenge anger expressed against medical or midwifery staff at this time. If the pregnant woman has family with her, they should be allowed time together to come to terms with the findings.

All units should have a clear protocol for the management and investigation of women with fetal death. It should encompass lines of responsibility so that steps are not inadvertently omitted or repeated.

It is important to establish the events leading up to the fetal death, as there may be factors that will impact on the next pregnancy. It does not take long to take a history of events, and mothers may forget important factors later. It is an important process for the mother; she may feel the need to go through events preceding the admission. Although some of the information that parents volunteer is not relevant, it should be listened to sympathetically and never dismissed as irrelevant.

## PROVIDING CHOICE AND ESTABLISHING THE SAFETY OF THE MOTHER

At this point, it is important to accede to mothers' choices in regard to management as long as these do not compromise safety.

Measurement of blood pressure and urinalysis should be undertaken to rule out significant pre-eclampsia. Where the fetal death is due to an abruption, clinical signs are usually apparent from the outset. If it is felt that the fetus has been dead for some time, a clotting screen should be performed to ensure that there is no coagulopathy.

## PREVENTION OF RHESUS (D) ISOIMMUNIZATION

Massive feto-maternal haemorrhage is one cause of fetal death and may have occurred hours or even days before clinical presentation. If the woman is Rhesus (D) negative, blood for Kleihauer testing should be taken soon after the diagnosis for an estimation of the volume of fetal–maternal transfusion. Anti-Rh (D) immunoglobulin should be given as soon as possible after presentation and not delayed. Delivery may not occur until after the 72-hour watershed beyond which immunoprophylaxis is less effective. A further dose of anti-Rh (D) immunoglobulin might be necessary once the Kleihauer result is known.

## HOW TO DELIVER

If the mother is well, the next step is to decide how and when to deliver her. Many women are horrified that a vaginal delivery is recommended. This must be approached in a sympathetic manner. Most women will understand that a straightforward vaginal delivery will minimize the length of postnatal inpatient time and speed their general recovery. There may be circumstances in which caesarean section has to be considered. These will include women for whom this management was previously planned, women with a major placenta praevia and women who simply cannot bear the concept of a vaginal delivery. There can be no hard and fast rules and each case must be individually managed. There have been no studies that have assessed the psychological impact of different delivery strategies in this context.

## DELIVERY

Women should be offered the choice of when they would like to deliver. The risk of coagulation problems secondary to a retained dead fetus is small. Estimated risk is 25 per cent if the fetus has been retained for 4 weeks. Therefore, given that over 90 per cent of women will deliver spontaneously following IUFD within 3 weeks, conservative management is an option that can be offered.[6] Some women will want to spend time at home before commencing induction and others will want to start the process as soon as possible.

Women should be cared for within the delivery suite in order that maternal safety is not compromised. In many units, a dedicated room is set aside for their management. It is good practice to allow partners and other family members to stay.

Women should have full access to analgesia as required. Diamorphine or morphine is a better option in this setting (as compared to pethidine) as both have a longer half-life. Epidural analgesia should be available for women with normal clotting, and patient-controlled analgesia may be useful for those who cannot receive epidural analgesia.

## INDUCTION OF LABOUR

If the woman appears to be physically well, her membranes are intact and there is no evidence of infection or bleeding, she should be offered a choice of immediate induction of labour or expectant management. If there is evidence of ruptured membranes, infection or bleeding, immediate induction of labour is the preferred management option.

There are various strategies that have been used for induction of labour after fetal death. Whichever method is used, it is important to remember that complications, such as uterine rupture and shoulder dystocia, can occur and management must be safe. Until relatively recently, third trimester induction was generally achieved with standard prostaglandin E$_2$ preparations. This was because of their safety profile in relation to uterine rupture. More recently, the combination of the antiprogesterone mifepristone and the prostaglandin analogue misoprostol has been used to good effect with low complication rates. The advantage of this protocol is that the induction to delivery time is shorter (median 8.5 hours). However, in order for the process to work efficiently, the mifepristone needs to be given 24–48 hours before starting misoprostol. Although this time can be spent at home, many women do not wish to delay starting, and in these women misoprostol alone or prostaglandin E$_2$ may be used. There is usually a longer time from induction to delivery in these cases [C].[6–8]

A standard protocol for mifepristone/misoprostol induction is shown below.

- Mifepristone: 200 mg 24–48 hours before induction.
- Misoprostol: 200 mg p.v. then 200 mg orally every 3–4 hours (maximum of four oral doses in 24 hours).

In gestations of 34 weeks or more, doses of 100 mg of misoprostol appear to be effective.

Extra-amniotic infusions are rarely used now, even in economically deprived areas, as misoprostol is safe and cheap. However, extra-amniotic saline has been shown to be reasonably effective as an alternative [B].[9] Where possible, membranes should be left intact for as long as possible as ascending infection can rapidly occur.

For women who have intrauterine fetal death and who have had a previous caesarean section, the risk of uterine rupture is increased. The dose of vaginal prostaglandin should be reduced accordingly, particularly in the third trimester.[8]

Postpartum haemorrhage is not uncommon, especially where there is pre-eclampsia, abruption, prolonged fetal death or infection. Prolonged chorioamnionitis and repeated small abruptions predispose to retained placenta. When this occurs, it should be dealt with quickly and antibiotic prophylaxis given.

## INVESTIGATIONS

It is important not to make assumptions about the cause of the IUFD that may deny parents full investigations. This is particularly so when a true knot or placental abruption is seen. Parents may wish to have a clear cause quickly identified, but it is the role of the medical and midwifery team to explain that only complete information can provide real answers.

The fetus should be carefully examined after birth. The birth weight should be recorded and the placenta weighed.

Any dysmorphic signs should be noted and if there is a suspected abnormality at this stage, an examination by a clinical geneticist or interested paediatrician can be helpful (this is particularly important if post-mortem is declined).

Sexing the baby is essential for identity and naming, but may be very difficult in early fetal deaths. Also, where there are dysmorphic features, there may be ambiguity. There must be no attempt to guess the sex by obstetricians or midwives as this may prove very damaging if the assessment is wrong. If necessary, it may be better to await the result of the initial post-mortem findings or karyotype.

No samples of any kind should be taken from the fetus without the consent of the parents (see below). When consent is obtained, several points should be considered but each case must be individually assessed as not all will be relevant (see Table 24.2).

Other information may become available later which may require further investigations. These would include parental karyotype if a fetal translocation were found or antiplatelet antibodies if intracranial haemorrhage is seen.

Karyotype analysis often fails. Where there are specific concerns, the genetic laboratory may be able to help with specific diagnoses by utilizing other techniques such as fluorescent *in-situ* hybridization or polymerase chain reaction. Fetal chondrocytes provide the most prolonged cell viability, and a small sample from the iliac crest or patella can sometimes provide a diagnosis. Some have recommended performing a fetal karyotype by transabdominal chorionic villus sampling or amniocentesis to avoid problems associated with delay and infection of the placenta during delivery. Whereas this may be ideal, it may be unacceptable to many mothers at this time. Fetal death where there are known abnormalities and no previous karyotype has been taken are the group most likely to benefit from this.

The Kleihauer test will become negative very quickly if there is ABO incompatibility. This test must therefore be performed as soon after confirmation of fetal death as possible and should not be delayed until after delivery. Mothers who have experienced huge feto-maternal transfusion may describe an episode of shivering, feeling unwell or rigors that may pinpoint the event; transfusion reactions have been described in this context.

Maternal glucose metabolism returns to normal almost as soon as the fetus dies. Blood sugar estimation is therefore generally unhelpful. Also, as the derangement is generally mild, HbA1c measurements are usually normal. A suspicion of disordered glucose metabolism may arise if the fetal weight is excessive and islet cell hyperplasia is

**Table 24.2** Investigations following IUFD

| Investigation | Aim |
|---|---|
| Kleihauer | Fetal-maternal haemorrhage |
| Full blood count with platelets | Baseline in case of bleeding; abnormalities may suggest pre-eclampsia or disseminated intravascular coagulation |
| Blood group, antibody screen | Isoimmunization |
| Anticardiolipin antibodies (IgG, IgM), lupus anticoagulant screen | Antiphospholipid syndrome |
| Haemoglobin $A_1C$ | Diabetes |
| Urea and creatinine | Renal disease/pre-eclampsia |
| Liver function tests, uric acid | Pre-eclampsia/obstetric cholestasis/acute fatty liver |
| Bile acids | Obstetric cholestasis |
| Syphilis, parvovirus, CMV, toxoplasmosis serology | Transplacental transmission of infection |
| High vaginal swab | Transcervical ascending infection (especially Group B *streptococcus*) |
| Placenta/fetal chondrocytes | Karyotypic abnormality |
| Placental pathology | Infection, infarction, abruption, trophoblast invasion failure, maternal or fetal vessel thrombosis |
| Post-mortem examination of fetus, limited investigation if PM declined: examination/x-rays/MRI | Structural or syndromic fetal abnormalities, growth restriction, infection |

confirmed (although other diagnoses such as Beckwith syndrome can also present in this manner). Women with unexplained stillbirth have a 4-fold increase in glucose abnormalities in subsequent pregnancies. Therefore, if this diagnosis is suspected, formal glucose testing should be undertaken in the next pregnancy [C].[10] It is established that antiphospholipid syndrome can lead to IUFD, and there is evidence that low-dose aspirin and low-molecular-weight heparin improve pregnancy outcome among those women who present with recurrent miscarriage (see Chapter 6.5, Haematological conditions). Thrombophilia may be associated with stillbirth in growth restricted fetuses and there may be placental features that point to an underlying thrombophilia.[9] It must be recognized that there are no studies to guide management in the subsequent pregnancy.

Obstetric cholestasis has been suggested as being implicated in as many as 40 per cent of fully investigated unexplained stillbirths. The diagnosis can be made by serum bile acid estimation. Measurement of liver function alone may miss the diagnosis in many cases. It is unclear how quickly the bile acids return to normal after fetal death but, given the high recurrence risk, it is worth performing this test as soon as possible.[5]

It is possible to screen maternal urine for the presence of illegal drugs. This should only be done with the consent of the mother and, in this author's experience, is unhelpful. Most mothers feel guilty enough if they think they have contributed to the death of their baby without needing concrete evidence. Those who divulge information about illicit drug use do not need the additional burden of proof. Those who do not provide this information are unlikely to consent to urine testing.

## POST-MORTEM

The uptake of post-mortem has declined recently following adverse publicity concerning organ retention. Many parents are unclear as to what a post-mortem entails and may have quite unjustified fears about the process.

Of all the investigations offered to parents, this is the most important. New information becomes available in as many as 40 per cent of cases, and even when an ultrasound diagnosis has been made, 25 per cent will have new or different findings. For many parents, this will be their best or only chance of finding out what happened [C].[11]

The issues to be discussed with parents must include the following.

### What the procedure is designed to do and how it is performed

Parents need to know that the person performing the examination is a dedicated perinatal pathologist. Unfortunately, and particularly recently, this may not be the case. Some regions perform their perinatal pathology in a main centre. When this is the case, parents should be told that the baby will need to be transferred and will be rapidly and safely returned. Babies classified as stillborn under UK law must be transferred by the undertaker.

The baby is always treated with dignity and respect. The incisions are closed and do not involve the face or limbs. In most cases the baby when dressed will look no different from the way it did before the post-mortem. The exception may be the very small macerated fetus whose skin is so thin that suturing is not possible. In these cases, the baby is wrapped.

## What tissues are kept

In general, the pathologist will not need to keep any organs. Samples for histology may be retained, but even these can be returned should the parents wish. Where a post-mortem is performed in the first trimester, organs are so small that occasionally whole organs need to be retained to make microscope slides. Again, these can be returned if wished.

Where there is a suspected central nervous system abnormality, the brain needs to be fixed before examination ideally. This can take many days, especially in a large term fetus. If this is an important aspect of the post-mortem (usually if there has been antenatal suspicion of abnormality), parents have three options:

1   to forego this extra information,
2   to delay funeral arrangements until this process is complete,
3   to allow the pathologist to retain the fetal brain and to proceed with funeral arrangements without the brain being returned.

Most parents who have given consent for post-mortem will want to wait and delay arrangements until the baby can be returned intact.

## Can anything else be offered to parents who do not want a post-mortem?

Placental pathology should be offered regardless of whether a full post-mortem is to be performed. However, it is important to be realistic about what information this can yield. Up to 48 hours after fetal death, placental morphology does not change very much, but after this time placental morphology changes such that it can be difficult to differentiate pre-existing from post-mortem changes. After 14 days from fetal death, placental pathology is unlikely to yield any useful information. It is important that the placental pathology is undertaken by an experienced perinatal pathologist, as ascribing causation based on placental changes is not a straightforward task.

Parents can be offered a limited post-mortem that examines specific areas. X-rays of the baby are useful, especially if there are dysmorphic features. Magnetic resonance imaging has been used to examine fetal morphology

post-mortem, and may have some advantages, especially with central nervous system lesions; however, it cannot replace a complete post-mortem examination.

Parents need careful counselling by someone who is experienced in dealing with this situation and who understands the processes involved. There has been much debate about whether the pathologist should obtain consent. The difficult logistics involved in this and the fact that most perinatal pathologists are currently only just coping with their workload are likely to preclude this. However, it is important that obstetricians are trained to seek consent in these cases and understand fully the issues involved. An excellent leaflet explaining post-mortem to parents is linked by the Human Tissue Authority at ‹www.hta.gov.uk/policiesandcodesofpractice/modelconsentforms.cfm›.

The final facet of obtaining good information at post-mortem is to give the pathologist all the relevant information. Where there are specific suspicions, the pathologist should be informed of these. It is usually helpful to speak directly with the pathologist about the case. This will also enable the doctor responsible for the case to attend the post-mortem if possible.

## AFTER DELIVERY

After delivery, there are many processes that need to be completed before discharge. The first and most important is to allow the parents as much (or as little) time with the baby as they need. Parents should be allowed to express their own wishes with regard to seeing and holding the baby. Some parents will want to come back to the hospital on a few occasions before they feel able to finally part from their lost baby; evidence from a case-controlled study showed that behaviours that promote contact with the stillborn infant were associated with worse outcome.[12] Women who had held their stillborn infant were more depressed than those who only saw the infant, while those who did not see the infant were least likely to be depressed – 13 of 33 (39 per cent), versus 3 of 14 (21 per cent), versus 1 of 17 (6 per cent) ($p = 0.03$). Women who had seen their stillborn infant had greater anxiety ($p = 0.02$) and higher symptoms of post-traumatic stress disorder than those who had not ($p = 0.02$). Women who had seen their infant were also more likely to show disorganized attachment behaviour towards their next infant – 18 of 43 (42 per cent), versus 1 of 12 (8 per cent) ($p = 0.04$). As these data were acquired from a case-controlled study, there may be many variables that are having an impact. Women who did not wish to see or hold their stillborn baby may have very different coping mechanisms from those who held the baby. Mothers who hold or see the baby may be a self-selected group who form attachments differently. However, these data do show that professionals should not unduly encourage women who do not wish to see or hold the baby to do so, as they may not benefit from this [C].

Parents should be offered the opportunity to have photographs taken and, if these are not wanted at the time, they can be kept, as many parents request them later (sometimes a long time later). The parents may want footprints or handprints of the baby to be taken.

Importantly, the above study indicated that having a funeral and keeping mementoes were not associated with further adverse outcomes, but the small numbers involved limited interpretation. Photographs should only be taken after seeking the parents' wishes, as in some cultures taking photographs of the dead is unacceptable.[13]

Most units have a bereavement team to take on the funeral arrangements with the parents. These teams are usually acutely aware of cultural requirements and may provide an important liaison between the family and the pathologist, especially where there is a need for funeral arrangements to proceed without delay. Unfortunately, it is often those who have the most to gain from postmortem who feel the most cultural pressure not to delay. Sympathetic discussion can often provide a way forward, and many pathologists will provide an out-of-hours service so that delays can be minimized.

Parents should be provided with the telephone numbers of organizations that may also offer support, such as the Stillbirth and Neonatal Death Society (SANDS), as they sometimes need to talk to people unconnected with the hospital. The bereavement team will also provide a contact number.

## Legal issues

It is necessary for parents to register the birth of any baby born after 24 weeks gestation. This is often a traumatic time for parents and the bereavement team can be helpful in assisting with this. The parents need the stillbirth certificate in order to register the baby. When the certificate is completed, it is important not to use abbreviations, and not to attempt to guess the cause of death. It is extremely difficult to have death certificates changed and parents can be deeply upset to find that a baby has a registered cause of death that is not accurate. The registrar's office may need to contact the doctor signing the death certificate, so it is always important to sign and print the name, and important information, such as recognized General Medical Council number and qualifications, must not be omitted. The less well the form is completed, the more time the bereaved parents will have to spend at the registrar's office while he or she tries to contact the doctor involved.

Clarification of the law by the Royal College of Obstetricians and Gynaecologists now means that fetuses that were known to have died before 24 weeks, or those where this is clearly the case on examination after delivery, are not designated as stillbirth and do not need to be registered.[2]

The law does not recognize fetal deaths before 24 weeks. The lack of legal recognition means that parents will not have a death certificate for these early fetal losses. It does not mean that they cannot arrange a funeral or cremation if they wish.

The coroner does not have any legal jurisdiction in cases of stillbirth (even intrapartum), and cases should not need to become the remit of the coroner.

## Suppression of lactation

The onset of lactation often catches women by surprise and is a source of considerable distress when it starts in earnest at about 48 hours. Although not all women need or want lactation suppression, discussion should take place so that advice can be given about how to cope. For most women, simply a good supportive bra, non-steroidal anti-inflammatory agents if there is discomfort, and time will be enough. However, for some women pharmacological measures are needed and a single dose of cabergoline, a long-acting dopamine agonist, is highly effective. Dopamine agonists for the inhibition of lactation should not be used in women with pre-eclampsia or a personal or strong family history of thromboembolic disease.

## Contraception

This subject is best covered by the general practitioner or consultant later, but women do need to know that they can conceive before their first period. A pregnancy conceived quickly may delay the grieving process and, before women go home, it does no harm to include a leaflet on contraception that will meet their needs.

## Going home

Although every effort is made to ensure women go home quickly, premature discharge must be avoided. It is undoubtedly more painful for women to have to return with problems, and safety is paramount. Many units have a bereavement suite or family room so that other family members can stay for support until discharge can safely be achieved.

Contact telephone numbers should be given to the woman or a companion, and there should be a contact who knows what has happened and who is easily available should problems occur. The community team will play a central role in the care of the family, and detailed communication with the general practitioner and community midwife is of paramount importance. They must be informed by telephone on the day of the woman's return to the community, and all antenatal appointments must be cancelled.

## Bereavement care

As perinatal death becomes less common, couples can feel increasingly isolated in their grief. The bereavement team and the community midwife and general practitioner need to be aware of the situation and to react quickly when problems appear to be mounting. It is particularly those couples with high expectations and little family or social support who can be most vulnerable at this time. It is helpful to ensure before discharge that provision is made for the partner to have some time off work, as he will often be forgotten at this time. Also, if the fetal loss has occurred early (20–24 weeks), the patient will need a sick note, as maternity leave will not be applicable.

Parents who have other children often wish to receive guidance about explaining the death of the baby to them. Children's books about death are available. Self-help groups (such as SANDS) also offer support that may sometimes be lacking from professionals. The couple's response to bereavement cannot be predicted by whether they already have children, or the gestation of the fetal loss. Couples respond in different ways and take different amounts of time to heal. The loss of a baby with a severe malformation should not be interpreted as a blessing; it may leave parents with significant fears for the future.

The death of one twin with the survival of the other is especially distressing for parents, who are faced with contradictory psychological processes. It is very difficult to celebrate the birth of one healthy baby and to grieve the death of the other. In this situation, mourning may get postponed or give rise to symptoms of failed grieving, which include the inability to care for and relate to the surviving child appropriately and may contribute to postnatal depression.

## Follow up

The obstetrician involved in the antenatal care is the usual choice to conduct the follow up. However, there may be occasions when the woman requests follow up by a different practitioner, and when this occurs it should not be questioned. It has traditionally been arranged for follow up to take place at around the time of the usual postnatal visit. In general, it is reasonable to try to schedule a visit once all information is available. Reporting times for PM vary and so it is important to know these before attempting to set a date for review.

Women often experience extreme anxiety coming back to the hospital where they have had such a devastating experience. If possible, a neutral venue should be chosen. In every case, there should be enough time to discuss events.

Ideally, the name of the baby should be ascertained before the interview. The bereavement team should be able to supply this. Not all parents will have named the baby.

Generally, parents need to have time to go through events as they recall them, to ask questions that are important to them, and to receive and understand the results of any tests that have been performed.

Often, the issues that are most troubling parents are not those that the medical team see as important, so it is vital to keep an open mind, to encourage parents to talk spontaneously and to be honest in replies. Parents may want to apportion blame to individuals or actions. When

this occurs, it is important to be honest and to offer apology where this is deemed necessary. Where there has been a failure of care, parents need to receive sincere apologies and reassurance that action to prevent a similar occurrence will take place. Being half-truthful or dishonest will not prevent or reduce litigation. However, where there has been no failure of care, it is important to support other colleagues' management in discussion with parents.

When an underlying cause for the fetal death has been identified, this must be clearly explained. There may be the need to involve other professionals, such as clinical geneticists, at a later date.

When no cause has been found, parents are often very frustrated. This is always difficult for professionals, as the wish to provide answers is one of our most ingrained rationales. It is important not to try to provide unfounded reassurance, but in all cases a clear plan of management for the next pregnancy should be outlined.

Parents often ask when they can try for another pregnancy. It must not be assumed that all couples will wish to do so, and this issue must be covered sensitively. In general, there are few sound medical reasons why couples should delay conception. However, it is important that the grieving process is complete (as much as can ever be so) before the next child. Mothers who conceive very quickly may have more problems with depression, post-traumatic stress disorder and disordered bonding after the next birth, although the evidence is very tenuous.[14]

It is helpful for parents if the issues discussed can be provided for them in a letter. Many women will not wish to book their next pregnancy at the same hospital, and a clear letter will help the future team to understand events. It is also helpful for parents as an aide memoire as they may not clearly remember some of the points covered. Finally, parents must be given the opportunity to come back if they are unclear about certain aspects and, for some, a preconceptual visit is helpful.

## MANAGEMENT OF THE NEXT PREGNANCY

It is beyond the remit of this chapter to discuss the potential management plans after fetal loss as the causes are very diverse and management must be individualized. The most important facet of management is to try to adhere to the plans that were formulated after the loss of the baby. It is unusual for professionals to disagree to such an extent that a previously agreed plan has to be changed. There may be minor differences of opinion, but it is better to put these aside in the interests of maintaining the faith of the patient in their care when at all possible. When the plan needs to be changed (such as may occur when new information comes to light), it is important to explain clearly why the changes need to be made and how this will improve the prospects of a healthy pregnancy.

After the birth of the next child, parents may require much reassurance that the baby is healthy. An examination by a senior paediatrician can do much to allay fears.

## SUMMARY

The management of women with fetal loss is an integral and important aspect of good obstetric care. If done well, it can help the grieving process.

- There is little that can be cited as evidence in this field. Most of the suggested management is based on the experience of various professionals and support groups.
- Regimens utilizing mefipristone/misoprostol in the third trimester appear safe and achieve shorter induction to delivery times but require pre-priming before induction, which adds to the total time before delivery [C].

## KEY POINTS

- Confirm fetal death quickly by ultrasound.
- Offer parents choice wherever possible.
- Do not make assumptions regarding the cause of death.
- The support of a bereavement team is an integral part of care.
- Do not discharge the mother home until it is safe to do so.
- Information should be provided at all stages in a form that parents can understand.
- Management of the next pregnancy should try to follow previously set plans.

## Key References

1. Registration of stillbirths and certification for pregnancy loss before 24 weeks of gestation. Good Practice No. 4. London: RCOG, January 2005.
2. Confidential Enquiry into Maternal and Child Health (CEMACH) *Perinatal Mortality 2007: United Kingdom*. London: CEMACH, 2009.
3. Gardosi J, Mul T, Mongelli M, Fagan D. Analysis of birthweight and gestational age in antepartum still-births. *Br J Obstet Gynaecol* 1998; **105**: 524–30.
4. NICE. *Diabetes in pregnancy: management of diabetes and its complications from preconception to the postnatal period*. National Collaborating Centre for Women's and Children's Health Commissioned by the National Institute for Health and Clinical Excellence, March 2008 (revised reprint July 2008).
5. Milkiewicz P, Elias E, Williamson C, Weaver J. Obstetric cholestasis. *BMJ* 2002; **324**: 123–4.
6. NICE. *Induction of labour*. NICE Clinical Guideline 70. National Collaborating Centre for Women's and Children's Health, June 2008.
7. El-Refaey H, Hinshaw K, Templeton A. The abortifacient effect of misoprostol in the second trimester. A randomised comparison with gemeprost in patients pre-treated with mifepristone (RU486). *Hum Reprod* 1993; **8**: 1744–6.
8. Wagaarachchi PT, Ashok PW, Narvekar NN *et al.* Medical management of late intrauterine death using a combination of mifepristone and misoprostol. *Br J Obstet Gynaecol* 2002; **109**: 443–7.
9. Mahomed K, Jayaguru AS. Extra-amniotic saline infusion for induction of labour in antepartum fetal death: a cost effective method worthy of wider use. *Br J Obstet Gynaecol* 1997; **104**: 1058–61.
10. Robson S, Chan A, Keane RJ, Luke CG. Subsequent birth outcomes after an unexplained stillbirth: preliminary population-based retrospective cohort study. *Aust NZ J Obstet Gynaecol* 2001; **41**: 29–35.
11. Weston MJ, Porter HJ, Andrews HS, Berry PJ. Correlation of antenatal ultrasonography and pathological examination in 153 malformed fetuses. *J Clin Ultrasound* 1993; **21**: 387–92.
12. Hughes P, Turton P, Hopper E, Evans CDH. Assessment of guidelines for good practice in psychosocial care of mothers after stillbirth: a cohort study. *Lancet* 2002; **360**: 114–18.
13. Gatrad AR, Sheikh A. Muslim birth customs. *Arch Dis Child Fetal Neonatal Ed* 2001; **84**: F6–8.
14. Turton P, Hughes P, Evans CDH, Fainman D. Incidence, correlates and predictors of post-traumatic stress disorder in the pregnancy after stillbirth. *Br J Psychiatry* 2001; **178**: 556–60.

# SECTION D
## First stage of labour

# Induction of labour

*Richard Hayman*

## MRCOG standards

- Candidates must be confident in performing an induction of labour within a wide range of clinical scenarios.
- Candidates should be able to counsel women in the antenatal clinic regarding the reasons for induction of labour and the risks and benefits.

In addition, we would suggest the following.

### Theoretical skills

- A revision of the knowledge of the process of normal parturition.
- An understanding of the relative merits of different methods of labour induction.
- An understanding of the setting of labour induction in the management of complicated and uncomplicated pregnancy.

## DEFINITION

An induction of labour (IOL) refers to the process of artificially initiating uterine contractions, prior to their spontaneous onset, with the intention to effect progressive effacement and dilatation of the cervix and, ultimately, delivery of a baby. The term 'induction of labour' generally refers to procedures performed in the third trimester, but occasionally may be applied to pregnancies at gestations greater than the legal definition of fetal viability (24 weeks in the UK) when fetal survival is an anticipated outcome. Any procedure performed prior to this gestation may be classified as a termination of pregnancy, and will not be discussed further in this chapter.

The management of labour induction remains a difficult problem for today's obstetrician. As a result of audit, clinical experience and evidence-based research, the National Institute for Health and Clinical Excellence (NICE) has issued formal guidelines for the management of IOL (CG070) based on those previously published by the Royal College of Obstetricians and Gynaecologists (RCOG). These should be read by all clinicians undertaking such interventions.[1]

## INCIDENCE

The induction of a labour is a common procedure and although it is currently employed in 15–20 per cent of all term pregnancies in the UK, this represents a fall from the peak levels of 40 per cent in the 1970s. These figures are not constant and have a wide variation, within and between regions which reflects differences in opinion and practice. The 'correct' level of intervention remains a matter of debate.

## INDICATIONS FOR INDUCTION OF LABOUR

The purpose of an induction is to achieve benefit to the health of the mother and/or baby, which must exceed that to be gained by continuing the pregnancy, excluding those situations for which delivery by planned caesarean section is prudent.

There are many reasons for IOL.[2] The commonly cited indications are detailed below. However, it is not the purpose of this chapter to outline all the possible reasons for induction, and many are not included.

- Pregnancy passing 41 completed weeks gestation.
- Pre-labour spontaneous rupture of membranes.
- Maternal disease, for example:
  - diabetes
  - hypertensive/renal disease
  - autoimmune disease, e.g. systemic lupus erythematosus.
- Pregnancy-related conditions:
  - pre-eclampsia
  - obstetric cholestasis
  - recurrent antepartum haemorrhage (APH)
  - APH at term
  - placental abruption.

- Fetal:
  - intrauterine growth restriction
  - oligohydramnios
  - isoimmunisation
  - intrauterine fetal demise.
- Maternal request.

It is also common to find that an IOL will be performed for cumulative reasons which if considered in isolation would not constitute a sufficient indication. It is vitally important that whatever the indication for induction, the gestational age must be calculated accurately so that appropriate resources and staff can be provided (including the administration of corticosteroids to promote fetal lung maturation; *in-utero* transfer to a unit suitable for neonatal care, etc.).

Pre-labour rupture of membranes is covered extensively in Chapter 22, Premature rupture of membranes, and will therefore not be dealt with further here.

Treatment and care should take into account a woman's individual needs and preferences. Women who are having or being offered IOL should have the opportunity to make informed decisions about their care and treatment in partnership with their healthcare professionals.[3] If a woman does not have the capacity to make decisions, healthcare professionals should follow the Department of Health guidelines – 'Reference guide to consent for examination or treatment' (available from ‹www.dh.gov.uk›). In addition, good communication between healthcare professionals and women is essential. It should be supported by evidence-based written information tailored to the needs of the individual woman. Treatment and care, and the information women are given about it, should be culturally appropriate. It should also be accessible to women, their partners and families, taking into account any additional needs such as physical or cognitive disabilities, and inability to speak or read English.

## INDUCTION OF LABOUR FOR POST-MATURITY

In the UK, the most common indication for labour induction is prolonged pregnancy. This accounts for approximately 70 per cent of all cases.

Until recently, most practitioners used the information obtained from a carefully taken history to calculate the expected period of confinement (37–42 weeks gestation). However, this approach proved inaccurate in the dating of up to 60 per cent of pregnancies and meant that many procedures (including screening for Down's syndrome and IOL for prolonged pregnancy) were inappropriately timed. Consequently, NICE and the National Screening Committee (NSC) recommend that all pregnant women should be offered an early ultrasound scan between 10 weeks 0 days and 13 weeks 6 days to determine

gestational age using a crown rump length measurement (and to detect multiple pregnancies). Such an approach helps to reduce the anxiety experienced by many women when they pass their 'expected date of delivery' and also reduces the requests for 'early' IOL. Where routine ultrasound dating is performed, less than 5 per cent of women will reach 42 weeks. However, women who have already experienced a prolonged pregnancy have a 30–40 per cent chance of doing so again.

At 41 weeks gestation, approximately 19 per cent of women remain undelivered. This drops to 3.5 per cent at 42 weeks. The timing of induction will thus have critical workload implications. The NICE and RCOG guidelines recommend offering induction beyond 41 weeks, but commencing further fetal surveillance at 42 weeks for women who do not wish induction. The later the induction is performed in the 41–42-week period, the fewer the number of inductions that will be needed [A].[1]

The recommended clinical practice in this area has been subject to a recent analysis comparing all the suitable controlled trials. It was concluded that IOL for gestations at or beyond 41 weeks (287 days) may reduce perinatal mortality and meconium aspiration syndrome and does not result in more caesarean deliveries when compared to expectant observational management, even among women whose cervix was not deemed to be favourable at the time of induction.[4]

However, it is important to remember that approximately 370 women will need to be induced to prevent a single stillbirth during this period of gestation. As such, a routine policy of offering an IOL for 'prolonged gestation' may generate an increase in the workload within any individual unit without significantly reducing the observed perinatal mortality.

## Assessment of the post-dates pregnancy

Many different tests of fetal well-being are performed for the assessment of the post-term fetus. These include:

- cardiotocography (CTG);
- ultrasonographic examination that includes:
  - amniotic fluid index,
  - a biophysical profile,
  - umbilical artery Doppler waveform analysis.

An amniotic fluid index of less than 5 cm, or maximum pool depth of less than 2 cm is associated with higher rates of fetal heart rate decelerations and meconium staining of amniotic fluid in labour and both are indications for delivery. Equally, a biophysical score of 6/10 (or less) or abnormal umbilical artery Dopplers would also suggest delivery over continued monitoring. The mechanism of fetal death in the late term pregnancy is poorly understood and these assessments of fetal well-being are likely to identify those fetuses that are compromised for reasons such as placental infarction/insufficiency. However, this is probably a different mechanism from that which is responsible for the death of many post-term fetuses. Consequently, obstetricians are unable to offer complete reassurance to the expectant mother who continues to await spontaneous onset of her labour based on the tests currently available. However, some form of monitoring additional to CTG must be offered from 42 weeks, if only to detect fetuses compromised in assessable ways. Currently, the guidelines recommend at least twice-weekly CTG and ultrasound for amniotic fluid volume as a minimum.[1]

## INDUCTION OF LABOUR FOR MATERNAL REQUEST

Induction of labour is sometimes performed for the convenience of the mother in the absence of any definite medical indication or clear health benefit (this is often described as a 'social induction'). Such inductions must be justified according to the particular circumstances, and any decision should be taken on an individual basis after full discussion of the potential benefits and disadvantages. As with any intervention in pregnancy, IOL is not free from unwanted side effects and should not be undertaken lightly (e.g. NICE document that: 'Induced labour has an impact on the birth experience of women. It may be less efficient and is usually more painful than spontaneous labour, and epidural analgesia and assisted delivery are more likely to be required').

The personal characteristics of women requesting elective, rather than selective, IOL have been extensively studied. Such patients often experience more problems in the antenatal period and appear to be more anxious with regard to labour and delivery than their counterparts. However, as advocated in *Changing Childbirth*, women should be allowed reasonable choices in their obstetric and midwifery care. If pregnancy has reached term and the cervix is favourable, there are no clear benefits for the fetus in delaying the onset of labour.

In multiparae with a favourable cervix, the risks are few; however, there is an increase in the incidence of instrumental deliveries and caesarean sections in nulliparae undergoing elective induction after 39 weeks [C]. Consequently, it should be explained that if an induction fails, the risks of delivery by caesarean section might outweigh any possible social benefits that may be gained, and thus an induction should not be commenced. Patients can only make an informed decision after careful consultation, with the risks and benefits clearly and appropriately presented.

A final comment is that a request for early IOL will sometimes present logistical problems to busy labour wards and the needs of women who require IOL for medical reasons must always be of paramount importance.

Occasionally, this needs to be explained when a request for induction cannot be met.

## OTHER INDICATIONS FOR INDUCTION OF LABOUR

Induction of labour may be considered for any number of indications. However, the evidence upon which the decision to induce is based is often poor, and unfortunately more often is absent. These include:

- Pre-labour rupture of membranes (PROM) at term (>37 completed weeks gestation): expedited delivery (induction commenced within 12 hours after PROM) reduces the incidence of chorioamnionitis, endometritis and admissions of a neonate to a neonatal care unit [B].[5]
- Preterm pre-labour rupture of the membranes: evidence for intervention not established. In addition, the optimal gestational age for IOL is not established.
- Suspected macrosomia: IOL does not improve the outcomes in the setting of suspected fetal macrosomia and in addition may have a negative impact on the incidence of delivery by lower segment caesarean section (LSCS) (evidence weak).[6]
- Twin pregnancy: the only RCT for twin's gestation at 37 weeks is not appropriately powered to determine the benefits and harms of induction.
- Oligohydramnios: Induction of labour for oligohydramnios at term is advocated by expert opinion to reduce the perinatal morbidity and mortality.
- Diabetes mellitus requiring insulin: a policy of routine IOL at 38 weeks reduces the incidence of fetal macrosomia in these patients. This may have an impact on the incidence of shoulder dystocia.
- Intrahepatic cholestatis of pregnancy: a small cohort study suggested that IOL may reduce intrauterine fetal death compared with expectantly managed controls; however, the evidence for this is weak.
- Maternal cardiac disease: no harmful or beneficial effects have been demonstrated for induction of labour for maternal cardiac disease.
- Suspected intrauterine growth restriction (IUGR):
  - In pre-term pregnancy with suspected IUGR, IOL does not reduce perinatal deaths or overall long-term disability. LSCS is less likely with expectant management.
  - The currently available RCT of IOL for suspected IUGR at term lacked statistical power to demonstrate any benefit or harm from IOL.
- Gastroschisis: There is no demonstrated benefit or harm for induction of labour at 36 weeks gestation for fetal gastroschisis.

A very recent randomized controlled trial has evaluated induction versus conservative management at 37 weeks onwards for women with mild pre-eclampsia or mild non-proteinuric hypertension. The primary endpoint was the development of severe maternal disease. This was significantly reduced in the induction group. There was no increase in caesarean section and no difference in neonatal outcomes, except that babies were slightly larger in the conservative management group. This study shows some benefit and no harm in induction at 37 weeks in women with mild pre-eclampsia or hypertension (see Table 25.1) [B].[7]

When faced with making a decision about an IOL, women should be able to access the best available information to enable them to make an informed choice. Clinicians, likewise, should use the best available evidence to support decision making. It should therefore be acknowledged that there is insufficient evidence to definitively guide care, with a number of commonly cited indications for labour induction not having a strong evidence base in practice. However, this does not mean that the indications cited are used without justification, only that further research is required to prove the balance of risks and benefits.

## MECHANISMS OF PARTURITION

Although many theories have been postulated, the exact mechanisms underlying the onset of parturition in humans are not fully understood. However, the initiation of human labour must involve a constellation of changes that leads to a swing in the balance between quiescence and activity within the uterus.

Some clues may be gleaned from animal models. In the sheep, the production of fetal cortisol causes an increase in the production of placental oestrogens and prostaglandins, which sensitize the myometrium to circulating oxytocics, and in turn initiate labour. These changes are mediated by the hypothalamic–pituitary axis. However, this situation appears dissimilar to that in humans, in whom anencephalic fetuses demonstrate no tendency to prolonged gestations.

This suggests that other processes are responsible, and although many mechanisms have been postulated, the exact role played by each of the suggested agents has not been clearly elucidated (Table 25.2).

**Table 25.1** Indications for induction of labour

| Indication[16] | Quality of Evidence | Benefits/ harm | Grade of Reccomendation |
|---|---|---|---|
| Post-term pregnancy | High | Net benefits | Strong |
| PROM | High | Net benefits | Strong |
| PPROM | Moderate | Uncertain | Weak |
| Macrosomia | Moderate | Uncertain | Weak (against IOL) |
| Twin gestation | Low | Uncertain | Weak |
| Oligohydramnios | Low | Uncertain | Weak |
| Diabetes | Moderate | Uncertain | Weak |
| IHCP | Very poor | Uncertain | Weak |
| Cardiac disease | Very poor | Uncertain | Weak |
| Mild pre-eclampsia | High | Net Benefits | Favours induction |
| Severe pre-eclampsia (preterm) IOL versus expectant management | Moderate | Uncertain | Weak (against IOL) |
| Severe pre-eclampsia (preterm) IOL versus LSCS | Very poor | Uncertain | Weak |
| Eclampsia (IOL versus LSCS) | Low | Uncertain | Weak |
| IUGR (pre-term) | High | Uncertain | Weak |
| IUGR (term) | Low | Uncertain | Weak |
| Gastroschisis | Low | Uncertain | Weak |

- IOL, induction of labour; IUGR, intrauterine growth restriction; LSCS, lower segment caesarean section; PROM, premature rupture of membranes; PPROM, preterm premature rupture of membranes.

**Table 25.2** Factors involved in the onset of labour

| Rise |
|---|
| Endogenous prostaglandins |
| Serum oestrogens |
| Oxytocin release |
| Dihydroepiandrostenedione |
| Basal cortisol |
| Interleukin-8 activity |
| **Fall** |
| Prostaglandin dehydrogenase |
| Serum progesterone |
| Cervical remodelling |
| Increase in uterine stretch receptors |
| Fetal ACTH |
| Upregulation of oxytocin receptors |
| **Other** |
| Fetal ACTH |
| Cervical remodelling |
| Increase in number and sensitivity of uterine stretch receptors |

- ACTH, adrenocorticotrophic hormone.

# INDUCTION OF LABOUR

The methods currently employed in labour induction modulate only a limited part of the labour processes. Induction does not usually involve just a single intervention, but a complex set of interventions that present challenges for clinicians and women. Therefore, it should not be surprising that induction of labour sometimes fails.

The methods currently employed include the following:

- Those employed by women that do not require formal medical prescription or involvement – ingestion of castor oil, acupuncture, herbal remedies, breast and nipple stimulation and sexual intercourse.
- Those that rely on mechanical forces to promote cervical effacement and dilatation and the initiation of uterine contractions – membrane sweeping, hygroscopic and mechanical dilators, extra-amniotic infusion of saline and amniotomy.
- Those that employ pharmacological agents to alter the cervical state, initiate uterine activity, or act by a combination of methods – prostaglandins, oxytocin, oestrogens, relaxin and antiprogestogens (mifepri-stone).

As a general rule, the more remote from term, the more difficult IOL will be, frequently requiring a combination of more than one technique over a period of a few days. There are fewer complications with methods employed closer to term as they precede the probable onset of spontaneous labour by only a few hours or days, when some of the receptor and biochemical changes are already mature.

## Assessment before induction commences

As with any intervention, before proceeding with an induction, it is important to ensure that the indication for induction still exists, and that any specific labour management issues that may occur as a consequence of the intervention are highlighted. The clinician must confirm the fetal lie and presentation by abdominal palpation, and assess the well-being of the fetus (commonly by electronic monitoring of the fetal heart rate).

The likelihood of either successful induction or its failure may be most specifically ascertained by assessing the condition of the cervix. A variety of clinical scoring techniques have been reported for the assessment of the cervix prior to induction; the most commonly employed is the Bishop's score, or a modification of this (Table 25.3). The most predictive elements in this system are the station of the presenting part, the length and dilatation of the cervix; as could be predicted, the shorter and more dilated the cervix, the shorter the intervention-to-delivery interval.

**Table 25.3** Modified Bishop's score

| Factor | Score | | | |
|---|---|---|---|---|
| | 0 | 1 | 2 | 3 |
| Cervical dilatation (cm) | <1 | 1–2 | 3–4 | >4 |
| Cervical length (cm) | >4 | 2–4 | 1–2 | <1 |
| Station of the head | –3 | –2 | –1 | 0 |
| Consistency | Firm | Average | Soft | |
| Position of the os | Posterior | Medium | Anterior | |

- The modified Bishop's score is the summation of the individual scores for each of the observations.

## Fetal fibronectin

Fetal fibronectin is released from the amniotic membranes into the cervical transudate, and concentrations >50 g/mL are associated with a favourable cervix and a decrease in intrapartum morbidity. The fibronectin concentration has also been shown to correlate more favourably with the outcome of labour induction, with a shorter induction-to-delivery interval and length of labour than may be predicted by clinical assessment of the cervical state alone.[8] Measurement of this glycoprotein may help tune the timing of labour induction by allowing a more accurate correlation between the state of the cervix, changes in uterine activity and the responsivity to prostaglandins. In general, however, as induction should always be clinically indicated, this test has limited additional benefit. Perhaps it has a role in dissuading those women requesting an early induction, when a negative fetal fibronectin test may indicate a higher chance of failure.

## Induction methods traditionally utilized by women

### Castor oil

This medication, when taken orally, stimulates contractions of the large and small intestine via an effect on the smooth muscle within the viscera. Accompanying this unpleasant 'side effect' is a stimulation of uterine activity, but much more common are profuse diarrhoea and abdominal cramps. Its safety profile for mothers and babies has never been fully investigated and its use should therefore be discouraged. It may potentially increase the incidence of meconium staining of liquor as it has an effect on a term fetus similar to that on the mother [D].

### Acupuncture

The use of acupuncture for labour induction is based on the traditions of Chinese medicine that date back at least

30 centuries. The published data from western literature are too small to address the issues of efficacy or safety, and its use outside the remits of clinical studies cannot be recommended.

## Herbal remedies

Traditional remedies employed to stimulate the onset of labour rely on products that contain ergot derivatives in various strengths that consequently exhibit a weak uterine stimulant effect. The dose and purity of these compounds are often variable, and there is not sufficient evidence to support their use. The efficacy of raspberry leaf tea, whose potential for labour induction stems from observations on brood mares, is equally dubious.

## Breast and nipple stimulation

Breast stimulation is thought to work by stimulating the release of oxytocin from the posterior pituitary. Although many different studies have attempted to standardize the 'treatment' provided (either through mechanical pumps or electrical stimulation), none has been shown to produce consistent and reproducible results.

There are case reports of nipple stimulation being associated with uterine hypertonus and fetal bradycardia. These same studies suggest that if nipple stimulation is to be advocated as a method of labour induction, continuous fetal monitoring should be employed at the same time. The studies that look at larger groups employing such techniques are fraught with technical difficulties and at best are difficult to interpret and at worst, meaningless.

## Sexual intercourse

Semen is rich in naturally occurring prostaglandins; however, there is little evidence to support the belief that sexual intercourse enhances cervical ripening.

## Medical interventions

## Mechanical

### Membrane sweeping

The practice of sweeping the membranes during vaginal examination has long been advocated as a method for stimulating the onset of labour. This procedure involves passing a finger through the cervical os, sweeping it around the internal surface of the cervix and gently pushing the membrane surface away.

It is recommended that all women be offered membrane sweeping prior to induction of labour (see below under Further reading), as it is associated with:

- increased likelihood of spontaneous labour within 48 hours (63.8 versus 83 per cent, relative risk (RR) 0.77, 95 per cent confidence interval (CI) 0.7–0.84, number needed to treat (NNT) 5);

- decreased incidence of prolonged pregnancy of 41 weeks or more (18.6 versus 29.9 per cent, RR 0.62, 95 per cent CI 0.49–0.79, NNT 8).

On a population basis, this may result in a decrease in the induction rate of 15 per cent, with no differences in maternal or fetal outcome [A].

However, it is important that before this is undertaken, women understand:

- the procedure is designed to impact as above;
- it may be a little uncomfortable;
- they may experience frequent contractions following the procedure;
- there may be a little vaginal bleeding following the procedure.

If the woman gives her consent for a membrane sweep, the procedure should be performed with gentleness and consideration. If consent is not given, the membranes should not be swept under any circumstances.

### Hygroscopic and mechanical dilators

When compared with their frequent use in the process of procuring a first or early second trimester abortion, cervical dilators have been employed with relative infrequency for the induction of labour.

Hygroscopic dilators work by absorbing water by osmosis, with a resulting change in their size and shape. When placed into the cervical canal over a period of hours (>12 hours – often overnight), they produce a mechanical dilatation, which then permits an amniotomy to be performed. These agents may also stimulate the local release of prostaglandins, which may have additional benefits on cervical ripening.

Balloon devices and Foley catheters placed within the cervical canal in an attempt to dilate the cervix mechanically have also been investigated. As with the hygroscopic devices, they have been shown to be effective in facilitating cervical dilatation, but overall have not improved the number of successful labour inductions.

With these devices, insertion is best performed with the patient in the lithotomy position, using an aseptic technique to visualize the cervix which must be exposed with a Cusco's speculum. One or more hygroscopic agents are then inserted into the cervical canal as judged appropriate by the cervical state, and left *in situ* for the period of time necessary to provide the required improvement in the cervical condition. Synthetic polyvinyl alcohol polymer sponges impregnated with magnesium sulphate (Lamicel) and the polyacrylonitrite tents are more rapidly effective than their naturally occurring counterpart (Laminaria Tent) [B].

Once the cervix has reached the required dilatation, the induction may be advanced by amniotomy and/or the administration of oxytocin. However, with any intra-cervical device, concerns regarding the introduction of iatrogenic infection have been raised. This risk probably increases in proportion to the duration of retention of any mechanical device, and consequently careful monitoring of the maternal pulse and temperature and the fetal heart rate must be undertaken.

While there may appear to be few indications for such interventions, as the efficacy, and safety, of prostaglandins make them almost redundant, their use in situations where prostaglandins have failed makes them a technique worth knowing about.

### Extra-amniotic infusion of saline

The infusion of 0.9 per cent saline solution into the extra-amniotic space via a Foley catheter has been used as a method of inducing labour. This technique appears to be equally effective at inducing labour as topical prostaglandins, with no difference in the incidence of maternal or neonatal infectious morbidity between the groups. There may be a trend towards an increase in the rate of caesarean section with the infusion intervention, although the studies to date have been too small to assess the clinical significance of this. Further studies are recommended.

### Amniotomy

Traditionally, amniotomy (rupturing of the amniotic membrane) has been either hindwater (performed with a Drew–Smythe catheter) or forewater (a procedure performed with an amniotomy hook – 'Amnihook' – or toothed forcep). The risks inherent with the hindwater approach – namely, uterine, placental and fetal trauma – make this intervention difficult to justify in modern obstetric practice. By comparison, the forewater procedure is safe. However, it still carries the risks of cord prolapse, placental abruption and the introduction of infection into the uterine cavity, as well as the potential for fetal trauma in over-enthusiastic hands.

Prior to any amniotomy, an abdominal palpation must be performed to confirm the fetal lie and presentation, as well as to allow auscultation of the fetal heart. Following this, the cervix is examined to confirm that the forewaters are intact. The station of the presenting part is noted and the membranes ruptured. This releases amniotic fluid, the quantity and colour of which should be noted (absence or presence of meconium). A check is made to ensure that the presentation/ station and position of the presenting part remain unchanged and that there is no prolapse of the umbilical cord. If required, a fetal scalp electrode may be sited.

The success of amniotomy is dependent upon the state of the cervix (dilatation and effacement), the parity of the woman and the station of the presenting part at the time of intervention. Up to 88 per cent of women with a favourable cervix will labour within 24 hours after amniotomy alone. Amniotomy, with the commencement of an early oxytocin infusion (commonly within 2–6 hours if prostaglandins have been used for cervical ripening), produces a significant reduction in the number of women remaining undelivered at 24 hours compared with those managed expectantly [B].

## Biochemical

### Prostaglandins

Prostaglandins are long-chain fatty acids derived from arachidonic acid via the cyclo-oxygenase-2 (COX-2) pathway, and exert a powerful effect on the cervix and myometrium at all stages of gestation. Not only do they modify the ground substance within the cervix, increasing its compliance, they also stimulate the onset of uterine contractions, and thus induce labour. They are therefore particularly useful for labour induction where the cervix is unfavourable.

Prostaglandins of the $E_2$ and $F_{2\alpha}$ class have been used to initiate labour, although there are few studies employing the latter in preference to the former. More recently, prostaglandin $E_1$ analogues (e.g. misoprostol) have received attention.

Prostaglandins may be given via the oral, intravaginal, intracervical or intravenous routes to good effect (Table 25.4). However, intracervical gel and intravaginal preparations have fewer systemic side effects compared with the other routes of administration. Meta-analyses have shown that there are advantages to the use of prostaglandins for ripening the cervix and for induction of labour, compared with oxytocin alone.[9] These are:

- increased successful vaginal delivery within 24 hours;
- decreased incidence of caesarean section;
- decreased risk of the cervix remaining unfavourable at 48 hours;
- reduced epidural usage.

This is at the expense of increased gastrointestinal side effects and uterine hypertonus, which occur in approximately 1 per cent of pregnant women receiving more than two 2 mg intravaginal gels.

Even in women with a favourable cervix, prostaglandins are associated with increased rates of successful vaginal delivery at 24 hours, though there are no differences in caesarean section or epidural rates [A].[9] It is recommended that prostaglandins are the first-line method for all women regardless of cervical score. Interestingly though, in the group with a favourable cervix, prostaglandins were associated with reduced levels of maternal satisfaction when compared to amniotomy with an oxytocin infusion.[1]

Intravaginal prostaglandin $E_2$ (either gel or tablets) appears to be marginally superior to intracervical preparations, with an increase in the success of induction and a decreased need for oxytocin. Failure rates of 10 per cent for the intracervical route versus <3 per cent for the intravaginal route have been quoted, although several studies have not demonstrated any difference.

There are theoretical advantages to the use of the gel over tablets; namely, that plasma levels are higher with the gel. Some studies suggested higher rates of instrumental vaginal delivery with gel in comparison to tablets, but this is not a universal finding. At present, given the lack of evidence for different clinical effects, the differential cost implications have led to the recommendation that tablets should be used.[1]

**Table 25.4** Route of administration for prostaglandins in induction of labour

| Route of administration | Prostaglandin type/dose and frequency | Benefits | Problems |
|---|---|---|---|
| Oral | $E_2$ tablets 0.5 mg hourly every 2 hours to a maximum of 2 mg | Avoids potential iatrogenic introduction of infection | Gastrointestinal side effects |
| Intravenous | $E_2$ infusions at 0.1 μg/min to a max of 4 μg/min | Enables titration against effect to be closely monitored | Gastrointestinal side effects |
|  | $F_{2\alpha}$ 3 μg/min to a max of 30 μg/min |  | Local tissue reactions (erythema) at infusion site |
| Intracervical | $E_2$ tablets | Reduced incidence of systemic side effects when compared with other routes of administration | Higher failure rate (10 versus 3 per cent), more difficult to administer and less efficient at ripening the cervix than intravaginal preparations |
|  |  |  | Potential iatrogenic introduction of infection |
| Intravaginal | $E_2$ tablets, viscous gel, wax pessary 2–5 mg in biodegradable form – latent period of 12 hours | Reduced incidence of systemic side effects when compared with other routes of administration | Potential iatrogenic introduction of infection |
|  | Sustained release preparations 5–10 mg in non-biodegradable form |  |  |

There are many randomized trials of prostaglandins but, as the populations, protocols, routes, dosages and dosage intervals are so heterogeneous, providing firm management conclusions is very difficult. Some protocols use repeated prostaglandin treatments at 6-hourly intervals for three doses, whereas others prescribe amniotomy and infusion of oxytocin 15 hours after a single prostaglandin treatment, unless labour is already established. There is only a marginal benefit in using more than three or four doses. Similarly, dosage intervals of 6 hours or doses of >4 mg (gel) or >6 mg (tablet) do not appear to be advantageous, although some women show little (if any response) to these doses (Table 25.5). Further clinical trials are therefore necessary to establish the most appropriate treatment regimen and maximal dose.

Prostaglandin $E_2$ is also available as a sustained release preparation (Propess, Ferring AB, Malmo, Sweden). This polymer-based vaginal insert contains 10 mg of prostaglandin $E_2$ that is released continuously over a 12-hour period, producing metabolite levels within the circulation that are similar to those found with 1 mg of intravaginal prostaglandin $E_2$ gel. A potential benefit of this preparation is that the insert can be removed from the vagina if uterine hypertonus or fetal distress develops. Although comparison with placebo indicates that it is probably a safe and effective induction agent, the preparation is expensive and its efficacy may be affected by the pH of the vagina. Further clinical trials are therefore necessary.

In summary, intravaginal PGE₂ is the preferred method of induction of labour, unless there are specific clinical

**Table 25.5** Recommended regimens for prostaglandin $E_2$ administration

| Type | Interval | Dose regimen | Total dose |
|---|---|---|---|
| Tablets | 6-hourly | 3 mg–3 mg | 6 mg all women |
| Gel | 6 hours | Nulliparae |  |
|  |  | 2 mg–1 mg | 3 mg |
|  |  | Multiparae |  |
|  |  | 1 mg–1 mg | 2 mg |

reasons for not using it (in particular the risk of uterine hyperstimulation) [A]. It should be administered as a gel, tablet or controlled-release pessary. Costs may vary over time, and trusts/units should take this into consideration when prescribing PGE₂.

The recommended regimens are:

- one cycle of vaginal PGE₂ tablets or gel: one dose, followed by a second dose after 6 hours if labour is not established (up to a maximum of two doses);
- one cycle of vaginal PGE₂ controlled-release pessary: one dose over 24 hours.

There is often debate about whether further doses can be given when women are experiencing mild tightenings in response to a gel given 6 hours previously. This is always a difficult area, and there are no studies on which to base practice. The manufacturer's leaflet suggests that uterine activity contraindicates a repeat dose, but this has to be a clinical decision. Where there is doubt, it is best to delay giving another dose if the cervix is unfavourable (if favourable, an amniotomy can be performed or the establishment of labour awaited). It may be best not to delay too long (especially not to leave women unassessed overnight), as this can lead to a very protracted and exhausting induction process. Usually it is apparent by 8–10 hours that labour is commencing or contractions are settling.

It is not clear from the available evidence as to the maximum dose of prostaglandin that may be administered to any individual patient. The national collaborating centre for women's and children's health instruct that vaginal PGE$_2$ products should be used in accordance with the manufacturers' recommendations. However, this is not of much help to the practising clinician facing the dilemma of how to manage an induction that has been commenced but appears not to be progressing despite the 'maximum' doses of prostaglandin having been administered.

NICE recommends that if an induction fails, the subsequent management options include:

- a further attempt to induce labour (the timing should depend on the clinical situation and the woman's wishes);
- caesarean section (refer to Chapter 31, Caesarean section [NICE clinical guideline 13];

It would therefore be advisable for clinicians to develop their own departmental protocols to advise staff on how best to manage such cases.

### Misoprostol

This prostaglandin E$_1$ analogue was initially developed for the treatment and prevention of peptic ulcer disease. It was subsequently noted to produce uterine contractions and has recently been utilized as an abortificant with marked success. In addition, misoprostol is cheaper and more easily stored than the other prostaglandins.

Several studies have shown that misoprostol appears to be as effective an induction agent as the currently available prostaglandin preparations in inducing labour in the third trimester, but the safest and most effective administration protocols have yet to be established.[10] It has been used in doses ranging from 50 μg (administered 4-hourly per vaginum to a maximum of five doses) to 100 μg (as single or repeat doses), and although the induction-to-delivery interval is reduced with increasing doses, this is often at the increased risk of uterine hypertonus. Oral doses appear to be safer than vaginal doses, but there is still not enough data to establish safety [A].[11]

There are considerable concerns regarding the rates of postpartum haemorrhage when misoprostol is used for induction, and of uterine dehiscence in women who have a previous caesarean section scar. Consequently, further work needs to be performed to establish a safe dosing regimen that carries a low risk of hypertonus and uterine dehiscence while maintaining an effect as a labour inductificant. Misoprostol remains unlicensed for labour induction and until the best dose regimen is determined, its use in labour induction should be confined to clinical trials.

### Oxytocin

Oxytocin is an octapeptide hormone secreted from the supraoptic and paraventricular nuclei of the hypothalamus. It is transported to the posterior pituitary along the axons of these neurons, where it is stored and then released in a pulsatile manner. Despite its short half-life in the circulation, oxytocin stimulates uterine activity, with the frequency and force of contractions being proportional to the oxytocin concentration in the plasma. Oxytocin also exhibits antidiuretic properties, a consequence of a structural similarity with vasopressin. Therefore, the possibility of fluid overload must always be borne in mind during administration in labour.

Although many different infusion regimens exist, it is generally recommended that oxytocin should be given via an infusion pump or syringe driver with a 'non-return valve', and the fluid load minimized. Most infusion regimens commence at low rates (1–2 mU/minute) and increase variably (titrated against contractions), arithmetically or logarithmically at intervals of between 10 and 30 minutes up to a maximum of approximately 32 mU/minute. The aim is to attain contractions at a frequency of 3–4 per 10 minutes, and in some cases this may be established with 12 mU/minute or less.

There is no evidence of benefit in using intervals of less than 30 minutes to increase the dose, as most, but not all, of the reports indicate that the use of longer intervals reduced uterine hypertonus, decreased maximum and total dose of oxytocin, and decreased the rate of caesarean section for fetal heart rate abnormalities.[11] This seems to be a logical approach as it takes 30–45 minutes for the plasma levels of oxytocin to reach a 'steady state'. Such a regimen also appears to have no adverse effects on induction–delivery intervals.

Pulsatile infusion regimens, in which boluses of oxytocin are given at 20–30-minute intervals, have been suggested to be more physiological, and more logical in view of the half-life of oxytocin and its receptor occupancy in labour. It is possible that such regimens require less oxytocin overall, with reduced risk of hyperstimulation, but so far there is little evidence to suggest they have any great advantage over those currently used.

The pregnant uterus is relatively insensitive to oxytocin and first requires priming with either endogenous or exogenous prostaglandins for oxytocin to have any substantial effect on uterine contractility. Consequently, medical priming with prostaglandin E$_2$ followed by an amniotomy (mechanical induction) and oxytocin infusion is the common sequence of interventions in an induction of labour. If oxytocin infusion is commenced at the time of amniotomy rather than delayed, there are advantages of a significantly shorter induction–delivery interval, reduced operative delivery rates and a reduction in postpartum haemorrhage. However, it is recommended that oxytocin should not be prescribed within 6 hours following the administration of vaginal prostaglandins. Whether these benefits outweigh the disadvantages of intravenous cannulation with consequent restricted mobility should be left to individual patients who, after appropriate counselling, can then make an informed choice.

## Agents currently being researched

### Nitric oxide donors
Nitric oxide donors stimulate cyclo-oygenase-2 (COX-2) activity. When administered per vaginum, they are believed to increase the production of prostaglandins within the cervix, and cause cervical remodelling and effacement. However, they may also exert a tocolytic effect on the term uterus, and may be associated with an increase in the induction-to-delivery interval and in the rates of caesarean section and postpartum haemorrhage. Further studies are required.

### Relaxin
In a few small clinical trials, this agent has been administered as a vaginal gel in an attempt to induce cervical ripening. At a dose of between 1 and 4 mg, the recombinant product of synthetic manufacture has been singularly unsuccessful in inducing labour when compared with placebo. It is possible that an increase in the prescribed dose or route of administration may provide different results.

### Antiprogestogens (mifepristone – RU486)
As an agent for ripening the cervix, this class of drugs exhibits great potential. In a prospective, randomized, controlled trial involving 120 women of mixed parity, 56 per cent of those given mifepristone commenced labour, compared with 22 per cent of the placebo group.[12] However, other outcomes between the two groups were no different; the incidence of delivery by caesarean section was equal in both groups. As mifepristone also crosses the placenta, and has the potential to cause disturbances in aldosterone and glucocorticoid metabolism, there exists the possibility of fetal or neonatal side effects, although none has so far been observed.

Due to the uncertainty concerning its safety it is currently recommended that mifepristone should only be offered as a method of induction of labour to women who have intrauterine fetal death.

### Interleukin-8
Interleukin-8 is a pro-inflammatory cytokine, produced *in vivo* by choriodecidual cells and implicated in the onset of spontaneous labour. Interleukin-8 production is stimulated by mifepristone and it has synergistic actions to the prostaglandins. This agent has good theoretical potential as a cervical collagenolytic and uterine stimulant, although its clinical application has yet to be investigated as research is currently limited to rabbits.

## PRACTICAL CONSIDERATIONS CONCERNING INDUCTION OF LABOUR

### Where should the initiation of induction of labour take place?

The main proviso for safe induction of labour is that it should be conducted in a setting in which there are adequate staffing levels to monitor both the fetus and mother where necessary. For prostaglandin administration, it may be that a ward area provides the necessary levels of surveillance. However, when induction is performed with a potentially compromised fetus or increased risks in the mother (prior caesarean section, pre-eclampsia, high parity, etc.), the extra level of surveillance provided by a labour ward should be the norm.

Once labour is established or oxytocin commenced, the labour ward is the appropriate setting, and women should be cared for on a one-to-one basis.

The 4th Annual Report of the Confidential Enquiry into Stillbirth and Deaths in Infancy (CESDI) cited an induction of labour as a contributory cause in 54 cases. The main problems identified were:

- inadequate monitoring and supervision in high-risk cases,
- lack of monitoring after prostaglandin induction,
- the use of prostaglandins in higher than recommended doses and for too long,
- repeated doses of prostaglandins (often without examination) causing hypertonus,
- use of oxytocin for too long despite lack of progress in labour,
- use of oxytocin despite evidence of good progress in labour,
- use of oxytocin despite clear signs of cephalo-pelvic disproportion or fetal compromise.

The report also highlighted the special care required when induction of labour is undertaken in a woman with a previous caesarean section, especially if the cervix is unfavourable and prostaglandin or oxytocin is employed.

CESDI's 4th Annual Report summarizing enquiry findings of the 873 intrapartum-related deaths in 1994–95 found that 52 per cent had received suboptimal care where 'different management would reasonably have been expected to have made a difference to the outcome'. It stressed the importance of teaching, assessment and supervision of all professionals caring for women in labour – a message that has been reiterated in subsequent annual reports.

Although published over a decade ago, these points are still of primary importance for the ongoing management of patients on the labour ward today. There have been initiatives nationally and locally in response to CESDI's findings. These have included a RCOG/RCM Working Party report 'Towards Safer Childbirth – Minimum Standards for the Organisation of Labour Wards' and the development of national evidence-based guidelines on induction of labour and the use and interpretation of electronic fetal monitoring.

## When to perform induction

Uterine contractility has a natural circadian rhythm, with the period of maximal activity occurring between 22:00 and 24:00 hours. The inference from this observation is that inductions of labour performed at this time would stand a greater chance of being successful than those commenced at other times. However, there are no data to support this hypothesis.

Many units have moved to a first dose of prostaglandin being inserted in the evening, with the aim of reducing the number of deliveries in the early hours. There are anecdotal reports that this is effective, but randomized trials have not been performed and as such NICE recommends that the first dose should be given in the morning.

# FETAL SURVEILLANCE FOLLOWING INDUCTION OF LABOUR

There are no trials that indicate the level of fetal surveillance required during an induction; however, as induction is a process most commonly undertaken when there are minimal risks to the fetus or mother, it would seem prudent to ascertain, as far as is possible, that the fetus is in good health before it is submitted to any stressful intervention. Therefore, when prostaglandins are used for cervical ripening, CTG should be performed for a minimum of 20 minutes before its administration and for 60 minutes thereafter and should be recommenced when contractions ensue.

After administration of vaginal PGE$_2$, when contractions begin, fetal well-being should be assessed with continuous electronic fetal monitoring. Once the cardiotocogram is confirmed as normal, intermittent auscultation should be used unless there are clear indications for continuous electronic fetal monitoring as described in 'Intrapartum care' (NICE clinical guideline 55). If the fetal heart rate is abnormal after administration of vaginal PGE$_2$, recommendations on management of fetal compromise in 'Intrapartum care' should be followed (see Chapter 29, Fetal compromise in the first stage of labour, for details). In women with risk factors for potential fetal compromise, electronic fetal monitoring should be commenced once contractions start.

# COMPLICATIONS OF INDUCTION OF LABOUR

## Failed induction of labour

It has been estimated that a 'failed induction' occurs in 3–5 per cent of cases in which prostaglandins have been used and in up to 35 per cent of cases induced with oxytocin alone. Overall, it is estimated that a failed induction in the presence of an unfavourable cervix is found in 15 per cent of cases. However, making a formal diagnosis of induction failure is frequently difficult as many different definitions exist and a consensus has yet to be reached.

Failed IOL must be differentiated from failure of labour progress due to cephalopelvic disproportion or malposition.

NICE define a failed induction as a failure to establish labour after one cycle of treatment, consisting of the insertion of two vaginal PGE2 tablets (3 mg) or gel (1–2 mg) at 6-hourly intervals, or one PGE2 controlled released pessary (10 mg) over 24 hours.

It may also be applied to cases in which the cervix fails to dilate beyond 3 cm during a period of appropriate stimulation with oxytocin – commonly quoted as 6 hours after the maximal infusion rate of syntocinon has been attained (although it should be remembered that this not an evidence-based recommendation).

These clinical scenarios present different dilemmas to the attendant obstetrician. Where the induction has involved the administration of prostaglandins alone, there is often little immediate risk to the mother or baby. The next stage of management must therefore be to question the indication for delivery and review the clinical scenario in this light. If the indication is weak, such as social convenience, a delay of a few days while awaiting the onset of spontaneous labour or a further attempt at induction may be indicated. In the interim, a suitable level of maternal and fetal surveillance must be undertaken, perhaps incorporating daily CTGs and twice-weekly biophysical scores. If the indication remains strong, however, there is little else to do but persist with the induction or deliver by caesarean section. This decision must be made at a senior level and in conjunction with the woman.

Where membrane rupture and oxytocin have been employed, the risks to both mother and baby are greatly increased. Not only are there risks of infection with prolonged rupture of the membranes, but also of:

- continued uterine stimulation and the effect on the fetal acid–base status,
- the antidiuretic effect of oxytocin on maternal and fetal electrolyte balance (especially if the indication for induction is pre-eclampsia),
- maternal, and paternal, exhaustion,
- rarely, uterine rupture.

NICE recommends that if an induction fails, healthcare professionals should discuss this with the woman and provide support. The woman's condition and the pregnancy in general should be fully reassessed, and fetal well-being should be assessed using electronic fetal monitoring.

If induction fails, the subsequent management options include:

- a further attempt to induce labour (the timing should depend on the clinical situation and the woman's wishes),
- resort to delivery by caesarean section (by far the easiest and perhaps safest option). However, a careful assessment (including confirming that the forewaters are indeed absent) may determine that a further period of observation should be employed. If no further change occurs after this time (e.g. 2 hours), delivery by caesarean section must be offered.

## Cord prolapse

An amniotomy performed without the presenting part located within or 'over' the pelvis runs the risk of cord prolapse. However, the occurrence of such a problem during labour induction is fortunately rare. Should the cord prolapse during such a procedure, pressure on the cord should be reduced by placing the patient in the knee/chest position/exaggerated left lateral position, the administration of 250 μg of terbutaline subcutaneously, and a doctor/midwife should displace the presenting part by the introduction of their hand within the vagina. Inserting a Foley catheter per urethram and filling the bladder with 400 mL normal saline may achieve a similar effect. Delivery must then be effected as quickly as possible to reduce the risks of hypoxia to the fetus.

## Abruption

A placental abruption may occur if rapid uterine decompression complicates an amniotomy. Care should therefore be taken if polyhydramnios is suspected and, if so, adequate precautions (e.g. intravenous access, theatre team aware, etc.) must be in place before the procedure is performed.

## Maternal

### Hyponatraemia

This avoidable complication often occurs as a consequence of prolonged intravenous oxytocin infusions. The fluid retention, electrolyte disturbance, coma, convulsions and death that may follow can be avoided by careful fluid balance management and by administering the oxytocin in an appropriate concentration (e.g. 40 IU in 50 mL 0.9 per cent 'normal' saline solution administered via a syringe driver). Similar electrolyte disturbances can occur in the neonate and in extreme cases lead to neonatal seizures.

## Uterine hyperstimulation

Any technique used to stimulate labour carries the potential risk of inducing uterine hyperstimulation – an inappropriate reaction of the myometrium to exogenous oxytocics, as a result of either drug hypersensitivity or drug overdose. Hyperstimulation is often the combination of both an increase in the frequency of uterine contractions and in the basal uterine tone. The resultant uterine hypertonus is associated with an elevation in the resting intrauterine pressure, which in turn may cause fetal hypoxia. The incidence of hyperstimulation appears to be related to the efficiency of the technique employed to stimulate labour. Misoprostol carries the greatest risk, whereas both prostaglandin $E_2$ and oxytocin appear to be less troublesome (each carrying a risk of hyperstimulation of approximately 1:500 inductions).

The potential management options include the following.

- In cases associated with oxytocin stimulation, the infusion should be decreased or discontinued.
- If there is evidence of fetal compromise, the administration of an intravenous bolus dose of a suitable tocolytic to reduce the hypertonus and allow the fetal heart to recover: e.g. terbutaline 250 μg subcutaneously (inhaled medication is of questionable benefit).
- Expedition of delivery (assisted vaginal delivery if fully dilated or delivery by caesarean section) within 30 minutes.

## Postpartum haemorrhage

Women delivered following labour induction have a higher incidence of postpartum haemorrhage than those delivering after a spontaneous onset of labour. These women may require a continuing oxytocin infusion for a few hours after delivery (at a higher dose and concentration than intrapartum).

## Fetal

### Prematurity

Situations in which an infant is born prematurely may be the consequence of a deliberate preterm induction, where the maternal or fetal condition merits intervention, for example pre-eclampsia. However, erroneous iatrogenic prematurity should not occur in modern obstetric practice, as ultrasound confirmation of the gestation will invariably have been performed, and all dates should be confirmed before an induction is undertaken. Where dates are uncertain, usually because of late presentation for antenatal care or missing early scans, fetal well-being should be established by ultrasound. Once it is established that the fetus is healthy, a policy of watchful waiting can be adopted. There may be a need to repeat tests of well-being. Induction can be planned once the cervix is favourable or if concerns arise regarding the mother or fetus.

**Table 25.6** Suggested methods for labour induction as guided by cervical status

| Bishop's score | Method of induction | Proven efficacy | Mechanism of action | Followed by |
|---|---|---|---|---|
| <5 | **Mechanical** | | Mechanical cervical dilatation | Amniotomy + oxytocin |
| | Catheters | X | | |
| | Balloons | X | | |
| | Hygroscopic dilators | X | | |
| | **Medical** | | | |
| | Prostaglandins | ✓ | Cervical modification and myometrial stimulation | Repeated doses if required – then amniotomy + oxytocin |
| | Anti-progestogens | ✓ | | |
| | Oestrogens | X | | |
| | DHEAS | X | | |
| | Relaxin | X | | |
| 5–8 | **Mechanical** | | | |
| | Amniotomy | ✓ | Cervical modification and myometrial stimulation | |
| | **Medical** | | | |
| | Prostaglandins (oral or vaginal) | ✓ | | Oxytocin infusion immediately or after a short delay |
| >8 | **Mechanical** | | | |
| | Amniotomy | ✓ | Cervical modification and myometrial stimulation | Repeated doses if required – then amniotomy + oxytocin infusion |
| | **Medical** | | | |
| | Prostaglandins | ✓ | | Oxytocin infusion immediately or after a short delay 2 hours before oxytocin if prostaglandins |

- DHEAS, dihydroepiandrostenedione.

## Hyperbilirubinaemia

Neonatal jaundice has been reported following the use of oxytocin, but not prostaglandin, during labour induction. In most cases, this jaundice is mild, short lived and does not require treatment.

## SPECIAL CASES

## Induction following caesarean section

This subject is covered extensively in Chapter 26, Management of previous Caesarean section. Decisions regarding induction should be made at a senior level.

## Grand multiparae

Induction of labour in the grand multipara is associated with an increased incidence of precipitate labour, uterine rupture and postpartum haemorrhage. Prostaglandins

are recommended as the first-line agent. In this group of women, it is reasonable to increase syntocinon more slowly, with 45-minute increments at the most. This appears to be safe in the majority of women.

## SUMMARY

A summary of the points covered in this chapter is shown in Table 25.6. An ultrasound to confirm gestation should be offered before 20 weeks gestation, as this reduces the need for induction for perceived post-term pregnancy. Women with uncomplicated pregnancies should be offered an induction of labour beyond 41 weeks. Prostaglandin should be used in preference to oxytocin when induction is undertaken in either nulliparous women or multiparous women with intact membranes, regardless of their cervical favourability. When induction is undertaken with prostaglandins, intravaginal prostaglandin $E_2$ tablets should be considered in preference to gel formulations or intracervical administration.

In the presence of abnormal fetal heart rate patterns and uterine hypercontractility (not secondary to oxytocin infusion), tocolysis should be considered. A suggested regimen is subcutaneous terbutaline 250 μg. Evidence suggests no benefit for prostaglandin gel over tablets for induction of labour. Tablets are cheaper and therefore recommended.

## KEY POINTS

- Induction of labour is a common procedure and is now performed in 15-20 per cent of all term pregnancies in the UK.
- Induction seldom involves a single intervention, but rather a complex set of interventions that can present challenges for both clinicians and patients.
- Many agents have had their role in the process of labour induction, established by carefully controlled trials, whereas others have been less formally assessed.
- The accurate assessment of each patient and her suitability for induction may help to increase the success rate of each intervention while decreasing the risk of iatrogenic problems.

## Key References

1. NICE. *Induction of Labour*. Clinical Guideline 70. London: National Institute for Health and Clinical Excellence, 2008.
2. Mozurkewich E, Chilimigras J, Koepke E *et al.* Indications for induction of labour: a best-evidence review. *BJOG* 2009; **116**: 626–36.
3. National Collaborating Centre for Women's and Children's Health. *Antenatal Care: Routine Care for the Healthy Pregnant Woman*, 2nd edn. London: RCOG Press, 2008.
4. Gulmezoglu AM, Crowther CA, Middleton P. Induction of labour for improving birth outcomes at or beyond term. *Cochrane Database Syst Rev* 2006: (**4**): CD004945.
5. Hannah ME, Hannah WJ, Hellman J *et al.* Induction of labour as compared with serial antenatal monitoring in post-term pregnancy. A randomized controlled trial. *N Engl J Med* 1992; **326**: 1587–92.
6. Chauhan SP, Grobman WA, Gherman RA *et al.* Suspicion and treatment of the macrosomic fetus: a review. *Am J Obstet Gynecol* 2005; **193**: 332–46.
7. Kloopmans C, Bijlenga D, Groen H *et al.* for the HYPITAT study. Induction of labour versus expectant monitoring for gestational hypertension or mild pre-eclampsia after 36 weeks gestation (HYPITAT): a multicentre, open-label randomised controlled trial. *Lancet* 2009; **374**: 979–88.
8. Garite TJ, Casal D, Garcia-Alonso A. Fetal fibronectin: a new tool for the prediction of successful induction of labour. *Am J Obstet Gynecol* 1996; **175**: 1516–21.
9. Kelly AJ, Kavanagh J, Thomas J. Vaginal prostaglandin (PGE2 and PGF2a) for induction of labour at term: *Cochrane Database Syst Rev* 2009; (**2**): CD003101.
10. Alfirevic Z, Weeks A. Oral misoprostol for induction of labour. *Cochrane Database Syst Rev* 2008; (**2**): CD001338.
11. Orhue AA. A randomized trial of 30-min and 15-min oxytocin infusion regimen for induction of labour at term in women of low parity. *Int J Gynaecol Obstet* 1993; **40**: 219–25.
12. Frydman R, Lelaidier C, Barton-Saint-Mleux C. Labour induction in women at term with mifepristone (RU486): a double-blind, randomized, placebo-controlled study. *Obstet Gynecol* 1992; **80**: 972–5.

# Management after previous caesarean section

*Lucy Kean*

---

## MRCOG standards

- Candidates are expected to be able to counsel women in the antenatal clinic regarding delivery after previous caesarean section.
- They should be able to manage the labour of a woman with a previous caesarean section, knowing how to advise accordingly, regarding both induction and augmentation of labour.
- Candidates should know the signs and symptoms of impending uterine rupture.

In addition, we would suggest the following:

- Know the rates of vaginal delivery in women undergoing labour after prior caesarean section in your unit.

## Practical skills

- Be able to recognize a morbidly adherent placenta at manual removal and manage with senior assistance.

## INTRODUCTION

Delivery by caesarean section accounted for 24.3 per cent of deliveries in England in 2006–07. In many units, emergency caesarean section rates for primigravidae of 24 per cent are seen. Consequently, the problem of management of women with a scarred uterus in subsequent pregnancies is one of the most common reasons for hospital referral in multigravida. It is a vital part of antenatal care that women are given a clear understanding of the plan of management from early in pregnancy, with the caveat that this may need to be adapted if the pregnancy presents unexpected problems.

## UNDERSTANDING THE RISKS

### Relative maternal morbidity and mortality

It is almost impossible to assess the relative mortality from caesarean section, as the indication for the caesarean section will undoubtedly impact on the outcome. There are no trials to instruct the practitioner in this and adapting information from published reports, such as the Confidential Enquiry into Maternal Deaths, is fraught with difficulty. In the most recent Confidential Enquiry into Maternal Deaths, 117 women died after caesarean section, but in only one case was the caesarean section performed for maternal request. In all of the other cases, there were compelling maternal or fetal indications for the procedure. Three women died following uterine rupture.[1]

Chapter 31, Caesarean section, discusses the risks of caesarean section in detail.

A good understanding of the risks of caesarean section is vital in counselling women with regard to subsequent delivery. The risks of both placenta praevia and placenta accreta increase exponentially with each repeat caesarean section, from a baseline risk of 0.26 and 0.01 per cent, respectively, in an unscarred uterus to 10 and 6.7 per cent after a fourth caesarean section (see Chapter 31).

In comparing elective repeat caesarean section (ERCS) with vaginal birth after caesarean section (VBAC), it is clear that the main maternal morbidity is encountered by women who need an emergency caesarean section for a failed VBAC. It is therefore vital that when discussing management with a patient, the individual risks and benefits must be considered.

The aim of this chapter is to attempt to quantify these risks, in order that, for each individual, appropriate counselling can be undertaken in planning the next delivery.

It is important to realize that women make decisions for a variety of reasons and that their choices may not always be those that we would make ourselves. The debate about choice with regard to delivery is not one that can be fully covered here, but it is apparent from the Sentinel Caesarean Section Audit that women are given far greater choice in planning their next delivery if their previous delivery was by caesarean section.[2]

There is remarkably little evidence to inform practice with regard to the management of previous caesarean section. There are no randomized trials comparing trial of labour with elective caesarean section, and most of the available data relate to observational studies.[3]

Candidates should be conversant with the Royal College of Obstetricians and Gynaecologists green top guideline 'Birth after previous caesarean birth'[4] and research that has been published since the guideline was produced.

## Repeat elective caesarean section: risks and benefits

### Maternal benefits

Caesarean section avoids labour with its risks of:

- perineal trauma (urinary and faecal problems),
- the need for emergency caesarean section,
- scar dehiscence or rupture with subsequent morbidity and mortality.

It also has the advantage of allowing a planned delivery.

### Maternal risks

- Prolonged recovery.
- Future pregnancies would probably require caesarean section for delivery.
- Increased risks of placenta praevia and accreta in subsequent pregnancies.

### Fetal benefit

- No risk from intrapartum scar rupture.

### Fetal risk

- Increased risk of transient tachypnoea/respiratory distress syndrome (1–3 per cent at 39 weeks, 6 per cent at 38 weeks).

## Planned VBAC: risks and benefits

### Maternal benefits

- Shorter hospital stay and convalescence.
- Potentially easier future deliveries.

### Maternal risks

- Increased risk of transfusion (relative risk 1.7, due to increased need in women with failed VBAC).
- Increased risk of endometritis (relative risk 1.6, due to increased risk in women with failed VBAC).
- Risk of uterine rupture (0.22–0.74 per cent which is stratified by need for intervention, i.e. highest risk with prostaglandin induction of labour, lowest risk for spontaneous delivery) [D].

### Fetal benefit

- Reduced risk of transient respiratory morbidity.

### Fetal risks

- 0.08 per cent risk of hypoxic ischaemic encephalopathy (similar to risk for nulliparous women).
- 0.04 per cent risk delivery-related death.

A large observational study from Scotland suggested that women with a previous caesarean section were at increased risk of stillbirth at term compared to women with an unscarred uterus. This study showed an absolute risk of 1.1/1000 women at or after 39 weeks for women previously delivered by caesarean section compared to a risk of 0.05 per cent for women with an unscarred uterus. The absolute risk of stillbirth after caesarean section is the same as that for the nulliparous population.[5] A subsequent large Canadian study of similar size showed no significant differences in antepartum stillbirth between the previous caesarean section and previous vaginal delivery groups.[6] The latter paper attempted to control for obesity, a risk factor for both caesarean section and stillbirth. It may be that obesity is the factor that increases the risk, rather than caesarean section [C].

## UTERINE RUPTURE RATE FOR WOMEN UNDERGOING LABOUR AFTER A SINGLE PRIOR CAESAREAN SECTION

Uterine rupture is accurately defined as a disruption of the uterine muscle extending to and involving the uterine serosa or disruption of the uterine muscle with extension into the bladder or broad ligament. A uterine dehiscence is defined as disruption of the uterine muscle with intact uterine serosa.[4]

Studies looking at rates of scar rupture are all observational. The most helpful study for informing UK practice reported 35 854 women with a single previous caesarean section, giving birth by means other than elective caesarean section at 37 or more weeks. Multiple births were excluded. This study showed that across the whole group the success rate for VBAC was 74.2 per cent. The uterine rupture rate was higher in women induced using prostaglandins, but not in women induced by other methods. The rupture rate was higher in women who had not previously also delivered vaginally. The overall risk of uterine rupture was 0.35 per cent. Women who had not previously delivered vaginally had a rupture risk of 1 in 210 if they did not undergo induction of labour with prostaglandins, and 1 in 71 if they were induced with prostaglandins. For women who had previously delivered vaginally, the risks were 1 in 514 and 1 in 175, respectively.[7]

The National Institute of Child Health and Human Development have produced a large multicentre prospective cohort study encompassing around 16 000 women undergoing ERCS compared to 18 000 women undergoing planned VBAC, mostly women delivering in tertiary centres. This study gave an overall risk of uterine rupture in the VBAC group of 0.74 per cent. Unsuccessful VBAC had the highest rupture rates of 2.3 per cent [D].[8]

The RCOG green top guideline suggests that women know that the risk of rupture is 22–74/10 000 compared to almost no risk for ERCS.[4]

## ADVISING WOMEN ABOUT INDIVIDUAL RISKS

When advising women on subsequent delivery, as much information about the previous caesarean section as possible should be sought. It is good practice to ask for a copy of the case notes of the previous surgery before making a final decision, as occasionally features may be seen that will alter management, such as extensions of the uterine incision, of which the woman may be unaware. It is also important to gain any available information about the circumstances leading to the caesarean section.

Good antenatal planning should individualize the risks and benefits for each woman for each type of delivery, allowing the woman to make the best choice for herself. Research suggests that most women do not have clear ideas about the best choice for delivery and want accurate information and advice individualized for their own set of circumstances.

## Type of scar, method of closure and previous operative morbidity

It is recognized that vertical upper segment uterine scars have a high risk of rupture, often with catastrophic results. Therefore, it is usual to recommend repeat prelabour caesarean section for women who are known to have undergone previous classical caesarean section. However, despite this, some women will arrive in labour. A scar rupture rate of 12 per cent has been seen in this group.[9] Lower segment vertical scars are associated with lower rates of uterine rupture of 2 per cent, but it is often very difficult to be sure that the scar did not encroach into the upper segment. With a full discussion of the risks and necessary precautions, women with a low uterine scar should be considered for VBAC.[4] It should not be assumed that a vertical abdominal incision means that the uterine incision will also be vertical; indeed, in most cases a vertical abdominal incision is associated with a transverse uterine incision. Given the extremely high rates of uterine rupture with vertical upper segment incisions, it is best to err on the side of caution whenever there is doubt.

J-shaped and inverted T-shaped incisions are associated with similar rupture rates to low vertical incisions of 1.9 per cent [D].

In the United States, a single layer uterine closure was the norm for some years. In the UK, this trend was not universally adopted and most women continued to undergo a traditional two-layer closure. The evidence on whether a single layer closure is associated with higher rates of subsequent rupture is conflicting. Because the only studies of rupture are either small or observational, the real risks are difficult to quantify. The largest study suggested an increase in risk with an odds ratio of 3.95 (95 per cent CI 1.35–11.9).[10]

One study addressed the issue of rupture related to intrapartum or post-partum pyrexia in the previous caesarean delivery. This study suggested an odds ratio of 4.02 in women experiencing both intrapartum and post-partum pyrexia. However, the study was small and the confidence intervals very wide (1.04–15.5) [D].

## Indication for previous caesarean section

The extent to which the reason for previous caesarean section impacts on subsequent successful trial of labour has been evaluated in a meta-analysis of observational studies [D].[11] The results are shown in Table 26.1.

## DOES CERVICAL DILATATION AT TIME OF PREVIOUS CAESAREAN SECTION IMPACT ON DELIVERY?

This question has been addressed through observational studies. Only women whose prior caesarean section was for 'failure to progress' were included (Table 26.2).[12]

These data accord with an overall rate of vaginal delivery for dystocia in the previous labour of 69 per cent, which compares well with the data from Rosen et al.,[9] and show that dilatation at arrest does not signify who will achieve successful delivery next time, although caesarean section for dystocia at any stage reduces the chance of successful VBAC [D].

**Table 26.1** Successful vaginal delivery in subsequent labour by reason for previous caesarean section (CS)

| Indication for previous CS | Success rate (%) |
|---|---|
| Malpresentation | 85 |
| Any reason + previous vaginal delivery | 84 |
| Fetal distress | 75 |
| Dystocia | 67 |
| Oxytocin in this labour | 63 |

First stage of labour

**Table 26.2** Successful vaginal delivery related to dilatation at arrest of the previous labour

| Dilatation at arrest (cm) | Vaginal delivery (%) |
|---|---|
| 0–5 | 61 |
| 6–9 | 80 |
| 10 | 69 |

## TRIAL OF LABOUR IN WOMEN WITH MORE THAN ONE PRIOR CAESAREAN SECTION

The NICHID study[8] used a multivariate approach to assess the rupture risk for women who have undergone two or more previous sections. The rupture rate was not higher for these women compared to women with a single previous caesarean section, but they did experience higher rates of transfusion and hysterectomy. Many other smaller observational studies have suggested an increase in risk of 2–3 in women with more than one previous caesarean section. Many of these studies were uncontrolled.

Success rates vary, but should be quoted as 62–75 per cent. Because of small numbers, the real risk for rupture in women with three or more sections is difficult to quantify. Small observational studies suggest that the rupture risk may be increased by a factor of 2 or 3.[4]

Women should therefore be counselled that a VBAC is an alternative and an individualized risk given where possible, based on all the available information.

## TRIAL OF LABOUR IN WOMEN WITH OBESITY

In the case of women with a scarred uterus and obesity, decision-making is often difficult. It is recognized that fetal birth weight is usually larger than average, and the prior caesarean section will often have been performed for poor progress in labour, as obesity appears to increase the risks of inefficient uterine activity. The wish to avoid a further abdominal delivery must be balanced against the increased morbidity that occurs if an emergency caesarean section is required. Observational data suggest that for women weighing in excess of 135 kg, the chance of vaginal delivery is very low (13 per cent) and elective caesarean section may be a better option in this very obese group.[13]

The rates of unsuccessful VBAC increase incrementally as body mass index (BMI) increases. Women with a body mass index above 30 have an odds ratio for failed VBAC of 2 (95 per cent CI 1.2–3.3).

## OTHER RISK FACTORS FOR UNSUCCESSFUL VBAC AND UTERINE RUPTURE

### Interdelivery interval

The interdelivery interval has been studied in three studies. All of the studies are retrospective and in all the analysis was limited to women with singleton pregnancies, at term, who had one prior cesarean birth and no prior vaginal births. This will therefore skew the data towards slightly higher rupture rates, as women with a previous vaginal birth form the lowest risk group for rupture. These studies are small. In one of the three, there was a slight increase in the risk of rupture in women with an interdelivery interval of less than 18 months, in the second a slight increase in risk for an interdelivery interval of less than 24 months and in the final small study no difference was found. The data are conflicting and uncontrolled. At most, the odds ratio increase in risk is 2–3.

### Maternal age

The success of vaginal birth in all women decreases as age increases regardless of whether the woman has previously undergone caesarean section. Studies have shown lower rates of successful VBAC in women over 35 years, but these studies have not controlled for confounding variables. Unsuccessful VBAC carries the highest rate of uterine rupture. It is not surprising, therefore, that a study has suggested a link between uterine rupture and maternal age.

### Other risk factors

Almost every factor known to be associated with lower chances of successful vaginal birth in any setting has been examined in relationship to VBAC and, unsurprisingly, those factors associated with overall lower rates of vaginal delivery are also associated with lower rates of successful VBAC. These include fetal macrosomia, delivery after 41 weeks, cervical dilatation of <4 cm at admission, non-white ethnicity, male infant and short maternal stature. When discussing choices with women, these factors can be borne in mind. Decision-making may therefore vary depending on the circumstances at the time, as some of these factors are dynamic.

## ANTENATAL MANAGEMENT

### Counselling and documentation

Wherever possible, the records of the delivery leading to caesarean section should be reviewed [E]. Occasionally, facts that the patient may be unaware of may come to light. It is especially important to review records where there is any doubt about the type of uterine scar used. Counselling the patient with regard to the likelihood of success is also important, and review of the previous labour is a necessary part of this counselling.

It is very important to document the discussion of the risks and benefits of both vaginal delivery and caesarean section with the patient carefully. Women should be provided with accurate information pertinent to their particular set of circumstances. The role of the doctor is to advise and guide where requested. The final choice rests with the woman. Women should be advised that the safest place to labour, should that be her wish, is in hospital. It is better to support a woman to labour in hospital, even if the clinician feels this is injudicious, than for her to feel unsupported and to labour at home.

If a woman is able to make her choice early in the pregnancy, her antenatal care can be tailored around this. If her choice is for VBAC and there are no other factors which place the pregnancy at risk, then a scheduled visit at 40 weeks to discuss a strategy should she pass 41 weeks is reasonable. Women can be offered an open appointment to return should they have further questions, but the provision of antenatal care can rest with the community midwife. For women with no identifiable pregnancy-related problems who choose ERCS, a date can be provided for caesarean section at 39 weeks so that the woman can prepare. This can be amended if circumstances change.

It is important to establish what choices women who choose ERCS would make should they labour before the date of planned caesarean section. Many, but not all, women would consider VBAC if spontaneous labour ensues before the planned date.

## PLANNING THE DELIVERY

### Value of pelvimetry

Pelvimetry performed either clinically or radiographically does not provide any useful information [A]. Four trials of more than 1000 women were included in the most recent Cochrane review. The trials were generally not of good quality. Women undergoing pelvimetry were more likely to be delivered by caesarean section (odds ratio 2.17, 95 per cent CI 1.63–2.88). No impact on perinatal outcome was detected.[14]

### Value of ultrasound for scar thickness

Ultrasound evaluation of the scar antenatally has been investigated as a method of determining women at higher risk of scar rupture during labour. Unfortunately, results do not give a high enough sensitivity for this modality to be used in everyday clinical practice.

## Documenting the plan and setting limits

Women are generally keen to avoid a repeat of the previous labour and so it may be reasonable to avoid the circumstances that led to problems in the previous labour, such as avoiding induction if the caesarean section was for failed induction. Women who underwent caesarean section for poor progress usually need reassurance that limits will be placed on their next labour so that they do not undergo a prolonged labour. Women are significantly more likely to request a repeat caesarean section if they had their initial surgery because of failure to progress in labour than if their initial caesarean section was because of suspected fetal compromise.

It is important when discussing delivery in the antenatal period to agree a clear plan of management and for this to be carefully documented and easily available to carers in labour. If the agreed plan is for delivery by elective caesarean section, it is good practice to give the patient a date for this, assuming an uncomplicated pregnancy. This can be made with the proviso that if circumstances change, it can be amended, but it does allow women to plan in advance and minimizes requests for early delivery later in pregnancy that can compromise neonatal well-being. In general, an elective caesarean section should be performed in the 39th week of pregnancy. It is possible to apply a little common sense where women have persistently laboured at 38 weeks, but it must be remembered that if women have a tendency to go well past their dates, even 39 weeks may be early for some babies.

## Assessment of the risk of placenta accreta

This is particularly pertinent in the management of women undergoing delivery after repeated caesarean sections. The risk is highest in women with a coexistent placenta praevia.

Findings suggestive but not diagnostic of a placenta accreta, on antenatal ultrasound include:

- loss of the normal hypoechoic rim of myometrial tissue beneath the placenta;
- loss of the normal hyperechoic uterine serosa–bladder wall interface;
- presence of tissue of placental echotexture extending beyond the uterine serosa, sometimes seen within the lumen of the bladder;
- sometimes multiple or large placental venous lakes are seen, giving the placenta a 'moth-eaten' appearance.

Magnetic resonance imaging (MRI) has been suggested as an alternative and possibly better method of imaging. Much depends on the experience of the person performing the scan. False negatives and positives occur with both modalities. Currently, in experienced hands, ultrasound alone is as good as MRI. If an accreta is suspected, then it is prudent to take precautions for major haemorrhage. Full consent and discussion of the potential outcomes should be undertaken.

For elective cases, precautions may include:

- the presence of a consultant obstetrician and consultant anaesthetist,
- provision of adequate blood and alerting the haematology laboratory to the case, so that extra haemostatic products can be made available if needed,
- consider cell saving for caesarean section,
- radiological input for siting arterial catheters for potential uterine artery embolization,
- an experienced surgeon in case hysterectomy is required,
- if bladder or bowel involvement is suspected, the attendance of the relevant surgical/urological team will be necessary.

## MANAGEMENT OF LABOUR

All carers on labour wards must be trained in the identification of the signs and symptoms of scar rupture. This is a requirement in the UK for accreditation at level 2 for the Clinical Negligence Scheme for Trusts (CNST).

### Signs and symptoms of scar rupture

The cardinal signs of imminent uterine rupture are:

- worsening cardiotocography (CTG) changes (especially prolonged variable or late decelerations),
- haematuria,
- secondary arrest,
- small amounts of vaginal bleeding,
- pain over the scar which persists between contractions.

Signs of uterine rupture are:

- fetal bradycardia,
- upward displacement of the presenting part,
- sudden loss of contractions,
- maternal hypotension,
- heavy vaginal bleeding.
- abdominal or shoulder pain.

If the fetus or placenta is extruded into the abdomen, there is very little time to salvage the fetus. Delivery needs to be accomplished within 10 minutes. Most fetuses in this situation are profoundly acidotic at the time of delivery.

### Conduct of the labour

#### General management
Some general steps can be taken on admission in labour to minimize the risks to the mother and fetus. These include:

- read the plan for labour in the notes and note any discussion points,
- site intravenous access (though this can be capped and flushed),

- group and save blood,
- discuss active management of the third stage,
- advise continuous electronic fetal monitoring once labour is established.

### Use of electronic fetal monitoring
There are no trials assessing the various modalities of monitoring of the fetus in labour. It is widely recognized that in most cases changes in the CTG precede uterine rupture; therefore the consensus opinion of the Expert Committee recommends continuous fetal monitoring in labour for women with a uterine scar [E].[15]

### Use of oxytocin to augment labour
The use of oxytocin in labour in women with previous caesarean section is contentious. There are no randomized studies to help and only observational data are available [D].

The potential for oxytocin to correct abnormal patterns of labour is the same in women with a previous caesarean section as it is in women without. However, given recent evidence that in nulliparous women oxytocin use does not reduce the rate of caesarean section, its use in the context of previous caesarean section might also be questioned.

Oxytocin augmentation appears to be associated with an increase in the risk of scar rupture of 2–3.[8]

It is vital that before considering Syntocinon, all steps are taken to optimize labour progress. With the advent of small fetal monitors and more mobility with epidural analgesia, it should be possible to allow women the opportunity to mobilize without compromising fetal surveillance. Forty per cent of women showing slow progress will respond to simple measures such as rehydration (see Chapter 27, Poor progress in labour). A more flexible approach should be adopted in women with a uterine scar, and consideration should be given for lower rates of progress before resorting to Syntocinon. When Syntocinon is thought to be necessary, the decision should be made at consultant level and the risks and benefits should be discussed with the mother [E]. Assessment of progress in labour should be ideally made by the same person and the frequency of vaginal examination may need to be increased as there is some evidence that early intervention for static progress over 2 hours after augmentation can be used to prevent uterine rupture.

## INDUCTION OF LABOUR

There have been many concerns voiced about induction of labour in women with a scarred uterus. Only four small, randomized trials assessing the method of induction have been performed. These trials are too small to provide any meaningful data. Several observational studies have been performed, but all of these have limitations.

Clearly, success rates for VBAC are lower if induction of labour is needed. The NICHD study showed a 33 per cent caesarean section rate in induced labours.[8] Other studies have suggested successful vaginal birth in 50–70 per cent of women with a previous vaginal birth undergoing induction of labour compared to 44–61 per cent in women who have not delivered vaginally previously.

## Membrane sweeping

Membrane sweeping is recommended for women where induction of labour is considered after 40 weeks. There are no trials assessing this approach in women with a previous caesarean section, but it seems a reasonable option and may reduce the need for intervention.

## Non-prostaglandin induction of labour

The NICHD study gave a risk for uterine rupture among women induced by non-prostaglandin methods of 89/10 000. This was almost exactly the same as the risk for women augmented in labour (87/10 000).[8] The data from Scotland did not show a significant increase in uterine rupture in women induced with artificial rupture of membranes and oxytocin with rates of 29/10 000.[7]

## Prostaglandin induction of labour

The NICHD study did not show a significantly higher risk of uterine rupture with prostaglandin induction of labour compared to non-prostaglandin methods of induction (140 versus 89/10 000).[8] The Scottish data showed a higher risk with prostaglandin induction of labour of 87 versus 29/10 000.[7] Interestingly, the figure for prostaglandin induction of labour in the Scottish study is identical to the risk of non-prostaglandin induction of labour in the NICHD study, and lower than the risk for prostaglandin induction of labour in the NICHD study.

Clearly, when deciding on the best strategy, the reason for induction must be considered and weighed against the risks of the procedure. Induction at 41 weeks is recommended to prevent the risk of stillbirth after this time. The risk of stillbirth at 41 weeks from epidemiological studies is 2–3/1000 [B]. The risks of perinatal death following induction of labour in women with a previous caesarean section is 1.1/1000 [D]. Given the possibility that stillbirth may be more common in women with previous caesarean section, the marginal benefit of induction past 41 weeks is still probably justified, but the benefits are not as clear cut as they are for women with an unscarred uterus.

An unfavourable cervix at the onset of induction is associated with higher rates of caesarean section, but not with any other adverse outcome [D].

Despite the potential increased risk of scar rupture with prostaglandin, the guideline development group who produced the most recent NICE guideline on induction of labour recommend that intravaginal $PGE_2$ be used as the preferred option in women with a previous caesarean section [E].[16]

## Documentation

- The involvement of a consultant obstetrician in decisions regarding mode of delivery, the need for induction and any decision to augment labour.
- Management plans should be fully documented.

Electronic fetal monitoring should be used once labour is established.

- Local guidelines should be developed.
- There should be adequate education of all staff, ensuring awareness of signs and symptoms of uterine rupture.

# MANAGEMENT OF THE THIRD STAGE

Postpartum haemorrhage is more common in women who have a scarred uterus, probably because of the inability of the scar tissue to contract and increased placental adherence. Therefore, a low threshold for very active management of the third stage should be implemented.

This should include:

- oxytocics at delivery of the shoulders,
- prompt delivery of the placenta after separation,
- consideration of continued Syntocinon infusion for 4 hours after delivery.

If the placenta is retained, the possibility of a placenta accreta must be borne in mind. Therefore, before proceeding to a manual removal, important steps must be taken.

- Establish the probable placental site from the previous scan reports. Accreta is much more likely if the placenta was noted to be anterior.
- Cross-match 4 units of blood.
- Obtain the woman's consent and note that the possibility of accreta has been discussed, with its potential problems and management options.
- Ensure that senior staff are aware and, if you are inexperienced, ask for help before you go to theatre.

If at the time of manual removal a clear plane of cleavage cannot be defined, placenta accreta is likely. Different management options have been tried with variable success.

## Hysterectomy

Two large studies have shown that maternal mortality is lower if an aggressive operative approach, i.e. hysterectomy, is instituted, and this must be considered as the safest approach where haemorrhage is severe [D]. However, because there are cases in which preservation of fertility is of overriding importance to the woman, several conservative measures have been reported.

## Leaving the entire placenta in place

This has been described where no plane of cleavage can be identified. Bleeding becomes much more likely once the placenta has been partially removed. Some units have used just expectant management or with additional methotrexate. Haemorrhage, sepsis and persistent placental retention are recognized complications, but successful pregnancies have been reported subsequently [D].

## Blunt dissection and curettage

This technique entails attempting to remove as much placenta as possible, utilizing oxytocin to help control bleeding and considering later curettage once bleeding is controlled. This approach has been successful in a few cases, but may lead to intractable haemorrhage and the need for hysterectomy.

## Conservative surgery

This encompasses local oversewing of bleeding areas or defects and uterine and internal iliac artery ligation. The degree of blood loss is likely to be great, and early recourse to hysterectomy should be instituted when blood loss is continuing.

Subendometrial vasopressin has been reported to be effective in one case in which all other measures had failed, and uterine artery embolization under radiographic control has also reportedly been effective in individual cases. Selective arterial ligation of the uterine or internal iliac vessels is occasionally helpful.

If a conservative option is chosen, meticulous observation must be instituted, and recourse to hysterectomy considered if haemorrhage persists.

## Radiological intervention

Embolization of the uterine arteries has met with some success in cases of accreta, but this option is often not available in an emergency situation. If a placenta accreta is suspected in advance of delivery by caesarean section, selective arterial catheterization can be undertaken at the beginning of the procedure and embolization undertaken if an accreta is confirmed and bleeding encountered.

## CONCLUSIONS

The current rates of caesarean section of 24 per cent in primiparae will inevitably lead to large numbers of women needing to choose the best method for delivery next time. Vaginal delivery after caesarean section is a safe option if precautions are taken. Induction of labour and augmentation lead to increased rates of scar rupture and must only be undertaken with caution. However, the risks of repeated caesarean section must also be considered, as it is recognized that placenta accreta increases in incidence exponentially with each repeat caesarean section (see Chapter 31, Caesarean section). Keeping primary caesarean section rates to a minimum will help to prevent the morbidity associated with both VBAC and repeated caesarean section.

### KEY POINTS

- A thorough history and examination of the notes should be made when booking a patient who has undergone a previous caesarean section.
- Where information is lacking, it should be sought.
- Vaginal delivery is a valid option after almost any prior lower segment caesarean section.
- After classical caesarean section, vaginal delivery should be avoided.
- Repeated caesarean sections carry exponentially increasing risks of placenta praevia and accreta, with significant maternal morbidity.
- The risk of scar rupture in labour after a single caesarean section is approximately 22–74/10 000.
- Oxytocin use in labour probably increases this risk by two to three times.
- Induction of labour may lead to at least a doubling in risk of scar problems, but it is possible that the magnitude of increase is higher if prostaglandins are needed.
- The risk of scar rupture may be two to three times higher after more than one caesarean section.
- Vigilance for scar rupture in labour is of paramount importance.
- Active management of the third stage should be standard.
- Placenta accreta must be considered if an anteriorly placed placenta is retained.

## Key References

1. Lewis G (ed.). The Confidential Enquiry into Maternal and Child Health (CEMACH). *Saving Mothers' Lives: Reviewing Maternal Deaths to Make Motherhood Safer – 2003–2005*. The Seventh Report on Confidential Enquiries into Maternal Deaths in the United Kingdom. London: CEMACH, 2007.

2. Thomas J, Paranjothy S, Royal College of Obstetricians and Gynaecologists Clinical Effectiveness Support Unit. *National Sentinel Caesarean Section Audit*. London: RCOG Press, 2001.

3. Dodd JM, Crowther CA, Huertas E *et al.* Planned elective repeat caesarean section versus planned vaginal birth

for women with a previous caesarean birth. *Cochrane Database Syst Rev* 2006; (**4**): CD004224.

4. Royal College of Obstetricians and Gynaecologists. Birth after previous caesarean birth. Green Top Guideline 45. London: RCOG, February 2007.

5. Smith GC, Pell JP, Dobbie R. Caesarean section and risk of unexplained stillbirth in subsequent pregnancy. *Lancet* 2003; **362**: 1779–84.

6. Wood SL, Chen S, Ross S, Sauve R. The risk of unexplained antepartum stillbirth in second pregnancies following caesarean section in the first pregnancy. *BJOG* 2008; **115**: 726–31.

7. Smith GC, Pell JP, Cameron AD, Dobbie R. Risk of perinatal death associated with labor after previous cesarean delivery in uncomplicated term pregnancies. *JAMA* 2002; **287**: 2684–90.

8. Landon MB, Hauth JC, Leveno KJ *et al*. Maternal and perinatal outcomes associated with a trial of labor after prior cesarean delivery. *N Engl J Med* 2004; **351**: 2581–9.

9. Rosen MG, Dickinson JC, Westhoff CL. Vaginal birth after caesarean: a meta-analysis of morbidity and mortality. *Obstet Gynecol* 1991; **77**: 465–70.

10. Bujold E, Bujold C, Gauthier R. Uterine rupture during a trial of labour after a one- versus two-layer closure of a low transverse caesarean. *Am J Obstet Gynecol* 2001; **184**: S18.

11. Rosen MG, Dickinson JC. Vaginal birth after caesarean: a meta-analysis of indicators for success. *Obstet Gynecol* 1994; **84**: 255–8.

12. Ollendorff D, Goldberg JM, Minogue JP, Socol ML. Vaginal birth after Caesarean section for arrest of labour: is success determined by maximum cervical dilatation during the prior labour? *Am J Obstet Gynecol* 1988; **159**: 636–9.

13. Chauhan SP, Magann EF, Carroll CS *et al*. Mode of delivery for the morbidly obese with prior Caesarean delivery: vaginal versus repeat Caesarean. *Am J Obstet Gynecol* 2001; **185**: 349–54.

14. Pattinson RC, Farrell E-ME. Pelvimetry for fetal cephalic presentations at or near term. *Cochrane Database Syst Rev* 2007; (**2**): CD000161.

15. Royal College of Obstetricians and Gynaecologists. *The Use of Electronic Fetal Monitoring*. Evidence-based Clinical Guideline No. 8. London: RCOG Press, 2001 NICE Clinical Guideline 70.

16. National Collaborating Centre for Women's and Children's Health. *Induction of Labour*. London: National Collaborating Centre for Women's and Children's Health, July 2008.

# Poor progress in labour

*Richard Hayman*

## INTRODUCTION

The management of labour and its complications is an issue of great importance worldwide. In low-income countries, prolonged labour is commonly associated with high levels of fetal and maternal morbidity and mortality as a consequence of inadequate levels of healthcare, obstructed labour, sepsis, uterine rupture and postpartum haemorrhage. Many of these problems might be overcome by the timely use of antibiotics and delivery by caesarean section, but unfortunately these are often unavailable. In the 'developed' world, deliveries are not problem free, although the consequences are of a lesser magnitude to society as a whole. In both settings, however, a careful and methodical approach to the management of labour and its abnormalities will be of considerable benefit to the individual mother and her baby.[1]

Augmentation of labour for 'poor progress' is now such a common event on labour wards in the UK that as many as 50 per cent of nulliparae may receive oxytocin in labour.

Policies incorporating such interventions in labour are not without consequences; across Europe the incidence of caesarean section in nulliparous women with a singleton, term, vertex fetus ranges from 10 to 35 per cent, with rates up to 23 per cent even for women in spontaneous labour. Although there is a multitude of indications for such interventions, many are performed for 'dystocia' or 'abnormal' patterns of labour. Many authorities argue that this level of intervention is too high. UNICEF, WHO and UNFPA guidelines recommend that, as a general rule, a minimum of 5 per cent of deliveries are likely to require a caesarean section in order to preserve the life and health of the mother or infant, and rates higher than 15 per cent indicate inappropriate use of the procedure. However, it is uncertain as to how these rates have been determined and consequently as to what the 'appropriate' rate should be. While it is irrefutably the case that delivery by caesarean section will contribute to the overall levels of maternal morbidity and mortality, especially when performed in an emergency situation, there is undoubtedly a place for caesarean sections in modern obstetric practice, albeit at a lower rate than that currently observed.

The ability to communicate succinctly and accurately is of paramount importance on any labour ward. It is therefore particularly important that all practitioners use standard definitions when conveying clinical information, especially when different staff members may perform serial examinations on the same patient – an inevitable consequence of the frequent shift changes that now occur.

## DEFINITIONS

**Effacement** relates to the length of the cervix. Recording effacement may be useful during the latent phase, during induction of labour and in threatened preterm labour.

It reflects cervical remodelling and is usually defined either as cervical length in centimetres or as no, partial, or full effacement.

**Dilatation**, the single feature on which most management decisions in labour are made, is defined in centimetres. By convention, full dilatation, where no cervix is palpable, is taken as 10 cm. Of course, this will be a variable that is dependent on the size of the fetal head, and consequently there may be large inter-observer differences. When management decisions need to be made, a series of repeated examinations by the same individual, or review by a more experienced member of staff, are important.

**Presentation** is the part of the fetus within the pelvis adjacent to the cervix. Presentations that can be delivered vaginally at term are:

- vertex,
- face (mento-anterior),
- breech.

**Malpresentations** are defined as anything other than a vertex. (Note that cephalic presentations will include face and brow, which are malpresentations.) Presentations that are not deliverable vaginally at term will include:

- face (mento-posterior),
- brow,
- shoulder.

A cord presentation may be delivered vaginally when diagnosed late in the second stage, and where it is anticipated that a quick vaginal delivery can be safely accomplished. It is also important to remember that all presentations may deliver vaginally if the fetus is very preterm.

**Position** is defined as the relationship of the denominator of the presenting part of the fetus to fixed points of the maternal pelvis.

The denominator is the most definable point of the presenting part:

- occiput for vertex presentations,
- sacrum for breech presentations,
- mentum for face presentations.

The fixed points on the maternal pelvis are:

- the symphysis pubis anteriorly,
- the sacrum posteriorly.

**Station** of the presenting part relates to descent within the pelvis. It should be first defined by abdominal palpation as number of fifths palpable. This is particularly important when there is moulding, as this may exaggerate the fetal head shape, with seemingly better descent on vaginal examination. Only after abdominal palpation should the station be defined vaginally. This is notoriously prone to inter-observer difference. By convention, station is defined in relationship to the ischial spines in centimetres above or below this landmark.

**Moulding** is an important part of a vaginal examination as it relates to the fit of the fetal head through the pelvis.

Various different methods have been used to define moulding. The easiest is to palpate the sagital suture and note the following:

- no moulding: sutures a little apart,
- 1+ sutures together with no gap,
- 2+ sutures overlap but reduce with gentle pressure,
- 3+ sutures overlap and do not reduce with gentle pressure.

**Caput** is a reflection of scalp oedema. Although it may be seen in prolonged labour, it may be present in normal labour and is not helpful in management planning.

All of the above features should be represented graphically on a partogram where possible and carefully documented at every vaginal examination.

## NORMAL LABOUR: STANDARDS FOR DEFINITION OF PROGRESS

The start of a normal labour is difficult to define precisely, although it is often cited as being from the onset of painful uterine contractions that are associated with effacement and dilatation of the cervix beyond 3 cm with descent of the head in a vertex presentation. This process culminates in the birth of a baby and is followed shortly afterwards by the delivery of a placenta.

Such a complex process has many interacting components, and the safe passage of the fetus through the pelvis is dependent less upon absolutes and more upon a series of unknown variables that include:

- cervical remodelling,
- the efficiency of uterine contraction,
- the flexibility of the bony and ligamentous pelvis,
- the moulding of the fetal head,
- the adaptability of the fetus' physiology.

Many observers have attempted to provide a simple and logical approach to analysing each of these areas and thus to untangle the intricate pathways involved.

Friedman's meticulous examination of patterns of progress in labour in the 1950s enabled clinicians to monitor each labour with reference to a 'known standard'. He noted that the first stage of parturition was usually a continuous process, extending from the time of admission to the labour ward to the full dilatation of the cervix.[2,3] This period could also be divided into latent and active phases (Figure 27.1).

As labour is only an accentuation of the uterine activity that is present throughout pregnancy, so defining the onset of labour is often problematic. During the latent phase, cervical change may be subtle and difficult to assess accurately. The cervical canal shortens from 3 cm in length to <0.5 cm, while dilating to 3 cm. This process encompasses little dilatation in comparison to the changes that occur within

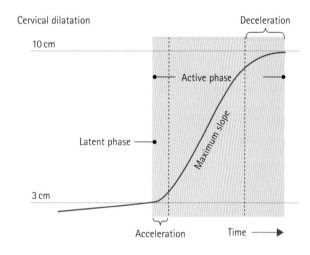

**Figure 27.1** Phases of normal labour

the cervical collagen content, the ground substance and the alignment with the birth canal. As a consequence, this is often the time that is most fraught with maternal frustration at the lack of tangible progress.

By comparison, the active phase is associated with changes in cervical dilatation, from 3 to 10 cm, and may be divided into:

- acceleration: between the latent phase and maximum slope;
- maximum slope: linear dilatation with time;
- deceleration phase: at the end of the active phase and prior to full dilatation.

Friedman's examination of such 'labour curves' in both multiparae and nulliparae suggested that a maximum slope dilatation of 1 cm/hour should be the minimum rate of progression. Although this value is often quoted, there are several problems with the universal acceptance of this figure as the 'gold standard', namely:

- the original data were not normally distributed, but skewed towards higher rates of dilatation;
- the lower limit of 1 cm/hour refers to the maximum slope phase, and not to the whole of the active phase of labour.

These figures were never intended as a method of choosing which labours needed augmentation (although they have subsequently been used for this purpose).

Several researchers have subsequently aimed to modify the original data to make them suitable for application to different demographic groups.[4–6] Although such analyses allowed the detection of labours with 'suboptimal' progress at an early stage, the claims that the instigation of appropriate management strategies would result in an improved outcome in the active management arm in comparison to the control population have not been met. In fact, many of these methods result in an increase in operative intervention when arbitrary delays in cervical dilatation are observed, without any improvement in the overall labour outcome.

Many of the perceived problems may actually be a result of:

- artefact inherent upon the misdiagnosis of the onset of labour,
- confounding variables, e.g. the Hawthorne effect (performing research may improve the outcome for reasons other than those under scrutiny),
- methodological flaws (rendering many of the findings unsuitable for application to the general population),
- failure to establish, test and substantiate 'norms and limits of biological variation' and not actual problems with labour itself.

## THE PASSAGES, THE PASSENGER AND THE POWERS

An improved understanding of the physiology of labour has enabled a more scientific approach to the management of the commonly encountered problems. Whereas specific patterns of deviation from the normal may be linked with possible pathologies, labour is still evaluated in the traditional terms of the passages, the passenger and the powers.

The passages relates to the bony components of the pelvis and the soft tissues within this semi-rigid structure. In developed countries where nutritional status in childhood is generally good, significant bony pelvic pathology is rare. However, the influence of the soft tissues on the outcome of labour is often ignored. Abnormalities of remodelling of the cervix and space-occupying viscera within the pelvis, such as impacted rectum, full bladder, cervical fibroids and ovarian cysts, may all lead to delay in the active phase. An impacted rectum and full bladder are problems easily remedied without resorting to surgical interventions, unlike the other scenarios for which delivery by caesarean section may be the safer of the options.

The passenger refers to the fetus. Although there is evidence to suggest that birth weights are rising in developed countries, the amount (30 g over 12 years) is unlikely to be of any biological significance. While induction of labour at term may seem logical to reduce the potential for macrosomia and its complications, positive benefits for either the mother or fetus have not been observed in the trials performed to date. The fetal head is designed to mould during labour to fit through the pelvis. Its smallest diameter (suboccipito-bregmatic) is that found with an occipito-anterior position in second stage. Larger diameters present when a fetal head does not rotate correctly during labour. Dystocia caused by malposition or malpresentation will be discussed later in this chapter.

The powers, i.e. uterine contractions, are the only component that can truly be manipulated. The forces that expel the baby and its placenta originate in the upper uterine segment, propagating through the myometrium towards the lower segment. This wave of activity is associated with the myometrial fibres located in this area contracting, relaxing and retracting, i.e. after relaxation they retain a length that is not as great as before the onset of the contraction. At the same time, the fibres of the lower uterine segment become elongated, thinned and incorporated into the supravaginal portions of the cervical canal. These factors interact to cause descent of the presenting part, and expulsion of the fetus.

Through the use of oxytocin, the frequency, intensity and duration of the contractions can be augmented. However, there are limits to the maximum effect that may be achieved, especially when the potential for inducing iatrogenic fetal compromise is taken into consideration. There is also little evidence to show that the outcome of labour, in terms of successful vaginal delivery, can be improved when the uterine activity is normal. There are groups of women who are more likely to have a dysfunctional labour than others, for example the obese, those of advanced maternal age, those with diabetes, multiple pregnancy, etc. While the mechanisms underlying the alterations in normal physiology is not yet fully understood within each of these groups, changes in myometrial activity, dysfunction of the gap junctions between cells and changes in the interaction between fetal and maternal factors undoubtedly play an important role.

## PATTERNS OF CERVICAL DILATATION

Graphical representation of cervical change over time may be charted on a partogram, along with other maternal and fetal observations.[7] Data presented in this way allow a rapid analysis of many inter-related facts, and although this may have many advantages, incorrect inclusion of the latent phase, inaccurate data recording and subjective assessment of the visual data may give an erroneous impression of sub-optimal progress and, in turn, increase the likelihood of operative intervention.

## DISORDERS OF LABOUR

Three major disorders of labour are often diagnosed. Once characterized, details concerning the aetiological factors, efficacy of modalities of treatment and prognostic outlook can be determined (Figure 27.2).

### Prolonged latent phase

During the latent phase, changes occur in the ground substance glycoprotein, collagen content and hydration state of the cervix, which result in the remodelling and efface-ment that may be observed during this period. Friedman described the latent phase as lasting up to 20 hours in nulliparae (median 8.6 hours) and 14 hours in multiparae (median 5.3 hours), although the absolute duration is dependent upon the definition of the onset of labour.

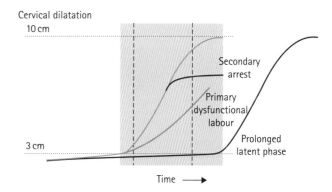

**Figure 27.2** Abnormal patterns of labour

During this period, women may experience painful contractions and need a great deal of support. However, it is important that unnecessary interventions to accelerate labour are not implemented at this point, as clinical studies have demonstrated that oxytocin augmentation during this phase does not result in an increase in the vaginal delivery rate, but rather a 10-fold increase in the incidence of caesarean delivery and a 3-fold increase in low Apgar scores [B].

In place of active intervention, careful explanation and the provision of adequate analgesia may be all that is required before the cervical changes complete and the active phase of labour is entered. Any decision to augment in the latent phase should be based on medical or obstetric indications. In such an event, management along the lines consistent with an induction of labour may be the most appropriate, although the risks of uterine hyperstimulation may be increased.

### Primary dysfunctional labour

Primary dysfunctional labour (PDL) is defined as poor progress during the active phase of labour. This affects up to 26 per cent of nulliparae and 8 per cent of multiparae and, whereas no single aetiology is responsible for all cases, 70 per cent of nulliparae and 80 per cent of multiparae will respond to oxytocin. This observation suggests that poor/inco-ordinate uterine activity is a significant factor, although an improvement in the rate of cervical dilatation does not necessarily correlate with an improved outcome in terms of vaginal delivery. Primary dysfunctional labour may culminate in an obstructed labour and is associated with higher rates of maternal infection, uterine rupture and postpartum haemorrhage [C].

Interventions for PDL include:

- optimization of maternal well-being (hydration, pain relief, etc.). It is important to note that in up to 40 per cent of women, progress will improve by simply improving maternal hydration;
- the provision of one-to-one care or a professional maternal companion if this is not already provided;

- a longer period of time to allow labour to progress;
- mobilization;
- augmentation with oxytocin;
- delivery by caesarean section.

The relative risks and benefits of each of these will be discussed below.

## Secondary arrest

Secondary arrest affects approximately 6 per cent of nulliparae and 2 per cent of multiparae, and may be defined as a cessation of cervical dilatation following a normal period of active-phase dilatation. Whereas any of the factors implicated in PDL may contribute to this abnormal labour pattern, secondary arrest is more likely to be associated with a significant underlying pathological process, with cephalo-pelvic disproportion (CPD), both relative and absolute, occasionally being encountered.

It should also be acknowledged that, up to the stage of arrest, the uterine activity has been sufficient to produce a normal response in terms of cervical effacement and dilatation. Thus, although augmentation may be considered, a diagnosis must be sought before such an intervention is commenced in order to reduce the complications associated with cases of absolute CPD. Nevertheless, in one series of patients with secondary arrest, 60 per cent of nulliparae and 70 per cent of multiparae demonstrated an improvement in progress with oxytocin. However, the caesarean section rate was ten times greater in the treatment arm than in the uncomplicated cohort. Cephalo-pelvic disproportion cannot usually be properly diagnosed until the latter stages of labour, and it is in these cases that particular care must be taken.

### Secondary arrest in the decelerative phase

Friedman observed that delay during the decelerative phase on a partogram, between cervical dilatations of 7 and 10 cm, was associated with an increased risk of failure to respond to oxytocin augmentation and difficulty in procuring a successful instrumental vaginal delivery. Before any intervention is considered, a careful clinical assessment must be performed, noting:

- an estimate of fetal size (a fetus measuring >40 cm on symphysis–fundal 'height' measurement at this stage of labour is likely to be large);
- the degree of engagement (fifths palpable per abdomen);
- position of the presenting part;
- signs of obstruction (moulding);
- presence of pelvic masses;
- descent of the presenting part with contractions;
- contraction frequency;
- fetal well-being.

Variable decelerations and a rising baseline are common in obstructed labour. Where fetal scalp sampling reveals a normal pH, the suspicion must be that the CTG changes could represent obstruction rather than fetal intolerance to labour.

Options at this stage are much as defined for PDL and are discussed below.

## Secondary arrest in the second stage of labour

The second stage of labour is the period from full cervical dilatation to delivery of the fetus, and is a continuum in the process of labour and not a static phase. It may also be divided into pelvic and perineal stages, representing the differences between full dilatation with the head high and the overwhelming sensation a patient feels when the presenting part is deep in the pelvis and exerting pressure on the rectum.

In the presence of a malposition, the second stage may become lengthened. The second stage may also lengthen when an epidural is present, an effect contributed to by relaxation of the pelvic floor and failure of the Ferguson reflex. As long as the fetal condition remains satisfactory, in the nullipara, an oxytocin infusion in combination with the provision of additional time for the co-ordination of maternal efforts with uterine activity can reduce the incidence of instrumental vaginal deliveries.

## INTERVENTIONS IN LABOUR

## Maternal hydration and pain relief

Data demonstrating that in primary dysfunctional labour approximately 40 per cent of nulliparae will respond to normal saline infusions (either before oxytocin is considered or after it has failed) highlight the fact that factors, such as maternal hydration, are vitally important in labour.

Pain relief and its effects on labour are discussed in Chapter 30, Obstetric anaesthesia. It is important that before augmentation is considered, pain relief is discussed with the patient. Although there is a transient reduction in contraction frequency after epidural analgesia is commenced, this usually resolves spontaneously and with careful management should not impact on the first stage of labour [A]. It is important to recognize that although epidural analgesia is associated with an increase in the rate of instrumental vaginal delivery, there is no evidence of an increased risk of delivery by caesarean section [A].

## The provision of one-to-one care

One-to-one care is the single most effective intervention to improve outcomes, both maternal and fetal, in labour. The carer does not have to be a midwife, but should not be the husband/partner (although of course his/her presence may be welcomed). Meta-analysis of randomized, controlled trials (RCTs) shows that the continuous presence of a caregiver reduces the likelihood of medication for pain relief, instrumental vaginal delivery, caesarean section and a 5-minute Apgar score <7. Continuous support is also associated with a slight reduction in the overall length of labour [A].[8]

## Mobilization

Much has been made of the contribution of mobility in the progress of labour, but in fact there is a remarkable paucity of good data. Only one good RCT is available that compares two types of epidural analgesia (mobile versus conventional). Although in the mobile epidural group, women were encouraged to walk, there was no difference in the length of labour, need for augmentation or type of delivery between the two groups [B].

## Amniotomy

Amniotomy has traditionally been practised to shorten the length of labour. Meta-analysis of the trials incorporating routine early amniotomy into the management of spontaneous labour shows that amniotomy is not associated with statistically significant reduction in duration of the first stage in nulliparous or multiparous women. The weighted mean difference for nulliraous women is 20.43 minutes (i.e. on average, the first stage would be 20 minutes shorter with amniotomy [A]).[9]

However, with early amniotomy there was a trend towards an increase in the risk of caesarean delivery (odds ratio (OR) 1.26; 95 per cent confidence interval (CI) 0.96–1.66)

Markers of neonatal well-being are similar between the two groups (Apgar scores, arterial cord pH, neonatal intensive care unit admissions).

Given that the reduction in length of labour is not large and not significant and that there is a potential for increase in the need for caesarean section, it has been suggested that amniotomy should be reserved for women with abnormal progress in labour.

## OXYTOCIN FOR LABOUR AUGMENTATION

- 'Inco-ordinate uterine activity' is a descriptive term for the observations from a tocographic recording.
- Inefficient uterine activity is a failure of the uterus to function in a way that results in normal progression of labour.
- Inco-ordinate uterine activity does not need to be specifically addressed if progress in labour is normal.

Despite widespread use in clinical practice, there is a huge paucity of evidence to demonstrate that the use of oxytocin to augment labour improves either the maternal or fetal outcomes. There have been few RCTs and those that have been performed are generally small. This is in part due to ethical committees not giving permission for a placebo arm, or poor trial recruitment in the presence of a placebo arm. In one small RCT assessing the use of oxytocin for PDL, improvement in progress of labour was seen, but this was not reflected in improved outcomes for mothers or babies. Although this trial did show that mothers randomized to oxytocin had higher satisfaction scores than those in the control arm, the numbers were too small to draw decisive conclusions.[10]

Comparative studies and one RCT demonstrate that 60–80 per cent of women will respond to syntocinon in terms of improved rates of cervical dilatation, but not other outcomes of labour.[11,12]

A multicentre RCT run in the north east of England concluded that among nulliparous women with primary dysfunctional labour, the early use of oxytocin did not reduce the incidence of caesarean section or short-term postnatal depression. However, early intervention was noted to shorten labour considerably with a trend towards a reduction in the number of operative vaginal deliveries required.[13]

Any decision to augment should be based on the clinical findings, and a full clinical assessment as described above must be made. This is mandatory when augmentation is to be considered in multiparous women. If CPD is thought to be present, delivery should be by caesarean section.

Augmentation of labour in multiparae is one of the greatest contributing factors to uterine rupture.[12] A decision to augment a multipara who presented in spontaneous labour must be made by an experienced person and only after a complete clinical re-evaluation of the case.

A full discussion should be undertaken with the woman before augmentation. It is reasonable not to augment and to allow labour to continue at a slower rate, but in all cases all other factors, such as maternal support and hydration, must be optimized.

## WHEN TO AUGMENT LABOUR

Augmentation with oxytocin has been advocated when the progress of labour falls behind that which would be considered optimal. This vague definition reflects the wide variations in clinical practice currently in operation. O'Driscoll et al.[12] advocated augmentation when labour was noted to be progressing at a rate of <1 cm/hour when reassessed 1 hour later. Others have employed 'action lines' – markers on the partogram drawn parallel but 2–4 hours behind the alert line (WHO recommends 4 hours, see Figure 27.3).[7]

Debate therefore exists about not only when oxytocin should be started, but also whether it should be used at all,

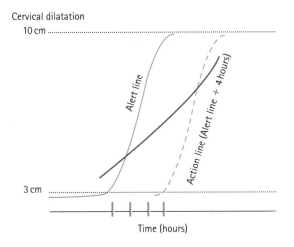

**Figure 27.3** Partogram showing ideal progress and slow labour crossing the WHO action line

especially where labour is progressing, albeit slowly. Part of the process of providing women with an informed choice is to acknowledge that, for some, simply accepting a slower rate of progress compared with the standard 'norm' is all that is required.

The Royal College of Obstetricians and Gynaecologists audit standards suggest that caesarean section should not be performed for poor progress in nulliparae before a trial of oxytocin. However, it should be realized that this recommendation is not based on any evidence from randomized trials and situations exist in which this advice should not be followed.

Once commenced, oxytocin should be titrated to provide a contraction frequency of four or five in 10 minutes, with each contraction lasting approximately 40 seconds. Such a regimen has been shown to be compatible with normal progress in labour (>1 cm/hour) with minimal adverse sequelae, as long as the appropriate action is taken if signs of maternal or fetal compromise develop. The frequency and duration of contractions may be assessed by either internal or external tocography; uterine tone and quantification of uterine activity can only be measured by internal tocography.

Advocates of intrauterine pressure monitoring claim that uterine hyperstimulation can be identified earlier and, in patients with a previous caesarean section scar, that dehiscence can be diagnosed more promptly with a consequent improvement in neonatal outcome. However, a prospective randomized study failed to show an improvement in the obstetric outcome when an intrauterine pressure catheter was employed in an augmented labour when compared with an external tocograph [B].[14] In clinical practice, it is undoubtedly easier, cheaper and less invasive to monitor uterine activity using an external monitor.

Given intravenously, oxytocin takes 30–45 minutes to reach steady-state levels. Increments for increase should not be performed more frequently than half-hourly. Many units use similar concentrations and maximum doses as for

induction of labour (NICE Clinical Guideline 70: Chapter 25, Induction of labour).

## HOW LONG TO AUGMENT

Debate continues about how long unsuccessful augmentation should continue before it can be confidently established that vaginal delivery will not be achieved. The data currently available suggest that a period of augmentation exceeding 8 hours' duration is unlikely to result in a successful vaginal delivery in the presence of persistent poor progress. However, it will not be appropriate to leave all women this long, and decisions must be taken in the context of full clinical assessment. Between 8 per cent of multiparae and 22 per cent of nulliparae will fail to respond to oxytocin and require delivery by caesarean section, although the majority of patients will deliver vaginally within this time with few risks of intrapartum injury [C]. It is important to recognize that as fetal compromise may result from augmentation of the forces, continuous monitoring of the fetus should be employed.

## ACTIVE MANAGEMENT OF LABOUR

In order to reduce the incidence of complications related to long labour, and to manage a clinical workload effectively, the concept of 'active management' of labour was formulated by O'Driscoll et al.[12] They adopted a pragmatic approach in which delay in nulliparae, whether due to inadequate uterine activity, relative CPD or other aberrant mechanisms, was treated by manipulation of the powers, as this was the only variable open to alteration. They observed that an oxytocin infusion in conjunction with a strict diagnosis of labour, early amniotomy and one-to-one care resulted in a marked reduction in the rate of interventional deliveries.

The Dublin team made every effort to ensure that it is understood that this strategy was not applicable to multiparae, though this message is often forgotten in other units. Active management is a package encompassing antenatal classes, one-to-one care, a strict diagnosis of labour, early amniotomy and oxytocin for slow progress and frequent vaginal assessment.

The low rates of caesarean section achieved in Dublin has not been matched in other units. Furthermore, the meta-analysis of the studies employing 'the complete' active management protocols fails to show an effective reduction in the rates of caesarean section and other operative vaginal deliveries. By contrast, the provision of continuous professional support in labour has been found to reduce both types of operative interventions, although the effect on the incidence of caesarean section was confined to those settings in which partners were excluded from the delivery room [A].

# OTHER CONTRIBUTORS TO POOR PROGRESS

## Relative cephalo-pelvic disproportion in cases of malposition

If the progress of labour remains unsatisfactory despite adequate augmentation of contractions, mechanical factors such as malposition or deflexion of the head may be found to contribute to the observed delay.

Rather than the presentation of the optimal suboccipito-bregmatic diameter (9.5 cm in an 'average' term fetus) in a well-flexed occipito-anterior position, the larger occipito-frontal diameter (11 cm) or other positions will result in relative CPD. However, the dynamic nature of labour will continuously alter the dimensions of the presenting part through flexion, rotation and moulding in relation to the pelvis. Likewise, the shape of the pelvis undergoes subtle changes and is not simply a static bony conduit. The relative combinations of the passenger and the passages to the delay may therefore be difficult to evaluate.

In cases of malposition, it is important to assess progress not only in terms of dilatation, but also in terms of rotation and descent. Therefore, accurate definition of position is very important when labour is not progressing Table 27.1 shows the potential fetal causes and associations with poor prognosis.

## Face presentation

A face presentation may be diagnosed by palpation of the chin, mouth, nose and orbital ridges per vaginum. The presenting diameters are those of the transverse biparietal (9.5 cm) and the saggital submento-bregmatic (9.5 cm). When the chin (mentum) is anterior, a face presentation may deliver spontaneously or following assistance with forceps, as a consequence of a presentation with 'favourable diameters' and the ability of the head to flex beneath the symphysis pubis while 'crowning'. In face presentations, a lower threshold for delivery by caesarean section is usually adopted, as avoidance of a difficult vaginal delivery is important.

**Table 27.1** Definitions and potential causes of poor progress

| Diagnosis | Fetal |
|---|---|
| Malposition | Occipito-posterior |
| | Occipito-lateral |
| | Deflexion |
| Malpresentation | Face (if mento-posterior) |
| | Congenital abnormality |
| Macrosomia | Diabetes |
| | Post-dates |

When the chin is posterior, the head is almost fully extended and unable to flex due to the sacral 'obstruction'. Although vaginal delivery may be possible if the head rotates during labour or with rotational forceps, in all but the most experienced hands, intervention by caesarean section is usually warranted.

## Contributory factors in absolute cephalo-pelvic disproportion

### Maternal causes

Pelvic abnormalities

#### Congenital
These are rare and include the following (Table 27.2).

- Incorporation of the sacrum into the fifth lumbar vertebrae: this results in the sacral promontory being higher than usual, with an apparent lengthening of the sacrum and an increase in the angle of inclination. Although women with sacralization of the fifth lumbar vertebra may successfully deliver vaginally, it contributes to CPD in a number of women.
- Protrusio acetabulae (the Otto pelvis): the acetabular heads protrude medially to distort the pelvic cavity and obstruct labour.

**Table 27.2** Contributory factors in absolute CPD

| Diagnosis | Maternal | Fetal |
|---|---|---|
| Bony abnormalities | Severe kyphosis | |
| | Severe scoliosis | |
| | Poliomyelitis | |
| | Maternal skeletal dysplasia | |
| | Rickets | |
| | Pelvic fracture | |
| Soft tissue abnormalities | Cervical fibroids | Hydrocephalus |
| | Ovarian tumour | Iniencephaly |
| | Pelvic kidney | Anencephaly |
| | Excessive fat | Conjoined twins |
| | Cervical cancer | |
| | Vaginal/vulval atresia | |
| | Vaginal septum | |
| | Gartner's duct cysts | |
| Malpresentation | | *Incidence at term* |
| | Face (if mento-posterior) | 1:500 |
| | Brow | 1:500 |
| | Shoulder | 1:1500 |
| | Compound presentations | 3:10 000 |

### Acquired

These are more common and include the following.

- Kyphoscoliosis: kyphosis of the thoracic spine promotes a compensatory lumbar lordosis, with consequent contractions in the pelvic anterior–posterior diameters. Scoliosis produces deformities of the pelvic inlet. Kyphoscoliosis combines these problems, and there may be additional maternal respiratory embarrassment.
- Pelvic fractures and disuse atrophy: direct pelvic trauma may result in a pelvis of any shape, which may or may not accommodate the passage of a fetus during childbirth. Rickets (vitamin D deficiency) may affect pelvic development in childhood, with a resultant narrowing of the pelvic inlet (sacral promontory pushed forward). This results in marked asynclitism of the presenting part and a significant risk of shoulder dystocia if the head is successfully delivered. Disuse atrophy may be the consequence of any primary pathology (poliomyelitis, spina bifida, tuberculosis, suppurative arthritis, etc.) and may result in a pelvis of any shape.

### Soft tissue abnormalities

Congenital abnormalities of the vagina are rarely a problem as the soft tissues will distort in the face of fetal descent and can often be pushed to one side, for example vaginal septum. Congenital or acquired strictures, on the other hand, may significantly impede descent and, because of the close proximity of the bladder anteriorly and the rectum posteriorly, delivery by caesarean section should be the treatment of choice.

## Fetal causes

### Brow presentation

A brow presentation is due to a deflexed head. The presenting diameters are those of the transverse biparietal (9.5 cm) and the saggital mento-verticular (13 cm). The mid-cavity of the pelvis measures only 12 by 12 cm in the average woman, and a brow is unlikely to negotiate its way through this passage unless it undergoes flexion to a vertex or extension to a face.

Diagnosis is usually made by a combination of:

- poor progress in labour (often apparent at early stages);
- at least two- to three-fifths of the head palpable per abdomen;
- vaginal station of –2 to –3 cm above the ischial spines;
- orbital ridges palpable on vaginal examination.

If a brow is diagnosed early in labour, two courses of action are acceptable.

1  Conservative: a short time (2–3 hours) may be allowed without oxytocin augmentation to see whether spontaneous flexion or extension occurs. This is the best strategy if uterine contractions are good and in multiparae.

2  Active: a short period of oxytocin augmentation may be allowed (1 hour) to see whether additional 'power' will resolve the problem. Caution must be taken with this line of management, especially in multiparae, and it should never be initiated in grande multiparae.

In either case, if there is no change in the presentation over the time allotted, the delivery should be by caesarean section.

The accoucheur should be aware that all malpresentations are more common preterm than at term. Therefore, they may not pose the same problems as the diameters of the fetal head are comparatively small. However, the same principles of management apply, and failure to progress should be dealt with in the safest manner (often by caesarean section).

Problems with fetal abnormalities and maternal abnormalities (see lists above) must always be considered when a malpresentation is identified.

Whatever the management of a poorly progressing labour, the possibility for a postpartum haemorrhage should always be anticipated by the attending team and managed accordingly.

## SUMMARY

- A latent phase of up to 20 hours in nulliparae (median 8.6 hours) and 14 hours in multiparae (median 5.3 hours) is normal, although absolute duration is dependent upon when the definition of the onset of labour is made. Oxytocin augmentation during this phase does not result in an increase in the vaginal delivery rate, but rather a 10-fold increase in the incidence of caesarean delivery and a 3-fold increase in low Apgar scores.
- PDL affects up to 26 per cent of nulliparae and 8 per cent of multiparae. While no single aetiology is responsible for all cases, 70 per cent of nulliparae and 80 per cent of multiparae will respond to oxytocin in terms of improvement in the rate of cervical dilatation.
- Secondary arrest affects approximately 6 per cent of nulliparae and 2 per cent of multiparae, and may be defined as a cessation of cervical dilatation following a normal period of active-phase dilatation. Sixty per cent of nulliparae and 70 per cent of multiparae demonstrated an improvement in progress with oxytocin.
- Improved rates of cervical dilatation with oxytocin do not necessarily lead to improved outcomes for mothers and babies.
- Meta-analysis of the studies employing the 'complete' active management protocols failed to show an effective reduction in the rates of caesarean section and other operative vaginal deliveries. By contrast, the provision of continuous professional support in labour reduces operative interventions and the need for pain relief, shortens labour and leads to infants being delivered in better condition.

## KEY POINTS

- Abnormalities of the progression of labour are common problems on the modern labour ward, due in part to classification systems that may overdiagnose these complications.
- Prolonged labour is not a diagnosis; it is an abnormality that may be detected during parturition, and for which a cause must be identified before treatment is instigated.
- Although the majority of cases of 'delay' will respond to uterine stimulation with oxytocin, this may not improve the outcomes and women should therefore choose whether to wait or to accept medical intervention.
- Cases of absolute CPD should be identified and managed accordingly.
- Delivery by caesarean section should not be regarded as a failure, but rather as an appropriate intervention after a full assessment.
- It is recommended that caesarean section should not be performed in nulliparae for delay in labour before oxytocin has been tried.
- Instrumental delivery may be challenging after correction of poor progress in labour and should only be performed by experienced practitioners.

## Key References

1. AbouZahr C, Wardlaw T. Maternal mortality at the end of a decade: signs of progress? *Bull WHO* 2001; **79**: 561–8.
2. Friedman EA. Primigravid labor. *Obstet Gynecol* 1955; **6**: 567–89.
3. Friedman EA. Labor in multiparae. *Obstet Gynecol* 1956; **8**: 691–703.
4. Studd J. Partograms and nomograms of cervical dilatation in management of primigravid labour. *BMJ* 1973; **4**: 451–5.
5. Cartmill RS, Thornton JG. Effect of presentation of partogram information on obstetric decision-making. *Lancet* 1992; **339**: 1520–22.
6. Cardozo LD, Gibb DM, Studd JW *et al.* Predictive value of cervicometric labour patterns in primigravidae. *Br J Obstet Gynaecol* 1982; **89**: 33–8.
7. World Health Organization. Maternal health and safe motherhood programme. World Health Organization partograph on management of labor. *Lancet* 1994; **343**: 1399–404.
8. Hodnett ED, Gates S, Hofmeyr GJ, Sakala C. Continuous support for women during childbirth. *Cochrane Database Syst Rev* 2007; (**3**): CD003766.
9. Smyth RMD, Alldred SK, Markham C. Amniotomy for shortening spontaneous labour. *Cochrane Database Syst Rev* 2007; (**4**): CD006167.
10. Blanch G, Lavender T, Walkinshaw S, Alfirevic Z. Dysfunctional labour: a randomised trial. *Br J Obstet Gynaecol* 1998; **105**: 117–20.
11. Bidgood KA, Steer PJ. A randomized control study of oxytocin augmentation of labour 1. Obstetric outcome. *Br J Obstet Gynaecol* 1987; **94**: 512–17.
12. O'Driscoll K, Stronge JM, Minogue M. Active management of labour. *BMJ* 1973; **31**: 135–7.
13. Hinshaw K, Simpson S, Cummings S *et al.* A randomised controlled trial of early versus delayed oxytocin augmentation to treat primary dysfunctional labour in nulliparous women. *BJOG* 2008; **115**: 1289–95.
14. Chua S, Kurup A, Arulkumaran S, Ratnam SS. Augmentation of labor: does internal tocography result in better obstetric outcome than external tocography? *Obstet Gynecol* 1990; **76**: 164–7.

# Meconium

*Andrew Currie*

---

## INTRODUCTION

The detection of meconium-stained amniotic fluid during labour often causes anxiety in the delivery room because of its association with increased perinatal mortality and morbidity.

Meconium is composed of swallowed amniotic fluid debris, bile pigment and the residue from intestinal secretions. It is a sterile, durable compound made up primarily of water (75 per cent), with mucous glycoproteins, lipids and proteases. Although meconium is sterile, its passage into amniotic fluid is important because of the risk of meconium aspiration syndrome (MAS) and its sequelae. Infants delivered through meconium-stained amniotic fluid are more likely to be depressed at birth and to require resuscitation and neonatal intensive care.[1]

## INCIDENCE

The passage of meconium *in utero* occurs in approximately 12–15 per cent of all fetuses, with the highest rates reported from North America.[2] Meconium-stained liquor is rare in premature infants (<5 per cent of preterm pregnancies); if it does occur, there is an association with infection and chorioamnionitis. Passage of meconium is increasingly common in infants >37 weeks gestation and occurs in up to 50 per cent of post-mature infants (>42 weeks).[2]

The incidence of MAS varies between 1 and 5 per cent of all deliveries where there has been meconium-stained liquor, with higher rates reported from North America compared to Europe. There are a number of factors associated with an increased risk of developing MAS; these include a lack of antenatal care, black race, male fetus, abnormal fetal heart rate monitoring, thick meconium, oligohydramnios, operative delivery, poor Apgar scores, no oropharyngeal suctioning and the presence of meconium in the trachea.[2]

## AETIOLOGY

Many theories have been proposed to explain the passage of meconium *in utero*; however, the precise mechanisms remain unclear. The fetal bowel has little peristaltic action and the anal sphincter is contracted. It is thought that hypoxia and acidaemia cause the anal sphincter to relax, while at the same time increasing the production of motilin, which promotes peristalsis.[3]

## PATHOPHYSIOLOGY

Meconium aspiration syndrome is a disease of term and post-term infants and its severity is inextricably linked to coexisting fetal asphyxia. Aspiration of meconium into the distal airways can occur either antenatally or postnatally, and in the majority of affected infants the exact timing is unclear.

Production of fetal lung fluid is a continuous process, with a net movement of fluid out of the lung. During normal fetal breathing, lung fluid is not usually drawn into the distal airway. It is suggested that prolonged fetal hypoxia stimulates fetal gasping and that the consequent acidaemia stimulates deep breathing – resulting in meconium being drawn into the distal airway of the fetus via the oropharynx and nasopharynx.

Aspiration is known to occur prior to delivery, as meconium has been found in the lungs of stillbirths and in infants delivered pre-labour by caesarean section without evidence of fetal distress. Perinatal inhalation can occur late in the second stage or immediately after delivery if the infant gasps or makes breathing movements while the oropharynx, nasopharynx or trachea contains meconium-stained liquor.

Meconium has a number of adverse effects on the neonatal lung, which may ultimately lead to the respiratory failure (and hypoxaemia) which characterizes MAS.[4] First, it causes mechanical obstruction of the airways with subsequent atelectasis and consolidation, as well as creating a ball-valve type effect, so that gas can pass over the meconium plug into the lung, but cannot be exhaled. This causes air trapping, hyperinflation and an increased risk of pneumothorax. Second, it acts as a chemical irritant causing pneumonitis, alveolar collapse and cell necrosis. The presence of organic material in the airway, although initially sterile, predisposes to secondary bacterial infection. Finally, meconium is known to inhibit the surface tension properties of surfactant at alveolar level, thus further increasing airway resistance.

# PREVENTION OF MECONIUM ASPIRATION SYNDROME

Given the potential morbidity and mortality from MAS (see below under Complications, morbidity and mortality), prevention would clearly be beneficial. This has led to a number of antenatal, intrapartum and postnatal preventative therapies being explored, with varying degrees of success. Many of these remain controversial and have not been subjected to the scrutiny of randomized, controlled trials.

## Antenatal therapies

### Amnioinfusion

This potential therapy was used in North America until recently. The rationale behind amnioinfusion is that by increasing the liquor volume, meconium will be diluted. In addition, in cases of oligohydramnios, the increased volume was felt to prevent cord compression, subsequent hypoxia, fetal gasping and passage of meconium. A previous meta-analysis of amnioinfusion trials showed that this therapy had a role in the prevention of MAS.[5] However, in 2005, a large multi-centre trial published in the *New England Journal of Medicine* recruited 1998 pregnant women to look at the use of amnioinfusion and found no improvement in outcome for severe meconium aspiration syndrome, perinatal death, or other major maternal and neonatal disorders,[6] as a result of which, this therapy cannot be recommended [A].

## Delivery by caesarean section

Although most studies suggest that infants with MAS are more likely to be delivered by caesarean section than by vaginal delivery, this is largely due to the suspicion or confirmation of fetal compromise. There is currently no evidence to suggest that MAS would be prevented by elective delivery by caesarean section of infants with meconium-stained liquor. Perhaps this is not surprising, as neither the conditions for, nor the timing of, aspiration can be predicted.

## Maternal sedation

It has been suggested that the administration of narcotics to labouring women will prevent fetal gasping *in utero* by suppressing fetal breathing. Although there has been success in the prevention of MAS in animal models, there are no data to support this therapy in humans. Moreover, the likely maternal and neonatal complications would preclude its use [E].

## Intrapartum/postpartum management

### Oropharyngeal suctioning

Suction of the oropharynx and nasopharynx before delivery of the shoulders and trunk was a well-established practice, used in the 1970s and 1980s. It seemed a reasonable assumption that suctioning in this way would minimize the amount of meconium in the upper airway and thus reduce the amount aspirated during the onset of respiration. This intervention was based on a non-randomized cohort study using historical controls and very small numbers. Subsequent studies using a similar suctioning approach have been unable to match the low incidence of MAS observed in the original study. More recently, a large randomized controlled trial into the use of oropharyngeal and nasopharyngeal suctioning for meconium before delivery of the shoulders showed no benefit for this practice.[7] As a result, this practice is no longer recommended and has been largely abandoned [B].

### Physical manoeuvres

It was also previously suggested that MAS may be prevented if the infant was prevented from breathing after delivery until the airway had been cleared. Methods advocated included thoracic compression, in which the thoracic cage of the infant was compressed by a healthcare professional in order to prevent respiration and subsequent aspiration of the contents of the upper airway, and cricoid pressure, in which external pressure is applied to the cricoid, thus preventing aspiration. This intervention was continued until a second resuscitator undertook oral and/or endotracheal suctioning. There is no evidence supporting the use of either of these methods in preventing MAS. In fact, both are potentially dangerous and cannot be recommended [E].

## Postnatal intervention

### Intratracheal suctioning

Until relatively recently, all infants with meconium-stained amniotic fluid underwent endotracheal intubation and suction immediately after birth, as this was known to reduce the incidence of MAS. More recently, evidence has suggested a change in practice depending on whether or not an infant is deemed vigorous. A Cochrane Library meta-analysis suggests that routine intubation of vigorous term infants in order to aspirate the lungs should be abandoned [A]. Suctioning of the oropharynx may be beneficial, but endotracheal suctioning should be reserved for depressed or non-vigorous infants or those who deteriorate following initial assessment.[8]

Aspiration of gastric contents to remove swallowed meconium is still practised in many centres. However, this practice has never been evaluated. The passage of an orogastric tube is likely to cause apnoea and/or bradycardia and is potentially harmful. This practice should be abandoned [E].

Saline lavage and physiotherapy are used in order to loosen meconium. No randomized studies have shown physiotherapy in infants with MAS to be beneficial. Saline lavage is potentially harmful, as saline will displace endogenous surfactant, which could in turn worsen the respiratory illness. In cases where saline lavage has been used, infants developed respiratory distress secondary to 'wet lung'.

## DELIVERY ROOM MANAGEMENT OF INFANTS BORN WITH MECONIUM-STAINED LIQUOR

It is important that a person experienced in neonatal resuscitation attends the delivery of all infants in whom thick meconium-stained liquor is noted, particularly if accompanied by suspected fetal compromise, as it is in these cases that MAS is likely to be a problem.

It is no longer recommended that the oropharynx should be suctioned with delivery of the head and before delivery of the shoulders and body. Instead, following delivery the infant should be transferred to a resuscitaire in the delivery room and then resuscitation should proceed according to the following:

If an infant is vigorous after delivery:

- No tracheal suctioning should be undertaken.
- Secretions should be cleared from the mouth and nose using a wide-bore suction catheter.
- Routine care should be given.

However, if an infant is not vigorous after birth (defined as depressed respirations, decreased muscle tone and/or heart rate <100 beats per minute):

- Direct endotracheal suctioning should be undertaken as soon as possible.

- Suction should be applied for no more than 5 seconds and the tube withdrawn.
- If meconium is aspirated from below the cords, the infant should be re-intubated and the process repeated, unless the infant has a profound bradycardia, in which case:
  - resuscitation should proceed with intermittent positive pressure ventilation (IPPV) without suctioning;
  - further suctioning can be attempted at a later stage.

If after the first suctioning no meconium is aspirated, no further suctioning should be attempted and the infant should be resuscitated using IPPV via an endotracheal tube.

These guidelines have also been incorporated into the UK Resuscitation Council's recommendations for newborn life support courses and are supported by ILCOR (International Liaison Committee on Resuscitation).

## CLINICAL MANIFESTATIONS OF MECONIUM ASPIRATION SYNDROME

Infants usually have signs of post-maturity, with dry, flaking skin that is often stained green/yellow by meconium. The most obvious feature of MAS is respiratory distress, characterized by tachypnoea with respiratory rates up to 100/minute, subcostal recession, nasal flaring and an expiratory grunt. As air trapping is a feature of this condition, hyperinflation of the chest is common. Meconium causes widespread crepitations throughout the chest on auscultation. Asphyxiated infants may be apnoeic, but exhibit identical physical signs once ventilated. The respiratory course varies depending on the severity of the MAS; however, the respiratory symptoms in most infants will have resolved by 14 days, and in some by 48 hours. Up to 60 per cent of infants with severe MAS will require mechanical ventilation[1,2] and many will have concomitant pulmonary hypertension of the newborn.[9] Infants with MAS may show signs of neonatal encephalopathy, depending on the degree of asphyxial insult. Jitteriness and irritability are common features and may last for several days. An early chest x-ray will show widespread patchy infiltrates with areas of hyperinflation interspersed with areas of atelectasis and consolidation. In mild cases, the x-ray may return to normal by 72 hours. In severe cases, the x-ray will show diffuse homogeneous opacification of the lung fields, reflecting the pneumonitis and interstitial oedema. Such changes may remain for up to 14 days or more.

## TREATMENT

No specific treatments are available for MAS. Infants should receive appropriate neonatal intensive care support until the meconium is cleared and respiratory function returns to normal. Special attention should be paid to the treatment of respiratory failure, acid-base status and secondary infection. Unless affected by coexisting asphyxia, many infants can be initially managed by administering humidified oxygen therapy via a headbox.

Continuous positive airway pressure (CPAP) is not indicated in these infants, as it increases the risk of pneumothorax and causes abdominal distension, which may lead to splinting of the diaphragm and exacerbate the respiratory symptoms [E].

Mechanical ventilation is often required.[2]

Intubation and ventilation are indicated if:

- the infant is asphyxiated and apnoeic;
- the infant is tiring;
- despite $FiO_2$ concentrations of 80 per cent, the infant remains hypoxic;
- the $PaCO_2$ increases above 8–9 kPa (60–67 mmHg).

Sedation with an opiate infusion is recommended in neonates who require ventilation as a result of meconium aspiration. Additionally, the use of muscle relaxants may be beneficial due to the need for high peak inspiratory pressures, to aid ventilatory management and reduce the risk of pneumothorax.

For infants who remain hypoxic on conventional ventilation, high-frequency oscillatory ventilation is a useful alternative. If despite good ventilatory management, there is continuing hypoxia and coexisting pulmonary hypertension of the newborn, the use of inhaled nitric oxide or extracorporeal membrane oxygenation (ECMO) is recommended. ECMO has been shown to improve the survival of infants with severe MAS [B].[10]

Surfactant has been used in a number of ways in MAS. First, surfactant replacement therapy has been shown to reduce the need for ECMO in infants with MAS [A].[11] Second, airway lavage with diluted surfactant has been used in an attempt to wash residual meconium from the airway [D]. Initial results are promising, but further work is needed.

In addition to good respiratory support, attention to support of other vital organs is mandatory. Meconium aspiration syndrome should be thought of as a multi-organ disease process. Cardiovascular support is vital, often requiring systemic pressures to be raised to help counteract the effects of right to left shunting through the patent ductus arteriosus due to persistent pulmonary hypertension of the newborn. Stringent attention to fluid balance is necessary as there is often renal impairment and if there is evidence indicating hypoxic ischaemic encephalopathy then consideration should be given to the use of therapeutic hypothermia as a neuroprotective treatment strategy.

## COMPLICATIONS, MORBIDITY AND MORTALITY

It is difficult to give precise details of morbidity in MAS, as complications and outcome are linked to concomitant neonatal encephalopathy and persistent pulmonary hypertension of the newborn.

Pneumothoraces are the most common complication of MAS and occur in up to 20 per cent of non-ventilated infants and up to 50 per cent of ventilated infants. Chronic lung disease is relatively uncommon, occurring in only 5 per cent of ventilated infants,[1] whereas up to 40 per cent of children who previously had MAS have asthma and about 50 per cent have abnormal lung function lasting many years.[13]

Persistent pulmonary hypertension of the newborn is a common complication, particularly in fatal cases.[11] Treatment includes ventilation plus the use of inhaled nitric oxide or ECMO.

Neurological morbidity is usually attributable to any co-existing neonatal encephalopathy, although damage may result from severe hypoxia secondary to the disease itself or to pulmonary air leaks. The neurological outcome for infants without neonatal encephalopathy is very good.

With improvements in neonatal care, the widespread availability of inhaled nitric oxide therapy and ECMO, deaths from MAS should now be rare. The mortality appears to have fallen from around 35 per cent in the 1970s to less than 5 per cent currently.[2] Most deaths are due to respiratory failure, but some are due to the renal or neurological sequelae of severe asphyxia.[12]

- There is no evidence supporting the use of saline lavage, chest physiotherapy, gastric aspiration or thoracic compression in the prevention of MAS.
- The routine suctioning of the oropharynx of the infant on the perineum (prior to delivery of the body) is no longer recommended and should be abandoned.
- Intratracheal suctioning after delivery should be reserved for the non-vigorous baby.
- The administration of surfactant in severe MAS reduces the need for ECMO.

### KEY POINTS

- Meconium-stained liquor is associated with increased morbidity and mortality in babies.
- MAS is linked to perinatal asphyxia.
- Good neonatal resuscitation skills reduce the incidence of MAS.

## ACKNOWLEDGEMENT

This chapter has been revised and updated. The author and editors acknowledge the contribution of Sandie Bohin to the chapter on this topic in the previous edition of the book.

First stage of labour

# Key References

1. Cleary GM, Wisewell TE. Meconium stained amniotic fluid and the meconium aspiration syndrome: an update. *Pediatr Clin North Am* 1998; **45**: 511–29.

2. Wisewell TE. Handling the meconium-stained infant. *Semin Neonatol* 2001; **6**: 225–31.

3. Lucas A, Christophides ND, Adrian TE *et al.* Fetal distress, meconium and motilin. *Lancet* 1979; **i**: 718.

4. Tyler DC, Murphy J, Cheney FW. Mechanical and chemical damage to lung tissue caused by meconium aspiration. *Pediatrics* 1978; **62**: 454–9.

5. Hofmeyr GJ. Amnioinfusion for meconium-stained liquor. *Curr Opin Obstet Gynecol* 2000; **12**: 129–32.

6. Fraser WD, Hofmeyer J, Lede R *et al.* Amnioinfusion for the prevention of the meconium aspiration syndrome. *New Engl J Med* 2005; **353**: 909–17.

7. Vain NE, Szyld EG, Prudent TE *et al.* for the Meconium Study Network. Oropharyngeal and nasopharyngeal suctioning of meconium-stained neonates before delivery of the shoulders: a multicentre, randomised controlled trial. *Lancet* 2004; **364**: 597–602.

8. Halliday HL, Sweet D. Endotracheal intubation at birth for preventing morbidity and mortality in vigorous, meconium-stained infants born at term. *Cochrane Database Syst Rev* 2001; (**1**): CD000500.

9. Wisewell TE, Tuggle JM, Turner BS. Meconium aspiration syndrome: have we made a difference? *Pediatrics* 1990; **85**: 715–21.

10. UK Collaborative ECMO Trial Group. UK collaborative randomised trial of neonatal extracorporeal membrane oxygenation. *Lancet* 1996; **348**: 75–82.

11. Soll RF, Dargavile P. Surfactant for meconium aspiration syndrome in full term infants. *Cochrane Database Syst Rev* 2007; (**1**): CD002054.

12. Swaminathan S, Quinn J, Stabile MW *et al.* Long-term pulmonary sequelae of meconium aspiration syndrome. *J Pediatr* 1989; **114**: 356–60.

# Chapter 29

# Fetal compromise in the first stage of labour

*Myles Taylor*

## MRCOG standards

- The ability to recognize, classify and act appropriately on cardiotocograph patterns.
- The ability to perform fetal blood sampling and to be able to interpret the results.

In addition, we would suggest the following:

### Theoretical skills

- Know the risk factors for fetal compromise and how they can be recognized either antenatally or in early labour.
- Understand the alterations in placental blood flow during contractions.
- Know the acute intrapartum complications that can lead to fetal compromise.
- Be aware of the different techniques available for assessing fetal well-being in labour, as well as their individual indications and limitations.
- Be able to quote the risk of serious neonatal morbidity and mortality.

### Practical skills

- Be confident in your ability to interpret a cardiotocograph, particularly with regard to recognizing those babies requiring immediate delivery.
- Be able to perform and interpret additional tests of fetal well-being for non-reassuring cardiotocographs that do not necessitate immediate delivery.
- Be able to apply a scalp electrode or perform a real-time ultrasound scan when it is not possible to obtain an adequate fetal heart rate trace using conventional Doppler techniques.

## INTRODUCTION

Members of the public, and indeed the legal profession, commonly relate childhood handicap to a 'difficult' labour and delivery. However, the Consensus Statement of the International Cerebral Palsy Task Force reported that intrapartum hypoxia could at most be responsible for only one in ten cases of cerebral palsy.[1] Nevertheless, as labour represents about 0.4 per cent (1/280) of the total duration of pregnancy, a 10 per cent contribution to suboptimal neonatal outcomes reminds us that it is a relatively 'high-risk' period. The fact that uterine perfusion is dramatically reduced during each contraction emphasizes the additional stress that labour places on fetuses.

## AIMS

The aim of monitoring fetal well-being during labour is to prevent birth asphyxia and so reduce perinatal mortality, morbidity and long-term handicap. Although all three of these outcomes are uncommon, the use of operative delivery for 'non-reassuring fetal status' remains an everyday occurrence on delivery suites in the United Kingdom. This is, in part, because of a wish to deliver on the downwards slope towards a poor outcome, before it actually occurs. The key question is what are the poor outcomes that we are trying to prevent? Currently, efforts are focused on reducing intermediate adverse outcomes in the hope that long-term permanent adverse outcomes (death and handicap) can be avoided. Such intermediate outcomes include neonatal intensive care unit (NICU) admissions at term, umbilical cord acidosis (pH <7.2) and base deficit >12 mmol/L, low Apgar scores and neonatal hypoxic ischaemic encephalopathy at term.

## ABSOLUTE OUTCOMES

### Perinatal mortality

This remains a widely accepted measure of maternity care, but such crude figures provide little help in assessing intrapartum monitoring. First, they are heavily distorted by very preterm births, in which fetal condition at birth is only one of many factors influencing outcome. Second, perinatal mortality rates also include stillbirths. It is self-evident that fetal monitoring can only be of use when the baby is alive at the onset of labour. Intrapartum term stillbirths may be a more appropriate mortality figure, as they are often related to events occurring during parturition. The intrapartum stillbirth rate in term singleton pregnancies is reported as only 0.3 per 1000.[2] The influence of fetal monitoring on such a rare event will remain difficult to study.

## Handicap

The achievement of normal long-term neurodevelopment is another major aim of intrapartum fetal assessment. The incidence of cerebral palsy is widely quoted as 2 per 1000. However, as mentioned previously, only in 10 per cent of cases (or 1 in 5000 births) are intrapartum events thought to have been of influence. Once again, the ability of fetal monitoring to impact on such a rarity is difficult to prove or disprove.

All obstetricians should therefore appreciate that intrapartum operative interventions carried out at term because of 'non-reassuring fetal status' are trying to prevent suboptimal outcomes seen in approximately 1 in 2000 births. It is necessary not only for obstetricians to react appropriately but also to avoid over-reaction.

## INTERMEDIATE OUTCOMES

### Apgar scores

To improve the recognition of intrapartum factors contributing to the absolute outcomes referred to above, markers of potential long-term morbidity have been used.

The influence of the condition of the baby at birth using Apgar scores taken at 1 and 5 minutes has been widely investigated, particularly in the earliest studies. All now agree that the 1-minute Apgar score purely reflects the need for neonatal resuscitation, regardless of aetiology. Unfortunately, the 5-minute Apgar score also appears to provide little predictive ability for long-term complications unless very low (<4) or moderately low (<7) and remaining so beyond 10 minutes of age.

There is not yet enough evidence to support the use of other similar markers, such as the need for intubation or ventilation.

### Arterial or capillary pH

Hypoxaemia will result when gas exchange across the placenta is impaired, with a gradual fetal accumulation of $CO_2$. This eventually leads to fetal acidaemia, which can be detected by analyzing fetal capillary or neonatal arterial pH. The widely accepted lower limit of normal for fetal or neonatal pH is 7.20. This represents two standard deviations below the mean fetal pH seen from intrapartum studies. It must be stressed that this value was chosen for statistical reasons, not primarily because of an association with neonatal morbidity. Clinical studies suggest that an umbilical arterial pH below 7.00 may be a more reliable marker of potential long-term problems, but the figure of 7.20 remains in everyday use to provide a wide margin of safety. The type of acidosis is also important. In a respiratory acidosis, the $PCO_2$ is elevated but the base excess is normal, a condition that will be easily resolved with the onset of neonatal respiration and gas exchange. Metabolic acidosis is associated with a transition to anaerobic metabolism and an accumulation of acids, such as lactate. It is defined by a base deficit >12 mmol/L and is a marker of moderate to severe neonatal morbidity in its own right.

## Neonatal encephalopathy

Neonatal behaviour and early-onset medical complications also provide some prognostic information. Neonatal encephalopathy refers to disturbed neurological function in the first week of life. Signs include difficulty maintaining respiration, depressed tone and reflexes, altered level of consciousness and seizures. Moderate to severe neonatal encephalopathy will be seen in most cases of brain damage secondary to intrapartum complications. However, neonatal encephalopathy has poor sensitivity with 75 per cent of cases having no clinical signs of intrapartum hypoxia.

## Criteria for intrapartum hypoxic events

No individual intermediate measure can precisely link intrapartum complications to absolute outcomes. Several groups have proposed pathways by which combinations of intermediate measures can help to define a causal intrapartum hypoxic event. The International Cerebral Palsy Task Force has listed criteria essential to link brain injury to an earlier intrapartum hypoxic event.[1] They include:

- evidence of a metabolic acidosis at birth (pH <7.00 and base deficit >12 mmol/L),
- early-onset moderate or severe encephalopathy,
- cerebral palsy of the spastic quadriplegic or dyskinetic type.

Other features that support an intrapartum hypoxic event include:

- a sentinel hypoxic event around the time of labour,
- a deterioration in the fetal heart rate pattern around the time of the sentinel event after a previously normal pattern,
- Apgar scores of <7 for longer than 5 minutes,
- early-onset multi-organ dysfunction,
- early imaging evidence of an acute cerebral abnormality.

## WHAT TYPE OF FETAL MONITORING IS BEST?

The Dublin Trial of Intermittent versus Continuous Monitoring remains the classic study in this field.[3] Despite subsequent studies, the conclusions have been largely unchallenged. In low-risk pregnancies, electronic continuous monitoring was better at detecting fetal acidosis and led to a reduced incidence of neonatal seizures. However, it did not appear to have any influence on the absolute outcomes of mortality and long-term handicap. Meta-analysis seems to support these conclusions, although it is recognized that the data are insufficient to detect a true difference in the rare absolute outcomes of death and handicap [A]. Most authorities agree that continuous monitoring leads to an increase in operative intervention, although this can be at least partially mitigated by the use of secondary tests of fetal well-being.

## WHAT IS A HIGH-RISK PREGNANCY?

The presence of any of the following risk factors at the onset of labour would label a fetus as being at 'high risk' of intrapartum hypoxia, for which the consensus is that continuous fetal monitoring should be offered:

- hypertension/pre-eclampsia,
- diabetes,
- antepartum haemorrhage (APH),
- significant maternal medical disease,
- intrauterine growth restriction (IUGR),
- preterm gestation,
- isoimmunization,
- multiple pregnancy,
- breech presentation,
- previous caesarean section,
- significant meconium staining of the amniotic fluid,
- pre-labour rupture of membranes for >24 hours,
- oligohydramnios abnormal umbilical artery Doppler studies,
- post-term pregnancy,
- epidural analgesia,
- induced or augmented labour.

Meconium staining of the amniotic fluid remains a marker of risk and is covered in more detail in Chapter 28, Meconium. In the Dublin trial, artificial rupture of the membranes was performed on admission, and the 5 per cent of women with either no fluid or significant meconium were excluded from the trial. Despite continuous monitoring and fetal blood sampling, the perinatal mortality rate in this group was 11 per 1000, compared to 2.1 per 1000 in the remaining trial participants. However, in the absence of fetal heart rate abnormalities, the presence of meconium is not an indication for fetal blood sampling.[4]

It is attractive to base intrapartum monitoring plans on a pre-labour assessment of risk. However, risk can change as labour progresses, with examples including the onset of vaginal bleeding, the development of meconium staining of the amniotic fluid or slow progress. Ongoing risk appraisal can assist the clinician in deciding how long to tolerate a suspicious (but not pathological) cardiotocograph (CTG) before employing secondary tests. It must be remembered that at least 40 per cent of cases of moderate to severe birth asphyxia in term pregnancies will occur to women in whom no antepartum risk factors were identified.[5]

## ADMISSION TESTS

Equally attractive to the pre-labour assignment of risk is an early labour re-assessment in low-risk pregnancies. In this situation, a screening test is applied to try to identify those fetuses that are more likely to develop intrapartum complications. Tools that have been used in this situation include CTGs, ultrasound assessment of amniotic fluid volume and umbilical artery Doppler. Research suggests that an abnormal admission test is associated with increased levels of obstetric intervention, but no significant reduction in adverse perinatal outcomes [B].[6,7] The RCOG/NICE guideline on intrapartum care does not recommend an admission test in women with uncomplicated pregnancies labouring at term.

## INTERMITTENT AUSCULTATION

In the low-risk situation, intermittent auscultation, either by Pinnard stethoscope or by hand-held Doppler, is often advocated. Current guidelines suggest auscultating the fetal heart rate every 15 minutes in the active phase of the first stage of labour. This should be for 60 seconds following a contraction, in order to detect significant decelerations. Maternal pulse should also be recorded by palpation to avoid confusion, particularly when a fetal heart rate abnormality is suspected.

The main criticisms of intermittent monitoring are that:

- The above standards are often not achievable on busy delivery suites.
- Gradual changes, such as an increasing baseline or falling variability, will be missed.
- There is no certification process for practitioners using intermittent monitoring.
- No hard record from the monitoring is generated and therefore it is impossible to audit any guidelines related to performing the technique.

First stage of labour

## CONTINUOUS ELECTRONIC FETAL MONITORING

The mainstay of 'high-risk' fetal assessment, electronic fetal monitoring (EFM), relies on several assumptions:

- that abnormal patterns in the fetal heart rate will be seen in the presence of compromise;
- that sufficient warning will be given to allow potentially beneficial interventions to be undertaken;
- that caregivers will recognize the abnormality and take appropriate action.

Many events, such as cord prolapse or abruption, may be so acute as to have no preceding period of deterioration in fetal well-being. Fetal monitoring may allow recognition of the problem, but no advance warning. A similar rapid deterioration may be seen in fetuses with diminished reserves at the onset of labour, such as those babies with IUGR. Alternatively, it has been suggested that a chronically compromised baby may not exhibit the same type of fetal heart rate changes when acute compromise is superimposed. CTG abnormalities in this situation may be subtle or even atypical. Low et al.[5] found that only 80 per cent of term births with metabolic acidosis exhibited a predictive fetal heart rate pattern. In other words, in one-fifth of cases, the obstetrician would have found the CTG acceptable. The pathophysiology behind other causes of neonatal harm, such as infection, may not be associated with severe or typical 'non-reassuring' fetal heart rate abnormalities until almost pre-terminal. Finally, events related to the actual delivery (trauma, shoulder dystocia, problems during resuscitation) contribute to morbidity and mortality, but cannot be predicted by intrapartum monitoring.

Some cases of abnormal intrapartum monitoring may have their roots in fetal development. Fetal cardiac anomalies are frequently undiagnosed antenatally and carry considerable morbidity and mortality. It is logical to assume that an abnormal heart will respond to the haemodynamic changes of labour atypically. Similarly, it can be difficult to disentangle prenatal neurological damage, occurring before the onset of labour, from that arising during labour. As the control of fetal heart rate involves higher centres, damage to these structures will lead to abnormal cardiovascular responses in labour. Thus, although it is tempting to assume that a poor neurological outcome is necessarily due to a stressful labour as reflected by an abnormal CTG, an alternative possibility needs to be considered, namely that pre-existing neurological damage led to an abnormal cardiovascular response to labour.

## WHAT IS A NORMAL CARDIOTOCOGRAPH?

A useful approach that helps to avoid over-reaction is initially to extract those features of a CTG that are normal by

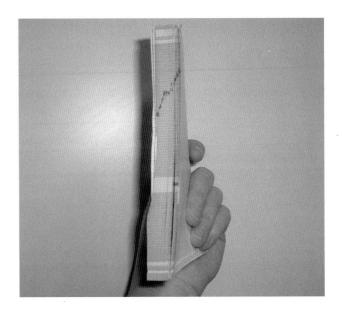

**Figure 29.1** Rising baseline

systematically reviewing baseline rate, heart rate variability and accelerations.[8]

- *Baseline*. The normal fetal baseline heart rate is 110–160 beats per minute (bpm). There is a small fall in baseline rate as gestation advances. A stable baseline over time is also important (Figure 29.1). Many women will also have had recent admissions, generating earlier CTGs for comparison.
- *Variability*. Fetal heart rate variability appears to result from a balance between sympathetic and parasympathetic influences. Therefore, a well-oxygenated nervous system is required for its full expression. Normal variability is >5 bpm. Short periods of reduced variability (particularly when associated with an inactive baby) can be entirely physiological, but in most cases variability will have recovered within 45 minutes.
- *Accelerations*. Fetal heart rate accelerations represent a response to many minor stresses. Commonly, this is fetal movement, but it also includes palpation or noise. It implies a fetus responsive to external stimuli and, therefore, intact neurocardiac pathways. Most authorities agree that accelerations are the hallmark of fetal well-being.

## WHAT IS AN ABNORMAL CARDIOTOCOGRAPH?

- *Baseline*. A continuous and progressive fetal bradycardia indicates fetal hypoxaemia. Fetal bradycardia can arise with any acute reduction in fetal oxygenation, such as cord compression, abruption or uterine hyperstimulation. If the bradycardia is moderate to severe or associated with other CTG abnormalities and the cause cannot be corrected promptly, urgent delivery will be necessary. An isolated tachycardia is rarely, if ever, associated with fetal compromise. Such a tachycardia may be appropriate in some situations. If the baby is very active, the mother will know and the variability will usually be excellent. A fetal tachycardia may arise secondary to a maternal tachycardia, often in response to pain. Clinicians must always be wary of an underlying diagnosis of chorioamnionitis as the fetus is in a hazardous environment that will not be reflected by scalp pH.

- *Variability.* A prolonged period of reduced variability, lasting >90 minutes, is clearly abnormal. The most concerning cause of decreased variability is fetal hypoxaemia, usually chronic, that has globally depressed central nervous system function. Other aetiologies include pre-existing neurological problems, maternal drugs and congenital heart block.
- *Accelerations.* These will rarely be seen in the presence of a compromised fetus.
- *Decelerations.* Decelerations arouse instant concern in many observers, particularly the less experienced. However, they should never be viewed in isolation, only

as a part of the whole clinical picture. Decelerations are usually divided into one of three types, but this can only be determined after observing a pattern repeating over time.

- *Early decelerations.* These decelerations begin with the onset of a contraction and mirror the shape of the contraction trace. They are usually thought to arise from vagal nerve stimulation secondary to cord compression. They are seen in approximately 1 in 20 first-stage CTGs and, in isolation, are rarely associated with fetal compromise (Figure 29.2).
- *Variable decelerations.* Variable decelerations are just that – variable. Each deceleration has a different shape and their timing with regard to contractions is unpredictable. They are the most common type of deceleration and are seen in up to one in eight first-stage traces (Figure 29.3). They are classically thought to arise from chemoreceptor stimulation secondary to cord compression. They may also result from head compression.
- *Late decelerations.* Late decelerations begin after the contraction, with the onset, nadir and recovery occurring after the onset, peak and end of a contraction (Figure 29.4). Only 1–2 per cent of labours

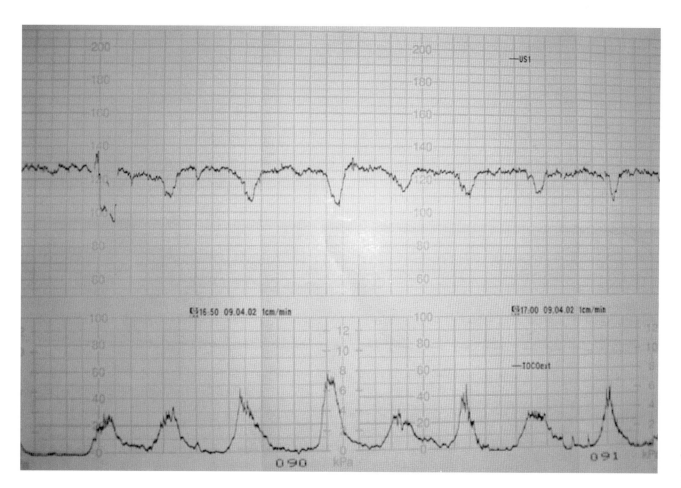

**Figure 29.2** Early decelerations

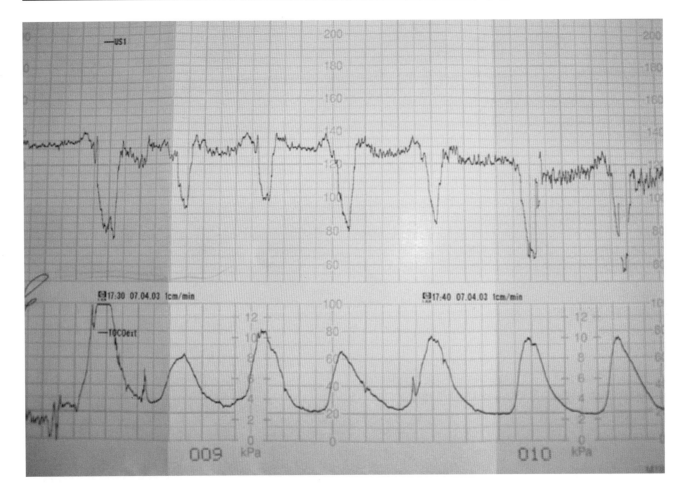

**Figure 29.3** Variable decelerations

demonstrate late decelerations in the first stage of labour. Late decelerations have been postulated to result from direct fetal myocardial depression secondary to hypoxaemia. There may be an additional contribution from chemoreceptor stimulation. Although isolated late decelerations with no other fetal heart rate abnormality are rarely associated with fetal compromise, the presence of any other coexisting abnormalities justifies secondary testing.

# CTG INTERPRETATION AND DOCUMENTATION

The RCOG and ACOG both recommend a three-tier system of interpretation of the CTG. In the UK, each CTG recording is interpreted as being either normal, suspicious or pathological (see Tables 29.1 and 29.2) and an appropriate management plan instigated in response. To assist this systematic approach, the use of a structured CTG proforma has been advocated.[9] This encourages a thorough analysis of the CTG in the clinical context, documentation of CTG findings and proposed management plan.

**Table 29.1** Categorization of fetal heart rate pattern (NICE Intrapartum Care Guideline 2007)

| Category | Definition |
| --- | --- |
| Normal | A FHR trace in which all four features are classified as reassuring |
| Suspicious | A FHR trace with one feature classified as non-reassuring and the remaining features classified as reassuring |
| Pathological | A FHR trace with two or more features classified as non-reassuring or one or more classified as abnormal |

● FHR, fetal heart rate.

No one element of the CTG should be interpreted in isolation. Regardless of how much intellectual activity is put into the interpretation of the CTG, it remains a screening test only. Even the most worrying pattern (late decelerations with reduced variability) is only associated with acidosis in 50 per cent of cases. Diagnostic or secondary tests are necessary to avoid unnecessary obstetric intervention.

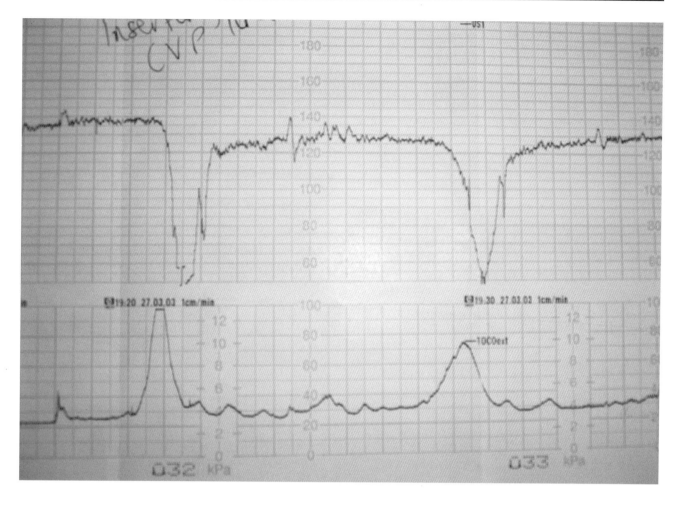

**Figure 29.4** Late decelerations

**Table 29.2** Classification of fetal heart rate trace features

| Feature | Baseline (bpm) | Variability (bpm) | Decelerations | Accelerations |
|---|---|---|---|---|
| Reassuring | 110–160 | ≥5 | None | Present |
| Non-reassuring | 100–109<br>161–180 | 40–90 min | Typical variable decelerations with over 50% of contractions, occurring for over 90 min. Single prolonged deceleration for up to 3 min | The absence of accelerations with otherwise normal trace is of uncertain significance |
| Abnormal | <100<br>>180<br>Sinusoidal pattern ≥10 min | <5 for 90 min | Either atypical variable decelerations with over 50% of contractions or late decelerations, both for over 30 min. Single prolonged deceleration for more than 3 min | |

## SECONDARY TESTS OF FETAL WELL-BEING

### Vibroacoustic stimulation

The use of vibroacoustic stimulation applied to the maternal abdomen in the presence of a non-reactive antenatal CTG is well documented.[10] The healthy fetus responds with an acceleration in fetal heart rate. The same technique has been applied in the intrapartum period. An acceleration evoked by vibroacoustic stimulation immediately prior to scalp sampling was never associated with a pH of <7.25. Vibroacoustic stimulation cannot completely eliminate the need for scalp sampling, as only 30 per cent of non-responders will be found to be acidotic. However, it can reduce the need for scalp sampling by up to 50 per cent [C].

First stage of labour

## Fetal blood sampling

Fetal scalp pH studies remain the principal secondary test of intrapartum fetal well-being. It is recommended that all units offering continuous EFM have facilities for fetal blood sampling (FBS). Fetal scalp pH lies between arterial and venous pH, but it cannot be determined to which it is closer in advance. As mentioned previously, the lower limit of normal is accepted as a pH of 7.20 in order to allow a wide margin of error. The recommended classification of fetal scalp pH is shown in Table 29.3.

- After a normal result, FBS should be repeated no more than 60 minutes later if the CTG remains pathological, or sooner if there are further abnormalities.
- After a borderline result, FBS should be repeated no more than 30 minutes later.
- An abnormal result should prompt urgent delivery.

Ideally, the base excess should also be measured to distinguish metabolic from respiratory acidosis. There is interest in simply measuring the capillary lactate levels, which provide similar information.[11] Testing systems have now been developed that require smaller volumes of fetal blood than conventional pH studies. This, in conjunction with the ability to sample at lesser dilatations, has led to a lower 'failure-to-sample' rate.

## Scalp stimulation

Most clinicians will have noted that fetuses that respond to scalp sampling with an acceleration almost always have a normal pH. This has been confirmed in formal studies, which showed 93 per cent of fetuses with a scalp pH >7.20 respond with an acceleration, compared to none of those that are acidotic.[12] This can be useful information when technical difficulties preclude sample collection. However, clinicians should always be wary of scalps that do not bleed, as this may reflect peripheral vasoconstriction in a compromised fetus.

## Fetal electrocardiogram

The knowledge that changes occur in both the fetal PR interval and ST segment of the fetal electrocardiogram (ECG) in response to hypoxaemia has prompted the use of computerized fetal ECG analysis in combination with conventional CTG to monitor the fetus in labour. Five randomized

**Table 29.3** Classification of fetal blood sample results (NICE Intrapartum Care Guideline 2007)

| Fetal blood sample result (pH) | Interpretation |
|---|---|
| ≥7.25 | Normal |
| 7.21–7.24 | Borderline |
| ≤7.20 | Abnormal |

controlled trials were included in a recent Cochrane review,[13] four examining ST segment analysis and one PR interval changes. Compared to conventional CTG, the combined used of ST analysis (STAN™) and CTG monitoring was associated with a lower risk of neonatal encephalopathy, a reduction in the number of fetal blood samplings, and fewer operative vaginal deliveries. However, there was no difference in the number of babies born with pH <7.05 or base deficit >12 mmol/L, caesarean section, or Apgar score <7 at 5 minutes. Monitoring with PR interval analysis did not appear to confer clinical benefit. This review concluded that ST analysis in labour shows promise, but there are a number of disadvantages. The technique requires the use of a spiral fetal scalp electrode and, if ST analysis is to be commenced where fetal heart rate abnormalities are present, it may be necessary to obtain the results of a fetal blood sample before commencing such monitoring.

Non-invasive fetal ECG acquisition, using abdominally sited electrodes is now technically possible[14] and in the future may become feasible in clinical practice. This technique avoids the use of a scalp electrode and also allows earlier fetal ECG monitoring in labour.

## Fetal pulse oximetry

There is no evidence that fetal pulse oximetry is of benefit in labour. The largest randomized controlled study to date failed to show any benefit in terms of caesarean section rate or neonatal condition.[15] Fetal pulse oximetry is not in use in the UK and it has not received the support of the ACOG in the United States.

# MANAGEMENT OF SUSPECTED FETAL COMPROMISE

## Improve placental blood supply

1  Correct maternal hypovolaemia and/or hypotension.
   a. Maternal positioning to avoid aorto-caval compression.
   b. Intravenous fluids when appropriate.
   c. Vasoconstrictors, such as ephedrine, for lower limb vasodilatation secondary to epidural analgesia.
2  Diminish uterine activity, particularly if excessive.
   a. Decrease or stop any oxytocin infusion.
   b. Remove vaginal prostaglandins if given recently. This may require vaginal lavage if gels have been used.
   c. Use bolus tocolytics (e.g. terbutaline 0.25 mg).

## Improve maternal oxygenation

Maternal oxygen therapy should not be used for more than a short period of time unless there is documented low maternal oxygen saturation. There is no evidence of benefit and a suggestion of possible detrimental effect when applied for more than a few minutes [A].

## Improve umbilical blood flow

Increase amniotic fluid volume. Transcervical amnioinfusion may reduce cord compression and frequently leads to an improvement in the fetal heart rate. One randomized trial showed a significant reduction in operative intervention and an improvement in cord pH at delivery.[16] Common protocols include infusing 500 mL of Hartmann's solution over 20–30 minutes followed by up to 250 mL/hour. To minimize the risk of amniotic fluid embolus and over-distension, the infusion should be gravity fed. It has also been suggested to improve fetal outcome by diluting meconium.

The decision of whether delivery is indicated, is based upon:

- clinical tests – such as the CTG and secondary tests of fetal well-being, including fetal blood sampling;
- the whole picture – including obstetric risk factors and progress in labour;
- untreatable fetal complications – such as abruption, cord prolapse and chorioamnionitis, scar dehiscence.

## A CLINICAL APPROACH TO REVIEWING INTRAPARTUM CTGs IN THE FIRST STAGE OF LABOUR

Does the abnormality require immediate delivery if it continues?

If **Yes** (think little, do lots):

1  Is there a possible precipitant?
   a. Cord prolapse/recent epidural/excessive uterine activity/bleeding/scar dehiscence, etc.
   b. If possible, rapidly take steps to correct any precipitants identified.
   c. If no corrective steps are possible or there is no response, deliver by caesarean section.

If **No** (do little, think lots):

1  For comparison, has there been a 'normal' CTG:
   a. earlier in labour?
   b. within a few weeks of admission?
2  On the current CTG, what normal features are present?
   a. stable baseline with normal rate,
   b. good variability.
   c. accelerations.
3  On the current CTG, what abnormal features are present?

Compare 1 and 2 with 3 to decide on the severity of any CTG abnormality and classify as *normal*, *suspicious* or *pathological* (see Table 29.1).

4  Is there a possible precipitant?
   a. Cord prolapse/cord compression/recent epidural/ excessive uterine activity/bleeding/scar dehiscence, etc.

If possible, take steps to correct any precipitants identified in 4.

5  What risk factors were present in the antenatal period?
6  Were there any recent changes immediately prior to labour?
   a. Maternal illness/reduced fetal activity, etc.
7  Have any risk factors developed during labour?
   a. Meconium/bleeding/poor progress/fever, etc.

Then use 5, 6 and 7 to decide:

- if and for how long this abnormality can be tolerated before delivering or employing secondary tests of fetal well-being (eg. fetal blood sampling), and
- when to next review the CTG – a deliberate plan is the best approach.

Always try to answer 'What is causing this CTG abnormality?'.

Do not forget 'benign' causes, such as recent narcotic analgesia or a rapidly progressing labour.

## ACKNOWLEDGEMENT

This chapter has been revised and updated. The author and editors acknowledge the contribution of Griff Jones to the chapter on this topic in the previous edition of the book.

### KEY POINTS

- Intrapartum events rarely lead to perinatal mortality or neurodevelopmental handicap after uncomplicated term pregnancies.
- Electronic fetal monitoring is a crude screening test with a poor predictive value for acidosis.
- Always review electronic fetal monitoring in the context of the whole pregnancy.
- Secondary tests of fetal well-being after non-reassuring CTGs are necessary to avoid over-intervention.
- Intrauterine therapy can improve non-reassuring CTGs and reduce operative delivery.

## Published Guidelines

National Institute for Health and Clinical Excellence. Intrapartum care – care of the healthy women and their babies during childbirth. London: NICE, September 2007.

First stage of labour

# Key References

1. MacLennan A. A template for defining a causal relation between acute intrapartum events and cerebral palsy: international consensus statement. *BMJ* 1999; **319**: 1054–9.
2. Smith GC. Life-table analysis of the risk of perinatal death at term and post term in singleton pregnancies. *Am J Obstet Gynecol* 2001; **184**: 489–96.
3. MacDonald D, Grant A, Sheridan-Pereira M *et al*. The Dublin randomized controlled trial of intrapartum fetal heart rate monitoring. *Am J Obstet Gynecol* 1985; **152**: 524–39.
4. Baker PN, Kilby MD, Murray H. An assessment of the use of meconium alone as an indication for fetal blood sampling. *Obstet Gynecol* 1992; **80**: 792–6.
5. Low JA, Pickersgill H, Killen H, Derrick EJ. The prediction and prevention of intrapartum fetal asphyxia in term pregnancies. *Am J Obstet Gynecol* 2001; **184**: 724–30.
6. Chauhan SP, Washburne JF, Magann EF *et al*. A randomized study to assess the efficacy of the amniotic fluid index as a fetal admission test. *Obstet Gynecol* 1995; **86**: 9–13.
7. Blix E, Reinar LM, Klovning A, Oian P. Prognostic value of the labour admission test and its effectiveness compared with auscultation only: a systematic review. *BJOG* 2005; **112**: 1595–604.
8. Macones GA, Hankins GD, Spong CY *et al*. The 2008 National Institute of Child Health and Human Development workshop report on electronic fetal monitoring: update on definitions, interpretation, and research guidelines. *Obstet Gynecol* 2008; **112**: 661–6.
9. Siassakos D. NICE training improves outcomes: making the right way the easiest way, 2008. Available from ‹www.nice.org.uk›.
10. Polzin GB, Blakemore KJ, Petrie RH, Amon E. Fetal vibro-acoustic stimulation: magnitude and duration of fetal heart rate accelerations as a marker of fetal health. *Obstet Gynecol* 1988; **72**: 621–6.
11. Wiberg-Itzel E, Lipponer C, Norman M *et al*. Determination of pH or lactate in fetal scalp blood in management of intrapartum fetal distress: randomised controlled multicentre trial. *BMJ* 2008; **336**: 1284–7.
12. Clark SL, Gimovsky ML, Miller FC. Fetal heart rate response to scalp blood sampling. *Am J Obstet Gynecol* 1982; **144**: 706–8.
13. Neilson JP. Fetal electrocardiogram (ECG) for fetal monitoring during labour. *Cochrane Database Syst Rev* 2006; (**3**): CD000116.
14. Taylor MJ, Thomas MJ, Smith MJ *et al*. Non-invasive intrapartum fetal ECG: preliminary report. *BJOG* 2005; **112**: 1016–21.
15. Bloom SL, Spong CY, Thom E *et al*. Fetal pulse oximetry and cesarean delivery. *N Engl J Med* 2006; **355**: 2195–202.
16. Schrimmer DB, Macri CJ, Paul RH. Prophylactic amnioinfusion as a treatment for oligohydramnios in laboring patients: a prospective, randomized trial. *Am J Obstet Gynecol* 1991; **165**: 972–5.

# Obstetric anaesthesia and analgesia

*David M Levy*

## INTRODUCTION

Obstetric *analgesia* is pain relief in labour; *anaesthesia* is the abolition of sufficient sensation to allow operative delivery.

Provision of analgesia is a key element of the modern management of labour. Women receive education antenatally about the options for analgesia in labour and often have very high expectations on admission to the delivery suite.

Regional (spinal, epidural or combined spinal–epidural) anaesthesia is now used for the vast majority of caesarean sections.

## ANALGESIA FOR LABOUR

Modes of analgesia include:

- relaxation therapy;
- immersion in warm water;
- aromatherapy;
- transcutaneous electrical nerve stimulation (TENS);
- inhalation of nitrous oxide – and other inhalational anaesthetics – in oxygen;
- parenteral opioids;
- regional analgesia.

The requirement for pharmacological pain relief in labour is reduced when a known practitioner provides continuous support throughout labour [A].[1] Immersion in water during the first stage of labour reduces analgesic requirements.[2] The evidence underpinning nonpharmacologic methods of pain relief in labour (including continuous support, bathing, upright position and massage) has been systematically reviewed.[3]

## Transcutaneous electrical nerve stimulation

Electrical impulses are applied to the skin via flexible carbon electrodes from a battery-powered stimulator. Stimulation of A-fibre transmission and local release of β-endorphins modulate pain, closing a postulated 'gate' in the dorsal horn of the spinal cord. The effect is similar to massage of the lower back by a birthing partner.

- Electrodes are placed over the T10–L1 dermatomes on either side of the spinous processes to provide analgesia for the first stage of labour. A second set of electrodes is placed over the S2–S4 dermatomes for second stage pain relief. Women can control the level of current delivered.
- There is no evidence that TENS provides better analgesia than placebo ('sham' TENS). However, TENS can diminish the need for other analgesic interventions, and is completely free from adverse effects.[4] TENS 'analgesia' seems to be rated more highly in retrospect than contemporaneously.

## Opioid analgesia

The analgesic efficacy of opioids in labour is limited, although sedation is almost invariable.[5]

- All opioids can cause decreased Apgar and neurobehavioural scores and neonatal respiratory depression, even when administered many hours before birth.
- Neonatal respiratory depression is readily reversible with naloxone, a specific opioid antagonist. The neonatal dose is 10 μg/kg i.m., repeated if necessary.

• Maternal gastric emptying is inhibited and the incidence of nausea and vomiting increased. An anti-emetic (e.g. cyclizine 50 mg or prochlorperazine 12.5 mg) should be given i.m. with the chosen opioid.

• Midwives can prescribe and administer controlled drugs in accordance with Nursing and Midwifery Council (Midwives) Rules and locally agreed policies and procedures. In the UK, pethidine is the most widely used i.m. opioid, although the use of diamorphine is increasing in the UK without evidence of greater efficacy.[6] Comparisons of pethidine 100 mg with diamorphine 5 mg, meptazinol 100 mg and tramadol 100 mg have failed to demonstrate superior analgesic efficacy or a more favourable side-effect profile associated with any one agent.

• Because of the additive risk of maternal respiratory depression, i.m. opioids should never be given in the event of inadequate regional analgesia without prior reassessment of the woman by an anaesthetist.

• A reduction in baseline cardiotocograph (CTG) variability can make interpretation difficult.

## Patient-controlled analgesia

Intravenous opioid by patient-controlled analgesia (PCA) system is useful in women with thrombocytopenia or other haematological reasons for avoiding regional analgesia or i.m. injections. The potency and rapidity of action of remifentanil can predispose to sudden respiratory depression – as labour pain is episodic as opposed to continuous, the therapeutic window is particularly narrow. There appears to be wide variation in the dose required for effective labour analgesia.

Despite a slower onset of action and less rapid clearance, fentanyl is perhaps the drug of choice, by 20–30 μg bolus and 5 min lockout period [E].

## Analgesia by inhalation

Sixty to 70 per cent of labouring women in the UK seek analgesia by inhalation of a 50:50 mixture of nitrous oxide and oxygen ($N_2O/O_2$). Marketed as Entonox® and Equanox®, the gas mixture is supplied in cylinders with a blue body and blue/white shoulders and is piped to labour rooms in many hospitals. The future availability of nitrous oxide is not assured. Protracted inhalation of $N_2O$ can inactivate vitamin $B_{12}$ and inhibit DNA synthesis. Isoflurane and sevoflurane, two fluorinated, potent inhalational anaesthetics, have been studied in labour at low doses, but not yet widely adopted.[5]

• $N_2O/O_2$ is self-administered by inspiration through a facemask or mouthpiece, which opens a demand valve. Diffusion from alveoli to pulmonary capillaries and delivery to the brain by the cardiac output are not instantaneous. Inhalation should therefore start as soon as a contraction begins, to allow maximum drug effect at the peak.

• The drug is non-cumulative and does not affect the fetus. $N_2O/O_2$ causes highly variable maternal sedation. Some women appear to be dreaming or drunk; others become somnolent or even briefly unrousable.

• Hyperventilation with $N_2O/O_2$ can be followed by a short period of apnoea; therefore, the woman should always hold the mouthpiece or mask herself. If she loses consciousness, she will let go. A few breaths of air eliminate the $N_2O$ and consciousness is invariably soon regained.

• A number of studies have questioned the analgesic effect of $N_2O/O_2$. Pain is often still perceived under the influence of the drug – it is merely rendered more bearable by the intoxicated state. Thirty to 40 per cent of women in labour derive no benefit.

• The risk of cross-contamination between patients sharing breathing systems dictates that mouthpieces and masks should be disposable, or sterilized between patients. Either a new disposable breathing system should be used for each patient, or a disposable breathing system filter interposed between the tubing and mouthpiece/mask.

## Regional analgesia for labour

Regional analgesia is the provision of pain relief by blockade of sensory nerves as they enter the spinal cord. Local anaesthetic and/or opioid can be introduced into epidural and/or subarachnoid (intrathecal) spaces.

Comparisons of regional analgesia regimens require careful scrutiny of which drugs have been introduced into which space(s) and their mode of administration (bolus or infusion).

Compared with other analgesic modalities, pain relief from regional blockade is undoubtedly superior.[7] Ninety per cent of consultant obstetric units in the UK provide a 24-hour regional analgesia service. The UK Obstetric Anaesthetists' Association (OAA) captured data in 2005 from 513 660 mothers in 166 units. The regional analgesia rate was 24.6 per cent. In the USA, the rate is 60 per cent.

Contraindications to regional blockade are outlined in Table 30.1. Subcutaneous low molecular weight heparin (LMWH) within the previous 10–12 hours is a relative contraindication. Scar tissue from previous spinal surgery can make identification of the epidural space difficult, and impede spread of local anaesthetic solution. However, catheterization of the subarachnoid space might nevertheless be feasible – early referral (ideally with the post-operative radiographs) should be made to an obstetric anaesthetist. Untreated pyrexia in labour raises the possibility of bacteraemia and seeding a vertebral canal abscess in the event of bleeding from an epidural vein. However, the likelihood of such a complication has to be weighed against the probably greater risks of general anaesthesia (e.g. anaphylaxis to succinylcholine) that might otherwise be avoided. Regional analgesia has been shown to cause pyrexia in labour in

**Table 30.1** Contraindications to regional analgesia, with associated risks

| Contraindication | Risk |
| --- | --- |
| Uncorrected anticoagulation or coagulopathy | Vertebral canal haematoma |
| Local or systemic sepsis (pyrexia >38°C not treated with antibiotics) | Vertebral canal abscess |
| Hypovolaemia or active haemorrhage | Cardiovascular collapse secondary to sympathetic blockade |
| Patient refusal | Legal action |
| Lack of sufficient trained midwives for continuous care and monitoring of mother and fetus for the duration of epidural blockade | Delayed recognition and treatment of maternal collapse/convulsion/ respiratory arrest or fetal compromise |

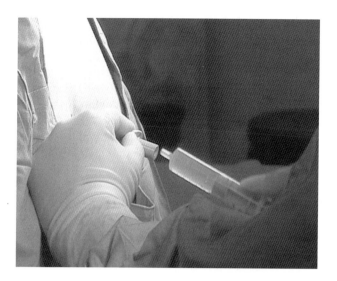

**Figure 30.1** Tuohy needle with loss-of-resistance syringe

around 15 per cent of women. Suggested mechanisms include abolition of hyperventilation and sweating (from the lower half of the body) and promotion of shivering. The potential importance is that maternal fever, particularly in association with fetal acidosis, greatly increases the risk of neonatal encephalopathy. Acetaminophen (paracetamol) and active cooling are indicated.

The link between epidural analgesia and backache has been thoroughly investigated and no evidence of causation found.[7] The risk of permanent neurological injury is probably less than 1:100 000. Obstetric palsies (e.g. compression of the lumbosacral trunk) are far more common.

Regional analgesia does not impair the initiation of breast feeding.

## Epidurals and spinals

The epidural space is identified by the loss of resistance to depression of a syringe plunger as a Tuohy needle is advanced (Figure 30.1) through the ligamentum flavum. A catheter is then threaded through the Tuohy needle (Figure 30.2) to facilitate bolus top-ups or a continuous infusion. The subarachnoid space, which contains cerebrospinal fluid (CSF), is a few millimetres deeper, inside the meninges. Needles used for deliberate spinal injection are much finer than Tuohy needles (Figure 30.3). Unlike local anaesthetics, which prevent the conduction of nerve impulses, opioids act on specific receptors in the spinal cord. Synergistic mixtures of local anaesthetic and opioids (usually fentanyl) have permitted significant reductions in the amount of local anaesthetic used. Side effects specific to opioids are respiratory depression (in the most unlikely event of cephalad spread of opioid to the brainstem) and pruritus.

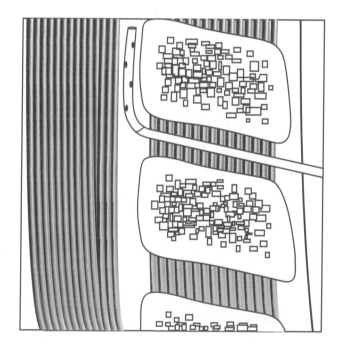

**Figure 30.2** Tuohy needle advanced through the ligamentum flavum, with the catheter in the epidural space

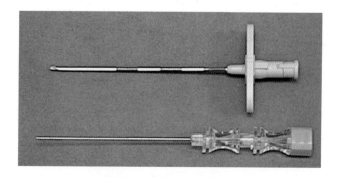

**Figure 30.3** Epidural Tuohy (above) and spinal needles

First stage of labour

## Dural tap

Accidental meningeal puncture with a Tuohy needle is called a 'dural tap'. Eighty-five per cent of women who have a dural tap will develop a severe, characteristically postural headache, caused by leakage of CSF. Only the presence of headache during labour is an indication for elective forceps or vacuum extraction at full dilatation. The definitive treatment is epidural injection of autologous blood (up to 20 mL) – a 'blood patch', best undertaken at 24–48 hours post-delivery. Occasionally, the patch has to be repeated. Women with persistent headache must be followed up until symptom-free. Intracranial hypotension (low CSF pressure) can be complicated (albeit very rarely) by cranial subdural haematoma secondary to tearing of a dural bridging vein.

## Total spinal

Five to ten times the dose of local anaesthetic is required for an equivalent effect after epidural as opposed to subarachnoid injection. Any communication between epidural and subarachnoid spaces introduces the risk of a large dose of local anaesthetic, intended for the epidural space, reaching the subarachnoid space. A block high enough to impair diaphragmatic innervation and cause respiratory arrest is known as a 'total spinal'. A total spinal should be a survivable event for mother and fetus. The mother will require emergency tracheal intubation and treatment of hypotension. The urgency of caesarean section will be dictated by the fetal heart rate pattern. Tracheal extubation should be feasible within 2–3 hours, once the high block has regressed.

## Local anaesthetic toxicity

If local anaesthetic is injected inadvertently into an epidural vein, symptoms and signs of local anaesthetic toxicity (Table 30.2) can arise from the effect of high concentrations of local anaesthetic in the central nervous system (CNS). Initial treatment follows the 'ABC' principle: airway, breathing and circulation (with relief of aorto-caval compression). A new, specific and effective treatment has been introduced for local anaesthetic-induced cardiac arrest: intravenous Intralipid™ 20 per cent. The dose for a 70 kg adult is 100 mL. All delivery suites should have a readily available emergency LipidRescue™ box, containing a 500 mL bag of Intralipid 20 per cent, 50 mL syringes and giving set. Details of evolving guidelines for this novel treatment are available at ‹www.lipidrescue.org›. One of the deaths in the most recent Report on Confidential Enquiries into Maternal Deaths[8] (accidental i.v. administration of bupivacaine from an infusion bag intended for epidural use) might have been averted had this therapy been available.

## Combined spinal–epidural analgesia

Combined spinal–epidural (CSE) analgesia entails an initial subarachnoid injection of fentanyl (in the UK) mixed with a small amount of local anaesthetic. The spinal injection makes the onset of analgesia considerably faster (5 minutes, as opposed to at least 20 minutes with an epidural). The resulting motor block is sufficiently minimal for women to retain sufficient muscle power to walk in labour. However, depending on the drug regimen, proprioception (information from joint receptors to maintain balance) might be impaired. The Comparative Obstetric Mobile Epidural Trial (COMET)[9] found that both low-dose infusion epidurals and CSE analgesia resulted in a lower incidence of instrumental vaginal deliveries compared to traditional intermittent (midwife-administered) bolus epidurals (Table 30.3) [B]. It is presumed that this is attributable to the preservation of motor tone and the bearing-down reflex, as mode of delivery was not influenced by whether or not women walked during the first stage of labour. The effect of mobility after full cervical dilatation remains equivocal.[10] A Cochrane review failed to find a difference in overall maternal satisfaction with CSE compared to epidural analgesia, despite the faster onset. CSEs were associated with more pruritus.[11]

## Patient-controlled epidural analgesia

Some units favour self-administration of epidural opioid and local anaesthetic: patient-controlled epidural analgesia (PCEA).[12] Compared with continuous infusion techniques, PCEA reduces the total administered dose of local anaesthetic, the degree of motor block and the number of anaesthetists' interventions. Some studies suggest that analgesia is improved by a continuous background infusion.

**Table 30.2** Symptoms and signs of local anaesthetic toxicity

| Symptoms | Signs |
| --- | --- |
| Numbness of tongue or lips | Slurring of speech |
| Tinnitus | Drowsiness |
| Light-headedness | Convulsions |
| Anxiety | Cardiorespiratory arrest |

**Table 30.3** COMET: analgesic regimen and mode of delivery

| Delivery | 'Traditional' epidural (n = 353) | Combined spinal epidural (n = 351) | Low-dose infusion epidural (n = 350) |
| --- | --- | --- | --- |
| Normal vaginal | 124 (35%) | 150 (43%) | 150 (43%) |
| Instrumental vaginal | 131 (37%) | 102 (29%) | 98 (28%) |
| Caesarean section | 98 (28%) | 99 (28%) | 102 (29%) |

- p = 0.04, 1DF (degree of freedom) for normal versus other deliveries.

## Regional analgesia and progress of labour

Regional analgesia can improve utero-placental blood flow in labour. However, a fall in blood pressure after a bolus dose of local anaesthetic can precipitate a fetal bradycardia. Adoption of full left-lateral position and treatment of hypotension by i.v. fluid bolus and/or vasopressor should resolve the fetal heart rate abnormality.

Despite better pain relief than other methods of analgesia, regional analgesia has been associated with longer first and second stages of labour, an increased incidence of fetal malposition, greater use of syntocinon®, and an increased risk of instrumental vaginal birth. No direct effect on the caesarean section rate has been demonstrated.[7]

A recent large, randomized controlled trial compared neuraxial (subarachnoid) fentanyl (at the initiation of CSE) with parenteral opioid (hydromorphone) at the first request for pain relief in labour, with deferral of regional analgesia.[13] Women who received early CSE experienced superior analgesia and a shorter duration of labour. The rates of caesarean section and instrumental delivery were similar (the study had 90 per cent power to detect a 50 per cent difference in caesarean section rate) [B].

There is no high level evidence upon which to withhold modern regional analgesia because an arbitrary degree of cervical dilatation has not yet been achieved.

## Instrumental delivery

When epidural analgesia is topped up for instrumental delivery, the block height and density should be adequate for caesarean section, in case the need arises to proceed swiftly to operative delivery if the instrument application fails.

## ANAESTHESIA FOR CAESAREAN SECTION

The OAA 2005 data collection identified a caesarean section rate of 23.9 per cent. Fifty-nine per cent were performed under single-shot spinal anaesthesia. Epidural anaesthesia was used in 23 per cent of cases (most were topped-up labour epidurals and CSEs). *De novo* CSEs accounted for 7 per cent of cases; the GA rate was 11 per cent (Figure 30.4). The UK National Institute for Health and Clinical Excellence (NICE) caesarean section guideline ‹www.nice.org.uk/Guidance/CG13› includes anaesthesia recommendations.

## Categorization of urgency

Good communication among obstetric, anaesthetic, midwifery and theatre staff is vital for a well-organized caesarean section. A four-point classification of urgency of caesarean section (Table 30.4), similar to that used by the National Confidential Enquiry into Patient Outcome and Death (NCEPOD), has been validated by close

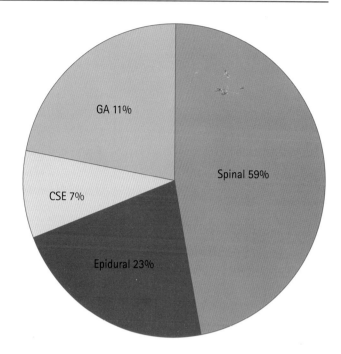

**Figure 30.4** UK caesarean sections, 2005. CSE, combined spinal-epidural; GA, general anaesthesia

**Table 30.4** Classification of urgency for caesarean section

| Category | Definition |
|---|---|
| Emergency (1) | Immediate threat to life of woman or fetus |
| Urgent (2) | Maternal or fetal compromise that is not immediately life threatening |
| Scheduled (3) | Needing early delivery but no maternal or fetal compromise |
| Elective (4) | At a time to suit the woman and maternity team |

agreement between anaesthetists' and obstetricians' gradings of more than 400 cases, and recently reassessed.[14] A decision-to-delivery interval of 30 minutes has become widely adopted as an audit standard, despite lack of any evidence that 30 minutes is a critical threshold in the development of intrapartum hypoxia. Spinal anaesthesia is often appropriate for urgent (Table 30.4) caesarean section, although a Confidential Enquiry into Stillbirths and Deaths in Infancy (CESDI) deemed repeated attempts at regional anaesthesia to be inadvisable in the absence of significant risk factors for general anaesthesia.[15] Auditable standards published by the Royal College of Anaesthetists (‹www.rcoa.ac.uk/docs/ARB-section8.pdf›) are listed in Table 30.5.

## *In utero* fetal resuscitation

Anaesthetists are increasingly attuned to contributing to the multidisciplinary management of *in utero* fetal

**Table 30.5** Audit recommendations: Royal College of Anaesthetists

| Proposed standard or target for best practice | >95% RA for elective (category 4) CS |
| --- | --- |
| | >85% RA for emergency (combined categories 1 to 3) CS |
| | <1% RA to GA conversion rate in elective CS |
| | <3% RA to GA conversion rate in emergency CS. (This figure of 3% includes regional anaesthetics for labour converted to GA for CS) |
| Suggested data to be collected | Number of CS, category of CS, type of anaesthetic and reason for its use |
| | Name and grade of anaesthetist and surgeon |
| | Conversion rate to GA and reason (e.g. technical difficulty, poor block, maternal request, fetal or surgical reasons) |
| | In particular, data collected should allow units to identify reasons for a low RA rate (or high RA to GA conversion rate) for category 1 CS, since this is the group most at risk from GA |

- CS, caesarean section; GA, general anaesthesia; RA, regional anaesthesia.

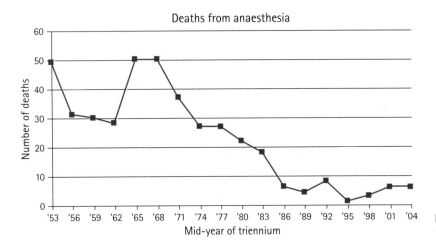

**Figure 30.5** Maternal mortality (number of deaths) from anaesthesia 1952–2005

compromise. The Bristol 'SPOILT' acronym is a useful aide memoire:

- **S**yntocinon® off
- **P**osition: full left lateral
- **O**xygen
- **I**.v. infusion of crystalloid
- **L**ow blood pressure: i.v. vasopressor
- **T**ocolysis: s.c. terbutaline 250 µg.

## Mortality

Maternal mortality attributed to anaesthesia has fallen considerably over the last 50 years (Figure 30.5). Capnography is arguably the most valuable component of physiological monitoring. Tracheal or oesophageal intubation can be confirmed immediately, with complete accuracy.

## Antacid prophylaxis

Fasting intervals of 6 hours for food and 2 hours for fluids (tea/coffee with semi-skimmed milk, or fruit squash) are appropriate for women scheduled for elective caesarean section. Ranitidine diminishes gastric acid secretion; sodium citrate neutralizes acid already in the stomach. Ranitidine 150 mg should be prescribed for 2 hours before an elective operation and administered 8-hourly to all women in labour with risk factors for caesarean section. Administration of a measure (30 mL) of sodium citrate 0.3 m immediately before caesarean section is almost universal practice. The risk of aspiration of gastric contents is not confined to general anaesthesia: protective laryngeal reflexes may be obtunded in the event of an excessively high regional block.

## Regional anaesthesia

### Single-shot spinal anaesthesia

Single-shot spinal anaesthesia has become the most popular anaesthetic technique for caesarean section (Figure 30.4), largely as a consequence of the widespread adoption of pencil-point tip needles (Figure 30.6). Compared to standard cutting bevel (or Quincke) needle tips, there is less leakage of CSF and a lower incidence of headache requiring epidural blood patch.

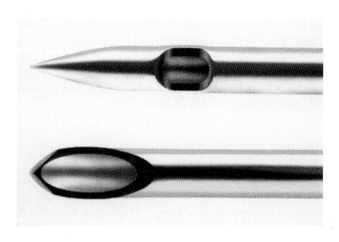

**Figure 30.6** Pencil-point (above) and cutting bevel-tip spinal needles

## Preload – or coload?

A crystalloid fluid preload has become recognized as an ineffective means of preventing hypotension after spinal injection. Its short intravascular half-life prevents a sustained increase in cardiac output before sympathetic blockade develops. Rather than infuse crystalloid before spinal blockade, fluid is best given (from pressurized infusion bag) as the block develops – hence 'coload'. Colloids, such as hydroxyethyl starch, have a longer intravascular half-life. They increase cardiac output and prevent hypotension more reliably than crystalloid. However, all colloids incur a risk of anaphylaxis, and concern has been raised that the further increase in cardiac output from autotransfusion of blood as the uterus contracts after delivery might precipitate circulatory overload.

Hypotension is best managed by:

- strict avoidance of aorto-caval compression;
- rapid infusion of crystalloid immediately after intrathecal injection;
- prompt boluses or infusion of vasopressor.

## Level of injection

Magnetic resonance imaging has shown that the conus medullaris of the spinal cord extends below the level of the body of L1 in 20 per cent of patients. Moreover, anaesthetists commonly underestimate the height of their approach. A series of case reports describing damage to the conus medullaris has led to an authoritative recommendation that spinal needles should not be inserted higher than the L3/4 interspinous space – practically, the space at or immediately above a line joining the highest points of the iliac crests.

## Dose of local anaesthetic

Most UK obstetric anaesthetists use hyperbaric bupivacaine 0.5 per cent. Gestation is important when deciding upon the dose for a single-shot spinal. In one study, loss of

cold sensation to T4 was achieved with 2.25 mL in all of a group of women at term, but only 16 per cent of women at 28–35 weeks gestation. The progressively gravid uterus causes increasing vena caval compression, epidural venous engorgement and consequent displacement of the dura and reduced subarachnoid space volume. Postural manoeuvres after intrathecal injection, such as moving from right to left lateral or flexing the knees and thighs, promote cephalad spread of the injectate by influencing vertebral canal blood volume.

Loss of light touch sensation to T5 is a better predictor of pain-free caesarean section under (opioid-free) spinal anaesthesia than loss of cold sensation. Light touch sensation is ascertained by asking if the woman has any appreciation of ethyl chloride dripped on to skin. The extent of the block and modality of testing should be recorded in case a subsequent claim of intraoperative pain has to be defended. The obstetrician must clarify with the anaesthetist that it is appropriate to start surgery.

Spinal anaesthesia can cause, within 5 minutes, a high block with precipitous fall in blood pressure – even despite i.v. coload and vasopressor. Relief of aortocaval compression by swift delivery of the baby will be required urgently. Obstetricians should not, therefore, leave the theatre suite during induction of spinal anaesthesia.

## Opioids

The addition of intrathecal fentanyl, diamorphine or morphine can reduce the incidence of intraoperative visceral pain, although fentanyl does not contribute significantly to post-operative analgesia. Reports of respiratory depression after intrathecal doses of opioids in obstetric practice are conspicuous by their absence. Intraoperative pain should be treated promptly by i.v. alfentanil (0.5 mg increments) or inhaled isoflurane or sevoflurane in an $N_2O/O_2$ 50:50 mixture, i.v. ketamine (20 mg increments) or conversion to general anaesthesia.

## Vasopressors

Ephedrine (alpha and beta sympathomimetic) was regarded as the vasopressor of choice in obstetrics for decades. Persisting reservations about the effects of alpha-agonists on uteroplacental blood flow were founded on studies of Columbian ewes, which did not undergo regional anaesthesia. Randomized comparisons of i.v. boluses of ephedrine and phenylephrine in women undergoing caesarean section found similar changes in maternal systolic pressure and cardiac output, but significantly lower UA pH in neonates whose mothers had received ephedrine. Increased fetal metabolic rate secondary to ephedrine-induced beta-adrenergic stimulation may be the explanation. Infusions of phenylephrine, compared with ephedrine, are associated with improved maternal haemodynamic control and less nausea and vomiting [B].[16] Phenylephrine is now widely regarded as the vasopressor of choice at caesarean section and should mitigate the slight fetal acidosis that was observed in a meta-analysis of spinals compared with epidurals or general anaesthetics.

## Spinal anaesthesia and pre-eclampsia

Over the last few years, it has become accepted by many that pre-eclampsia is not necessarily a contraindication to single-shot spinal anaesthesia; if the abnormal systemic vasoconstriction is of humoral rather than neural aetiology, sympathetic blockade should not, logically, cause precipitous hypotension. Prior vasodilatation by effective antihypertensive treatment (e.g. oral methyldopa or i.v. hydralazine) with limited intravascular volume expansion seems to avert problematic hypotension. Judicious fluid boluses and small increments of either ephedrine or phenylephrine will correct hypotension. Pre-emptive infusions of vasopressor are best avoided to avoid arterial pressure overshoot.

## Post-operative analgesia

Supplementation of intrathecal diamorphine or morphine by regular oral, rectal or i.v. paracetamol (1 g 6-hourly) and diclofenac (50 mg 8-hourly, 12 hours after an initial 100 mg post-operative dose), with oral dihydrocodeine if required (60 mg 4-hourly), makes patient-controlled i.v. morphine unnecessary for most women. Non-steroidal anti-inflammatory drugs (NSAIDs) are contraindicated in the initial post-operative period if caesarean section has been complicated by excessive bleeding or there is concern about the adequacy of haemostasis (e.g. uterine atony). In pre-eclampsia, prescription of NSAIDs should be deferred until 24 hours postpartum and confirmation

of normal renal function. Transversus abdominis plane (TAP) blocks (Figure 30.7) have emerged as highly effective adjuncts to other analgesic modalities. Morphine requirements (as evidenced by PCA morphine consumption) can be markedly reduced, if no long-acting intrathecal opioid has been administered.[17]

## Epidural anaesthesia

Few elective caesarean sections are now performed under epidural anaesthesia, because the quality of anaesthesia is generally poorer than that afforded by subarachnoid block. The rate of conversion to general anaesthesia for epidurals is consistently greater than that for spinals. *De novo* epidural anaesthesia is still favoured by some when gradual establishment of block is desired to minimize hypotension. In severe pre-eclampsia, postoperative infusion of epidural bupivacaine/fentanyl in a high-dependency area will confer optimal analgesia and contribute to blood pressure control. A South African study demonstrated that women who were fully conscious and co-operative after an eclamptic seizure could safely undergo caesarean section under epidural anaesthesia. All women had platelet counts $>100 \times 10^9$/L and had been treated with magnesium sulphate.[18]

## Conversion of labour analgesia

In women in labour deemed high risk for caesarean section – and those with potentially difficult airways – consideration should be given to instituting epidural analgesia early. It should be established that the block is working well, without missed segments. If analgesia in labour has been poor, it is unlikely that anaesthesia for caesarean section will be satisfactory. Conversion

LS - Lumbar spine
LD - Latissimus dorsi
PM - Psoas major
QL - Quadratus lumborum
MM - Mulitfidus, Iliocostalis
TA - Transverse abdominis
IO - Internal oblique
EO - External oblique
N - 50mm blunt tipped needle
ST - Subcutaneous tissue

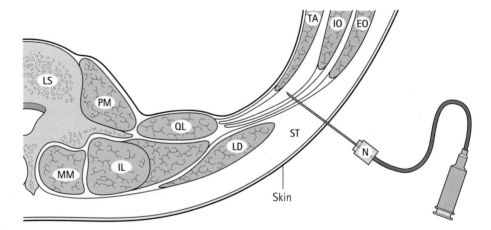

**Figure 30.7** Transversus abdominis plane block. Line drawing of a transverse section through the abdominal wall at the level of the lumbar triangle of Petit (TOP). The floor of the triangle is composed, from superficial to deep, of the fascial extensions of external oblique, internal oblique, and transversus abdominis, respectively, and the peritoneum. The needle is inserted through the triangle, using the loss-of-resistance technique. The needle is shown in the transversus abdominis plane, and the fascial layers have separated as a result of the injection of local anesthetic

of analgesia for labour to surgical anaesthesia for cae-sarean section takes around 20 minutes. In contrast to single-shot spinal anaesthesia, abrupt changes in blood pressure are unusual. Good communication among mid-wives, obstetricians and anaesthetists should make general anaesthesia for the woman with a working epidural a rarity. Even in the event of cord prolapse, traditionally managed without question by general anaesthesia, there might be time for an epidural top-up, provided upward displacement of the presenting part is effective in avoiding cord compression.

## Combined spinal–epidural anaesthesia

Some units have adopted CSE anaesthesia as their standard technique for caesarean section, despite lack of evidence of overall superiority compared with single-shot spinals. CSE anaesthesia is useful when there is a possibility that surgery might outlast a single-shot spinal block – a standard intrathecal dose of local anaesthetic lasts typically around 90 minutes. In the event of protracted surgery (e.g. caesarean hysterectomy in a woman with placenta praevia), an epidural catheter will allow extension of the block. However, the initial spinal anaesthetic block precludes ascertainment of correct positioning of the epidural catheter.

## Continuous spinal anaesthesia

Threading a fine gauge catheter into the subarachnoid space can permit repeated fractionated bolus doses directly into the CSF compartment, allowing high quality anaesthesia which can be extended if surgery is protracted. The technique has been reserved for women with cardiovascular risk factors (e.g. complex cardiac disease) for whom abrupt sympathetic blockade might be deleterious.

The US Food and Drug Administration banned microspinal catheters (27 g or smaller) in 1992, in response to a cluster of cases of cauda equina syndrome. The cause was, in all likelihood, pooling of hyperbaric 5 per cent lidocaine (not available in the UK) in the sacral area, as opposed to morbidity associated with the catheter *per se*. A multicentre comparison of continuous intrathecal labour analgesia versus continuous epidural labour analgesia was published in 2008, powered to detect a >1 per cent incidence of neurological complications related to use of the intrathecal catheter [B].[19] There were no permanent neurological deficits in either group.

## Placenta praevia and antepartum haemorrhage

Regional anaesthesia has been associated with reduced estimated blood loss and transfusion requirements at caesarean section with placenta praevia. Although the evidence is not high level, the commonly held obstetric view that placenta praevia mandates general anaesthesia is not supported. Individual risk factors must be considered

in every case. Anterior placenta praevia in a woman over 35 who has undergone previous caesarean sections suggests a particularly high risk of placenta accreta and massive haemorrhage. General anaesthesia with intraoperative red cell salvage and provision for post-operative ICU admission might be considered prudent.

An important distinction must be made between women with the potential for major intraoperative haemorrhage (as in placenta praevia) but who are normovolaemic (i.e. have not bled), and those who present with antepartum haemorrhage. Pregnant women can compensate for significant blood loss by vasoconstriction, which will be abolished by regional anaesthesia. *Any woman who has bled and is pale and tachycardic is not suitable for regional anaesthesia, regardless of the blood pressure.*

Regional anaesthesia might be ideal for advanced placement of uterine artery balloons immediately before caesarean section, but totally inappropriate for interventional radiological management of haemorrhage.

## General anaesthesia

General anesthesia may be indicated for 'emergency' caesarean sections (Table 30.4) and for other cases for which a regional block is absolutely contraindicated (e.g. uncorrected coagulopathy) or has failed.

Good communication between the anaesthetist and obstetrician is vital in these cases, and the safety of the mother must always remain of paramount importance.

If the history or evaluation of the airway suggests that tracheal intubation might be difficult, awake fibre-optic intubation should be considered. The principal risks of general anaesthesia are:

- airway problems (e.g. failed tracheal intubation);
- aspiration of gastric contents;
- anaphylaxis (principally to succinylcholine).

In the event of anaphylaxis, adrenaline (epinephrine) is likely to improve rather than reduce utero-placental blood flow. Rapid operative delivery while the anaesthetist administers pharmacological treatment will aid maternal resuscitation.

## Depth of anaesthesia

The regimen of thiopental, succinylcholine and intubation has remained standard and largely unchanged since it superseded ether by facemask 50 years ago, and has permitted a lighter plane of inhalational general anaesthesia. General anaesthesia is 'innocuous and reversible' for the baby, provided maternal oxygenation and normocarbia are maintained, aorto-caval compression is avoided and a paediatrician is present to support neonatal ventilation. If uterine hyperstimulation has been contributory to fetal compromise, uterine relaxation conferred by a volatile agent might be therapeutic. In contrast, a maternal stress response to excessively light general anaesthesia will be to the detriment of uteroplacental blood flow. With inhalational agent monitoring now universally available, the risk of awareness in obstetric anaesthesia should have been consigned to history. Cases of explicit awareness are attributable to failures of basic anaesthetic practice (i.e. inadequate anaesthesia during neuromuscular blockade).[20]

The introduction of sugammadex, a specific antagonist for rocuronium, has offered the possibility of discontinuing the use of succinylcholine (the muscle relaxant with worst side-effect profile), 50 years after its introduction.

### Special considerations in pre-eclampsia

Any dubious notion of light general anaesthesia for the baby's benefit should be over-ridden by efforts to protect the mother's cerebral circulation. A death in the 2003–2005 Confidential Enquiries[8] was attributable to intracerebral haemorrhage sustained in the course of a predictable pressor response to difficult tracheal intubation. A generous bolus dose of opioid should be given to supplement the i.v. induction. Prior communication with a paediatrician is essential in order for preparation to be made for antagonism of opioid and provision of ventilatory support for the neonate.

The onset and duration of succinylcholine are unaffected by therapeutic serum magnesium concentrations. However, the durations of action of all non-depolarizing drugs are potentiated, and the use of a peripheral nerve stimulator is essential to ensure adequate reversal at the end of surgery. There should be a low threshold for blood pressure monitoring by radial arterial line, both in theatre and post-operatively in the high-dependency unit.

Any patient whose larynx was noted to be swollen at laryngoscopy, or in whom intubation was traumatic, is at particular risk of laryngeal oedema. Postoperative care must be undertaken in an ICU or high-dependency area with an anaesthetist immediately available. The ominous significance of stridor (impending airway obstruction) must be understood, and vigilance maintained. Should stridor develop, an anaesthetist must be called immediately.

### Special considerations for maternal cardiac disease

In labour, the sympathetic blockade consequent upon high-dose, intermittent bolus doses of epidural local anaesthetic must be avoided. Low-dose regimens can be embraced and topped up slowly and carefully if required for operative delivery [E].

Compared to regional anaesthesia, opioid-based general anaesthesia affords greater preservation of systemic vascular resistance. Regional anaesthesia avoids myocardial depression but can lead to unpredictable decreases in preload and/or afterload. General anaesthesia might therefore be preferable for caesarean section in women with fixed cardiac output states. If acute peri-operative deterioration is potentially amenable to surgical remedy (e.g. emergency valve replacement), caesarean section might best be undertaken in a cardiac theatre, with extracorporeal circulatory support immediately available.

## Pre-assessment and the role of the anaesthetist

All units should have a referral system between obstetricians and obstetric anaesthetists. Trainees and non-consultant anaesthetists providing out-of-hours cover should never be presented with complex cases 'out of the blue'. Obstetric referrals to a specialist physician's clinic (e.g. cardiology) should be brought to the attention of a consultant obstetric anaesthetist.

Anaesthetists' principal concerns are:

- the feasibility of regional block – which depends on flexion of the lumbar spine and normal coagulation;
- whether tracheal intubation at emergency caesarean section might be hazardous, e.g. because of limited neck flexion/mouth opening;
- the influence of medical conditions and their treatment on the safe conduct of regional or general anaesthesia.

The presence of morbidly obese women admitted in labour or to the antenatal ward should be brought to the attention of the duty obstetric anaesthetist. Morbid obesity should ring as many alarm bells as does severe pre-eclampsia. Regional blockade will almost certainly be a challenge, and general anaesthesia hazardous. A summary care plan with '6 Rs' mnemonic has been introduced at the Royal Berkshire NHS Foundation Trust:

1  Early review by anaesthetist on arrival on labour ward or once established labour has started;
2  Ranitidine throughout labour;
3  Early venous cannulation;
4  Regional block – consider early;
5  Heparin thromboprophylaxis – strongly consider for all but straightforward vaginal births;
6  Senior help will be needed for GA.

Criteria for referral are listed in Table 30.6.

### EBM

- The need for analgesia in labour is reduced by the continuous support of a known practitioner.
- Regional blockade is superior to other modalities of analgesia.
- Regional analgesia entails an extremely low risk of neurological complication, and does not increase the incidence of postnatal backache.
- Regional analgesia has been associated with an increased requirement for instrumental vaginal delivery, but not caesarean section.
- Continuous low-dose epidural infusions and CSEs are associated with a lower risk of instrumental vaginal delivery than conventional bolus epidural analgesia.

**Table 30.6** Criteria for antenatal anaesthetic referral

| |
| --- |
| **Cardiovascular problems** |
| Congenital heart disease |
| Valvular heart disease |
| Arrhythmias |
| Cardiomyopathy |
| Poorly controlled hypertension |
| **Respiratory problems** |
| Severe asthma (requiring steroids or hospital admission) |
| Breathlessness which limits daily activity |
| Cystic fibrosis, or any other chronic pulmonary disease |
| **Neurological/musculoskeletal problems** |
| Any spinal surgery, e.g. laminectomy, scoliosis correction |
| Congenital conditions, e.g. spina bifida |
| Muscular dystrophy, myotonia |
| Myasthenia gravis |
| Demyelinating disease (multiple sclerosis) |
| Spinal cord injury |
| Rheumatoid arthritis or any condition affecting neck/jaw |
| Cerebrovascular disease, e.g. aneurysm, arteriovenous malformation |
| **Haematological problems** |
| Anticoagulation |
| Coagulation/platelet disorders, hepatic disease |
| Patients who have been treated for malignancy, e.g. lymphoma, leukaemia (cardiorespiratory legacy of radiotherapy/chemotherapy) |
| **Airway problems** |
| Previous difficult tracheal intubation |
| Inability to open mouth or move jaw or head normally |
| **Drug-related problems** |
| Cholinesterase abnormalities – succinylcholine (Scoline) apnoea |
| Allergy or adverse reaction to anaesthetic drugs |
| Malignant hyperthermia |
| Drug misusers – with no peripheral venous access |
| **Other** |
| Morbid obesity – body mass index (weight ÷ height squared) >40 kg/m² |
| Needle phobia |
| Panic attacks |
| Any obscure eponymous syndrome that no one seems to have heard of ... which may pose problems if emergency anaesthesia is needed |
| Any women with concerns regarding analgesia or anaesthesia, e.g. previous problems with inadequate epidural for labour, or pain/awareness during caesarean section |
| Jehovah's Witnesses |

## KEY POINTS

- Opioids confer more sedation than analgesia; no one agent is superior.
- Compared to intermittent bolus epidurals, low-dose epidural infusions and combined spinal–epidural analgesia result in a lower incidence of instrumental vaginal deliveries.
- Intravenous Intralipid™ can reverse local anaesthetic-induced cardiac arrest.
- Almost 90 per cent of caesarean sections in the UK are performed under regional anaesthesia.
- Single-shot spinals are the most common regional technique for caesarean section. The addition of opioid to the local anaesthetic can reduce the incidence of intraoperative pain and provide post-operative analgesia.
- Epidural anaesthesia is generally of poorer quality than spinal anaesthesia. A combined spinal–epidural technique is useful when it is anticipated that surgery might be protracted.
- General anaesthesia is indicated for the majority of caesarean sections where there is immediate threat to the life of the mother or fetus and a regional technique is absolutely contraindicated or has failed.
- The principal risks of general anaesthesia are airway problems, aspiration of gastric contents and anaphylaxis.
- Ranitidine should be prescribed for women in labour with risk factors for caesarean section.
- Placenta praevia does not necessarily dictate general anaesthesia for caesarean section. Regional anaesthesia is inappropriate for women with signs of significant haemorrhage.
- All units should have a referral system between obstetricians and anaesthetists.

## Key References

1. Hodnett ED, Gates S, Hofmeyr GJ, Sakala C. Continuous support for women during childbirth. *Cochrane Database Syst Rev* 2007; (**3**): CD003766.
2. Cluett ER, Burns E. Immersion in water in labour and birth. *Cochrane Database Syst Rev* 2009; (**2**): CD000111.
3. Simkin PP, O'Hara MA. Nonpharmacologic relief of pain during labor: systematic review of five methods. *Am J Obstet Gynecol* 2002; **186**: S131–59.
4. Dowswell T, Bedwell C, Lavender T, Neilson JP. Transcutaneous electrical nerve stimulation (TENS) for pain relief in labour. *Cochrane Database Syst Rev* 2009; (**2**): CD007214.
5. Wee M. Analgesia in labour: inhalational and parenteral. *Anaesth Int Care Med* 2007; **8**: 276–8.
6. Tuckey JP, Prout RE, Wee MYK. Prescribing intramuscular opioids for labour analgesia in consultant-led

maternity units: a survey of UK practice. *Int J Obst Anesth* 2008; **17**: 3–8.

7. Anim-Somuah M, Smyth RMD, Howell CJ. Epidural versus non-epidural or no analgesia in labour. *Cochrane Database Syst Rev* 2005; (**4**): CD000331.

8. Lewis, G (ed.) *The Confidential Enquiry into Maternal and Child Health (CEMACH). Saving Mothers' Lives: reviewing maternal deaths to make motherhood safer – 2003–2005.* The Seventh Report on Confidential Enquiries into Maternal Deaths in the United Kingdom. London: CEMACH, 2007: www.cemach.org.uk.

9. Comparative Obstetric Mobile Epidural Trial (COMET) Study Group UK. Effect of low-dose versus traditional epidural techniques on mode of delivery: a randomised controlled trial. *Lancet* 2001; **358**: 19–23.

10. Wilson MJA, MacArthur C, Cooper GM *et al.* Ambulation in labour and delivery mode: a randomised controlled trial of high-dose vs mobile epidural analgesia. *Anaesthesia* 2009; **64**: 266–72.

11. Simmons SW, Cyna AM, Dennis AT, Hughes D. Combined spinal-epidural versus epidural analgesia in labour. *Cochrane Database Syst Rev* 2007; (**3**): CD003401.

12. Halpern S, Carvalho B. Patient-controlled epidural analgesia for labor. *Anesth Analg* 2009; **108**: 921–8.

13. Wong CA, Scavone BM, Peaceman AM *et al.* The risk of caesarean delivery with neuraxial analgesia given early versus late in labor. *N Engl J Med* 2005; **352**: 655–65.

14. Kinsella SM, Scrutton MJL. Assessment of a modified four-category classification of urgency of caesarean section. *J Obstet Gynaecol* 2009; **29**: 110–13.

15. Focus Group. Obstetric anaesthesia delays and complications. In: *Confidential Enquiry into Stillbirths and Deaths in Infancy, 7th Annual Report.* London: Maternal and Child Health Research Consortium, 2000: 41–52.

16. Ngan Kee WD, Lee A, Khaw KS *et al.* A randomised double-blinded comparison of phenylephrine and ephedrine infusion combinations to maintain blood pressure during spinal anesthesia for caesarean delivery: the effects on fetal acid-base status and hemodynamic control. *Anesth Analg* 2008; **107**: 1295–302.

17. McDonnell JG, Curley G, Carney J *et al.* The analgesic efficacy of transversus abdominis plane block after caesarean delivery: a randomised controlled trial. *Anesth Analg* 2008; **106**: 186–91.

18. Moodley J, Jjuuko G, Rout C. Epidural compared with general anaesthesia for caesarean delivery in conscious women with eclampsia. *Br J Obstet Gynaecol* 2001; **108**: 378–82.

19. Arkoosh VA, Palmer CM, Yun EM *et al.* A randomized, double-masked, multicenter comparison of the safety of continous intrathecal labor analgesia using a 28-gauge catheter versus continuous epidural labor analgesia. *Anesthesiology* 2008; **108**: 286–98.

20. Paech MJ, Scott KL, Clavisi OM *et al.*, the ANZCA Trials Group. A prospective study of awareness and recall associated with general anaesthesia for caesarean section. *Int J Obst Anesth* 2008; **17**: 298–303.

# Chapter 31

# Caesarean section

*Richard Hayman*

---

## MRCOG standards

### Theoretical skills

Candidates are expected to:

- Have attended a basic surgical skills course.
- Have a thorough knowledge of abdominal and pelvic anatomy.
- Understand the setting of caesarean section in the context of abnormal labour and its management.
- Be able to counsel a woman regarding the pros and cons of caesarean section for a variety of different reasons.
- Be able to counsel a woman in a subsequent pregnancy concerning a trial of vaginal delivery.

### Practical skills

- Be confident to perform a delivery by caesarean section in a wide range of clinical scenarios.
- Where possible, have seen a classical caesarean section and have witnessed a caesarean hysterectomy.

## INTRODUCTION

Delivery by caesarean section (CS) has been part of human culture since ancient times, but despite rare references to operations on living women, the initial purpose was essentially to retrieve the infant from a dead or dying mother as a measure of last resort. It was not until much later that intervention with a good outcome for both mother and baby became possible. Birth by CS has become a commonplace intervention on the modern labour ward and has now, according to some, reached epidemic proportions. Consequently, a dramatic rethink of all midwifery and obstetric management is being called for, mainly by those outside the profession.

## Today's clinical setting

The national Sentinel Caesarean Section Audit reported that the overall CS rate in 2001 was 21.5 per cent (England and Wales) accounting for approximately 120 000 births per year. While the CS rates for maternity units ranged from 10 to 65 per cent (interquartile range (IQR): 18 and 24 per cent); 10 per cent of women had CS before labour (range between maternity units 4–59 per cent (IQR: 8 and 12 per cent)), and 12 per cent of women who went into labour had a CS (range between maternity units 2–22 per cent (IQR: 10 and, 14 per cent)).[1,2]

It is believed that some of the differences in CS rates observed may be explained by differences in the demographic and clinical characteristics of the population, such as maternal age, ethnicity, previous CS, breech presentation, prematurity and induction of labour.

Although CS rates have increased over the last 10–15 years, the four major clinical determinants of the CS rate have not changed.

Common primary indications reported for women having a primary CS (first CS) were: failure to progress in labour (25 per cent), presumed fetal compromise (28 per cent) and breech presentation (14 per cent).

The most common indications for women having a repeat CS were previous CS (44 per cent), maternal request as reported by clinicians (12 per cent), failure to progress (10 per cent), presumed fetal compromise (9 per cent) and breech presentation (3 per cent).[2]

Currently, in the UK, slightly more than one in seven women experiences complications during labour that provides an indication for surgical delivery. These problems can be life threatening for the mother and/or baby (e.g. eclampsia, abruptio placenta) and, in approximately 40 per cent of such cases, a caesarean section provides the safest route for delivery. In all cases, the principal aims must be to ensure that those women and babies who need delivery by CS are so delivered, and that those who do not are saved from an unnecessary intervention. In 1985, concern regarding the increasing frequency of CS led the World Health Organization (WHO) to hold a Consensus Conference. This conference concluded that there were no health benefits above a CS rate of 10–15 per cent. The Scandinavian countries managed to hold CS rates at this level during the 1990s, with outcomes comparable to or better than those of countries with higher CS rates. However, this is no longer the case and CS rates in these countries have now increased towards those of the other developed nations.

Although many factors have been associated with an increase in the CS rate, not all have been to the detriment of the mother or baby. Interestingly, while the CS rate has risen over the two preceding decades, the instrumental vaginal delivery rate has remained relatively constant, at approximately 10 per cent.

## FACTORS THAT MAY CONTRIBUTE TO AN INCREASE IN THE RATES OF CAESAREAN SECTION

### Dating the pregnancy

Until recently, most practitioners used the information obtained from a carefully taken history to calculate the expected period of confinement (37–42 weeks gestation). However, this approach proved inaccurate in the dating of up to 60 per cent of pregnancies and meant that many procedures (including screening for Down's syndrome and induction of labour for prolonged pregnancy) were inappropriately timed. Consequently, the National institute for Health and Clinical Excellence (NICE) and the National Screening Committee (NSC) recommend that all pregnant women should be offered an early ultrasound scan between 10 weeks 0 days and 13 weeks 6 days to determine gestational age using a crown rump length measurement (and to detect multiple pregnancies).

### Fetal monitoring

Following its introduction in the 1970s, electronic fetal monitoring (EFM) was universally implemented without the appropriate trials. This resulted in an increase in the incidence of CS without a demonstrable improvement in perinatal outcome. Undoubtedly, inappropriate monitoring increases the rate of interventions and current recommendations are for intermittent auscultation to be performed in all 'low-risk pregnancies', with continuous EFM in those pregnancies deemed to be 'high risk' or 'low risk with additional risk factors' (see Chapter 29, Fetal compromise in the first stage of labour).

### Analgesia in labour

Epidural analgesia has become increasing available and utilized on labour wards in the UK. Several studies have reported an increase in the incidence of instrumental vaginal deliveries when epidural analgesia is provided to more than 50 per cent of parturients. However, epidural analgesia has not been associated with a higher rate of CS (9.6 per cent in the epidural cohort versus 13.6 per cent in the opioid group – relative risk (RR) 0.70; 95 per cent confidence interval (CI) 0.38–1.31)[A].[3]

### Macrosomia

Maternal concern about fetal size is a common problem that frequently engenders anxiety among obstetricians and midwives. Although there is evidence to suggest that birth weights are rising in developed countries, the amount (30 g over 12 years) is unlikely to be of any biological significance. Unfortunately, both clinical and ultrasonographic estimations of fetal size are prone to inaccuracy (especially in large term infants), and many unnecessary inductions of labour and caesarean deliveries are performed as a consequence. Currently, there is no evidence to support induction of labour for suspected fetal macrosomia in the non-diabetic woman (see Chapter 25, Induction of labour).

### Maternal request

Traditionally, caesarean sections have been reserved for situations guided by standard clinical indications. However, requests for delivery by an elective CS where there is not a compelling obstetric indication are becoming more common.

Maternal request was given as the primary reason for 7 per cent of caesarean deliveries in the UK in 2001. There is, however, huge heterogeneity in studies examining the effect of maternal request on CS rates. Study results range from 1.5 to 28 per cent in the contribution of request as the primary reason for section, and this is due, in major part, to the differing definitions of 'request'. The arguments surrounding this area are complex and combine ethical dilemmas, the fetal and maternal risks of vaginal and surgical deliveries and the financial consequences of permitting such a preference.

During the antenatal period, the dialogue between patients and their doctors has increased over recent years. *Changing Childbirth* enshrined in practice the principle of total involvement of the pregnant woman in her own care. Implicit in this is the consideration of her wishes relating to delivery.[4] Therefore, discussions must be accompanied by the careful imparting of information, counselling and advice, but should the patient's opinions differ from those of her healthcare providers, these cannot simply be ignored. The risks of CS and labour are different, and the risks of recurrent caesarean deliveries are additive (increasing risk of placenta praevia, accreta, operative complications, etc.). However, if these risks are fully explained to the woman, she should be allowed to accept one set of risks over the other. Consequently, for a fully informed patient, an elective CS should not be viewed as bad practice, but rather as an appropriate management plan. Where maternal request is the sole reason, care should be taken to explore the request and a second opinion can be sought.

A woman's request for CS appears to be treated more favourably if she has previously undergone CS, although this may not necessarily be a valid approach.

## INDICATIONS

There are many different reasons for performing a delivery by CS. The four major indications accounting for more than 70 per cent of operations are: previous CS, dystocia, malpresentation and suspected fetal compromise. Other indications, such as multi-fetal pregnancy, abruptio placenta, placenta praevia, fetal disease and maternal disease, are less common. No list can be truly comprehensive and, whatever the indication, the over-riding principle is that whenever the risk to the mother and/or the fetus from vaginal delivery exceeds that from operative intervention, a CS should be undertaken.

Absolute indications for recommending delivery by CS are few; almost all indications are relative and there will be circumstances in which CS may be best for one woman but not another. Lack of consent by a woman with the capacity to give consent will prohibit CS regardless of the clinical need, as discussed below.

### Indications for which elective caesarean section would be the strongly recommended means of delivery

- Past obstetric history:
  - previous classical CS,
  - interval pelvic floor or anal sphincter repair,
  - previous severe shoulder dystocia with significant neonatal injury.

- Current pregnancy events:
  - significant fetal disease likely to lead to poor tolerance of labour,
  - monoamniotic twins,
  - placenta praevia,
  - obstructing pelvic mass,
  - active primary herpes at onset of labour.

- Intrapartum events:
  - fetal compromise in the first stage,
  - maternal disease for which delay in delivery may compromise the safety of the mother,
  - absolute cephalo-pelvic disproportion (brow presentations, etc.).

There are many other reasons why a CS may be recommended that are too numerous to list; in almost every case there will be practitioners who believe that vaginal delivery is feasible or a better option, and therefore each woman deserves a personal evaluation of her individual needs.

**Table 31.1** RCOG definition of type of caesarean section

| Type | Definition |
|---|---|
| Emergency | Immediate threat to life of woman or fetus |
| Urgent | Maternal or fetal compromise which is not immediately life threatening |
| Scheduled | Needing early delivery but no maternal or fetal compromise |
| Elective | At a time to suit the patient and the maternity team |
| Perimortem | Carried out in extremis while the mother is undergoing active resuscitation |
| Post-mortem | Carried out after the death of the mother in order to try to save the fetus. |

## URGENCY OF CAESAREAN SECTION

NICE have recommended that the urgency of CS should be documented using the following standardized scheme in order to aid clear communication between healthcare professionals about the urgency of a CS (see Table 31.1):

1. immediate threat to the life of the woman or fetus;
2. maternal or fetal compromise which is not immediately life-threatening;
3. no maternal or fetal compromise but needs early delivery;
4. delivery timed to suit woman or staff.[1]

## MORBIDITY AND MORTALITY

Although CS is becoming increasingly safe and evidence is mounting regarding the risks of labour and vaginal delivery, pregnant women, their midwives and doctors need to understand and appreciate the maternal risks associated with the different modes of delivery. Some maternal deaths following CS are not attributable to the procedure itself, but rather to medical or obstetric disorders that led to the decision to deliver using this approach. Many women who deliver vaginally encounter the same problems.

The Confidential Enquiries enable the risks associated with each method of delivery to be analysed. A comparison of fatality rates can be useful, but it is preferable to restrict the analysis to direct deaths, as many women whose deaths were classified as indirect had pre-existing illness. Direct deaths are specifically those that result from obstetric complications of the pregnant state, from interventions, omissions or incorrect treatment, or from a chain of events that occur after any of the above. The number of maternal deaths by mode of delivery at 24 or more completed weeks of gestation, United Kingdom 2003–2005 are shown in Table 31.2.

First stage of labour

**Table 31.2** Number of maternal deaths by mode of delivery at 24 or more completed weeks of gestation; United Kingdom 2003-2005

| Mode of delivery | Direct deaths | Indirect deaths | Direct and Indirect deaths | | Coincidental | Late | All | |
|---|---|---|---|---|---|---|---|---|
| | (n) | (n) | (n) | (%) | (n) | (n) | (n) | (%) |
| Unassisted vaginal | 24 | 33 | 57 | (30) | 8 | 5 | 70 | (30) |
| Ventouse | 3 | 3 | 6 | (3) | 0 | 0 | 6 | (3) |
| Forceps | 7 | 3 | 10 | (5) | 1 | 0 | 11 | (5) |
| Vaginal breech | 0 | 2 | 2 | (1) | 0 | 0 | 2 | (1) |
| Caesarean section | 55 | 62 | 117 | (61) | 18 | 5 | 141 | (61) |
| Emergency | 28 | 23 | 51 | (27) | 2 | 1 | 54 | (23) |
| Urgent | 3 | 3 | 6 | (3) | 1 | 3 | 10 | (4) |
| Scheduled | 2 | 5 | 7 | (4) | 5 | 1 | 13 | (6) |
| Elective | 4 | 9 | 13 | (7) | 2 | 0 | 15 | (7) |
| Peri or postmortem | 18 | 22 | 40 | (21) | 8 | 1 | 49 | (21) |
| Total delivered | 89 | 103 | 192 | (100) | 27 | 11 | 230 | (100) |

**Table 31.3** Direct death rates per million maternities by mode of delivery in UK, 1997-1999

| Mode of delivery | Calculated maternities (×1000) | Direct deaths | Death rate per million maternities |
|---|---|---|---|
| Vaginal | 1710 | 29 | 16.9 |
| Caesarean section | 413 | 34 | 82.3 |
| Elective | 130 | 5 | 38.5 |
| Emergency | 69 | 14 | 202.9 |
| Urgent | 137 | 14 | 102.2 |
| Scheduled | 78 | 1 | 12.8 |
| All maternities | 2123 | 63 | 29.7 |

**Table 31.4** Estimated direct death rates per million maternities by mode of delivery in UK, 2003-2005

| Mode of delivery | Calculated maternities (×1000) | Direct deaths | Death rate per million maternities |
|---|---|---|---|
| Vaginal | 1487.5 | 24 | 16.1 |
| Caesarean section | 419.5 | 55 | 131.1 |
| Elective | 242.2 | 4 | 16.5 |
| Emergency | 177.3 | 33 | 186.1 |
| All maternities | 1907 | 89 | 46.7 |

Using hospital episode statistics data, it is possible to estimate the overall number of caesarean sections that took place in the UK between 1997 and 1999.[5] Estimated case fatality rates can thus be calculated and are shown in Table 31.3. Although figures are not available in such detail for more recent years, it is possible to calculate the direct death mortality rates for 2003–2005 using figures available from the Office of National Statistics. These estimate that the average delivery rate by elective CS to be 9.3 per cent of all deliveries and emergency CS to be 12.7 per cent (giving an overall LSCS rate of 22 per cent of all deliveries) and are shown in Table 31.4.

It can be seen that the case fatality rate for all caesarean sections is at least five times that for vaginal delivery, and for emergency caesarean delivery this may be 12 times greater. These differences are likely to be highly significant. In the absence of other evidence (e.g. from randomized,

controlled trials of different modes of delivery), it is not appropriate to be dogmatic about best practice, although any decision to undertake major surgery with an associated mortality should be taken very seriously by all concerned. The Confidential Enquiry continues to emphasize that a CS constitutes major surgery.

## REPEAT CAESAREAN SECTION

Providing the first operation was carried out for a non-recurrent cause, and providing the obstetric situation close to term in the succeeding pregnancy is favourable, a trial of vaginal delivery is appropriate. The factors to be weighed when determining the recommended mode of delivery depend on the balance between the desires of the mother, the risks of a repeat operation, the risks to her child of labour, and the risk of labour on the strength of the old scar (see Chapter 26, Management of previous caesarean section).

# PROCEDURE

## Informed consent

Full informed consent must always be obtained prior to operation. The level of information discussed must be commensurate with the urgency of the procedure, and a commonsense approach is needed. Although it is often difficult to impart complete and thorough information when caesarean sections are performed as emergency procedures, mothers must understand what is being planned and why. Where possible, all women must be educated in pregnancy about CS and the circumstances in which it may be urgently needed. It is important to remember that no adult may give consent for another (although it is good practice to keep relatives fully informed). Where there is incapacity to consent (as may occur with conditions such as eclampsia), the doctor is expected to act in the patient's best interests, remembering that the patient is the mother and not the fetus.

Resistance to a recommended emergency CS is rare, as long as the indications for delivery are discussed in an appropriate and considerate manner. When it occurs, it is often the consequence of a failure in communication. Full documentation of the recommendation and its refusal is mandatory, but no healthcare provider can force a competent adult to undergo surgery against her will. One must always respect the wishes of the patient and her cultural and religious beliefs, no matter how challenging the consequences appear. In an elective or unhurried atmosphere, where there is significant doubt about capacity to consent, two medical opinions are required to over-ride patient wishes. It is advised, though not mandatory, that one of these should be obtained from a psychiatrist. The national consent forms require both the risks and benefits to be discussed with patients and recorded on the consent form. It is suggested that the top copy of the form should be offered to the patient, although in some situations this may not be appropriate.

Although it is usual to obtain written consent, it is important to remember that verbal consent is equally valid and in an emergency situation may be more appropriate. Common medical practice is to highlight risks but not benefits, but it is important to remember that the operation is being offered because of the perceived benefits, which in many cases are both maternal and fetal.

## Surgical basics

Following on from Munro Kerr's description of the lower segment procedure in the early twentieth century, more than 90 per cent of caesarean sections are performed using adaptations of this technique.

Routine pre-operative preparation with suprapubic shaving should be undertaken. The bladder should be emptied. It is the policy in many units for a catheter to remain *in situ* peri-operatively and for a defined period thereafter (commonly 24 hours or until the patient is mobile). Although this approach may improve patient comfort post-operatively and reduce the incidence of over-distension of the bladder (a complication of regional anaesthesia), such a policy runs the risk of introducing an iatrogenic urinary tract infection.

A left lateral tilt minimizes compression of the maternal inferior vena cava and reduces the incidence of hypotension (with its consequent reductions in placental perfusion). The patient should then be draped in the standard manner. Plastic adhesive drapes may prove more effective than standard drapes in the prevention of wound infections.

The choice of incision and closure should be individualized to the characteristics of the woman and the circumstances demanding operative intervention.

## Skin incisions

Two basic skin incisions are used – suprapubic and midline vertical.

The transverse incision has the advantages of improved cosmetic results, decreased inter-operative and post-operative analgesic requirements and thus less pulmonary compromise and superior wound strength postpartum.[6,7]

The vertical incision, on the other hand, provides greater ease of access to the pelvic and intra-abdominal organs and may be enlarged more easily. Haeri demonstrated no difference between the two incisions when comparing overall operative time, post-operative haemoglobins of <10 g/dL, or post-operative febrile morbidity [D].[6] However, Mowatt and Bonnar[7] reported an 8-fold increase in the incidence of wound dehiscence with the midline incision when compared to a transverse abdominal approach (this difference may be reduced by mass closure techniques) [D].

### The Pfannenstiel incision

The skin and subcutaneous tissues are incised using a transverse curvilinear incision at a level of two fingerbreadths above the symphysis pubis, extending from and to points lateral to the lateral margins of the abdominal rectus muscles. The subcutaneous tissues are separated by blunt dissection and the rectus sheath is incised transversely along the middle 2 cm. This incision is then extended with scissors or blunt dissection before the fascial sheath is separated from the underlying muscle. Separation is performed cephalad to permit adequate exposure of the peritoneum in a longitudinal plane and perforating blood vessels should be cauterized to minimize the risks of development of subrectus haematomas. The recti are separated from each other, the peritoneum incised and the abdominal cavity entered.

### The Cohen incision

This incision is similar to the Pfannenstiel incision, but permits a more rapid and bloodless entry into the peritoneal cavity. A straight transverse incision is made between two points inferior and medial to the anterior superior iliac spine, the subcutaneous tissues are divided in the midline for 3 cm and the central rectus sheath is similarly divided. By blunt dissection and vertical traction, the subfascial space is opened, the peritoneum exposed and the abdominal cavity entered high above the bladder. Entry with this technique into the abdominal cavity is often not suitable for repeat caesarean sections, where scarring may distort the underlying fascial planes.

## The infra-umbilical incision

The vertical skin incision is specifically indicated in cases of extreme maternal obesity, if the need for CS is coupled with the suspicion of other intra-abdominal pathology necessitating surgical intervention, or where access to the uterine fundus may be required (classical CS).

The lower midline incision is made from the lower border of the umbilicus to the symphysis pubis, and may be extended caudally towards the xiphisternum if required. Sharp dissection to the level of the anterior rectus sheath is performed, which is then freed of subcutaneous fat in the midline. The rectus sheath is then incised, taking care to avoid damage to any underlying bowel, and extended inferiorly to the vesical peritoneal reflection and superiorly to the upper limit of the abdominal incision.

## Uterine incisions

As with the skin incision, the nature of the uterine incision is determined by the clinical situation. A low transverse uterine incision is used in more than 95 per cent of caesarean deliveries due to ease of repair, reduced blood loss and lower incidence of dehiscence or rupture in subsequent pregnancies when compared with the alternative incisions.

There are relatively few absolute indications for classical section. However, these include a lower uterine segment containing fibroids or a lower segment covered with dense adhesions, both of which may make entry difficult. Such obstruction may be associated with heavy bleeding or may distort the anatomy to such an extent that the lower segment approach is not safe. Other indications include grade IV placenta praevia, transverse lie with the back down and especially when associated with prolapse of a fetal arm (a more satisfactory delivery will be achieved through a lower segment incision after correction of the lie), fetal abnormality (e.g. conjoined twins), or CS in the presence of a carcinoma of the cervix (so as to avoid damage to the cervix and its vascular and lymphatic supplies).

The uterus is palpated to identify the size and presenting part of the fetus and to determine the direction and degree of rotation of the uterus. A Doynes or similar retractor blade is inserted inferiorly and the loose reflection of vesico-uterine serosa overlying the uterus picked up with toothed forceps, opened with scissors and divided laterally.

The underlying lower uterine segment is reflected with blunt dissection, and the developed bladder flap held rostrally with the retractor. The uterus is then opened in a transverse plane for a distance of 1–2 cm; the incision may be extended laterally with either blunt dissection (lateral and upward pressure with the index fingers) or scissors. Such an incision should be adequate to allow delivery of the fetus without extension into the broad ligament or uterine vessels. If necessary, cutting the incision upward unilaterally (J-incision) or bilaterally (U-shape) will avoid such an extension and provide extra room. Damage to the uterine vessels or broad ligament, when it occurs, is associated with an increase in maternal morbidity (especially blood loss) and prolonged hospitalization. If a midline extension is required, the T-incision, in future pregnancies vaginal delivery will be contraindicated because of an increased risk of uterine rupture [C].

A modified classical or De Lee incision should also be in the surgeon's repertoire. This entry is vertical on the uterus in the sagittal plane, is extended to the level of entry of the round ligaments, but is not taken onto the fundus (unlike a true classical section). Although delivery through this incision decreases the risk of rupture in subsequent pregnancies compared with a classical incision, most would recommend future deliveries by elective CS.

The fetal lie is then stabilized, the membranes are ruptured if still intact, and the accoucheur's hand is positioned below the presenting part. If cephalic, the head is flexed and delivered by elevation though the uterine incision, either manually or with forceps. Fundal pressure is then applied to aid the delivery. However, this should not be commenced until the presenting part is located within the incision – for fear of converting the lie from longitudinal to transverse.

Specific manoeuvres must be employed at CS, prior to membrane rupture for stabilization of transverse or oblique lies, and for delivery of the breech.

Once the fetus is delivered, an oxytocic (e.g. 5 IU syntocinon i.v.) is administered to aid uterine contraction and placental separation.[8] Prophylactic antibiotics should be administered to reduce the incidence of postoperative endometritis, and although no one regimen has been shown to have a clear advantage over any other, a single dose of either a first-generation or second-generation cephalosporin + metronidazole, or ampicillin with clavulanic acid, would be suitable [A].[9] There is no evidence to suggest that a prolonged course of antibiotics is more beneficial than a single dose when used for prophylaxis [A].[10]

The placenta should be delivered by combined cord traction; manual removal significantly increases the intraoperative blood loss and post-operative infectious morbidity [A].[8] The uterus should then be inspected to ensure complete removal of the placenta and membranes. Some authors advise confirmation of a patent cervical canal to ensure a patent passage for the drainage of lochia, although this is not necessary in labouring women.

Repair of the incision may be performed with the uterus *in situ* or following exteriorization. Exteriorization is not routinely necessary, but enhances visualization of the lower segment and thus facilitates surgical repair; especially when there have been lateral extensions to the incision margins. Evidence comparing blood loss between the two techniques is contradictory. One trial reported a decrease in the haematocrit fall with exteriorization compared with intraperitoneal procedures, whereas another did not. The main problems with exteriorization are increases in maternal pain, vagal-induced vomiting and the incidence of venous air emboli, although the incidence of infectious morbidity is not altered. There is currently not enough information to adequately evaluate the routine use of exteriorization of the uterus for repair of the uterine incision.

## Uterine closure

Placement of Green–Armytage forceps on the inferior uterine edge in addition to each angle improves visualization and reduces blood loss further, especially in the presence of bleeding venous sinuses. Closure should be performed in either single or double layers with continuous or interrupted sutures. The initial suture should be placed just lateral to the incision angle, and the closure continued to a point just lateral to the angle on the opposite side. A running stitch is often employed and this may be locked to improve haemostasis. If a second layer is used, an inverting suture or horizontal suture should overlap the myometrium. There are only two reported randomized, controlled trials comparing single-layer versus two-layer closure. A single-layer closure is associated with reduced operating time, with no statistically significant differences in the use of extra haemostatic sutures, incidence of endometritis, decrease in post-operative haematocrit or use of blood transfusion [B]. There have recently been some concerns regarding single-layer closure, as one widely reported observational study of scar dehiscence in subsequent labours showed a higher incidence than previously reported. One possible aetiological factor that has been suggested is the move to single-layer closure during the period studied. The effectiveness and safety of single layer closure of the uterine incision is therefore uncertain and, except within a research context, the uterine incision should be sutured with two layers.[1,11]

In cases associated with extended 'tears', once the uterine angles are secure, the defect should be repaired as a primary procedure prior to uterine closure. Lacerations involving uterine tissue are usually repaired without difficulty. However, vertical lacerations into the vagina or lateral extensions into the broad ligament may be associated with substantial blood loss and the potential for ureteric damage. To minimize bleeding from the perforated myometrial vessels in such cases, the needle must be positioned just distal to the apex of the laceration and, once inserted, should not be withdrawn.

Once repaired, the incision is assessed for haemostasis and 'figure-of-eight' sutures can be employed to control bleeding. The uterus, tubes and ovaries are inspected, elective or emergency adnexal procedures performed (e.g. tubal ligation ovarian cystectomy for dermoid cyst), and the paracolic gutters cleaned. Peritoneal closure is unnecessary and may result in a higher incidence of adhesion formation than would otherwise occur [A]. Many surgeons routinely place drains in the subfascial space to reduce haematoma formation, but such management is most appropriate in the presence of infection or in the obese, where a large 'space' is potentially left. In all cases, attention to haemostasis is the key.

## Abdominal closure

Closure is performed in the anatomical planes with high-strength, low-reactivity materials such as polyglycolic acid or polyglactin (Dexon® and Vicryl®). Interlocking of the sutures should be avoided as this can devascularize the tissues and delay the healing process. Closure of a midline incision differs at the level of the rectus sheath. Here, repair should be effected with a running continuous suture of polyglycolic acid, large-bore monofilament polypropylene or nylon, which have delayed/prolonged absorption characteristics.

In any patient with an increased risk of haematoma formation, such as severe pre-eclampsia, HELLP syndrome or morbid obesity, a closed drainage system located anterior to the rectus sheath may be required. Subcutaneous sutures to approximate Camper's fascia should be used in women with more than 2 cm of subcutaneous fat, as they have been shown to reduce the incidence of wound disruption and seroma formation, and potentially may lower the overt infection rate [C]. The skin may be closed using any number of techniques. The most common involve surgical staples, subcuticular stitches or tension sutures (interrupted or continuous/polyglycolic acid, large-bore monofilament polypropylene or nylon). However, lower transverse abdominal skin incisions closed with a subcuticular stitch result in less post-operative discomfort and are more cosmetically appealing at the 6-week post-operative visit when compared to incisions closed with staples. [B]

## COMPLICATIONS

Caesarean section is a major abdominal surgical procedure and carries with it all the risks inherent in such an approach.

## Intra-operative complications

### Bowel damage

Bowel damage is rare at CS, but may occur during a repeat procedure or if adhesions are present from previous surgery. Damage is often recognized by smell or the observation of faecal soiling. The management is dependent on the site of the injury, and is best conducted in conjunction with a general surgeon. Small bowel damage is repaired using a two-layer closure with 2-0 Vicryl® or equivalent. Large

First stage of labour

bowel damage is managed likewise, but in addition a temporary defunctioning colostomy may be required. Post-repair peritoneal lavage is mandatory, as is a treatment course with broad-spectrum antibiotics, for example a cephalosporin and metronidazole.

## Haemorrhage

Haemorrhage accounts for 6 per cent of deaths associated with CS and an unknown proportion of operative morbidity. This complication may be due to the operative procedure as a consequence of damage to the uterine vessels, or may be incidental as a consequence of uterine atony or placenta praevia. There are many manoeuvres that may be employed to manage such cases, which range from bimanual compression, infusions of oxytocin and administration of 15-methyl prostaglandin $F_{2\alpha}$ to conservative surgical procedures such as uterine compression sutures, to the more radical, but life-saving, hysterectomy.

## Placenta praevia

The proportion of patients with a placenta praevia is increasing as a consequence of CS. The incidence increases almost linearly after each previous CS (Table 31.5), and as the risks of such a complication increase with increasing parity, future reproductive intentions are very relevant to any individual decision for operative delivery.

Clark et al.[12] also reported that 25 per cent of women undergoing caesarean delivery for placenta praevia in the presence of one or more uterine scars subsequently underwent caesarean hysterectomy for placenta accreta.

In patients with an anticipated high risk of haemorrhage, for example known cases of placenta praevia, at least four units of blood should be routinely cross-matched, and must be available in theatre before the procedure is commenced. A combined approach to the management of such patients, with the anaesthetists, haematologists and obstetricians working together, will result in the best standard of care.

**Table 31.5** Risk of placenta praevia and accreta with repeat caesarean

| Number of previous caesarean sections | Incidence of placenta accreta (%) (total 0.3%) | Incidence of placenta accreta in those with placenta praevia (%) | Overall risk of placenta accreta (%) |
|---|---|---|---|
| 0 | 0.26 | 5 | 0.01 |
| 1 | 0.65 | 24 | 0.16 |
| 2 | 1.8 | 47 | 0.85 |
| 3 | 3 | 40 | 1.2 |
| 4 | 10 | 67 | 6.7 |

## Urinary tract damage

Direct injury to the bladder is not uncommon during CS. The transverse lower abdominal incision carries the risk of cystotomy, especially after prolonged labours where the bladder is displaced caudally, after previous CS where scarring obliterates the vesico-uterine space, or where a vertical extension to the uterine incision has occurred. Pre-operative catheterization in association with careful operative technique should reduce the likelihood of damage occurring. If damage to the bladder is suspected, transurethral instillation of methylene blue-coloured saline will help to delineate the extent of the defect. When such an injury is observed, a repair with 2-0 Vicryl® as a single continuous or interrupted layer is appropriate. The urinary catheter will need to remain in situ for 7–10 days and prophylactic antibiotics prescribed.

Damage to the ureters is uncommon, as reflection of the bladder displaces them rostrally, but if suspected, the ureters should be investigated and repaired in conjunction with a urological surgeon.

## Caesarean hysterectomy

The most common indication for caesarean hysterectomy is uncontrollable maternal haemorrhage, a situation not infrequently associated with a morbidly adherent placenta. This operation, while a major undertaking, should not be left too late as the risk of operative complications, maternal morbidity and mortality increase with increasing haemorrhage.

Although postpartum haemorrhage is relatively common (occurring after about 1 per cent of deliveries), life-threatening haemorrhage requiring immediate treatment affects only 1 in 1000 deliveries. There is no 'clinical standard' at which intervention by hysterectomy is recommended, so local protocols must be formulated to address this specific issue and to guide the individual clinician to intevene if the loss remains uncontrollable after, for example, 2.5 L. It is important to note that the Confidential Enquiries continue to cite delays in performing definitive surgery, for example a hysterectomy, as an avoidable cause of maternal mortality.[3]

The most important risk factor for emergency postpartum hysterectomy is a previous CS, especially when the placenta overlies the old scar and increases the risks of placenta accreta. This complication alone accounts for 30 per cent of emergency caesarean hysterectomies.[12]

From the early stages, such cases should be managed by an experienced obstetrician and anaesthetist. It is also important to counsel such patients accordingly, and to gain consent pre-operatively for caesarean hysterectomy when appropriate.

Other common indications for hysterectomy are:

- atony (43 per cent);
- uterine rupture (13 per cent);
- extension of a low transverse incision (10 per cent);
- leiomyomata preventing uterine closure and haemostasis (4 per cent).

Hysterectomies performed for atony are significantly associated with the following factors when compared to hysterectomies performed for other indications:

- amnionitis;
- CS for labour arrest;
- oxytocin augmentation of labour;
- magnesium sulphate infusion;
- excessive fetal weight.

It should be remembered that the pelvic tissues in the pregnant woman are lax, with increased vascularity. They are therefore prone to bleed more freely than in the non-pregnant state, and extra care must be taken to ensure the pedicles are correctly ligated. Identification of the lower margin of the cervix may be exceedingly difficult, and a subtotal procedure may need to be considered.

## Documentation

Good documentation of the procedure is of paramount importance. This should include the categorization of the degree of urgency of the procedure and critical timings, i.e. the time of decision to deliver, skin incision, delivery of the baby. The type of suture material used, the procedure and any complications must be recorded. The surgeon should include a note that the cavity of the uterus was checked and empty and that ovaries and tubes were inspected. The blood loss must be noted and for all emergency procedures the cord gas results should be recorded.[1]

It is the surgeon's responsibility to ensure that the post-operative precautions such as antibiotics and anti-thrombotic measures are undertaken. Clear post-operative instructions should include a note on suture removal (or not) and, if there are any specific instructions, these must be clearly recorded and communicated to the midwife caring for the woman.[1]

## Post-operative complications

### Infection and endometritis

The single most important risk factor for postpartum maternal infection is caesarean delivery, and women undergoing caesarean section have a 5–20-fold greater risk of an infectious complication when compared with a vaginal delivery [D]. These complications include fever, wound infection, endometritis, bacteraemia, other serious infection (including pelvic abscess, septic shock, necrotizing fasciitis and septic pelvic vein thrombophlebitis) and urinary tract infection. Such sequelae are an important and substantial cause of maternal morbidity and are often associated with a significant increase in the length of the hospital stay. It should be remembered that fever can occur after any operative procedure, and a low-grade fever following a caesarean delivery may not necessarily be a marker of infection. Other common causes that enter the differential

diagnosis include haematoma, atelectasis and deep vein thrombosis (see Table 31.6).

The incidence of post-operative wound infection has been quoted to be between 1 and 9 per cent. The following factors are associated with an increased risk of post-operative infection:

- preterm labour;
- ruptured membranes;
- prolonged labour;
- delivery by an inexperienced surgeon;
- the number of vaginal examinations;
- internal fetal monitoring;
- urinary tract infection;
- anaemia, blood loss;
- diabetes;
- general anaesthesia;
- obesity;
- low socioeconomic status.

Labour, its duration and the presence of ruptured membranes appear to be the most important factors, with obesity playing a particularly important role in the occurrence of wound infections.

The most important source of microorganisms responsible for post-caesarean section infection is the genital tract, particularly if the membranes are ruptured preoperatively. Even in the presence of intact membranes, microbial invasion of the intrauterine cavity is common, especially with preterm labour. Infections are commonly polymicrobial.

The pathogens isolated from infected wounds and the endometrium include:

- *Escherichia coli* and other aerobic Gram-negative rods;
- group B *Streptococcus*;
- other *Streptococcus* species;
- *Enterococcus faecalis*;
- *Staphylococcus aureus*;
- coagulase-negative staphylococci;
- anaerobes (including *Peptostreptococcus* species and *Bacteroides* species);
- *Gardnerella vaginalis* and genital mycoplasmas.

Although *Ureaplasma urealyticum* is commonly isolated from the upper genital tract and infected wounds, it is unclear whether it is a pathogen in this setting. Wound infections caused by *Staphylococcus aureus* and coagulase-negative staphylococci arise from contamination of the wound with the endogenous flora of the skin at the time of surgery.

The general principles for the prevention of any surgical infection include careful surgical technique, skin antisepsis and antimicrobial prophylaxis. Without prophylaxis, the incidence of endometritis is reported to range from 20 to 85 per cent and the rates of wound infection and serious infectious complications may be as high as 25 per cent. The reduction in the risk of endometritis with antibiotics appears to be similar across a spectrum of patient groups:

**Table 31.6** Summary of effects on maternal health of CS when compared with vaginal birth (taken from the NICE report: Caesarean Section 2004)

| Effect around the time of birth | Absolute risk % | | Relative risk (95% CI) CS compared with vaginal birth | Evidence level |
|---|---|---|---|---|
| | CS | Vaginal birth | | |
| Reduced after a planned CS | | | | |
|    Perineal pain | 2 | 5 | 0.3 (0.2, 0.6) | [B] |
| Increased after a planned CS | | | | |
|    Abdominal pain | 9 | 5 | 1.9 (1.3, 2.8) | [B] |
|    Bladder injury | 0.1 | 0.003 | 36.6 (10.4, 128.4) | [D] |
|    Ureteric injury | 0.03 | 0.001 | 25.2 (2.6, 243.5) | [D] |
|    Hysterectomy | 0.8 | 0.01 | 95.5 (67.7, 136.9) | [C] |
|    Length of hospital stay | 3–4 days | 1–2 days | | [B] |
|    Maternal death | 82.3 per million | 16.9 per million | 4.9 (3.0, 8.0) | [D] |
| Not different | | | | |
|    Haemorrhage (in excess of 1000 mL) | 0.5 | 0.7 | 0.8 (0.4, 4.4) | [A] |
|    Infection (wound or endometritis) | 6.4 | 4.9 | 1.3 (1.0, 1.7) | [A] |
| Long-term effects | | | | |
|    Reduced after a planned LSCS | | | | |
|       Urinary incontinence (3 months postpartum) | 4.5 | 7.3 | 0.6 (0.4, 0.9) | [B] |
|       Utero-vaginal prolapse | 1 | 5 | 0.6 (0.5, 0.9) | [C] |
|    Not different (3 months postpartum) | | | | |
|       Faecal incontinence | 0.8 | 1.5 | 0.5 (0.2, 1.6) | [B] |
|       Back pain | 11.3 | 12.2 | 0.9 (0.7, 1.2) | [B] |
|       Postnatal depression | 10.1 | 10.8 | 0.9 (0.7, 1.2) | [B] |
|       Dyspareunia | 17.0 | 18.7 | 0.9 (0.7, 1.1) | [B] |
| Implications for future pregnancies increased after CS | | | | |
|    Having no more children | 42 | 29 | 1.5 (1.1, 2.0) | [C] |
|    Placenta praevia | See Table 31.5 | See Table 31.5 | | [C] |
|    Uterine rupture | 0.4 | 0.01 | 42.2 (31.1, 57.2) | [C] |
|    Antepartum stillbirth | 0.4 | 0.2 | 1.6 (1.2, 2.3) | [C] |

- elective caesarean section: RR = 0.24 (95 per cent CI = 0.11–0.48);
- emergency caesarean section: RR = 0.30 (95 per cent CI = 0.25–0.35);
- undefined or all patients: RR = 0.29 (95 per cent CI = 0.26–0.33) [A].[9]

Overall, the use of prophylactic antibiotics at CS results in a major, clinically important and statistically significant reduction in the incidence of episodes of fever, endometritis, wound infection, urinary tract infection and serious infections.

The common regimens have been subjected to a number of trials and have been summarized by meta-analysis [A]. Almost all trials included endometritis, febrile morbidity, wound infection and urinary tract infection as outcome measures. In only three trials were antibiotics given pre-operatively, making comparison of the timing of the first dose impossible.

The analysis examined types of antibiotic prophylaxis, single-dose versus multiple-dose regimens and method of administration (systemic versus peritoneal lavage).

The drug regimens compared included comparisons of different types of cephalosporins, extended spectrum penicillins, ampicillin and ampicillin plus gentamicin.

No drug regimen was superior to any other, with the exception that second- or third-generation cephalosporins were associated with fewer urinary tract infections than extended spectrum penicillins (odds ratio (OR) 0.38, 95 per cent CI 0.17–0.83). Multiple-dose regimens did not reduce the rates of febrile morbidity (OR 1.32, 95 per cent CI

0.95–1.84), endometritis (OR 0.92, 95 per cent CI 0.7–1.23) or wound infection (OR 0.91, 95 per cent CI 0.58–1.43). However, fewer urinary tract infections were seen in the multiple-dose group (OR 0.6, 95 per cent CI 0.43–0.83).[9,10]

There continues to be some debate about the necessity of antibiotics in women at very low risk undergoing elective CS. The most recent large randomized, controlled trial (not included in the meta-analysis) suggested again that prophylactic antibiotics might be unnecessary [B]. Four hundred and eighty women undergoing elective CS had cefoxitin or placebo. Wound infection occurred in 13.3 and 12.5 per cent of women in the placebo and cefoxitin groups, respectively. Prophylactic antibiotics did not decrease febrile morbidity, wound infection, endometritis, urinary tract infection and pneumonia. Hospital stay was on average a day less than for those who received placebo. Putting the data from this trial into the meta-analysis gives a relative risk for endometritis in the treatment group of 0.4 (95 per cent CI 0.2–0.79), suggesting that prophylactic antibiotics do reduce the risk of endometritis after elective CS, but do not reduce incidence of other infective morbidity.

The best guidance is that, at the very least, antibiotics should be used whenever there are risk factors in women undergoing CS.

## Pulmonary emboli and deep vein thrombosis (venous thromboembolism)

Pulmonary embolism (PE) remains a leading direct cause of maternal death. However, there has been a dramatic fall in deaths from PE after CS following criticism made in the 1994–97 Confidential Enquiry into Maternal Deaths and the subsequent Royal College of Obstetricians and Gynaecologists (RCOG) recommendations for thromboprophylaxis. It is also likely that the inclusion of thromboembolism prophylaxis guidelines as part of the Clinical Negligence Scheme for Trusts standards has contributed to the widespread application of these guidelines. In the last reported triennium, 33 deaths from PE were reported and only nine were after CS. The major areas for attention now encompass recognition of thromboembolism in women presenting to general practitioners or in accident and emergency departments, and the ongoing issue of prescribing appropriate treatment for those women who are obese, both prior to, and after delivery by CS.

It is difficult to be specific about the incidence of non-fatal PEs post-caesarean section, as these are notoriously difficult to record due to presentation at different times and to many different professionals. Everyone dealing with pregnant or recently pregnant women needs to be aware of the following symptoms.

- Deep vein thromboembolism (DVT): leg pain or discomfort (especially in the left leg), complaints of pulled muscles or muscle strain, swelling, tenderness, increased temperature and oedema, lower abdominal pain and elevated white cell count. One or many of these symptoms may present.

- PE: dyspnoea, collapse, chest pain, cough, haemoptysis, faintness, raised jugular venous pressure, focal signs in chest, and symptoms and signs associated with DVT. Remember that pelvic veins account for most post-caesarean section PEs and leg signs may not be present.

The subjective, clinical assessment of DVT and PE is unreliable, and less than half of the women with clinically suspected venous thromboembolism have the diagnosis confirmed when objective testing is employed. However, the index of suspicion must be high, and consequently treatment should be commenced while awaiting diagnostic confirmation.

The incidence of such complications can undoubtedly be reduced by the peri-operative administration of prophylactic heparin and the prompt initiation of treatment, when required, in accordance with the guidelines issued by the RCOG (see Chapter 6.5, Haematological conditions).

## Psychological sequelae

The spontaneous birth of a live infant can convey a huge degree of both satisfaction and achievement for both the mother and her partner. Although all women entering labour face the risks of an emergency delivery, the majority will achieve a normal vaginal delivery without complications. Whatever the outcome, pain, exhaustion and the demands of a newborn baby can complicate the recovery and, when combined with fear of the unknown and a sense of 'loss of control', may have dramatic effects on the woman both in the long and the short term. The recovery period after labour thus depends on a large number of interacting factors.

It is commonly believed that the general recovery after CS is more prolonged than after vaginal delivery and it is recognized that all difficult deliveries carry increased maternal psychological and physical morbidity. Recent evidence suggests that the compromised postpartum psychological functioning in women delivered by CS may be secondary to delayed contact with the baby. This is important, as it is a factor that in most cases should be amenable to remedy.

## SUMMARY

- Effective thromboembolism prophylaxis has reduced the number of deaths from pulmonary embolism after CS and should be a routine part of CS management.
- Repeat caesarean sections increase the risks of placenta praevia and accreta.
- There is a significant reduction in the risk of endometritis with antibiotics across a spectrum of patient groups:
  - elective caesarean section: RR = 0.24 (95 per cent CI = 0.11–0.48);

- emergency caesarean section: RR = 0.30 (95 per cent CI = 0.25–0.35);
- undefined or all patients: RR = 0.29 (95 per cent CI = 0.26–0.33).

- Repeated courses of antibiotics for routine prophylaxis are not necessary.
- Antibiotic drug regimens covering the common organisms are equally as effective as prophylaxis.
- Manual removal of the placenta at CS increases the risk of endometritis.
- Single-layer closure of the uterus is as effective as a two-layer closure but the trial numbers are relatively small and the question of uterine dehiscence has not been addressed in relationship to this technique.
- Peritoneal closure is not necessary routinely.

## KEY POINTS

- The rate of delivery by CS continues to be an issue of great concern to many midwives, obstetricians, politicians and society as a whole, but should not be considered in isolation from other changes taking place in society.
- Maternal satisfaction is an important part of childbirth and must be taken into consideration when implementing any changes in childbirth policy. There is no evidence that there will be a widespread increase in maternal requests for CS.
- There is a real need for national debate about whether maternal choice is a valid indication and, if agreed, this should be fully funded.
- Placenta praevia, particularly in patients with a previous uterine scar, may be associated with uncontrollable uterine haemorrhage at delivery, and caesarean hysterectomy may be necessary. A very experienced operator is essential and a consultant must be readily available.
- Every unit must have a protocol for the management of massive haemorrhage.

## Key References

1. NICE clinical guideline CG013. *Caesarean section.* London: NICE, April 2004.
2. Thomas J, Paranjothy S, Royal College of Obstetricians and Gynaecologists Clinical Effectiveness Support Unit. *National Sentinel Caesarean Section Audit.* London: RCOG Press, 2001.
3. Howell CJ. Epidural versus non-epidural analgesia for pain relief in labour. *Cochrane Database Syst Rev* 2000; (**2**): CD000331.
4. Report of the Expert Maternity Group. *Changing Childbirth.* London: HMSO, 1993.
5. The Confidential Enquiries into Maternal Deaths in the United Kingdom. *Why Mothers Die 1997–1999.* London: RCOG Press, 2001.
6. Haeri AD. Comparison of transverse and vertical skin incisions for Caesarean section. *S Afr Med J* 1976; **52**: 33–4.
7. Mowatt J, Bonnar J. Abdominal wound dehiscence after Caesarean section. *BMJ* 1971; **2**: 256–7.
8. Wilkinson C, Enkin MW. Manual removal of placenta at caesarean section. *Cochrane Database Syst Rev* 2000; (**2**): CD000130.
9. Hofmeyr GJ, Smaill F. Antibiotic prophylaxis regimens and drugs for cesarean section. *Cochrane Database Syst Rev* 2000; (**2**): CD001136.
10. Bagratee JS, Moodley J, Kleinschmidt I, Zawilski W. A randomised controlled trial of antibiotic prophylaxis in elective Caesarean delivery. *Br J Obstet Gynaecol* 2001; **108**: 143–8.
11. Enkin MW, Wilkinson C. Single versus two layer suturing for closing the uterine incision at Caesarean section. *Cochrane Database Syst Rev* 2007; (**3**): CD000192.
12. Clark SL, Yeh SY, Phelan J *et al.* Emergency hysterectomy for obstetric haemorrhage. *Obstet Gynecol* 1984; **64**: 376–80.

# SECTION E
Second stage of labour

# Fetal compromise in the second stage of labour

*Myles Taylor*

## INTRODUCTION

The management of suspected fetal compromise in the second stage of labour demands considerable skill, in terms of both decision-making and practical ability. Uterine contractions have peaked in terms of strength and frequency, and the resulting intrauterine and uterine wall pressures are further increased by maternal pushing. These pressures will frequently be greater than maternal arterial blood pressure, temporarily abolishing placental perfusion. Compression of the fetal head and umbilical cord is at its greatest, as the amniotic fluid volume has reached a nadir and passage through the rigid bony pelvis has begun. After many hours of stressful labour, fetal reserves may also be reduced or depleted. All these factors combine to make fetal heart rate abnormalities particularly common, although many of these abnormalities will be entirely benign. Having reached full dilatation, there is also an expectation that vaginal birth will be achieved.

Despite the factors detailed above, clinicians must remain wary of undertaking difficult assisted vaginal deliveries in the presence of fetal compromise. For this reason, secondary tests of fetal well-being still have a place in the second stage of labour. Such tests can give reassurance that further time for head descent and/or rotation can be allowed, converting a difficult delivery into an easier one or even a spontaneous birth.

## DEFINITIONS

See Chapter 29, Fetal compromise in the first stage.

## WHAT TYPE OF FETAL MONITORING IS BEST IN THE SECOND STAGE?

The debate over the advantages and disadvantages of intermittent auscultation versus continuous electronic monitoring in the first stage of labour also arises when considering fetal monitoring in the second stage. Unfortunately, there is little evidence to inform this discussion. However, an obvious practical disadvantage of intermittent monitoring in the second stage is that it is difficult for an obstetrician called to undertake an assisted delivery to confirm fetal well-being. Instead, any concern regarding a difficult delivery should be met with either a short period of electronic fetal monitoring or fetal scalp blood sampling.

### Intermittent auscultation

In the low-risk situation, intermittent auscultation, either by Pinnard stethoscope or by hand-held Doppler, remains popular. Conventional guidelines, such as those issued in 2007 by the Royal College of Obstetricians and Gynaecologists (RCOG), suggest auscultating the fetal heart rate for at least 1 minute at least every 5 minutes in the second stage and the maternal pulse should also be recorded [E].

## WHAT IS A NORMAL SECOND STAGE CARDIOTOCOGRAPH?

In an early large study of 1755 second stage heart rate traces, 75 per cent maintained a normal baseline rate, with about 5 per cent becoming tachycardic.[1] The remaining 20 per cent of traces developed a baseline bradycardia that was transient in one-third, persistent in one-third and progressive in the remaining third.

Overall, a normal baseline in combination with an absence of decelerations was seen in only one-quarter of second stage heart rate tracings. However, 60 per cent of these 'normal' traces either exhibited no accelerations or poor variability, resulting in 90 per cent of all second stage cardiotocographs (CTGs) showing some degree of abnormality.

Therefore, the definition of a normal second stage CTG is difficult. Using standards applied for antenatal or even first stage CTGs, a normal CTG would appear to be rare in the second stage of labour.

Early studies of second stage CTG abnormalities related neonatal outcome to Apgar scores rather than cord pH. Provided the baseline heart rate remained normal, only 2 per cent of neonates ended up with a 5-minute Apgar score <7 [C].[1] Later studies found a similar risk of metabolic acidosis in this situation.[2–5]

## WHAT IS AN ABNORMAL SECOND STAGE CARDIOTOCOGRAPH?

*Baseline.* Apart from late decelerations, the only fetal heart rate pattern that is strongly suggestive of fetal hypoxaemia is a continuous or progressive bradycardia.

Approximately 10 per cent of persistent or progressive bradycardias in the second stage will lead to 5-minute Apgar scores <7.[1] Neither superimposed early nor variable decelerations influence these figures. In later studies, fetal bradycardia was linked with neonatal acidosis.[3–5] Both Piquard et al.[6] and Cardoso et al.[5] found the mean umbilical artery pH to be lower in the presence of a fetal bradycardia. The severity of the bradycardia also correlates with perinatal risk. Acidosis was found in 30–40 per cent of moderate to severely bradycardic fetuses;[3,4] in more than half of the cases there was a metabolic acidosis. One study found that a fetal heart rate of <70 beats per minute (bpm) increased the risk of acidosis 26-fold and the risk of metabolic acidosis 5-fold.[2]

A baseline tachycardia is reportedly associated with low 5-minute Apgar scores in 6 per cent of cases[1] and with neonatal acidaemia in up to 20 per cent.[3,4] However, it is rarely linked with a base excess >12 mmol/L.[4]

*Variability.* The work of Gilstrap et al.[3] suggested that absent variability dramatically increased the risk of neonatal acidosis, even in the presence of an otherwise normal CTG. A cord pH <7.20 was seen in 24 per cent of cases with isolated absent variability, compared to 3 per cent of completely normal second stage traces. Gull et al.[7] investigated the inter-relationship between baseline bradycardias and variability. In the presence of a baseline heart rate <100 bpm, the risk of neonatal metabolic acidaemia increased as the interval before loss of variability shortened and as the duration of loss of variability increased. This suggests that loss of variability corresponds to fetal decompensation.

*Accelerations.* These are not commonly present in the second stage.

*Decelerations.* Decelerations are remarkably common, and are seen in more than 70 per cent of second stage heart rate traces.

- *Early decelerations* occur in 14 per cent of second stage traces. They do not appear to increase the risk of a low 5-minute Apgar score,[1] and should be viewed as benign – regardless of baseline rate.
- *Variable decelerations* are much more common, being seen in approximately half of second stage CTGs. After taking into account the baseline heart rate, mild variable decelerations have little influence on the incidence of low Apgar scores.[1] However, deep variable decelerations, with a drop in fetal heart rate of <70 bpm, are associated with a 10-fold increase in the risk of metabolic acidosis [C].[2]
- *Late decelerations* are relatively uncommon in the second stage, being seen in only 5 per cent of traces. However, their presence dramatically increases the chances of a low 5-minute Apgar score, regardless of baseline rate.[1] If the baseline rate is normal, a 5-minute Apgar score <7 is seen in 10 per cent of cases. This increases to 20–25 per cent when superimposed on a persistent or progressive baseline bradycardia. The combination of a baseline tachycardia and late decelerations is associated with a 14 per cent risk of low Apgar scores. The presence of late decelerations increases the risk of metabolic acidosis 17-fold.[2]

## ACTIVE VERSUS PASSIVE SECOND STAGE

Many clinicians now divide the second stage of labour into a passive and an active phase. During the former, continued descent of the fetal head occurs with neither maternal effort nor urge to push. The risks of acidosis in this passive phase are probably similar to those of the active first stage. Certainly, Nordstrom *et al.*[8] showed fetal scalp lactate to increase in parallel with the length of active pushing in the second stage [C].

## SECONDARY TESTS OF FETAL WELL-BEING

### Fetal blood sampling

Fetal scalp pH studies remain the principal secondary test of fetal well-being in the second stage of labour. There is no evidence that their accuracy falls, and they are usually technically very easy.

### Other secondary tests

There has been little investigation into the prognostic ability of other secondary tests of fetal well-being, such as vibroacoustic stimulation, scalp stimulation, fetal electrocardiogram (ECG) or pulse oximetry in the second stage of labour. Combining ST analysis (STAN™) with CTG monitoring has the advantage of reducing operative vaginal delivery rates by 10 per cent (see Chapter 29, Fetal distress in the first stage) [A].[9] However, recent guidelines on the use of STAN have emphasized that ST monitoring should not be commenced in the second stage as this risks missing ST changes which have already occurred in cases of pre-existing fetal hypoxia.[10]

## THE MANAGEMENT OF SUSPECTED FETAL COMPROMISE IN THE SECOND STAGE OF LABOUR

- Improve placental blood supply.
  - Maternal positioning to avoid aorto-caval compression.
  - Intravenous fluids when appropriate.
  - Vasoconstrictors, such as ephedrine, for lower limb vasodilatation secondary to epidural analgesia.
- Improve maternal oxygenation.
  - Maternal oxygen therapy may be helpful if used for a short period while other measures are instituted. However, the routine use of oxygen therapy in the second stage was found to lead to an increase in newborn acidosis [A].[11]
- Diminish uterine activity if excessive.
  - Decrease or stop any oxytocin infusion. In the second stage, bolus intravenous tocolytics have been associated with an increase in instrumental delivery, but no improvement in fetal outcome [A].[12] Their use in this situation should be restricted to cases where a

short delay is expected before operative delivery can be undertaken.
- Decide if delivery is indicated, based upon:
  - the severity of the CTG abnormality and results of any secondary tests of fetal well-being;
  - response to the above interventions to improve the situation;
  - the whole clinical picture, including obstetric risk factors, progress in labour and potential assisted delivery;
  - untreatable fetal complications such as abruption, cord prolapse and chorioamnionitis, and scar dehiscence.

There is little evidence to support the use of amnioinfusion in the second stage of labour to reduce cord compression and improve umbilical blood flow.

## ACKNOWLEDGEMENT

This chapter has been revised and updated. The author and editors acknowledge the contribution of Griff Jones to the chapter on this topic in the previous edition of the book.

---

**A clinical approach to reviewing abnormal second stage CTGS**

Always ask yourself:

What factors are present that increase the neonatal risk of instrumental delivery? For example, meconium/macrosomia/malposition/mid-cavity arrest/diabetes/previous shoulder dystocia.

Does the abnormality require immediate delivery?
**Yes**
Is an assisted delivery likely to be easy?
- **Yes** - occiput anterior (OA)/low station/little caput or moulding
- **Deliver in room**
- **No** - malposition/mid-cavity arrest/major moulding or caput
  - Undertake delivery in theatre either as trial or directly by caesarean section
  - Strongly consider fetal blood sampling before trial of instrumental delivery

**No**
Is an assisted delivery likely to be easy?
- **Yes** - OA/low station/little caput or moulding
Has progress been steady in active second stage?
- **Yes**: offer mother choice of continued pushing for set time before recommending assisted delivery.
- **No**: consider oxytocin (consider fetal blood sampling beforehand) if mother wishes to avoid assisted delivery
If no intervention possible to improve situation, recommend assisted delivery in room

- **No** - malposition/mid-cavity arrest/major moulding or caput)

Has progress been steady in active second stage?

- **Yes:** consider fetal blood sampling to allow more time and convert to an easier delivery
- **No:** consider fetal blood sampling and then oxytocin

  - If inappropriate to intervene to improve progress, recommend delivery
  - In theatre either as a trial or directly by caesarean section, strongly consider fetal blood sampling before trial of instrumental delivery

## KEY POINTS

- CTG abnormalities are very common in the second stage, but many are benign.
- Particular attention should be paid to marked bradycardias, any bradycardia with reduced variability and late or severe variable decelerations.
- Use fetal scalp sampling to avoid potentially difficult instrumental deliveries in the presence of pre-existing fetal compromise.

## Published Guidelines

National Institute for Health and Clinical Excellence: *Intrapartum care – care of the healthy women and their babies during childbirth*. London: NICE, September 2007.

## Key References

1. Krebs HB, Petres RE, Dunn LJ. Intrapartum fetal heart rate monitoring. V. Fetal heart rate patterns in the second stage of labor. *Am J Obstet Gynecol* 1981; **140**: 435–9.

2. Sheiner E, Hadar A, Hallak M *et al*. Clinical significance of fetal heart rate tracings during the second stage of labor. *Obstet Gynecol* 2001; **97**: 747–52.

3. Gilstrap LC 3rd, Hauth JC, Toussaint S. Second stage fetal heart rate abnormalities and neonatal acidosis. *Obstet Gynecol* 1984; **63**: 209–13.

4. Gilstrap LC 3rd, Hauth JC, Hankins GD, Beck AW. Second-stage fetal heart rate abnormalities and type of neonatal acidemia. *Obstet Gynecol* 1987; **70**: 191–5.

5. Cardoso CG, Graca LM, Clode N. A study on second stage cardiotocographic patterns and umbilical acid-base balance in cases with first stage normal fetal heart rates. *J Matern Fetal Invest* 1995; **5**: 144–9.

6. Piquard F, Hsiung R, Mettauer M *et al*. The validity of fetal heart rate monitoring during the second stage of labor. *Obstet Gynecol* 1988; **72**: 746–51.

7. Gull I, Jaffa AJ, Oren M *et al*. Acid accumulation during end-stage bradycardia in term fetuses: how long is too long? *Br J Obstet Gynaecol* 1996; **103**: 1096–101.

8. Nordstrom L, Achanna S, Naka K, Arulkumaran S. Fetal and maternal lactate increase during active second stage of labour. *Br J Obstet Gynaecol* 2001; **108**: 263–8.

9. Neilson JP. Fetal electrocardiogram (ECG) for fetal monitoring during labour. *Cochrane Database Syst Rev* 2006; (**3**): CD000116.

10. Amer-Wahlin I, Arulkumaran S, Hagberg H *et al*. Fetal electrocardiogram: ST waveform analysis in intrapartum surveillance. *Br J Obstet Gynaecol* 2007; **114**: 1191–3.

11. Thorp JA, Trobough T, Evans R *et al*. The effect of maternal oxygen administration during the second stage of labor on umbilical cord blood gas values: a randomized controlled prospective trial. *Am J Obstet Gynecol* 1995; **172**: 465–74.

12. Campbell J, Anderson I, Chang A, Wood C. The use of ritodrine in the management of the fetus during the second stage of labour. *Aust NZ J Obstet Gynaecol* 1978; **18**: 100–13.

# Shoulder dystocia

*Myles Taylor*

## INTRODUCTION

Shoulder dystocia is an acute obstetric emergency requiring rapid intervention to prevent neonatal morbidity and mortality. The relative infrequency of shoulder dystocia means that few obstetricians are truly experienced in the management of this complication. However, the high perinatal mortality and morbidity associated with this condition means that all labour ward practitioners must possess a detailed knowledge of the condition and how to overcome it.

## DEFINITION

Classically, shoulder dystocia is recognized when the fetal chin retracts firmly back on to the perineum immediately after delivery of the head, the so-called 'turtleneck' sign. A widely used, but not universally accepted, definition of shoulder dystocia is a delivery that requires additional obstetric manoeuvres to release the shoulders after gentle downward traction has failed.[1]

A logical approach to the assessment of severity of an earlier shoulder dystocia is essential. Events surrounding the delivery should be considered under three headings.

1 Additional manoeuvres:
   a. What steps were required to effect delivery? See below under the headings: First-line: simple measures, Second-line: advanced measures and Third-line measures.
2 Fetal complications:
   a. Apgar scores and degree of resuscitation required,
   b. neonatal unit admission,
   c. direct fetal trauma (Erb's palsy, fractures),
   d. long-term handicap (neurodevelopmental, palsy).
3 Maternal complications:
   a. perineal trauma (extended episiotomy or tear, third degree tear),
   b. postpartum haemorrhage.

## INCIDENCE

The lack of a universally agreed definition for shoulder dystocia hampers any estimate of incidence. As a rough guide, approximately 1 per cent of deliveries are complicated by shoulder dystocia.

# COMPLICATIONS

## Fetal

Short-term complications, such as fractures of the humerus or clavicle, are not uncommon; however, these heal well and have an excellent prognosis. Transient brachial plexus injury, such as Erb's palsy, is also relatively common. Fortunately, with early recognition, prompt physiotherapy and even neurosurgical treatment, most improve over time, leaving only 1–2 per cent of shoulder dystocia cases with long-term dysfunction. Hypoxic–ischaemic encephalopathy may develop after severe cases and carries a risk of later neurodevelopmental handicap. Perinatal mortality secondary to shoulder dystocia was reported in 56 cases in the United Kingdom in 1994–95, an incidence of approximately 1 in 25 000 births.[2]

## Maternal

Excessive blood loss from extensive perineal, vaginal and even cervical lacerations is possible. Extension of perineal trauma into third or fourth degree tears is also recognized.

# AETIOLOGY

The mechanics underlying shoulder dystocia have been reviewed by Johnstone and Myerscough.[3] Although the bisacromial diameter is larger than the biparietal diameter, the shoulders have the advantage of inherent mobility. As the fetal head passes through the pelvic outlet, the shoulders simultaneously enter the pelvic inlet. Ideally, the shoulders should enter the pelvis transversely, although they are usually oblique, with the posterior shoulder moving towards the sacrosciatic notch. As restitution of the fetal head occurs, the shoulders rotate through the pelvis and the anterior shoulder presents under the symphysis pubis.

In cases of true shoulder dystocia, either the anterior shoulder or, in severe forms, both the anterior and posterior shoulders are arrested at the pelvic inlet. It is a common misconception that the pelvic outlet and perineum contribute to shoulder dystocia. This is in part fuelled by the advice to perform an extended episiotomy which serves only to create the space necessary for vaginal manipulations.

# PREDISPOSING FACTORS

## Excessive fetal size

The incidence of shoulder dystocia is known to increase in line with birth weight. Below 3.5 kg, the reported incidence is 0.2–0.8 per cent, rising to 5–23 per cent with birth weights above 4.5 kg.[4,5]

Despite this relationship, half of all shoulder dystocia cases occur with babies of normal birth weight. This may be because some babies that fail to meet an absolute criterion for macrosomia (such as a birth weight >4.0 kg) are actually relatively large for gestation for that particular woman. Unfortunately, it is difficult to know in advance the 'intended' birth weight for any individual woman's offspring. However, customized fetal growth charts are increasingly available; these use maternal ethnic origin, build and parity to individualize predicted fetal weight at any gestation.

Clinicians must remain wary of any clinical situation or condition that is likely to increase fetal weight abnormally. Maternal diabetes, long known to be associated with a risk of excessive fetal growth, is a major risk factor [B].[6] Other causes of fetal macrosomia, either relative or absolute, include maternal obesity, multiparity and post-dates pregnancies.

## Intrapartum events

Relative disproportion is often suggested by poor progress in labour, but this is a poor predictor of subsequent shoulder dystocia.[6,7] Shoulder dystocia has been associated with mid-cavity instrumental deliveries,[7] but since this reflects a significant failure of descent, it is again highlighting poor progress in labour.

Parturition has long been linked with the three Ps – the passages, the passenger and the powers. It may be that inefficient uterine contractile activity underlies some cases of shoulder dystocia. It has been suggested that the endogenous powers pushing the shoulders through the birth canal in cases of shoulder dystocia are actually more important than the traction forces generated by the obstetrician.[8] An aetiological role for the 'powers' is also suggested by the increased incidence of shoulder dystocia found in induced labours, associated with an increased risk of dysfunctional labour and operative delivery.[5,7,9]

# MANAGEMENT

## Antenatal assessment

### Recurrence risks

Overall recurrence risks for shoulder dystocia are approximately 10–15 per cent.[10,11] These may underestimate the risks, since caesarean section may have been advised for those pregnancies where a poor outcome occurred after shoulder dystocia. The above studies suggest increased risks in overweight women or with large or 'larger' babies in the subsequent pregnancy.

### Review of previous delivery

A careful review of the events surrounding an earlier delivery is essential, using the system outlined above under Incidence. This must include a review of the previous maternity notes, which may necessitate correspondence with other units.

### Screening for gestation diabetes

If there is any suspicion of excessive fetal growth in a previous pregnancy (regardless of birth weight), a glucose tolerance test should be arranged for 28 weeks gestation. If impaired glucose tolerance is found, measures should be implemented to minimize any fetal effects [C].

### Pelvimetry

There is no evidence to support the routine use of pelvimetry in this situation [B]. Its use should be highly selective. Examples of situations in which it might be considered include a predisposing factor for pelvic contraction, such as a previous significant fracture.

## Antenatal intervention

### Identification of fetal macrosomia

The prediction of fetal weight, either clinically or by ultrasound, is inaccurate in the third trimester where the margin of error in predicting birthweight exceeds 10 per cent. Thus, information gained from prenatal assessment of size can only be used as one risk factor in the overall clinical picture. It facilitates advance planning and preparation but, in isolation, should not dictate any particular management. The recognition of significant macrosomia in association with other risk factors, particularly diabetes or a previous birth with shoulder dystocia, requires careful assessment.

### Early induction

Evidence from observational and randomized trials does not support the use of induction to prevent shoulder dystocia in suspected macrosomia (ACOG Practice Bulletin 22 Guideline) [B].[9,12,13] As mentioned previously, induced labours are reported to have a higher incidence of shoulder dystocia.

### Elective caesarean section

The American College of Obstetricians and Gynecologists (ACOG Practice Bulletin 22 guideline) recommends considering elective caesarean section when the birth weight is predicted to be greater than 5 kg in non-diabetics or 4.5 kg in diabetics [D].[14] Despite this, it acknowledges that such a policy would result in 443 caesarean sections in diabetic women to prevent a single permanent newborn injury.

These calculations are strongly influenced by our inability to reliably predict macrosomia antenatally. At present, there are few grounds on which to recommend elective caesarean section on the basis of fetal size alone. Decisions should be individualized, based on an appreciation of all risk factors present.

### Diabetic control

It is logical to suppose that tight diabetic control may reduce the incidence of fetal macrosomia. At present, there is a small body of evidence to support this assumption [C].

## Intrapartum management

### Advance planning

Antenatal risk factors for shoulder dystocia should be noted.

- Reassessment of risk should be carried out if there is poor progress in labour. In women believed to be at significant risk, advance preparation is essential.
- Midwifery and medical staff should establish a contingency plan involving:
  - who needs to be aware of the potential problem,
  - who will be present at the delivery, and
  - what steps will be taken should difficulties arise.

In mothers who have failure of descent in the second stage, the presence of other risk factors for shoulder dystocia will influence not only if, but also where, and by whom, an instrumental delivery is attempted. Although a trial of instrumental delivery in theatre does not reduce the risk of shoulder dystocia, it ensures the presence of adequate staffing to deal with it efficiently.

An epidural should always be considered in situations in which there is judged to be a considerable risk of shoulder dystocia, particularly if it is felt that maternal distress may interfere with co-operation.

Early diagnosis allows prompt intervention. The 'turtle sign' is usually obvious, but if there is delay in delivery of the shoulders, examination to define the location of the anterior shoulder (above or below the symphysis) can be helpful.

## TREATMENT

There are no randomized trials to provide guidance for the management of this obstetric emergency. In women judged to be at particularly high risk, obstetricians should consider the prophylactic use of some of the simple measures described below in order to avoid delay in delivery of the shoulders. In this situation, it is probably still worth waiting for the next contraction before completing the delivery.

Help should always be summoned as soon as a problem is recognized. As well as additional midwives, neonatology and anaesthetic staff should be called. Manipulations to overcome shoulder dystocia cannot be learnt from a book. Practical training in obstetric emergencies must be undertaken, as offered on an ALSO© course or similar. Manipulations should be considered under three headings.

An episiotomy should be considered, but it is not mandatory (RCOG guideline No. 42).

## First-line: simple measures

These measures should always be tried first and will be successful in 90 per cent of cases. Remember to maintain the head in a neutral position, avoiding excessive lateral traction. In the absence of medical staff, midwives will have often already tried placing the mother in a lateral position, which is reported to have some benefit.

- McRoberts manoeuvre involves hyperflexion of the maternal thighs on to the maternal abdomen, either by the mother herself or by a pair of assistants. It has been shown radiographically to flatten the lumbosacral curve and lessen any obstruction from the sacral promontory.
- Suprapubic pressure is often used simultaneously. Using a stance similar to that of cardiopulmonary resuscitation (CPR), pressure is exerted obliquely on the posterior aspect of the anterior shoulder. The aim is to move the shoulders into the wider oblique diameter of the pelvis and force the anterior shoulder under the symphysis pubis.
- Consideration should be given to expediting in the all-fours position.[15] The decision to move the mother into this position will depend on the individual accoucheur and the feasibility of moving the mother.
- Identify a 'scribe' to note times of staff attendance and manoeuvres performed.

Fundal pressure is not recommended as this can cause uterine rupture. Maternal pushing should be discouraged as this may lead to further impaction of the shoulders.

## Second-line: advanced measures

Failing correction of the problem with simple measures, more aggressive manipulations will be required either by internal rotational manoeuvres or by delivery of the posterior arm. These may involve considerable discomfort to the mother (and distress to her partner) and warning should be given. In order that a hand can be introduced into the vagina, a generous episiotomy may be required.

### Internal rotational manoeuvres

- *Rubin's manoeuvre* – By approaching the anterior shoulder from behind, attempts should be made to rotate the shoulders into the oblique diameter of the pelvis, using

a finger hooked into one axilla. Ideally, one should attempt to move the fetus in a direction that allows the shoulder to move inwards towards the chest, which will decrease the dimensions of the shoulders. Once disimpacted, traction can again be tried.
- *Wood's screw manoeuvre* – If simple rotation fails and the posterior shoulder is below the sacral promontory, Wood's screw manoeuvre should be attempted. Approach the posterior fetal shoulder from the front and rotate the posterior shoulder through 180° so that it becomes the anterior shoulder. By simultaneously combining this with a degree of downward traction, the rotated shoulder remains within the pelvis and appears under the symphysis.
- *Reverse Wood's screw manoeuvre* – Approach the posterior shoulder from behind and rotate the fetus in the opposite direction from Rubin or Wood's screw manoeuvres. This may be successful when previous manoeuvres have failed.

### Delivery of the posterior arm

- By advancing a hand into the uterus posteriorly and finding the fetal hand, delivery of the posterior fetal arm can be achieved by sweeping it across the fetal chest.

## Third-line measures

If all the above measures have been tried and retried and the baby is still alive, third-line measures could be considered. However, the likelihood of any individual obstetrician gaining experience of these techniques within the UK is remote. Furthermore, publication bias means that clinicians often only report their successes. It is likely that heroic measures have, on many occasions, been followed by stillbirth, neonatal death or profound handicap, at a cost of considerable maternal morbidity.

- *Cleidotomy.* Deliberately fracturing the fetal clavicle(s) can be used to shorten the biacromial diameter. However, this can be difficult to perform and can lead to injury of the underlying vascular and pulmonary structures.
- *Zavenelli manoeuvre.* The fetal head is replaced into the uterus by reversing the steps of parturition. This may require additional uterine relaxation, using either bolus tocolytics or general anaesthesia. Abdominal rescue describes intrauterine manipulation through a transabdominal hysterotomy to facilitate vaginal delivery.
- *Symphysiotomy.* This can lead to a 2–3 cm increase in the bony pelvic diameters. However, there is a significant risk of long-term maternal morbidity. Special skills and equipment are required, including a solid-bladed scalpel. The urethra must be catheterized and displaced laterally. In the absence of an epidural, local anaesthesia is needed. It is likely that the fetus will have been severely compromised by the time a symphysiotomy could be safely performed on most UK labour wards.

# DOCUMENTATION

After a delivery complicated by shoulder dystocia, it is important that the details surrounding the delivery are accurately recorded. This is important for medico-legal reasons – for example, where Erb's palsy is present, it is important to determine whether the affected shoulder was anterior or posterior, since trauma to the posterior shoulder plexus is not due to action by the accoucheur (RCOG guideline No. 42). Good documentation is also useful for helping form a plan in any subsequent pregnancy.

It is important to record the following:

- time of the delivery of the head,
- direction of the head is facing after restitution,
- manoeuvres performed, their timings and order,
- time of the delivery of the body,
- staff in attendance,
- condition of the baby and Apgar scores and cord pH blood levels.

In terms of psychological benefit, the role of maternal debriefing remains controversial. However, mothers must understand what went wrong, both to minimize inappropriate blame of themselves or others and so that they may alert their caregivers in their next pregnancy.

# ACKNOWLEDGEMENT

This chapter has been revised and updated. The author and editors acknowledge the contribution of Griff Jones to the chapter on this topic in the previous edition of the book.

## KEY POINTS

- Neither fetal macrosomia nor shoulder dystocia can be reliably predicted.
- Most strategies to prevent shoulder dystocia are either ineffective (early induction) or lead to excessive intervention (elective caesarean section).
- The presence of known risk factors, particularly two or more, should trigger advance preparations to deal with or avoid the situation, before it actually arises.
- Since shoulder dystocia will often occur without warning, obstetricians must have well-rehearsed strategies to overcome it.

## Published Guidelines

American College of Obstetricians and gynecologists. ACOG Practice Bulletin Number 22. *Fetal Macrosomia*. Clinical Management Guidelines for Obstetricians/ Gynecologists. November 2000.

Focus Group – Shoulder dystocia. In: *Confidential Enquiry into Stillbirths and Deaths in Infancy*, 5th annual report, Section 8, Focus Group – Shoulder Dystocia. London: HMSO, 1996.

Royal College of Obstetricians and Gynaecologists. RCOG guideline No. 42, Shoulder Dystocia, December 2005.

## Key References

1. Resnik R. Management of shoulder girdle dystocia. *Clin Obstet Gynecol* 1980; **23**: 559–64.
2. Hope P, Breslin S, Lamont L *et al*. Fatal shoulder dystocia: a review of 56 cases reported to the Confidential Enquiry into Stillbirths and Deaths in Infancy. *Br J Obstet Gynaecol* 1998; **105**: 1256–61.
3. Johnstone FD, Myerscough PR. Shoulder dystocia. *Br J Obstet Gynaecol* 1998; **105**: 811–15.
4. Mocanu EV, Greene RA, Byrne BM, Turner MJ. Obstetric and neonatal outcome of babies weighing more than 4.5 kg: an analysis by parity. *Eur J Obstet Gynecol Reprod Biol* 2000; **92**: 229–33.
5. Acker DB, Sachs BP, Friedman EA. Risk factors for shoulder dystocia in the average-weight infant. *Obstet Gynecol* 1986; **67**: 614–18.
6. Acker DB, Sachs BP, Friedman EA. Risk factors for shoulder dystocia. *Obstet Gynecol* 1985; **66**: 762–8.
7. McFarland M, Hod M, Piper JM *et al*. Are labor abnormalities more common in shoulder dystocia? *Am J Obstet Gynecol* 1995; **173**: 1211–14.
8. Gonik B, Walker A, Grimm M. Mathematic modeling of forces associated with shoulder dystocia: a comparison of endogenous and exogenous sources. *Am J Obstet Gynecol* 2000; **182**: 689–91.
9. Dublin S, Lydon-Rochelle M, Kaplan RC *et al*. Maternal and neonatal outcomes after induction of labor without an identified indication. *Am J Obstet Gynecol* 2000; **183**: 986–94.
10. Smith RB, Lane C, Pearson JF. Shoulder dystocia: what happens at the next delivery? *Br J Obstet Gynaecol* 1994; **101**: 713–15.
11. Lewis DF, Raymond RC, Perkins MB *et al*. Recurrence rate of shoulder dystocia. *Am J Obstet Gynecol* 1995; **172**: 1369–71.
12. Combs CA, Singh NB, Khoury JC. Elective induction versus spontaneous labor after sonographic diagnosis of fetal macrosomia. *Obstet Gynecol* 1993; **81**: 492–6.
13. Gonen O, Rosen DJ, Dolfin Z *et al*. Induction of labor versus expectant management in macrosomia: a randomized study. *Obstet Gynecol* 1997; **89**: 913–17.
14. Sokol RJ, Blackwell SC. ACOG practice bulletin: Shoulder dystocia. Number 40, November 2002. *Int J Gynaecol Obstet* 2003; **80**: 87–92.
15. Bruner JP, Drummond SB, Meenan AL, Gaskin IM. All-fours maneuver for reducing shoulder dystocia during labor. *J Reprod Med* 1998; **43**: 439–43.

# Instrumental vaginal delivery

*Richard Hayman*

## INTRODUCTION

While initially reserved for the delivery of dead infants, from as early as 1500BC there exist reports of successful deliveries of live infants in obstructed labours. Chamberlain's development of the modern obstetric forceps in the late sixteenth century dramatically changed the aim of intrapartum intervention in favour of delivery of a live infant, and following from William Smellie's description of the use of forceps in midwifery, instrumental intervention in the process of labour has become an integral part of obstetric care.

During 2005–2006, of the 593 400 births recorded in the UK, 65 867 (11.1 per cent) were assisted with forceps/ventouse. However, the incidence of instrumental intervention varies widely both between and within countries and may be performed as infrequently as 1.5 per cent or as often as 26 per cent. Such differences may be linked to the alternative management strategies that are employed on individual labour wards, and various techniques have been implemented to help lower the rates of assisted delivery.[1]

Operative vaginal delivery has been identified as a major risk factor for fetal morbidity and mortality, as well as early and late maternal morbidity (including faecal incontinence). Consequently, the Royal College of Obstetricians and Gynaecologists (RCOG) have issued clinical guidelines regarding the use of instruments to aid vaginal delivery,

stating that 'the operator must have the knowledge, experience and skills necessary to use the instruments and manage complications that may arise'. The guideline emphasizes the relative merits of the two instruments, the indications for their use and their associated complications, the conclusion being that 'the careful well-trained operator will select the instrument best suited to the individual circumstances'.[2,3]

## STRATEGIES FOR REDUCING THE NEED FOR INSTRUMENTAL VAGINAL DELIVERY

Many different strategies have been employed to help lower the rates of assisted delivery. However, only a few of these are evidence based.

- Provision of a caregiver in labour. This is associated with a reduction in the need for operative vaginal delivery (odds ratio (OR) 0.77) [A].
- Active management of the second stage with syntocinon in nulliparous women with epidural analgesia [B].
- Delayed pushing in nulliparous women with epidural analgesia [B].[4]

When the onset of active pushing is delayed by the introduction of a passive second stage, the chance of a spontaneous delivery is slightly increased. It is also important to recognize that the incidence of difficult deliveries is reduced (relative risk (RR) 0.79) with a specific reduction being noted in mid-pelvic procedures (RR 0.72).[4] The practice of assessing fetal well-being by fetal blood sampling in the second stage may also provide the confidence to both mother, midwives and obstetricians to delay the onset of 'active parturition' rather than intervene too eagerly.

Other techniques that are commonly used to reduce the incidence of intervention in the second stage, but have no evidence to support their practice, are upright positions in labour[5] and allowing the effect of an epidural to 'wear off' before any expulsive efforts are commenced [C]. Indeed, allowing a previously effective epidural to wear off to the point that the mother has considerable pain is likely to be detrimental to a successful second stage rather than helpful, and seems unnecessarily cruel.[6]

## INDICATIONS FOR ASSISTED VAGINAL DELIVERY

There are two basic categories into which the indications for assisted vaginal delivery may be placed.

### Fetal

- Fetal head malpositions (occipito-lateral and occipito-posterior).
- Presumed fetal compromise.
- Elective instrumental intervention.
- Vaginal breech delivery: forceps can be applied to the after-coming head to control the delivery of the vertex, a situation where the ventouse is contraindicated.

The most common fetal indications are those concerning malpositions of the fetal head (occipito-transverse and occipito-posterior). This occurs more frequently with regional anaesthesia, as a consequence of alterations in the tone of the pelvic floor that impede spontaneous rotation to the optimal occipito-anterior position. Epidural analgesia has been shown to be associated with longer first and second stages of labour, increased incidence of fetal malposition, increased use of oxytocin and increased incidence of instrumental vaginal deliveries. It is possible that the increasing incidence of instrumental deliveries may reflect the rising demand for regional anaesthesia.

Fetal distress is a commonly cited indication for instrumental intervention, although it is infrequently the fetus that is actually distressed. Presumed fetal compromise is a more comprehensive term, especially when employed in conjunction with a precise description of the situation surrounding the intervention in order to validate the decision.

The use of elective instrumental intervention for infants of reduced weight is more controversial. In infants of less than 1.5 kg, delivery with forceps offers no advantage over spontaneous delivery and may, in fact, increase the incidence of intracranial haemorrhage [C]. Ventouse carries the same risks, but in addition should be avoided in infants of less than 35 completed weeks of gestation.[2,7]

### Maternal

- Maternal distress, exhaustion, or prolongation of the second stage of labour (>2 hours in a primigravida (3 hours if an epidural is *in situ*); or >1 hour in a multipara (2 hours if an epidural is *in situ*)).
- Medically significant conditions, such as aortic valve disease with significant outflow obstruction; myasthenia

gravis; significant APH due to placental abruption or vasa praevia; severe hypertensive disease; and previous caesarean section (to minimize the risk of scar rupture) are less common.

The reasons cited for intervention are often imprecise as one or more factors may interact, for example delay in the second stage as a consequence of poor maternal effort combined with a transitional malposition. Determining which is the more important may be a case of semantics as independently or conjointly, they are an indication for delivery. However, they are not necessarily an indication for delivery by a specific instrument.

Delivery options in the second stage include caesarean section and this should particularly be considered if there is a high 'index of suspicion' of delivery failure. It is therefore suggested that most mid-cavity procedures, which by their nature have a higher rate of complications than outlet or low deliveries, should be performed in theatre. However, the psychological consequences of transferring a patient to an operating theatre in the second stage should not be underestimated.

## INSTRUMENT CHOICE AND MANAGEMENT OPTIONS

The choice of instrument employed by the accoucheur should be based on a combination of indication, experience and training, and it is the last two of these issues that must be formally addressed in light of today's changes in junior 'doctors' hours' and working practices. It is certainly the case that only adequately trained or supervised practitioners should undertake any vacuum or forceps delivery.

Systematic review has shown the vacuum extractor, when compared to the forceps, to be:

- Significantly more likely to [A]:
  - fail at achieving a vaginal delivery (OR 1.7; 95 per cent confidence interval (CI) 1.3–2.2; NNH 20)
  - be associated with a cephalohaematoma (OR 2.4; 95 per cent CI 1.7–3.4; NNH 17)
  - be associated with retinal haemorrhage (OR 2.0; 95 per cent CI 1.3–3.0; NNH 50)
  - be associated with maternal worries about the baby (OR 2.2; 95 per cent CI 1.2–3.9; NNH 17)
  - (NNH 5 number needed to harm, i.e. for every 20 vacuum deliveries there is one 'extra' failure, compared with forceps).
- Significantly less likely to be associated with [A]:
  - use of maternal regional/general anaesthesia (OR 0.6; 95 per cent CI 0.5–0.7; NNT 12)
  - significant maternal perineal and vaginal trauma (OR 0.4; 95 per cent CI 0.3–0.5; NNT 10). Anal sphincter injury in particular is half as common with a ventouse delivery.

- severe perineal pain at 24 hours (OR 0.54; 95 per cent CI 0.31–0.93; NNT 17)
  - (NNT 5 number needed to treat, i.e. for every ten ventouse deliveries one less case of significant maternal perineal trauma will occur).
- Equally likely to be associated with [A]:
  - delivery by caesarean section (OR 0.6; 95 per cent CI 0.3–1.02)
  - low 5-minute Apgar scores (OR 1.7; 95 per cent CI 0.99–2.8)
  - the need for phototherapy (OR 1.08; 95 per cent CI 0.7–1.8).[8]

Unfortunately, there is a paucity of long-term follow-up data for both the mother and the baby. However, one of the largest randomized controlled trials demonstrated no difference between the groups delivered by forceps or ventouse when the women were assessed at approximately 5 years postpartum. Bowel urgency was more common in the ventouse group (26 versus 15 per cent, $p = 0.06$), but this just failed to reach statistical significance. This study also demonstrated no differences at this age in the infants delivered by each method.[9]

Although the degree of rotation required is a significant indicator of the potential difficulty of the delivery, the data currently available from the published trials cannot be analysed separately to compare the use of ventouse and forceps (e.g. Kiellands) for rotational deliveries.

To enable benchmarking, audit and comparison between studies, a standard definition of the types of operative delivery should be used. The American College of Obstetricians and Gynecologists criteria are adapted in Table 34.1 and define the delivery by the station and position.

## ROTATIONAL INSTRUMENTAL VAGINAL DELIVERY VERSUS CAESAREAN SECTION

Often the decision facing the obstetrician is whether to perform a 'difficult' vaginal delivery or a caesarean section. Caesarean section has often been viewed as the less harmful of the two interventions, however, there are limited data comparing the morbidity of second stage caesarean section with instrumental vaginal delivery. One prospective cohort study of 393 women with term, singleton, liveborn, cephalic pregnancies requiring operative delivery in theatre at full dilatation showed that factors increasing the likelihood of caesarean section included:

- maternal body mass index (BMI) >30,
- neonatal birth weight >4.0 kg,
- occipito-posterior position.

Women who were delivered by caesarean section were more likely to have a major haemorrhage of more than 1 L

**Table 34.1** Classification for operative vaginal delivery (adapted from ACOG, 2000)

| Term | Definition |
|------|------------|
| Outlet | Fetal scalp visible without separating the labia |
| | Fetal skull has reached the pelvic floor |
| | Sagittal suture is in the antero-posterior diameter or right or left occiput anterior or posterior position(rotation does not exceed 45 degrees) |
| | Fetal head is at or on the perineum |
| Low | Leading point of the skull (not caput) is at station plus 2 cm or more and not on the pelvic floor |
| | Two subdivisions: |
| | (a) rotation of 45 degrees or less |
| | (b) rotation more than 45 degrees |
| Mid | Fetal head is one-fifth palpable per abdomen |
| | Leading point of the skull is above station plus 2 cm but not above the ischial spines |
| | Two subdivisions: |
| | (a) rotation of 45 degrees or less |
| | (b) rotation more than 45 degrees |
| High | Not included in classification |

and to need a hospital stay of more than 5 days. On the other hand, babies delivered by caesarean section were less likely to have trauma than babies delivered by forceps but more likely to require admission for intensive care.[10] It is important to note that serious trauma was not limited to the vaginally delivered group, and that the experience of the operator was directly related to the chance of major haemorrhage whatever the mode of delivery. It should therefore be the aim at this stage in labour to deliver women vaginally, unless there are clear signs of cephalo-pelvic disproportion. It is undoubtedly the case that skilled obstetricians should supervise complex operative deliveries, whatever time of day they occur [C].

### Pre-requisites for any instrumental delivery

- Confirmed rupture of the membranes.
- The cervix must be fully dilated (except second twin and rare other situations – see below).
- Vertex presentation with identification of the position.
- For occipito-anterior and transverse positions, no part of the fetal head should be palpable abdominally. For occipito-posterior positions, it is acceptable that one-fifth of the head may be palpable per abdomen. The presenting part should be at +1 or more below the ischial spines.
- Adequate analgesia/anaesthesia.

- Empty bladder/no obstruction below the fetal head (contracted pelvis/pelvic kidney/ovarian cyst, etc.).
- A knowledgeable and experienced operator with adequate preparation to proceed with an alternative approach if necessary.
- An adequately informed and consented patient (consent must be obtained though written consent is not necessary).

For forceps, all the pre-requisites above apply but, in addition, it is essential that the operator checks the pair of forceps to ensure that a matching pair has been provided and that the blades lock with ease (both before and after application).

## Basic rules

It has been suggested that failure rates of less than 1 per cent should be achieved with well-maintained apparatus and the use of the correct technique. However, many feel that this is an unrealistic target, an observation illustrated by the study of Johanson et al.[11] who achieved a vaginal delivery with the first instrument in only 86 per cent of cases.

The following factors were cited as contributing to delivery failure.[11–13]

- Failure to select the correct cup type: inappropriate use of the silastic cup (especially in the presence of deflexion of the fetal head, excess caput, a macrosomic infant or prolonged second stage of labour).
- Inadequate initial case assessment: high head, misdiagnosis of the position and attitude of the head.
- Incorrect cup placement: positioning either too anterior or lateral.
- Traction along the wrong plane.
- Poor maternal effort, with inadequate use of syntocinon to aid expulsive efforts in the second stage.

## Patient evaluation

Before embarking on an instrumental vaginal delivery an abdominal palpation should be performed. The fetal head should be at the very most one-fifth palpable and it is wise to measure the symphysis fundal height (SFH). A SFH measurement of >40 cm is above the 97th centile for term in the second stage of labour. A careful pelvic examination is essential to determine whether there are any 'architectural' contraindications to performing an instrumental vaginal delivery. If, for example, a contracted pelvis is the cause of failure to progress in the second stage, due consideration must be paid to determining the type of instrument to be employed, or whether it may in fact be more prudent to perform a caesarean section. The shape of the subpubic arch, the curve of the sacral hollow and the presence of flat or prominent ischial spines all contribute to the decision as to whether a vaginal delivery may be safely performed. Anthropoid (narrow), android (male/funnel-shaped), or platypelloid (squashed) pelvises all make instrumental deliveries more difficult and may preclude the use of rotational forceps.

With any difficult instrumental delivery the risk, of a shoulder dystocia occurring after successful delivery of the fetal head should always be born in mind, as should the subsequent and probable postpartum haemorrhage that will follow. As a consequence, the accoucheur must be able to develop the skills necessary to anticipate all such events and to manage the consequences in a logical and calm manner.

## CONTRAINDICATIONS

The ventouse should not be used:

- in gestations of ≤35 completed weeks because of the risk of cephalohaematoma and intracranial haemorrhage;
- in cases of face presentation.

There is minimal risk of fetal haemorrhage if the vacuum extractor is employed following fetal blood sampling or application of a spiral scalp electrode, and no excess incidence of fetal trauma (bleeding) was reported in two randomized trials comparing deliveries performed with forceps or ventouse.

Forceps and vacuum extractor deliveries before full dilatation of the cervix are contraindicated, although possible exceptions occur with the vacuum delivery of a second twin where the cervix has contracted or with a prolapsed cord at 9 cm if rapid delivery is anticipated [E].

## ANALGESIA

Analgesic requirements are greater for a forceps than for a ventouse delivery. Where rotational forceps are needed, regional analgesia is preferred. For a rigid cup ventouse delivery, a pudendal block with perineal infiltration may be all that is needed and, if a soft cup is used, analgesic requirements may be minimal. A requirement for haste should not preclude the use of analgesia. No operator would consider performing a caesarean section without the appropriate anaesthesia, and the same should be true for a vaginal delivery.

## POSITIONING

Instrumental deliveries are traditionally performed with the patient in the lithotomy position and using as aseptic a technique as is possible. The angle of traction needed requires that the foot of the bed be removed. For patients with limited movements, such as those with symphysis dysfunction, it may be necessary to limit abduction of the thighs to a minimum. It is the accoucheur's duty to ensure that the bladder is emptied.

# INSTRUMENT TYPES

## Ventouse/vacuum extractors

The basic premise of such instruments is that a suction cup, of a silastic or rigid construction, is connected, via tubing, to a vacuum source (Figure 34.1). Either directly through the tubing, or via a connecting 'chain', direct traction can then be applied to the presenting part to expedite delivery. Recent developments have removed the need for cumbersome external suction generators and have incorporated the vacuum mechanism into 'hand held' pumps, e.g. Kiwi OmniCup™. Such devices have been shown to be safe and may be useful for rotational deliveries, especially as they are low profile and are easily manoeuvred into the correct position. However, they have been shown to have a significantly higher failure rate than the conventional ventouse, with cup detachments occurring more frequently than the 'standard equipment'. This may not, however, reflect a problem with the equipment, but rather a combination of increasing inexperience of the accoucheur on the labour ward, poor case selection (the inappropriate use of a ventouse *per se* where a forceps delivery would be preferable), and a failure to compare 'like with like' (simple outlet deliveries compared with rotational deliveries).

## Choosing the type of cup

The soft cups are appropriate for straightforward deliveries with an occipito-anterior position. However, soft cups are significantly more likely to fail to achieve vaginal delivery than rigid cups. Although they are associated with less scalp injury for the fetus (OR 0.45) [A], there appears to be no difference in terms of maternal injury between the groups. Metal cups appear to be more suitable for 'occipito-posterior', transverse and difficult 'occipito-anterior' position deliveries where the infant is larger or there is a marked caput.[12,13]

The vacuum extractor can be used during the delivery of a second twin (this also being the only routine situation where application of an instrument with the cervix less than fully dilated is permitted), but should never be used with a breech presentation.

## Technique

For successful use of the ventouse, determination of the flexion point is vital. This is located at the vertex, which, in an average term infant, is on the saggital suture 3 cm anterior to the posterior fontanelle and thus 6 cm posterior to the anterior fontanelle. The centre of the cup should be positioned directly over this, as failure to do so will lead to a progressive deflexion of the fetal head during traction, with an increased risk that the baby will not be deliverable vaginally [B].

The operating vacuum pressure for nearly all ventouse is between 20.6 and 20.8 kg/cm$^2$ (260–280 kPa/500–800 cm H$_2$O). No evidence exists that incremental 'step-wise'

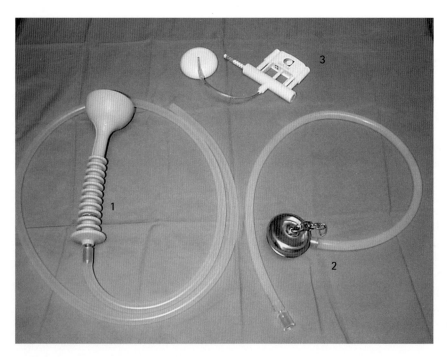

**Figure 34.1** Three different types of ventouse. (a) A siliastic cup ventouse, and (b) a metal cup ventouse for posterior application – the 'Bird cup'. Both of these require external vacuum generators. (c) A hand-held ventouse (with a pump incorporated in the handle)

increases in pressure improve the rate of success of delivery when compared with a linear increase. Using the latter technique with a silastic cup, a caput secundum is formed instantly, and with the metal cup, an adequate chignon is produced in less than 2 minutes. The standard teaching has been that the largest cup that can be placed should be; however, in practice a 5 cm cup is suitable for nearly all deliveries. It is prudent to increase the suction to $0.2\,\mathrm{kg/cm^2}$ first and then to recheck that no maternal tissue is caught under the cup edge. When this is confirmed, the suction can then be increased.

Traction must occur in the plane of least resistance along the axis of the pelvis – the traction plane. This will usually be at exactly 90 degrees to the cup, and the operator should keep a thumb and forefinger on the cup at the traction insertion to ensure that the traction direction is correct and to feel for slippage. Safe and gentle traction is then applied in concert with uterine contractions and voluntary expulsive efforts. This minimizes undue traction and the risk of trauma to the fetus. With the ventouse, the operator should allow no more than two episodes of breaking the suction in any vacuum delivery; and the maximum time from application to delivery should ideally be less than 15 minutes. If there is no evidence of descent with the first pull, the patient should be reassessed to ascertain the reason for failure to progress (Figure 34.2). This may simply be a failure of the equipment to provide adequate traction as a consequence of a leakage of the vacuum or the presence of a large caput. Inclusion of maternal soft tissues within the cup, traction along the incorrect plane, misdiagnosis of the position of the fetal head with incorrect equipment placement, choice of the wrong instrument, and cephalo-pelvic disproportion are other reasons for failure of delivery.

Rotation is achieved by the natural progression of the head through the pelvis. The operator must never try to assist rotation by turning the cup manually, as this is unhelpful and can lead to severe scalp lacerations [D].

It is not acceptable to use a ventouse when:

- the position of the fetal head is unknown;
- there is a significant degree of caput that may either preclude correct placement of the cup or, more sinisterly, indicate a substantial degree of cephalo-pelvic disproportion;
- the operator is inexperienced in the use of the instrument.

## Forceps

### Types of forceps

The basic forceps design has not radically changed over many years and all types in use today consist of two blades with shanks, joined together at a lock, with handles to provide a point for traction. However, the specific details of construction vary between the instruments. The blades may be fenestrated (open), pseudofenestrated (open with a protruding ridge), or solid. Likewise, the length of the shanks, the design of the lock (convergent, divergent or sliding) and the fashioning of the handles are instrument specific (Figure 34.3).

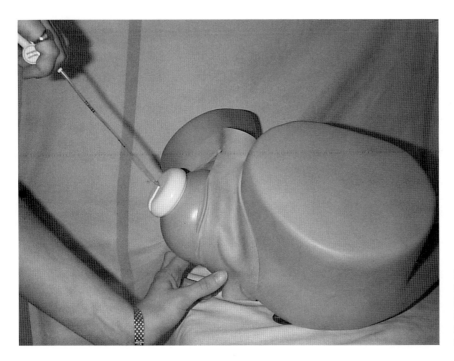

**Figure 34.2** Application of a hand-held ventouse (Kiwi OmniCup). The cup should be positioned over the flexion point to ensure optimal delivery technique. Manipulation of the cup during crowning of a fetus in an occipito-anterior position is shown

Second stage of labour

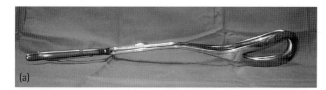

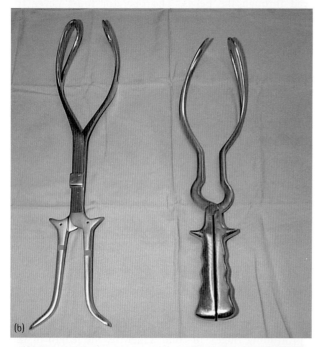

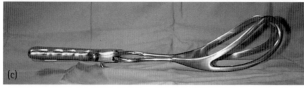

**Figure 34.3** Rotational (a and b; left) and non-rotational (b; right and c) obstetric forceps

## Technique

Once the patient has been optimally positioned, the pelvis must be examined to establish the positions and station of the vertex and the contours of the pelvis. At this stage, the accoucheur should always be prepared to abandon the vaginal route of delivery if a caesarean section is deemed safer. The forceps should be discretely held in front of the patient so as to visualize how they will be inserted per vaginum and placed around the fetal head.

It is appropriate to use non-rotational forceps when the head is occipito-anterior <15°. Where the head is positioned >15° from the vertical, rotation must be accomplished before traction (which for minor degrees may often be accomplished by manual rotation).

By convention, the left blade is inserted before the right with the accoucheurs hand protecting the vaginal wall from direct trauma. With proper placement of the forceps blades, they come to lie parallel to the axis of the fetal head and between the fetal head and the pelvic wall. The operator

then articulates and locks the blades, checking their application before applying traction. If the application is not correct, the blades must be repositioned or the procedure abandoned.

Traction should be applied intermittently in concert with uterine contractions and maternal expulsive efforts. The axis of traction changes during the delivery and is guided along the J-shaped curve of the pelvis. As the head begins to crown, the blades are directed to the vertical, a Ritgen manoeuvre is performed or an episiotomy fashioned (Figure 34.4). Once the head is delivered, the forceps are removed in the reverse order to which they were inserted, and the delivery is completed in the normal fashion.

Kiellands forceps are the most commonly utilized instrument for rotational forceps deliveries and, as specific techniques are required, only those who have been properly trained in their use should employ them. These forceps are unique in their design, having a minimal pelvic curve to allow rotation around a fixed axis, and a sliding lock to enable correction of asynclitism.

The method of application of the Kiellands blades to a head in the transverse position, which need not be employed for direct occipito-posterior positions, differs from the standard forceps technique and is commonly described as the 'wandering method'. As with the standard technique, the forceps are assembled and held in position to enable visualization of their final position prior to their application. The anterior blade is chosen, introduced in the standard manner, but subsequently manoeuvred over the fetal face until it comes to lie over the parietal bone. The internal hand is used for guidance and protects the maternal soft tissues from trauma. The posterior blade, which occupies the sacral hollow, can be directly inserted in most instances, but if this proves not to be possible, application in the manner of the anterior blade should be performed, but in reverse. Rotation should be performed between contractions and may be accomplished by pushing the head 'up' to the level of the pelvic mid-cavity, or by gentle traction at the level at which the head has reached.

With Kiellands, the axis of traction is more toward 'the vertical' in the first instance and then proceeds as previously described. It is especially important that extra care be taken towards the end of the delivery as the much reduced pelvic curve design of the forceps makes perineal damage more likely. Rotational forceps deliveries have been abandoned in many institutions as they have been associated with spiral tears of the vagina and other soft tissue injuries, and in some cases uterine rupture. However, for those experienced in their use, they still have a role, as the ventouse is associated with a higher incidence of failure of delivery in occipito-posterior and occipito-transverse positions.

## Episiotomy

It has been recommended that an episiotomy be cut whenever an instrumental vaginal delivery is performed [E].

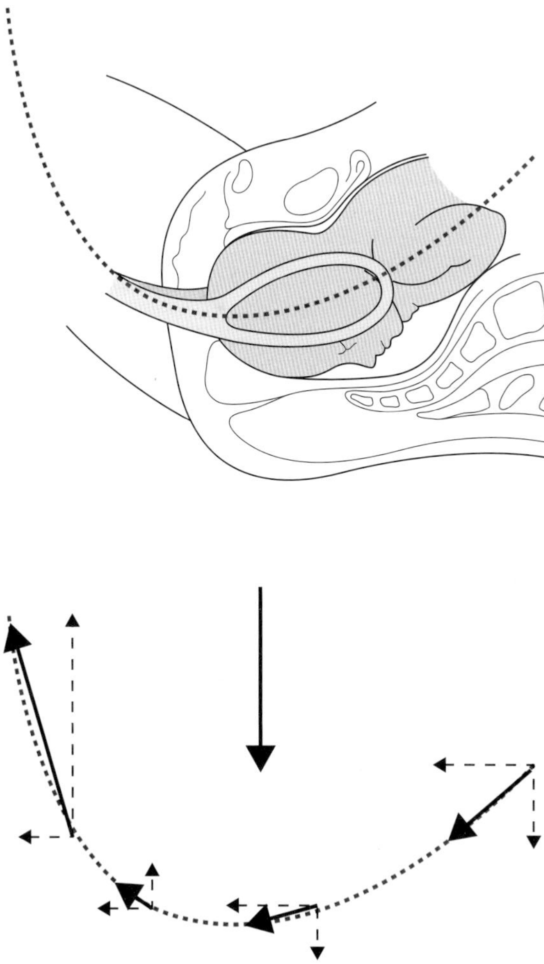

**Figure 34.4** Axis of traction. (a) The traction axis is dependent on the station of the presenting part and changes during delivery. This J-shape curve is independent of the instrument chosen. (b)–(e) Illustrations of the direction of the forces required during delivery of a fetus in an occipito-anterior position

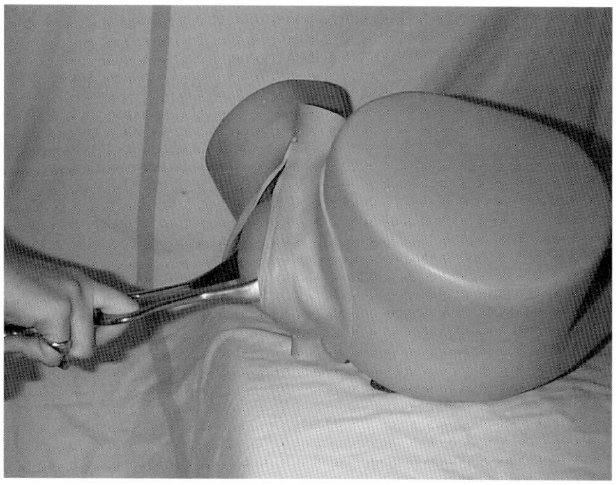

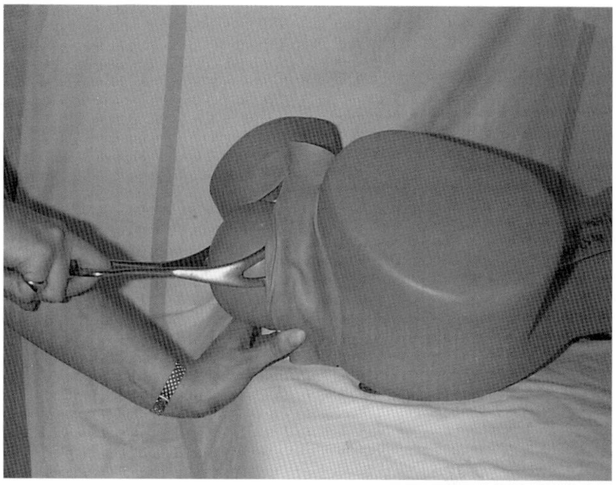

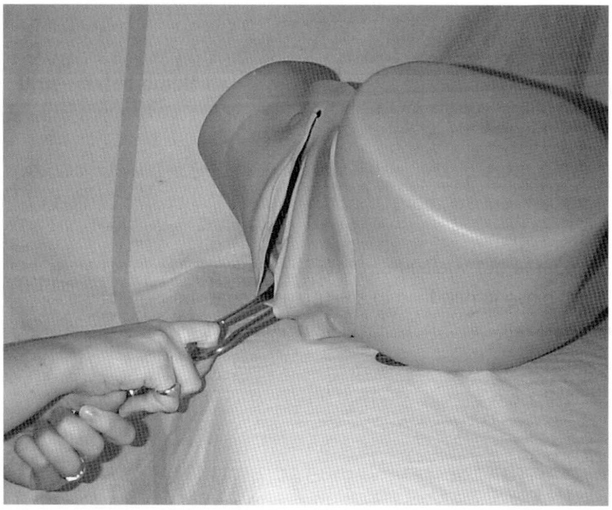

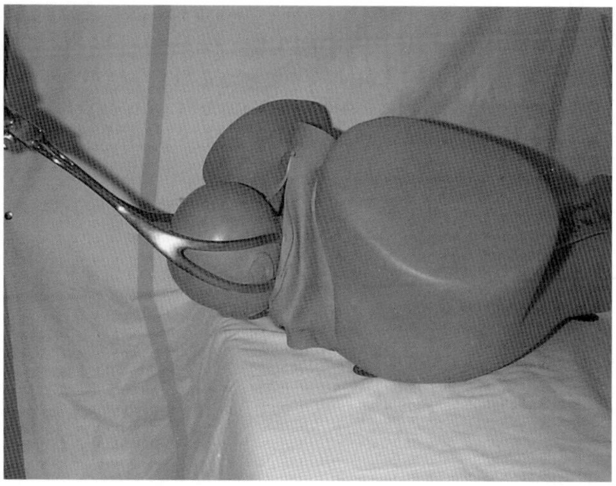

This is not based on any robust evidence. Perineal trauma will occur in most nulliparous women undergoing instrumental vaginal delivery, and episiotomy should be considered in these women in order to limit multiple lacerations. In multiparae, particularly those requiring only a simple ventouse, an episiotomy may not be needed. It should be noted, however, that with assisted vaginal deliveries an episiotomy does not protect against third-degree and fourth-degree tears.

## Special considerations

### Failure of the chosen instrument

Failures can occur when the choice of instrument is wrong (e.g. a silastic cup ventouse for a rotational delivery), when the positioning of the ventouse cup is wrong or when the position has been wrongly defined, leading to larger diameters presenting to the pelvis in occipito-posterior positions. Failure is also more common if the fetus is large or maternal effort poor. Fourteen to 27 per cent of deliveries will not be accomplished when the ventouse is the instrument of first choice. The lower figures are achieved when a rigid posterior cup is used for rotational deliveries. If forceps are chosen first, up to 10 per cent of deliveries may not be accomplished.

In many circumstances, the head may then have descended to a point at which caesarean section becomes even more hazardous. Unfortunately, there have been no appropriately performed randomized studies to guide the best approach when such a circumstance occurs. Observational studies show that the outcomes for babies are worse with the application of a second instrument than if the instrument of first choice is successful, but this is hardly surprising.[14] In addition, the rates of third-degree and fourth-degree tears are higher when a second instrument is used.[15]

Unfortunately, there are no easy answers. A policy of delivering all such women by caesarean section will undoubtedly also lead to an increase in maternal morbidity and perhaps mortality. The art of obstetrics is not to find oneself in such a position to start with. By diligently assessing the patient (using ultrasound to confirm the fetal position if necessary), choosing the correct instrument and using it properly such risks should be minimized.

Where the first instrument fails, the following scenarios may be appropriate.

- The reason for cup failure was detachment (the reason for failure in 40 per cent of ventouse deliveries attempted), but the head is occipito-anterior and on the perineum. A full reassessment should be made. If it is confirmed that this is still the case (i.e. occipito-anterior with the head on the perineum), a simple lift-out forceps is acceptable. If there are any concerns, senior help must be sought before using a second instrument.
- The instrument failed because there was little or no descent with the first pull. Where there has been little or no descent, delivery must be by caesarean section.

- The instrument failed because the position was wrongly defined. In this case, the next option will be either a rotational forceps or caesarean section. Already the fetus will have been subjected to traction, probably with minimal descent. Only after a full assessment by a senior person in theatre could a further instrumentation be considered. In many cases, delivery by caesarean section may be the safer option for the fetus.

## ROTATIONAL DELIVERIES IN CASES OF SUSPECTED FETAL COMPROMISE

Concern has been expressed that the risk incumbent with rotational delivery for fetal compromise, especially with Kiellands forceps, should persuade the accoucheur to opt for delivery by caesarean section instead. Such advice is based on little evidence, and mainly reflects the views of one study in which there was observed to be a significant difference in base deficit in cord venous blood, but no difference in pH, in infants delivered by rotational when compared to non-rotational deliveries.[16] The main factor to consider must be the ease with which delivery will be accomplished. This will relate to the fetal position, station and size, the progress of the labour, the degree of analgesia and the experience of the operator. Each case must be judged on an individual basis. An easy forceps will be preferable to a difficult caesarean section, and vice versa.

## Complications

Assisted deliveries with both vacuum and forceps can be associated with significant maternal and fetal complications.

In the most recent report of the Confidential Enquiries into Maternal Deaths (2003–2005), there were seven direct deaths in patients delivered by forceps and three in those delivered by ventouse; however, there were no deaths directly attributable to the method of delivery. Previously, there have been reports of two maternal deaths associated with cervical tears in women delivered by ventouse prior to the attainment of full cervical dilatation, and one secondary to a traumatic uterine rupture following a forceps delivery.

Traumatic vaginal delivery is considered the most important risk factor for faecal incontinence in women and may occur not only after recognized third- and fourth-degree perineal tears, but also after apparently non-traumatic vaginal delivery [B]. The incidence of such damage is increased by intervention with any instrument, rising from an approximate baseline incidence of 10–25 per cent following ventouse and 40 per cent following forceps. Studies using endo-anal ultrasonography have shown that persisting sphincter defects are the main cause of faecal incontinence and not, as was previously believed, neurological damage. However, at 5-year follow up, there are no discernible differences in symptoms between women delivered by forceps and those delivered by ventouse.[9] Successful delivery by the instrument of first choice will limit damage as will good technique as a consequence of adequate training.

Postpartum haemorrhage is more common in women needing instrumental vaginal delivery compared to women who deliver spontaneously, but less common than in women delivered by caesarean section in the second stage. The three common causes of 'tone', 'tissue' and 'trauma' should always be borne in mind and measures to limit any loss include:

- The prophylactic administration of an appropriate oxytocic post delivery:
  - Syntometrine i.m. (1 ampoule)
  - Syntocinon bolus i.v. (five units) or infusion (40 units in 50 mL 0.9 per cent NaCl solution over 4 hours) or 10 IU i.m. as a stat dose
  - Misoprostol 800 μg p.r.
- Prompt identification and repair of cervical, vaginal and perineal trauma (Note: suturing may be commenced prior to completion of the third stage of labour.
- Diligent examination of the placenta and membranes.

Underestimation of blood loss at instrumental vaginal delivery is common, and so, where possible, loss should be measured through the weighing of swabs and towels.

Fetal complications are no less important; however, combined evidence from all available controlled trials (1175 babies in the vacuum extractor groups and 1155 babies in the forceps groups) allows conclusions to be drawn only about the relatively common neonatal outcomes. Although concerns about risks of intracranial and subgaleal haemorrhage remain, in a recent review of 583 340 live-born singleton infants born to nulliparous women, the rate of subdural or cerebral haemorrhage in vacuum deliveries did not differ significantly from that associated with forceps use or caesarean section during labour.[17] Overall, the risks of perinatal trauma using the vacuum extractor correlate with [B]:

- the duration of application;
- the station of the fetal head at the commencement of the delivery;
- the difficulty of the delivery;
- the condition of the baby at the time of commencement of the procedure.

As discussed previously, it is important to remember that the risks of such damage significantly increase among babies who are exposed to multiple attempts at both vacuum and forceps delivery.

## Documentation

Clear documentation of the procedure is of paramount importance. This must include the indication for the delivery, evidence of a full maternal and fetal assessment including abdominal palpation, as well as the findings on vaginal examination. As for caesarean section, critical timings should be recorded, this is especially important for ventouse delivery, when the time of establishment of the vacuum and time to effect delivery should be noted. The procedure should be accurately recorded, including the management of the third stage. Documentation of perineal trauma and repair must be documented and standards for this are covered in Chapter 36, Perineal trauma. The blood loss must be critically assessed and, where possible, measured. Post-operative precautions should be noted and a full reassessment of the thrombotic risk undertaken. Where appropriate, thromboembolism prevention measures should be instituted.

Cord blood gas analysis should be undertaken and the results recorded.

## CLINICAL RISK MANAGEMENT IN OBSTETRICS

Instrumental vaginal delivery has never been free from criticism, and is certainly not without risks, although most instrumental deliveries have normal outcomes and give no reason for complaint. However, in today's litigious society, the risks of litigation against accoucheurs or the hospital in which they practise are increased by a poor outcome.

Common allegations against practitioners that are cited in lawsuits include (amongst others): inadequate indication; failure to exclude cephalo-pelvic disproportion; improper use of instruments with excessive use of force resulting in fetal or maternal injury; lack of informed consent (although this may not be fully possible in an emergency situation); and inadequate supervision.

Consequently, the basis of any defence following an adverse outcome is based upon the quality of the record keeping and evidence of appropriate training (OSATS). Proper documentation is a critical part of the surgeon's responsibility in performing any operative delivery and should include, as a basic minimum:

- a statement of the indication for the procedure;
- the anaesthesia used;
- the examination findings prior to commencement of the procedure;
- the personnel involved and an outline of the procedure performed;
- the difficulty of the extraction;
- the performance of rotation;
- fetal injuries;
- maternal soft-tissue trauma and their repair;
- an estimate of the blood loss.

The fear of litigation must not dictate good medical practice, and assisted vaginal deliveries remain an appropriate intervention when practised with the appropriate safeguards. It should be remembered that although both intrapartum asphyxia and, to a lesser degree, intrapartum trauma contribute to neonatal morbidity, abnormal fetal growth, prematurity, chromosomal abnormalities, intrauterine infection and other non-genetic chromosomal disorders contribute a far more significant degree to permanent neonatal complications.

## TRAINING OBSTETRICIANS IN PRACTICAL SKILLS

Good outcomes are achieved if training is thorough and supervision is requested when any delivery is thought to be potentially more difficult than the operator is used to.

Accurate application of the forceps or the vacuum extractor and close adherence to standard techniques are essential in the safe performance of all instrumental deliveries. The RCOG now recommend that trainees are experienced in assisting spontaneous vaginal deliveries before attempting to execute instrumental deliveries, and competence in the use of ventouse and forceps should be achieved prior to conducting unsupervised deliveries. Practical procedures can be learnt only in action, and descriptions are a poor substitute for seeing and doing them. However, comprehensive descriptions of the techniques of forceps and ventouse deliveries are accessible and should be read.

With many of the 'more difficult' vaginal deliveries being abandoned in many institutions, and a generalized de-skilling in their use, training in some centres may be deemed to be less than comprehensive. As a profession, we are in danger of abandoning methods of procuring a successful vaginal delivery because of the perceived danger of specific instruments, when the danger lies, not with the instrument, but in the inadequate training and competence of the accoucheur.

## CONCLUSIONS

Despite the known risks, instrumental vaginal delivery undoubtedly continues to have a role in the management of the second stage of labour. Caesarean sections performed at this stage are not infrequently traumatic for both patients and staff, and are themselves associated with a significant morbidity and mortality.

- Failure rates are higher with soft than with rigid cups and with ventouse than with forceps.
- Soft cups should not be used for rotational deliveries.
- Use of a second instrument increases the risks of fetal and maternal damage.
- Caesarean section in the second stage is associated with higher rates of haemorrhage than instrumental delivery.

### KEY POINTS

- Careful assessment of each patient, combining history and examination, must be performed before any intervention is undertaken. Ultrasound has a vital role in helping the accoucheur identify any fetal malposition.
- *Sang froid* should be the motto of choice, and the accoucheur should always consider the available alternative.
- Instruments should only be used by those trained to do so.

## Key References

1. Stephenson PA. *International Differences in the Use of Obstetrical Interventions.* Copenhagen: WHO (EUR/ICP/MCH), 1992.
2. Strachan BK, Murphy DJ. *Instrumental Vaginal Delivery.* Clinical Green Top Guidelines No. 26. London: RCOG Press, 2005.
3. Hodnett ED, Gates S, Hofmeyr GJ, Sakala C. Continuous support for women during childbirth. *Cochrane Database Syst Rev* 2007; (**3**): CD003766.
4. Fraser WD, Marcoux S, Krauss I *et al.* Multicenter, randomized, controlled trial of delayed pushing for nulliparous women in the second stage of labor with continuous epidural analgesia. The PEOPLE (Pushing Early or Pushing Late with Epidural) Study Group. *Am J Obstet Gynecol* 2000; **182**: 1165–72.
5. Gupta JK, Hofmeyr GJ. Position for women during second stage of labour. *Cochrane Database Syst Rev* 2004; (**1**): CD2006.
6. Anim-Somuah, Smyth RMD, Howell CJ. Epidural versus non-epidural or no analgesia in labour. *Cochrane Database Syst Rev* 2005; (**4**): CD000331.
7. American College of Obstetricians and Gynecologists. *Operative Vaginal Delivery.* Technical Bulletin No. 196. Washington DC: American College of Obstetricians and Gynecologists, 1994.
8. Johanson RB, Menon BKV. Vacuum extraction vs. forceps delivery. *Cochrane Database Syst Rev* 2000; (**2**): CD000224.
9. Johanson RB, Heycock E, Carter J *et al.* Maternal and child health after assisted vaginal delivery: five year follow-up of a randomised controlled study comparing forceps and ventouse. *Br J Obstet Gynaecol* 1999; **106**: 544–9.
10. Murphy DJ, Liebling RE, Verity L *et al.* Early maternal and neonatal morbidity associated with operative delivery in second stage of labour: a cohort study. *Lancet* 2001; **358**: 1203–7.
11. Johanson RB, Rice C, Doyle M *et al.* A randomised prospective study comparing the new vacuum extractor policy with forceps delivery. *Br J Obstet Gynaecol* 1993; **100**: 524–30.

12. Vacca A. The trouble with vacuum extraction. *Curr Obstet Gynaecol* 1999; **9**: 41–55.

13. Johanson R, Menon V. Soft versus rigid vacuum extractor cups for assisted vaginal delivery. *Cochrane Database Syst Rev* 2000; (**2**): CD000446.

14. Gardella C, Taylor M, Benedetti T *et al*. The effect of sequential use of vacuum and forceps for assisted vaginal delivery on neonatal and maternal outcomes. *Am J Obstet Gynecol* 2001; **185**: 896–902.

15. Sultan AH, Kamm MA, Hudson CN. Anal sphincter disruption during vaginal delivery. *N Engl J Med* 1993; **329**: 1905–11.

16. Baker PN, Johnson IR. A study of the effect of rotational forceps delivery on fetal acid–base balance. *Acta Obstet Gynecol Scand* 1994; **73**: 787–9.

17. Towner D, Castro MA, Eby-Wilkens E, Gilbert WM. Effect of mode of delivery in nulliparous women on neonatal intracranial injury. *N Engl J Med* 1999; **341**: 1709–14.

Second stage of labour

# Breech presentation

*Richard Hayman*

## MRCOG standards

- Candidates are expected to be proficient in vaginal breech delivery and the management of twin deliveries for which breech delivery/extraction may be required.
- Knowledge of the relative risks and benefits is expected such that the candidate can counsel women with regard to breech delivery and external cephalic version (ECV).

### Theoretical skills

- Revise your knowledge of the process of parturition with a breech presentation.
- Plan the management when confronted with a breech presentation both prior to and during labour.
- Have seen an external cephalic version.

## INTRODUCTION

The management of a fetus presenting by the breech has been an area of great controversy and changing practice. From a situation in which the breech was considered advantageous, presumably because the midwife could pull on the legs to expedite delivery, to 'once a breech, always a caesarean section', changes in observed practice have frequently reflected the attitudes of the attendant birth professionals rather than following principles determined by suitable randomized, controlled trials.

Although the Term Breech Study has done much to clarify thinking around delivery of the breech infant at term, some management issues still remain controversial.

## AETIOLOGY

The incidence of breech presentation varies with gestational age, and is between 14 and 20 per cent at 28 weeks and 2.2 and 3.7 per cent at term. Thus a major reason for breech presentation in labour is preterm delivery, as most fetuses will turn spontaneously towards term. There is unfortunately, a higher perinatal mortality and morbidity with breech presentation when compared with gestation matched cephalic-presenting contemporaries. This is principally due to an increased risk from birth asphyxia or trauma.[1]

Another important cause for a breech presentation is a maternal or fetal abnormality. Up to 18 per cent of preterm and 5 per cent of term breeches have congenital abnormalities as compared with 2.5 per cent of term cephalic babies.

Thus, breech presentation is a signal for potential fetal problems and this should inform antenatal, intrapartum and neonatal management. Caesarean section for breech presentation has been suggested as a way of reducing the associated fetal problems, and in many countries in northern Europe and North America, caesarean section has become the normal mode of delivery in this situation. However, it is important to remember that the perinatal mortality remains increased even when the delivery is by caesarean section and corrected for gestation, congenital defects and birth weight.[1]

Maternal and fetal abnormalities associated with breech presentation are discussed in Chapter 18, Malpresentation.

## DIAGNOSIS

Three clinical breech presentations are recognized.

1 Extended (frank): the legs of the fetus are flexed at the hip and extended at the knee. Such a presentation occurs in 60–70 per cent of all breech presentations at term, and carries the lowest risks of cord prolapse and feto-pelvic disproportion.
2 Flexed (complete): the hips and knees are flexed so the feet present to the pelvis. (Feeling a foot at the cervix does not constitute a footling; most are flexed breeches.)
3 Footling (incomplete): at least one leg extended at the hip and knee, the buttocks therefore not being within the pelvis at all. This presentation carries the highest risks of cord prolapse and feto-pelvic disproportion.

Clinical diagnosis of the breech presentation may be difficult by palpation alone. Suggestive features are:

- A history of subcostal discomfort, with the palpation of a 'solid' fetal pole at the uterine fundus.
- Auscultation of the fetal heart sounds above the umbilicus.
- Palpation of the fetal ischial tuberosities, sacrum and anus during vaginal examination. (Differentiation from a face presentation may be difficult, but in a face presentation careful palpation will frequently distinguish the bony landmarks of the malar eminences, mentum and mouth with its obvious bony margin.)

Such observations are frequently imprecise, and it is estimated that 30 per cent of breech presentations are not diagnosed until the onset of labour. As abdominal palpation has been shown to have a sensitivity of 28 per cent and specificity of 94 per cent, confirmation by ultrasound scan must therefore be regarded as the 'gold standard'.

## MANAGEMENT OPTIONS FOR BREECH PRESENTATION

When determining the mode of delivery that is most suitable, many factors must be taken into consideration. The main comparison must be between maternal and fetal risks and benefits, a difficult equation to calculate, even at the best of times.

In all studies of breech presentation, maternal morbidity is increased in women delivered by caesarean section when compared to those having a vaginal delivery. Such morbidity includes haemorrhage, hysterectomy, uterine and wound haematomas and infections, urinary tract infection and deep vein thrombosis and pulmonary embolism.[1] The risks associated with future deliveries are also not inconsiderable, especially with preterm breech deliveries through a vertical uterine incision, and should feature in any risk versus benefits equation.[2,3] The fetal risks of occipital diastasis, intraventricular and periventricular injury, anoxic risk and skeletal trauma are well documented and are discussed in more detail below. However, it is inappropriate to compare maternal risks and fetal/neonatal risks directly, as the potential adverse consequences of each complication affect the recipient in vastly different ways. Only the mother can determine where the balance lies, and it should be the role of the attendant clinician to empower her to reach a carefully formulated and clinically sound decision. It is important to remember that elective caesarean section compares favourably to vaginal birth, with the highest morbidity being in women undergoing emergency caesarean section after the onset of labour.

### Preterm: 26–36 completed weeks

- Approximately 25 per cent of all babies delivered at these gestations will be by the breech.

- The overall incidence of breech presentation between these gestations is 0.5 per cent.

When compared with vertex-presenting counterparts, the premature breech often:

- is small for gestational age,
- has a higher head to body circumference ratio,
- has a higher association with antepartum stillbirth and neonatal demise.

Caesarean delivery is not always an atraumatic option for the fetus, and a preterm breech infant faces some formidable difficulties whatever the mode of delivery. During a vaginal breech delivery, the occipital bone of the fetus is particularly exposed to damage due to its impact upon the maternal pubis during decent of the fetal head in the second stage of labour. Such forces may act to separate the central portion of the occipital bone from the lateral part (occipital diastasis), with potential damage to the cerebellum and herniation of brain tissue through the foramen magnum. If this does not result in stillbirth or early neonatal death, the diagnosis may be delayed until the child is older, when signs of ataxic cerebral palsy may develop. Fortunately, this is a rare occurrence.

More frequently, problems of intraventricular and periventricular damage due to hypoxia or haemorrhage during the antenatal, peripartum, intrapartum and postpartum courses may occur. Although these injuries may be related to the mechanics of vaginal delivery, avoiding such circumstances may not prevent them occurring.

Other common problems faced by the breech fetus include the following:

- Damage to the internal organs, transection of the spinal cord, nerve palsies and fractures of the long bones – these frequently result from the injudicious use of traction on the presenting parts [D].[4]
- Entrapment of the after-coming head. The risk of such a problem increases when the active second stage is begun before full cervical dilatation is achieved (more common with footling than with other presentations). Although prevention is preferable to intervention, should this problem occur, incising the cervix at 4 and 8 o'clock with a pair of scissors may result in its resolution. A complete examination must be performed following delivery, the haemorrhage must be arrested and the defect repaired.

The preterm breech usually presents in labour. Although routine external cephalic version (ECV) before term has not been shown to confer any advantages in such a case, ECV could be considered if the membranes are intact.

Although the majority of obstetricians use delivery by caesarean section for the uncomplicated preterm breech, only a minority believe that there is sufficient evidence to justify this policy. There is general acknowledgement (included in some reports) that the numerous retrospective studies that suggest that caesarean section confers a better outcome in this situation have been subject to bias.

The poor outcome for very low birth weight infants is mainly related to complications of prematurity and not to the mode of delivery.[2] Grant reviewed the controlled trials assessing the value of elective versus selective caesarean delivery of the 'small baby'.[5] He concluded that the data 'are not sufficient to justify a policy of elective caesarean section', and, in the absence of good evidence that a preterm baby needs to be delivered by caesarean section, the decision about the mode of delivery should be made after close consultation with the labouring woman and her partner. Attempts have been made to answer the questions concerning preterm breech delivery, but clinicians were unwilling to randomize women, leading to the abandonment of the trial.

## Management of the preterm breech in labour

When a woman is not in labour and an indication exists for expediting delivery, the preferred route will usually be by caesarean section. When time permits, such an intervention should always be preceded by the mother being given a course of antenatal steroids.

In labour, the management depends on:

- an accurate diagnosis of labour (50 per cent of cases of presumed preterm labours settle spontaneously);
- consideration of the administration of tocolysis to delay labour while steroids are administered or transfer to another unit is arranged;
- confirmation of the presentation;
- exclusion of a fetal abnormality (a detailed ultrasound scan should be performed if one has not been completed previously and if time and labour permit).

As with all preterm labours, many will be precipitate and several will be associated with antecedents that are often pathological. The decision regarding the best method of delivery must take into account the following:

- Gestation: the very preterm infant is unlikely to benefit from caesarean section and maternal risks will be higher.
- Fetal abnormality.
- The progress of labour: this is often very quick, and caesarean section may not be realistic.
- Fetal status: at gestations with expected good outcomes, non-reassuring fetal status may indicate caesarean section.

Full discussion with the parents, with realistic evaluation of the fetal and maternal risks, should take place with an obstetrician and neonatologist.

## Procedure: preterm breech delivery

An experienced obstetrician should supervise vaginal delivery of the breech. Ideally, an epidural should be sited and effective, to prevent pushing prior to full cervical dilatation. This will also enable intradelivery manipulations, the painless application of forceps to the after-coming head, or rapid recourse to operative delivery. As with all preterm deliveries, a paediatrician should be present and an anaesthetist available. Delivery with the membranes intact has been shown to confer some advantage to the fetus [D].[3]

Should the cervix clamp down around the fetal head following delivery of the body, gentle flexion by insertion of the index finger into the fetal mouth may be advantageous. If this does not succeed, incision of the cervix should be performed as previously described.

Caesarean delivery can nearly always be performed through a transverse lower abdominal incision. The nature of the most beneficial uterine incision is less certain, although from a maternal viewpoint, a J-shaped extension to the lower uterine incision has many advantages over a classical/De Lee or inverted-T approach. However, with a fetal mortality of up to 80 per cent with breech presentations below 28 weeks, it may not be in the mother's best interests to compromise her future childbearing by employing a classical approach.

## Presentation at term

The decline in the incidence of breech presentations towards term suggests that spontaneous version is a common occurrence, with approximately 57 per cent turning between 32 and 36 weeks and 25 per cent thereafter. Even if a primigravid patient with a fetus in an extended breech presentation (one of the least favourable for spontaneous version) is to be delivered by caesarean section, the presentation should be confirmed by ultrasound scan, as the chance of spontaneous version at this stage is not insignificant. This is even more important in multiparous patients offered this management.

### Reducing the incidence of breech presentation at term

#### Posture
Four randomized trials have been undertaken to establish whether or not postural management (knee–chest position for up to 10 minutes a day) is effective in converting breech to cephalic presentations. No significant benefits were found in these studies, and there is therefore no evidence to support routine recommendation of the knee–chest position [A].[5]

#### External cephalic version
External cephalic version has been practised since the time of Hippocrates and has been demonstrated to be associated with a significant reduction in the risk of caesarean section (odds ratio (OR) 0.4; 95 per cent confidence interval (CI) 0.3–0.6) without any increased risk to the baby. It is current best practice that all women with an uncomplicated breech pregnancy at term (37–42 weeks) should be offered ECV [A].[6,7]

Although primarily intended for the management of the uncomplicated breech pregnancy at term, ECV has also been carried out successfully during early labour. It can be performed in women who have had a prior caesarean section and appears to be safe, though trials are not randomized and are only small. This may be acceptable to some women as, if the fetus stays breech, many will decide on caesarean section for delivery, which makes the choices much more limited should they have future pregnancies.[6,7]

Further discussion of the benefits, risks, contraindications and complications of ECV is detailed in Chapter 18, Malpresentation.

## Elective caesarean section versus planned vaginal breech delivery at term

At term, the first question that must be addressed when confronted by a breech presentation is 'Where is the placenta?' Once this question has been successfully answered, a rational approach may be applied to further management.

For the fetus, the best method of delivering a term frank or complete breech singleton is by planned caesarean section [A].[8,9]

Before 2001, much of the evidence supporting elective caesarean section in preference to vaginal breech delivery was obtained from two small randomized trials and data from hospital audit. These studies, which revealed outcomes for vaginal delivery and delivery by caesarean section rather than comparing a policy of intended caesarean section with a policy of intended vaginal birth, showed no differences in mortality between the groups. However, an increase in short-term morbidity was noted among those babies delivered vaginally.[11]

The Canadian Medical Research Council (MRC) funded an international multicentre randomized, controlled trial of planned vaginal delivery versus planned elective caesarean section for the uncomplicated term breech.[10]

Subanalysis was undertaken after excluding deliveries that occurred:

- after a prolonged labour;
- after labours induced or augmented with oxytocin or prostaglandins;
- in cases where there was a footling or uncertain type of breech presentation at delivery;
- in cases for which there was no skilled or experienced clinician present at the birth.

In this subanalysis, the risk of the combined outcome of perinatal mortality, neonatal mortality or serious neonatal morbidity with planned caesarean section compared with planned vaginal birth was 16/1006 (1.6 per cent), compared with 23/704 (3.3 per cent) (relative risk (RR) 0.49; 95 per cent CI 0.26–0.91; $p < 0.02$).[6]

In a further subanalysis, results were separated into those obtained from countries with higher perinatal mortality (>20/1000) and those from countries with a lower perinatal mortality (<20/1000). The findings suggested that the benefits of delivery by caesarean section became even more significant in countries with a low perinatal mortality rate, but were not as significant in countries with a higher perinatal mortality rate. It is important to remember that there were no differences between any of the groups in terms of maternal mortality or serious early maternal morbidity.

However, this study did not evaluate long-term outcomes for child or mother, and many have raised serious questions about the study design.[11] Although it is possible that careful exclusion of growth-restricted infants, better intrapartum monitoring and full clinical pelvimetry and umbilical cord assessment might have improved the prospects for a vaginal breech delivery, the results of the Term Breech Trial led the Royal College of Obstetricians and Gynaecologists (RCOG) to the recommendation that 'the best method of delivering a singleton fetus at term with an extended or flexed breech presentation is by planned LSCS'. This information should be disseminated to pregnant women, their families and all clinicians involved in maternity care.[8]

It has been suggested that the Term Breech Trial, by reflecting conventional 'expert' views, sanctioned the conventional positioning of the patient in the dorsal lithotomy position for delivery and thereby missed an opportunity to evaluate labour and delivery in upright positions (considered by some to be physiologically and anatomically more sound). However, this view has not been substantiated with clinical evidence. More recently, an observational prospective study with an intent-to-treat analysis concluded that, in units where planned vaginal delivery is a common practice and when strict criteria are met before and during labour, planned vaginal delivery of singleton fetuses in breech presentation at term remains a safe option that can be offered to women. In the latter study, of the 2526 women with planned vaginal deliveries, 1796 delivered vaginally (71 per cent). The rate of neonatal morbidity or death was considerably lower than the 5 per cent in the Term Breech Trial (1.60 per cent; 95 per cent CI 1.14–2.17), and not significantly different from the planned caesarean section group.[11]

A two-year follow up was conducted at the Term Breech Trial centres which expected to be able to achieve follow-up rates of about 80 per cent. The primary outcome, death or neurodevelopmental delay at age two years, was similar between the two groups (RR 1.09, 95 per cent CI 0.52–2.30). The smaller number of perinatal deaths with planned caesarean section was balanced by a greater number of babies with neurodevelopmental delay. This was unexpected, as there had been fewer babies in the planned caesarean section group with severe perinatal morbidity. In addition, mothers in the planned caesarean section group expressed less worry about their babies' health. Planned caesarean section was surprisingly found to be less costly than planned vaginal breech births (excluding possible future costs related to complications of a scarred uterus).[12]

It has been estimated that for every infant potentially saved by a caesarean section, one woman will experience a uterine rupture during a subsequent pregnancy (in a setting in which vaginal birth after caesarean is practised). A study from the Netherlands estimated that, in the four years following publication of the Term Breech Trial, the increase of approximately 8500 elective caesarean sections probably prevented 19 perinatal deaths. However, it also resulted in four maternal deaths that may have been avoidable. It is estimated that, in future pregnancies, nine perinatal deaths would be expected and 140 women would have potentially life-threatening complications as a result of rupture of the uterine scar.[13]

It remains likely that some women will choose to deliver vaginally and that some women for whom a caesarean section is planned will labour too quickly for the operation to be undertaken (nearly 10 per cent of women assigned to deliver by caesarean section in the Term Breech Trial delivered vaginally). It therefore remains important that clinicians and hospitals are prepared for vaginal breech delivery.

## Criteria for the selection of patients in whom a trial of vaginal delivery may be appropriate

Issues to be considered when counselling a woman planning a vaginal birth are:

- the careful selection of patients;
- appropriate intrapartum management;
- the skill, experience and judgement of the intrapartum attendant.

It is undisputed that a trial of labour should be precluded in the presence of medical or obstetric complications that are likely to be associated with mechanical difficulties at delivery. Likewise, a trial of vaginal breech delivery is more likely to be successful if both mother and baby are of 'normal' proportions.[14]

When contemplating a trial of vaginal breech delivery, the fetal presentation should be either extended (frank) or flexed (complete), with no evidence of feto-pelvic dispro-portion and a clinically 'adequate' pelvis. Although clinical judgement is subjective, no other form of pelvimetry has been proven to be of increased benefit and does not need to be used routinely. X-ray pelvimetry has figured prominently in protocols for planned vaginal birth, but none of these studies was able to confirm the value of this examination in selecting women who were more likely to succeed in a trial of labour or in having any effect on peri-natal outcome. In another subanalysis of the Term Breech Trial, the use of radiological pelvimetry was not linked to improved outcome [B].[10]

Ultrasonographic estimation of the fetal weight should be undertaken. Women expecting infants with an estimated weight of >3800 g should be counselled that caesarean section is a safer option. By performing such a scan, fetuses with severe abnormalities, hyperextension of the fetal neck or presenting with a footling breech may be excluded.

See figure 18.1, p. 274 for a management algorithm for breech presentation.

## Intrapartum management

Should the patient choose to opt for a trial of vaginal deli-very, careful and continuous monitoring of fetal well-being must be ensured. In the 7th Annual Confidential Enquiry into Stillbirth and Deaths in Infancy (CESDI) report, the single and most avoidable factor associated with breech stillbirths and deaths among breech babies was suboptimal care in labour. Fetal acid-base status may be ascertained by sampling blood from the fetal buttocks when the fetal heart rate trace is suspect.[15] However, should fetal blood sampling be required to facilitate the management during a breech delivery, intervention by caesarean section should be seriously considered.

It is important to note that despite the 'rigid' entry crite-ria of the Term Breech Trial, there were still frequent inci-dents of suboptimal care, including the misinterpretation of suspicious or pathological CTGs, delays in asking for senior help and clinical inexperience at the time of delivery that may well have exacerbated the risks for an already hypoxic baby.[16]

## Procedure: vaginal term breech delivery

Ultrasonographic examination of the fetus is essential in determining those infants suitable for trial of vaginal delivery.

- An estimation of the fetal weight, within its limitations of ±15 per cent at term, may exclude those fetuses for whom a vaginal delivery would be somewhat more haz-ardous. A cut-off of 3.8 kg has been suggested (a figure not based on any specific scientific evaluation), but it should be remembered that the error of ultrasound esti-mation of fetal weight is greater in the breech than in the vertex-presenting fetus.
- The presence of a 'star gazing' or hyperextended fetal neck is an important finding associated with spinal cord and brain injuries during birth. Although the aetiology is not known, proposed causative factors include a nuchal cord (cord around the fetal neck), fundal placenta, spasm of the fetal neck musculature and uterine abnor-malities. Extension >90° is associated with a particularly poor prognosis, and delivery by caesarean section is to be recommended with such findings.

It is probably wise to perform a clinical examination of the pelvis to exclude the obvious deformities associated with a contracted pelvis, but more formal estimation of the pelvic structures is of limited value.

Close consultation with the mother and her partner and counselling about the implications of the choice of vaginal breech delivery versus delivery by caesarean section are some of the most important issues to be addressed.

## Risks of vaginal breech delivery

All risks to both the mother and fetus must be by comparison with the alternative method of delivery available, specifically caesarean section. Whereas short-term problems are often obvious, many of the more subtle long-term problems encountered may actually be due to the fact that breech presentation itself may be a poor prognostic variable, and that being breech at term is risky regardless of the route of delivery (Table 35.1). In the Term Breech Trial, the excess neonatal morbidity was approximately 1 per cent and the neonatal morbidity 15 per cent.

## Procedure: breech delivery

The principle of vaginal breech delivery is to allow the spontaneous delivery of the fetus through the combination of uterine activity and maternal expulsive efforts. Operator intervention should be limited to a few well-timed manoeuvres, with injudicious traction on the fetal body or limbs avoided at all costs. Not only can traction lead to direct injury, such interventions may also increase displacement of the fetal limbs from their normal attitude, increasing the relative disproportion between fetus and pelvis that may already exist.

The mechanism of delivery is divided into three stages: delivery of the fetal hips (bitrochanteric diameter); delivery of the shoulders (biacromial diameter); and delivery of the head (biparietal diameter).

With a breech, the presenting part usually engages with the bitrochanteric diameter occupying the oblique

**Table 35.1** Fetal and maternal morbidity as a result of breech delivery

| Fetal | Low Apgar scores at birth reflecting poor 'overall' condition |
|---|---|
| | Intracranial haemorrhage |
| | Medullary coning |
| | Occipital diastasis |
| | Severance of the spinal cord |
| | Hypopituitarism |
| | Brachial plexus injury |
| | Long-term neurological damage |
| | Fracture of the fetal long bones and epiphyseal separation |
| | Rupture of the internal organs |
| | Genital damage in the male |
| | Damage to the mouth and pharynx |
| Maternal | Soft tissue injuries to genital tract with increased morbidity |

or transverse plane at the pelvic inlet. With the sacrum anterior, the anterior hip leads and, on meeting the pelvic floor, is rotated anteriorly beneath the pubic arch. Should the posterior hip reach the pelvic floor first, it undergoes long anterior rotation. The breech is then held up behind the pubic arch, lateral flexion allowing the posterior hip to be born first. The fetus then straightens as the anterior hip is delivered, the legs and feet following. As the shoulders enter the brim in the oblique or transverse diameters, the trunk undergoes external rotation. The shoulders then descend and undergo internal rotation, which brings them into the antero-posterior diameter of the pelvic outlet. The third and final part to enter the pelvis is the fetal head. This rotates until the posterior part of the neck becomes fixed under the subpubic arch and the head is born by flexion.

### Management during the first stage

Labour should be conducted in a setting that allows rapid intervention by caesarean section should the clinical situation demand it (in the Term Breech Trial, 50 per cent of emergency caesarean deliveries were for failure to progress and 29 per cent for fetal distress).[9,10] On arrival on the labour ward, the diagnosis of labour and presentation of the fetus by the breech should be confirmed, intravenous access established and fetal monitoring commenced.

An epidural anaesthetic may be recommended in order to prevent involuntary expulsive efforts prior to full cervical dilatation, and to permit emergency delivery by caesarean section should the clinical situation demand it. However, epidural anaesthesia is not essential, and in fact there may be a higher chance of obtaining a successful vaginal delivery without it [D].[17] The use of oxytocin to stimulate uterine contractions should be discouraged in the light of the Term Breech Trial findings, and any failure to make the expected progress in cervical dilatation or for the breech to descend appropriately in the first stage of labour should prompt careful consideration of whether caesarean section is advisable. However, augmentation of uterine activity may still have a place in the management of a few select cases, but only after careful review of the facts, senior obstetric advice and, most importantly, discussion with the mother and her partner concerning their wishes.

### Management during the second stage

The active second stage of labour only begins with full cervical dilatation and visualization of the fetal anus at the perineum, and must be managed by an operator trained in the delivery of the breech. There are different opinions about the best way to manage a breech delivery and there is no evidence to support one method above the other. In some countries (such as The Netherlands), spontaneous breech delivery is the norm. In the UK assisted delivery is taught, and in some parts of the USA the Bracht manoeuvre is popular.

In an assisted breech delivery, the lithotomy position should be adopted, supine hypotension being avoided by

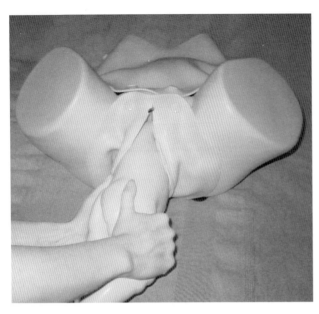

**Figure 35.1** Breech delivery

lateral tilt by insertion of a wedge. A pudendal block can be provided if an epidural is not *in situ*. An episiotomy may be performed at this stage as it will facilitate the manual and forceps manipulation of the after-coming head and may be exceedingly difficult to perform at a later stage of the delivery process.

The breech should be allowed to deliver spontaneously to the level of the umbilicus, rotation of the fetus to sacro-anterior being the only correction permitted if it is not in this position already (Figure 35.1). Flexion of the fetal knee by pressure in the popliteal fossa associated with abduction of the thigh will aid delivery of the legs, which should then be supported. A loop of cord is then 'brought down' to minimize traction and the risks of traumatic cord injury. Ideally, the remainder of the delivery from this stage should be achieved with the minimum of interference, although this is seldom the case.

Once the legs and abdomen have emerged, the fetus should be allowed to hang from the perineum until the wings of the posterior scapula are seen. The arms are frequently folded across the fetal chest, and require no particular manoeuvres to expedite their delivery. No attempt should be made to deliver an arm until the scapula and one axilla are visible. If injudicious traction is employed, extension of the arms above the fetal head may require Lovset's manoeuvre to free them. In this case, the fetus is grasped over the bony pelvis, with the accoucheur's thumbs along the sacrum, and turned so as to bring the posterior arm anterior (Figure 35.2a). The elbow will appear below the symphysis pubis and that arm is subsequently delivered by sweeping it across the fetal body (Figure 35.2b). This manoeuvre should then be repeated with the other arm.

A nuchal arm – the arm lying above and behind the fetal head (flexed at the elbow and extended at the shoulder) – is

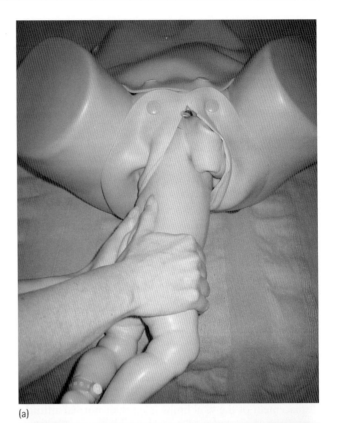

(a)

(b)

**Figure 35.2** Lovset's manoeuvre. (a) The fetus is grasped over the bony pelvis with the accoucheur's thumbs along the sacrum. The fetus is then turned so as to bring the posterior arm anterior. (b) The elbow will appear below the symphysis pubis and that arm is subsequently delivered by sweeping it across the fetal body

often the consequence of inappropriate traction on the breech. It is best dealt with in one of the following ways:

- A modified Lovset's manoeuvre – rotating the fetal back in the direction of the trapped arm, thus forcing the elbow towards the fetal face and over the fetal head.

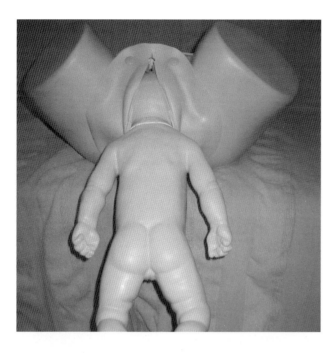

**Figure 35.3** Once the legs and abdomen have emerged, the fetus should be allowed to hang from the perineum until the wings of the posterior scapula are seen

Once 'free', a more traditional Lovset's intervention may then be performed.

- If this technique fails, grasping the arm by hooking a finger over it may result in its delivery – but is also likely to result in a humeral fracture.
- If this does not work, as a last resort, general anaesthesia should be induced, the body of the fetus 'pushed up' the hand passed along the ventral surface and the most accessible arm brought down.

The fetus should then be allowed to hang from the vulva for a few seconds – 'as long as it takes the accoucheur to wash their hands' (Figure 35.3) – until the nape of the neck is visible at the anterior vulva. This allows the head to descend into the pelvis and avoid the complications of hyperextension that can occur with traction at this stage. The duration of time that should be allowed to lapse from the visualization of the umbilicus to the fetal mouth clearing the perineum should be maximally 10–15 minutes – this is not based on any specific evidence, rather a pragmatic approach to minimize the duration of the second stage.

## Delivery of the fetal head

### The Burns–Marshall technique
The operator's assistant should grasp the ankles of the fetus and raise the body vertically above the mother's abdomen. This promotes flexion of the fetal head and encourages it into the anterior–posterior diameter of the pelvic outlet (Figure 35.4). This often allows spontaneous delivery of the fetal head without further intervention,

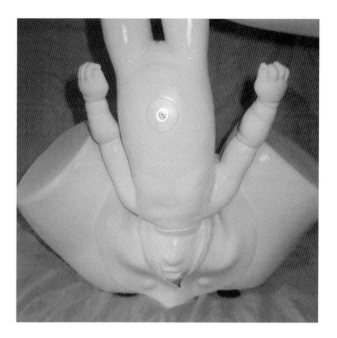

**Figure 35.4** The Burns-Marshall technique

and it is therefore advisable to protect the perineum, by covering it with a hand, to prevent precipitate delivery and severe perineal trauma. Forceps may be applied in the usual fashion to facilitate and slow delivery of the fetal head. Too rapid an extraction may result in decompression forces on the fetal skull inducing intracranial bleeding or tentorial tears.

### Mauriceau–Smellie–Veit manoeuvre
With the fetus supported on the right forearm of the accoucheur, the middle finger is placed into the fetal throat and the forefinger and ring finger are placed either on the malar eminences. Pressure is applied to the fetal tongue to encourage flexion of the head and thus present the favourable suboccipito-bregmatic diameters to the pelvis. The accoucheur's left hand is then employed to exert pressure on the fetal occiput to encourage further flexion (Figure 35.5).

### Forceps application
The application of forceps may be required to aid delivery of the head. Straight forceps, such as Kielland forceps, are often easier to apply than Neville–Barnes or Andersons (Piper's forceps are specifically designed for this task but are unavailable in most obstetric units in the UK). These should be applied in the usual fashion but must be placed below the fetal body (Figure 35.6). As the smallest part of the fetal head is lowest in the vagina, the accoucheur must ensure that the forceps blades accommodate the occiput. Premature straightening of the blades may not only result in undue pressures on the fetal head, but may also expose the maternal soft tissues to the perils of instrumental trauma.

Second stage of labour

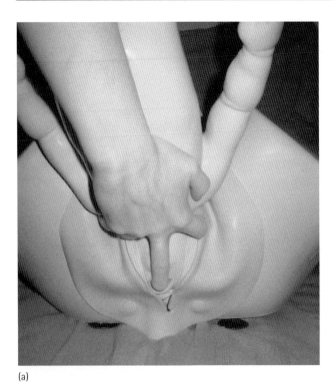

(a)

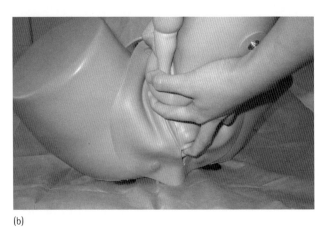

(b)

**Figure 35.5** The Mauriceau–Smellie–Veit manoeuvre

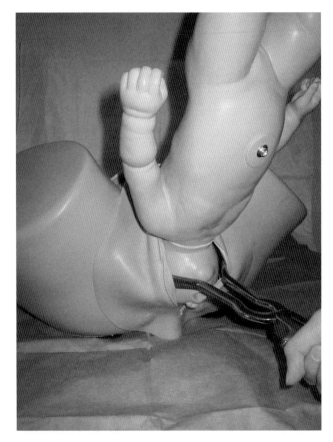

**Figure 35.6** The application of forceps

Whatever technique is employed, the fetal head should be delivered slowly to reduce the chances of decompression injuries occurring to the fetal skull and brain.

Should the head fail to descend into the pelvis following delivery of the shoulders:

- the body of the fetus should be turned sideways and suprapubic pressure applied to increase flexion and encourage entry through the pelvic inlet in the occipito-lateral position; a McRobert's manoeuvre may help;
- consideration must be given to incising the cervix (preferably at 4 and 8 o'clock) should descent have begun before full cervical dilatation is achieved;
- consideration must be given to the possibility of fetal abnormalities such as hydrocephalus – ultrasound

confirmation may be helpful; vaginal delivery may only be possible in cases of hydrocephalus by drainage of cerebrospinal fluid aspiration through the foramen magnum.

Although these manoeuvres have been practised for many years, they actually bear little resemblance to what happens during a spontaneous breech delivery. Bracht has described an alternative set of manoeuvres, which not only appear to be safe for the mother and baby, but are also less complicated for the accoucheur to perform.[18]

Whatever the approach, a paediatrician should always be present at delivery.

## Breech extraction

With breech extraction, the obstetrician delivers the infant with little or no assistance from the mother. The only indication for performing a breech extraction is to deliver a second twin. Before starting, the accoucheur must ensure that the cervix is fully dilated and that there are no mechanical obstacles to delivery. A footling presentation is frequently easier to extract than a flexed or extended breech, and in such a case Pinard's manoeuvre should be employed to deliver the foot. Groin traction is performed to draw the breech over the perineum, Lovset's manoeuvre to facilitate delivery of the arm, and downward traction to bring the fetal head into the pelvis.

## Caesarean section

Both elective and emergency caesarean delivery for the term breech should present few problems for the obstetrician, although extension of the uterine incision into a J shape may be required to facilitate access (see Chapter 31, Caesarean section). However, performance of a caesarean section does not prevent the possibility of birth injury, especially with injuries concerning the fetal abdominal organs, spine and head, and precautions similar to those undertaken with a vaginal breech delivery should be observed.

## Training

There have been major changes in the organization of junior doctors' work patterns over the last few years and coincidentally in the management of breech pregnancies. Over a ten-year period it appears that there has been a 10-fold reduction in vaginal breech delivery experience for UK registrars. As this number can be expected to fall further following the conclusions of the Term Breech Trial, alternative methods of training urgently need to be introduced (e.g. videos, models and scenario teaching) and regular updates performed.

It is therefore imperative that any woman who gives birth to a breech vaginally should be cared for by an attendant(s) with suitable experience.

## Management of the twin breech

In the majority of studies to date, the major problems associated with vaginal breech delivery relate to fetal distress in labour and difficult delivery. However, these trials only include singleton pregnancies and do not specifically address the problems for twins. Nevertheless, the plan for delivery will need careful consideration and full discussion with the parents, preferably before the onset of labour.

Although many clinicians choose caesarean section when the first twin presents as a breech because of concern about 'interlocking', this complication is extremely rare. It is equally as important to realize that no changes in neonatal morbidity or mortality in breech-presenting twins (first and second) were noted in one study over a time period during which the caesarean section rate increased dramatically (21 per cent to almost 95 per cent) [D].[19] There was, however, an increase in maternal mortality in association with caesarean delivery during the same interval.

Where the second twin is non-vertex (about 40 per cent of twins), it is the consensus opinion that vaginal delivery is safe [E]; studies show no difference in 5-minute Apgar scores or in any other indices of neonatal morbidity or mortality between the two groups.

## Documentation

It is essential that all details of care be clearly documented, including:

- the risks and benefits to both the mother and baby of each management plan discussed;
- the agreed management plan for labour;
- clear contemporaneous documentation of the events of labour;
- the identity of all those involved in the procedures;
- postnatal cord blood pH records.

---

### EBM

- Thirty per cent of breech presentations are not diagnosed until the onset of labour. Abdominal palpation has been shown to have a sensitivity of 28 per cent and specificity of 94 per cent. Confirmation of the presentation by ultrasound scan should be regarded as the 'gold standard'.
- ECV has been demonstrated to be associated with a significant reduction in the risk of caesarean section (OR 0.4; 95 per cent CI 0.3–0.6).
- The Term Breech Trial confirmed that vaginal delivery is more hazardous than elective caesarean section, with the overall risk of perinatal death for the term frank/complete breech fetus when delivered by planned caesarean birth being reduced by 75 per cent (RR 0.23; 95 per cent CI 0.07–0.8).
- In a subanalysis of the Term Breech Trial, the risk of the combined outcome of perinatal mortality, neonatal mortality or serious neonatal morbidity with planned caesarean section compared with planned vaginal birth was 16/1006 (1.6 per cent) compared with 23/704 (3.3 per cent) (RR 0.49; 95 per cent CI 0.26–0.91; $p < 0.02$).

---

### KEY POINTS

- Breech presentation, whatever the mode of delivery, is a signal for potential fetal handicap and this should inform antenatal, intrapartum and neonatal management. Each patient requires individualized attention and evaluation.
- At term, the first question that must be addressed when confronted by a breech presentation is 'Where is the placenta?' The second is 'Is the fetus healthy?'
- All women with an uncomplicated breech pregnancy at term (37–42 weeks) should be offered ECV.
- Planned caesarean section greatly reduces both perinatal/ neonatal mortality and neonatal morbidity, at the expense of somewhat increased maternal morbidity. The questions of long-term morbidity and the cost implications of implementing a policy of caesarean section for all breech deliveries have not been addressed.

- Evidence from the Term Breech Trial cannot be directly extrapolated to preterm breech delivery. As a consequence, the management of the preterm breech remains an area of clinical controversy. ECV before term has not been shown to offer any benefits.
- The most experienced obstetrician available should manage labour, with continuous fetal monitoring as standard. Epidural anaesthesia may be provided if the mother so wishes, but is not compulsory. Premature expulsive efforts must be discouraged, as these can lead to head entrapment, nuchal arms and hyperextension of the fetal head.

## Key References

1. Cheng MH. Breech delivery at term: a critical review of the literature. *Obstet Gynecol* 1993; **82**: 605–18.

2. Danielian PJ, Wang J, Hall MH. Long-term outcome by method of delivery of fetuses in breech presentation at term: population-based follow up. *BMJ* 1996; **312**: 1451–3.

3. Penn ZJ. Breech presentation. In: James DK, Steer PJ, Weiner CP, Gonik B (eds). *High Risk Pregnancy, Management Options*. London: WB Saunders, 2006: 1334–59.

4. Mazor M, Hagay ZJ, Leiberman J *et al.* Fetal abnormalities associated with breech delivery. *J Reprod Med* 1985; **30**: 884–6.

5. Grant A. Elective versus selective caesarean section delivery of the small baby. *Cochrane Database Syst Rev* 2001; (**2**): CD000078.

6. Hofmeyr GJ, Hannah HM. Planned caesarean section for the term breech delivery. *Cochrane Database Syst Rev* 2003; (**3**): CD000166.

7. Hofmeyr GJ, Kulier R. External cephalic version for breech presentation before term. *Cochrane Database Syst Rev* 2006; (**1**): CD000084.

8. Royal College of Obstetricians and Gynaecologists. *The Management of Breech Presentation*, Guideline No. 20b. London: RCOG Press, 2006.

9. Tatum RK, Orr JW, Soong S, Huddleston JF. Vaginal breech delivery of selected infants weighing more than 2000 g. A retrospective analysis of 7 years of experience. *Am J Obstet Gynecol* 1985; **152**: 145–55.

10. Hannah ME, Hannah WJ, Hewson SA *et al.* Term Breech Trial Collaborative Group. Planned caesarean section versus planned vaginal birth for breech presentation at term: a randomised multicentre trial. *Lancet* 2000; **356**: 1375–83.

11. Goffinet F, Carayol M, Foidart JM *et al.* Is planned vaginal delivery for breech presentation at term still an option? Results of an observational prospective survey in France and Belgium. *Am J Obstet Gynecol* 2006; **194**: 1002–11.

12. Doyle NM, Riggs JW, Ramin SM *et al.* Outcomes of term vaginal breech delivery. *Am J Perinatol* 2005; **22**: 325–8.

13. Rietberg CCT, Elferink-Stinkens PM, Visser GHA. The effect of the Term Breech Trial on medical intervention behaviour and neonatal outcome in The Netherland: an analysis of 35453 term breech infants. *BJOG* 2005; **112**: 205–9.

14. Recommendations of the FIGO Committee on Perinatal Health on Guidelines for the Management of Breech Delivery. *Eur J Obstet Gynecol Reprod Biol* 1995; **58**: 89–92.

15. Brady K, Duff P, Read JA, Harlass FE. Reliability of fetal buttock sampling in assessing the acid–base balance of the breech fetus. *Obstet Gynecol* 1989; **74**: 886–8.

16. Lumley J. Any room left for disagreement about assisting breech births at term? *Lancet* 2000; **356**: 1368–9.

17. Chadha YC, Mahmood TA, Dick MJ *et al.* Breech delivery and epidural analgesia. *Br J Obstet Gynaecol* 1992; **99**: 96–100.

18. Edelstone DI. Breech presentation. In: Kean LH, Baker PN, Edelstone DI (eds). *Best Practice in Labor Ward Management*. Edinburgh: WB Saunders, 2000: 141–65.

19. Oettinger M, Ophir E, Markovitz J *et al.* Is caesarean section necessary for delivery of a breech first twin? *Gynecol Obstet Invest* 1993; **35**: 38–43.

# Perineal trauma

*Lucy Kean*

## INTRODUCTION

Perineal trauma is a common event in first labours, affecting up to 90 per cent of first-time mothers. It is a cause for concern for many women and in some countries has led to a large increase in the numbers of women requesting elective caesarean section. Considerable postnatal morbidity and occasionally mortality can be attributed to this, and therefore a clear understanding of the best management of perineal trauma is mandatory for every clinician working in obstetrics.

## ANATOMY OF THE PELVIC FLOOR AND DEFINITIONS OF TRAUMA

In order to understand the pathophysiology of perineal trauma, an understanding of the anatomy of the pelvic floor is required.

First-degree trauma is defined as injury to the perineal skin alone. Second-degree trauma involves injury to the perineum, including the perineal muscles, but not involving the anal sphincter. Figure 36.1 shows the muscles of the perineum and the usual extensions of mediolateral and midline episiotomy.

Third-degree extensions involve any part of the anal sphincter complex (external and internal sphincters) and fourth-degree encompasses extension into the rectal mucosa.

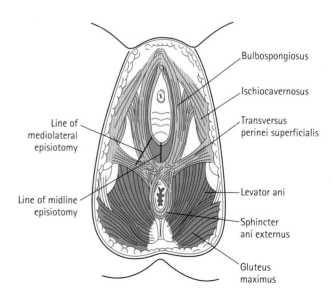

**Figure 36.1** Muscles of the perineum

The Royal College of Obstetricians and Gynaecologists (RCOG) of the United Kingdom recommends classifying anal sphincter damage as follows.[1]

- 3a: less than 50 per cent of the external anal sphincter (EAS) is torn.
- 3b: more than 50 per cent of the external anal sphincter is torn.
- 3c: tear involving the internal anal sphincter (almost always involves complete disruption of the external sphincter).
- Fourth degree: injury to the both the external and internal anal sphincter complex extending into the rectal mucosa.

## FIRST- AND SECOND-DEGREE PERINEAL TRAUMA

In a first pregnancy, perineal trauma affects up to 90 per cent of women, with episiotomy rates of 40–60 per cent being common in many countries. The perineum following delivery is often the source of much discomfort and pain for many women. Morbidity to the perineum may persist for weeks to years post-delivery. This can result in a cascade of events such as dyspareunia, psychosexual dysfunction, maladjustment to motherhood and relationship breakdown. Minimizing the risk of perineal trauma should therefore be at the forefront of care during labour.

## RISK FACTORS FOR PERINEAL TRAUMA

It is recognized that perineal trauma is associated with:

- larger infants,
- prolonged labour,
- instrumental delivery.

Instrumental delivery and forceps delivery carry a particularly large increase in the risk of extended trauma, with as many as 60 per cent of women experiencing ultrasonographically visible anal sphincter defects in research studies.[2] Long second stage also appears to contribute to perineal damage. Malposition of the fetal head in labour is a risk factor for long labour and instrumental delivery and thus perineal trauma.

## REDUCING THE RISK OF PERINEAL TRAUMA

### The role of episiotomy

Liberal use of mediolateral episiotomy does not appear to reduce the incidence of third-degree tears, with the exception of two small trials. Midline episiotomy certainly increases the risk of extended trauma, with a reported odds ratio (OR) of 4.5–6 for third- or fourth-degree tears. It is important to recognize that there are significant differences in extension rates for mediolateral and midline episiotomies. Meta-analyses that do not make this distinction are unlikely to adequately assess the effect of episiotomy. Where episiotomy is restricted, some, but not all trials have shown an increase in anterior vaginal trauma, but this does not equate to an increase in urinary problems.

Combining trials of restrictive policy for episiotomy compared with standard care gives the following results:[3]

- severe perineal trauma (third- and fourth-degree tears): RR 0.74 (95 per cent confidence interval (CI) 0.42–1.28)
- any posterior perineal trauma: RR 0.87 (95 per cent CI 0.83–0.91)
- anterior trauma: RR 1.75 (95 per cent CI 1.52–2.01)
- Apgar score <7 at 1 minute: RR 1.05 (95 per cent CI 0.76–1.45).

Combining trials for examination of pain after delivery was not possible because of the heterogeneity of reported outcomes, but it is clear that pain scores in the short term were generally lower in all trials in the restricted episiotomy groups (42.5 per cent usual care versus 30.7 per cent restricted episiotomy, at discharge in the largest trial).

Women in the restrictive episiotomy groups were likely to resume sexual intercourse earlier.

NICE have recommended that:

- There is considerable high-level evidence that the routine use of episiotomy (trial mean 71.6 per cent; range 44.9–93.7 per cent) is not of benefit to women either in the short or longer term, compared with restricted use (trial mean 29.1 per cent; range 7.6–53.0 per cent) [A].
- Where an episiotomy is performed, the recommended technique is a mediolateral episiotomy originating at the vaginal fourchette and usually directed to the right side. The angle to the vertical axis should be between 45 and 60° at the time of the episiotomy [A].

This final point is an important practice point, as a common error made by inexperienced practitioners is to angle the episiotomy too medially. Perineal stretching at crowning makes the perineum appear broader and therefore a much more horizontal angle of incision is required than would be expected.

### Conduct of normal birth

In nulliparae during the weeks before giving birth, perineal massage appears to protect against perineal trauma (risk difference −0.08, 95 per cent CI −0.12, −0.04) [B].[4] However, massage of the perineum in the second stage has no influence.

The conduct of delivery has also been examined in three studies. Changing established practice is obviously difficult, as in one study there was only 73 per cent compliance in the 'hands poised' group (versus 95 per cent in 'hands on').[5] Across the three studies the rates of perineal trauma were similar in both groups: 29 per cent first-degree trauma and 37 per cent second-degree trauma. Thus, conduct of the delivery in terms of a hands-on or hands-off approach showed no advantage of one method over the other.

The use of lidocaine spray has been evaluated and shown to have no effect on pain, but possibly a small reduction in trauma rates [B].[3]

Birth position in women without an epidural does not influence perineal trauma rates (increased spontaneous trauma), but reduced episiotomy rates in women who were not supine. Non-supine positions were also associated with higher rates of bleeding, but fewer fetal heart rate abnormalities, a marginally shorter second stage (by 4.28 minutes) and less pain [A].[6]

## Mode of delivery

Mode of delivery has a large impact on rates of perineal trauma. Of course, elective caesarean section prevents damage to the perineum from labour-related events, and reducing the rates of instrumental vaginal delivery will reduce the incidence of perineal trauma.

Ventouse delivery appears to be associated with less perineal trauma (see Chapter 34, Instrumental vaginal delivery). Ventouse delivery (risk difference −0.06, 95 per cent CI −0.10, −0.02) and spontaneous birth (−0.11, 95 per cent CI −0.18, −0.04) causes less anal sphincter trauma than forceps delivery.[4,7] However, at five-year follow up, there is no difference in reported symptoms in women delivered by either ventouse or forceps. Therefore, given that the highest rates of severe perineal damage occur in women for whom two instruments are needed to achieve delivery, the first choice must be the instrument most likely to deliver the baby safely and with which the obstetrician is experienced.[7,8]

Episiotomy has been recommended when instrumental vaginal delivery is performed. This is not based on any evidence, and a more flexible approach is needed. Ventouse delivery in a multiparous woman may not require any episiotomy, and an intact perineum may result. However, a forceps delivery in a nulliparous woman is likely to require episiotomy (although even for this, there is no evidence that episiotomy reduces the likelihood of extended trauma).[7]

## Epidural analgesia and prolonged second stage

The issue of epidural analgesia and instrumental delivery are closely linked and trials that attempt to divide the two are difficult to perform. Epidural analgesia has been shown to be associated with an increased risk of instrumental vaginal delivery, with the attendant perineal morbidity.[9] There is an association between long second stage and perineal trauma, with increased risk of severe trauma in women experiencing long second stages. However, it has been shown that allowing a passive second stage in nulliparae with continuous epidural analgesia reduces the incidence of difficult instrumental delivery (RR, 0.79; 95 per cent CI, 0.66–0.95). Spontaneous delivery is also slightly more likely among women who delay pushing (RR, 1.09; 95 per cent CI, 1.00–1.18).[10] Given that instrumental delivery represents the greatest risk to the perineum, it is probably better to allow descent of the head with a passive second stage and to consider augmentation with oxytocics in nulliparae, but further research is needed to evaluate the risks and benefits fully.

# REPAIR TECHNIQUES FOR FIRST- AND SECOND-DEGREE TRAUMA

Adequate lighting, analgesia and any necessary assistance are mandatory before attempting to repair a tear or episiotomy. It is unacceptable to perform a perineal repair with inadequate anaesthesia, just as performing a caesarean section without adequate anaesthesia would be considered unacceptable.

Before commencing a repair, a full examination should take place. The vaginal apex must be identified and the anal sphincter inspected. If the practitioner is inexperienced in the examination of the anal sphincter, someone with experience should be called at this stage. One study has shown that when the practitioner is uncertain, re-examination by a trained person identifies significantly more anal sphincter ruptures.

Minor first-degree trauma that is not bleeding and where the skin edges are opposed does not need closure; however, a careful examination should be undertaken to ensure there is no damage to the perineal muscles.

Women should be advised that second-degree trauma should be sutured, as this leads to faster healing and less gaping of the perineum.

Some authors use a continuous suture technique to perform the entire repair, finishing with a subcuticular skin suture. It is vital to ensure that the apex of the vaginal component is secured, as paravaginal haematoma formation can occur if the apex is missed. When individual bleeding arteries are identified, they should be ligated separately. Once the repair is complete, it is important to perform the following:

- Remove any vaginal tampon placed to aid visualization.
- Count swabs and ensure none is retained.
- Count and dispose carefully of any needles.
- Inspect the repair to ensure vascular haemostasis.
- Perform a rectal examination to ensure no sutures have breached the rectal mucosa and to palpate the anal sphincter to ensure it is intact.
- Prescribe analgesia.
- Document the repair, using a diagram if necessary.
- Document that the swab and needle count is correct.

## Evidence for suture technique

The Cochrane review showed that continuous suture techniques compared with interrupted sutures for perineal closure (all layers or perineal skin only) are associated with less pain for up to ten days postpartum (RR 0.70, 95 per cent CI 0.64–0.76). A greater reduction in pain was seen when continuous suturing techniques were used for all layers (RR 0.65, 95 per cent CI 0.60–0.71). There was an overall reduction in analgesia use with the continuous subcutaneous skin suture compared to interrupted sutures for closure of perineal skin (RR 0.70, 95 per cent CI 0.58–0.84). Women were less likely to experience dyspareunia if they had continuous suturing for all layers (RR 0.83, 95 per cent CI 0.70–0.98). Fewer women required suture removal in the continuous suturing groups versus interrupted (RR 0.54, 95 per cent CI 0.45–0.65), but no significant differences were seen in the need for resuturing of wounds or long-term pain.[11]

The Ipswich Childbirth Study randomized women to either a two- or three-stage repair (two stages are closure of vagina and perineal tissue but not skin, as long as the skin edges can be approximated to within 5 mm). A two-stage repair was associated with less long-term perineal dysaesthesia (30 versus 40 per cent; RR 0.75, 95 per cent CI 0.61–0.91) and less discomfort when sexual intercourse was resumed [B].[12] A recent study showed no difference between a continuous technique and a three-stage repair, using a non-locking vaginal suture; however, less suture material was needed for the continuous technique. Therefore, a technique utilizing a continuous technique is likely to produce results as good as any other, with a minimal use of suture material, reducing infection risk.[13]

## Evidence for suture material

Much effort has been dedicated towards comparing different types of suture material. Catgut has been widely compared with polyglycolic acid sutures (Dexon™ and Vicryl™) and the conclusion is that catgut was associated with more short-term pain. However, in the United Kingdom, the manufacturers have now withdrawn catgut. The above study assessing technique also addressed the issue of short versus medium half-life polyglactin sutures (Vicryl versus Vicryl Rapide, Ethicon, UK). The primary end-point for the study of pain at ten days showed no difference between the two suture types, though more women with standard Vicryl sutures required analgesia in the preceding 24 hours and more women experienced pain on walking. Suture material was much less likely to need removal at a later stage in the group sutured with the more rapidly absorbed polyglactin suture. At ten days, the midwives were more likely to comment that the wound was gaping in the group sutured with the rapidly absorbed suture (6.1 versus 3.4 per cent; 95 per cent CI 1.14–2.92), although at three months the outcomes were no different [B].[14]

Braided sutures have not been compared with monofilament sutures.

## Follow up

In general, most first- and second-degree perineal repairs will heal without problems. Important issues relate to the failure to identify anal sphincter damage, which may only become apparent later. Women who have experienced difficult vaginal deliveries may value the opportunity to discuss their delivery at a later date.

The ideal setting for follow up for women experiencing persistent problems after delivery is a dedicated perineal dysfunction clinic. Where this is not available, a team approach involving obstetricians and physiotherapists, with access to appropriate investigative techniques, such as endoanal ultrasound and manometry, is important. Urinary problems are amenable to biofeedback techniques, and physiotherapy input is vital to ensure that these are appropriately taught and reinforced.

# THIRD- AND FOURTH-DEGREE TRAUMA

## Incidence

Internal anal sphincter incompetence results in insensible faecal incontinence, whereas external anal sphincter incompetence causes faecal urgency. Third-degree tears are reported in approximately 2.8 per cent of primigravidae and 0.4 per cent of multigravidae. The reported rates will vary among units with different rates of instrumental delivery. New-onset symptoms of faecal incontinence are reported in 10 per cent of primigravidae undergoing instrumental vaginal delivery at ten months, and in 3 per cent of primigravidae undergoing spontaneous vaginal delivery. Some of these new symptoms are attributable to pudendal neuropathy, as 5 per cent of women report new symptoms after emergency caesarean section, whereas new onset bowel symptoms are very uncommon after elective caesarean section. Some degree of faecal urgency probably related to occult anal sphincter damage is much more common, with 44 per cent of women reporting this at five years following instrumental delivery of their first baby.

Ultrasonographically visible anal sphincter defects are apparent in 82 per cent of women undergoing forceps delivery and in 48 per cent of ventouse deliveries.[2] However, most women report infrequent problems, and there is no difference in long-term follow up between forceps and ventouse delivery.[8]

Research studies investigating anal sphincter damage have demonstrated sphincter defects visible on ultrasound in 40 per cent of women after vaginal delivery of their first baby, although two-thirds of these will be asymptomatic.[15] The much higher incidence of problems demonstrated in research studies underlines two important facts:

1 Women are embarrassed about faecal problems after childbirth,
2 Ultrasonographically demonstrated lesions do not translate into confirmed problems of faecal continence.

Anal sphincter damage is mainly limited to first deliveries, whereas pudendal nerve damage can be cumulative. Pudendal nerve damage occurs during labour as the nerve becomes compressed and stretched. Delivery late in the first stage or second stage by caesarean section does not prevent this. It has also been shown that ultrasonographically visible anal sphincter defects can be demonstrated in women who were demonstrated to have an intact anal sphincter at the time of delivery. The mechanism for this late disruption is unclear. It may be related to infection or haematoma formation, or possibly to partial unrecognized sphincter ruptures.

# Risk factors for third- and fourth-degree tears

The risk factors for third-degree and fourth-degree tears are shown in Table 36.1.

Risk factors are cumulative, and in some cases the risks may be greater than the sum of two individual risks, for instance the risk of severe trauma when two instruments are needed is much greater than the summed risks for each individual instrument.

# Repair

## Identification of extent of damage

All women sustaining perineal trauma should be carefully examined to assess the severity of damage to the perineum, vagina and rectum. All staff performing perineal repair must be confident in their ability to diagnose anal sphincter injury. It is imperative to examine carefully for rectal extension, as small buttonhole tears can be overlooked and lead to fistula formation.

When disrupted, the anal sphincter retracts, forming a dimple on either side of the anal canal. Rupture of the rectal mucosa will almost always involve damage to both the internal and external anal sphincters.

**Table 36.1** Factors associated with increased risk of third-degree tears

|  | Odds ratio |
| --- | --- |
| Primigravida | 2–7 |
| Second stage of labour of >60 minutes (including passive second stage) | 2 |
| Instrumental vaginal delivery | 1.7–7 |
| Midline episiotomy | 5–11 |
| Macrosomia (>4 kg) | 2.9 |
| Persistent occipitoposterior position | 1.7 |
| Epidural analgesia | 1.5 |
| Prior third-degree tear | 4 |
| Induction of labour | 2 |
| Shoulder dystocia | 4 |

A good repair of the sphincter is imperative, as this is the factor most strongly associated with future faecal continence.

## Conduct of the repair

The most recent Cochrane review of three eligible trials involving 279 women showed that the overlap technique was associated with a significantly lower incidence in faecal urgency (RR 0.12, 95 per cent CI 0.02–0.86) and lower anal incontinence score (weighted mean difference −1.70, 95 per cent CI −3.03 to −0.37). The overlap technique was also associated with a lower risk of deterioration of anal incontinence symptoms over 12 months (RR 0.26, 95 per cent CI 0.09–0.79). There was no difference in perineal pain (RR 0.08, 95 per cent CI 0.00–1.45), dyspareunia (RR 0.62, 95 per cent CI 0.11–3.39), flatus incontinence (RR 0.93, 95 per cent CI 0.26–3.31) and faecal incontinence (RR 0.07, 95 per cent CI 0.00–1.21) between the two repair techniques at 12 months. There was no significant difference in quality of life.[16]

There have been two subsequent trials demonstrating no differences in outcome. It must also be recognized that one of the trials included in the Cochrane review included repairs done by one of two trained specialists, making the findings unlikely to be generalizable. The RCOG guideline suggests that there is no evidence to suggest that an overlap technique is better than end-to-end approximation of the muscle [A].[1]

Whichever method is used, it is important to ensure that the muscle is correctly approximated with long-acting sutures so that it is given adequate time to heal. 3a tears will always be repaired using an end-to-end technique as the majority of the sphincter fibres remain intact. In the case of 3b tears, some practitioners have advocated cutting the remaining fibres to perform an overlap repair.

The repair must be performed or directly supervised by a practitioner trained in the repair of third- and fourth-degree trauma. There must be adequate analgesia. In practice, this means either a regional or general anaesthetic, as local infiltration does not allow sufficient relaxation of the sphincter to allow a satisfactory repair. The lighting must be adequate and an assistant is usually needed. This means in practice that repair should be undertaken in the operating theatre.

Repair of the rectal mucosa should be performed first. 2:0 polyglycolic acid interrupted sutures with the knots placed on the mucosal side are commonly used. Next, the layers of the internal sphincter should be replicated across the defect with interrupted sutures of 2:0 or 3:0 Vicryl or polydioxanone suture (PDS). The torn external sphincter is then repaired. This should be re-approximated with either three or four figure-of-eight sutures, or an overlap technique.

A 2.0 or 3.0 PDS is ideal. Polyglycolic acid is also used. A single study comparing the two showed no difference in outcomes at 12 months [B]. However, the longer tensile retention of PDS and its monofilament characteristics make it especially suitable. Short half-life treated polyglactin sutures (Vicryl Rapide) are not acceptable as they do not have a long enough half-life to ensure muscle healing. Also, non-absorbable sutures should not be used in the acute setting as these can form a focus for infection, requiring removal. The knots should be buried beneath the superficial perineal muscles, to minimize knot migration.

The remainder of the perineal repair is undertaken as for second-degree trauma. It is imperative to ensure that a good repair of the perineal muscles is performed, as a short or deficient perineum make injury in future deliveries more likely.

Retention of urine secondary to the anaesthesia or repair is common and a urinary catheter should be inserted until spontaneous voiding is achieved.

## Post-operative precautions

It is common practice after delayed anal sphincter repair to use a constipating regimen to allow the repair to heal before stools are passed. This is difficult in recently delivered women who have very different needs from those of the surgical patient. Constipative regimens have been compared with stool-softening regimens. It is concluded that constipative management leads to more pain and a longer post-operative stay compared to stool-softening regimens, but with no difference in repair success. Lactulose and a bulk agent, such as Fybogel, are recommended for 5–10 days.

It is common sense to give a broad-spectrum antibiotic. It is important to include an antibiotic that will cover possible anaerobic contamination, such as metronidazole. This should be prescribed orally rather than *per rectum*.

Adequate oral analgesia should be prescribed. Paracetamol, non-steroidal anti-inflammatory drugs and opioid analgesia are acceptable. However, opioids used alone can exacerbate constipation, and thus the former should be used first.

Before the woman goes home,

- ensure that she has had a chance to discuss the delivery with a senior member of the team;
- prescribe necessary analgesia and stool softeners;
- advise on perineal hygiene;
- counsel that 60–80 per cent of women will be asymptomatic following healing of the repair;
- provide a contact number in case problems occur;
- make an initial plan for short-term management with a physiotherapist;
- counsel that sutures occasionally migrate and fragments may be passed *per vaginum* or, occasionally, *per rectum*; help should be sought if there are concerns;
- give an appointment for follow up.

## Follow up

All women who have sustained a third- or fourth-degree tear should be offered follow up by someone interested in this field. A team approach as outlined earlier is best. Physiotherapy should include augmented biofeedback, as this has been shown to improve continence.

At 6–12 weeks, a full evaluation of the degree of symptoms should take place. This must include careful questioning with regard to faecal and urinary symptoms. A standard questionnaire for women to complete before attending is helpful in precisely delineating the degree of symptoms. Symptomatic women should be offered investigation, including endoanal ultrasound and manometry.

Asymptomatic women with low squeeze pressures and a demonstrable sphincter defect of more than a quadrant should be counselled regarding the pros and cons of future deliveries. Women with ongoing severe symptoms should be considered for secondary surgery. As pudendal neuropathy can take at least six months to improve, any further surgical intervention is best deferred until at least this time; however, in exceptional cases in which sphincter disruption is demonstrated and faecal incontinence is debilitating, surgery may be required earlier.

Women with mild symptoms should be advised to avoid gas-producing foods and bulking agents, constipating agents and biofeedback offered.

## Counselling about subsequent delivery

Women can be divided into one of three or four groups with regard to their next delivery.

## Previous third/fourth-degree tear, no ongoing symptoms

These women should be counselled that there is approximately a 4 per cent risk of further anal sphincter damage in a subsequent vaginal delivery. This recurrence is not predictable antenatally. Women who were transiently incontinent after their first delivery are particularly at risk of worsening of symptoms, and 17–24 per cent may develop worsening symptoms after subsequent delivery.[17]

When women opt for subsequent vaginal delivery, every effort should be made to avoid instrumental vaginal delivery. There is no evidence that episiotomy prevents muscle damage, and most women appreciate an intact perineum if that can be achieved. The second stage should not be prolonged. Women need careful counselling about epidural analgesia with reference to both the type of delivery and length of second stage. Where anal sphincter damage does not occur, new-onset symptoms are usually attributable to pudendal neuropathy, which usually improves with time. Transient flatus incontinence is reported by 10 per cent of women delivered without further sphincter damage.

## Women who continue to be symptomatic

The majority of these women will have a demonstrable defect on ultrasound. There is a risk of worsening of symptoms, which may then make life much more difficult. Women should be carefully counselled with regard to the additional effects of worsening pudendal damage and the small risk of further muscle damage. The majority of women in this group may opt for caesarean section, but for those choosing vaginal delivery, every effort should be made to avoid operative vaginal delivery and lengthy second stage.

## Women who have undergone a secondary anal sphincter repair

The consensus is that these women should be delivered by caesarean section [E]. However, there are no data to advise women who wish to try for a vaginal delivery. Again, instrumental delivery and long second stage should be avoided where possible.

## Women who are asymptomatic, but have demonstrable anal sphincter defects or abnormal manometry on testing

This is a difficult group to manage, as there are few data to advise management. These women are at risk of new symptoms following subsequent delivery. Those at most risk appear to be women with a full quadrant defect, and these women may wish to choose caesarean section next time [C].[18]

The plan for delivery must be clearly documented in the case notes.

## Perineal trauma and female genital mutilation (circumcision)

Female genital mutilation (FGM) is defined as all procedures involving partial or total removal of the external female genitalia or other injury to the female genital organs, whether for cultural or other non-therapeutic reasons. The practice of female circumcision is very common in parts of the Middle East and Africa, but also to some extent in India and Indonesia. Somalia, Egypt and Sudan are the countries with the highest rates of FGM. It is important to note that the practice is not limited to particular cultural or religious groups and all women from areas of risk must be sensitively questioned and examined.

For most women, the procedure will have been undertaken when they were children. Some women may not have any recollection of the procedure, and for most women it will be seen by them as a normal thing to have happened. It is vital, therefore, that questioning is undertaken with sensitivity. It is usually easier to refer to the practice as 'cutting' as most women understand what is meant by this.

The practice involves removal of parts of the female genital organs, including the labia minora, infundibulum, clitoris and, in some cases, the labia majora. It is important to ascertain the extent of the FGM, as complications are more likely with type III FGM (Table 36.2). Ninety per

**Table 36.2** Classification of types of female genital mutilation procedures (World Health Organization)

| Type | Definition |
| --- | --- |
| I | Partial or total removal of the clitoris and/or the prepuce (clitoridectomy) |
| II | Partial or total removal of the clitoris and the labia minora, with or without excision of the labia majora (excision) |
| III | Narrowing of the vaginal orifice with creation of a covering seal by cutting and appositioning the labia minora and/or the labia majora, with or without excision of the clitoris (infibulation) |
| IV | All other harmful procedures to the female genitalia for non-medical purposes, e.g. pricking, piercing,[a] incising, scraping and cauterizing |

[a] Piercing is part of this WHO classification but the legal status of this is unclear in the UK.

cent of women who have undergone FGM will have types I, II or IV.

Under the 1985 and 2003 Acts, it is illegal in the UK to perform FGM for traditional or ritual reasons, and is punishable by imprisonment for up to 14 years. It is also illegal to remove an individual to another country for the purposes of FGM. Interestingly, responsibility for decisions regarding surgical reduction of the labia for cosmetic/comfort reasons has been derogated to doctors. It is advised that where a doctor is unsure of the legal position of any request, ethical committee and a legal opinion is sought.

If a healthcare worker is concerned regarding a child who may be at risk of FGM the appropriate child-protection measures should be undertaken (usually via the nominated child-protection officer or social services).

In the main, the issues seen with FGM are those related to the sequelae of the procedure. Type III is most often associated with physical problems, but all women are at risk of the psychological problems related to FGM.

Physical problems include:

- urinary tract infection,
- chronic inflammation and scarring,
- clitoral dermoid cysts (which can become infected),
- fistulae.

Psychological problems are common with one-third to one-half of women displaying symptoms of post-traumatic stress disorder, depression, fear of childbirth and other anxiety states.

Obstetric complications are more likely with the more severe types of FGM. An increase in the rates of caesarean section, postpartum haemorrhage, neonatal resuscitation and stillbirth are seen with types II and III FGM, with type III posing the highest risk.

In settings where high quality intrapartum care is available, FGM does not appear to lead to a longer second stage, but perineal tears and the need for episiotomy is much more common.

When women who are likely to have undergone FGM are seen in the antenatal clinic, it is vital that they are sensitively questioned and examined and that a careful plan of management is made for delivery. Psychological support may be needed. A discussion regarding whether defibulation is advised antenatally or intrapartum should be undertaken by a senior professional with experience in this area.

If vaginal access is very limited, defibulation at about 20 weeks may be the best option for a safe labour. If vaginal access is adequate, then defibulation in the first stage under epidural anaesthesia or in the second stage as the head crowns is reasonable. Usually, a midline anterior episiotomy (division of the labia) is required. A catheter may need to be passed to identify the urethra when the anterior episiotomy is performed. A carefully placed posterior mediolateral episiotomy will be needed if there is rigid scar tissue. Great care must be taken when performing the posterior mediolateral episiotomy, as the presence of the scar tissue can lead to extensive tears if not appropriately managed.

Following delivery, the labial edges should be oversewn if they are bleeding. It is not acceptable to re-infibulate by sewing the labial edges together. The Royal College of Obstetricians and Gynaecologists guideline[19] states that:

*Any repair carried out after birth, whether following spontaneous laceration or deliberate defibulation, should be sufficient to appose raw edges and control bleeding, but must not result in a vaginal opening that makes intercourse difficult or impossible.*

Postnatal care should include regular inspection of the perineum to ensure healing, as poor or delayed healing is not uncommon. Women who have had defibulation performed during pregnancy or delivery should be re-examined in any future pregnancy, as re-infibulation between pregnancies is not uncommon.

# ACUTE HAEMATOMA

## Incidence

The reported incidence of puerperal haematomas varies widely, ranging from one in 1500 to one in 309. However, large and clinically significant haematomas complicate between one in 1000 and one in 4000 deliveries.

## Aetiological factors

- Episiotomy (85–90 per cent of cases).
- Instrumental vaginal delivery.

- Primiparity.
- Hypertensive disorders.

Multiple pregnancy, vulval varicosities, macrosomic infants and prolonged second stage have all been implicated, but their contribution is probably small.

In two-thirds of haematomas, failure to achieve perfect haemostasis at the time of repair, particularly at the upper end of the incision, has been implicated. However, haematomas can occur without any perineal laceration, due to stretching and avulsion of vessels during delivery.

The anatomy of the perineum and vagina plays an important part in the limitation or extension of haematoma formation. Infralevator haematomas, most commonly associated with vaginal delivery, are limited superiorly by the levator ani, medially by the perineal body and from extension on to the thigh by Colles fascia and the fascia lata. These may extend into the ischiorectal fossa. They usually arise from small vulvar or labial vessels, branches of the inferior rectal, inferior vesical or vaginal branch of the uterine arteries. They usually present as vulval pain out of proportion to that expected from an episiotomy, with an ischiorectal mass and discoloration. Continued bleeding or urinary retention may also occur.

In contrast, supralevator haematomas have no fibrous boundaries. They may be paravaginal or supravaginal. They arise from branches of the uterine artery, the inferior vesical and pudendal artery. Bleeding can track into the broad ligament, the retroperitoneal and presacral spaces. Thus, they present as rectal pain and pressure, an enlarging rectal or vaginal mass or with hypovolaemic shock.

Broad ligament haematomas will cause upward and lateral displacement of the uterus. The uterus feels well contracted and there may be little revealed vaginal bleeding. As these haematomas are above the pelvic diaphragm, they are more rarely associated with vaginal delivery, although they can occur if genital trauma extends into the fornices or if a cervical tear is sustained. They may also occur in cases of uterine rupture or scar dehiscence.

Following delivery, the vulvar and paravaginal tissues are loose and oedematous. They can accommodate large amounts of blood before a haematoma becomes obvious and gives rise to symptoms (500–1500 mL). Blood loss estimation is therefore extremely difficult and is usually grossly underestimated.

## Presenting symptoms

### Infralevator haematomas
- Vaginal swelling.
- Continued vaginal bleeding.
- Severe rectal/vaginal pain.
- Urinary retention.

If postpartum blood loss was moderate, bleeding into the haematoma may produce signs of shock.

## Supralevator haematomas

- Cardiovascular collapse.
- Uterine displacement.
- Abdominal or rectal pain.
- Continued vaginal bleeding.

Urgent magnetic resonance imaging (MRI) or computed tomography (CT) scanning may help in the identification of supravaginal haematomas.

## Management

Small, non-expanding haematomas of less than 3 cm can be managed conservatively. Larger or expanding haematomas require surgical management to prevent pressure necrosis, septicaemia, haemorrhage and death. Full maternal resuscitation in conjunction with anaesthetic colleagues is vital. Blood loss is likely to be significantly underestimated and early recourse to transfusion is necessary. As for repair of genital trauma, adequate analgesia, assistance and lighting are needed.

If the haematoma lies beneath a repair, this should be taken down. If no repair was made, an incision in the inferior portion of the mass near the introitus should be made. Clot is evacuated and the area involved is irrigated with saline. Individual bleeding points should be ligated, although it is more common to find diffuse ooze from very friable haemorrhagic paravaginal tissue. If the tissues allow, a layered closure or primary closure should be undertaken; however, the tissues are generally very difficult to place sutures into, as they are extremely friable. If sutures appear to be tearing out, closing the defect over a soft suction drain such as a Jackson–Pratt drain with a tight pack in the vagina for 12–24 hours may achieve the necessary reduction of dead space and control of bleeding. A urethral catheter will be needed, both to allow effective bladder emptying and to monitor urinary output. Prophylactic broad-spectrum antibiotics should be given, as the risk of subsequent infection is reasonably high and late problems are often attributable to infection. There must be a high index of suspicion if repeated symptoms occur, as the risk of recurrence in the first 12–48 hours is high (approximately 10 per cent). Special vigilance after pack removal is particularly important.

Large paravaginal and supravaginal haematomas can be much more complicated. Extension into the retroperitoneal space or broad ligament can be life threatening. The cervix should be carefully examined to assess cervical lacerations. This is best accomplished by grasping the cervix with a sponge holder, starting at 12 o'clock. A second sponge holder is placed at 2 o'clock and the cervix examined between the two. If intact, the first holder is moved to 4 o'clock. By working around the cervix in this way the whole circumference can be examined and tears identified. Tears must be repaired with full-thickness interrupted sutures, ensuring that the apex is identified. A combined vaginal and abdominal approach may be needed to evacuate clot, identify bleeding and secure haemostasis.

An abdominal approach is always needed for tears of the cervix or upper vagina where the apex cannot be identified and bleeding is occurring. Ureteric injury can result from blindly placed deep sutures in the fornix.

Internal iliac artery ligation, hysterectomy and radiological embolization techniques have all been described to control intractable bleeding.

Careful observation in a high dependency area is required for 12–24 hours, as recurrence of the haematoma may occur in up to 10 per cent of cases. These women are likely to have lost very large amounts of blood and the strategy for major obstetric haemorrhage should be followed. Early recourse to surgery, antibiotics and transfusion has improved maternal mortality in this life-threatening situation.

It is important that measures to reduce thromboembolism are not ignored in these women, as they have a high risk of thrombosis. While many surgeons may wish to defer heparins until the risk of recurrence is lessened, other measures such as full-length thromboembolic stockings, compression boots and leg exercises can all be safely implemented without increasing the risk of recurrence.

## DOCUMENTATION

Clear written notes in black ink must be made following any perineal trauma. These must include:

- a clear record of the extent of trauma,
- type of analgesia/anaesthesia,
- comprehensive notes of the procedure undertaken and suture material used (including evidence of anal sphincter examination),
- documentation of a swab and needle count before and after the procedure,
- estimated blood loss,
- post-operative instructions covering all aspects (fluid replacement, extra monitoring, antibiotics, thromboprophylaxis, stool softeners),
- pre-discharge instructions as necessary,
- follow-up needs.

The notes must be signed, with the date and time. The operator's name should be printed and a contact or pager number given if possible.

## SUMMARY

- Episiotomy does not prevent third- and fourth-degree tears. Midline episiotomy increases the risk of such trauma.
- Perineal massage antepartum reduces the risk of third- and fourth-degree trauma in primiparae by a small amount.
- There are higher rates of ultrasonographically visible anal sphincter defects after forceps compared with ventouse, but no difference in maternal symptoms at five years.

Second stage of labour

- Leaving the perineal skin approximated, but not closed, is associated with less perineal dysaesthesia. If the skin is sutured, a subcuticular suture causes less short-term pain.
- A loose continuous repair without locking the vaginal component is associated with less short-term pain.
- Rapidly absorbed sutures are associated with as good results as standard polyglactin sutures, but require removal far less frequently.
- Overlap and end-to-end approximation of the anal sphincter produce similar results after repair of third-degree tears.

## KEY POINTS

- Perineal trauma is a source of post-delivery morbidity in a large number of women, especially primiparae.
- Suture techniques can be employed that minimize pain.
- The anal sphincter must be examined whenever a perineal repair is undertaken, as many sphincter ruptures are missed.
- Third- and fourth-degree repairs should be performed in optimal surroundings by a suitably trained operator.
- Follow up should be conducted by a team with an interest in the management of perineal trauma.
- Documentation should include all aspects of the repair, with clear post-repair instructions.
- Women from countries of high incidence should be asked about FGM and a careful plan for delivery documented.
- Women with haematomas need vigilance for recurrence in the first 24 hours after drainage.

## Key References

1. Royal College of Obstetricians and Gynaecologists. *Management of Third- and Fourth-Degree Perineal Tears*. Clinical Green Top Guideline No. 29. London: RCOG Press, 2007.
2. Sultan AH, Johanson RB, Carter JE. Occult anal sphincter trauma following randomized forceps and vacuum delivery. *Int J Obstet Gynecol* 1998; **61**: 113–19.
3. Intrapartum Care. Care of healthy women and their babies. Clinical guideline 55. London: National Institute for Health and Clinical Excellence, 2007.
4. Eason E, Labrecque M, Wells G, Feldman P. Preventing perineal trauma during childbirth: a systematic review. *Obstet Gynecol* 2000; **95**: 464–71.
5. McCandlish R, Bowler U, Van Asten H *et al.* A randomised controlled trial of care of the perineum during second stage of normal labour. *Br J Obstet Gynaecol* 1998; **105**: 1262–72.
6. Gupta JK, Hofmeyr GJ, Smyth RMD. Position in the second stage of labour for women without epidural anaesthesia. *Cochrane Database Syst Rev* 2005; (**3**): CD002006.
7. Royal College of Obstetricians and Gynaecologists. *Instrumental Vaginal Delivery*. Clinical Green Top Guideline No. 26. London: RCOG Press, 1999.
8. Johanson RB, Heycock E, Carter J *et al.* Maternal and child health after assisted vaginal delivery: five year follow-up of a randomised controlled study comparing forceps and ventouse. *Br J Obstet Gynaecol* 1999; **106**: 544–9.
9. Anim-Somuah M, Smyth RMD, Howell CJ. Epidural versus non-epidural or no analgesia in labour. *Cochrane Database Syst Rev* 2005; (**3**): CD000331.
10. Fraser WD, Marcoux S, Krauss I *et al.* Multicenter, randomized, controlled trial of delayed pushing for nulliparous women in the second stage of labor with continuous epidural analgesia. The PEOPLE (Pushing Early or Pushing Late with Epidural) Study Group. *Am J Obstet Gynecol* 2000; **182**: 1165–72.
11. Kettle C, Hills RK, Ismail KMK. Continuous versus interrupted sutures for repair of episiotomy or second degree tears. *Cochrane Database Syst Rev* 2007; (**3**): CD000947.
12. Gordon B, Mackrodt C, Fern E *et al.* The Ipswich Childbirth Study: 1. A randomised evaluation of two stage postpartum perineal repair leaving the skin unsutured. *Br J Obstet Gynaecol* 1998; **105**: 435–40.
13. Valenzuela P, Saiz Puente M, Valero J *et al.* Continuous versus interrupted sutures for repair of episiotomy or second-degree perineal tears: a randomised controlled trial. *BJOG* 2009; **116**: 436–441.
14. Kettle C, Hills RK, Jones P *et al.* Continuous versus interrupted repair with standard or rapidly absorbed sutures after spontaneous vaginal birth: a randomised controlled trial. *Lancet* 2002; **359**: 2217–23.
15. Fynes M, O'Herilhy C. The influence of mode of delivery on anal sphincter injury and faecal incontinence. *Obstet Gynecol* 2001; **3**: 120–5.
16. Fernando RJ, Sultan AHH, Kettle C *et al.* Methods of repair for obstetric anal sphincter injury. *Cochrane Database Syst Rev* 2006; (**3**): CD002866.
17. Fitzpatrick M, Behan M, O'Connell PR, O'Herlihy C. A randomised clinical trial comparing primary overlap with approximation repair of third degree tears. *Am J Obstet Gynecol* 2000; **183**: 1220–4.
18. Fynes M, Donnelly V, Behan M *et al.* Effect of second vaginal delivery on ano-rectal physiology and fecal continence. *Lancet* 1999; **354**: 983–6.
19. Royal College of Obstetricians and Gynaecologists. *Female Genital Mutilation and its Management*. Clinical Green Top Guideline No. 53. London: RCOG Press, 2009.

# SECTION F

## Postpartum complications: neonatal

# Perinatal asphyxia

*Andrew Currie*

## INTRODUCTION

Perinatal asphyxia is an important cause of death and disability in the term neonate. Although the pathophysiology of the asphyxial process is understood, there are currently few interventions available that preserve brain function and few treatment modalities have been subject to randomized, controlled trials. Mild therapeutic hypothermia has recently shown positive results and is discussed later in the chapter.

A number of clinical, biochemical and radiological markers of hypoxic–ischaemic damage are available, but their use in predicting outcome requires caution.

Perinatal asphyxia can lead to the neonatal condition called 'hypoxic–ischaemic encephalopathy'. Neonatal encephalopathies are a heterogenous group of disorders clinically defined by a disturbance in the neurological function of the neonate in the early days of life. They are the result of a number of causes including hypoxic–ischaemic insults, metabolic disorders, sepsis, drug exposure, intracranial bleeds, neurological malformations, etc. Neonatal encephalopathies are usually grouped into mild moderate or severe (or alternatively stage I, II and III) depending on the severity of symptoms and signs. These range from mild hyperalertness in very mild cases through to stupor, severe hypotonia, seizures and respiratory embarrassment in severe cases.

The most common single cause for neonatal encephalopathy is hypoxic–ischaemic encephalopathy, secondary to some perinatal asphyxial process. However, it is important to understand both from a clinical point of view and a medicolegal perspective that not all neonatal encephalopathies are the result of hypoxia or asphyxia and other causes should be ruled out, especially when the clinical history is ambiguous. Thus, it is more appropriate to use the term 'neonatal encephalopathy' without ascribing a particular cause until appropriate investigations have been undertaken.

## DEFINITION

The terms 'birth asphyxia' and 'perinatal asphyxia' are widely used to describe an intrapartum hypoxic–ischaemic insult in a term infant. However, the precise clinical definition varies, making interpretation of data on incidence, clinical manifestations and outcome difficult.

It is unclear if premature infants, with their immature central nervous system, exhibit the same responses to hypoxic–ischaemic insults as term infants. Preterm infants are of course at higher risk of cerebral insults outside the intrapartum period.

## INCIDENCE OF HYPOXIC–ISCHAEMIC INJURY

The incidence varies depending on the definition used and whether preterm infants are included. The incidence appears to be higher in developing countries, although preterm infants are often included in published data. With improvements in antenatal and intrapartum monitoring, the incidence appears to have fallen in some published UK studies, from 6.0 per 1000 live births in the early 1980s[1] to 1.0 per 1000 live births in the mid-1990s. Subsequently, population surveys in the United Kingdom show the rates appear to have stabilized over recent years at around 1.2 per 1000 live births [C].[2]

## PREVENTION

In order to prevent brain injury caused by hypoxia–ischaemia, there needs to be awareness as to when and under what conditions the injury might occur. Most available information relates to the detection of problems during the intrapartum period. However, it is clear that not all hypoxic–ischaemic insults occur intrapartum and that many occur prior to labour and delivery [C].[3] In recent years, major advances in antenatal assessment have been made and a number of tools for the antenatal assessment of fetal well-being are now widely used, including monitoring fetal movements, fetal heart rate, biophysical profiles, fetal growth and blood flow velocity in umbilical and fetal blood vessels (see Chapter 14, Tests of fetal well-being).

The aim of intrapartum monitoring is to detect 'fetal compromise'; this is often used as a marker for hypoxia–ischaemia. Detection of fetal compromise does not help in timing the hypoxic insult, as it may reflect the infant's inability to mount a normal physiological response to an earlier hypoxic event. Intrapartum assessments of fetal well-being/fetal compromise include:

- monitoring of fetal heart rate, either intermittently or continuously,
- assessment of fetal acid-base status,
- passage of meconium *in utero*.

It should be noted that the detection of fetal compromise is a poor predictor of hypoxic–ischaemic encephalopathy (HIE) or later cerebral palsy.

Once concerns have been raised regarding the well-being of the infant, in order to ensure optimum resuscitation, it is vital that communication is made to neonatal staff prior to delivery. It is essential that staff attending the delivery are appropriately trained in neonatal resuscitation and are given any relevant details in the maternal history that may affect resuscitation; for example, placental abruption, for which the infant may require blood during the resuscitation.

## PATHOPHYSIOLOGY OF BRAIN INJURY

Perinatal asphyxia occurs when a lack of oxygen and acidosis cause organ impairment. Deprivation of oxygen to the brain can occur in two ways:

1 **hypoxaemia** – a reduction in the amount of oxygen in the blood,
2 **ischaemia** – a reduction in the amount of blood perfusing the brain.

Although brain injury occurs at the time of the hypoxic–ischaemic insult, it is now well established that neuronal damage is an ongoing process which starts at the time of the primary injury and following a 'latent' period continues, despite resuscitation, into the recovery phase (secondary injury).

This is supported clinically by the delay of up to 24–48 hours before typical signs of encephalopathy are observed, with further delays before radiological changes are seen on either ultrasound or magnetic resonance imaging (MRI) [C].[4]

Following a hypoxic–ischaemic insult, cell death occurs in two phases. The mechanisms involved are different and are influenced by the severity and nature of the original insult. The neuronal injury resulting from hypoxic–ischaemic insult in a term infant is 'selective neuronal necrosis'. It is unaffected by resuscitation and occurs 5–30 minutes after the onset of ischaemia. Primary neuronal death predominantly affects the watershed areas of the cerebral cortex, is bilateral and usually symmetrical. Many neurons do not die during this primary phase; they do, however, appear vulnerable to further injury and death as a result of severe cerebrovascular dysfunction. This appears to trigger a series of biochemical events resulting in secondary neuronal death as a result of apoptosis. Evidence from animal and early clinical studies indicates that a therapeutic window exists between the primary and secondary phases when intervention may prevent secondary neuronal death and subsequently improve neurological outcome.[5]

## AETIOLOGY

Perinatal asphyxia may be the result of an acute event or may occur as a result of chronic hypoxia (Table 37.1). It is important to note that in many cases no single factor is identified and that asphyxia may be caused by several antenatal factors or antenatal and intrapartum factors coexisting. It is difficult to accurately quantify the timing of hypoxic–ischaemic insults, as reported studies differ widely in their definitions, methodologies and inclusion criteria. It has been estimated that approximately 20 per cent of insults occur antenatally, 35 per cent occur intrapartum, and, in a further 35 per cent, there are both antenatal and intrapartum factors involved.[3] In the remaining cases, the timing is difficult to define. It is clear that despite differences in definition, intrapartum events contribute to a significant proportion of cases.

## CLINICAL FEATURES AND MANAGEMENT OF HYPOXIC–ISCHAEMIC ENCEPHALOPATHY

Despite the subjective nature of the scoring system, the universal method employed to assess an infant's well-being at birth is the Apgar score. Infants who have been exposed to a hypoxic insult will invariably have low Apgar scores beyond 1 minute; however, other factors not associated with asphyxia can also lower the Apgar score, for example anaesthetic agents and prematurity. Despite this, there

**Table 37.1** Causes of and associations with perinatal asphyxia

**Impaired maternal oxygenation**

Maternal cardiovascular disease

**Impaired uterine blood flow**

Vascular disturbance, pre-eclampsia, diabetes

Maternal hypotension/hypovolaemia

**Impaired placental function**

Placental infarction

Abruption

Post-maturity

Infection

**Impaired blood flow to cord, e.g. cord compression/prolapse**

**Abnormal fetal haemoglobin**

Rhesus haemolytic disease

Twin–twin transfusion

Feto-maternal transfusion

**Maternal drugs**

Cocaine

**Failure to establish adequate cardiopulmonary circulation after birth**

**Meconium aspiration**

**Congenital cardiorespiratory disease**

**Table 37.2** Clinical grading for hypoxic-ischaemic encephalopathy[7]

| Grade I (mild) | Grade II (moderate) | Grade III (severe) |
|---|---|---|
| Irritability | Lethargy | Comatose |
| Mild hypotonia | Marked abnormalities in tone | Severe hypotonia |
| Poor suck | Requires tube feeds | Failure to maintain spontaneous respiration |
| Hyperalert | Seizures | Prolonged seizures |

flaccid and unresponsive. The clinical signs progress over the first 24–48 hours before gradual improvement is seen. The severity of HIE can be graded clinically as mild, moderate or severe, as shown in Table 37.2.[1] The management after hypoxia–ischaemia is crucial, as the affected infant is still at risk of reperfusion injury.[5] Transfer to a neonatal intensive care unit with facilities for cerebral and systemic monitoring is of the utmost importance. Full supportive care is required, with great attention to detail. As well as general intensive care, specific neurological monitoring and care should also be given.

## General management

During episodes of hypoxia, blood flow is distributed in order to preserve blood supplies to vital organs, namely the brain, heart and adrenals. This leaves other organs, particularly the kidney, liver and gut, prone to ischaemic damage. With this in mind, blood pressure should be continuously monitored and hypotension avoided in order to ensure cerebral perfusion and to prevent further underperfusion of other organs. Hypotension is common and usually due to myocardial dysfunction rather than hypovolaemia. It should be treated promptly with volume expansion and/or inotropes as clinically indicated. Care should be taken not to overload infants with fluid, as acute tubular necrosis and inappropriate antidiuretic hormone release are common sequelae. Maintenance fluids should be restricted by 25 per cent for the first 48 hours or so, based on regular clinical assessment of hydration, serum and urinary electrolytes, urine output and specific gravity and the infant's weight.

Asphyxiated infants are at risk of developing necrotizing enterocolitis and therefore oral feeds should be introduced with caution. Prevention of tissue catabolism is important and thus nutritional support should be provided by parenteral nutrition until feeds are established.

Respiratory support with endotracheal intubation should only be undertaken if hypercapnia develops, if the infant has prolonged or frequent convulsions or if there is coexisting respiratory disease. Hyperventilation is not

is good evidence that prolonged depression of the Apgar score is associated with death or major neurological disability [C].[6]

It is essential that personnel trained in neonatal resuscitation are present prior to the delivery of an asphyxiated infant. Resuscitation should establish a secure airway, ensure adequate oxygenation and restore circulation. Some severely affected infants will require endotracheal intubation and ventilation in the delivery room; however, others will require little in the way of initial resuscitation, but will deteriorate after the first 24 hours. Intravenous fluids, and in particular colloid, should be used with caution in restoring the circulation in severe asphyxia, the exception being where there is a clear history of antepartum haemorrhage or placental abruption; in such cases, O-negative blood should be administered in the delivery room.

If, despite appropriate resuscitation, there is no spontaneous cardiac output by 10 minutes or respiratory activity by 30 minutes, the outlook for both term and preterm infants is poor.

## Post-resuscitation management

Infants who have experienced an asphyxial insult develop the clinical syndrome known as hypoxic–ischaemic encephalopathy. After resuscitation, the infant may be recommended, as hypocapnia reduces cerebral perfusion and may compound the ischaemic insult. Respiratory support is guided by regular arterial blood gas analysis. Hypoxia should be avoided and the $PaO_2$ kept between 8 and 12 kPa (60–90 mmHg).

Neonatal meningitis may present in a similar way to HIE and therefore if there is any doubt, a lumbar puncture should be performed and treatment commenced. Routine antibiotics have no part to play in the treatment of HIE.

Disseminated intravascular coagulation is not uncommon in severe cases of HIE, and therefore regular assessments of clotting status should be made. Treatment includes additional vitamin K, platelets, cryoprecipitate and/or fresh frozen plasma infusions.

## Neurological management

Much of the management after hypoxic–ischaemic insults has not been subject to randomized, controlled trials. Probably the one major exception to this is the series of recent multi-centre studies investigating mild hypothermia as a neuroprotective measure (see below under Therapeutic hypothermia for treatment of HIE).

In severe HIE, cerebral oedema and raised intracranial pressure (ICP) are commonly observed. Management strategies to lower ICP have included the administration of hyperosmolar agents and lowering $PaCO_2$. There is no evidence that hyperventilation and the ensuing hypocarbia are beneficial in reducing ICP, and therefore accepted practice is to maintain the $PaCO_2$ within the normal range [E].

The use of hypertonic saline has been shown to be beneficial in lowering ICP in animal models and in adults. Its use has not been evaluated in the neonate and it cannot be recommended. There is no evidence for the use of mannitol, frusemide or steroids in the treatment of cerebral oedema in neonates.[7]

Seizures are a salient feature of HIE. Frequent and prolonged clinically evident seizures should be treated promptly with anticonvulsant(s). Phenobarbitone is the drug of choice, as recent evidence suggests that the use of phenytoin, diazepam or chloral hydrate confers no benefit [A].[7] Anticonvulsants can be stopped once seizures are controlled. The use of early prophylactic phenobarbitone as a 'neuroprotector' in HIE has been subject to a meta-analysis, which concluded that routine use is not recommended in perinatal asphyxia [A].[8]

Glucose metabolism in HIE has been extensively studied and yet is still not fully understood. Normoglycaemia should be maintained, as there is evidence that both hypoglycaemia and hyperglycaemia may worsen brain injury.

## New neuroprotective strategies

A number of new neuroprotective strategies have evolved in recent years.[5,7] Most have been used in animal models, with only a few trials in the human neonate. The rationale behind these interventions is in the prevention of reperfusion injury. Interventions have included magnesium sulphate, calcium channel blockers, allopurinol as a free radical scavenger, the Chinese herb *Salvia miltiorrhizae*, naloxone and hypothermia. Of these alternatives, selective hypothermia is the only strategy that has shown positive results.

## Therapeutic hypothermia for treatment of HIE

As mentioned earlier, neuronal cell death is the result of a combination of primary and secondary cellular energy failure. There is little that can be done to prevent primary neuronal cell death; however, between these two phases there is a latent period of several hours which may serve as a therapeutic window to prevent the secondary energy failure.

There is clear evidence that fever on top of HIE results in a worse outcome.[9] In addition, a number of animal studies have shown that cooling ameliorated the delayed energy failure and inhibited neuronal cell apoptosis. As a result, over recent years, a number of large clinical trials have taken place studying the effects of therapeutic hypothermia in HIE. A recent meta-analysis of these studies has concluded that induced mild hypothermia to a core temperature of 33.5°C resulted in a reduction in the combined outcome of mortality and neurodevelopmental disability at 18 months in term infants with moderate or severe hypoxic–ischaemic encephalopathy. As a result of this and a more recent multi-centre clinical study confirming these results, it is generally agreed that therapeutic hypothermia should be offered in cases of moderate and severe HIE.

The treatment is primarily a preventative strategy treatment, so it is important that cooling is commenced as soon as HIE is suspected, and ideally within 6 hours of birth before clinical evidence of secondary neuronal cell death (such as seizures) appears.

## INVESTIGATIONS

Continuous integrated single-channel electroencephalogram (EEG) monitoring is now in widespread use and is very useful both from a clinical treatment point of view and prognostically.

The value of neuroimaging is limited in the first 24–48 hours of life. Ultrasound evidence of lesions in the thalami and basal ganglia, focal infarctions and changes in periventricular white matter are usually seen after the first 48 hours of life. Their presence before this suggests an antenatal insult.

Magnetic resonance imaging is useful in asphyxiated infants. Early scans characteristically show brain swelling and abnormal signal intensity within the basal ganglia, periventricular white matter, subcortical white matter and cortex. Late MRI findings associated with poor outcome include delayed myelination as a marker for neuronal loss and extensive white matter changes.

## OUTCOME

Determining the outcome after perinatal asphyxia is difficult for a number of reasons:

- The definition of asphyxia varies.
- There is variation in the outcomes assessed – mortality, motor, behavioural, etc.
- There is varied inclusion/exclusion of preterm infants.
- The age at time of assessment varies.

What is clear, however, is that the neurological outcome depends on the severity of the insult. It is well recognized that term infants with grade I HIE (mild) have no long-term developmental problems, whereas severe HIE is associated with a poor outcome. It is more difficult to predict the outcome of moderate HIE as there are few readily available reliable markers of long-term impairment. One early predictor of adverse outcome is the severity of the neurological abnormalities found on clinical examination, particularly in association with discontinuous activity on EEG. Severe acidosis associated with poor Apgar scores, multi-organ failure and encephalopathy immediately after birth are also markers of poor outcome [C].[10]

The major neurological sequelae in surviving infants are motor deficits and, in particular, spastic quadriplegia and dyskinetic cerebral palsy. There may also be associated visual or intellectual impairment or epilepsy. It is important to note that not all cerebral palsy is the result of perinatal asphyxia and not all asphyxiated infants develop cerebral palsy [C].[11]

## SUMMARY

- Phenobarbitone is the drug of choice for convulsions secondary to HIE.
- There is as yet no evidence to support routine seizure prophylaxis in infants with HIE.
- Most infants with severe HIE will develop neurological sequelae. Most infants with mild HIE will have no long-term sequelae. Infants in the moderate category remain the most difficult in whom to predict outcome.
- Therapeutic hypothermia has been proven to improve outcomes in IIIE and should be offered as early as possible as part of these infants' intensive care.

## ACKNOWLEDGEMENT

This chapter has been revised and updated. The author and editors acknowledge the contribution of Sandie Bohin to the chapter on this topic in the previous edition of the book.

## KEY POINTS

- Most cases of HIE have an intrapartum element.
- However, not all infants with HIE develop cerebral palsy, and not all children with cerebral palsy demonstrate HIE.
- Damage due to HIE occurs in two phases: the initial insult and then further reperfusion injury (primary and secondary cellular energy failure).
- Damage is usually symmetrical and affects watershed areas.
- A persistently depressed Apgar score is generally associated with poor outcomes.
- Mild therapeutic hypothermia is now recognized as an important part of the management of moderate to severe HIE.

## Key References

1. Levene MI, Kornberg J, Williams THC. The incidence and severity of post-asphyxial encephalopathy in full term infants. *Early Hum Dev* 1985; **11**: 21–6.
2. Trent Neonatal Survey Report 2007. Trent Infant Mortality and Morbidity Studies. Leicester University, 2005–2007.
3. Volpe JJ. Hypoxic–ischaemic encephalopathy: clinical aspects. In: *Neurology of the Newborn*, 3rd edn. Philadelphia: WB Saunders, 1995.
4. Sie LT, Van der Knapp MS, Van Wezel-Meyler G *et al.* Early MR features of hypoxic–ischaemic brain injury in neonates with periventricular densities on sonogram. *Am J Neuroradiol* 2000; **21**: 852–61.
5. Cornette L, Levene MI. Post-resuscitative management of the asphyxiated term infant. *Semin Neonatol* 2001; **6**: 271–82.
6. Nelson KB, Ellenberg JH. Apgar scores as predictors of chronic neurological disability. *Pediatrics* 1981; **68**: 36–44.
7. Whitelaw A. Systematic review of therapy after hypoxic–ischaemic brain injury in the perinatal period. *Semin Neonatol* 2000; **5**: 33–44.
8. Evans DJ, Levene MI. Anticonvulsants for preventing mortality and morbidity in full-term newborns with perinatal asphyxia. *Cochrane Database Syst Rev* 2007; (**3**): CD001240.
9. Lieberman E, Eichenwald E, Mathur G *et al.* Intrapartum fever and unexplained seizures in term infants. *Pediatrics* 2000; **106**: 983–8.
10. Yudkin PL, Johnson A, Clover LM, Murphy KW. Clustering of perinatal markers of birth asphyxia and outcome at age five years. *Br J Obstet Gynaecol* 1994; **101**: 774–81.
11. Blair F, Stanley FJ. Intrapartum asphyxia: a rare cause of cerebral palsy. *J Pediatrics* 1988; **112**: 515–19.

Postpartum complications: neonatal

# Neonatal resuscitation

*Andrew Currie*

## INTRODUCTION

Health professionals involved with childbirth should be capable of providing life support to the newly born when the need arises.

To facilitate this, various professional bodies have been developed, including the UK Resuscitation Council, the European Resuscitation Council and the International Liaison Committee on Resuscitation (ILCOR).[1–3] Each professional body has produced guidelines and training programmes to improve resuscitation practices.

Much of resuscitation procedures is based on 'best practice', with very little evidence-based medicine to support it. This is hardly surprising given the ethical dilemmas that would be created by trying to perform randomized, controlled studies of resuscitation techniques.

This chapter concentrates on the essential steps required to provide safe and appropriate resuscitation to the newborn. It draws on recommendations from the above resuscitation bodies and, where possible, the evidence is reviewed.

## INCIDENCE

Most studies show that approximately 90–95 per cent of all births require no resuscitation. The other 5–10 per cent need some form of respiratory support, with possibly up to 1–2 per cent requiring full cardiopulmonary resuscitation.[4]

## PHYSIOLOGICAL CHANGES

Many physiological adaptations occur to the infant at birth.[5] The most important involve the cardiovascular system, respiratory system and thermoregulatory mechanisms.

## Respiratory

*In utero*, the lungs are full of fluid (30–35 mL/kg in term infants). Pulmonary pressures are suprasystemic, thus reducing blood flow to the fetal lung. To adapt to extrauterine life, lung fluid production reduces near term. In addition, the mechanics of birth include the birth canal exerting an immense extrathoracic pressure on the infant during its descent, squeezing lung fluid from the trachea and upper airways. With delivery, a natural 'recoil' of the airways (along with the infant's first respiratory efforts) helps to inflate the lungs. Subsequent breaths become progressively easier, due to development of a functional residual capacity and improving lung compliance. Dispersal of surfactant to form a monolayer within the alveolar system further improves lung mechanics by lowering surface tension and ensuring alveoli remain open, even in expiration.

## Cardiovascular

Major features of the fetal cardiovascular system include high pulmonary pressures and a series of three anatomical right-to-left shunts.

1 The ductus venosus carries blood from the placenta back to the fetus (effectively connecting the umbilical vein to the inferior vena cava).
2 The foramen ovale is important in diverting blood from the right atrium to the left, thus bypassing the lungs.
3 The ductus arteriosus diverts blood from the pulmonary artery to the aorta.

Following birth, the pulmonary pressures fall. This is as much to do with changes at a cellular level (including the effects of cytokines, prostaglandins and the influence of endogenous nitric oxide) as with the mechanics of lung inflation. The ductus venosus closes soon after clamping of the umbilical cord, with establishment of the normal venous circulation. The fall in pulmonary pressures allows greater blood flow into the pulmonary circulation. This increases the blood volume returning to the left atrium, with consequent closure of the foramen ovale and increased systemic pressures; these in turn reverse the shunting across the ductus arteriosus. The ductus arteriosus subsequently closes under the influence of increasing oxygen concentrations and prostaglandins. As a result, the normal neonatal circulation is established. The conversion of the fetal to the neonatal circulation may take several days to complete.

## Thermoregulation

The infant is born naked and wet into a hostile environment. Immature thermoregulatory mechanisms can lead to cold stress with serious morbidity, such as acidosis, hypoglycaemia and respiratory distress. Equally, pyrexia may be as dangerous, studies showing that it worsens cerebral hypoxic injury.[6] Hence, an essential part of neonatal resuscitation is maintenance of a normal body temperature.

## AETIOLOGY

Many causes have been associated with a potentially compromised infant at birth. These can be divided into maternal, fetal and intrapartum. A list of the more common is shown in Table 38.1.

## MANAGEMENT OF THE RESUSCITATION

### Basic principles (fundamental to optimize patient outcome)

- As with any resuscitation, the ABC (airway, breathing, circulation) approach is the most appropriate. The vast majority of neonatal 'arrests' arc primarily due to respiratory problems. Hence, heavy emphasis is placed on ensuring an adequate airway and efficient ventilation delivery to the child.
- Good preparation is essential to optimize clinical management.
- Resuscitation of the newborn is a team approach. Clear communication is essential.
- The ability to assess a situation and act accordingly on a regular basis is crucial. The ability to use basic knowledge in a safe, logical and adaptive manner makes resuscitation of the patient a more rewarding process.

**Table 38.1** Common causes for a compromised newborn infant

| **Maternal** |
| --- |
| Chronic ill-health |
| Drug ingestion (legal and illegal) |
| Hypertension |
| Diabetes mellitus |
| Anatomical abnormalities |
| Placenta praevia |
| **Fetal** |
| Multiple pregnancies |
| Prematurity |
| Post-term (>42/52) |
| Intrauterine growth restriction |
| Congenital abnormalities |
| Liquor disturbances (oligohydramnios/polyhydramnios) |
| Hydrops |
| Isoimmunization |
| Intrauterine infection |
| **Intrapartum** |
| Fetal distress |
| Abnormal presentation |
| Prolapsed cord |
| Antepartum haemorrhage |
| Prolonged rupture of membranes |
| Thick meconium |
| Instrumental deliverie |

### Preparation

Good preparation is as important to a successful outcome as the actual resuscitation itself. Preparation involves more than getting equipment ready.

### Medical history

Accurate medical information is invaluable. Although a detailed medical history is ideal, time is often against this. It is vital to establish key facts quickly.

Useful questions that may influence the actual resuscitation process include the following:

- How many infants should we expect? This will dictate numbers of personnel and amount of equipment, as well as help inform likelihood of complications.
- What is the gestation? While the basics of resuscitation remain the same, priorities and expectations will differ and may influence the approach taken.

- Are there any congenital anomalies (e.g. congenital diaphragmatic hernia)? Specific conditions do influence the approach taken to resuscitation.
- Has the mother had any relevant medication in the last few hours (e.g. opiates)? This may affect the infant's response to resuscitation.
- Has there been any meconium prior to delivery? Again, this will influence the approach taken to the resuscitation procedure (see below under Meconium).

## Personnel

All workers involved in birth should be able to provide basic neonatal life support, and regular updates of skills should be undertaken. Ideally, somebody trained in advanced neonatal life support should also be readily available.

Resuscitation is a team event. Individuals should understand their roles. Ideally, two to three people make an effective team: one to look after the airway, one to look after the cardiovascular circulation and the third to assist with drugs, fluids and additional equipment. One person should take the role of leader; this ensures clarity of the roles and efficient team working.

Other important tasks that may be delegated in the acute situation include informing neonatal unit staff who will be looking after the infant following resuscitation and communicating with the parents, who need to be informed of events as early and fully as possible.

## Communication and documentation

Often, the source of mishaps and complaints is poor communication. In addition, poor documentation makes post-hoc reviews very difficult. The importance of accurate information gathering, documentation and communication cannot be emphasized enough. Accurate timing must be recorded and all records (midwifery, obstetric and neonatal) should be consistent. In the acute situation, if sufficient staff are available, one team member should be asked to keep a record of times and procedures.

## Environment

A brightly lit, warm and draft-free room is ideal. As well as reducing morbidity due to heat loss, an appropriate environment ensures that attendants can see and assess the infant.

The infant's temperature should be kept in the normothermic range. Hyperthermia is associated with increased neuronal damage in cases of perinatal hypoxia. Hypothermia is equally associated with increased morbidity, particularly in the premature infant. However, recent multicentre trials showing that induced mild hypothermia is neuroprotective in term infants with moderate or severe perinatal asphyxial hypoxia, have slightly clouded the issue of avoiding hypothermia in the delivery room.[7] These studies managed infants with core temperatures at 33.5°C for up to 72 hours.

It is speculative to relate these studies to the acute resuscitation when often the clinical picture is unclear; however, it has been suggested that in the presence of possible perinatal hypoxia in a term infant, consideration should be given over to turning off the radiant warmer on the resuscitaire. It is unlikely this quandary will be resolved and so currently the recommendation remains that for the acute resuscitation situation, maintenance of normothermia and certainly prevention of hyperthermia, should be the rule [E].[7]

## Equipment

Having the right equipment, which is reliable, is paramount to a successful resuscitation. Table 38.2 shows a list of essential equipment.

Within the hospital setting, all essential equipment is found on a resuscitaire – best described as a mobile, open cot. The heat and warmth sources are located above a firm, flat surface. A clock is attached. There are usually two sources of oxygen (piped and cylinders), with two outlets. Air supplies should also be available on resuscitaires. Studies have indicated that resuscitation with air is as effective as oxygen[8] in term infants [A]. There is also

**Table 38.2** Essential equipment for neonatal resuscitation

| Equipment |
| --- |
| Light source |
| Source of warmth (heater and/or warmed linen) |
| Flat surface (±firm mattress) |
| Clock |
| Suction apparatus (able to deliver suction up to 100 mmHg) |
| Suction catheters |
| Oxygen supply |
| Ventilation system (either 'bag-valve-mask' or 'mask and T-piece', or both) |
| Endotracheal tubes (various sizes from 2.5 to 4.0 mm internal diameter) |
| Introductory stylet |
| Fixation kit for endotracheal tube |
| Laryngoscopes (with straight blades and spare bulbs) |
| Oropharyngeal airways |
| Nasogastric tubes |
| Umbilical venous catheters |
| Scalpel |
| Intravenous cannulae |
| Intraosseous cannula |
| Syringes and needles |
| Fluids and medications |

increasing concern about the detrimental effects of hyper-oxia to the lungs and eyes in the preterm infant. Thus, it is increasingly felt that the initial approach to resuscitation of the newborn should be with the use of air and only if there is a poor response to this should introduction of oxygen be considered. The availability of an air/oxygen blender to bet-ter manage the concentration of oxygen used is considered to be a better approach.

Suction apparatus is intrinsic in the resuscitaire. The rest of the equipment should be readily available, stored in vari-ous drawers mounted on the resuscitaire.

The resuscitaire should be situated in the delivery room.

Fluids and medications may or may not be stored with the resuscitaire. If not, they should be in a readily accessible place for emergency use.

It is the responsibility of the individuals using equipment for resuscitation to ensure that they are competent with its use and that it is working properly. All resuscitation equip-ment should be checked daily, as well as before and after each use.

## THE RESUSCITATION PROCESS

This section assumes birth is taking place in a maternity suite with a resuscitaire; however, the principles can be applied to any setting.

Figure 38.1 shows a step-by-step approach. Each step is explained in more detail below.

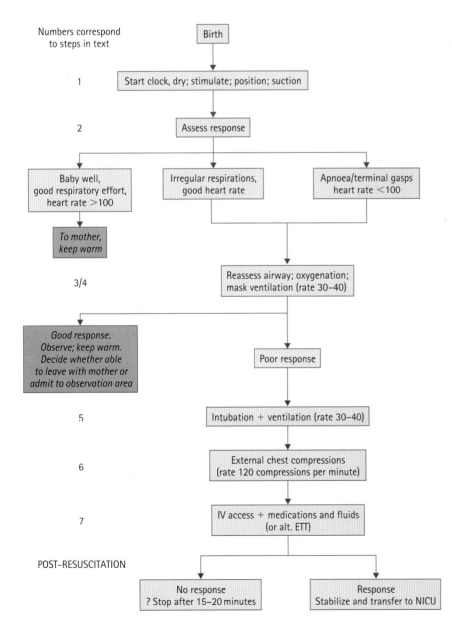

**Figure 38.1** Neonatal resuscitation in the delivery room. ETT, endotracheal tube

## Step 1

With the birth of the whole baby, the clock is started and the infant is transferred to the resuscitaire. The infant is placed with the head in the 'neutral position', towards the resuscitator. The neutral position involves the head being placed so that the eyes are looking directly upward. This position helps maintain airway patency.

The infant should be kept warm. For the term infant and larger preterm infant, this may be achieved by drying with a warm towel. A vigorous, not aggressive, rub with the towel serves the dual purpose of drying the infant and stimulating breathing. The infant is then wrapped in a second, warm towel. Evidence indicates that for the premature infant in the delivery suite (less than 30 weeks gestation) heat loss is best managed by placing it directly into a plastic bag, without drying, under a radiant heat source.

The airway must be correctly positioned and also needs to be clear. Babies have secretions in their oropharynx at birth. Assuming these are not copious and the infant is vigorous, the infant will clear them independently. Routine oropharyngeal suctioning is to be avoided [E].

Infants with excessive secretions, or those with thick meconium (see below under Special situations) and/or blood, need suctioning. A suction catheter can be placed in the oropharynx; care must be taken not to push the catheter too far back, and some authorities advocate not inserting it further than 5 cm. A suction pressure of 100 mmHg is appropriate. Excessive toileting of the oropharynx causes reflex bardycardia and laryngospasm.

These initial steps should take no more than 20–30 seconds.

## Step 2

The infant is then assessed. Initial assessment should include heart rate, respiratory effort and colour. This should have occurred by 30 seconds of age.

Assessment (and reassessment) is vital to a successful outcome. Many workers use the Apgar score (Table 38.3) to aid them. This was originally described by Virginia

**Table 38.3** Apgar scoring system

| Parameter | Score | | |
|---|---|---|---|
| | 0 | 1 | 2 |
| Heart rate | 0 | <100 | >100 |
| Breathing | Apnoeic | Irregular | Good |
| Colour | White | Blue | Pink |
| Muscle tone | Floppy | Some movement | Active |
| Reflex response | None | Grimace | Cough, cry, sneeze |

Apgar, an anaesthesiologist, in 1953. Whilst this is a useful tool, it has its limitations. Apgar scores are carried out at 1 minute and 5 minutes of life. Further scores may be done at 5-minute intervals depending on subsequent progress. It is an internationally recognized assessment tool, giving an indication of the neonate's condition after birth. However, it would be inappropriate to delay resuscitating an apnoeic infant with a profound bradycardia at birth, while waiting for a low 1-minute Apgar score.

From the initial assessment, the infant will fall into one of three groups.

1 Well, healthy and vigorous. The child has a good respiratory effort, is pink centrally, and the heart rate is >100 beats per minute (bpm). This infant can be wrapped up and given to the parents.
2 Cyanosed, poor respiratory effort, with or without a heart rate <100 bpm. This infant needs further intervention.
3 White, apnoeic or terminal gasps, with absent heart beat or profound bradycardia (<60 bpm). This infant needs full intensive resuscitation.

If the child's condition is still a cause for concern, the previous interventions should be checked.

- Is the airway clear and positioned correctly?
- Has the child responded to stimulation?

## Step 3

Next, use of supplementary oxygen may be considered. How this is delivered, and in what concentration, depends on a number of factors including the state of the respiratory effort: an apnoeic infant will not respond to wafting oxygen over its face; however, it may be inappropriate to jump to mask ventilation to deliver oxygen in a child with reasonable respiratory effort who is only mildly cyanosed and will probably respond to continued stimulation plus facial oxygen.

Recent studies looking at use of air versus oxygen for resuscitation have questioned the previously accepted best practice of using 100 per cent oxygen for resuscitation. Animal and clinical trials indicate that resuscitation with air in the term infant is as effective as 100 per cent oxygen and may even be advantageous [C].[9] Concerns exist relating to the effects of oxygen on the respiratory centres, as well as its direct effects on lungs by means of free radical production. Such effects are even more contentious in the preterm infant. As a result, some workers have advocated commencing resuscitation with air and using blended oxygen mixtures to try to minimize any side effects.

Recent guidelines from ILCOR and the UK Resuscitation Council have emphasized the importance of adequate airway and ventilation, leaving the decision to use oxygen to be considered depending on the clinical situation [E].[3]

# Step 4

Following this intervention, the infant's response should be reassessed. If there is still concern, ventilation should be commenced.

Indications for ventilation are:

- an apnoeic infant, or one with gasping respirations despite the above interventions;
- an infant that remains cyanosed despite adequate oxygen delivery.

At this stage in the rescusitation, the infant should be no more than 1 minute of age. This is time enough to know if simple interventions are going to work, without causing further insult by undue delay.

Ventilation is performed either with a bag–valve–mask (bvm) apparatus or a face-mask plus T-piece connector.

- The bag–valve–mask is attached to a gas supply (air plus oxygen) and should have a reservoir bag attached. This helps to increase the concentration of oxygen to near 100 per cent if needed. (In practice it is probably nearer 60–80 per cent with a refill bag, as opposed to 30–40 per cent without; 100 per cent oxygen concentration is difficult to achieve with bvm devices due to leakage at various points.) It is recommended that 500-mL bags be used to aid efficient delivery of ventilatory breaths. These devices have a 'pop-off' valve, which is set to between 20 and 30 cmH$_2$O. (The 'pop-off' valve reduces the risk of excessive peak pressures, which could cause overinflation.) The face mask is applied over the nose and mouth. For neonates, a circular face mask forms the best seal. Positive pressure is applied by squeezing the bag fully, then allowing it to reinflate before the next breath.
- The face-mask plus T-piece is also attached to an appropriate air and oxygen supply. Again the face mask is applied over the nose and mouth to form a seal. Above the face mask is a hole over which the resuscitator's thumb is applied to create a positive pressure. The peak pressure can be set using a pressure gauge.

Both techniques are easily learnt, although the T-piece plus face mask probably results in more reliable delivery of a set positive pressure compared to the bvm technique. Certain types of T-piece plus face mask apparatus can also deliver positive end-expiratory pressure (PEEP), which is advantageous in helping to create and maintain a functional residual capacity.

When starting ventilation, five 'rescue' breaths should be administered. These are more sustained breaths, designed to overcome the high airways resistance present in the lungs of the infant who has not breathed. This is much easier to achieve using the T-piece plus face mask technique, in which the thumb can be applied for 1–2 seconds at a set pressure. With the bvm technique, prolonged breaths are difficult to achieve, but higher pressures can be applied by locking the 'pop-off' valve.

Following these initial rescue breaths, the infant's response should be assessed. If there is still concern regarding respiration, regular ventilation should be commenced. This is delivered at a rate of 30–40 breaths per minute, with each breath lasting approximately 0.5 seconds. The peak pressure should be set to achieve adequate lung expansion without overdistension. Clinically, this can be assessed by chest movement, breath sounds, colour and heart rate, as well as improving spontaneous respiratory effort. Ventilation should be stopped once good, spontaneous, respiratory effort is achieved.

# Step 5

After another 30–60 seconds of face mask ventilation, if there is still inadequate response, endotracheal intubation for more efficient ventilation should be considered.

Indications for intubation include:

- poor respiratory effort despite appropriate interventions as above,
- thick meconium at delivery,
- anticipated need for long-term ventilatory support.

Intubation is achieved using a straight-bladed laryngoscope held in the left hand and an endotracheal tube held in the right hand. The laryngoscope blade size can be chosen to suit the infant. Thus a size 1 blade is suitable for term infants, whereas a size 0 is better suited to preterm infants. A size 00 is available for extremely premature infants with small mouths.

The blade is inserted into the mouth in the midline and the laryngoscope is pulled forward and upward, thus bringing the lower jaw and tongue up and forward until the uvula is visible. At this point it may be necessary to suction the oropharynx using a suction catheter in the right hand. The blade is then advanced over the back of the tongue into the venecular and pulled forward. This elevates the epiglottis, revealing the glottis and vocal cords. It should be remembered that the larynx in the newborn is more 'floppy' than in adults, hence to aid vision, external downward pressure over the cricoid cartilage may be needed to help bring the vocal cords into view. An alternative technique is to place the laryngoscope in the oropharynx as far as it will go, pull the lower jaw and tongue forward and upward to maximize vision and then gradually withdraw the laryngoscope until the epiglottis slips into view, with the vocal cords visible below. This is quicker, but can be more traumatic if not performed carefully.

Once the vocal cords are visualized, the endotracheal tube can be inserted. There is a choice between a straight-sided and a shouldered endotracheal tube (Coles tube). The shouldered tube is stiffer, to help intubation. An introductory stylet can be used to help stiffen whichever endotracheal tube is used.

For resuscitation purposes, oropharyngeal intubation is best practised [E], as this is simpler and quicker than nasopharyngeal intubation – a technically more demanding skill.

Once the endotracheal tube has been positioned, the ventilatory circuit can be attached and ventilatory breaths delivered. Adequate air entry should be confirmed (equal chest movement, breath sounds, appropriate colour and heart rate). If there is any doubt about whether the tube is in the correct position, it should be removed and the infant ventilated with a face-mask system whilst the situation is reassessed.

The act of intubation should take no longer than 20–30 seconds from the time of inserting the laryngoscope blade in the mouth until the endotracheal tube is attached to the ventilatory circuit. While performing this action, the infant is effectively being asphyxiated, thus undue delay is unacceptable.

> Endotracheal intubation should not be attempted by inexperienced practitioners without appropriate supervision.

Ventilation breaths are delivered at a rate of 30–40/minute, the same as for mask ventilation. Slightly higher rates (up to 60 breaths/minute) may be used for premature infants.

Once intubation has been established, the practitioner must be alert to potential complications, such as a blocked or displaced endotracheal tube, equipment failure and pneumothorax.

## Step 6

Once the airway and breathing have been addressed, the next step is to assess the circulation. The heart rate and pulses should be checked. Useful sites include the base of the umbilical cord or brachial pulse, as other pulses can be difficult to elicit. Infants with a heart rate of <60 bpm which have not responded to appropriate ventilation require external chest compressions. This is performed by depressing the lower half of the sternum by one-third of the anteroposterior diameter of the chest. In practice, for most infants this equates to 1–2 cm.

Chest compressions can be performed either using both thumbs over the lower sternum, with the hands wrapped around the chest, or by placing the index and middle fingers over the lower sternum. It is more important that appropriate sternal compressions are performed, regardless of which technique is preferred. A rate of 120 chest compressions per minute (two per second) should be attained. If ventilation is being undertaken at the same time, a ratio of three chest compressions to one breath is appropriate. Chest compressions should be stopped once the cardiac rate is >60–80 bpm.

## Step 7

This step involves vascular access, use of medication and volume expansion.

- Vascular access may be needed for advanced resuscitation. Use of the umbilical vein is the quickest and most effective

means of achieving access. An umbilical catheter, primed with 0.9 per cent saline, should be inserted to a depth of approximately 5 cm. Alternative forms of access include the use of peripheral intravenous cannulae (but only if a peripheral vein is readily accessible) or an intraosseous needle. The endotracheal tube can also be used for quick access for certain medications (e.g. adrenaline).
- Medication:
  - **Adrenaline** (epinephrine) is probably the most important medication available. It can be given via any route, most commonly intravenous or endotracheal. The recommended dose is 0.1–0.3 mL/kg of 1:10 000 solution (or 10–30 mcg/kg). Following administration, 1–2 minutes of ventilation and chest compressions are performed. This dose may be repeated every 1–2 minutes. Higher doses (i.e. 100–300 mcg/kg or 0.1–0.3 mL/kg of 1:1000 solution) are no longer recommended as there is no evidence that this is beneficial and, indeed, some studies suggest higher doses of adrenaline may be detrimental to the infant [B].[3]
  - **Sodium bicarbonate** remains controversial. It may be useful in prolonged resuscitations when sustained cellular acidosis may affect myocardial contractility. If used, administration should be limited to a 4.2 per cent solution in aliquots of 1.0–2.0 mL/kg intravenously. The aim is to improve acidic conditions in the heart and thus improve myocardial contractility, as well as facilitating the beneficial effects of adrenaline.
  - **Naloxone** may be used in the infant with respiratory depression as a result of maternal intrapartum opiate analgesia. The dose is 200 µg intramuscularly. Naloxone is not a substitute for appropriate resuscitation, which should always take precedent. Also, it is best avoided in infants of drug-dependent mothers, as it can result in a severe withdrawal state in these infants. Finally, the caregiver should note that naloxone has a shorter half-life than most opiates and doses may need to be repeated.
  - **Dextrose.** Hypoglycaemia is a major problem in prolonged resuscitations. Hence, small aliquots of dextrose may be required. A dose of 2–3 mL/kg of 10 per cent dextrose should be adequate.
  - Use of volume replacement.
  - **Blood.** If there is any suggestion of haemorrhage, O-negative blood should be used: 10–20 mL/kg can be given as a bolus and the response assessed.
  - For other causes of circulatory disturbance, volume replacement with a crystalloid or colloid can be useful in the resuscitation scenario. The dose is again 10–20 mL/kg. Following a Cochrane review[10] that found the use of albumin to be detrimental, most authorities recommend crystalloids, such as 0.9 per cent saline [A].

> Glucose solutions must not be used for volume replacement.

# POST-RESUSCITATION

## Continuing care

Once the infant has been successfully resuscitated, it is essential that provision for ongoing care be provided. This may simply involve handing a well infant to the mother to keep warm and feed, with attendants available to ensure there is no deterioration, or transfer of the sick infant to a neonatal intensive care unit for ongoing intensive care.

Before any transfer, the infant should be reassessed clinically. All lines, including endotracheal tubes, intravenous cannulae, nasogastric tubes and monitoring leads, should be secured. The need for ongoing medication and fluids should be considered.

Comprehensive documentation, including interventions, responses and subsequent management plans, should be completed and signed legibly. The family should be fully informed of events.

## Discontinuing care

Unfortunately, not all resuscitation attempts are successful and the decision to stop resuscitative attempts can be extremely difficult. As a guide, it is appropriate to consider discontinuing attempts if there is no spontaneous circulation by 15 minutes [E].

## Non-initiation of resuscitation

This can also be a contentious issue and it is important that units develop guidance in this area. Most practitioners would accept that it is inappropriate to routinely attempt resuscitation in infants less than 23 weeks gestation or 400 g birth weight. Equally, it is ethically acceptable not to resuscitate infants with lethal anomalies, such as anencephaly or trisomy 13 and 18.

In cases of uncertainty, an alternative approach is to commence resuscitation, and withdraw intensive care only once more information is available. However, it should be remembered that both withdrawal and withholding of intensive care are ethically equivalent.

With such decisions, the family should be fully informed and involved, as they will have to live with the consequences.

# SPECIAL SITUATIONS

## Extreme prematurity

These infants have much greater difficulties due to their immature physiology. Their lungs are poorly developed, lack surfactant and have poor lung compliance. They thus experience greater degrees of respiratory distress. Many infants less than 30 weeks gestation require early ventilation, with administration of surfactant. Indeed, some practitioners advocate 'elective' intubation of all infants less than 28 weeks. This has become contentious with greater awareness of the damage caused by barotrauma and oxygen toxicity.

Premature infants have a much greater surface area to body mass ratio, and thus lose heat much more quickly than term infants. Their cardiovascular systems are also immature, with poor autoregulation of the cerebral circulation. Care should be exercised when administering volume expanders.

The major practical differences in the approach to resuscitation of a premature infant include: use of a sterile plastic bag and a radiant heat source instead of drying with warm towels; consideration of elective early intubation and administration of surfactant to minimize lung injury; special attention to avoid excessively high oxygen concentrations.

## Meconium

Whereas it was previously taught that all infants with meconium present prior to delivery should have their airway viewed and suctioned under direct vision, it is now accepted that this approach can be detrimental in the majority of cases (see Chapter 28, Meconium) [A].[11] As a rule, infants born in good condition with good respiratory effort do not require airway visualization or oropharyngeal suctioning. Infants with depressed respiratory effort at birth should have their airway inspected and cleared prior to any other resuscitative efforts. The aim of this is to prevent inhalation of any meconium into the lungs of the compromised infant, as this can cause mechanical problems with breathing, as well as a chemical peumonitis.

## Hydrops

The main problem at birth, regardless of the cause, is the presence of large effusions (pleural, pericardial and peritoneal). These often need draining as a matter of urgency at delivery. Probably the quickest method is the use of an 18 or 20 FG cannula attached to a syringe. This can be advanced into the effusion to be drained, while maintaining gentle negative pressure on the syringe. As soon as fluid is aspirated, the cannula should be advanced over the needle, which is removed. In this way, the cannula can act as a temporary drain until a more permanent one can be inserted.

## Congenital diaphragmatic hernia

At birth, the major concerns relate to the degree of lung hypoplasia and amount of bowel and other abdominal content in the chest. Early control of the infant's ventilation in addition to preventing the infant swallowing air and thus inflating the stomach in the chest is generally felt to be best practice. To this end, the infant may be best managed with early intubation and muscle relaxation soon after birth. A large-bore nasogastric tube is inserted to keep the bowel empty.

Owing to lung hypoplasia, caution with positive pressure ventilation must be exercised to prevent pneumothorax.

## Congenital cardiac disease

Management depends on the lesion. There are too many to discuss in this chapter, except to say that infants with duct-dependent lesions should be commenced on a low-dose prostaglandin infusion early after birth. Otherwise, for the purposes of early neonatal resuscitation, there is no need for other special measures.

## Polyhydramnios

The main difference over the usual resuscitation process in this circumstance is to exclude a possible oesophageal atresia by inserting a large-bore nasogastric tube.

## SUMMARY

This chapter briefly discusses the process of resuscitating the newborn infant. It emphasizes the ABC approach, with a need for continual appraisal of a situation. It should be stressed that the vast majority of infants require no, or minimal, intervention. Equally, for those who do need help, most problems are related to the respiratory system, and attention to detail with regard to the airway and ventilation will be all that is required.

- Resuscitation should initially start with managing temperature control and ensuring a patent airway [E].
- In the term baby, air is as good as 100 per cent oxygen for resuscitation and may have additional benefits [B].
- High doses of adrenaline are no longer recommended as they confer no additional advantage and may be detrimental [C].

### KEY POINTS

- The vast majority of infants need nothing more active than keeping warm at birth.
- Nearly all neonatal resuscitations involve respiratory failure as the primary event.
- Optimizing airway patency is the most important part of neonatal resuscitation.
- Always remember the ABC approach.
- Do not forget to keep the infant warm.

## ACKNOWLEDGEMENT

This chapter has been revised and updated. The author and editors acknowledge the contribution of Sandie Bohin to the chapter on this topic in the previous edition of the book.

## Key References

1. Royal College of Paediatrics and Child Health and Royal College of Obstetricians and Gynaecologists. *Resuscitation of Babies at Birth*. London: BMJ Publishing Group, 1997.
2. Phillips B, Zideman D, Wyllie J *et al*. European Resuscitation Council Guidelines 2000 for Newly Born Life Support. A statement from the Paediatric Life Support Working Group and approved by the Executive Committee of the European Resuscitation Council. *Resuscitation* 2001; **48**: 235–9.
3. International Consensus Conference on Cardiopulmonary Resuscitation and Emergency Cardiovascular Care Science with Treatment Recommendations. *Circulation* 2005; **112**: 111–99.
4. Kattwinkel J, Niermeyer S, Nadkarni V *et al*. Resuscitation of the newly born infant. *Circulation* 1999; **99**: 1927–38.
5. Bhutani VK. Extrauterine adaptations in the newborn. *Semin Neonatol* 1997; **2**: 1–12.
6. Gunn AJ, Bennet L. Is temperature important in delivery room resuscitation? *Semin Neonatol* 2001; **6**: 241–9.
7. Jacobs SE, Hunt R, Tarnow-Mordi WO *et al*. Cooling for newborns with hypoxic ischaemic encephalopathy. *Cochrane Database Syst Rev* 2007; (**4**): CD003311.
8. Rabi Y, Rabi D, Yee W. Room air resuscitation of the depressed newborn: A systematic review and meta-analysis. *Resuscitation* 2007; **72**: 353–63.
9. Saugstad OD. Resuscitation of newborn infants with room air or oxygen. *Semin Neonatol* 2001; **6**: 233–9.
10. Alderson P, Schierhout G, Roberts I, Bunn F. Colloids versus crystalloids for fluid resuscitation in critically ill patients. *Cochrane Database Syst Rev* 2000; (**2**): CD000567.
11. Halliday HL, Sweet DG. Endotracheal intubation at birth in vigorous term meconium-stained babies. *Cochrane Database Syst Rev* 2002; (**4**): CD000500.

# Common neonatal problems

*Andrew Currie*

## INTRODUCTION

Most infants are born healthy and remain so throughout their lives. However, they can develop a number of common problems which, while not necessarily life threatening, may nonetheless cause significant morbidity and parental anxiety.

This chapter introduces the reader to the most common problems encountered at or shortly after birth, concentrating in the main on those relating to the term infant.

At the end of this chapter, there is a brief summary of the more complicated problems associated with prematurity.

## INCIDENCE

There are no reliable figures relating to how often paediatricians are asked to review infants for anything other than a newborn check.

Infants requiring paediatric input fall into two main groups. The first group comprises those that require acute care. These infants are primarily seen within the delivery suite shortly after birth. Paediatricians are called either to the resuscitation or for acute problems such as 'the grunting infant'.

The other group comprises infants seen on the postnatal wards. They are usually several hours of age, and any concern is less acute. Table 39.1 summarizes an audit of common, non-life-threatening problems seen within one unit during a one-year period, and gives an indication of the concerns paediatricians are asked to respond to on the postnatal wards. The birth population was approximately 5500 births per year. Routine newborn examinations and acutely ill infants have been excluded.

It can be seen from this table that many common problems in the newborn period are not serious health issues, but nonetheless can cause considerable morbidity and anxiety.

**Table 39.1** Numbers of infants presenting with common problems on the postnatal wards over a 12-month period, in a birth population of 5500 per year

| Clinical condition(s) | Total number |
| --- | --- |
| Hips | 213 |
| Jaundice | 99 |
| Cardiac murmurs | 33 |
| Antenatal anomalies | 25 |
| Birth trauma | 16 |
| Surgical | 23 |
| Hypothermia | 2 |
| Hypoglycaemia | 5 |
| Vomiting | 2 |
| Infection | 23 |
| Maternal infection | 34 |
| Other maternal conditions | 23 |
| Family history | 64 |
| Genetic | 15 |
| Skin lesions | 31 |

# COMMON NEONATAL COMPLICATIONS PRESENTING IN THE FIRST 24 HOURS

## Respiratory/grunting (transient tachypnoea of the newborn)

One of the most common problems that paediatricians review is acute respiratory embarrassment. Tachypnoea and 'grunting' are the most common concerns. 'Grunting' is the descriptive term given to the noise made by forced expiration against a closed glottis. It is essentially a sign of alveolar disease: the alveoli do not open adequately, hence the infant tries to open them by increasing his or her intrathoracic pressure. Most commonly, 'grunting' and tachypnoea are caused by excess lung fluid, which has not fully cleared following birth. These signs usually appear within the first few hours after birth and settle within 24–48 hours. The infant is otherwise well and observation is usually all that is required. This condition is often referred to as transient tachypnoea of the newborn (TTN). It must be remembered that this is a diagnosis of exclusion. More serious conditions, such as sepsis, aspiration, pneumothorax or respiratory distress syndrome, should be excluded. The signs of acute respiratory embarrassment are the same for many aetiologies;[1] thus, such infants should be seen by a paediatrician. If the signs are not settling quickly (i.e. within a few hours), if they worsen or if there are other risk factors in the history, the infant should be admitted to a neonatal unit for further investigation and management. This complication is common among babies delivered by elective caesarean section, with as many as 15 per cent of neonates being affected [B].[1]

## Hypoglycaemia

This subject causes much anxiety and continues to generate much controversy.[2] It is now accepted that many newborn infants go through a period of relatively low blood glucose levels shortly after birth. Assuming they are otherwise well, they can utilize alternative fuel sources, such as ketones and lactate, in the short term. This means that for term infants of average birth weight, it is unnecessary to monitor blood glucose and start invasive treatments. They should be left alone to establish breast or bottle feeding normally. The importance of hypoglycaemia is to identify and treat the 'at-risk' infant. Examples include:

- preterm infants (<36 weeks),
- growth-restricted babies,
- the infants of diabetics,
- infants with perinatal asphyxia,
- septic infants,
- infants with inborn errors of metabolism.

In these groups, a blood glucose <2.6 mmol/L is generally accepted to indicate hypoglycaemia [E]. Any infant presenting with low blood glucose must be carefully examined for the underlying cause and treated accordingly. The treatment of hypoglycaemia involves the administration of glucose. In the well infant, feeding with milk should be the first-line treatment. If this is not successful, or if there are indicators to suggest the infant is unwell, intravenous dextrose may be needed (a 10 per cent solution should be used initially). It may be necessary to give intravenous bolus doses (small boluses of 2–3 mL/kg of 10 per cent dextrose, followed by an infusion). All infants requiring additional glucose should be admitted to a neonatal unit.

## Hypothermia

This can be defined as a rectal temperature <36°C. It is most commonly seen in growth-restricted and preterm small infants, or as part of the clinical picture in the sick infant. Newborn infants are born exposed and wet, and can lose heat very quickly if not dried and covered adequately. Hypothermia can cause significant morbidity; infants are lethargic and feed poorly. More seriously, hypothermia is associated with hypoglycaemia, metabolic acidosis and respiratory distress.

The septic infant may also present with hypothermia rather than pyrexia. Hence, when dealing with the cold newborn, the first concern is to look for the underlying cause. Once this has been dealt with, specific measures to warm the child include a warm environment (this may seem obvious, but it is often found that delivery rooms are environmentally unfriendly for the newborn infant), drying the infant adequately and dressing him or her in warm clothes (including skin-to-skin contact with the mother and warm towels, covers), and the use of a radiant heater or warming mattresses. For extreme hypothermia, more invasive measures, such as reheating with warmed plasma expanders or exchange transfusions with warmed blood, have been used. However, it is debatable whether these convey any benefit over the use of a radiant heater and warming mattress.

## Fractures

These are not common. Fracture of the clavicle is the most frequently seen, followed by the humerus, femur and skull bones. Fractures usually result from traumatic deliveries, for example in association with shoulder dystocia and difficult instrumental deliveries [D].[3] However, this is not inevitably the case and certainly the medical literature gives examples of apparently unexplained fractures.

Clavicular fractures are best treated conservatively and have an excellent prognosis. Mild analgesia may be helpful.

Fractures of long bones may require some form of simple splinting to immobilize the limb and thus reduce pain.

Skull fractures are more serious, and the possibility of underlying haemorrhage must be considered.

The majority of neonatal fractures will heal uneventfully with conservative treatment.

## Cephalohaematomas

These result from bleeding between the periosteum and skull bones, and take the shape of the underlying skull bone. As they resolve, they may exacerbate jaundice, and the possibility of associated injury (such as skull fracture or intracranial bleeding) should be ruled out. Most cephalohaematomas are benign and resolve without problems. During resolution, the swelling may increase in size; this is usually due to fluid shift into the haemorrhage by osmosis as the clot breaks down. The carers should be warned of this, as it can cause concern.

## Nerve palsies

Erbs palsy and facial palsy are the most common nerve palsies. Erbs palsy is due to damage to the brachial plexus (cervical roots C5, 6 and 7), and is commonly associated with traction on the neck and shoulders during difficult deliveries,[3] although cases occurring in infants delivered by caesarean section have been reported. The result is usually a flaccid arm held in a pronated and internally rotated position. Recovery rates vary according to different studies. Between 49 and 94 per cent make a full recovery, with most improving by 12 months of age.[4] Early physiotherapy can help, and surgical treatment techniques to repair damaged nerves are now available for those cases that do not resolve spontaneously. Such cases should be referred early.

Facial palsies are commonly ascribed to obstetric manoeuvres, such as the use of forceps causing pressure damage; however, facial palsies also occur in infants delivered normally.[3] Most are probably the result of external pressure causing a lower motor neuron injury, and the prognosis is excellent. If an upper motor neuron lesion is suspected, the infant should be investigated for possible cerebral injury or congenital disorders. There is no specific treatment required.

## Sternomastoid tumours

These are the result of bleeding into the sternomastoid muscle. They are not normally recognized at birth, and do not become obvious until a few weeks of age. Physiotherapy is required to prevent contracture of the muscle. The prognosis is good.

## Traumatic cyanosis

This is a petechial rash present over the face and head, and may extend to the upper body, although the rest of the child is usually spared. It is probably the result of venous congestion, resolves spontaneously and is only of importance because it has been mistaken for true cyanosis. Simple reassurance is all that is required.

## Lacerations

Occasionally, the infant may suffer skin lacerations during delivery, usually during caesarean section. They are usually superficial and heal without problems. Suturing or use of steristrips may be needed for deeper wounds.

## THE NEWBORN EXAMINATION

This is included in this chapter because it plays a major role in the care of the newborn. It entails a clinical examination of the infant, carried out in the first week of life. It is meant as a screening health check, although there has been much controversy concerning its usefulness. At least 80 per cent of mothers find it a useful and reassuring process.[5]

It is probably not worth performing this examination within the first 24 hours of life, as there is a high chance of both false-negative and false-positive findings. Equally, assuming the infant is well, a 24-hour interval provides a chance for the infant to recover from the stresses of birth, and allows bonding to occur.

The newborn examination should be performed in a well-lit, warm room to prevent the exposed infant getting cold.

As with all medical examinations, it helps to have a routine system. By convention, the neonatal check is performed from the head and working down. Auscultation of the heart is opportunistic, as the infant needs to be quiet. A full explanation of the examination process would be lengthy, and the reader is referred to any of the standard textbooks of neonatology for this. A few points to remember include the need for proper hand hygiene when examining infants, and that the infant should not be left exposed for prolonged periods of time. It is often best to leave the nappy area until last. As part of the newborn check, parents should be asked about the passage of urine and stool, as well as any feeding concerns. In addition, a check should be made of the weight and head circumference.

## COMMON NEONATAL PROBLEMS PRESENTING ON THE POSTNATAL WARD

## Feeding

This is a huge subject and is one of the most common causes of anxiety in mothers.

There are two methods of feeding infants: breastfeeding and the use of formula milk feeds. Breastfeeding is clearly the best choice for a number of reasons, including the following:

- It adapts to the infant's nutritional needs.
- It has anti-infective properties.
- It helps with bonding.
- It helps the mother lose weight.
- It aids contraception.
- It is convenient and free.

However, there are a few problems associated with breastfeeding. Contrary to many mothers' preconceptions, breastfeeding is not always established readily. This can lead to a sense of failure and to the abandonment of breastfeeding if no support is available. Ill and preterm infants do not readily feed. In this situation, facilities should be available to help with the expression of breast milk until such time as the child is ready to suckle. There are often concerns about milk volumes; these are usually helped by support and reassurance. Test weighing has previously been used to try to quantify the amount of milk an infant is getting; however, this is not only unhelpful, but indeed can be positively detrimental to breastfeeding as it often instils a further sense of failure in the mother.

Other problems include concern about inverted nipples, cracked nipples, engorged breasts, overfeeding and weaning. These concerns should be easily addressed with the right support and information. Mastitis can also cause problems, but is not a reason to stop breastfeeding. Antibiotics or non-steroidal anti-inflammatory agents may be indicated.

There are very few contraindications to breastfeeding. Probably the most common are chronic ill-health in the mother (such as cystic fibrosis), potential infective risk (e.g. human immunodeficiency virus (HIV) in developed countries), acute ill-health in both the mother and infant, and certain metabolic disorders in the infant (such as phenylketonuria and galactosaemia).

Artificial feeding with formula milk is the alternative. Problems specific to this include:

- poor preparation of feeds,
- inadequate sterilization,
- cost.

Other problems common to both methods include problems with sucking and swallowing co-ordination. These may be due to anatomical factors, such as cleft palates or large tongues, as well as physiological factors, such as immaturity of the sucking reflexes.

Vomiting can be a major problem, and is most commonly due to gastro-oesophageal reflux. Assuming that the infant is well and growing, reassurance is usually all that is needed. Examination to exclude other causes of vomiting, such as pyloric stenosis and sepsis, should be performed. Failure to thrive is often due to feeding problems, but usually presents later in life. Bilious vomiting is pathological until proven otherwise, and should always prompt the search for a cause.

## Urine/stools

It is not uncommon for neonatologists to be asked to review an infant who has either not passed urine or not opened his/her bowels. Either situation is usually benign. A detailed history, including review of the antenatal progress and birth, is important. The external genitalia and anus should be examined as part of the assessment.

Most infants pass urine within the first 24 hours. This is often missed if it occurs at the time of birth. If there is any doubt but the infant otherwise appears well, it is worth placing cotton wool ball(s) in the nappy. An infant who has not passed urine within the first couple of days or in whom there is any other concern may need further investigation to exclude either obstruction (such as posterior urethral valves in males) or renal disease.

An infant who has not opened his or her bowels within the first 2–3 days should also be reviewed. Obstruction due to anal atresia should be obvious shortly after birth; however, conditions such as anal stenosis and Hirschprung's disease are easily missed if not considered. Investigation in such situations may involve gentle rectal examination, radiological tests and possibly rectal biopsy. Advice should be sought from a neonatologist and/or paediatric surgeon.

## Weight loss

It is normal for infants to lose weight in the first week of life. This is predominantly due to water loss. Breastfed infants tend to lose slightly more weight than bottle-fed infants. By 1 week of age, infants should start putting weight on. The average weight gain is 20–30 g/day in term infants. Weight loss in excess of 10 per cent is unusual and needs further investigation. There is a long list of causes of excess weight loss, ranging from inadequate intake, through inadequate nutritional content, to feed intolerance and ill-health.

## Skin lesions

Skin lesions are a common cause of concern in the otherwise well newborn infant. They include the following:

- *Birthmarks* such as the flammeus naevus (or 'stork mark') and port wine stains. It should be noted that strawberry birthmarks do not appear until a few weeks of age. Another birthmark is the Mongolian blue spot (very common in Asian and Afro-Caribbean babies), which consists of blue macules found over the back and is caused by melanocytes in the deep dermal layers.
- *Skin defects*, such as the aplasia cutis lesion. This is a congenital absence of the skin over the scalp. It usually has a punched-out appearance, with a healed edge, and it is important to distinguish it from trauma. These lesions usually heal spontaneously, by granulation. Plastic surgery, when older, is required for larger lesions.

- *Rashes.* Common rashes include erythema toxicum neonatorum, a red maculopapular rash, which comes and goes in the first few days and is of no clinical significance. Miliaria may also cause concern; this rash is caused by obstruction of sweat glands. Pustular rashes are common; most are sterile, but possible infection needs to be excluded. Nappy rashes include napkin dermatitis and candidiasis, both of which are very common and cause considerable anxiety.
- *Skin tags.* These can occur anywhere on the body; common sites are around the ears, anus and vagina. Pre-auricular skin tags have classically been associated with renal disorders, although the evidence is tenuous.

## Facial problems

- *Clefts of the lip* are usually obvious at birth. With better antenatal screening, many are now diagnosed on antenatal ultrasonography. The possibility of an associated chromosomal disorder should be considered, although most are independent of any other disorder. Although cosmetically they may look very abnormal, the surgical results are excellent. Parents need careful counselling from an early stage, including the use of 'before and after surgery' photographs for reassurance. During the neonatal period, the main concern is one of feeding, and referral for specialist advice at an early stage is paramount.
- Isolated *clefts of the palate* are almost never detected antenatally. They may be detected at a newborn check or can present in the early neonatal period as difficulty in feeding, apnoeas, choking episodes, poor feeding and chest infection. They are often associated with syndromes, and a meticulous neonatal examination should be performed. Referral to a geneticist may be indicated if there are other dysmorphic features. The specialist cleft lip and palate centre should be involved at an early stage.
- *Soft palate defects* can be particularly difficult to diagnose and may not be detected until late in childhood. They can result in feeding problems, as well as speech difficulties, and it is thus important that the palate is visualized to the back of the mouth, as well as palpated as part of the newborn examination.

## Orthopaedic

- *Talipes* ('club foot') is a common referral for paediatric assessment. It is important to differentiate between fixed talipes and positional talipes. The former needs referral to orthopaedic surgeons and physiotherapy, whereas the latter is of no consequence and the parents can be reassured.
- Examination of the *hips* is performed to detect dislocation. The hip should be held in a flexed, slightly internally rotated position, between index finger and thumb, while the knee is stabilized within the palm of the hand. The hip is then downwardly displaced to see if it can be dislocated. It is then externally rotated and upward pressure is exerted on to the outer trochanter of the hip with a view to reducing a dislocated hip. These are essentially the Ortolani and Barlow manoeuvres and are designed to diagnose a dislocatable or dislocated hip (in which case a 'clunk' should be felt). This is to be distinguished from a clicky hip, which is usually either due to poor examination technique or lax ligaments around the joint. Dislocated and dislocatable hips need referral to the orthopaedic team. Ultrasonography is useful to discriminate where there is uncertainty. It is also indicated in babies at greater risk of dislocated hips (breech deliveries, positive family histories). The use of double nappies is no longer recommended.

## Accessory digits

It is not uncommon for infants to be born with accessory fingers and toes. Most of these are pre-axial and not associated with any other problems. The infant should be thoroughly examined for other anomalies. Most accessory digits are attached by a thread of skin, and are easily dealt with by tying off with a suture. Those with thicker bases should be referred to a plastic surgeon.

## Surgical

- *Hernias.* Common hernial sites include umbilicus and inguinal canal. Umbilical hernias are easily reducible and usually resolve spontaneously. They are more common in Afro-Caribbean and Asian infants. Inguinal hernias are more serious. They are up to six times more common in males than females and there is an increased incidence of complications in the newborn. Early referral to a paediatric surgeon for operative correction is advised. Premature infants more commonly develop inguinal hernias than term infants.
- *Bilious vomiting* always needs investigating; although it may be innocent, the risk of intestinal obstruction or other serious pathology must be considered.
- *Hydrocoeles* are due to fluid accumulation in the scrotum as a result of incomplete closure of the processus vaginalis. They can be differentiated from inguinal hernias because it is possible to get above them and they transilluminate. Most hydrocoeles resolve spontaneously.
- *Hypospadias* occurs in approximately 1:300 male infants. It is characterized by a congenitally short urethra that opens on to the ventral surface of the penis, an abnormally formed foreskin, and chordee of the penis. Referral to a paediatric urologist is required. The parents should be advised not to have the child circumcized, as the foreskin is vital in any reconstructive surgery. The possibility of chromosomal abnormalities

(especially sex chromosome problems) needs to be considered in severe cases.

- *Undescended testes* are common in the newborn male. Most are unilateral, and reassurance that descent will occur is all that is required. If the testicle has not descended by one year of age, referral to a paediatric surgeon is warranted. Bilaterally undescended testicles are much more unusual and require further investigation to exclude underlying disorders, such as intersex or hormonal disorders of the pituitary–adrenal–testicular axis.

## Genetic

Paediatricians are commonly asked to review an infant whose appearance has given cause for concern. Most of the time, simple reassurance is all that is required. However, in all cases the child should be carefully and thoroughly examined. There are many dysmorphic features – too numerous to list here. In cases where doubt exists, further advice should be sought from a clinical geneticist. Chromosomal tests, as well as other investigations (dictated by the presenting condition), may be needed. It is important that the parents are carefully counselled. If doubt exists, this should be explained, to avoid erroneous conclusions being made.

## Eyes

- The vast majority of 'sticky eyes' are due to blocked tear ducts; simple toileting with lukewarm sterile water and cotton wool or gauze is all that is required. If the discharge persists, or is particularly copious, infections should be considered, and a swab sent for microbiological culture and sensitivity. The eyes should then be treated with topical antibiotics. Staphylococcal infections are the most common and are usually successfully treated with either topical gentamicin or neomycin. Chloramphenicol eye drops are also available and popular, but can mask chlamydial infection. Chlamydial infection should be considered if the discharge is copious or persistent. *Chlamydia* requires special culture mediums to grow, and is treated with chlortetracycline eye ointment plus systemic erythromycin.
- Congenital *cataracts* are rare. The newborn check is designed to detect them by looking for the normal red reflex with an ophthalmoscope. If a cataract is present, the red reflex will be absent, or partially obscured, depending on the size of the cataract. In this situation, urgent referral to an ophthalmologist is required. With early intervention, it is possible to improve subsequent vision.

## Cardiac murmurs

Heart murmurs are a common finding in newborn infants; however, most cardiac murmurs in the newborn infant are innocent flow murmurs – these are especially audible in the first days of life. As a general rule, identification of a cardiac murmur should lead to a careful clinical examination, an electrocardiogram (ECG) and measurement of limb oxygen saturations in the right arm and lower limbs (i.e. pre-ductal and post-ductal oxygen saturations). The majority of infants will be found to have a soft systolic murmur (i.e. with a grading of 1–2/6), a normal cardiovascular examination, no significant change in pre-ductal and post-ductal oxygen saturations, and a normal ECG. These infants can be reviewed in 4–6 weeks, as the chance of a significant cardiac lesion is very small. Parents should be warned of the small risk of a cardiac defect; if they have any concerns, such as the child getting breathless, tired, not feeding or going blue, they should seek medical advice urgently.

Infants who do not meet these criteria should be referred to a paediatric cardiologist for further investigation.

## Maternal group B streptococcal infection

It is generally accepted that infants of group B streptococcus (GBS) carriers are at greater risk of infection. However, quantifying that risk is difficult. Equally, given the high carriage rate amongst the normal population (estimated between 30 and 50 per cent), it is difficult to ascertain the best treatment approach.

Group B streptococcal disease is divided into early and late onset.

*Early-onset disease* is caused by passage of the infant through the genital tract in a carrier mother (many women are carriers and few babies are affected). It may present as:

- a clinical picture which mimics severe perinatal asphyxia,
- severe respiratory failure at birth,
- signs of early neonatal sepsis, such as temperature instability, lethargy, irritability, respiratory signs and tachycardia.

It is a neonatal emergency with potentially life-threatening consequences.

Universal pregnancy screening programmes and the use of prophylactic antibiotics are not recommended in the UK (see Chapter 22, Premature rupture of membranes).

In an attempt to identify at-risk babies, it is recommended that infants born to mothers who are GBS carriers and have one or more of the following features deserve special attention:

- previous infant born with GBS disease,
- spontaneous onset of premature labour,
- prolonged rupture of membranes,
- evidence of invasive GBS disease in the mother.

If mothers are given sufficient antibiotics early enough in the labour, the infant should be adequately covered [A].[6]

If this does not occur, or the infant is in any way unwell, he or she should be screened and treated with intravenous antibiotics. Subsequent management will depend on the clinical course and the results of cultures.

*Late-onset GBS disease* is probably related to infection after birth from a carrier mother. It can be present days or weeks later, most commonly with pneumonia or meningitis.

## Renal

In addition to determining whether or not a baby has passed urine (see above under Urine/stools), other renal problems usually relate to infants who have been found to have renal anomalies during antenatal ultrasound screening. Assuming the infant is well, repeated scanning can be performed within the first few weeks of life; many anomalies will have resolved. If there are continuing abnormalities, further investigation is required to delineate the nature of the anomaly.

Infants with significant bilateral renal anomalies on antenatal ultrasound (e.g. bilateral dysplastic, cystic kidneys or bilaterally dilated ureters) need more urgent investigation. They should also be monitored for failing renal function.

## Metabolic

The Guthrie test is a screening test performed on all newborn infants within the first week of life. It involves the collection of blood drops from a heel prick, and screens for:

- hypothyroidism,
- phenylketonuria,
- cystic fibrosis (in certain parts of the UK, immunoreactive trypsin levels are measured).

In addition, a few parts of the UK are also using the test to screen for sickle cell disease and medium chain acylcoenzyme A dehydrogenase deficiency (MCAD). The test should be performed once the infant has been established on feeds for a few days.

## Sacral dimples

Sacral dimples are a common finding, usually at the base of the spinal column. It is also important to ask about bowel actions and urine excretion and to check the lower limbs for normal movements and power. Assuming the base is easily seen and there are no other abnormalities, simple reassurance is all that is required. If the base is not visualized, or if the sacral dimples are larger than 0.5 cm diameter or associated with other features, such as tufts of hair, ultrasound investigation and paediatric review are indicated.

The most commonly associated problem is tethering of the spinal cord, which usually presents later in life.

## Umbilical cord

The umbilical cord is a common source of concern. The cord stump usually falls off within a few days.

- The most serious problem is one of *infection*. It is common for the cord stump itself to become colonized with commensal organisms, resulting in a 'sticky' or 'smelly' cord stump. Assuming the infant is otherwise well, with no signs of ascending infection, simple toileting with sterile saline or water is all that is needed [A].[7] Should there be any signs of spreading infection or systemic illness, the infant must be treated immediately. Ascending infection from the cord stump is usually due to *Escherichia coli*, other Gram-negative organisms or *Staphylococcus aureus*, and is a neonatal emergency requiring intravenous antibiotics.
- Umbilical stump *granulomas* do not present until after the cord stump has separated. Most resolve, although some practitioners treat them with application of a silver nitrate stick. Great care should be exercised so as not to cause chemical burns to the surrounding skin. They must be differentiated from a patent urachus which is an embryological remnant connecting the bladder to the base of the umbilical cord and can result in passage of urine. It requires surgical correction.

## Jaundice

Jaundice is a common, and potentially serious, problem with numerous causes:

- physiological jaundice, due to overloading of the immature hepatic system as a result of excessive red blood cell breakdown: the infant develops an unconjugated hyperbilirubinaemia between the second and fifth days, settling by a week of age;
- sepsis;
- haemolysis due to Rhesus or ABO incompatibility.

Acute haemolytic disease usually presents within the first 24–48 hours of life, thus any baby appearing jaundiced within this time must be investigated.

Treatment may not be necessary. The most important reason for treating jaundice is to prevent kernicterus, which is associated with severe unconjugated hyperbilirubinaemia and may result in death or major neurological sequelae. Most infants can be treated with simple phototherapy, although for more serious cases exchange transfusions are needed.

Prolonged jaundice is also of concern in the neonate. As a general rule, any term infant with evidence of jaundice beyond 10–14 days of age, or a preterm infant after 3 weeks of age, should be considered as having prolonged jaundice. There are numerous causes, of which the most common is 'breast milk jaundice' (a diagnosis of exclusion). All infants with prolonged jaundice should be investigated. It is particularly important to exclude a conjugated hyperbilirubinaemia, as this may be due to obstruction (e.g. biliary atresia), which can be treated successfully with surgical intervention if diagnosed early.[8]

## PROBLEMS ASSOCIATED WITH PREMATURITY

Respiratory distress syndrome (also known as hyaline membrane disease) is due to a lack of surfactant in the lungs, leading to acute respiratory failure. The severity varies from mild respiratory symptoms, requiring minimal input, to severe respiratory failure, requiring full intensive care and complex ventilator strategies.

Respiratory distress syndrome can either recover or develop into chronic lung disease (bronchopulmonary dysplasia). Other complications include pulmonary interstitial emphysema and other airleak syndromes.

Effectively, every system in the premature infant is at greater risk of problems. Premature infants are at risk of cardiovascular instability and hypotension requiring treatment. They are susceptible to cerebral insults, especially intraventricular haemorrhage and periventricular leukomalacia (the development of cysts in the periventricular areas at a few weeks of age) due to ischaemic injury. Their immature immune systems put them at higher risk of sepsis. They easily become anaemic, due to marrow immaturity, as well as the need for frequent phlebotomy. Their gastrointestinal system is vulnerable. They often show feed intolerance initially, and there is a high risk of necrotizing enterocolitis. (Necrotizing enterocolitis is a serious condition, which affects the lining of the bowel; it probably results from infection superimposed on bowel that has suffered an ischaemic insult.)

Premature infants also have a higher risk of long-term sequelae, including poor growth, neurodevelopmental disabilities and chronic lung disease.

## CONCLUSION

This chapter highlights some of the more common problems faced with the newborn infant. It concentrates on common acute problems occurring in the delivery suite shortly after birth and subsequently on common concerns that subsequently present on the postnatal wards. Most of the common problems occurring after the first hours following birth are not life threatening, but do cause significant anxiety and morbidity.

## ACKNOWLEDGEMENT

This chapter has been revised and updated. The author and editors acknowledge the contribution of Sandie Bohin to the chapter on this topic in the previous edition of the book.

### KEY POINTS

- Most common neonatal problems are non-life threatening.
- Recognizing the sick infant from the well infant is vital to avoid disaster.
- The newborn examination is a clinical screening test, and as such its limitations should be borne in mind.

## Key References

1. Dani C, Reali MF, Bertini G *et al*. Risk factors for the development of respiratory distress syndrome and transient tachypnoea in newborn infants. Italian Group of Neonatal Pneumology. *Eur Respir J* 1999; **14**: 155–9.
2. Cornblath M, Hawdon JM, Williams AF *et al*. Controversies regarding definition of neonatal hypoglycemia: suggested operational thresholds. *Pediatrics* 2000; **105**: 1141–5.
3. Perlow JH, Wigton T, Hart J *et al*. Birth trauma. A five-year review of incidence and associated perinatal factors. *J Reprod Med* 1996; **41**: 754–60.
4. Pollack RN, Buchman AS, Yaffe H, Divon MY. Obstetrical brachial palsy: pathogenesis, risk factors, and prevention. *Clin Obstet Gynecol* 2000; **43**: 236–46.
5. Wolke D, Dave S, Hayes J *et al*. Routine examination of the newborn and maternal satisfaction: a randomised controlled trial. *Arch Dis Child Fetal Neonatal Ed* 2002; **86**: F155–60.
6. Smaill F. Intrapartum antibiotics for Group B streptococcal colonisation. *Cochrane Database Syst Rev* 2002; (**3**): CD000115.
7. Zupan J, Garner P. Topical umbilical cord care at birth. *Cochrane Database Syst Rev* 2002; (**3**): CD001057.
8. Johnson LH, Bhutani VK, Brown AK. System-based approach to management of neonatal jaundice and prevention of kernicterus. *J Pediatr* 2002; **140**: 396–403.

# Perinatal mortality

*James Drife*

## INTRODUCTION

Babies may die at any time during pregnancy or after birth, and obstetric complications, such as preterm labour, may result in death of the infant several weeks after delivery. Perinatal mortality, however, is strictly defined as stillbirths and deaths of babies in the first week of life. In all countries the perinatal mortality rate (PMR), even with this relatively limited definition, is much higher than the maternal mortality rate. In the United Kingdom in 2007, the PMR (7.7 per 1000 live and stillbirths) was over 50 times higher than the maternal mortality rate (14/100 000 maternities), though exact comparison is difficult because of the different denominators.[1]

The PMR is widely used as an indicator of the quality of obstetric care and enables comparisons to be made among nations, regions and indeed individual hospitals. Nevertheless, perinatal mortality includes a wide range of conditions – from preterm labour to sudden infant death syndrome – with a wide range of underlying causes. For useful clinical lessons to be learned, perinatal mortality must be subdivided by the time of the death and by the causes.

## DEFINITIONS

The following definitions are those used in the UK and published in the annual reports of the Centre for Maternal and Child Enquiries (CMACE), which took over in 2009 from the Confidential Enquiry into Maternal and Child Health (CEMACH). CEMACH reports are available at ‹www.cmace.org.uk› and its work is described later in this chapter.

- *Stillbirth.* The legal definition in England and Wales is 'A child which has issued forth from its mother after the 24th week of pregnancy and which did not at any time after being completely expelled from its mother breathe or show any other signs of life'.
- *Early neonatal death.* Death of a liveborn infant occurring less than 7 completed days (168 hours) from the time of birth.
- *Perinatal mortality rate.* The number of stillbirths and early neonatal deaths (those occurring in the first week of life) per 1000 live and stillbirths.

CEMACH also gathers data on deaths that fall outside the strict definition of perinatal mortality. In some regions, for example, late fetal deaths are notified. Other categories and definitions are as follows:

- *Late fetal loss.* Death occurring between 20 weeks + 0 days and 23 weeks + 6 days. If gestation is not known or not sure, all births of at least 300 g are reported.
- *Neonatal death.* Death before the age of 28 completed days following live live birth.
- *Late neonatal death.* Death from age 7 days to 27 completed days of life.
- *Post-neonatal death.* Death at age 28 days and over, but under one year.
- *Infant death.* Death in the first year following live birth, on or before the 365th day of life (366th in a leap year). Infant deaths therefore include early and late neonatal deaths and post-neonatal deaths.

When infant and neonatal death rates are calculated, the denominator is 'per 1000 live births'. This is slightly different from the denominator 'per 1000 live and still-births' which is used to calculate the late fetal loss rate, the stillbirth rate and the PMR.

## Definitions of 'stillbirth'

Miscarriages are not included in the PMR. In the UK, it is legally necessary to register stillbirths – i.e. babies born dead after 24 weeks – but registration of miscarriage is not required. The dividing line between miscarriage and still-birth, however, is arbitrary and may vary from country to country. In the United States, for example, there is no single definition used in all states, although guidelines recommend reporting deaths after 20 weeks gestation.

In the UK, the dividing line was 28 weeks until 1992. When it was lowered to 24 weeks, the official stillbirth rate rose by nearly 30 per cent. The change was made because, with modern neonatal care, many fetuses born alive at under 28 weeks can now survive. Indeed, survival is possible even below 24 weeks, but this was retained as the dividing line in the UK partly because, under British law, therapeutic abortion for social reasons is allowed up to 24 weeks gestation.

The World Health Organization (WHO) has chosen a dividing line of 22 weeks, but in many parts of the world it may be difficult to define gestation exactly and therefore fetal weight is the main basis of the WHO definition of stillbirth:

*The death of a fetus weighing at least 500 g (or when birth weight is unavailable, after 22 completed weeks of gestation or with a crown–heel length of 25 cm or more), before the complete expulsion or extraction from its mother.*

In all countries, if a baby is born alive and dies soon after delivery, this is classified as a neonatal death irrespective of the gestation. This may lead to some anomalies. For example, in the UK, a baby born at 23 weeks gestation will be included in the national statistics if death occurs after delivery, but not if death occurs before delivery.

## CONFIDENTIAL ENQUIRIES INTO PERINATAL DEATHS

### History

In England and Wales, the Confidential Enquiry into Maternal Deaths (CEMD) has been running continuously since 1952. This method was extended to the deaths of babies in 1992, when the Confidential Enquiry into Stillbirths and Deaths in Infancy (CESDI) was set up. Its aim was to improve understanding of the risks of death from 20 weeks of pregnancy to one year after birth, and

of how these might be reduced. From 1996, CESDI was managed by a consortium of four Royal Colleges – those of Midwives, Obstetricians and Gynaecologists, Paediatrics and Child Health, and Pathology. In 2002, CEMD and CESDI joined to form the Confidential Enquiries into Maternal and Child Health (CEMACH) which was part of the National Institute for Health and Clinical Excellence (NICE). In 2009, CEMACH became the Centre for Maternal and Child Enquiries (CMACE), an independent charity funded mainly by the National Patient Safety Agency (NPSA).

Although these developments produced a bewildering proliferation of acronyms, the basic aims have not changed. Obstetricians should be pleased that the 'confidential enquiry' method of improving care is now being more widely used, after being pioneered 60 years ago by the RCOG and the (then) Ministry of Health when they set up the CEMD. Enquiries into perinatal deaths require a larger infrastructure than the CEMD. Every year in England, Wales and Northern Ireland, there are over 5000 perinatal deaths, compared with about 100 maternal deaths. CESDI and CEMACH therefore have full-time regional co-ordinators and support staff, and there are separate arrangements for Wales and Northern Ireland.

### Methods

Every maternity unit in England, Wales and Northern Ireland has a CEMACH co-ordinator who notifies the regional office of each death using a 'Perinatal Death Notification Form'. This form contains details of the mother's background, previous pregnancies and medical history, the current pregnancy and delivery, and the outcome including the cause of death. (Post-mortem data are not required.) In addition, deaths are reported to CEMACH by pathologists, coroners, child health systems and local congenital anomaly registers, leading to a very high level of ascertainment. Collaboration with the equivalent organization in Scotland (NHS Quality Improvement Scotland) provides UK-wide statistics and the National Perinatal Mortality Surveillance programme publishes a report every year. Data are cross-checked with registration data from the Office of National Statistics and missing cases are tracked down. As well as the national report, CEMACH produces individual reports for Trusts and Strategic Health Authorities, while still maintaining anonymity of cases.

### The work programmes of CEMACH

CESDI reported on specific subjects, such as intrapartum-related deaths, sudden unexpected deaths in infancy and deaths around the limits of fetal viability, and CEMACH does the same. Its work programme is divided into two subprogrammes. One is the Child Health Enquiry, which began in 2004 and examines health outcomes for children aged from 28 days to 18 years. Its first project was a review of child deaths occurring in 2006 and its current study, on head injury, will run until 2012. The other subprogramme is the Maternal and Perinatal Enquiry. As well as the ongoing CEMD and perinatal mortality surveillance, this includes a study of obesity in pregnancy (to run until 2011) and an audit of intrapartum care focussing on avoidable factors relating to stillbirth, neonatal death and neonatal encephalopathy (to run until 2013).

## Perinatal post-mortem examination

The enquiry does not depend on post-mortem results. Perinatal post-mortem rates have fallen in recent years, partly because of 'organ retention' controversies in the UK and other countries in the 1990s, when it came to light that organs had been retained after post-mortem without the permission of parents having been specifically sought. Several bodies produced guidelines[2] to ensure that parents are better informed, and that those who discuss post-mortems with parents understand the process so that consent is full and informed. The Chief Medical Officer recommended that all Trusts should designate a named individual to provide information to families, but this person is not always available. In 2004, the Human Tissue Act came into force and the Human Tissue Authority (HTA) was set up. Autopsies can only be done in premises licensed by the HTA, which in 2006 published its code of practice for consent.[3] All this had the effect of discouraging doctors from requesting consent for post-mortem, although the number of cases in which post-mortem is offered is now increasing again. There is increasing interest in 'minimally invasive' autopsy using techniques such as magnetic resonance imaging.[4]

## INCIDENCE

### Worldwide

Of the 130 million babies born every year, about four million die in the first 4 weeks of life, and a similar number are stillborn.[5] Three-quarters of all neonatal deaths happen in the first week and the risk is highest on the first day of life. Low-income and middle-income countries account for 99 per cent of the world's neonatal deaths, with the highest numbers in south-central Asian countries and the highest rates generally in sub-Saharan Africa. WHO estimates that the global PMR is between 50 and 60 per 1000 births (compared to 7.7 in the UK). Accurate data, however, are often lacking, and the Director-General of WHO summed up the problem in developing countries as follows:

*There are between 7 and 8 million perinatal deaths, but we do not know exactly how many are stillbirths and how many are early neonatal deaths. In many cases, births of infants who die soon after birth are neither recorded nor counted. ... Although the exact medical*

*causes in countries may differ, the problem is simple: the common denominator for these deaths is the lack of appropriate and quality services, confounded by poverty.*

There are wide differences among countries. In parts of South-east Asia, 40 per cent of children die by their fourth year. The underlying reason is often malnutrition, which makes children more susceptible to infection and affects particularly those born into large and poorly spaced families. There are also differences within the developed world. In Europe, the PMR in some countries is double that in others. By comparison, differences in PMRs due to minor variations in the definition of stillbirth are relatively unimportant.

## The United Kingdom

Data on perinatal mortality have been collected in the UK for the last 60 years. During this time, there has been a dramatic reduction in perinatal deaths. This has mainly been due to the improved health of the population, better nutrition and wider education, although the role of the healthcare services is also important, particularly in recent years. In 1963 in England and Wales, the stillbirth rate was >17 per 1000 total births and the neonatal death rate was >14 per 1000 live births. By 1999, these rates had fallen to 5.0 and 3.9, respectively. In 2007, however, the respective figures were 5.2 and 3.3 (see Table 40.1). The neonatal mortality rate continued to fall, but there was no change in the stillbirth rate, which indeed has remained largely unaltered since 1992, when the 24-week definition of stillbirth was introduced. The CEMACH report for 2005 commented that 'This lack of progress in reducing the stillbirth rate is a matter of public concern'.[6]

## AETIOLOGY

### General risk factors

In the UK, the risk factors for perinatal mortality include the extremes of maternal age.[1] In 2007, neonatal mortality was highest among teenage mothers, at 4.4/1000 live births, while

**Table 40.1** Numbers of perinatal deaths in the UK in 2007[1]

| Total births | 776 852 |
|---|---|
| Stillbirths | 4037 |
| Early neonatal deaths | 1979 |
| Late neonatal deaths | 555 |
| Total number of perinatal deaths | 6016 |
| Perinatal mortality rate (per 1000 total births) | 7.7 |
| Stillbirth rate (per 1000 total births) | 5.2 |
| Neonatal mortality rate (per 1000 live births) | 3.3 |

stillbirth rates were highest in women over 40, at 7.7/1000 births. Other risk factors are ethnicity, with a doubling of perinatal mortality among Black and Asian mothers, and social deprivation, with the most deprived quintile of the population having double the rate of neonatal deaths compared to the least deprived. The effects of ethnicity and social class on perinatal mortality are less marked than their effects on maternal mortality, but the same groups are at risk. Being underweight or overweight is also thought to be a risk factor, but no conclusions could be drawn from recent data and further information is awaited from the CEMACH study on obesity.

## Classification systems

For many years there have been three systems of classification of perinatal deaths, based on a mixture of obstetric and neonatal perspectives. CEMACH has now developed a new classification of its own, aimed at providing more insight into why babies die and identifying better intervention strategies. Its most recent report, however, uses the long-established systems: the extended Wigglesworth classification, the Obstetric (Aberdeen) classification, and the Fetal and Neonatal Factor classification.

### Extended Wigglesworth classification

There are nine categories in this classification. The first four categories are the main ones as far as the UK is concerned and are discussed in more detail below.

- Category 1. Congenital defect or malformation (lethal or severe).
- Category 2. Unexplained antepartum fetal death.
- Category 3. Death from intrapartum asphyxia, anoxia or trauma.
- Category 4. Immaturity.
- Category 5. Infection. This applies when there is clear microbiological evidence of infection – e.g. group B streptococci.
- Category 6. Other specific causes. Some conditions are not covered in the main four categories, e.g.
  - fetal conditions, such as hydrops fetalis
  - neonatal conditions, such as pulmonary hypoplasia
  - paediatric conditions, such as malignancy.
- Category 7. Accident or non-intrapartum trauma. This includes confirmed non-accidental injury.
- Category 8. Sudden infant death, cause unknown. This category includes all infants in whom the cause was unknown at the time of death. Information from post-mortem may be added later.
- Category 9. Unclassifiable. This category may be used, but only as a last resort.

### Obstetric (Aberdeen) classification

This system includes 22 categories grouped under the following headings.

- Congenital anomaly
- Isoimmunization
- Pre-eclampsia
- Antepartum haemorrhage
- Mechanical (e.g. cord prolapse or malpresentation)
- Maternal disorder
- Miscellaneous
- Unexplained.

### Fetal and Neonatal Factor classification

This system includes 24 categories grouped under the following headings.

- Congenital anomaly
- Isoimmunization
- Asphyxia before birth
- Birth trauma
- Severe pulmonary immaturity
- Hyaline membrane disease
- Intracranial haemorrhage
- Infection
- Miscellaneous
- Unclassifiable or unknown.

In the Fetal and Neonatal Factor classification, as in the Obstetric (Aberdeen) classification, only one category can be applied to any one death, and categories at the head of the list take priority over those lower down. For example, a baby who dies of intracranial haemorrhage (number 7 on the above list) would be categorized by the cause, such as birth trauma (number 4) or hyaline membrane disease (number 6).

## Causes of perinatal mortality

Table 40.2 shows the causes of perinatal mortality in the UK in 2007 according to the Wigglesworth classification. Stillbirths account for more than two-thirds of all perinatal deaths, which may surprise some professionals. Compared to conditions such as premature labour, little research is being done on causes of stillbirth, and compared to problems such as sudden infant death syndrome ('cot death') stillbirths are rarely discussed in the media. Mothers who experienced stillbirth say they did not know the problem still existed, and in 2009 a campaign was launched by the Stillbirth and Neonatal Deaths Society (SANDS) to raise awareness and promote research. The name of the campaign, 'Why 17?', draws attention to the fact that on average there are 17 perinatal deaths each day in the UK – ten times the number of cot deaths.

Table 40.3 shows that almost 75 per cent of stillbirths are 'unexplained' according to the Wigglesworth criteria, illustrating why a new classification is needed. The 2007 report[1] analyzed the weights of the 'unexplained' stillbirths and found that 38 per cent were less than the tenth centile for gestational age, suggesting that intrauterine growth retardation (IUGR) may be part of the explanation for some stillbirths.

**Table 40.2** Causes of death: England, Wales, Northern Ireland, Channel Islands and Isle of Man (2007)[1] (Wigglesworth classification)

| | Number | Percentage |
|---|---|---|
| **Stillbirths** | | |
| Antepartum fetal death | 2397 | 76.1 |
| Congenital malformation | 265 | 8.2 |
| Intrapartum anoxia | 205 | 6.4 |
| Infection | 113 | 3.5 |
| Others | 288 | 5.8 |
| Total | 3268 | 100 |
| **Neonatal deaths** | | |
| Immaturity | 963 | 44.3 |
| Congenital malformation | 537 | 24.7 |
| Intrapartum anoxia | 232 | 10.7 |
| Infection | 212 | 9.8 |
| Sudden infant death | 39 | 1.8 |
| Others | 287 | 8.7 |
| Total | 2270 | 100 |

**Table 40.3** Stillbirths 'unexplained' by Wigglesworth classification: England, Wales, Northern Ireland, Channel Islands and Isle of Man, 2007[1] (Obstetric classification)

| | Percentage |
|---|---|
| Unexplained | 74.4 |
| Antepartum haemorrhage | 10.7 |
| Maternal disorder | 8.1 |
| Pre-eclampsia | 4.9 |
| Others | 1.9 |

Intrapartum anoxia accounted for 437 of the 5538 perinatal deaths in 2007 (Table 40.2). This proportion (8 per cent) has not changed since 1999, despite the attention paid by risk managers to intrapartum fetal surveillance. This cause for concern was highlighted in the *2006 Annual Report of the Chief Medical Officer on the State of the Public Health*, in a chapter entitled '500 missed opportunities'.

# PREVENTION

## Worldwide

At the Millennium Summit in New York in 2000, world heads of state named reducing child mortality and improving maternal health among the Millennium Development Goals. The target for 2015 is to reduce by two-thirds the under-5 mortality ratio and by three-quarters the maternal mortality ratio from their 1990 levels. Strategies for reducing perinatal mortality overlap with those for reducing maternal mortality and a shared theme is the need for a functioning health system which can provide emergency obstetric care.

The reduction in intrapartum stillbirths in developed regions during the last 50 years means that in countries like the UK most stillbirths occur in the antepartum period. By contrast, in low-resource countries, there is a preponderance of late pre-term, term and intrapartum stillbirths, which could be prevented by known risk assessment methods and prompt delivery, often by caesarean section.[7] There is clear evidence that interventions are effective in reducing stillbirths, but a functioning health service is needed so that these interventions can be implemented.

Other improvements can be made. Family size throughout the world has been reduced by improving access to contraception, and some reduction in perinatal mortality can be achieved by basic hygiene, access to trained health workers and simple, well-tried technology. Promotion of breastfeeding is particularly important in developing countries. Not only does it provide appropriate nourishment for the newborn, but it also reduces the risk of infection from artificial feeding, provides passive immunity through maternal antibodies, and acts as a natural contraceptive to ensure adequate pregnancy spacing.

## The United Kingdom

Perinatal mortality can be reduced only if there is a will to do so, and this currently seems to be lacking.[8] The potential will be discussed under the four main categories of the Wigglesworth classification.

### Category 1. Congenital malformation

Congenital abnormalities accounted for 14 per cent of perinatal deaths in 2007. Current screening for congenital abnormalities includes universal fetal anatomy scanning in mid-pregnancy, and screening for chromosomal abnormalities through ultrasound and/or biochemical tests in the public and private sectors. Down's syndrome, the most common chromosomal abnormality, does not usually cause neonatal death, and therefore the biochemical screening programme has little effect on perinatal mortality.

Around 18 per cent of lethal congenital anomalies at birth are cardiovascular and these constitute the leading cause of death in this category. The cardiovascular system, however, is difficult to visualize adequately at routine ultrasound screening. Specialist cardiac screening is carried out for fetuses at high risk, but is too expensive in terms of personnel and equipment to be offered routinely.

Postpartum complications: neonatal

The fetal spine is easier to visualize, and most neural tube defects (NTDs) are identified at a gestation at which the woman can be offered termination of pregnancy. This has resulted in a decrease in perinatal mortality from this condition, but an increase in therapeutic termination. Ideally, congenital malformations would be prevented rather than being diagnosed early enough for termination, but this is difficult to achieve. The government has advised that all women should take periconceptual folic acid to reduce the incidence of NTDs, but only a minority do so.

## Category 2. Antepartum fetal death

Antepartum fetal death accounted for 43 per cent of perinatal deaths in 2007, but it causes surprisingly little soul-searching among obstetricians. In the 1990s, a CESDI study of antepartum term stillbirth showed that of 86 cases, 22 were associated with IUGR and many of the mothers had noticed a change in fetal movements. A CESDI study of stillbirths in 1996–97 found that 45 per cent were associated with suboptimal care. It recommended better screening for IUGR (using symphysis–fundal height measurements) and better communication with mothers so that those with concerns about reduced fetal movements can be seen promptly for checks on fetal well-being (See Box 40.1).[2] Its findings are worth reviewing, in view of the very limited improvement in the stillbirth rate since the 1990s.

> ### Box 40.1 Nature of suboptimal care (from CEDSI stillbirth enquiry, 1996–97)[2]
>
> - Risk recognition
>   - Failure to recognize high-risk woman at booking
> - Growth
>   - Inadequate monitoring of growth
>   - Failure to recognize intrauterine growth restriction
>   - Failure to act on intrauterine growth restriction
> - Fetal movement
>   - Failure of professional to act on decreased fetal movements
>   - Importance of changes in fetal movement not explained to woman
>   - Decreased fetal movements not reported by mother until after delivery
> - Management
>   - Failure to act on high-risk situation/history
>   - Failure to act on raised blood pressure and/or proteinuria
>   - No plan of care/management
>   - Failure to act on suspicious antenatal CTG
>   - Failure to do or repeat glucose tolerance test
>   - Poor diabetic management
>   - Inappropriate grade of staff involved in care
> - Communication
>   - Poor documentation
>   - Poor communication – oral and written
> - Lifestyle
>   - Maternal smoking
>   - Poor attendance for antenatal checks
> - Post-delivery
>   - Inadequate screening following stillbirth
>   - Post-mortems – quality issues, failure to send samples
>   - Bereavement support.

Women at risk need particular attention. Studies in Scandinavia have shown that the increased perinatal mortality among ethnic minority women is due to suboptimal perinatal care, including delay in seeking antenatal care, inadequate management of IUGR, misinterpretation of CTGs and poor communication.[9] Such studies have not been carried out in the UK.

For all women, routine antenatal care too often fails to identify IUGR. Current UK guidelines recommend screening by fundal height measurement, despite a Cochrane review showing no evidence of benefit. Its sensitivity may be improved by using customized growth charts. Another approach would be routine ultrasound scanning in the third trimester, which is normal practice in France. In the UK, however, scanning is done in the first and second trimesters, but third trimester scanning is seen as too expensive, despite evidence that it may be worthwhile.[10]

## Category 3. Intrapartum asphyxia

In 2007 the total number of births in the UK was 776 852 (almost 100 000 more than in 2000). The 437 deaths from intrapartum anoxia translate to a risk of one in 1778, which may represent an improvement since 1994–95, when the risk of death from intrapartum-related events was one in 1561. Nevertheless, there has been no detailed study of intrapartum-related deaths since 1994–95, when over 78 per cent of the cases were criticized for suboptimal care – alternative management 'might' (25 per cent) or 'would reasonably be expected to' (52 per cent) have made a difference to the outcome.[11] The main problem before labour was failure to recognize risk factors, and during labour was inadequate assessment of the fetus by heart rate monitoring and blood sampling.

Prompted partly by these findings, the Royal Colleges of Midwives and of Obstetricians and Gynaecologists published guidelines for improved standards of care in labour. These recommended, among other things, more involvement of consultant obstetricians in the day-to-day running of delivery suites, and have subsequently been updated.[12] National evidence-based guidelines were also produced on induction of labour and the use and interpretation of electronic fetal monitoring (EFM). There was a gratifying response at local level and in 2002 the CESDI report included the following statement:[2]

> It is therefore extremely encouraging to see that intrapartum-related mortality has now decreased significantly from 0.95 (1994) to 0.62 (1999) per 1000 live births and stillbirths. Although it is not possible to predict if this is a continuing downward trend, it is hoped that by maintaining efforts to achieve the highest possible standard of intrapartum care this will prove to be the case.

In 2007, intrapartum-related mortality was 0.56 per 1000 live births and stillbirths, which does represent a downward trend, although a much slower one than in the late 1990s. The emphasis in recent years has been on identifying 'low risk' women and promoting normal birth, but there have been persistent concerns about the levels of staffing in UK labour wards. Pressure on staff has come not only from a 15 per cent increase in the number of deliveries between 2000 and 2007, but also from the high proportion of deliveries to women born outside the UK – now almost 25 per cent nationally and over 70 per cent in some parts of London. These women are at higher risk and require extra care.

## Category 4. Immaturity

At least 17 per cent of perinatal deaths are due to immaturity (Table 40.2). The immediate causes of death include respiratory distress syndrome, infection, neurological causes and gastrointestinal causes. Advances in neonatal care have improved the survival of premature infants to a remarkable degree. Survival rates for babies born at 27–28 weeks gestation are now around 90 per cent, although around 20 per cent of these infants survive with some degree of impairment. It is now well recognized that antenatal steroids given to the mother will reduce the risk of perinatal mortality from respiratory distress syndrome, but they must be given at least 24 hours before delivery and sometimes it is impossible to delay delivery long enough for them to work.

An increasing variety of tocolytic drugs is now available for the treatment of premature labour, but the ideal solution is prevention rather than cure. Many researchers are pursuing the elusive goal of identifying high-risk groups and finding effective preventive treatment, and the use of progestogens appears promising.[13]

## Clinical risk management

For many years it has been standard practice for maternity hospitals to hold perinatal mortality meetings to review cases of perinatal death. The clinical history and pathological findings are examined and the implications for the management of similar cases are discussed. Many hospitals have extended this method to include 'near-miss' incidents. It is essential that such discussions take place in a blame-free atmosphere, so that constructive suggestions can be made for improving care.

These meetings are examples of the 'person approach', recognizing the importance of individuals, but there is now increasing emphasis on the 'systems approach' to risk management, relating the safety steps described by the NPSA to the labour ward.[14] This system recognizes and indeed expects staff to make errors and concentrates on improving the system to reduce the chance of errors occurring, to recognize them when they do occur and to prevent adverse consequences. The emphasis is on support for staff rather than blame. There are signs that this approach is beginning to reduce litigation and it is to be hoped that a reduction in perinatal mortality will follow.

## SUMMARY

Worldwide, there are between 7 and 8 million perinatal deaths annually, 99 per cent of which occur in developing countries, where the main causes are poverty, malnutrition and lack of access to healthcare. Improvements could be made by basic hygiene, access to trained healthcare workers, and promotion of breastfeeding, but reduction in perinatal mortality requires functioning healthcare systems delivering emergency obstetric care.

In the UK, perinatal mortality is low by comparison, but could be reduced still further. Intrapartum management has been improved with better training in the interpretation of electronic monitoring and more involvement of senior staff. Congenital malformations can be detected during pregnancy, but the ideal strategy is prevention. Prevention of preterm labour remains a considerable challenge, but neonatal care continues to improve survival rates. Antepartum fetal death is the major contributor to perinatal mortality and its reduction requires meticulous antenatal care, with better detection and management of intrauterine growth restriction. In this regard, particular attention must be paid to at-risk groups, such as poor women and those from ethnic minorities.

---

### EBM

- Maternal steroid administration before preterm delivery reduces perinatal mortality [A].
- The evidence does not support the routine use of electronic fetal monitoring in low-risk labours.
- Dietary supplementation in chronically malnourished women reduces perinatal mortality [B].

## KEY POINTS

- The perinatal mortality rate is the number of stillbirths and deaths in the first week of life per 1000 live and stillbirths.
- Globally, the perinatal mortality rate is around 50–60.
- Worldwide, perinatal mortality is due to poverty, malnutrition and infection, and lack of emergency obstetric care. It can be reduced by better hygiene and better access to healthcare.
- In the United Kingdom, the perinatal mortality rate is currently 7.7.
- The main causes in the UK are antepartum stillbirth (43 per cent), immaturity (17 per cent), congenital malformations (15 per cent) and intrapartum asphyxia (8 per cent).
- Deaths from intrapartum asphyxia have fallen only slightly in the last 15 years.
- Antepartum stillbirths, by far the leading cause, could be reduced by more focused antenatal care, concentrating on the detection of intrauterine growth restriction and on better communication with at-risk women.
- Perinatal post-mortems require fully informed consent from parents, and sensitive counselling is very important.

## Key References

1. Confidential Enquiry into Maternal and Child Health (CEMACH). *Perinatal Mortality 2007: United Kingdom.* London: CEMACH, 2009.
2. Confidential Enquiry into Stillbirths and Deaths in Infancy. Eighth Annual Report. London: Maternal and Child Health Research Consortium, 2002.
3. Human Tissue Authority. Code of Practice – Consent. London: HTA, 2006.
4. Thayyii S, Cleary JO, Sebire NJ *et al.* Post-mortem examination of human fetuses: a comparison of whole-body high-field MRI at 9.4T with conventional MRI and invasive autopsy. *Lancet* 2009; **374**: 467–75.
5. Lawn JE, Cousens S, Zupan J, for the Lancet Neonatal Survival Steering Team. 4 million neonatal deaths: When? Where? Why? *Lancet* 2005; **365**: 891–900.
6. Confidential Enquiry into Maternal and Child Health (CEMACH). *Perinatal Mortality 2005: England, Wales and Northern Ireland.* London: CEMACH, 2007.
7. Goldenberg RL, McClure EM, Belizan JM. Commentary: reducing the world's stillbirths. *BMC Pregnancy Childbirth* 2009; **9** (Suppl. 1): S1.
8. Drife J. Can we reduce perinatal mortality in the UK? *Expert Rev Obstet Gynecol* 2008; **3**: 1–3.
9. Saastad E, Vangen S, Froen JF. Suboptimal care in stillbirths – a retrospective audit study. *Acta Obstet Gynecol Scand* 2007; **86**: 444–50.
10. McKenna D, Dornan J. Who's looking for the high-risk fetus in the low-risk mother? *Obstet Gynaecol* 2005; **7**: 50–1.
11. Confidential Enquiry into Stillbirths and Deaths in Infancy. *Fourth Annual Report: Concentrating on Intrapartum Deaths 1994–95.* London: Maternal and Child Health Research Consortium, 1997.
12. Royal College of Obstetricians and Gynaecologists, Royal College of Midwives, Royal College of Anaesthetists, Royal College of Paediatrics and Child Health. *Safer Childbirth: Minimum Standards for the Organisation and Delivery of Care in Labour.* London: RCOG Press, 2007.
13. Simhan HN, Caritis SN. Prevention of preterm delivery. *New Engl J Med* 2007; **357**: 477–87.
14. Strachan BK. Reducing risk on the labour ward. *Obstet Gynaecol* 2005; **7**: 103–7.

# SECTION G
Postpartum complications: maternal

# Postpartum collapse

*Peter J Thompson*

## INTRODUCTION

Postpartum collapse is a major cause of maternal mortality and morbidity in both the developed and developing worlds. Although the most common causes of postpartum collapse are not confined to the immediate postpartum period, because of the rapid haemodynamic, hormonal and anatomical changes occurring at this time, there is an increased prevalence of these conditions.

Although many of these conditions require specific management plans, the generic treatment of a shocked patient, i.e. airway protection, administration of oxygen and gaining intravenous access, is common to all.

## DEFINITION

Postpartum collapse is the onset of shock in the immediate period following delivery of the fetus.

## INCIDENCE

There are no good denominator data available to accurately determine the incidence of this condition.

## AETIOLOGY

There are many causes of postpartum collapse, with the most common and most important being listed in Table 41.1. Many of these aetiologies have common pathways via hypovolaemia, whether it be absolute hypovolaemia, as in haemorrhage, or relative hypovolaemia secondary to changes in the autonomic nervous system, as in uterine inversion. It is noteworthy that with the exception of psychiatric cases all the main conditions that contribute to both direct and indirect maternal mortality in the UK are represented in this list.

The management of many of these conditions has been described elsewhere in this book, and will therefore not be addressed here. This chapter concentrates on the causes of postpartum collapse marked with an asterisk in Table 41.1.

### Vaso-vagal attacks

Vaso-vagal attacks are relatively common occurrences and are induced by many external stimuli, which result in extreme emotions, such as fright, anxiety or phobias. They are frequently preceded by a prodromal state consisting

**Table 41.1** Aetiology of postpartum collapse

| Pulmonary emboli | Vaso-vagal attacks* | Uterine inversion* |
|---|---|---|
| Septic shock | Epileptic convulsions | Cardiac arrest* |
| Haemorrhage | Cerebrovascular accident | Cardiac arrhythmias |
| Amniotic fluid embolus* | Eclampsia | Iatrogenic* |

*See text for explanation.

of dizziness, nausea, sweating, tinnitus and yawning. The aetiology is one of vasodilatation, leading to a pooling of blood and therefore a relative hypovolaemia. As a result, the heart begins to empty, stimulating mechanoreceptors in the wall of its left ventricle. This, in turn, acts centrally to initiate further vasodilatation and a bradycardia. These attacks usually resolve spontaneously, although it is advisable to position the patient flat and then elevate her legs to encourage central venous return and hence adequate filling of the heart [E]. Similar syncopal episodes may also be present in patients with cardiac disease, specifically those women who have arrhythmias or obstructive heart disease.

## Cardiac arrest

Cardiac arrest during the postnatal period is usually associated with hypovolaemia, obstructive heart disease or complex congenital heart disease. However, with increasing maternal age at the time of delivery, ischaemic heart disease is now seen more commonly. Indeed, in the last Confidential Enquiry into Maternal Mortality 2003–2005,[1] 12 women died following myocardial infarction (eight of these cases were secondary to ischaemic heart disease) and a further four women died of ischaemic heart disease where no evidence of myocardial infarction was found at autopsy. The rate of myocardial infarction is usually quoted as one in 10 000 births. The interprim publications from the UK Obstetric Surveillance System (UKOSS) have only found one case per 143 000 maternities, with further efforts being made to ascertain if this is a true incidence or if it represents under reporting.[2] Reversible causes of cardiac arrest are listed in Table 41.2.

Resuscitation of women who have had a cardiac arrest in pregnancy is usually complicated by the fact that, when supine, a gravid uterus will compress the inferior vena cava, decreasing venous return. Emptying the uterus, by delivering the fetus, will improve stroke volume by 60 per cent and is therefore mandatory if resuscitation has not been successful within 5 minutes [D]. Although this latter problem is not present in the immediate postpartum period, the uterus may still be of sufficient size to cause significant aortocaval compression and therefore resuscitation should be conducted with the patient on a left lateral tilt [D]. This results in an increased cardiac output of 25 per cent when compared to a supine patient.[3,4] The optimum tilt is a left

lateral tilt at an angle of 27°. This angle was calculated by Rees and Willis,[5] who examined all angles between 0 and 90°, comparing their efficiency for chest compression and their propensity to increase central impedance to venous return. At this angle, it is possible to exert 80 per cent of the mechanical pressure on the chest that one would if the patient were flat. As a result of this study, the Cardiff Resuscitation Wedge was designed and manufactured.

Management therefore consists of diagnosing and treating any reversible cause of the arrest, while simultaneously following the European Resuscitation Council Guidelines 2005 for Adult Advanced Life Support.[6] These are summarized in Figure 41.1. Once a cardiac arrest has been diagnosed, a precordial thump may be administered by a trained healthcare professional, although its success rate is low if the arrest has already lasted longer than 30 seconds [D]. Basic life support should begin once the airway is secured, with chest compression at a rate of 100 per minute and a compression to ventilation ratio of 30:2. The most recent guidelines suggest that chest compression begins before rescue breaths are given as in these initial moments of a non-asphyxial cardiac arrest oxygenation of the blood is high, but delivery of oxygen to the myocardium and brain is poor. Chest compression is often performed suboptimally and the person leading the resuscitation needs to rotate the person performing chest compressions regularly, approximately every 2 minutes.

Post-resuscitation care should include transfer of the patient to a critical care unit or coronary care unit [D]. Patients who are hypothermic should not be warmed and those who are pyrexial should receive antipyretics [C].

## Amniotic fluid embolus

Amniotic fluid embolism is rare, with estimates of the incidence varying between 1.3 and 12.5 per 100 000.[7] Good denominator data are at present being collected by UKOSS and these preliminary results show an incidence of 1.8 per 100 000 (CI 1.3–2.4) with a mortality rate of 24 per cent, lower than previously thought.[2] Due to its high mortality rate, there were 17 direct maternal deaths attributable to amniotic fluid embolism in the years 2003–2005.[1] The aetiology is still debated, but appears to be an anaphylactic reaction to the passage of amniotic fluid and particulate matter into the lungs. This results in a biphasic model where initially patients develop pulmonary hypertension and hypoxia presenting as respiratory distress, central cyanosis and circulatory collapse, with survivors undergoing a resolution of the pulmonary hypertension and subsequent development of left ventricular failure.[8] Approximately half of the patients who survive the initial insult develop disseminated intravascular coagulation.

Diagnosis of the condition is suspected when patients suddenly collapse either in labour or shortly after delivery with signs of central cyanosis, although confirmation of the diagnosis can be made on examination of lung tissue at

**Table 41.2** Reversible causes of cardiac arrest

| Four 'H's | Four 'T's |
|---|---|
| Hypovolaemia | Tension pneumothorax |
| Hypoxia | Cardiac tamponade |
| Hyper/hypokalaemia, hypocalcaemia, acidaemia | Thromboembolic or mechanical obstruction |
| Hypothermia | Toxic or therapeutic substances in overdose |

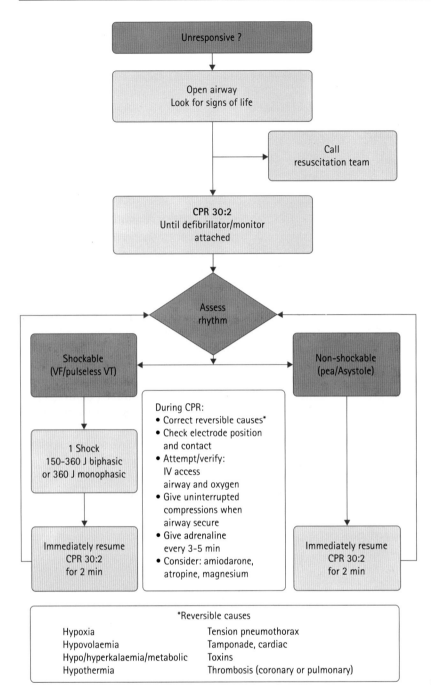

**Figure 41.1** European Resuscitation Council Algorithm for Adult Advanced Life Support

post-mortem, or on examination of blood films for the presence of squames or fetal hair. Management of these patients revolves around the generic treatment of shock and coagulopathies, with the former often requiring the information provided by pulmonary artery wedge pressures to guide inotropic interventions [D]. Although high-dose hydrocortisone has been suggested as an appropriate treatment, no studies have examined this.

## Uterine inversion

Uterine inversion is a rare condition, occurring with an incidence of one in 10 000 pregnancies. Although maternal death secondary to uterine inversion is well recognized, in the last Confidential Enquiry into Maternal Mortality 2003–2005,[1] no such deaths were documented. The degree with which the fundus of the uterus inverts is variable, with the mildest form being dimpling of the fundus and the most severe being complete inversion, where the fundus of the uterus passes through the cervix. There is no agreement on the aetiology of this condition, although several factors appear to be associated with its occurrence. These include:

- mismanagement of the third stage of labour, either by inappropriate traction during controlled cord traction or too rapid removal of the placenta during manual removal;

- maternal age >25 years;
- a sudden rise in intra-abdominal pressure in the presence of a relaxed uterus;
- a fundally placed placenta with a short umbilical cord.

Patients present with a picture of shock in the absence of visible blood loss. This shock appears to be of neurogenic origin secondary to traction on structures adjacent to the uterus. The fundus of the uterus may be visible at the introitus; however, if not, it will be detected on vaginal examination. This latter examination is mandatory in all patients who appear to be shocked in the immediate postpartum period in the absence of visible blood loss [E]. Not only can this lead to the exclusion of a diagnosis of an inverted uterus, but a diagnosis of a supralevator haematoma will also be excluded.

Treatment is based on the principles of managing a shocked patient and then replacing the uterus as soon as possible. If the diagnosis is made immediately, the uterus can often be replaced manually prior to the onset of shock. However, once the uterus has been inverted for only a few minutes, the tissues surrounding it constrict, preventing its replacement. In this circumstance, manual replacement may be possible using general anaesthesia [D]. If this fails, O'Sullivan's hydrostatic technique may be attempted: the vagina is filled with warm saline while being blocked at the introitus with the attendant's fist. The hydrostatic pressure resulting from the instillation of 4–5 L of saline may be sufficient to balloon the vagina and reverse the inversion [D].

Should neither of these techniques result in replacement of the uterus, a laparotomy and Haultain's procedure should be performed before the uterus becomes ischaemic from obstruction of its blood supply. At laparotomy, traction is placed on the round ligaments and an incision is made through the muscular ring in the posterior uterine wall. Continued manual pressure on the fundus from the vagina and traction of the round ligaments will allow replacement of the uterus, and the incision is closed [D]. In all these treatment options, it needs to be remembered that if the placenta is still attached it should not be removed until the uterus has been replaced, as the uterus will be unable to contract and constrict the placental bed blood vessels and therefore major haemorrhage may ensue [E].

In all the previously described management options, once the uterus is correctly sited, a Syntocinon infusion should be commenced to encourage contraction of the uterus [E]. It should be noted that a recurrence rate of approximately 30 per cent has been quoted in the literature, although recent figures are unavailable.

## Iatrogenic causes

Iatrogenic causes of loss of consciousness in the postnatal period include inappropriate advice on positioning the woman, with a resultant syncopal episode, and reactions to the administration of drugs. Although any drugs may be administered at this time, those that are most frequently used include Syntocinon, Ergometrine and local anaesthetics.

Syntocinon may cause sudden hypotension and, in women who are supine and have recently haemorrhaged, can be sufficient to result in loss of consciousness. This situation should be managed as for any shocked patient, with the appropriate positioning of the woman, protection of the airway and the administration of oxygen and intravenous fluids. In the previous Confidential Enquiries into Maternal Mortality, it has been reiterated that Syntocinon should be used with care in such situations. Ergometrine, which is usually administered along with Syntocinon, is a powerful smooth muscle constrictor and is contraindicated in women with severe hypertension, as it may precipitate a hypertensive crisis and haemorrhagic cerebrovascular accident.

In women with inadequate analgesia, infiltration of the perineum with a local anaesthetic is mandatory prior to surgical repair of the perineum. Lidocaine, the most widely used local anaesthetic for this purpose, is ideally suited, with an onset and duration of action after infiltration of 5 minutes and 1 hour, respectively (maximum plasma concentrations occur at 25 minutes). Overdosage usually presents as lightheadedness, sedation, paraesthesia, twitching and convulsions. However, if the drug is administered intravenously, it may result in the precipitation of cardiac arrhythmias and cardiac arrest. This is one of the reversible causes of cardiac arrest and should be managed according to the guidelines described by the European Resuscitation Council [E].[5]

It is therefore imperative for all healthcare professionals who infiltrate with lidocaine to ensure that injections are not intravenous and to be aware of the maximum dose of lidocaine that can be administered safely. This will depend, among other things, upon the patient's size and the degree of vascularity of the area being infiltrated. This latter variable can be altered by the administration of a vasoconstrictors to the local anaesthetic. The recommended maximum dose of lidocaine is 200 mg (500 mg, if administered with adrenaline). However, this situation is complicated by the fact that most local anaesthetics are labelled in percentage solutions and hence professionals need to understand how much lidocaine there is in a specified percentage solution. This equation is shown below.

One litre of a 100 per cent solution contains 1 kg of the active ingredient. Therefore, 10 mL of 0.5 per cent lidocaine contains:

$$\frac{1000 \text{ g} \times 10 \text{ mL} \times 0.5}{1000 \text{ mL} \times 100} = 0.05 \text{ g} = 50 \text{ mg}$$

---

### EBM

- There are few randomized, controlled trials of the management of acute postpartum collapse.
- There are, however, internationally accepted evidence-based guidelines for adult resuscitation.

## KEY POINTS

- All healthcare practitioners should be aware of the local guidelines to treat the shocked patient.
- European guidelines are available for resuscitation following cardiac arrest.
- Pregnant women who have had a cardiac arrest need to be placed in a left lateral tilt at an angle of 27°.
- Prompt replacement of an inverted uterus may be life saving.
- Local anaesthetic solutions are labelled in per cent and can easily be converted into milligrams.
- Local and national guidelines are essential for the management of these conditions.
- Good denominator data for many of the conditions that cause postpartum collapse are being collated by the UK Obstetric Surveillance System.

## Key References

1. Department of Health. *Saving Mother's Lives: 2003–2005.* London: CEMACH, 2007.

2. Knight M, Kurinczuk JJ, Spark P *et al.* on behalf of UKOSS. United Kingdom Obstetric Surveillance System (UKOSS) Annual report 2008. Oxford: National Perinatal Epidemiology Unit, 2008.

3. Lee RV, Rodgers LD, White LM, Harvey AC. Cardiopulmonary resuscitation of the pregnant woman. *Am J Med* 1986; **81**: 311–18.

4. Uckland K, Novy MJ, Peterson EN. Maternal cardiopulmonary dynamics IV. The influence of gestational age on the maternal cardiovascular response to posture and exercise. *Am J Obstet Gynecol* 1969; **104**: 856–64.

5. Rees GAD, Willis BA. Resuscitation in pregnancy. *Anesthesia* 1998; **43**: 347–9.

6. Nolan JP, Deakin CD, Soar J *et al.* European Resuscitation Council Guidelines for resuscitation 2005 Section 4. Adult Advanced Life Support. A statement from the Advanced Life Support Working Group (1) and approved by the Executive Committee of the European Resuscitation Council. *Resuscitation* 2005; **67** (Suppl. 1): S39–S86.

7. Gilbert WM, Danielsen B. Amniotic fluid embolism: decreased mortality in a population-based study. *Obstet Gynecol* 1999; **93**: 973–7.

8. Clark SL. New concepts of amniotic fluid embolism: a review. *Obstet Gynecolsurv* 1990; **45**: 360–8.

# Postpartum haemorrhage

*Peter J Thompson*

## INTRODUCTION

Haemorrhage is still one of the leading causes of maternal mortality in the United Kingdom with postpartum haemorrhage playing a significant role in the deaths of nine women in the last triennial report.[1] Any discussion of postpartum haemorrhage must cover both the primary and secondary conditions, although the majority of this chapter is aimed at the management of primary postpartum haemorrhage. It should be noted that the new Confidential Enquiry into maternal deaths will be published in 2010.

## DEFINITIONS

The differentiation between primary and secondary postpartum haemorrhage is more than an academic discussion, as the aetiology, clinical presentation, treatment and prognosis of the two conditions are very different.

Postpartum haemorrhage is subclassified as follows:

- Primary postpartum haemorrhage is defined as the loss of 500 mL of blood from the genital tract following, but within the first 24 hours of, the delivery of the baby. A caveat is added in that if the blood loss is <500 mL, but is sufficient to cause hypovolaemic shock in the patient, this is also classified as a primary postpartum haemorrhage. A new definition of massive postpartum haemorrhage has been introduced, being the loss of greater than 1000, 1500 or 2500 mL of blood. Owing to the relatively low risks of blood loss below these levels, this is thought to be of greater clinical relevance. The incidence of this complication is being used in some units as an indicator of the standard of maternity care and is being promoted by the Royal College of Obstetricians and Gynaecologists as one of their clinical indicators on the maternity scorecard.[2,3]
- Secondary postpartum haemorrhage is more of a subjective diagnosis, as its definition is blood loss from the genital tract of a volume greater than expected after the first 24 hours, but within the first 6 weeks of delivery.

## INCIDENCE

The incidence of primary postpartum haemorrhage in the developed world is approximately 5 per cent of all deliveries.[4] The incidence of massive postpartum haemorrhage in the United Kingdom has been reported as 6.7 per 1000.[2] This figure was obtained by analysis of a cohort of 48 865 women who delivered in a one-year period. Although significant morbidity will be associated with this condition, other data concerning its incidence are limited. However, the risk of mortality from postpartum haemorrhage was calculated to be 0.42 per 100 000 maternities in the last triennial report on maternal mortalities in the UK.[1]

## AETIOLOGY

The most common aetiology of primary postpartum haemorrhage is uterine atony, followed by genital tract trauma.

Uterine atony may have many causes, including retained placental fragments, and is associated with prolonged labour, multiple pregnancies, polyhydramnios, instrumental deliveries and grand multiparity. Other somewhat rarer causes include coagulopathies, pathological placentation (e.g. placenta accreta) and uterine inversion. These rarer causes retain a significant level of importance because of their relative over-representation among severe cases of haemorrhage.

The major aetiological factors associated with secondary postpartum haemorrhage are retained placental fragments and endometritis.

# MANAGEMENT

It is important to discuss the options for the prevention of postpartum haemorrhage with women antenatally. It has been well established that active management of the third stage of labour, with the administration of Syntometrine at the time of delivery of the infant's anterior shoulder followed by controlled cord traction, is associated with a relative risk of postpartum haemorrhage of 0.38 (95 per cent confidence interval (CI) 0.32–0.46) [A].[5] However, there is a substantial increase in the risk of maternal side effects, such as nausea with active management of the third stage of labour when compared to physiological management.[5] Women at risk of a postpartum haemorrhage should also have an intravenous cannula inserted during labour and blood taken for estimation of the haemoglobin concentration, and serum should be grouped and saved [E]. Such women include those in the risk categories mentioned above, as well as women who have had a previous postpartum haemorrhage, who have a risk of recurrence of approximately 25 per cent. Examination of the placenta post-delivery should identify a proportion of women who have retained placental fragments and who will require manual removal of the placenta.

Significant postpartum haemorrhage is an obstetric emergency that requires a multi-disciplinary team for optimum management [E]. Initial management is dependent upon rapid diagnosis. This is difficult, as it is well recognized that both obstetricians and midwives are poor at accurately estimating blood loss at the time of delivery. This can be further confounded by the ability of fit young women to maintain their blood pressure, either with or without a tachycardia, until they have lost approximately 15 per cent of their blood volume.

## Resuscitation

Immediate management will involve resuscitation of the hypovolaemic patient with the siting of two large-bore (16 G) intravenous cannulae, fluid administration, the application of facial oxygen, and examination to determine the aetiology of the haemorrhage, often performing uterine massage [E]. Although for many years clinical teaching has been that fluid replacement by colloid is superior to the use of a crystalloid, examination of randomized, controlled trials in patients with hypovolaemia has failed to show any benefit with the preferential use of colloids [A].[6] Although these studies are in the non-pregnant population, it is reasonable to extrapolate this conclusion to fit pregnant women. In this early stage of resuscitation, it is important to obtain blood for a full blood count, clotting studies and group and cross-matching.

## Disseminated intravascular coagulation

Disseminated intravascular coagulation (DIC) is a life-threatening complication of massive haemorrhage. Regardless of the aetiology, the management should revolve around maintaining an adequate intravascular volume and treating the underlying cause, in this case stopping the haemorrhage. This condition is discussed in more detail in Chapter 23, Antepartum haemorrhage. However, one should aim to follow four basic principles:

1 to maintain the intravascular volume,
2 to administer fresh frozen plasma (FFP) at a rate to keep the activated partial thromboplastin:control ratio <1.5,
3 to administer packed platelets to maintain a platelet count $>75 \times 10^9$/L,
4 to administer cryoprecipitate to keep the fibrinogen level >1 g/dL.

Although administration of blood components should be guided by haematological results, as described above, this should not be delayed until the patient is moribund, as successive Confidential Enquiries into maternal mortalities have identified delay in transfusion as a significant contributor to maternal mortality [D].

## Specific management strategies

Uterine atony can be managed pharmacologically or by a combination of pharmacological and surgical intervention. If the placenta is thought to be complete, the uterus is clinically atonic and there are no significant signs of genital tract trauma, an examination in theatre may be avoided by the administration of ergometrine followed by a Syntocinon infusion. Although the former has significant side effects, including nausea, vomiting and hypertension, its tonic action on the uterine muscle is a valuable adjunct to therapy with Syntocinon alone. However, caution is necessary in patients with pre-eclampsia, who may suffer episodes of severe hypertension following the administration of ergometrine.

Should these efforts fail to control the bleeding, examination of the genital tract needs to be performed with adequate lighting and patient analgesia. This usually means examination in an operating theatre with the patient having a regional or general anaesthetic. If the bleeding is significant, this examination should not be delayed in order to obtain blood results; if the anaesthetist is concerned about the risks of siting a regional anaesthetic in the presence of a possible coagulopathy or hypotension, then immediate resuscitation should be followed by the administration of a general anaesthetic [E].

Examination under anaesthesia should include examination of the vagina, cervix and, in the case of continued bleeding, exploration of the uterine cavity digitally to identify and remove any retained fragments of the placenta. If the uterine cavity is explored digitally, this should be covered by the administration of a broad-spectrum antibiotic. At this time, if no other cause for the haemorrhage has been identified, administration of prostaglandin analogues, either intramuscularly (if carboprost is available) or rectally (if only misoprostol or gemeprost is available), is advisable. The success of carboprost administration was as high as 88 per cent in one study.[7] Misoprostol administration has also been thought to be effective in decreasing blood loss in cases of primary postpartum haemorrhage, although there are limited data on optimal dosage, route and efficacy.[8] Suggested dosages of these uterotonics can be seen in Table 42.1. Bimanual compression of the uterus may also need to be performed at this stage; this decreases blood loss partly because of the fact that it puts the uterine arteries under tension. In addition to uterotonics, drugs that promote coagulation can be administered, such as tranexamic acid and recombinant factor VIIa. These drugs are not, however, without risk, with recombinant factor VIIa in particular having a recognized risk of thrombotic cerebrovascular accidents and myocardial infarction.

If these pharmacological and basic surgical steps have not achieved haemostasis, the uterus can be packed by either a traditional technique using gauze[9] or, as has more recently

**Table 42.1** Suggested dosages for uterotonics

| Uterotonic | Route of administration | Dosage |
|---|---|---|
| Syntocinon | i.v. | Bolus dose of 5 iu, followed if necessary by an infusion of 40 iu in 40 mL of saline run at 10 mL/hour |
| Syntometrine | i.m. | 1 mL |
| Ergometrine | i.v./i.m. | 250–500 µg |
| Carboprost | i.m. | 250 µg every 15–90 minutes, to a maximum of 2 mg (eight doses) |
| Misoprostol | p.r. | 800 µg |
| Gemeprost | Intrauterine | 1–2 mg |

been described, balloon insufflation.[10,11] This technique can be employed regardless of whether the abdomen is open or closed, and may therefore avoid the need for open laparotomy [D]. Indeed, the provisional data on the use of balloon insufflation using a Rusch urological balloon appear very encouraging, although there are problems related to when and by how much the balloon should be deflated.

Should these steps fail, the patient will require a laparotomy. At that time, either unilateral or bilateral uterine artery ligation can be performed, with success rates reported of more than 90 per cent [D].[12]

This technique involves placement of a suture through the broad ligament to include 2–3 cm of myometrium. The suture should be placed approximately 2 cm above the point where an incision for a lower segment caesarean section would be, thus ligating the ascending branch of the uterine artery and avoiding inclusion of the ureter in the suture.

Arterial ligation has been modified into a series of stepwise procedures producing uterine devascularization. This technique, described in Egypt, involves five steps: unilateral ligation of the uterine artery at the level of the lower segment; bilateral ligation of the uterine artery at the level of the lower segment; low ligation of the uterine artery after mobilization of the bladder; unilateral ovarian vessel ligation; and bilateral ovarian vessel ligation [D].[13] The first two of these steps resulted in haemostasis in more than 80 per cent of cases in the original report. Although ligation of the internal iliac arteries has been well described in the literature, it requires a high level of surgical skill and is reported as avoiding hysterectomy in only 50 per cent of cases.[14] The surgical time and complication rate in this series were also higher than when a hysterectomy was performed. After all these levels of uterine devascularization, subsequent menstruation and successful pregnancies have been reported.

The use of compression sutures of the uterus has been reported from Switzerland and the United Kingdom,[15,16] although their exact role in the treatment of postpartum haemorrhage has yet to be established. Compression sutures are only of possible benefit if bimanual compression of the uterus results in significant decrease in blood loss. Initially, the operation described by B-Lynch involves inserting a compression suture through a lower uterine segment incision, either the caesarean section incision or making a new incision. The suture is placed 3 cm below the incision and 3 cm in from its lateral border, through the uterine wall and cavity, exiting through a similar position on the superior aspect of the incision 3 cm above and 4 cm in from the lateral border. It then passes over the uterine fundus 3–4 cm from the right cornua and passes posteriorly down the uterus to enter the posterior uterine wall at the same level as the upper anterior entry point. The suture is then placed under moderate tension, while an assistant compresses the uterus. It is then placed back through the posterior wall on the left at a similar point as on the right. The suture is passed back over the fundus and then inserted through the upper and lower incisions on the left in a similar fashion as on the right. It is then tied. Initially, this technique was described using a 2-catgut suture on a 70 mm round-bodied hand needle. However, since the withdrawal of catgut, an alternative suture would be 1-monocryl.

A modification of the technique without opening a previously intact uterus has also been described.

Other options, such as arterial embolization and the use of recombinant factor VIIa, have been successfully described; however, good denominator data on the success rates of these are not available at this time.[17,18] The importance of good denominator data is demonstrated by the UK Obstetric Surveillance Survey (UKOSS), where rare conditions are identified and registered with a central co-ordinating body. One such study into the prevalence of peripartum hysterectomy showed that 50 women who subsequently went on to have a hysterectomy had had a B-Lynch suture inserted, which compares to the nine cases in the world literature where this procedure failed.[19] Data on all three of these procedures are now being collected by UKOSS.

Hysterectomy with ovarian conservation may be required as a life-saving procedure. In the UK, it has a reported incidence of approximately 4.1 per 10 000 deliveries.[19] Experienced obstetricians need to be involved in the decision-making process during this cascade of events and, where possible, the patient and her relatives should be kept fully informed.

Selective arterial embolization has been described both prior to hysterectomy and for persistent bleeding following hysterectomy. However, as mentioned above, its efficacy is still unknown and at the present time its use is limited by its availability.

The post-operative management of these patients may include the use of critical care units, with careful monitoring of central venous pressure being a recommendation from consecutive maternal mortality reports [D]. In the long term, these patients may also need professional counselling, especially if they have undergone a hysterectomy, and a debriefing with the lead clinician in charge of the patient's care is likely to improve patient understanding and satisfaction [E].

The management of secondary postpartum haemorrhage may, if severe, follow similar lines to the above. However, if milder, the management will depend upon the aetiology of the condition, with patients with suspected endometritis being treated with broad-spectrum antibiotics and those with suspected retained fragments of the placenta by uterine exploration. Because of the high incidence of infection, it is important that any uterine instrumentation is covered by administration of a broad-spectrum antibiotic [E]. In this situation, the role of ultrasound in the detection of retained products of conception is limited, because of the difficulty in distinguishing between placental tissue and an organized blood clot on ultrasonographic examination [E].

## EBM

- A systematic review of randomized, controlled trials shows that active management of the third stage of labour decreases the incidence of postpartum haemorrhage.
- A systematic review of the optimal choice of fluid for resuscitation shows no advantage in choosing a colloid before a crystalloid.
- No high order avoidance exists to support one form of surgical management of postpartum haemorrhage over any other.
- There are few randomized, controlled trials of the management of postpartum haemorrhage.
- A series of retrospective and prospective studies has shown that even with severe haemorrhage, a combination of medical and surgical treatment should avoid the need for hysterectomy in the vast majority of cases.
- The efficacy of different therapies for peripartum haemorrhage is being assessed by the UK Obstetric Surveillance Survey.

## KEY POINTS

- Postpartum haemorrhage is still a cause of maternal mortality in the United Kingdom.
- Active management of the third stage of labour decreases the risk of postpartum haemorrhage.
- Early identification of postpartum haemorrhage with accurate estimation of blood loss is essential.
- Acute management requires a multi-disciplinary approach with the involvement of senior clinicians.
- It is important to monitor central venous pressure in severe cases.
- Early transfusion and correction of coagulopathy is fundamental.
- All units need their own detailed protocols for the management of massive postpartum haemorrhage.

## Key References

1. Department of Health. *Saving Mother's Lives: 2003–2005*. London: CEMACH 2007.
2. Waterstone M, Bewley S, Charles Wolfe C. Incidence and predictors of severe obstetric morbidity: case–control study. *BMJ* 2001; **322**: 1089–94.
3. Arulkumaran S, Chandraharan E, Mahmood T *et al.* Maternity dashboard clinical performance and governance score card. Good Practice No 7. London: RCOG, 2008.
4. Anonymous. The management of postpartum haemorrhage. *Drug Ther Bull* 1992; **30**: 89–92.

5.  Prendiville WJ, Elbourne D, McDonald S. Active versus expectant management in the third stage of labour. *Cochrane Database Syst Rev* 2001; (**4**): CD000007.

6.  Perel P, Roberts IG. Colloids versus crystalloids for fluid resuscitation in critically ill patients. *Cochrane Database Syst Rev* 2007; (**4**): CD000567.

7.  Oleen MA, Mariano JP. Controlling refractory atonic postpartum hemorrhage with Hemabate sterile solution. *Am J Obstet Gynecol* 1990; **162**: 205–8.

8.  Mousa HA, Alfirevic Z. Treatment for primary postpartum haemorrhage. *Cochrane Database Syst Rev* 2007; (**1**): CD003249.

9.  Maier RC. Control of postpartum hemorrhage with uterine packing. *Am J Obstet Gynecol* 1993; **169**: 317–23.

10. Katesmark M, Brown R, Raju K. Successful use of a Sengstaken–Blakemore tube to control massive postpartum haemorrhage. *Br J Obstet Gynaecol* 1994; **101**: 259–60.

11. Johanson R, Kumar M, Obhrai M, Young P. Management of massive postpartum haemorrhage: use of a hydrostatic balloon catheter to avoid laparotomy. *Br J Obstet Gynaecol* 2001; **108**: 420–2.

12. O'Leary JA. Uterine artery ligation in the control of post cesarean hemorrhage. *J Reprod Med* 1995; **40**: 189–93.

13. Abd Rabbo SA. Stepwise uterine devascularization: a novel technique for management of uncontrolled postpartum hemorrhage with preservation of the uterus. *Am J Obstet Gynecol* 1994; **171**: 694–700.

14. Anonymous. Postpartum haemorrhage. *Clin Obstet Gynecol* 1994; **37**: 824–30.

15. Schnarwller B, Passweg D, von Castleberg B. Erfolgreiche Behandlung einr medikamentos refraktaren Uterusatonie durch Funduskompressionsnahte [Successful treatment of drug refractory uterine atony by fundus compression sutures]. *Geburtshilfe Frauenheilkd* 1996; **56**: 151–3.

16. B-Lynch C, Coker A, Lawal AH *et al*. The B-Lynch surgical technique for the control of massive postpartum haemorrhage: an alternative to hysterectomy? Five cases reported. *Br J Obstet Gynaecol* 1997; **104**: 372–5.

17. Ahonen J, Jokela R. Recombinant factor VIIa for life-threatening post-partum haemorrhage. *Br J Anaesth* 2005; **94**: 592–5.

18. Badawy SZ, Etman A, Singh M *et al*. Uterine artery embolization: the role in obstetrics and gynecology. *Clin Imaging* 2001; **25**: 288–95.

19. Knight M on behalf of UKOSS. Peripartum hysterectomy in the UK: management and outcomes of the associated haemorrhage. *BJOG* 2007; **114**: 1380–7.

# Postpartum pyrexia

*Peter J Thompson*

## INTRODUCTION

Historically, postpartum sepsis was most commonly secondary to infection with group A *Streptococcus*, and the prognosis was poor. Although the advent of antimicrobial therapy has significantly improved the prognosis, the last triennial report demonstrates that puerperal sepsis is not a disease of the past. Indeed, in this report, maternal mortality from genital tract sepsis was identified as the cause of direct maternal deaths in 18 women, with eight of these deaths being due to group A streptococcal infection, as were all three postpartum cases.[1]

## DEFINITIONS

Normal core body temperature is 37–37.5°C, with a diurnal variation of body temperature resulting in evening temperatures being 0.5–1°C higher than those in the morning. Oral and axillary temperatures are usually 0.4 and 1°C lower than core temperature, respectively. Persistent elevation of body temperature above those normal levels is termed 'pyrexia' or fever. The standard definition for puerperal fever used for reporting rates of puerperal morbidity is an oral temperature of 38.0°C or more on any two of the first ten days postpartum, or 38.7°C or higher during the first 24 hours postpartum.

## INCIDENCE

Following delivery, pyrexia is common, with fever secondary to disorders of the breast occurring in approximately 18 per cent of healthy mothers.[2,3] Benign fever with resolution in the first 24 hours occurs with an incidence of 3 per cent.[4] Fever associated with infection is more common, with urinary tract infections occurring in 2–4 per cent of women following delivery and endometritis in 1.6 per cent. Infections of the lower genital tract are uncommon and account for only approximately 1 per cent of cases of puerperal infection.[5]

## AETIOLOGY

The aetiology of pyrexia following delivery can be separated into four broad categories:

1. benign fever,
2. breast engorgement,
3. infections of the urogenital tract,
4. distant infections.

The most common infections of the urogenital tract are endometritis, urinary tract infections and infections of perineal repairs. Although not all pyrexias are of an infective origin, infection is the most important diagnosis and a thorough examination to search for a possible site of infection should be made. Rare causes of infection should be borne in mind in those patients who have recently been in tropical countries. Specific infections in the puerperium are caused by the same organisms that cause these infections at other times.

The development of endometritis is secondary to contamination of the uterine cavity with vaginal organisms during labour and delivery, with subsequent invasion of the myometrium. Endometritis is usually a polymicrobial infection associated with mixed aerobic and anaerobic flora. Bacteraemia may be present in 10–20 per cent of cases. The organisms that contribute to this condition include groups A and B beta-haemolytic *Streptococci*, aerobic Gram-negative rods, *Neisseria gonorrhoeae* and certain anaerobic bacteria.

Regardless of the aetiology of the pyrexia, the common pathway appears to be the production of endogenous pyrogens released by leukocytes in response to an antigenic stimulus. These then act on the hypothalamus, which in turn acts on the vasomotor centre, resulting in an increased production of heat and a decrease in heat loss.

## MANAGEMENT

### Prophylaxis

Prophylaxis against infections in the puerperium is particularly important in the case of delivery by caesarean section [A],[6] although there is no good evidence supporting the use of antibiotics at the time of instrumental delivery [A][7] and recent publications from the National Institute for Health and Clinical Excellence (NICE) suggest that women with congenital heart disease do not require antibiotic prophylaxis against infectious endocarditis.[8] If, however, women with congenital heart disease develop pyrexia, then this must be excluded and close liaison with local cardiologists should be maintained [E], as in the last triennial report into maternal mortality there were two indirect deaths attributable to infectious endocarditis.[1]

### General management

Management will depend upon the origin of the pyrexia. Because of the diverse nature of aetiologies mentioned above, a thorough history and examination need to be performed, with particular attention to examination of the breasts, chest and any wound sites. This includes an abdominal examination of the uterus for tenderness, a sign of endometritis. The endometrial cavity should be thought of as a wound site in this situation [E]. Features that are more typical of a benign fever are the presence of early low-grade pyrexia in the absence of any other symptomatology.

Appropriate cultures should be taken and, depending on the clinical features present, these may include wound and vaginal swabs, midstream specimens of urine, sputum samples and blood cultures. Management should consist of supportive therapy to ensure hydration and, where necessary,

the administration of regular paracetamol, which acts as an antipyretic and will improve patient comfort, while not altering the course of the disease process [B].[9] In cases of severe septicaemia, transfer to a critical care unit may be required so that inotropic support can be initiated.

## Specific management

This should be aimed at the administration of an appropriate antibiotic, which may need to be given intravenously in the first instance. In line with controls assurance standards, all hospitals should have an antibiotic policy determined by examination of the antibiotic sensitivities of organisms that have been detected within that unit. An example of one such policy from Birmingham Women's Hospital is included in Table 43.1. Once the relevant culture results are available, it is essential that any empirical antibiotic therapy commenced is reviewed in light of the known antibiotic sensitivities.

**Table 43.1** First-line antibiotic treatment for obstetric complications at Birmingham Women's Hospital

| Condition | First-line treatment | Second-line treatments |
|---|---|---|
| Chest infection | Amoxycillin and await cultures | Trimethoprim or clarithromycin or i.v. cefuroxime |
| Infective endocarditis prophylaxis | Treat relevant cardiac conditions with the prophylaxis policy in the BNF 'as for special risk' | |
| Wound infection | Flucloxacillin | Erythromycin or trimethoprim |
| Wound infection with cellulitis | Benzylpenicillin i.v. and flucloxacillin i.v | Contact microbiology for advice |
| Septicaemia post-surgery | Cefuroxime i.v. and metronidazole p.r. | Contact microbiology for advice |
| Septicaemia: antenatal | Augmentin | Cefuroxime i.v. and metronidazole p.r. |
| Septicaemia: postnatal | Cefuroxime i.v. and metronidazole p.r. | Contact microbiology for advice |
| Endometritis | Augmentin oral | Trimethoprim ± metronidazole |
| Urinary tract infection | Await cultures unless systemically unwell, if so cefuroxime i.v. | |
| Prophylaxis for caesarean section | Augmentin i.v. | Cefuroxime i.v. and metronidazole p.r./i.v |

● BNF, British National Fomulary.

The management of proven endometritis has been shown to be optimal if antibiotics that cover *Bacteroides fragilis* and other penicillin-resistant anaerobic bacteria are used. When uncomplicated endometritis is clinically improving on intravenous therapy, there appears to be no advantage in continuing oral therapy [A].[10] As no single antibiotic regimen has yet been shown to be superior to others in the treatment of urinary tract infections, therapy should be determined by policies based on the antibiotic sensitivities of bacteria isolated locally [A].[11]

Recently, the Health Protection Agency in England has noted an estimated 62 per cent increase in the incidence of invasive group A streptococcal infections, with a reported increased mortality rate of 25 per cent. While not all these cases were in postpartum women, some fatalities were. A high index of suspicion should be maintained when patients present with symptoms suggestive of invasive group A streptococcal sepsis, such as general malaise, high fever, severe muscle aches, dizziness, hypotension, confusion, unexplained diarrhoea and vomiting, localized muscle tenderness, pain out of proportion to external signs and a flat red rash over large areas of the body. Where group A streptococcal sepsis is suspected, immediate liaison with a consultant microbiologist is required, the Health Protection Unit informed and any contacts that show signs or symptoms of non-invasive group A streptococcal infection should be treated with penicillin V or, if allergic, azithromycin.[12]

Wound infections and endometritis may both be complicated by abscess formation. In these circumstances, antibiotic therapy alone is insufficient, and surgical drainage will be required [E]. The long-term complications of endometritis include subfertility [D].

The management of fever associated with breast problems is detailed elsewhere (see Chapter 45, Problems with breastfeeding). Suspected cases of invasive group A streptococcal septicaemia require prompt treatment.

## EBM

- Systematic reviews of randomized, controlled trials show:
  - a decrease in infective morbidity following caesarean section if prophylactic antibiotics are used;
    in cases of endometritis, antibiotics that cover *Bacteroides fragilis* and other penicillin-resistant anaerobic bacteria should be used;
  - if the endometritis is uncomplicated, oral therapy following intravenous therapy is unnecessary.
- Randomized, controlled trials show that the administration of paracetamol to pyrexial patients increases their comfort and does not affect the progress of the disease.
- Expert opinion regarding controls assurance suggests that all hospitals should have their own antibiotic policy.

## KEY POINTS

- Puerperal sepsis is still a significant cause of maternal mortality.
- A thorough examination and acquisition of appropriate cultures are mandatory.
- The National Health Service Executive have produced guidelines regarding controls assurance which suggest that all hospitals should have their own antibiotic policy.
- Paracetamol administration is safe and improves patient comfort.

## Key References

1. Department of Health. *Saving Mother's Lives: 2003-2005.* London: CEMACH, 2007.
2. Almeida OD Jr, Kitay DZ. Lactation suppression and puerperal fever. *Am J Obstet Gynecol* 1986; **154**: 940–1.
3. Marshall BR, Hepper JK, Zirbel CC. Sporadic puerperal mastitis. An infection that need not interrupt lactation. *J Am Med Assoc* 1975; **233**: 1377–9.
4. Ely JW, Dawson JD, Townsend AS *et al.* Benign fever following vaginal delivery. *J Fam Pract* 1996; **43**: 146–51.
5. Sweet RL, Ledger WJ. Puerperal infectious morbidity: a two-year review. *Am J Obstet Gynecol* 1973; **117**: 1093–100.
6. Hofmeyr GJ, Smaill FM. Antibiotic prophylaxis for cesarean section. *Cochrane Database Syst Rev* 2002; (**3**): CD000933.
7. Liabsuetrakul T, Choobun T, Peeyananjarassri K, Islam QM. Antibiotic prophylaxis for operative vaginal delivery. *Cochrane Database Syst Rev* 2004; (**3**): CD004455.
8. National Institute for Health and Clinical Excellence. Prophylaxis against infectious endocarditis, Guideline 64. NICE, 2008.
9. Prescott LF. Paracetamol: past, present, and future (review). *Am J Ther* 2000; 7: 143–7.
10. French L, Smaill FM. Antibiotic regimens for endometritis after delivery. *Cochrane Database Syst Rev* 2004; (**4**): CD001067.
11. Vazquez JC, Villar J. Treatments for symptomatic urinary tract infections during pregnancy. *Cochrane Database Syst Rev* 2001; (**4**): CD002256.
12. Duerden BI. Increase in invasive group A streptococcal infections in England. Department of Health, Central Alerting System April 2009, gateway reference 11632.

# Disturbed mood

*Peter J Thompson*

---

## INTRODUCTION

There is significant morbidity and mortality associated with mood disorders in pregnancy, with the morbidity being in both social and physical terms. In the past, it was felt that pregnancy had a protective affect with fewer women committing suicide than would be expected;[1] however, this has been contradicted by reports into maternal mortality in the United Kingdom. In the last triennial report examining maternal mortality, there were 12 indirect deaths caused by suicide, with another 22 late maternal deaths. Of these women, five were suffering with a psychosis and seven with a severe depressive illness. All except two of these 12 deaths occurred following delivery and the majority had a previous history of depressive illness or puerperal psychosis.[2] Antenatal disorders of mood tend to involve the management of pre-existing psychiatric conditions, while although any psychiatric condition can arise either as a recurrence or *de novo*, there are specific postnatal disorders of mood. These fall into three broad categories: 'baby blues', postnatal depression and puerperal psychosis. This section aims to cover all four of these areas.

## DEFINITIONS

'Baby blues' (or postpartum blues) is the term used to describe the transient experience of tearfulness, anxiety and irritability that frequently occurs in the first few days following delivery.

In comparison, postpartum psychosis is a disorder defined as a severe mental disorder usually occurring in the first 4 weeks of delivery, characterized by the presence of irrational ideas and unusual reactions to the baby. In addition, these patients also suffer fewer specific symptoms, such as restlessness, irritability, insomnia and lability of mood.

The symptoms of postnatal depression do not differ from the symptoms of depression at other times of life, but a temporal association with childbirth distinguishes it from other forms of depression. There does, however, seem to be little agreement on what the limits of this temporal relationship are, which makes assessment of the literature more difficult. Most studies are limited to depression with onset within three months of delivery, although some studies extend this limit to six months.

## INCIDENCE

As antenatal disorders of mood disturbance are usually due to pre-existing psychiatric conditions, the incidence is approximately the same as amongst non-gravid women of a similar age.

More than 50 per cent of women suffer from postpartum blues, usually commencing on the fourth or fifth postnatal day.[3] The incidence of postnatal depression is approximately 10–15 per cent,[4] whereas postnatal psychosis is rare, occurring in 0.1 per cent of cases.[5]

## AETIOLOGY

### Antenatal conditions

As already mentioned, although antenatal mood disorders are usually secondary to pre-existing conditions, they can be precipitated for the first time by a significant life event – the pregnancy. Pregnancy can place an additional strain on many relationships, not to mention the worries of future financial burdens, which may be sufficient to destabilize a susceptible individual. Therefore, these conditions may be secondary to the social implications of pregnancy rather than the pregnancy itself.

## Baby blues

As the immediate postnatal period is a time of significant physiological and social change, it is not surprising that a significant number of mothers suffer from disorders of mood. Baby blues is a self-limiting condition that has not been associated with any specific metabolic or endocrinological disturbance. It is more common in women following their first delivery, and sufferers are not more likely to have a past psychiatric history than non-sufferers. Other factors such as lack of sleep, hospitalization and pain have been implicated in the aetiology of this condition.

## Postnatal depression

The social and physiological changes seen at this time are also relevant to postnatal depression and puerperal psychosis. Although it is still true that no specific endocrinological change has been associated with the onset of postnatal depression, it has previously been hypothesized that the fall in both progesterone and oestrogen concentrations are implicated, as these hormones are known to have psychoactive properties. Unlike baby blues, postnatal depression is associated with a past history of psychiatric illness. One of the problems with determining the aetiology of this condition is that not all experts even recognize it as a separate disease entity.

## Puerperal psychosis

Whether puerperal psychosis is a discrete disease entity or a rapidly evolving affective psychosis is a matter of much debate. The aetiology of puerperal psychosis is poorly understood; however, it does appear to be more common following the first delivery, in patients with previous bipolar disorders and is recognized as having a 25 per cent risk of recurrence in subsequent pregnancies. Many patients also suffer from recurrent relapsing affective disorders for the remainder of their lives.[6]

## MANAGEMENT

## Antenatal conditions

Management of psychiatric illnesses during pregnancy is similar to that outside pregnancy. The main concerns are the effects that psychotropic drugs may have on the fetus, due to their high transplacental transfer rates. Indeed, although these drugs are not licensed for use in pregnancy, it is well established that if medication is withdrawn for mood disorders, there are high rates of relapse during pregnancy, anxiety disorders and schizophrenia. In view of this, several reviews have been published examining the possible teratogenic effects of these drugs (see Chapter 8, Medication in pregnancy). However, as new data are established on the adverse effect of drugs daily, readers are encouraged to search for the latest systematic reviews and teratology databases for themselves, e.g. ‹http://toxbase.u5e.com/›.

Overall, antidepressants as a group have not been associated with an increase in major malformations, although in the case of paroxetine, and more recently fluoxitene, both the relevant drug company and the Food and Drug Administration in the United States of America issued a warning regarding cardiac malformations following paroxetine usage in the first trimester [D].[7]

Following treatment in the first trimester of pregnancy, benzodiazepines, antipsychotic medication and lithium have all been associated with small but significantly increased risks of teratogenicity in the offspring. Therefore, women with a psychiatric disorder who are pregnant or who are trying to conceive should be counselled regarding the relative risks of disease relapse and fetal exposure to medication, and where appropriate an alternative, safer drug may be prescribed [C].

Women with a past history of psychiatric problems are at an increased risk of developing postnatal depression, and should therefore be identified and offered increased professional support following delivery [E]. However, to date, antenatal screening programmes have been unsuccessful and are not recommended in the National Institute for Health and Clinical Excellence (NICE) guideline on antenatal and postnatal mental health.[8]

## Baby blues

Research into the management of this condition is limited, with the only significant research being focused on an attempt to identify women who are at increased risk of developing either postnatal depression or puerperal psychosis. Management consists of providing a supportive environment for the new mother, with both professionals (particularly midwives) and the family working together [E]. Drug therapy is not indicated, as the condition is usually self-limiting. Those women in whom the condition persists beyond 10–14 days[9] and those who have marital difficulties appear to have an increased risk of developing puerperal psychosis.

NICE have recommended in their guideline on postnatal care of women that resolution of these symptoms should be confirmed between 10 and 14 days post-delivery, and if they have not resolved, assessment for postnatal depression performed and where appropriate further referral instigated [E].[10]

# Postnatal depression

Whether or not postnatal depression is a separate disease entity from depression, there is no doubt that it can have significant long-term effects on the mother–infant relationship and the development of the infant. Therefore, early detection and appropriate treatment are essential. The Edinburgh Postnatal Depression Score is a self-report scale that has ten items relating to symptoms of depression. The detection rates of postnatal depression in the community can be improved by implementation of the Edinburgh Postnatal Depression Score at a 6 weeks postnatal check [C].[11]

The treatment of postnatal depression in the past has mainly revolved around social support and supportive therapy, the administration of sex hormones (oestrogen and progesterone) and the prescription of antidepressants. In the case of sex hormone therapy, a systematic review of studies that used oestrogen or progesterone to treat women with postnatal depression showed discouraging results. Treatment with high doses of oestrogen did appear to reduce the depression scores of women with severe postnatal depression, but the potential side effects of thromboembolic disease, endometrial hyperplasia and inhibition of lactation make this an unattractive therapy for women to take. Progesterone therapy was associated with a higher incidence of postnatal depression than placebo. This could be because the mood elevation seen with natural progesterone is not an effect of synthetic progestogens.[12] Therefore, these medications cannot be recommended for women with postnatal depression [A]. Modern therapy, therefore, revolves around supportive therapy and pharmacological treatments.

Early involvement of a psychiatrist with experience in this condition is essential [E] and if the patient requires hospitalization, it is preferable to avoid separation from the baby, which will necessitate admission to a specialized mother and baby unit [D]. Ten trials have been included in a systematic review of the treatment of postnatal depression with psychosocial and psychological interventions as compared with the usual postpartum care.[13] This review showed a risk ratio of 0.44 (CI 0.24–0.88) for the evidence of depression at 1 year in favour of the interventions [A].

There are sparse data where the role of antidepressants for the treatment of this condition has been investigated in the context of a randomized controlled trial, though a systematic review of treatment of depression in pregnancy and the postpartum period showed the largest treatment effect was seen in those treated with antidepressants with or without the addition of cognitive–behavioural therapy [A].[14] NICE have recommended that for women with a new onset of mild to moderate depression in the postnatal period, self-help strategies, non-directive counselling and brief courses of cognitive–behavioural therapy or interpersonal psychotherapy should be offered first, with antidepressant medication reserved for those who are resistant to the above, those with a history of severe depression and

those who decline psychological treatment. For those with moderate depression with a history of a depressive episode or those with severe depression during the postnatal period, treatment should be structured psychological treatment or, if the patient has a preference for them, with antidepressants. If either of these treatments fail, a combination of the two treatments should be considered [E].[8]

# Puerperal psychosis

This is a psychiatric emergency and its treatment requires hospitalization. As it is preferable to avoid separation of the mother from her infant, admission to a specialized mother and baby unit should be arranged, where antidepressant and neuroleptic medication can be initiated and supervised by psychiatrists [C]. Failure to treat the condition aggressively is associated with rates of infanticide as high as 4 per cent [C].[15] This aggressive treatment may include electroconvulsive therapy [D].

## EBM

- Systematic review of two randomized, controlled trials shows progesterone therapy to be of no benefit, although oestrogen therapy may decrease the severity of depression when used as adjunctive therapy.
- A randomized, controlled trial has shown that fluoxetine is as effective as cognitive–behavioural therapy for the treatment of postnatal depression.
- Cohort studies show that the Edinburgh Postnatal Depression Score is effective in detecting women at risk of postnatal mood disorders.
- Retrospective cohort studies show that most drugs used to treat psychiatric conditions are relatively safe to use in pregnancy.
- NICE do not recommend screening for mental health disorders in the antenatal period for those at risk of mild to moderate postnatal depression.

## KEY POINTS

- Most drugs used to treat psychiatric disorders are relatively safe to use in pregnancy.
- Postnatal screening for postnatal depression using the Edinburgh Postnatal Depression Score is effective.
- The best treatment for postnatal depression appears to be cognitive–behavioural therapy, with the administration of antidepressants where necessary.
- Puerperal psychosis is a psychiatric emergency.
- Most women who commit suicide following or during pregnancy have a significant history of mental health disorders.

# Key References

1. Appleby L. Suicidal behaviour in childbearing women. *Int Rev Psychiatry* 1996; **8**: 107–15.

2. Department of Health. *Saving Mother's Lives: 2003–2005*. London: CEMACH, 2007.

3. Kendell RE, McGuire RJ, Connor Y, Cox JL. Mood changes in the first three weeks after childbirth. *J Affect Disord* 1981; **3**: 317–26.

4. Cox JL, Murray D, Chapman G. A controlled study of the onset, duration and prevalence of postnatal depression. *Br J Psychiatry* 1993; **163**: 27–31.

5. Kumar R, Robson KM. A prospective study of emotional disorders in childbearing women. *Br J Psychiatry* 1984; **144**: 35–47.

6. Davidson J, Robertson E. A follow-up study of postpartum illness, 1946–1978. *Acta Psychiatr Scand* 1985; **71**: 451–7.

7. National Teratology Information Service (NTIS). *Use of Paroxetine in Pregnancy*. Newcastle upon Tyne: NTIS, Regional Drug and Therapeutics Centre, 2005.

8. National Institute for Health and Clinical Excellence. *Antenatal and Postnatal Mental Health. Clinical Management and Service Guidance. NICE Clinical Guideline 45*. London: NICE, 2007. Available from: ‹www.nice.org.uk/guidance/CG45/niceguidance/pdf/English›.

9. Robinson GE, Stewart DE. Postpartum psychiatric disorders. *CMAJ* 1986; **134**: 31–7.

10. Demott K, Bick D, Norman R *et al*. *Clinical Guidelines and Evidence Review for Post Natal Care: Routine Post Natal Care of Recently Delivered Women and their Babies*. London: National Collaborating Centre for Primary Care and Royal College Of General Practitioners, 2006.

11. Georgiopoulos AM, Bryan TL, Wollan P, Yawn BP. Routine screening for postpartum depression. *J Fam Pract* 2001; **50**: 117–22.

12. Dennis CL, Ross LE, Herxheimer A. Oestrogens and progestins for preventing and treating postpartum depression. *Cochrane Database Syst Rev* 2008; (**4**): CD001690.

13. Dennis CL, Hodnett ED. Psychosocial and psychological interventions for treating postpartum depression. *Cochrane Database Syst Rev* 2007; (**4**): CD006116.

14. Bledsoe SE, Grotne NK. Treating depression during pregnancy and the postpartum: a preliminary meta-analysis. *Res Soc Work Pract* 2006; **16**: 109–120.

15. D'Orban PT. Women who kill their children. *Br J Psychiatry* 1979; **134**: 560–71.

# Problems with breastfeeding

*Peter J Thompson*

## INTRODUCTION

Although a physiological process, breastfeeding is an action that women perform for only a small part of their lives. For it to be successful, not only do the correct physiological processes have to occur, but both the mother and neonate need to adapt to this situation, and whereas some mothers and babies seem to be able to establish it without any problems, others do not. Increasingly, the proportion of women breastfeeding has been identified as a high priority for the government in their white paper 'Our Healthier Nation'.[1] Indeed, the World Health Organization recommends exclusive breastfeeding until the age of six months.[2] For these targets to be reached, interventions of proven benefit need to be employed throughout the health service. To this aim, UNICEF have developed a programme whereby maternity services that employ their Ten Steps to Successful Breast Feeding can apply for Baby-Friendly status. These ten steps are evidence-based standards designed to promote, protect and support breastfeeding. These steps cover topics including the establishment of local policies, training of staff, antenatal and postnatal education of women and the establishment for support groups. As an incentive to maternity services, many primary care trusts in England are insisting on their acute trusts achieving Baby-Friendly status.

## DEFINITIONS

There are extensive data in the literature supporting the concept that the optimum food for babies is breast milk. The benefits bestowed upon the infant are pertinent in both the short and long term. Included in these benefits is reduced morbidity from respiratory, gastrointestinal, urinary tract and middle ear infections, as well as a decreased tendency towards atopy and obesity. For the mother, there are both health benefits, such as a decrease in the incidence of epithelial ovarian cancer and premenopausal breast cancer, as well as financial benefits. Therefore, conditions that interfere with breast-feeding constitute important epidemiological health issues.

## INCIDENCE

The last national audit in 2005 showed that following delivery approximately 76 per cent of women in the United Kingdom commence breastfeeding. Breastfeeding is much more common among women from social class I than amongst those in socioeconomic class V and in England than other parts of the United Kingdom.[3] However, in the UK, these rates fall to approximately 48 per cent at 6 weeks and 25 per cent at six months, with less than 1 per cent exclusively breastfeeding at six months postpartum. These figures represent a significant increase on previous national audits.

## AETIOLOGY

The establishment of lactation is dependent upon a variety of influences, including the production of prolactin from the anterior pituitary gland and oxytocin from the posterior pituitary gland. These hormones stimulate milk production and ejection, respectively. However, problems with lactation are rarely due to pituitary–hypothalamic axis dysfunction. Indeed, the main reasons why women neither initiate breastfeeding nor continue it as long as in other European countries appear to relate to social and cultural issues. This section does not attempt to discuss these, but concentrates on the management of mastitis, breast abscess formation, enforced separation of mother and baby, and poor infant feeding. Many of these problems are interrelated and it has been suggested that the majority can be avoided by using a technique of feeding on demand and attaching the baby to the nipple in the correct position from the first feed onwards.[4]

# MANAGEMENT

## Mastitis

Mastalgia is defined as painful breasts. In the first week after birth, mastalgia is the third most common cause cited by women for the discontinuation of breastfeeding, with 24 per cent of women who discontinue giving this reason.[3] The aetiology of this condition revolves around the imbalance between the production of milk and infant consumption that occurs in a small proportion of women. When milk production exceeds the infant's requirements, the alveolar spaces within the breasts become distended, with the breast feeling hot, swollen and tender. This swelling leads to compression of the capillaries, which in turn increases the arterial pressure to the breasts, causing compression of the connective tissues and a decrease in lymphatic drainage. This results in the formation of oedema and engorgement of the breast (obstructive mastitis), which may develop into infective mastitis.

Five factors have been associated with the development of breast engorgement: delayed initiation of feeds, infrequent feeds, time-limited feeds, a late shift from colostrum to milk production, and the habit of administering supplementary feeds.[5] Therefore, avoidance of these will significantly decrease the incidence of this problem.

Many interventions have been proposed for the treatment of breast engorgement, some of which have been the subject of systematic reviews, which have examined both traditional and modern treatments. The most effective treatments tested involved the use of anti-inflammatory agents [B]. The agents tested are not available in the UK, and it is uncertain whether these results are applicable to similar agents. Interventions, such as the topical application of cabbage leaves, the use of gel packs and ultrasound treatment, all showed an improvement in symptoms, though not to a greater extent than placebo. It has been postulated that these improvements are secondary to warming and physically massaging the breast [A].[6]

As previously mentioned, breast engorgement may become complicated by infection, leading to infective mastitis. The most common causative organism is *Staphylococcus aureus*, with others occasionally being implicated, including *Staphylococcus epidermidis*, groups A, B and F beta-haemolytic *Streptococcus*, *Haemophilus influenzae* and *Escherichia coli*. Management consists of the administration of an antibiotic that is effective against beta-lactamase-producing bacteria

and encouraging the mother to continue breastfeeding or manually expressing milk [B].

## Breast abscess formation

Although uncommon, the exact prevalence of this condition is not well reported, with the better estimates being in the region of 0.1 per cent.[7] It does, however, appear to be more common in women over 30 years of age, primiparous women and particularly following mastitis, with a reported incidence of 5–11 per cent most commonly following inadequate treatment of the mastitis.[8] Not surprisingly, therefore, the prevention of abscess formation is achieved by the avoidance of milk stasis.[9,10] However, unlike for infective mastitis, most authors would recommend that feeding from the affected breast ceases when pus is draining from the nipple [C]. Once formed, abscesses requires either surgical drainage, usually under general anaesthesia[11] or preferably needle aspiration with or without ultrasound control,[12,13] with the administration of broad-spectrum antibiotics [C]. When surgical drainage is performed, choice of incision for the drainage is controversial; circumferential incisions give optimum cosmetic results, but radial incisions carry a smaller risk of damage to other lactiferous ducts. Therefore, it would seem sensible to perform circumferential incisions to drain superficial abscesses, whereas deep abscesses should be drained via a radial incision [E].

## Enforced separation of mother and baby

Separation of mother and baby, usually secondary to the ill health of one or both parties, may have a significant impact on the establishment of breastfeeding. The successful long-term establishment of breastfeeding is dependent upon frequent feeding,[6] and this is obviously complicated when the parties are physically separated or when one or other party is too ill to feed. Indeed, ensuring that mothers and babies are together 24 hours a day is one of the '10 Steps to Successful Breastfeeding' promoted by UNICEF. However, systematic reviews have failed to show improved prevalence of long-term breastfeeding in groups of women who commence feeding early (within 30 minutes) when compared to those who commence feeding their infants between 4 and 8 hours post-delivery [A].[14]

If breastfeeding is to be established in these circumstances, the expression of breast milk, in place of frequent feeds, is essential [D]. This can be done by hand or mechanically, with collection of the milk in a container to feed the infant at a later date.

This problem is seen commonly in babies admitted to a neonatal unit and, because of the many advantages of breastfeeding such children, many units have established milk banks to store this milk. There are occasions when breastfeeding may be contraindicated, for example maternal human immunodeficiency virus (HIV) infection or relatively contraindicated, for example severe maternal ill health. In such conditions, it may be appropriate to prescribe a dopamine antagonist, such as cabergoline, which will cause the production of milk to stop.

## Poor infant feeding

Poor infant feeding secondary to ill health has already been considered above. Poor technique of breastfeeding is another cause of poor feeding. A systematic review of increased support for mothers by healthcare professionals has shown a significantly decreased risk of discontinuation of breastfeeding. This effect was larger when there was both professional and lay support and the effect increased further when these supporters were UNICEF trained [A].[15]

---

### EBM

Systematic reviews of randomized, controlled trials show that:

- prolonged breastfeeding is not more prevalent in women who perform the first feed within 30 minutes of birth;
- support from a professional person increases the likelihood of a woman exclusively breastfeeding;
- the treatment of choice for breast engorgement is an anti-inflammatory agent.

There are few randomized, controlled trials on the management of the other breast pathologies mentioned above, with most evidence coming from cohort or retrospective studies.

---

### KEY POINTS

- Breastfeeding is beneficial to both mother and infant.
- A high proportion of women never commence breastfeeding and, of those who do, fewer than half will still be breastfeeding at six months.
- Women with obstructive and infective mastitis should continue to breastfeed.
- Women with breast abscesses should discontinue breastfeeding and will require needle aspiration or surgical drainage.

## Key References

1. Department of Health. *Our Healthier Nation.* London: HMSO, 1998.
2. World Health Organization. Global Strategy for Infant and Young Child Feeding. 2003. Available from: ‹www.who.int/nutrition/publications/infantfeeding/en/index.html›.
3. The infant feeding survey 2005. The information Centre 2007. Available from: ‹www.ic.nhs.uk/statistics-and-data-collections/health-and-lifestyles-related-surveys/infant-feeding-survey/infant-feeding-survey-2005›.
4. Inch S, Renfrew MJ. Common breastfeeding problems. In: Iain Chalmers I, Enkin M, Keirse MJNC (eds). *Effective Care in Pregnancy and Childbirth*, vol. 2. Oxford: Oxford University Press, 1989: 1375–89.
5. Moon JL, Humenick SS. Breast engorgement: contributing variables and variables amenable to nursing intervention. *J Obstet Gynecol Neonatal Nurs* 1989; **18**: 309–15.
6. Snowden HM, Renfrew MJ, Woolridge MW. Treatments for breast engorgement during lactation. *Cochrane Database Syst Rev* 2001; (**2**): CD000046.
7. Dener C, Inan A. Breast abscess in lactating women. *World J Surg* 2003; **27**: 130–3.
8. Berens PD. Prenatal, intrapartum and postpartum support of the lactating mother. *Paediatr Clin North Am* 2001; **48**: 365–75.
9. Thomsen AC, Hansen KB, Moller BR. Leukocyte counts and microbiologic cultivation in the diagnosis of puerperal mastitis. *Am J Obstet Gynecol* 1983; **146**: 938–41.
10. Thomsen AC, Espersen T, Maigaard S. Course and treatment of milk stasis, noninfectious inflammation of the breast, and infectious mastitis in nursing women. *Am J Obstet Gynecol* 1984; **149**: 492–5.
11. Benson EA. Management of breast abscesses. *World J Surg* 1989; **13**: 753–6.
12. Karstrup S, Solvia J, Nolose CP *et al.* Acute puerperal breast abscesses: US-guided drainage. *Radiology* 1993; **188**: 807–9.
13. Schwarz RJ, Shrestha R. Needle aspiration of breast abscess. *Am J Surg* 2001; **182**: 117–19.
14. Renfrew MJ, Lang S, Woolridge MW. Early versus delayed initiation of breastfeeding. Cochrane Database Syst Rev 2000; (**3**): CD000043.
15. Britton C, McCormick FM, Renfrew MJ *et al.* Support for breastfeeding mothers. *Cochrane Database Syst Rev* 2007; (**1**): CD001141.

# PART THREE

# Gynaecology

# SECTION A
## Reproductive medicine

# Normal and abnormal development of the genitalia

*Rebecca Deans, Catherine Minto and Sarah M Creighton*

## MRCOG standards

### Theoretical skills

- Revise your knowledge of the embryological development of the male and female urogenital system.
- Understand the situations in which a disruption in these pathways can lead to disorders of sex development, Müllerian anomalies and Wolffian duct remnants.
- Understand the classification of Müllerian anomalies.
- Know about first-line investigations for disorders of sex development and Müllerian anomalies and treatments available in tertiary referral centres.

### Practical skills

- Be able to take an appropriate history.
- Be able to initiate appropriate investigations to enable a diagnosis and/or tertiary referral.

## INTRODUCTION

Fetal development of the gonads, external genitalia, Müllerian ducts and Wolffian ducts can be disrupted at a variety of points, leading to a wide range of conditions with a large spectrum of clinical presentations. Disorders of sex development (DSD) occur when there is a disruption of either gonadal differentiation or fetal sex steroid production or action. Müllerian anomalies and Wolffian duct remnants occur when there is disruption of the embryological development of these systems. An understanding of embryology, as well as molecular genetics, helps us determine the biological basis of these conditions. Many of these cases present in infancy, with initial investigations and treatment performed by paediatric endocrinologists. Some will present for the first time to the gynaecologist and fertility subspecialist with primary amenorrhoea or infertility. Paediatric and urological surgeons may

have initially treated others. Patients with DSDs may have co-existing medical problems and require thorough evaluation. As well as anatomical and fertility concerns for these patients, there are often many psychological issues, therefore management in a multidisciplinary team (MDT) is essential for the management of more complex cases. In some conditions, the optimal operative management is still uncertain, and there is currently debate regarding the optimal timing or need for genital surgery in patients with DSD conditions who present in childhood.

## NORMAL EMBRYOLOGICAL DEVELOPMENT OF THE INTERNAL AND EXTERNAL GENITALIA

Genetic sex is determined at the moment of conception by the presence or absence of the Y chromosome, and after week 6 should guide the subsequent development of the fetus down one of two standard pathways – male or female. Until this time, development is the same in all fetuses. Primordial germ cells (the precursors of gametes) can be seen at 3 weeks in the endoderm of the yolk sac wall. During weeks 5 and 6, they migrate by amoeboid movement to the genital ridge (future gonad), an area of mesenchyme medial to the developing mesonephros and Wolffian (or mesonephric) duct. During week 6, primitive sex cords form around the germ cells in the indifferent gonad. The two Müllerian (or paramesonephric) ducts also appear lateral to the Wolffian ducts. At the same time, at the caudal end of the fetus, the cloacal membrane folds and is separated into the anterior urogenital and posterior anal parts. The urogenital section with the genital tubercle will become the future external genitalia, and by week 7 consists of a genital tubercle, urogenital membrane, urogenital folds and, more laterally, labioscrotal swellings. At the end of week 7, the urogenital membrane has degenerated and the urogenital sinus freely communicates with the amniotic fluid.

The first noticeable divergence in male and female fetuses is the differentiation of gonadal structure. The indifferent gonad has the potential for testicular or ovarian development. The presence of intact germ cells seems necessary for the ovary to develop, but this is not required for testicular development. The gonad remains undifferentiated until around 42 days. After gonadal differentiation has occurred, the presence or absence of gonadal hormone production and other fetal factors then guides the development of the Müllerian ducts, Wolffian ducts and external genitalia. Sertoli cells in the fetal testis secrete anti-Müllerian hormone (AMH – also called Müllerian inhibiting substance, MIS), leading to active regression of the Müllerian ducts, and early Leydig cells commence production of testosterone which acts through the androgen receptor on the Wolffian ducts, leading to the development of the vas deferens, seminal vesicle and epididymis. Testosterone is converted to its active metabolite dihydrotototestosterone (DHT). The fetal ovaries do not secrete androgen or AMH, and therefore there is female external genital development, growth of the Müllerian ducts and spontaneous regression of the Wolffian ducts.

## STANDARD MALE PATHWAY

In an XY fetus, activation of the SRY (sex-determining region of the Y chromosome) gene at the end of week 6 guides the indifferent gonad to commence development into a testis.[1] Other autosomal genes (e.g. WT1, SOX9, SF-1) are also involved in this genetic cascade.[2] The medullary sex cord cells become Sertoli cells, surrounding the primitive germ cells. At puberty, these will become the seminiferous tubules surrounding the spermatozoa. Sertoli cells produce AMH, which acts locally to cause apoptotic regression of the adjacent Müllerian ducts from 7 weeks. The appendix testis and prostatic utricle are usually all that remain of the Müllerian ducts in the male.

At around weeks 8–10, Leydig cells appear in the testis and start to secrete testosterone. The control of testosterone production may be independent initially, then under the control of placental human chorionic gonadotrophin (hCG) through the shared leutinizing hormone/hCG receptor (LHCRG), and subsequently by 20 weeks the hypothalamic pituitary (gonadotrope) axis becomes active and fetal leutinizing hormone (LH) production controls steroidogenesis. Testosterone acts through the androgen receptor and causes development of the Wolffian ducts into the vasa deferentia, and later the seminal vesicles and epididymides. Testosterone is also released into the circulation and undergoes peripheral conversion to its more active metabolite DHT by the enzyme 5α reductase type 2, and acts on the target tissues of the perineum resulting in development and growth of the genital tubercle, urogenital sinus, urogenital folds and labioscrotal swellings into the glans penis, penile shaft, urethral tube and scrotum, respectively. The penis is similar in size to the clitoris at 14 weeks and, under the influence of DHT,

continues growing until birth. Testicular descent is mediated by the Leydig cells under the influence of the hypothalamic pituitary (gonadotrope) axis and commences at 12 weeks, and is usually complete by week 34.

## STANDARD FEMALE PATHWAY

Traditionally, ovarian development in an XX fetus has been considered a 'default pathway', however, emerging research indicates that a distinct set of genes are expressed in the developing ovary required for maintaining ovarian integrity and actively opposing testicular development (DAX1, WNT4/RSPO1), termed 'anti-testis' genes.[3–5] These genes, in combination with the absence of the SRY gene, cause the indifferent gonad to commence ovarian differentiation at around week 7. The sex cord cells degenerate and secondary sex cords form and surround the primordial germ cells. Between 5 and 24 weeks, rapid mitotic expansion of primordial oogonia occurs, followed by first meiotic division (8–36 weeks), and subsequently meiotic arrest as primordial follicles. The presence of ovaries is not required for regression of the Wolffian ducts, and it is the absence of local testosterone that causes their regression at 10 weeks. The paroophoron, epoophoron and Gartner's cysts are all that may remain of the Wolffian ducts in the female. The absence of circulating testosterone also leads to an absence of peripheral DHT and directs the genital tubercle, urogenital sinus, urogenital folds and labioscrotal swellings to develop into the clitoris, lower vagina, labia minora and labia majora, respectively.

As AMH is not produced by the fetal ovary, the Müllerian ducts continue to develop. These paired mesodermal ducts originate in week 5, lateral to the Wolffian ducts at the third to fifth thoracic segment. They are thought to be associated with the basement membrane of the Wolffian ducts and grow caudally guided by them. The cranial ends of the Müllerian ducts are independent of the Wolffian ducts and remain separate as the Fallopian tubes. At the pelvis, the Müllerian ducts cross the Wolffian ducts anteriorly to lie medially next to each other. At weeks 8–10, the pelvic Müllerian ducts have fused and subsequent breakdown of their medial walls leads to a single tube, which will become the upper vagina, cervix and the uterine epithelium and glands. Surrounding mesenchymal tissue will become the myometrium and stroma. At their caudal end, the fused Müllerian ducts form the Müllerian tubercle, which connects with a thickened area of the urogenital sinus that develops into the paired sinovaginal bulbs. This connection of the endodermal urogenital sinus and mesodermal Müllerian ducts forms the vaginal plate – a column of squamous tissue. It remains unknown how much of each tissue (and possibly some of the Wolffian duct) contributes to this developing vagina. Over weeks 10–16, the vaginal plate enlarges and develops a cavity, which is separated from the urogenital sinus by an endodermal membrane. Gradual change of the lower Müllerian duct epithelium from columnar to stratified squamous epithelium occurs, ending at the future external cervical os. By month 5, the urethra and vagina are separated by a septum, and the endodermal membrane between the vagina and urogenital sinus breaks down to form the hymen. The urogenital sinus forms the vaginal vestibule.

## HUMAN SEX DEVEOPMENT

Human sex development can be divided into three main parts:

1   Chromosomal sex (presence of X and/or Y chromosome).
2   Gonadal sex (development of the gonad into either testis or ovary).
3   Phenotypic or anatomic sex (the appearance of the internal and external genitalia).

This differs from the concept of gender or 'brain sex', which encompasses gender identity which is one's self representation, gender role behaviour and sexual orientation. Occasionally, there is discordance between sex and gender, as well as the elements of gender. It is important to note that no single category dictates someone's sex, and it is important to consider all components of sex when managing the patient with DSD.

## KEY POINTS

- The *SRY* gene directs the gonad to become a testis.
- The absence of the *SRY* gene in combination with 'anti-testis' genes differentiate the gonad to the ovary.
- The presence or absence of androgen acting via androgen receptors determines external genital development.
- The presence of gonadal testosterone production leads to Wolffian duct differentiation into vas deferens, epididymis and seminal vesicle.
- The presence of gonadal AMH production leads to Müllerian duct regression.
- The absence of gonadal AMH production allows Müllerian duct differentiation into the upper vagina, cervix, uterine glands and epithelium and Fallopian tubes.
- The absence of gonadal testosterone production allows Wolffian duct regression.
- The genital and urinary system are closely associated and therefore abnormalities that occur in the Müllerian system commonly affect the renal system.
- Definition of sex encompasses chromosomal sex, gonadal sex, and phenotypic sex. Gender relates to psychosexual development.

## ABNORMAL EMBRYOLOGICAL DEVELOPMENT – DISORDERS OF SEX DEVELOPMENT

### Definition and classification

Over the last 20 years, there has been a significant increase in the understanding of the underlying aetiology of many forms of abnormal embryological development. Clinicians were becoming increasingly aware that traditional terms, such as intersex, true hermaphroditism, female pseudohermaphroditism and male pseudohermaphroditism, are confusing, inaccurate and often considered negative by the patients involved. Therefore, a consensus meeting was held in 2005, and one of the main elements to emerge was a new nomenclature system for this group of disorders, which is more generic, diagnostically accurate and less derogatory.[6–8] The term 'disorders of sex development' or DSD was established to describe congenital conditions with atypical development of chromosomal, gonadal or anatomic sex. This encompasses a blend of the physically defining features associated with males or females, i.e. karyotype, gonadal structure, internal genitalia and external genitalia, and covers a diverse range of conditions including individuals with standard male or female genitalia, who may have a variety of internal genital organs and karyotype, and also those with ambiguous external genitalia. In addition, an updated classification system was proposed (Table 46.1) which divides conditions into:

- sex chromosome DSD,
- 46XY DSD,
- 46XX DSD.

**Table 46.1** Updated nomenclature for disorders of sex development

| Terminology used previously | Proposed new terminology |
| --- | --- |
| Intersex | Disorders of Sex Development (DSD) |
| **Male pseudohermaphrodite** | |
| Undervirilization XY male | |
| Undermasculinization XY male | 46, XY DSD |
| **Female pseudohermaphrodite** | |
| Overvirilization of an XX female | |
| Masculinization of an XX female | 46, XX DSD |
| True hermaphrodite | Ovotesticular DSD |
| XX male or XX sex reversal | 46 XX testicular DSD |
| XY sex reversal | 46 XY complete gonadal dysgenesis |

- Adapted from Ref. 6, with permission.

Reproductive medicine

This new classification system also embodies a wider range of disorders, for instance sex chromosome DSD includes Turner syndrome (45X), and Kleinfelter syndrome (47XXY), which were not previously considered 'intersex' conditions. Similarly, female patients with congenital adrenal hyperplasia (CAH) who were traditionally considered to have an adrenal disease are now included as 46XX DSD due to the surgical and reproductive consequences associated with this disorder. Although there are a large number of DSD conditions, only the more common conditions have been considered in this chapter (Table 46.2).

With new knowledge concerning fetal sexual differentiation and development, greater awareness and understanding of female sexual function and a more patient-centred emphasis on condition management, it is hoped that patient care will be improved in this group of individuals. Although there are no randomized trials or even adequate long-term data to inform DSD condition management, currently expert opinion and a few small cohort studies and retrospective, uncontrolled trials form the basis of management.[9] Disclosure of important aspects of the patient's condition (karyotype, gonadal status, fertility potential) is essential.[10]

## Incidence

The incidence of DSD conditions in the UK is unknown. An estimate for the prevalence is one in 2000.[11] Conditions with autosomal recessive inheritance are more common in communities in which consanguinity is common.

## Aetiology

Most DSD conditions occur due to a genetic or environmental disruption to the pathway of fetal sexual development. This disruption can be to gonadal differentiation or development, sex steroid production, sex steroid conversion or tissue utilization of sex steroids.

## Presentation and investigation

Every DSD condition has a spectrum of severity and therefore may present in a variety of ways:

- ambiguous genitalia at birth;
- mismatch of fetal chromosomal results, such as amniocentesis or chorionic villus sample with phenotype at birth;

**Table 46.2** Key features of DSD conditions

| DSD condition | Karyotype | External genitalia | Internal genitalia | Special features |
|---|---|---|---|---|
| Congenital adrenal hyperplasia (CAH) | XX | Masculinized | Uterus and ovaries | Co-existing glucocorticoid (and sometimes also mineralocorticoid) deficiency requiring steroid replacement therapy |
| Complete androgen insensitivity syndrome (CAIS) | XY | Female | Testes | Absent pubic and axillary hair; at risk of osteoporosis; gonadal malignancy risk small until after 50 years of age |
| Swyer syndrome | XY | Female | Streak gonads and uterus | High risk of gonadal malignancy; poor breast development; normal axillary and pubic hair |
| 5-α-reductase deficiency | XY | Female or ambiguous at birth, masculinizing at puberty | Testes | In those with testes *in situ*, 60–80 per cent undergo change of gender from female to male at some point from late childhood onwards |
| 17-β-hydroxysteroid dehydrogenase – type 3 deficiency | XY | Variable; often female or ambiguous at birth, masculinizing at puberty | Testes | In those with testes *in situ*, 60–80 per cent undergo change of gender from female to male at some point from late childhood onwards |
| 46 XX/XY ovotesticular DSD | 71 per cent XX 20 per cent XX/XY 7 per cent XY 2 per cent other | Often ambiguous | Mix of ovary and/or testis and/or ovotestes; uterus or male ducts | Fertility described as both males fathering a child and females carrying a pregnancy |

- salt-losing crisis in neonatal life (congenital adrenal hyperplasia);
- sibling history of intersex;
- ambiguity of the genitalia developing in childhood or puberty;
- inguinal hernia with unexpected gonad;
- pelvic mass with gonadal tumour;
- primary amenorrhoea or pubertal delay;
- infertility;
- sexual dysfunction;
- part of a syndrome with other anomalies (e.g. renal anomalies in Denys–Drash syndrome).

Initial investigation will depend on presentation, but should include karyotype, testosterone, LH, follicle-stimulating hormone (FSH), 17-hydroxyprogesterone and pelvic ultrasound scan. Further investigation will depend on initial findings, external genital appearance and clinical presentation, and may include androstenedione, DHT, oestradiol, 24-hour urinary collection for steroid metabolites, hCG stimulation test, synacthen test, renal ultrasound scan, magnetic resonance imaging (MRI) and DNA for genetic testing.

## Management

The areas to consider in intersex management are:

- accurate diagnosis,
- need for hormone replacement therapy,
- screening for associated medical conditions,
- provision of condition information,
- psychological treatments,
- disclosure of diagnosis,
- genetic counselling for other family members,
- sex assignment for children,
- gonadal malignancy risk,
- fertility options,
- genital surgery options for ambiguous genitalia,
- vaginal enlargement options,
- access to peer support.

Accurate diagnosis at presentation is essential, and referral to an appropriate paediatric or adult multidisciplinary DSD service (endocrinology, gynaecology, surgery and psychology expertise), where available, is ideal. Individuals with different DSD conditions may require specific medical and surgical treatments; however, all should have access to experienced clinical psychologists and peer support via the relevant national support organizations. Over the past decade, a major shift in management has been the recognition that all patients have a right to information concerning their condition details, and the provision of this information and the options available need sensitive communication in a supported environment. Ideally, this should be with the expertise of a trained clinical psychologist. It is no longer considered good practice to withhold condition

details from the patient.[8,10] There is no evidence other than clinical experience and ethical evaluation on which to base this management, as there have been no studies evaluating long-term psychological outcomes with concealed or revealed diagnosis information; however, it is considered that disclosure should be planned with the opportunity for ongoing dialogue,[12] and in general disclosure is associated with enhanced psychosocial adaptation.[10] Gonadal malignancy and fertility options vary with the different DSD conditions.[8]

Cases presenting at birth or in childhood may be seen by a paediatric gynaecologist as part of a DSD team, but more often will be under the care of a paediatric endocrinologist, paediatric surgeon or paediatric urologist. The majority of these cases will have presented due to ambiguous genitalia. After thorough evaluation and diagnosis, sex of rearing is assigned and cosmetic genital surgery is considered where relevant. Currently, many neonates with ambiguous genitalia are assigned as females. The rationale for early feminizing genital surgery for the more severely virilized cases includes relative technical ease of surgery, negating the need to disclose the disorder with patient, and an assumed 'one stage' procedure with the theoretical aim of initially aiding parental acceptance of the child's assigned gender, and later improving the psychological outcomes for the child.[13,14] All of the indications for genital surgery are now being re-evaluated, and current management based upon clinical audits and vocal adult patient support groups have led to recommendations to delay unnecessary genital surgery till an age of informed consent, and to individualize care.[8] At present, it remains unknown whether infant genital surgery has an effect on parental acceptance of assigned gender or on later psychological outcomes for the child. Small cohort studies suggest that the majority of infants undergoing genital surgery will require repeat genital treatment (surgery or vaginal dilatation therapy) at or after puberty, mainly for vaginal introital stenosis but also for cosmesis.[15,16] Sexual function following feminizing genital surgery suggest that women's sexual and reproductive outcomes are impaired.[17] Small observational studies of adults who had undergone clitoral reduction surgery in childhood have suggested that orgasm is reduced[14,18,19] and that genital surgery may contribute to adult sexual dysfunction.[20–22]

Gynaecologists are more often involved in the care of the older child developing ambiguous genitalia at puberty, or in follow up of adults who underwent feminizing genital surgery as children. In many subjects born with ambiguous genitalia, there will be vaginal hypoplasia or agenesis, and the gynaecologist will need to discuss the treatment options at the appropriate time. Where childhood surgery has been performed, there is a strong possibility that repeat surgery may be required for vaginal stenosis, hypoplasia or genital cosmesis. This treatment is indicated to improve psychological and sexual outcomes; however, there have been no studies to provide evidence that improvements in these outcomes are achieved.

Enlargement procedures for vaginal hypoplasia include self-dilatation therapy or surgical vaginoplasty. These interventions are offered to improve psychological and sexual outcomes. There is disagreement about both the optimal timing and the intervention to use; however, it is recommended that these should be performed during or after adolescence.[8,23] There is a consensus now that vaginal dilatation therapy is the treatment of choice for vaginal hypoplasia due to the absence of surgical risk, including the later risk of malignancy in vaginal graft material. In a retrospective study, the success of dilators were as high as 86 per cent for achieving normal vaginal length, and 81 per cent of patients were able to have intercourse free of pain,[24] but success depends on the motivation of the patient, and the appropriate time to start treatment must be individualised. Concomitant psychological support may improve outcomes. The surgical vaginoplasty method depends on the genital configuration and surgeon's expertise. In some cases, the aim of vaginoplasty is to open up the lower vagina, with the upper vagina being normally developed. A pull-through vaginoplasty with complete separation of the vagina from the urethra may be required where the vagina does not reach the perineum but instead has joined the urethra near to the bladder, forming a single urogenital perineal opening (the high confluence vagina). In conditions in which the entire vagina is hypoplastic or absent, there are many vaginoplasty techniques: laparoscopic tension via an external traction device, peritoneal grafting, amnion grafting, skin grafting, bowel grafting, muscle flaps, labial expansion flaps, etc. Each method has different risks and benefits. The surgical risks include malignancy (in graft material), contracture leading to introital stenosis or loss of vaginal length, vaginal prolapse, dry vagina or excessive vaginal discharge.

## EBM: Genital surgery for ambiguous genitalia

- There is only minimal evidence to inform management.
- There have been few studies of psychological outcomes after childhood clitoral and genital surgery.
- Cohort studies include beneficial effects of surgery and minimizing families concerns and distress.[14,15]
- Cohort studies suggest the cosmetic and anatomical outcomes of vaginal and clitoral childhood surgery may be poor.[15]
- Control-matched cohort studies of adult female sexual function suggest that childhood cosmetic clitoral surgery impairs sexual function but does not prevent orgasm.[14,18,19]

## EBM: Vaginal enlargement procedures for vaginal agenesis or hypoplasia

- The treatment of choice is dilator therapy and should be first line in the absence of previous surgery.
- Vaginal dilator therapy should be reserved for adolescent and adult patients and avoided in children.
- Studies suggest that vaginal enlargement self-dilatation therapy is successful in up to 86 per cent of cases.[24,25]
- Studies show that childhood vaginal enlargement surgery may require revision in up to 90 per cent of cases.[15,16]
- There are no randomized, controlled trials of the outcomes of different vaginoplasty techniques.
- Retrospective uncontrolled studies have not shown one method of vaginoplasty surgery to have superior results to another method.

## 46 XX DSD – ABNORMAL EMBRYOLOGICAL DEVELOPMENT OF THE MÜLLERIAN DUCTS AND PERSISTENCE OF WOLFFIAN STRUCTURES

Abnormal development of the Müllerian ducts can lead to a wide range of conditions. Many are subtle variations of normal Müllerian anatomy, and often remain asymptomatic or require no treatment. Others are transverse or longitudinal structural abnormalities or agenesis of parts of the Müllerian ducts, and may present to the gynaecologist in a variety of ways. An understanding of the timing and sequence of embryological development of the entire urogenital system helps in understanding the range of conditions that occur. Occasionally, Müllerian anomalies may be associated with other conditions such as renal or spinal abnormalities or, more rarely, developmental defects of the cloaca such as bladder exstrophy, cloacal anomalies or anorectal anomalies. Ovarian development is independent of Müllerian duct development. Also considered in this section are lower transverse vaginal septae and the imperforate hymen (which derive from the urogenital sinus endoderm) and persistence of Wolffian duct remnants.

### Müllerian anomalies

#### Definitions

There have been many attempts to classify Müllerian abnormalities, and the American Fertility Society classification is the most widely used (Figure 46.1). Congenital Müllerian abnormalities generally fall into one of three

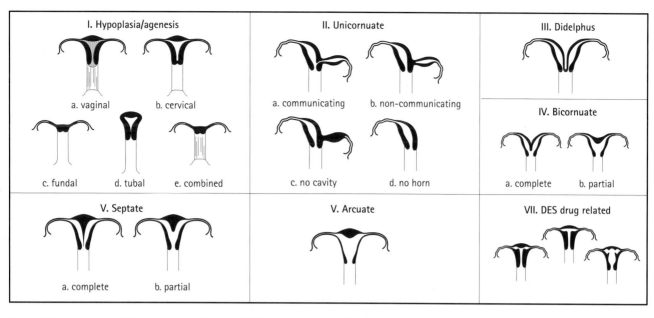

**Figure 46.1** American Fertility Society classification of Müllerian anomalies. (From The American Fertility Society classifications of adnexal adhesions, distal tubal occlusion, tubal occlusion secondary to tubal ligation, tubal pregnancies, Müllerian anomalies and intrauterine adhesions. *Fertil Steril* 1988; *49*: 944–55.) Reproduced with permission of the American Society for Reproductive Medicine. DES, diethylstilbestrol

groups: normally fused single Müllerian system with agenesis of one or more parts; unicornuate systems (unilateral hypoplasia or agenesis of one Müllerian duct); or lateral fusion failures (including didelphic and bicornuate anomalies). Rokitansky syndrome (agenesis of the uterus and vagina) is considered separately later in this section.

## Incidence

The prevalence is thought to be 0.5 per cent in the female population.[26] The incidence in women with infertility is substantially higher. The most common are septate and bicornuate anomalies.

## Aetiology

The cause of Müllerian anomalies is unknown; they may be due to genetic errors, teratogenic events, or a combination of these. Only a minority of cases appear to have a family history. It is assumed that there has been failure of fusion of the two Müllerian ducts, failure of one or both ducts to develop, or failure of resorption of the areas of Müllerian duct fusion. The causes of transverse vaginal septae are unknown.

## Presentation and investigation

The spectrum of anomalies is wide and around 75 per cent of these women will remain asymptomatic. The remaining 25 per cent will present in a variety of ways. Secondary sexual development is normal as ovarian development and function are independent of Müllerian duct and urogenital sinus growth.

### Presentation of Müllerian anomalies

- primary amenorrhoea;
- cyclical abdominal pain (obstruction to menstruation);
- severe dysmenorrhoea (obstruction to menstrual drainage from one Müllerian duct, e.g. the non-communicating rudimentary horn associated with a unicornuate uterus);
- pelvic mass – haematocolpos (vagina distended with menstrual blood) or haematometra (uterus distended with menstrual blood);
- menorrhagia;
- dyspareunia (transverse or longitudinal vaginal septae);
- infertility and recurrent miscarriage;
- ectopic pregnancy;
- obstetric complications, e.g. preterm birth, abnormal lie and uterine rupture.

### Investigation of Müllerian anomalies

This includes an assessment of the internal and external uterine contours. Ultrasound, MRI and hysterosalpingogram are often used, sometimes in association with laparoscopy or hysteroscopy. Imaging of the renal tract is also indicated.

## Management

Management of these anomalies depends on the type of anomaly and the presenting features. Symptomatic uterine and longitudinal vaginal septae can be resected hysteroscopically. The horns of a bicornuate uterus can be joined together into one cavity by an abdominal metroplasty. Any form of obstruction to menstrual flow requires surgery to relieve the obstruction and prevent pain and endometriosis. The didelphic uterus is often associated with vaginal septae that can lead to unilateral obstruction and requires careful vaginal surgery to remove the septum. Transverse vaginal septae can be of varying thicknesses, and complete removal is essential to try to prevent a stenotic ring at the site of surgery. For thick transverse vaginal septae, a combined abdomino-perineal procedure is often required.

The hymen usually opens after the fifth month of fetal life. An imperforate hymen presents either in neonatal life with a mucocolpos or at puberty with haematocolpos. A purple-blue bulge at the introitus associated with primary amenorrhoea is diagnostic. Surgery to create an adequate window for vaginal drainage cures the problem.

## Rokitansky syndrome (also called Mayer–Rokitansky–Kuster–Hauser (MRKH) syndrome)

### Definition and incidence

This condition is agenesis or hypoplasia of the vagina and uterus. The uterus is either absent or consists of a small central rudimentary uterine bud or bilateral uterine buds on the pelvic side walls. The incidence in the UK is estimated as between one in 4000 and one in 6000 females.

The aetiology remains unknown. The control mechanisms leading to Müllerian duct regression in males and Müllerian duct survival and growth in females are not well defined.

### Presentation and management

The usual presentation is primary amenorrhoea with normal secondary sex characteristics. Occasionally, the condition is identified in childhood. Investigation is as standard for primary amenorrhoea, and should exclude intersex conditions and include renal tract imaging due to the 30–40 per cent incidence of associated renal anomalies.

Management needs to encompass both psychological interventions, to help with aspects such as accepting the diagnosis, living with the condition, forming relationships and improving sexual function and quality of life outcomes, and interventions that can be used to enlarge or create the vagina. The aim of vaginal enlargement techniques (both surgical vaginoplasty and self-applied vaginal dilatation therapy) is to improve sexual function; however, there have been no studies to assess the effectiveness of these interventions on this outcome. Vaginoplasty surgery and dilators should not be used in childhood. Uterine transplant is not an option for the foreseeable future, although tissue engineering techniques may eventually provide new treatment options. As ovarian function is normal, fertility is possible via surrogacy.

## Incomplete regression of the Wolffian system

Parts of the Wolffian duct may fail to regress completely in females, presenting as cysts lateral to the Müllerian duct. Usually these are incidental findings and most are asymptomatic, although they can grow to be large. The epoophoron and paraoophoron can be found beside the ovary in the mesosalpinx. Gartner's duct (the lower part of the Wolffian duct) cysts can occur anywhere from the broad ligament down to the vagina, and may present as vulval or vaginal masses. Wolffian remnants are also seen in the cervix. Very rarely, the Wolffian system may persist as the primitive mesonephric system draining functioning glomeruli, and an extra ureter can be found emptying into the vagina.

### KEY POINTS

- Abnormalities of the Müllerian system are asymptomatic in 75 per cent of women.
- Imaging of the renal tract should be performed whenever abnormalities of the Müllerian system are found.
- This condition should be considered high on the list of differential diagnosis in patients presenting with painless amenorrhoea, and normal secondary sexual development.

## 46XX DSD – Congenital adrenal hyperplasia

This condition occurs in an XX fetus due to an enzyme deficiency (usually 21 hydroxylase) in the adrenal gland. The XX fetus proceeds down the female development pathway, with ovarian formation and development of the Müllerian ducts into uterus, cervix and upper vagina. Owing to the adrenal enzyme deficiency, cortisone production is deficient, and so the adrenal gland undergoes hyperplasia to try to produce sufficient cortisol. A byproduct of this survival mechanism is the production of large quantities of androgens. These high circulating androgen levels lead to masculinizing effects at the external genitalia, and ambiguous genitalia or normal-looking male genitalia at birth.

This is one of the most common DSD conditions, with a UK population prevalence estimated at one in 10 000, of whom half are female. It is the only DSD condition that can be life threatening, as unrecognized cortisol deficiency can lead to a salt-wasting crisis in the neonate. Management aims to correct the cortisol deficiency and excess androgen production. Gender assignment at birth is usually female due to the presence of ovaries and uterus with fertility potential. Genital surgery to cosmetically feminize the appearance has been standard practice in the past, although there is now controversy concerning the benefits and risks of this procedure.[8] Adolescents and adults considering surgery to reduce the size of the clitoris, for cosmetic concerns or due to pain during sexual intercourse, are counselled that the actual risk of damage to clitoral orgasm is unknown, but is estimated at 20–25 per cent. At puberty, a review of the vagina is necessary to identify obstruction, stenosis or hypoplasia.

## Other causes of XX fetal virilization

In a manner similar to that of congenital adrenal hyperplasia, other exogenous causes of androgens (e.g. maternal androgen-secreting tumours or the use of virilizing drugs such as danazol in pregnancy) may rarely lead to masculinizing of the external genitalia in an XX fetus.

## 46XY DSD – Androgen receptor defects - Complete androgen insensitivity syndrome

Androgen insensitivity syndrome (CAIS) occurs due to the complete inability of the body to respond androgens. The cause is a disruption of the androgen receptor gene on the long arm of the X chromosome. Previously the condition was called testicular feminization, due to the erroneous assumption that the testes must be producing a feminizing factor. In this condition, an XY fetus proceeds initially down the pathway of male fetal sexual determination. The SRY gene leads to normal testicular development, and both AMH and testosterone are normally produced. The AMH ensures regression of the Müllerian duct; however, due to the lack of ability of all body cells to respond to androgen, female external genitalia develop and female central nervous system organization occurs. The result is an XY female with absent Müllerian structures, normal female genitalia, variable vaginal hypoplasia, absent or sparce pubic and axillary hair, normal breast development, normal female behaviour and gender identity and intra-abdominal testes that produce high levels of circulating testosterone.

Androgen insensitivity syndrome can also occur as a partial form (partial androgen insensitivity syndrome, PAIS) in which some response to androgens occurs. The aetiology of this condition is less well understood, although some cases have a disruption in the androgen receptor gene allowing some function. Presentation is a spectrum from ambiguous genitalia to a normal male phenotype with infertility. For those cases identified in early infancy, assignment of sex of rearing is difficult, with no data concerning outcome. Future sexual function as male or female is unknown, with physical growth of the genitalia being unpredictable and a lack of scientific knowledge about how sexual orientation and gender identity develop. It is likely that both male- and female-type behaviours and gender identity are at least partly pre-programmed by the fetal sex steroid environment, and in PAIS the fetal sex steroid environment is unknown.

## 46 XY DSD – Gonadal dysgenesis

In this condition (also known as Swyer syndrome), disruption at the very start of the male sex determination pathway causes an XY fetus to divert to the female development pathway. In 15–30 per cent of cases, the fault lies with the SRY gene, and gonadal testicular differentiation does not occur. In the remaining cases, disruption of other testis-determining genes is assumed to be the cause. In the absence of SRY activation, ovarian determination probably occurs, but cannot be sustained due to the lack of a second X chromosome. The result is a dysgenetic (abnormally formed) streak gonad. As this gonad produces neither AMH nor testosterone, the external genital development is female and the Müllerian ducts develop into the vagina, uterus and cervix.

The streak gonad again fails to produce hormones at puberty, leading to the usual clinical presentation of primary amenorrhoea with poor breast development. In contrast to CAIS, these women have normal pubic and axillary hair and the presence of a normal uterus. Investigation will show raised gonadotrophins and low testosterone and oestradiol levels. Menstruation usually commences with hormone replacement therapy (oestrogen and progesterone are necessary), and pregnancy is possible with donor oocytes. Gonadectomy is recommended due to the high malignancy risk of dysgenetic gonads.

Other forms of XY gonadal dysgenesis that can lead to DSD conditions are less well understood. Partial gonadal dysgenesis with some testicular function, and mixed gonadal dysgenesis (a unilateral testis and a contralateral streak gonad) are conditions that usually present with variable degrees of genital masculinization or ambiguity. Regression of each Müllerian duct depends on the local concentration of AMH produced by the fetal gonad on each side, and unilateral uterine development can occur if one gonad is more dysgenetic and hence produces less AMH than the contralateral gonad (see Chapter 47, Karyotypic abnormalities).

## 46XY DSD – Androgen biosynthetic defects (5-Alpha-reductase type 2 deficiency and 17-beta-hydroxysteroid dehydrogenase type 3 deficiency)

These conditions may present in a similar fashion with genital ambiguity at birth. In the past, most cases were assigned to a female sex of rearing; however, this management is currently under review and now each case is individually considered.[8] Both are autosomal recessive conditions in which an XY fetus initially starts down the male development pathway with normal testis development. However, there is a deficiency of enzymes involved in androgen synthesis, leading to mainly female external genital development. If left untreated in childhood, both conditions will result in increasing masculinization at puberty, and possibly a change in gender identity from female to male for some individuals. 5-Alpha-reductase-type 2 is the enzyme responsible for the peripheral conversion of testosterone to the more potent androgen DHT required for fetal genital masculinization. 17-Beta-hydroxysteroid dehydrogenase type 3 is the gonadal enzyme needed for the final step in testosterone production in the fetal testis, i.e. conversion of androstenedione to testosterone. Each of these enzymes has more than one isoenzyme, and it is likely that activation of other isoenzymes is responsible for the virilization seen at puberty.

Clinical presentation of both these conditions is usually mild ambiguity of the genitalia (clitoromegaly) at birth or early childhood in an XY female. However, the presentation can be variable, and a number of these patients will present to a gynaecologist with virilization at puberty. Müllerian structures are absent and Wolffian structures are present. The testes are intra-abdominal in childhood, and often descend to the inguinal canal or labioscrotal folds after puberty. Without childhood intervention, secondary sexual development is usually masculine, with poor breast development and normal pubic and axillary hair. The incidence of these conditions is unknown, but with the new scientific knowledge of these enzymes over the past decade, 17-beta-hydroxysteroid dehydrogenase type 3 deficiency is now being diagnosed in some cases previously labelled as CAIS. In cases diagnosed in childhood, the management and assignment of gender are difficult. There have been insufficient cohorts raised as either males or females from childhood to evaluate the outcomes of adult gender identity, sexual function, psychological outcomes and quality of life. Fertility may be possible as a male, although infertility is common. Diagnosis is by DNA serum samples, and urinary steroid profile (either 24 hour or spot sample).

## 46 XX/46 XY DSD

This condition is defined by the presence of both ovarian tissue with Gräafian follicles and testicular tissue containing distinct tubules in one person. It is said to be the rarest DSD condition, but has a higher prevalence in some areas, such as Africa. The gonads can be any mix of ovary, testes and ovotestes. The aetiology is unknown.

Most cases present with ambiguous genitalia, although clinical presentation is very variable. The degree of genital masculinization is thought to be a reflection of the amount of functional testicular tissue. The spectrum of internal genital development is influenced by the composition of the adjacent gonad, with up to 80 per cent having internal female organs and therefore being potentially fertile. The karyotype is 46XX in the majority, with a smaller proportion having a mosaic XX/XY karyotype, and only a minority having a 46XY karyotype. At present, there are insufficient data from cohort studies to advise on optimal management in terms of gender assignment in childhood.

# Key References

1. Harley VR, Clarkson MJ, Argentaro A. The molecular action and regulation of the testis-determining factors, SRY (sex-determining region of the Y chromosome) and SOX9 [SRY-related high-mobility group (HMG) box 9]. *Endocr Rev* 2003; **24**: 466–87.

2. Warne GL, Zajac JD. Disorders of sexual differentiation. *Endocrinol Metab Clin North Am* 1998; **27**: 945–67.

3. Nef S, Schaad O, Stallings NR *et al.* Gene expression during sex determination reveals a robust female genetic program at the onset of ovarian development. *Dev Biol* 2005; **287**: 361–7.

4. Beverdam A, Koopman P. Expression profiling of purified mouse gonadal somatic cells during the critical time window of sex determination reveals novel candidate genes for human sexual dysgenesis syndromes. *Hum Mol Genet* 2006; **15**: 417–31.

5. Parma P, Radi O, Vidal V *et al.* R-spondin1 is essential in sex determination, skin differentiation and malignancy. *Nat Genet* 2006; **38**: 1304–9.

6. Hughes IA, Houk C, Ahmed SF, Lee PA. LWPES Consensus Group; ESPE Consensus Group. Consensus statement on management of intersex conditions. *Arch Dis Child* 2006; **91**: 554–63.

7. Lee PA, Houk CP, Ahmed SF, Hughes IA. Writing Group for the International Intersex Consensus Conference. *Pediatrics* 2006; **118**: 753–7.

8. Houk CP, Hughes IA, Ahmed SF, Lee PA. Summary of consensus statement on intersex disorders and their management. *Pediatrics* 2006; **118**: 753–7.

9. Creighton S, Minto C. Managing intersex. *BMJ* 2001; **323**: 1264–5.

10. Liao LM, Green H, Creighton SM, Conway GS. Patient experiences in obtaining and giving information about disorders of sex development. *Br J Obstet Gynaecol* 2010; **117**: 193–9.

11. Blackless M, Charuvastra A, Derryck A *et al.* How sexually dimorphic are we? Review and synthesis. *Am J Hum Biol* 2000; **12**: 151–66.

12. Carmichael P, Ransley P. Telling children about a physical intersex condition. *Dialogues Pediatr Urol* 2002; **25**: 7–8.

13. Warne G, Grover S, Hutson J *et al.* A long-term outcome study of intersex conditions. *J Pediatr Endocrinol Metab* 2005; **18**: 555–67.

14. Crouch NS, Minto CL, Liao LM *et al.* Sexual function and genital sensation after feminizing genitoplasty for congenital adrenal hyperplasia: a pilot study. *BJU Int* 2004; **93**: 135–8.

15. Creighton SM, Minto CL, Steele SJ. Objective cosmetic and anatomical outcomes at adolescence of feminising surgery for ambiguous genitalia done in childhood. *Lancet* 2001; **358**: 124–5.

16. Alizai NK, Thomas DFM, Lilford RJ *et al.* Feminizing genitoplasty for congenital adrenal hyperplasia: what happens at puberty? *J Urol* 1999; **161**: 1588.

17. Gastraud F, Bouvattier C, Duranteau L *et al.* Impaired sexual and reproductive outcomes in women with classical forms of congenital adrenal hyperplasia. *J Clin End Metab* 2007; **92**: 1391–6.

18. Randolph J, Hung W, Rathlev MC. Clitoroplasty for females born with ambiguous genitalia: a long-term study of 37 patients. *J Pediatr Surg* 1981; **16**: 882–7.

19. Newman K, Randolph J, Parson S. Functional results in young women having clitoral reconstruction as infants. *J Pediatr Surg* 1992; **27**: 180–83.

20. May B, Boyle M, Grant D. A comparative study of sexual experiences. *J Health Psychol* 1996; **1**: 479–92.

21. Dittmann RW, Kappes ME, Kappes MH. Sexual behavior in adolescent and adult females with congenital adrenal hyperplasia. *Psychoneuroendocrinology* 1992; **17**: 153–70.

22. Nordenskold A, Holmdahl G, Frisen L *et al.* Type of mutation and surgical procedure affect long term quality of life for women with congenital adrenal hyperplasia. *J Clin Endocrinol Metab* 2008; **93**: 380–86.

23. Statement of the British Association of Paediatric Surgeons Working Party on the Surgical Management of Children Born with Ambiguous Genitalia, July 2001. Available at ⟨http://www.baps.org.uk/⟩.

24. Ismail-Pratt IS, Bikoo M, Liao LM *et al.* Normalisation of the vagina by dilator treatment alone in Complete Androgen Insensitivity Syndrome and Mayer-Rokitansky-Kuster-Hauser Syndrome. *Hum Reprod* 2007; **22**: 2020–24.

25. Robson S, Oliver GD. Management of vaginal agenesis: review of 10 years practice at a tertiary referral centre. *Aust NZ J Obstet Gynaecol* 2000; **40**: 430–33.

26. Nahum GG. Uterine anomalies. How common are they and what is their distribution among subtypes? *J Reprod Med 1998*; **43**: 877–87.

# Karyotypic abnormalities

*Diana Fothergill*

## INTRODUCTION

There are a number of karyotypic abnormalities that may present to the gynaecologist with an initial complaint of primary amenorrhoea. Others will have been diagnosed in childhood but are referred on for further management by paediatricians and endocrinologists. Some karyotypic abnormalities have little impact on gynaecological problems, but those affecting the sex chromosomes are covered briefly. This is a rapidly changing field of medicine, and more sophisticated tests can lead to refinements in original diagnoses, so it may be appropriate to repeat genetic investigations or to test other cell lines.

## TURNER SYNDROME (45X AND MOSAICS)

This is the most common abnormality in females involving the sex chromosomes: 1 in 2500 live-born girls are affected, although most pregnancies with this abnormality are miscarried, probably secondary to major cardiac defects. It is estimated that 15 per cent of all miscarriages have a 45X karyotype. The incidence does not rise with increasing maternal age, but screening early pregnancies for increased nuchal thickness has led to more cases being diagnosed antenatally, as cystic hygroma and non-immune hydrops

are frequently features of Turner syndrome. Over half of these girls will have some form of mosaicism. The rate of detection is partly dependent on how hard it is looked for, as the cell lines may vary in different tissues.[1] If Turner syndrome is clinically suspected but the blood karyotype is normal, it is advisable to check a second tissue such as a skin biopsy.

Over two-thirds of Turner syndrome cases result from loss of a paternal sex chromosome; in some there are fragments of a sex chromosome still present. If this is a Y chromosome, there is a 7–10 per cent risk of gonadoblastoma development, and gonadectomy is usually advised.[2] If this has not been performed, regular ultrasound examination of the gonad may be prudent.

### Physical abnormalities associated with Turner syndrome

- Growth failure: low birth weight and short stature.
- Ovarian failure: no secondary sexual development in most cases, occasionally secondary amenorrhoea in mosaics.
- Inverted, widely spaced nipples, shield chest.
- Webbed neck.
- Puffy hands and feet in babies due to lymphoedema.
- Low hairline.
- Cubitus valgus.
- High, arched palate, micrognathia and defective dental development.
- Renal dysgenesis.
- Cardiac malformations, including coarctation of the aorta.
- Distortion of the Eustachian tube leading to otitis media.
- Nail dysplasia.
- Eye deformities.

Intelligence is usually normal, but there is an increased risk of impairment of nonverbal skills, for example maths and visuospatial.[3] The phenotypic abnormalities result in most cases being diagnosed in infancy and childhood. The girls are then usually referred to a gynaecologist after optimal growth potential has been achieved using growth hormone, for advice about long-term hormone replacement therapy (HRT). In most girls, ovarian failure has occurred early in life; although they have a uterus and vagina, they will not develop any secondary sexual characteristics without hormonal supplements. A low dose of oestrogen is given initially to encourage steady growth of the breasts; this is usually started after the age of 12 years, as the administration of oestrogen promotes epiphyseal fusion, which stops further growth. The dose of oestrogen is gradually increased over two years. The uterus will respond to oestrogen therapy, so after two years it is necessary to add progestogens cyclically to produce regular endometrial shedding, or in a continuous combined regime to suppress endometrial development. Hormonal therapy may be by the oral or transdermal route. Many girls are maintained on oral contraceptive preparations that have the benefit of being socially acceptable, as well as not incurring National Health Service (NHS) prescription charges. HRT should be continued until at least the age of 50 years.

There are a number of long-term health issues which affect women with Turner syndrome:

- hypertension,
- coarctation of the aorta – 11 per cent and bicuspid aortic valve – 16 per cent, which increase the incidence of dissecting aneurysm,
- diabetes – 25 per cent,
- hypothyroidism – 25–30 per cent,
- coeliac disease – 4–6 per cent,
- sensorineural hearing loss – 50 per cent,
- renal disease,
- eye problems – red green colour blindness in 8 per cent, and increased risk of amblyopia,
- osteoporosis.

Mortality in women with Turner syndrome is 3-fold higher than in the general population.[4] The gynaecologist may be the only point of regular medical contact and needs to be aware of these issues, particularly when pregnancy is desired. A full cardiological assessment is advisable before referral to an assisted conception unit for counselling about treatment with donor oocytes.[5] Clinical pregnancy rates are reported to be comparable to those of other women with primary ovarian failure (up to 46 per cent per embryo transfer), but miscarriage rates are higher.[6] There is an increased risk of complications including diabetes and hypertension in the pregnancy, and delivery by caesarean section may be required because of the woman's short stature. Spontaneous conceptions have been reported, usually in women with mosaicism or structural abnormalities of the X chromosome which have led to short stature, but whose ovaries have been preserved. These pregnancies have a high rate of miscarriage and malformation, resulting in a healthy child being born in less than 40 per cent of pregnancies.[7]

> ## EBM
>
> - There is little published evidence of the effects of long-term HRT in Turner women and on the optimal preparation to be used.
> - Oestrogen therapy has been shown to increase bone mineral density.

Patients with Noonan syndrome have a similar phenotypic appearance to Turner, but this is an autosomal dominant trait with no abnormality of the sex chromosomes and there is no effect on ovarian function.

## 47XXX

These girls are not often referred to gynaecologists, although 47XXX occurs in about one in 1000 live-born females. They may have genitourinary abnormalities but are of normal height, and sexual development occurs normally. Academic performance is usually below average. The ovaries often fail prematurely and women may present with secondary amenorrhoea and require HRT. Somewhat surprisingly, most women give birth to chromosomally normal children, but prenatal diagnosis should be considered.

## 48XXXX, 49XXXXX

Almost all girls with these karyotypes are of subnormal intelligence. Ovarian dysfunction is quite common.

## 46XY

Characteristically, this diagnosis is made when a phenotypically normal girl presents with primary amenorrhoea or delayed puberty. There are a variety of conditions that are associated with this karyotype, which are described more fully earlier in this section.

In androgen insensitivity syndrome, the problem lies with the end-organ response to testosterone. The testes are functional and Müllerian inhibition factor is produced, so the uterus and vagina do not develop. Breast development usually takes place as circulating testosterone is peripherally converted to oestrogen, but there is absent pubic hair due to the abnormal androgen receptors.

In Swyer syndrome, or pure gonadal dysgenesis, there is a lack of functional gonadal tissue and, as a consequence, Müllerian structures persist and a normal uterus and vagina are found. Breast development does not normally

Reproductive medicine

occur and typically girls present above average height with delayed puberty. Pubic and axillary hair may be present due to the effect of peripherally produced androgens. Treatment is similar to that for Turner syndrome, with oestrogen to develop the breasts and the addition of progestogens to cause withdrawal bleeds. Donor egg and embryo pregnancies have been reported.[8] Streak gonads may be present and there is concern that these have a high incidence of malignant change.[9]

# STRUCTURAL ABNORMALITIES OF THE X CHROMOSOME

There are many abnormalities that can occur in the X chromosome. The most common is an isochromosome for the long arm, most often found in mosaic form with 45X. Deletions of part of the long or short arm have variable effects depending on the level at which the deletion has occurred. If the short arm is missing, most girls will be of short stature; if the long arm is missing, there is usually gonadal dysgenesis. It is of interest to note that although one X chromosome is inactivated, it is necessary to have two normal X chromosomes to maintain fertility.

## KEY POINTS

- Karyotypic abnormalities are a common cause of primary amenorrhoea.
- HRT is required in all patients with ovarian failure.
- Ovum donation may be an option for fertility.
- Turner syndrome has long-term health implications.

## Key References

1. Ranke MB, Saenger P. Turner's syndrome. *Lancet* 2001; **358**: 309–14.
2. Gravholt CH, Fedder J, Naeraa RW, Muller J. Occurrence of gonadoblastoma in females with Turner syndrome and Y chromosome material: a population study. *J Clin Endocrinol Metab* 2000; **85**: 3199–202.
3. Bondy CA Care of girls and women with Turner syndrome: a guideline of the Turner syndrome study group. *J Clin Endocrinol Metab* 2007; **92**: 10–25.
4. Schoemaker MJ, Swerdlow AJ, Higgins CD *et al.* Mortality in women with Turner syndrome in Great Britain: a national cohort study. *J Clin Endocrinol Metab* 2008; **93**: 4735–42.
5. The Practice Committee of the American Society for Reproductive Medicine Increased maternal cardiovascular mortality associated with pregnancy in women with Turner syndrome. *Fertil Steril* 2005; **83**: 1074–5.
6. Foudila T, Soderstrom-Anttila V, Hovatta O. Turner's syndrome and pregnancies after oocyte donation. *Hum Reprod* 1999; **14**: 532–5.
7. Tarani L, Lampariello S, Raguso G *et al.* Pregnancy in patients with Turner's syndrome: six new cases and a review of literature. *Gynecol Endocrinol* 1999; **12**: 83–7.
8. Sauer MV, Lobo RA, Paulson RJ. Successful twin pregnancy after embryo donation to a patient with XY gonadal dysgenesis. *Am J Obstet Gynecol* 1989; **161**: 380–1.
9. Lukusa T, Fryns JP, Kleczkowska A *et al.* Role of gonadal dysgenesis in gonadoblastoma induction in 46,XY individuals. The Leuven experience in 46,XY pure gonadal dysgenesis and testicular feminization syndromes. *Genet Couns* 1991; **2**: 9–16.

# Menarche and adolescent gynaecology

*Diana Fothergill*

## MRCOG standards

### Theoretical skills

- Know the normal sequence of events in puberty to be able to recognize when investigation is appropriate.
- Know the causes of delayed puberty and how to establish the diagnosis.
- Know how the management of excessive menstruation differs from in adulthood.

### Practical skills

- Be able to assess the stage of development of secondary sexual characteristics.
- Have observed consultations with the girl and parent, and be able to obtain the history and counsel about management.

## INTRODUCTION

Puberty marks the change from childhood to adolescence, with the development of breasts and secondary sexual hair and the onset of menstruation. At the same time, there is a period of accelerated growth. The gynaecologist is most often consulted when these events are delayed. The paediatrician will see more cases of precocious puberty.

### Causes of precocious puberty

- Idiopathic.
- McCune Albright syndrome (café-au-lait spots and polyostotic fibrous dysplasia).
- Tumours of the adrenal or ovary producing steroids.
- Cerebral tumours.
- Ingestion of exogenous oestrogens.

The age at which the changes take place is variable, but it is abnormal for there to be no sign of secondary sexual development at the age of 14 years.

The trigger for the changes to start is an increasing frequency and amplitude of pulses of gonadotrophin release. The ovaries are then stimulated to begin to produce oestrogen, which acts on the breast tissue to promote growth. This usually begins at around the age of 9 and takes about five years to be completed. There is evidence to suggest that this is occurring at a younger age, particularly in African-American girls, prompting a reassessment of the age at which precocious puberty should be investigated.[1] Pubic hair growth is stimulated by androgens released by the ovary and the adrenal gland. Breast and pubic hair development is described in five stages following the classification by Marshall and Tanner (Table 48.1).[2] Growth charts indicate the range of normal ages at which these stages are attained. In most girls, breast development starts before the growth of pubic hair.

Even before these changes are obvious, there is acceleration of growth, which is frequently accompanied by a rapid increase in shoe size. The peak height velocity, of approximately 8 cm/year, occurs just before the onset of menses – on average around the age of 12 years. Oestrogen promotes closure of the epiphyses, so final height is usually attained about two years after menarche.

Menarche occurs 2.3 ± 1 years after the onset of breast development. The average age of menarche has declined and is now 12.52 years in white girls and 12.06 years in African-Americans.[3] The factors involved include improved nutrition and genetic influences: daughters often undergo menarche at a similar age to their mothers. Initial menstrual cycles are usually anovulatory and often irregular for several years.

## DELAYED PUBERTY

Most referrals to gynaecologists are because of concern about delay in the onset of menstruation. In order to determine the likely cause for this it is first important to establish whether puberty itself is delayed. A detailed history should be taken, asking about general health, the age at which breast and pubic hair development started, and if the girl has had a growth spurt or still appears to be growing. Any chronic illness may lead to constitutional delay in puberty. Teenage girls may

**Table 48.1** Marshall and Tanner staging

| Stage | Breast | Pubic hair |
|---|---|---|
| I | Pre-adolescent, elevation of papilla only | No pubic hair |
| II | Breast bud - elevation of breast and papilla as small mound; enlargement of areolar diameter | Sparse growth of long downy hair along the labia |
| III | Further enlargement but no separation of the contours | Hair coarser, darker and more curled; over mons |
| IV | Projection of the areola and papilla to form a secondary mound above the level of the breast | Adult-type hair but no spread to thighs |
| V | Mature; areola recessed to general contour of breast | Adult, with horizontal upper border and spread to thighs |

be reluctant to answer questions and the mother frequently gives much of the history, but it is important to address the girl rather than talking directly to the mother. Examination should include accurate measurement of height, together with assessment of the stage of breast and pubic hair development, and these should be plotted on growth charts. The examination should be sensitively performed – ask the girl if she wishes her mother to be present, as some feel more embarrassed with the mother there – and only expose one part of the body at a time. An internal examination should not be performed; inspection of the external genitalia is all that is necessary, as further assessment of the internal organs will be achieved by ultrasound scanning of the pelvis.

Investigations usually include:

- measurement of gonadotrophins – follicle-stimulating hormone (FSH) and luteinizing hormone (LH) – and oestrogen,
- karyotyping,
- ultrasound scan of the pelvis to confirm the presence of the uterus and ovaries,
- possibly x-ray to determine bone age.

Additional biochemical tests to assess thyroid function, prolactin and 17-α-hydroxyprogesterone may also be appropriate.

## ABSENT BREAST AND PUBIC HAIR

### Hypogonadotrophic hypogonadism

The majority of girls with low gonadotrophins have constitutional delay in puberty. This may be secondary to chronic illness, for example cystic fibrosis. Improvement in the underlying condition usually results in catch-up growth.

Girls with anorexia nervosa have low levels of gonadotrophins and, if the problem starts at a young age, will have absent or poorly developed secondary sexual characteristics. A similar situation is found in many athletic girls, the classic example being gymnasts, who have a low body weight and very low body fat. This can lead to the 'female athletic triad', with disordered eating, amenorrhoea and osteopenia, and an increased risk of stress fractures.[4]

Congenital deficiency of gonadotrophins is more rarely encountered; this problem is more often seen in boys with delayed puberty. It may also be associated with anosmia due to hypoplasia of the olfactory lobes, when it is known as Kallman's syndrome. Brain imaging will be necessary to establish this diagnosis.

Acquired deficiency may follow damage to the hypothalamus or pituitary as a result of trauma, tumour such as a craniopharyngioma, irradiation, or infection – frequently secondary to hydrocephalus. Infiltration of these organs can also occur in haemochromatosis, which may be secondary to transfusions for sickle cell disease or thalassaemia and to Wilson's disease.

In all these conditions, ultrasound will confirm the presence of an immature uterus and small, inactive ovaries. The bone age will help to differentiate cases of constitutional delay, as it will be behind chronological and height age.

Treatment may be required if there are no signs of spontaneous onset of puberty, although most girls with constitutional delay will proceed to normal development if left untreated. A study conducted on untreated girls indicated that they experienced considerable distress, which affected their success at school, work or socially; 50 per cent would have preferred to receive treatment.[5] Pulsatile gonadotrophins have been used but are very difficult to sustain as they require a subcutaneous injection attached to a portable pump for several months. The more widely used approach is to give low doses of ethinyl oestradiol 1–2 μg per day for 3–6 months. Frequently, spontaneous sexual maturation then occurs, but if not, the dose is gradually increased over several years.[6]

### Hypergonadotrophic hypogonadism

This occurs when there is failure of gonadal development. The normal release of gonadotrophins occurs, but as there is no response from the gonad, there is no negative feedback to control gonadotrophin levels. The most common cause is Turner syndrome (45X) or other genetic problems (see Chapter 47, Karyotypic abnormalities). Other causes include damage to the ovaries by irradiation, surgery, chemotherapy or infection. Galactosaemia is also associated with ovarian failure and its management presents a challenge as oral preparations of oestrogen and progesterone contain lactose. Autoimmune ovarian failure may be associated with other autoimmune disorders such as Addison's disease, vitiligo and hypothyroidism.

One of the less common causes of congenital adrenal hyperplasia is the deficiency of 17-α-hydroxylase. This enzyme is required to produce both oestrogen and testosterone, so virilization does not occur at birth, but there is also a failure of development of secondary sexual characteristics.

The treatment consists of gradually increasing levels of oestrogen replacement, combined with progesterone to induce withdrawal bleed once doses stimulate endometrial development.

## NORMAL BREAST AND PUBIC HAIR DEVELOPMENT

### Anatomical causes

If puberty has progressed normally but the girl has failed to menstruate, the most common cause is an anatomical abnormality. It is uncommon for girls with an imperforate hymen or transverse vaginal septum to present to an outpatient clinic; they usually present as an emergency with cyclical abdominal pain, possibly with a palpable abdominal mass. The blockage prevents the flow of menstrual blood and there is usually a tense blue bulge seen at the introitus. Ultrasound scanning may show a distended vagina containing blood, and normal ovaries. Where there is a thin imperforate hymen, treatment is straightforward, as incision will allow the blood to drain and the mass will resolve. Treatment of a thicker and possibly higher septum is more complex and is best dealt within a tertiary referral centre, as injudicious excision can result in stricture formation which is difficult to treat and will lead to considerable problems with intercourse.

The most common cause is Müllerian agenesis, which is described in detail in Chapter 46, Normal and abnormal development of the genitalia.

### Hyperprolactinaemia

This is more often a cause of secondary amenorrhoea, but can present as primary amenorrhoea and there may not be any galactorrhoea. A high prolactin level should prompt investigation for a pituitary adenoma. Treatment is the same as in the older female, with dopamine agonists such as cabergoline, which will result in the onset of menstruation.

### Congenital adrenal hyperplasia

Menarche is often delayed in this condition, and when menstruation starts it may be erratic. Poor control of the condition, often due to poor compliance with treatment, may be the cause. The ovaries also often have a polycystic appearance on scan. Fertility rates in these women are poor for a number of reasons: infrequent ovulation,

difficulties in achieving penetrative sex and failure to form relationships.[7]

## NORMAL BREAST BUT SCANTY OR ABSENT PUBIC HAIR DEVELOPMENT

This is the classical presentation of androgen insensitivity syndrome. The karyotype will be XY. Pubic hair fails to grow because of end-organ insensitivity to androgens, but breast development occurs due to peripheral conversion of androgens to oestrogen. No hormonal treatment is required (see Chapter 46, Normal and abnormal development of the genitalia).

## MENORRHAGIA AND DYSMENORRHOEA

As initial menstrual cycles are usually anovular, they are normally painless, but bleeding may be prolonged.

Girls are often referred to gynaecologists because of concern about missing school, particularly when studying for state examinations, due to heavy and painful periods. Almost invariably they are accompanied by a mother who will tell you about the problems she had with her periods. It is very important to speak to the girl herself to try to establish if there is a genuine problem, and to make some effort to quantify the loss by the degree of soakage of the pads used. The number of pads used per day may be quite misleading, and as most women do not know what amount of loss is normal, it can be very difficult for a girl to know whether she is actually experiencing an abnormal amount of bleeding.

Excessive menstrual loss will usually result in a fall in the haemoglobin level, and occasionally the loss can be so great that emergency admission and transfusion are required. Many of these girls will have an underlying medical disorder. It is most important to exclude a coagulation disorder, such as von Willebrand's disease, or a platelet dysfunction, which may be present in a third of these cases.[8,9] There may be no previous personal or family history of bleeding symptoms. If such a disorder is found, it may be possible to treat the girl with desmopressin on a cyclical basis.[10] The oral contraceptive pill is usually prescribed and, where blood loss is recurrently excessive, it can be helpful to prescribe this continuously for three or more cycles to reduce the frequency of withdrawal bleeds. However, several studies have reported than the number of days of bleeding is not statistically different from conventional cyclic dosing.[11]

Occasionally, girls present with life-threatening haemorrhage. The options for treatment include medroxyprogesterone acetate 5 mg orally every 1–2 hours for 24 hours and then 20 mg daily for 10 days, or a 50 μg oral contraceptive pill taken 6-hourly for 48 hours, then reduced to once daily over the next 3 days.[12] Intravenous oestrogen has also been used (40 mg 4-hourly for 24 hours) combined with a highly progestational oral contraceptive pill, but is not readily available in many pharmacies. It is rarely necessary to perform a diagnostic curettage.

---

**EBM**

All girls with menorrhagia who are found to be anaemic should be investigated for a bleeding disorder, including testing for von Willebrand's disease and platelet function defects.

---

Dysmenorrhoea usually responds to simple analgesia or oral contraceptives. However, where these measures fail, it is important to bear in mind the possibility of partial obstruction of menstrual flow. There are a number of reported cases of obstructed hemivagina and uterine horn associated with ipsilateral renal agenesis.[13] These usually present with severe cyclical pain and an abdominal mass due to a hemihaematometra and haematocolpos. Removal of the occluded vaginal septum allows drainage and relief of symptoms. Endometriosis occurs in many of these patients, presumably secondary to the enforced retrograde menstrual flow.

There are many causes of chronic pelvic pain in young women, including psychosomatic factors. It is important to realize that endometriosis should be excluded in chronic pelvic pain that has not responded to simple measures. Laparoscopy may be indicated. The symptoms are often not those typically encountered in older women.[14]

---

**KEY POINTS**

- Secondary sexual characteristics have started to develop in most girls by the age of 14 years.
- Menarche normally occurs two years after breast development has commenced.
- Ovarian failure is the most common cause of delayed puberty – karyotyping and gonadotrophins are essential investigations.
- Tests for bleeding disorders should be performed for any girl with moderate to severe menorrhagia.
- Endometriosis can occur in teenagers.

---

# Key References

1. Kaplowitz PB, Oberfield SE. Reexamination of the age limit for defining when puberty is precocious in girls in the United States: implications for evaluation and treatment. The Drug and Therapeutics and Executive Committees of the Lawson Wilkins Pediatric Endocrine Society. *Pediatrics* 1999; **104**: 936–41.

2. Marshall WA, Tanner JM. Variations in pattern of pubertal changes in girls. *Arch Dis Child* 1969; **44**: 291.

3. Anderson SE, Must A. Interpreting the continued decline in the average age at menarche: results from two nationally representative surveys of U.S. girls studied 10 years apart. *J Pediatr* 2005; **147**: 753–60.

4. Warren MP, Stiehl AL. Exercise and female adolescents: effects on the reproductive and skeletal systems. *J Am Med Womens Assoc* 1999; **54**: 115–20.

5. Crowne FC, Shalet SM, Wallace WH *et al*. Final height in girls with untreated constitutional delay in growth and puberty. *Eur J Pediatr* 1991; **150**: 708–12.

6. Albanese A, Stanhope R. Investigation of delayed puberty. *Clin Endocrinol* 1995; **43**: 105–10.

7. Mulaikal RM, Migeon CJ, Rock JA. Fertility rates in female patients with congenital adrenal hyperplasia due to 21-hydroxylase deficiency. *N Engl J Med* 1987; **316**: 178–82.

8. Smith YR, Quint EH, Hertzberg RB. Menorrhagia in adolescents requiring hospitalization. *J Pediatr Adolesc Gynecol* 1998; **11**: 13–15.

9. Bevan JA, Maloney KW, Hillery CA *et al*. Bleeding disorders: a common cause of menorrhagia in adolescents. *J Pediatr* 2001; **138**: 856–61.

10. Lee CA, Chi C, Pavord SR *et al*. The obstetric and gynaecological management of women with inherited bleeding disorders – review with guidelines produced by a taskforce of UK Haemophilia Centre Doctors' Organization. *Haemophilia* 2006; **12**: 301–36.

11. Edelmann A, Gallo MF, Nichols MD *et al*. Continuous versus cyclic use of combined oral contraceptives for contraception: systematic Cochrane review of randomized controlled trials. *Hum Reprod* 2006; **21**: 573–8.

12. Slap GB. Menstrual disorders in adolescence. *Best Pract Res Clin Obstet Gynaecol* 2003; **17**: 75–92.

13. Stassart JP, Nagel TC, Prem KA *et al*. Uterus didelphys, obstructed hemivagina, and ipsilateral renal agenesis: the University of Minnesota experience. *Fertil Steril* 1992; **57**: 756–61.

14. Propst AM, Laufer MR. Endometriosis in adolescents. Incidence, diagnosis and treatment. *J Reprod Med* 1999; **44**: 751–8.

# Ovarian and menstrual cycles

*William L Ledger*

## MRCOG standards

- Have a thorough understanding of the physiology of the menstrual cycle.
- Be able to explain disturbances in the cycle (e.g. anovulation, premature menopause) with reference to ovarian and uterine physiology.
- Understand the mechanism of action of drugs that affect the cycle.

## INTRODUCTION

Efficient reproduction is essential to the continuance of any species and is the most basic drive to existence. Humans are relatively inefficient reproducers, but have still managed to over-populate the planet within only a few tens of thousands of years. Knowledge of the basic physiology of the processes by which the development of the ovarian follicle, ovulation, fertilization and implantation occur is an essential prerequisite to an understanding of the events which lead to malfunction of the system, for example in hypothalamic amenorrhoea, premature ovarian failure and polycystic ovary syndrome. Knowledge of ovarian and endometrial physiology underpins the pharmacological interventions applied in many common gynaecological conditions, including menorrhagia, hyperandrogenic disorders, endometriosis and infertility.

## THE OVARIAN CYCLE

The human premenopausal ovary consists of a central dense collagenous stroma surrounded by a thin outer cortex. The cortex contains thousands of primordial follicles, each containing a germ cell surrounded by a single layer of granulosa/theca cells. The germ cell is arrested at the diplotene stage of prophase of the first meiotic division. The primordial follicle may remain at this point for many years, until a change in the local environment within the ovary allows it to resume meiosis and grow. The primordial follicle will then develop into a pre-antral follicle in which the separate theca and granulosa cell layers become discernable, and will then develop a cavity, or antrum, to become an antral follicle. The earliest stages of development of the follicle are independent of the gonadotrophins – luteinizing hormone (LH) and follicle-stimulating hormone (FSH) and may possibly be regulated by locally released growth factors within the ovary, such as bone morphogenic proteins (BMPs), activins or GDF 9. The process by which individual primordial follicles re-enter the growth phase occurs throughout late fetal life, during childhood, through puberty and pregnancy and is not affected by drugs such as the oral contraceptive pill or gonadotrophin-releasing hormone (GnRH) analogues. More than 99 per cent of all follicles will fail to ovulate, instead being destroyed and becoming atretic within the ovary, as a result of apoptosis (programmed cell death). The immutable nature of this process of follicle depletion helps in the understanding of the phenomenon of 'idiopathic' premature ovarian failure (premature menopause). A woman with early menopause probably received a lower than average number of primordial follicles during fetal life, leading to her 'running out' of her ovarian reserve more rapidly than others.

Each month, a cohort of antral follicles begins to develop from the primary follicle stage. The initial stages of antrum development are independent of FSH. The early antral follicles secrete glycoproteins including inhibin B and anti-Müllerian hormone (AMH), also known as Müllerian inhibitory substance (MIS) into the circulation. AMH secretion declines as the large antral, FSH-dependent stage is reached, whereas inhibin B continues to be secreted by the leading follicle. The point at which the lead antral follicle grows and reaches the stage of sensitivity to FSH and LH coincides with the time of the intercycle rise in FSH, the small but significant elevation in circulating FSH level that is seen during the menstrual phase of the cycle. One follicle (or occasionally two follicles) is at the correct stage of development to respond to FSH and LH by enlarging and continuing to grow. The outer theca cell layer of the follicle has receptors for LH and the necessary enzymes to synthesize androgens, while the inner granulosa cell layer, which is intimately connected to the oocyte, responds to FSH by developing aromatase, the enzyme which synthesizes oestrogens from androgens. Hence the theca/granulosa cell layers have to act in concert to synthesize oestrogens by responding individually to different gonadotrophins – the two cell, two gonadotrophins theory.

By secreting oestradiol into the circulation, the growing follicle reduces the circulating level of FSH by negative feedback on the hypothalamus and pituitary. Hence, other follicles in the cohort are not exposed to a sufficiently high level of FSH to allow them to continue to develop, and they become atretic. Thus, a single follicle each month becomes dominant, and is destined to ovulate some 10 to 12 days later. As the follicle grows, the granulosa cells secrete more oestradiol into the circulation and also secrete a complex mixture of peptide and glycoprotein growth factors into the oestrogen-rich follicular fluid that bathes the oocyte. As the follicular diameter reaches approximately 18 mm, the rising concentrations of oestradiol trigger a coordinated secretion of LH from the anterior pituitary – the LH surge. The LH surge triggers the final maturation of the oocyte, with completion of meiosis and extrusion of the first polar body, which contains one of the two haploid sets of chromosomes from the oocyte. At the same time, the LH surge also induces an inflammatory reaction within the wall of the follicle adjacent to the mouth of the Fallopian tube. Rapid formation of new capillary blood vessels and release of interleukins, prostaglandins and other cytokines result in follicular rupture and ovulation some 38 hours after the initiation of the LH surge.

Following release of the oocyte, further neovascularization and enzyme induction within the luteinized theca/granulosa cells produce progesterone, which appears rapidly in the circulation after ovulation. Progesterone from the corpus luteum acts on the endometrium to induce secretory changes, and suppresses secretion of FSH from the pituitary, preventing development of a further dominant follicle. The processes of synthesis and secretion of progesterone are maintained by LH and later, if pregnancy occurs, by human chorionic gonadotrophin (hCG) from the trophoblast. In the absence of 'rescue' by hCG, the corpus luteum involutes after 12–14 days, resulting in a decline in concentrations of progesterone in the circulation, with concomitant menstruation as a result of progesterone withdrawal (Figure 49.1).

## THE MENSTRUAL CYCLE

Each month, the endometrium must become receptive to implantation of the early embryo at the correct time of the cycle, in coordination with the arrival of the newly fertilized embryo in the uterine cavity. The pattern of events during the menstrual cycle reflects the necessity for close coordination of ovulation, fertilization and endometrial receptivity. Initially, the endometrium must regrow from the basalis layer, which remains after shedding of the more superficial layers of endometrium at menstruation. As the new endometrium grows, formation of spiral arteries provides the necessary vascular supply for later development of the maternal side of the placenta, should implantation occur. The proliferative endometrium grows in the first half of the menstrual cycle, being driven by oestradiol secreted into the circulation by the developing follicle. Hence follicular growth and endometrial growth are closely coordinated. After the LH surge, the follicle secretes large amounts of progesterone, which induces morphological changes in the endometrium. The glandular elements within the endometrium now proliferate and the superficial epithelial layer of the endometrium secretes a number of adhesion molecules, including glycodelin and integrins, which mediate the attachment, adhesion and initial stages of implantation of the embryo on to the endometrium. These proteins are only expressed for 1–2 days in the midluteal phase of the cycle, defining the implantation window.

Once it has hatched from the blastocyst, the embryo attaches some 6 days after fertilization. Trophoblast cells invade into the endometrium to establish the early placenta, while the inner cell mass begins to differentiate into the new fetus. One of the earliest signs of the establishment of pregnancy is the identification of hCG from trophoblast in the maternal circulation. This hormone maintains the secretion of progesterone from the corpus luteum and thereby prevents breakdown of the endometrium, with menstruation. The presence of hCG is essential for the maintenance of early pregnancy, until the luteo-placental shift at 10–12 weeks gestation, at which point the feto-placental unit becomes autonomous and luteal progesterone secretion is supplanted by production by placental cells.

## INHIBINS IN THE OVARIAN CYCLE

Inhibins are heterodimeric glycoproteins consisting of alpha and beta chains linked by disulphide bonds (Figure 49.2). They are secreted from the granulosa cell layer of the follicle and the theca/granulosa of the corpus luteum. Inhibin A, with alpha and beta A subunits, is secreted from the mature dominant follicle and in large amounts from the corpus luteum. Inhibin B, with alpha and beta B subunits, is released from the developing cohort of antral follicles in the early follicular phase of the cycle, and from the early dominant follicle. Inhibin B is not detectable in the luteal phase of the cycle or in pregnancy, whereas inhibin A secretion is maintained from the placenta during pregnancy and in labour. It seems likely that inhibin B from the dominant follicle acts with oestradiol to inhibit growth of other members of the cohort,

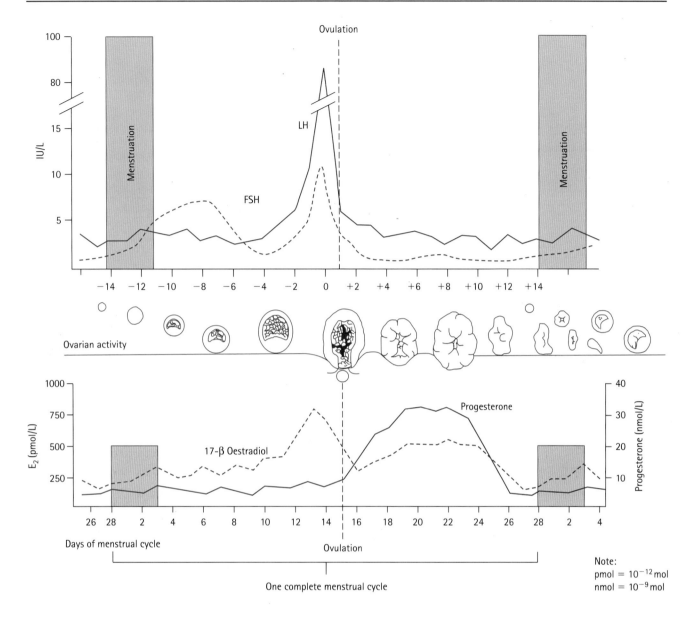

**Figure 49.1** Ovarian and pituitary hormones and growth of endometrium during the cycle. LH, luteinizing hormone

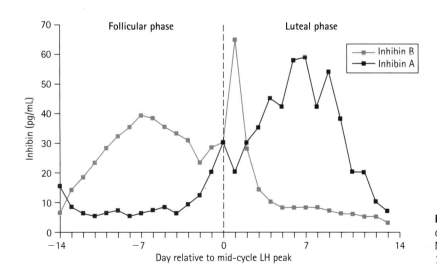

**Figure 49.2** Inhibin A and B during the menstrual cycle. (Reproduced with permission from Groome NP, Illingworth PJ, O'Brien M *et al. JCEM* 1996; **81**: 1401-5. © The Endocrine Society.)

preventing the risk of multiple pregnancy, while inhibin A may participate in the regulation of the LH surge and maintenance of the corpus luteum.

# APPLICATIONS OF THE PHYSIOLOGY OF THE OVARIAN AND MENSTRUAL CYCLES

## Investigation of anovular infertility

Accurate and rapid measurements of ovarian and pituitary hormones in peripheral blood samples have become the mainstay of the investigation of anovulation. Women who are anovular generally report an irregular or absent menstrual cycle and may have stigmata of polycystic ovary syndrome, hyperprolactinaemia or anorexia. Pituitary function in such cases is usually assessed by measurement of LH, FSH, prolactin and thyroid function on day 2 or 3 of a menstrual period. If periods are absent or infrequent, menses can usually be induced by a short course of progestogen (e.g. 10 days of Provera, 10 mg twice daily). This regime will induce a withdrawal bleed if the endometrium is adequately oestrogenized. If no bleed occurs, the patient is pregnant, has damaged or absent basalis layer of the endometrium or lacks sufficient oestrogen to 'prime' the endometrium. Lack of oestrogen may result from hypogonadal hypogonadism or reduced circulating levels of FSH and LH commonly due to anorexia or over-exercise.

More commonly, levels of FSH and LH may be within the normal range, possibly with an elevation of LH. This will suggest a diagnosis of polycystic ovary syndrome, confirmed by measurement of serum androgens and sex hormone-binding globulin and ovarian ultrasound. Patients with polycystic ovary syndrome may also exhibit mild elevation in levels of prolactin, but elevated levels of prolactin must always be assumed to be caused by a pituitary prolactinoma until proven otherwise. A clinical history of galactorrhoea and tunnel vision with amenorrhoea and headache should prompt imaging of the pituitary fossa, which is probably best done by magnetic resonance imaging (MRI).

If both FSH and LH are elevated, there is the possibility of premature ovarian failure. The patient may give a history of menopausal symptoms and may have a family history of early menopause. There may also have been exposure to pelvic irradiation or chemotherapy – more and more patients are surviving childhood cancers, such as leukaemias and lymphomas, but at the cost of loss of ovarian function. A diagnosis of premature ovarian failure should always be confirmed by repeated measurement of gonadotrophins and oestradiol, a karyotype to rule out chromosomal abnormalities, such as mosaic Turner's syndrome, and advice regarding hormone replacement therapy. Beware of results of measurements of LH and FSH being made in mid-cycle:

samples may have been collected during the LH surge, possibly leading to a healthy ovular patient being erroneously diagnosed as having ovarian failure.

Recently, measurement of AMH has been introduced as an alternative marker of ovarian reserve to FSH. AMH measurement has the advantage of being independent of the stage of the cycle – there is little cyclicity of secretion and hence a blood sample can be taken on any day of the month. AMH secretion is also not significantly affected by use of the oral contraceptive pill or hormone replacement therapy, and, unlike FSH, AMH release is not pulsatile. A high AMH is seen in cases of polycystic ovary syndrome and concentrations decline as the ovaries age, with low levels being seen as menopause approaches.

## Principles of treatment of anovular infertility

A sound knowledge of the regulation of the ovarian cycle helps understanding of the principles of treatment of anovulation. Clomiphene citrate has been the first line of treatment for anovulation associated with polycystic ovary syndrome for many years. Clomiphene has a complex action on the ovary, being a mixture of two isomers, one strongly anti-oestrogenic and the other weakly pro-oestrogenic. In essence, exposure to clomiphene citrate results in elevation of FSH levels in the circulation, by altering the set point of the feedback loop between oestradiol and FSH – a reduction in oestradiol caused by clomiphene resulting in an elevation in FSH. Higher levels of FSH may in turn induce a follicle to grow and ovulate, although at a cost of the risk of multiple pregnancy.

Similarly, daily injection of FSH can now be given to induce ovulation in clomiphene-resistant patients. This treatment over-rides the natural mechanism of follicle selection, which works by oestrogen and inhibin from the dominant follicle acting on the pituitary to reduce circulating levels of FSH, resulting in other members of the cohort of antral follicles becoming atretic. Maintenance of high levels of FSH by injection allows all members of the cohort to grow. In a young patient, more than 20 follicles may grow in synchrony, reflecting the large size of the antral follicle pool. Even larger numbers of follicles may be seen if FSH is given to a patient with polycystic ovary syndrome, leading to the risk of ovarian hyperstimulation syndrome (OHSS). In older patients treated with similar doses of FSH, only two or three follicles may appear, demonstrating the decline in ovarian reserve that generally occurs after 35 years of age.

Measurement of AMH or inhibin B in the early follicular phase of the cycle may also be helpful in assessing ovarian reserve. A high level of AMH or inhibin B is suggestive of preservation of a large cohort of follicles, with 'good' ovarian reserve, whereas a low inhibin B suggests depletion of the follicle pool. A combination of high FSH and low AMH and inhibin B has been used in assisted conception to predict poor ovarian response to superovulation, while a high AMH and inhibin B is suggestive of risk of over-response to superovulation with ovarian hyperstimulation syndrome.

In the early days of superovulation with injected FSH, the hormone was derived from human pituitary, and later from the urine of postmenopausal women (who have high levels of FSH as a result of loss of ovarian oestradiol feedback on the pituitary). Such urinary preparations of FSH invariably also contain LH. More recently, the genes for the alpha and beta subunits of FSH have been transfected into a Chinese hamster ovarian cell line, which expresses human FSH protein in culture. Such 'recombinant' FSH is devoid of LH action. Most *in vitro* fertilization (IVF) cycles are now conducted using FSH superovulation after pituitary down-regulation with a GnRH agonist, resulting in a profound suppression of endogenous LH production. Use of recombinant FSH following GnRH agonist downregulation results in the growth of a cohort of follicles in an almost LH-free environment. The demonstration that such cycles generate healthy oocytes that can fertilize and produce pregnancies shows that only small amounts of LH are necessary for the maintenance of function of the theca cells in the follicle. However, studies with patients with Kallmann syndrome, who have essentially no LH, have shown that recombinant FSH will induce growth of follicles but not secretion of oestradiol, resulting in the absence of growth of the endometrium. Hence, a basal secretion of LH is necessary for successful coordination of the ovarian and endometrial cycles, supporting the two cell, two gonadotrophin hypothesis.

## Ovarian physiology in assisted reproduction

Progress in assisted reproduction has largely come about from an improved understanding of ovarian physiology and early embryology. Early IVF treatment required laparoscopic aspiration of the single dominant follicle present in the natural cycle, the development of which was followed by assay of metabolites of oestrogens in urine and LH in serum. As soon as the onset of the LH surge was detected, oocyte collection was undertaken, often at night-time or at weekends. The procedure was 'hit or miss', with many attempts failing to obtain an oocyte. Introduction of 'superovulation' with FSH injection allowed the growth of a cohort of follicles, improving the chances of obtaining oocytes, but the high levels of oestradiol secreted from the multiple growing follicles produced the risk of a premature LH surge with loss of oocytes by ovulation before oocyte collection could be undertaken. The introduction in the mid-1980s of GnRH agonist pre-treatment before superovulation almost completely removed this risk. Pituitary downregulation prevented the release of LH in response to rising levels of oestradiol, greatly improving

the efficiency of superovulation and allowing day-time scheduling of oocyte collection.

More recently, the 'long' protocol of ovarian stimulation in which daily injection of FSH was preceded by 2–3 weeks of pituitary downregulation with GnRH agonists has been superceded by the 'antagonist' protocol in which FSH injection is started on day 2 or 3 of the natural menstrual period. The GnRH antagonist is then introduced after 5 or 6 days of FSH. This protocol is much quicker than the 'long', involving 9 or 10 days of injection rather than 3 or 4 weeks. This is made possible by the rapid onset of action when GnRH antagonists are used, since they directly block the GnRH receptor, whereas use of the agonist produces an initial 'flare' in FSH secretion followed some days later by the desired suppression as receptor desensitization emerges.

## Management of problems in early pregnancy

The principle of luteal 'rescue' by hCG secreted from the developing feto-placental unit resulting in maintenance of high circulating levels of progesterone has had considerable impact on the management of the luteal phase in downregulated IVF cycles and on the treatment of recurrent early pregnancy failure. Measurement of hCG in serum or urine forms the basis of early detection of pregnancy, and suboptimal rises or falls in hCG levels are associated with impending miscarriage or ectopic pregnancy. Pituitary downregulation in IVF cycles has prevented the problem of premature LH surges, but results in low levels of LH being present in the luteal phase of the cycle, with a negative effect on the function of the corpus luteum. 'Luteal phase support' in the form of hCG injection or, more recently, progestogenic compounds given by injection or as vaginal pessaries is routinely given to IVF patients after embryo transfer, to overcome any adverse impact of low progesterone levels on the establishment of pregnancy. Similarly, patients with recurrent miscarriage have traditionally been given progesterone or hCG treatment in an attempt to prevent miscarriage, although the benefit of such an approach has not been demonstrated in randomized, controlled trials.

## SUMMARY

This chapter outlines the events that regulate the ovarian and menstrual cycles. An understanding of the interplay between the pituitary gonadotrophins and ovarian steroids and glycoproteins has underpinned many of the recent developments in reproductive medicine. Knowledge of ovarian and uterine physiology helps the understanding of diagnostic and therapeutic approaches to patients with infertility and ovarian failure.

Reproductive medicine

## KEY POINTS

- The ovarian and uterine cycles are tightly coordinated in order to ensure receptive endometrium at the time at which the embryo is ready to implant.
- The pituitary hormones LH and FSH are regulated by feedback from the ovary by sex steroids (oestrogens and progesterone) and peptides (inhibins).
- Knowledge of pituitary–ovarian physiology has allowed rational development of drugs to influence the cycle, including GnRH agonists and antagonists to suppress the LH surge and prevent premature ovulation, and injectable gonadotrophins to stimulate multiple follicular development for IVF.
- The causes of anovulation can usually be elucidated quickly using timed measurements of FSH, LH, progesterone and oestradiol, sometimes with additional measurement of prolactin and thyroid function.

# Contraception, sterilization and termination of pregnancy

*Kulsum Jaffer*

## MRCOG standards

### Learning outcomes

- To understand and demonstrate the appropriate knowledge, skills and attitudes in relation to fertility control – contraception, sterilization and termination of pregnancy.

### Theoretical skills

- Thorough understanding of all methods of contraception – reversible, irreversible and emergency contraception.
- Methods, risks and laws relating to termination of pregnancy.

### Practical skills

- Candidates should be able to take an appropriate history and counsel patients requesting contraceptive advice, sterilization and termination of pregnancy.
- Diploma of the Faculty of Sexual and Reproductive Healthcare (DFSRH), Letter of Competence in Intrauterine Techniques (LoC IUT) and Letter of Competence in Subdermal Implant Techniques (LoC SDI) are highly recommended.

## INTRODUCTION

Many factors determine the method of contraception a person chooses. To be effective, contraception must be used correctly and consistently.

Contraceptive effectiveness is usually presented in terms of failure rates rather than success rates and are expressed as failure rates per 100 woman years (WY). One woman year is equal to 13 cycles.

Most contraceptive users are medically fit and can use any contraceptive method safely. However, some medical conditions are associated with increased health risks when certain contraceptives are used, either because the method adversely affects the condition or because the condition or its treatment affects the contraceptive.

The World Health Organization (WHO) published the WHO Medical Eligibility Criteria (WHOMEC)[1] for contraceptive use which relates to the safety (in terms of direct health risk) of using a contraceptive method by women with certain medical conditions or using certain drugs.

The UK Medical Eligibility Criteria (UKMEC),[2] reproduced in Table 50.1, were adapted from WHOMEC for use by UK clinicians in line with national health policies, needs, priorities and resources.

**Table 50.1** Definition of UKMEC category

| UKMEC | Definition of category |
|---|---|
| 1 | A condition for which there is no restriction for the use of the contraceptive method |
| 2 | A condition where the advantages of using the method generally outweigh the theoretical or proven risks |
| 3 | A condition where the theoretical or proven risks usually outweigh the advantages of using the method. The provision of a method requires expert clinical judgement and/or referral to a specialist contraceptive provider, since use of the method is not usually recommended unless other more appropriate methods are not available or not acceptable |
| 4 | A condition which represents an unacceptable health risk if the contraceptive method is used |

- Reproduced with permission from reference 2.

# FERTILITY AWARENESS METHODS

Fertility awareness (FA) methods are more commonly known as natural family planning (NFP). They have been defined by the WHO as 'the voluntary avoidance of intercourse by a couple during the fertile phase of the menstrual cycle in order to avoid a pregnancy'.[3] Fertility awareness methods are associated with higher failure rates than other available methods of contraception. They are often perceived as being better for women's health than hormonal and intrauterine methods. Some choose natural methods on moral or religious grounds, others because they have experienced, or have concerns about, the side effects of artificial methods or because they have medical conditions which limit their contraceptive choice.[4]

Fertility awareness methods rely on the fact that there are only certain days during the menstrual cycle when conception can occur. Following ovulation, the ovum is viable within the reproductive tract for a maximum of 24 hours. However, the life span of the sperm is considerably longer, in the region of 3–7 days. These methods require long periods of sexual abstinence. They provide low and varying levels of efficacy and do not provide any protection against sexually transmitted infections (STIs).

## Cycle or rhythm method

Cycle length is recorded for a minimum of six cycles. Likely fertile days are then calculated allowing for the survival time of sperm and ova, using the following formula:

First fertile day = shortest cycle minus 20
Last fertile day = longest cycle minus 10

This method requires a significant period of sexual abstinence; for example, in the case of a regular 28-day cycle, 10 days of sexual abstinence are required during each cycle.

## Temperature method

Following ovulation, there is a rise in the progesterone levels which produces a rise in the basal body temperature of 0.2–0.4°C, which is maintained until the onset of menstruation. The fertile phase ends after three consecutive high temperatures are recorded (>0.2°C above the six preceding recordings). This is known as the '3 over 6' rule. Intercourse is avoided from the onset of menstruation until the day on which the third higher level temperature has been recorded. Intercourse is then allowed until the onset of the next menstruation.

In the example of a 28-day cycle, abstinence is required for about 18 days per cycle. Infection, illness and medication can affect the body temperature and interfere with the method.

A failure rate of 2.0 per 100 WY has been reported.[5]

## Cervical mucus method (Billing's method)

During the follicular phase of the cycle, the cervical mucus appears like raw egg white, i.e. it is clear, slippery and stretchy (spinbarkeit phenomenon). The final day of the 'fertile mucus' is considered to be the day when ovulation is most likely to occur. Abstinence must be maintained from the day when fertile mucus is first identified until 3 days after the peak day. The end of the fertile period is characterized by the appearance of 'infertile mucus', which is scanty and viscous.

Semen, sexual excitement, spermicides, lubricants, bleeding and vaginal infections can confuse mucus assessment.

The actual failure rate for typical use has been reported as 22 per 100 WY.[6]

## Cervical palpation method

Daily self-palpation of the cervix helps to detect the changes occurring in the size of the external os and its position relative to the introitus. The cervix rises during the follicular phase of the cycle. At ovulation, it reaches peak height from the introitus with maximum softness and the os admits a finger tip. The cervix then descends, becomes closed and firm and is closer to the vulva towards the end of the luteal phase.

## Minor clinical indicators of fertility

Ovulation pain (mittelschmerz), mid-cycle show of blood, onset of breast symptoms, skin and mood changes can occur in some women. When present, they can be helpful in confirming the major signs.

Various combinations of FA methods can be used to increase the accuracy of identification of the fertile and infertile periods.

## Personal fertility monitors

Persona (Unipath, UK) is a small hand-held device that is able to detect urine concentrations of oestrone-3-glucuronide (E3G) and luteinizing hormone (LH) and thus signifies the start and end of the fertile period. On potentially fertile days, a red light indicates the need for abstinence from intercourse. Safe days are indicated by a green light and a yellow light implies that a urine sample is required. Following the urine test, a red or green light will be displayed depending on the LH and E3G ratio.

Persona can be used for cycle lengths between 23 and 35 days. It cannot be used if a woman is experiencing menopausal symptoms, while breastfeeding, soon after childbirth, is taking hormones or is on tetracyclines.

Failure rate is around six per 100 WY.

## Lactational amenorrhoea method

A woman who is fully breastfeeding and is amenorrhoeic during the first six months after childbirth has a 2 per cent chance of getting pregnant [B]. Hence, the lactational amenorrhoea method (LAM) is categorized as one of the natural family planning methods.[7]

> ### KEY POINTS
>
> **Fertility awareness methods**
> - The fertility awareness methods help to identify the fertile and infertile phases of the menstrual cycle.
> - They require long periods of sexual abstinence.
> - They provide low levels of contraceptive efficacy.

## BARRIER METHODS

Barrier methods provide a physical barrier which stops the sperm from getting into the vagina or upper genital tract.

There are many types available including male and female condoms, caps, diaphragms, sponges and spermicides.

They provide varying degrees of protection from STIs, including the human immunodeficiency virus (HIV) and premalignant and malignant disease of the cervix.

## Male condoms

The majority of male condoms are made from fine latex rubber. Those who suffer from latex sensitivity can use polyurethane condoms [C]. Oil-based lubricants and vaginal preparations drastically reduce the strength of the condom [C].

Failure rates for condoms range from three to 23 per 100 WY.

## Female condoms (Femidom)

The female condom is a 15 cm long and 7.5 cm diameter polyurethane sheath with rings at either end. It is stronger than the male latex condoms with a less risk of splitting and is not weakened by oil-based lubricants and vaginal preparations.

Failure rates are in the region of 5–21 per 100 WY.

## Occlusive caps

Occlusive caps comprise of diaphragms, cervical and vault caps and the vimule. They should be used in combination with spermicides to provide maximum protection [C]. Occlusive devices are available in a range of sizes and initially need to be fitted by trained personnel. They require a high degree of motivation for successful use, which is reflected in the varying rates of efficacy. Women should be reassessed for the size of the diaphragm or cap if they have gained or lost 3 kg (7 lb) in weight [C].

## Diaphragms

A diaphragm is a thin latex rubber or silicone hemisphere. The rim of which is reinforced by a flexible flat or coiled metal spring. The flat spring diaphragm is for the normal vagina, whereas the coil and arcing spring ones are for the tight and lax vaginae, respectively. Their external diameters range from 55 to 95 mm, with 5 mm increments. The diaphragm should lie across the cervix extending from the posterior vaginal fornix to behind the symphysis pubis.

Urinary tract infections are more common in diaphragm users. Inflammatory reactions, abrasions or even frank ulcers can also be caused by local pressure.

## Cervical caps

Since October 2007, only one cervical cap, i.e. the Femcap, has been available in the UK. It fits snugly onto the cervix by suction.

## Vaginal sponges

These are made of polyurethane foam and impregnated with spermicide. They are inserted into the vagina to cover the cervix. They act as carriers for spermicide and absorb semen.

'Today' and 'Protectaid' contraceptive sponges have recently been withdrawn from the UK market.

## Spermicides

These are chemicals that bring about sperm death by causing osmotic changes in the sperm. The most common spermicide is Nonoxinol '9'. It can cause vaginal irritation and ulceration and may increase the risk of HIV transmission [C]. Spermicides are used in conjunction with barrier methods.

> ### KEY POINTS
>
> **Barrier methods**
> - The strength of the latex condoms is considerably reduced by oil-based lubricants and vaginal preparations. However, these do not have any affect on the polyurethane ones.
> - They provide varying degrees of protection from STIs and premalignant and malignant disease of the cervix.
> - Spermicides are usually used in conjunction with the barrier methods.
> - Nonoxinol 9 can cause vaginal irritation and ulceration and may increase the risk of HIV transmission.

## COITUS INTERRUPTUS

This is the withdrawal of the penis from the vagina before ejaculation takes place and therefore requires considerable control on the part of the man.

Failure rates of about 10 per 100 WY have been quoted.[8]

## COMBINED HORMONAL CONTRACEPTION

Combined hormonal contraception (CHC) includes the combined oral contraceptive (COC) pill, the transdermal patch and the vaginal ring. The patch and the ring are no different from the pill in terms of mechanism of action, safety and efficacy. However, there are no data regarding the major side effects of the ring and the patch, therefore at present it is advisable that data for COCs also applies to the NuvaRing and the Evra Patch.

## Mechanism of action

All CHCs inhibit ovulation. The vaginal and cervical mucus becomes scanty and viscous and inhibits sperm transport. The endometrium becomes atrophic and is unreceptive for implantation.

## Non-contraceptive benefits

Combined hormonal contraceptives decrease menstrual pain and blood loss. There is a decrease in the incidence of functional ovarian cysts, benign ovarian tumours, benign breast disease, pelvic inflammatory disease and acne. There is also a 50 per cent reduction of ovarian and endometrial cancers which continues for 15 years after stopping the CHC. There is a possible protective effect against rheumatoid arthritis, thyroid disease and duodenal ulceration.

## Major side effects

### Venous thrombo-embolism

The most common serious risk of CHC is venous thrombo-embolism (VTE). This risk is greatest during the first year of CHC use. If a woman is not on any CHC, the risk of VTE is five per 100 000 WY. If she is on a pill containing second generation progestogens, for example levonorgestrel (LNG), then this risk increases to 15 per 100 000 WY. This risk is further increased to 25 per 100 000 WY with pills containing third generation progestogens, for example desogestrel and gestodene. However, with pregnancy the VTE risk is 60 per 100 000 WY [B]. The Danish retrospective study[9] and the MEGA case controlled study[10] have not only found an increased relative risk for VTE with desogestrel and gestodene, but also with cyproterone acetate and drosperinone compared to LNG. Pill users who have a Factor V Leiden mutation have up to 20 times the risk of VTE compared to non-pill users.

### Myocardial infarction

A meta-analysis of 23 studies has shown that the relative risk for users is 2.5 when compared to never users.[11] This risk increases with smoking and hypertension.

### Stroke

The risk of ischaemic stroke is increased among current users of COC (RR 2.7) [B]. This risk is further increased with smoking and hypertension and in migraine sufferers.

### Migraine

The risk of ischaemic stroke is increased in migraine sufferers and the use of CHC further increases this risk. Migraine with aura at any age is a UKMEC 4 category for CHC use.

### Cancer

Breast cancer
There is a small increase in the risk of developing breast cancer while women are on CHC – from 10 per 1000 non-pill users to 11 per 1000 pill users [B].[12] This increased risk decreases to the background risk after discontinuation of the CHC for ten years.

Cervical cancer
There is a slight increased risk of cervical intra-epithelial neoplasia, cervical cancer and also the morbidity from it with COC use [B].

Liver cancer
With CHC use, there is a slight increase in benign and malignant tumours of the liver.

## Combined oral contraceptive pill

It is almost 99 per cent effective. Combined oral contraceptive formulations are either fixed dose or phasic, when the dose of the oestrogen and progestogen changes during the cycle. Phasic preparations are designed to mimic the body's cyclical variation in hormone levels.

Yasmin and Qlaira are relatively new COCs.

## Yasmin

Yasmin contains 30 µg of ethinyl oestradiol and 3 mg of drosperinone. Drosperinone acts like a natural progestogen and displays progestogenic, antiandrogenic and antimineralocorticoid activities. It blocks androgen receptors and inhibits sebum production. It therefore has a beneficial effect on the skin and on premenstrual symptoms.

## Qlaira

Qlaira is a new COC containing oestradiol valerate (E2V) and dienogest (D) in the following doses:

| Days | 2 | 5 | 17 | 2 | 2 |
|------|------|------|------|------|---|
| E2V  | 3 mg | 2 mg | 2 mg | 1 mg | 0 |
| D    | 0    | 2 mg | 3 mg | 0    | 0 |

It contains 26 active and two placebo tablets. Hence the pill-free interval is reduced to 2 days. Reducing the pill-free interval has been shown to decrease mood changes, headaches, menstrual loss and pelvic pain. Therefore, it may be suitable for women who complain of oestrogen withdrawal symptoms (as mentioned above).

In situations when extra precautions are needed, 9 days of extra precautions are needed for Qlaira instead of the 7 days for conventional COCs.

Oestradiol valerate is a body identical oestrogen. Studies have shown that it has less effect on the haemostatic parameters and lipid profile than Microgynon 30 and Logynon. It may therefore prove useful for women over 35 and those with uncomplicated diabetes.[13]

Pearl index is 0.4 per 100 WY which is similar to those reported for other COCs.

Qlaira has different missed pill guidelines to the other COCs. The following guidelines should be followed if one pill is missed for more than 12 hours.

- Day 1–17. Take the missed pill immediately and the next tablet at the usual time (even if it means taking two on the same day)
  - Continue with the tablet taking in the normal way
  - Abstain or use an additional contraceptive method for 9 days

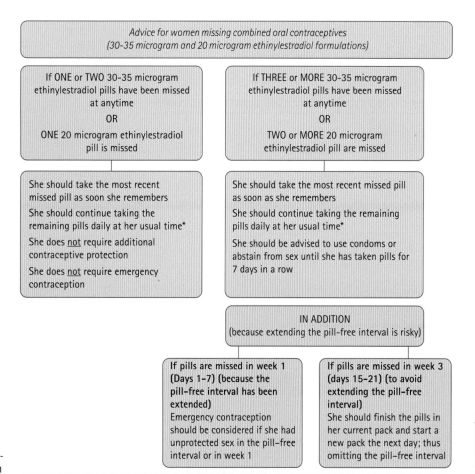

**Figure 50.1** Missed pill guidelines for combined oral contraceptives. Reproduced from FFPRHC/FSRH guidance – Combined Oral Contraception – Missed Pills, April 2005

- Day 18–24. Discard the rest of the packet
  - Start taking the day 1 pill from a new packet immediately and continue taking these pills at the correct time
  - Abstain or use an additional contraceptive method for 9 days
- Day 25–26. Take the missed tablet immediately and the next tablet at the usual time (even if it means taking two tablets on the same day)
  - Additional contraception is not necessary
- Day 27–28. Discard the forgotten tablet and continue tablet taking in the normal way
  - Additional contraception is not necessary

### Dianette

Dianette contains 35 μg of ethinyl oestradiol and 2 mg of cyproterone acetate. It is not licensed as an oral contraceptive but is used as one. It is used for treating moderate to severe acne and hirsutism. There is an increased incidence of VTE in Dianette users more than the second generation COCs. A few cases of severe depression have been reported with Dianette. Therefore it has been advised by the Committee on Safety of Medicines (CSM) that it should be withdrawn 3–4 cycles after the condition/s for which it was prescribed initially have resolved.

## Other combined hormonal contraceptives

### Evra patch

Twenty microgrammes of ethinyl oestradiol and 150 μg of norelgestromin are released per 24 hours. It is the first transdermal contraceptive applied once weekly for 3 weeks followed by a patch-free week (3 weeks on, 1 week off).

Pearl index is 1.24 per 100 WY. It has been reported that contraceptive efficacy is reduced in women weighing over 90 kg.

It provides a new delivery system and another contraceptive choice for women. Efficacy, cycle control and safety profile are similar to COCs.

### Nuva ring

The Nuva ring is a flexible, latex-free ring made of plastic and ethylene vinyl acetate which releases 120 μg of etonogestrel and 15 μg of ethinyl oestrdiol daily. It is 54 mm in diameter and 4 mm thick. It is placed vaginally once every 3 weeks and following a 1 week ring-free interval, a new ring is inserted.

Efficacy and cycle control are comparable to the COCs. The side-effect profile is also similar to that of COCs. However, women have reported more vaginal symptoms of vaginitis, leucorrhoea, foreign body sensation, coital problems and expulsion.[14] It provides another useful contraceptive for women.

## CHC - UKMEC Category 3 – Risks generally outweigh benefits

- **Breastfeeding** – between 6 weeks and 6 months postpartum and fully or almost fully breastfeeding
- **Postpartum** – <21 days postpartum
- **Smoking** – aged ≥35 years and smoking <15 cigarettes per day, or stopped smoking <1 year ago
- **Obesity** – BMI ≥35 kg/m²
- **Cardiovascular disease** – multiple risk factors for arterial cardiovascular disease
- **Hypertension** – elevated blood pressure >140 to 159 mmHg systolic or >90 to 94 mmHg diastolic. Also adequately controlled hypertension
- **Family history of VTE in a first-degree relative aged <45 years**
- **Immobility (unrelated to surgery)** – e.g. wheelchair use, debilitating illness
- **Known hyperlipidaemias** – e.g. familial hypercholesterolaemia
- **Migraine without aura, at any age** – continuation of the method
- **Past history (≥5 years ago) of migraine with aura at any age**
- **Undiagnosed breast mass** – initiation of the method.
- **Past history of breast cancer and no evidence of recurrence for five years; carriers of known gene mutations associated with breast cancer (e.g. BRCA1)**
- **Diabetes** – with nephropathy/retinopathy/neuropathy; or other vascular disease
- **Gallbladder disease** – symptomatic medically treated or current
- **History of cholestasis** – past COC-related
- **Viral Hepatitis** – acute or flare
- **HIV** – on anti-retroviral therapy (drug interactions)
- **Drugs which induce liver enzymes** – e.g. rifampicin, rifabutin, ritonovir, St John's Wort and certain anticonvulsants (i.e. phenytoin, carbamazepine, barbiturates, primidone, topiramate, oxcarbazepine)and lamotrigine
- **Undiagnosed breast mass** – initiation of the method.
- **Past history of breast cancer and no evidence of recurrence for five years; carriers of known gene mutations associated with breast cancer (e.g. BRCA1)**
- **Diabetes** – with nephropathy/retinopathy/neuropathy; or other vascular disease
- **Gallbladder disease** – symptomatic medically treated or current
- **History of cholestasis** – past COC-related
- **Viral Hepatitis** – acute or flare
- **HIV** – on anti-retroviral therapy (drug interactions)
- **Drugs which induce liver enzymes** – e.g. rifampicin, rifabutin, ritonovir, St John's Wort and certain anticonvulsants (i.e. phenytoin, carbamazepine, barbiturates, primidone, topiramate, oxcarbazepine)and lamotrigine

## CHC - UKMEC Category 4 - Unacceptable health risk and should not be used

- **Breastfeeding** - <6 weeks postpartum
- **Smoking** - aged ≥35 years and smoking ≥15 cigarettes per day
- **Cardiovascular disease** - multiple risk factors for arterial cardiovascular disease
- **Hypertension** - blood pressure ≥160 mmHg systolic and/or ≥95 mmHg diastolic; or vascular disease
- **VTE** - current (on anticoagulants) or past history
- **Major surgery with prolonged immobilization**
- **Known thrombogenic mutations**
- **Current and history of ischaemic heart disease**
- **Stroke**
- **Valvular and congenital heart disease** - complicated by pulmonary hypertension, atrial fibrillation, history of sub-acute bacterial endocarditis
- **Migraine headaches** - with aura at any age
- **Breast disease** - current breast cancer
- **Diabetes** - with nephropathy, retinopathy, neuropathy or other vascular disease
- **Viral hepatitis** - active or flare
- **Cirrhosis** - severe decompensated disease
- **Liver tumours** - benign, hepatocellular adenoma and malignant- hepatoma
- **Systemic lupus erythematosus** (SLE) - positive or unknown antiphospholipid antibodies

## KEY POINTS

### Combined hormonal contraception

- The Nuva ring and the Evra patch are the relatively new forms of CHC. They are no different from the COC pill in terms of mechanism of action, safety and efficacy.
- VTE is a serious risk of CHC use. It is most during the first year of use. Pill users who have a Factor V Leiden mutation have up to 20 times the risk of VTE compared to non-pill users
- Migraine with aura is a UKMEC 4 for CHC use.
- There is a slightly increased risk of developing breast, liver and cervical cancers with CHC use.
- Qlaira is the first 26 day pill reducing the pill-free interval to 2 days.

## PROGESTOGEN-ONLY PILLS

## Mode of action

Progestogen-only pills (POPs) alter cervical mucus and prevent sperm penetration. The endometrium is altered so that it is not conducive for implantation. In addition, traditional POPs can inhibit ovulation but this can be variable – up to 60 per cent, whereas in the case of a desogestrel-only pill – Cerazette – 97 per cent of the cycles are anovulatory. Therefore, inhibition of ovulation is the main mode of action of Cerazette [C].

## Effectiveness

Failure rates for traditional POPs vary from 0.3 to 8.0 per 100 WY, but are lower for women aged over 40 years (0.3 per 100 WY) compared to younger women. The failure rates of the traditional pills and Cerazette are similar [B]. There is no evidence to suggest that the efficacy of any POP is reduced in women weighing >70 kg and therefore one pill per day is advised as per licence [B].

## Side effects

Changes in the bleeding pattern are common. Two in ten women are amenorrhoeic, whereas four in ten have regular bleeding and another four in ten have irregular bleeding. Mood changes can occur with POP use.

## Risks

There is no causal association between POP use and cardiovascular disease (VTE, myocardial infarction and stroke) or breast cancer.

Women of any age with a history of migraine (with or without aura) can safely use POPs.

Missed pill guidelines for all POPs are given in Figure 50.2.

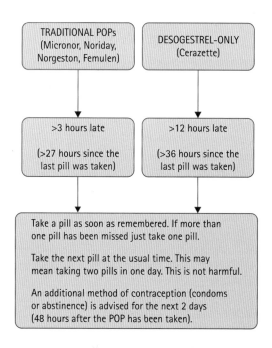

**Figure 50.2** Missed pill guidelines for all progestogen-only pills. Reproduced from FFPRHC/FSRH - Clinical guidance Progestogen-only Pill, November 2008 [C]

## POP – UKMEC Category 3 – Risks generally outweigh benefits

- Current and history of ischaemic heart disease and stroke – continuation of the method
- Past history of breast cancer and no evidence of recurrence for five years
- HIV – on anti-retroviral therapy (drug interactions)
- Cirrhosis – severe (decompensated)
- Liver tumours – hepatocellular adenoma and malignant hepatoma
- SLE – positive or unknown antiphospholipid antibodies

## POP – UKMEC Category 4 – Unacceptable health risk and should not be used

- Breast disease – current breast cancer

## KEY POINTS

### Progestogen-only pill

- Traditional POPs have a 3-hour window period, whereas Cerazette has 12 hours before the missed pill guidelines have to be implemented.
- They can be safely used by women who suffer from migraines (with or without aura).

# LONG-ACTING REVERSIBLE CONTRACEPTION

Long-active reversible contraception (LARC) methods require administering less than once per cycle or month:

- they are more cost effective than COCs even at one year of use;
- intrauterine contraceptive devices (IUCD), intrauterine systems (LNG-IUS) and implants are more cost effective than injectables;
- increased uptake will reduce unintended pregnancies;
- in 2003/2004, LARCs were used by 8 per cent of women aged 16–49 years.

The LARC methods are:

- Non-hormonal: intrauterine contraceptive device (IUCD or Cu-IUD)
- Hormonal: intrauterine system (LNG-IUS); progestogen-only injectable contraception (POIC); progestogen-only implants (POI).

# INTRAUTERINE CONTRACEPTION – IUCD AND LNG-IUS

The gold standard IUCDs are the T-shaped IUCDs with banded copper on the arms and containing at least 380 mm² of copper. They last for ten years whereas other Cu-IUDs and LNG-IUSs are for five years [C].

A Cu-IUD inserted in a woman at the age of 40 years or over can be retained for one year after the last menstrual period if aged over 50 years or two years if under 50 years or until contraception is no longer required [C].

The LARC guideline recommends that women who have the LNG-IUS inserted at or after the age of 45 years and are amenorrhoeic may retain the LNG-IUS until the menopause [E].

## Effectiveness

Failure rates are less than 2 per cent with TCu380A and TCu380S coils and less than 1 per cent for LNG-IUS [C].

## Mode of action

Intrauterine devices work by inhibiting fertilization by direct toxicity [B]. An inflammatory reaction within the endometrium can also have an anti-implantation effect. Copper is toxic to the ovum and the sperm and the copper content of the cervical mucus inhibits sperm penetration as well.

LNG-IUS works primarily by its effect on the endometrium, preventing implantation. In addition, its effects on cervical mucus reduces sperm penetration [B].

## Insertion and removal prerequisites

A sexual history should be taken from all women attending for IUCD/IUS insertions to assess the risk of STIs. Prior to IUCD/IUS insertion, women at higher risk of STIs (age <25 years, change in sexual partner, or more than one partner in the last year) should be offered screening for Chlamydia trachomatis as a minimum [C]. For women assessed as being at higher risk of STIs, and results of screening are not available at the time of the insertion, then the use of prophylactic antibiotics to cover Chlamydia should be considered (good practice point).

Additional protection is not needed at IUCD insertion, as the mode of action is by inhibition of fertilization and implantation and these effects are immediate after insertion. However, it is required before IUCD removal, as viable ova or sperm may be present in the female genital tract before removal. The woman is therefore advised to abstain, use condoms or start another method 7 days before removal [C].

Antibiotic prophylaxis for the prevention of infective endocarditis is not recommended in women undergoing intrauterine insertion or removal.[15]

## Discontinuation

The most common reasons for discontinuation of intrauterine contraception are unacceptable vaginal bleeding and pain. Another reason is PID/infection. Discontinuation rates for all reasons are similar for different IUCDs – framed or frameless and for LNG-IUS [A].

# Risks

## Expulsion

Expulsion of intrauterine contraception occurs in approximately one in 20 women and is most common in the first three months after insertion and often during menstruation [B].

A Cochrane review found a small excess in expulsions with Multiload Cu375 compared to TCu380A in the fourth and subsequent years. The expulsion rate for a frameless Cu-IUD was higher than the TCu380A at one year. Early expulsions with a frameless device (GyneFix) are common.[16]

In general, there are no differences in the rates of expulsion of the various IUCDs and between IUCD and IUS [A].

## Pelvic inflammatory disease

Although there is a 6-fold increase in the risk of PID in the 20 days after the insertion of intrauterine contraception, the overall risk is low unless there is exposure to STIs [B].

Management

In a woman with an intrauterine contraceptive *in situ* and the signs and symptoms are suggestive of pelvic infection, then appropriate antibiotics should be commenced. Where possible, triple swabs should be taken prior to commencing antibiotic therapy. There is no need to remove the device at this stage. The intrauterine method can be removed if symptoms fail to improve after commencement of antibiotics for 72 hours.

The removal should be carried out at an appropriate time (see above under insertion and removal prerequisites). There may even be a need to give emergency hormonal contraception following the removal.

The woman should be followed up to ensure resolution of symptoms, counselling for safer sex and partner notification.

The partner also needs to be treated with appropriate antibiotics.

## Presence of actinomyces-like organisms (ALOs)

Actinomyces-like organisms (ALOs) can be detected on smears in women who have intrauterine contraception *in situ*.

Management

If there are no signs or symptoms suggestive of pelvic infection, then there is no need to remove the device. Neither is there any need for subsequent screening.

If symptoms of infection develop, then the woman should be advised to seek medical advice. Other causes of infection, for example STIs, should be considered at this stage.

## Perforation

The risk of uterine perforation associated with intrauterine contraception is up to two per 1000 insertions [B]. It is more common at the time of insertion. Women should be informed about signs and symptoms of uterine perforation and infection. There should be a 6-week interval after an asymptomatic, suspected perforation before an IUCD/IUS insertion is attempted again.

Management

If perforation is suspected at the time of insertion, the procedure should be stopped and vital signs (blood pressure and pulse rate) and level of discomfort monitored until they are stable.

An ultrasound scan and/or plain abdominal x-ray should be organized to locate the device if it has been left *in situ*.

## Ectopic pregnancy

The annual ectopic pregnancy rate for Cu-IUD users is 0.02 per 100 woman-years (0.3–0.5 per 100 woman-years for those not using contraception) [A].

## Bleeding patterns and pain

Spotting, light bleeding, heavier or longer periods are common in the first 3–6 months following Cu-IUD insertion [C]. These bleeding patterns usually decrease with time.

Irregular bleeding and spotting is common during the first 6–8 months of LNG-IUS insertion. By one year, amenorrhoea or light bleeding ensues [B].

Management

Women who experience problematic bleeding while using an intrauterine contraceptive should have a sexual history taken to establish STI risk and/or be investigated for gynaecological pathology if clinically indicated. When these have been excluded in the case of LNG-IUS, bleeding problems can be treated with mefenamic acid or ethinylestradiol (alone or as an oral contraceptive) provided there are no contraindications to oestrogen therapy. Non-steroidal anti-inflammatory drugs (NSAIDs) or antifibrinolytics, for example tranexamic acid, can be used to treat abnormal bleeding with Cu-IUDs.

## Vasovagal syncope

The incidence of vasovagal syncope at intrauterine contraception insertions is between 0.2 and 2.1 per cent. The signs of syncope are sweating, pallor and bradycardia – pulse of <60 beats/minute.

Management

- Abandon procedure, lower head or raise legs
- Remove instruments ± coil
- Monitor BP and pulse
- Administer oxygen (FSRH – essential for intrauterine contraception inserting clinics)

Medication

- Atropine i.v. (0.6 mg/mL). (Bradycardia – heart rate <40 beats/min or systolic BP <90 mmHg.) Repeat every few minutes up to a dose of 3 mg.

## Lost threads

Management

Women should be advised to use another method until it is confirmed that the device is *in situ*. The cervical canal can be explored with a thread retriever or a Spencer Wells forceps to bring the threads down if they are in the canal. If this is not successful then an ultrasound scan of the pelvis should be organized. If the intrauterine device is not located on ultrasound, then a plain x-ray of the abdomen should be arranged to identify an extrauterine location. If radiological investigations fail to reveal the device it then is presumed to have been expelled.

## Pregnancy

### Management
An ectopic pregnancy should be excluded. If the threads of the device are visible then the IUCD should be removed up to 12 weeks gestation. Women who become pregnant with an IUCD *in situ* should be informed of the increased risks of second-trimester miscarriage, preterm delivery and infection if the intrauterine device is left *in situ*. Removal would reduce adverse outcomes but is associated with a small risk of miscarriage

## Hormonal side effects
Due to the systemic absorption of LNG (though very small amounts), progestogenic side effects, headaches, mood changes, acne, breast tenderness or change in libido, can occur with LNG-IUS [C].

## Ovarian cysts
There is a slightly increased incidence of functional ovarian cysts in LNG-IUS users compared to IUCD users [B].[17]

### IUCD – UKMEC Category 3 – Risks generally outweigh benefits
- Postpartum – between 48 hours and <4 weeks
- VTE – current (on anticoagulants)
- Ovarian cancer – initiation of the method
- Pelvic tuberculosis – continuation of the method
- AIDs – initiation of the method
- SLE – initiation of the method in women with severe thrombocytopenia

### IUCD – UKMEC Category 4 – Unacceptable health risk and should not be used
- Pregnancy, puerperal sepsis and immediate post-septic abortion
- Unexplained vaginal bleeding – initiation of the method
- GTD – persistently elevated beta HCG levels or malignant disease
- Cervical cancer – initiation of the method in women awaiting treatment
- Endometrial cancer – initiation of the method
- Ovarian cancer – initiation of the method
- Current PID, symptomatic and asymptomatic chlamydial infection or purulent cervicitis or gonorrhoea – initiation of the method
- Pelvic tuberculosis – initiation of the method

### LNG-IUS – UKMEC Category 3 – Risks generally outweigh benefits
- Postpartum – between 48 hours and <4 weeks
- Current and past history of IHD – continuation of the method
- Stroke – continuation of the method
- Pelvic tuberculosis – continuation of the method
- AIDs – initiation of the method
- Cirrhosis – severe, decompensated
- Liver tumours – hepatocellular adenoma and malignant hepatoma
- SLE – positive or unknown antiphospholipid antibodies

### LNG-IUS – UKMEC Category 4 – Unacceptable health risk and should not be used
- Puerperal sepsis
- Post-septic abortion
- Unexplained vaginal bleeding – initiation of the method
- GTD – persistently elevated beta HCG levels or malignant disease
- Cervical cancer – initiation of the method in women awaiting treatment
- Endometrial cancer – initiation of the method
- Ovarian cancer – initiation of the method
- Breast cancer – current
- Current PID, symptomatic and asymptomatic chlamydial infection or purulent cervicitis or gonorrhoea – initiation of the method
- Pelvic tuberculosis – initiation of the method

## KEY POINTS

### Intrauterine contraception
- Gold standard IUCD is the T-shaped IUD with banded copper on the arms and containing at least 380 mm$^2$ of copper.
- The most common reasons for discontinuation are bleeding irregularities and pain.
- There is no difference in the rates of expulsions of various IUCDs and between IUCD and IUS.
- There is an increased risk of PID in the first 20 days after insertion.
- Vasovagal syncope can occur with intrauterine contraception insertions. Intravenous atropine should be given when the HR falls below 40 beats/min or systolic BP is less than 90 mmHg.
- An IUD fitted after the age of 40 and an IUS after the age of 45 (provided she is amenorrhoeic) can be left *in situ* until the menopause.
- The device should be removed (provided the threads are visible at the external os) if a woman gets pregnant with a coil/Mirena *in situ*. There is a slightly increased risk of miscarriage with the removal.

## Non-contraceptive benefits

LNG-IUS reduces menstrual blood loss and decreases pain and is therefore used in the treatment of heavy menstrual bleeding. It provides endometrial protection from the stimulatory effects of oestrogens and is used along with oestrogen therapy in the management of menopausal symptoms [B]. It can also be used in the management of endometriosis.

## PROGRESTOGEN-ONLY INJECTABLE CONTRACEPTION

Two POICs are available in the UK. They are:

- Depot medroxy progesterone acetate (DMPA) given intramuscularly every 12 weeks. It is the most commonly used POIC in the UK.
- Norethisterone enanthate (NET-EN), licensed for short-term use. It is also given intramuscularly but 8-weekly.

## Mode of action

The main mode of action is inhibition of ovulation [C]. Thickening of the cervical mucus prevents sperm penetration into the upper reproductive tract. It also brings about changes in the endometrium making the environment unfavourable for implantation.

## Effectiveness

The failure rate of DMPA is <4 in 1000 over two years [A].

## Return of fertility

There is a delay in the return of fertility of up to one year with POIC [C]. However, there is no evidence to suggest that fertility is reduced long term.

## Discontinuation

Fifty per cent of POIC users will discontinue the method within one year. The main reasons for discontinuation are bleeding problems and weight gain [B].[18]

## Side effects

### Bleeding problems

Amenorrhoea, spotting, infrequent bleeding or prolonged bleeding can occur with POICs. Amenorrhoea is more likely as duration of use increases. A third of the women are amenorrhoeic at three months and 70 per cent by 12 months of use [B].[18]

Management

Women who experience problematic bleeding while using a POIC should have a sexual history taken to determine if there is a STI risk and/or be investigated for gynaecological pathology if clinically indicated. When these have been excluded, bleeding problems can be treated with mefenamic acid or ethinylestradiol (alone or as an oral contraceptive), provided there are no contraindications to oestrogen therapy [C]. Sometimes, giving the injection 2 weeks earlier helps with the bleeding, but this is not evidence based.

## Weight gain

The average weight gain among women using DMPA is between 2 and 6 kg. It tends to be more in women with a BMI of ≥30 than those with a BMI of <25.

## Health concerns

### Cardiovascular disease

POICs do not appear to be associated with an increased risk of stroke, VTE or myocardial infarction [C]. They are medically safe for women when oestrogens are contraindicated.

### Bone mineral density

Concerns have been raised about the potential detrimental effects of DMPA on bone mineral density (BMD). There has been particular concern about use of DMPA in women aged <18 years (who have not yet attained their peak bone mass) and among older women (who are approaching the menopause when bone loss will occur). DMPA is associated with a small loss of BMD which mostly recovers when DMPA is discontinued [B]. There is no evidence that DMPA increases fracture risk in present or past users [E].

The Department of Health and Medicines and Healthcare products Regulatory Agency (MHRA)[19] issued guidance that was endorsed by the Faculty of Sexual and Reproductive Healthcare (FSRH) on the use of DMPA as follows:

- In women aged under 18 years, DMPA may be used as first-line contraception after all options have been discussed and considered unsuitable or unacceptable [C].
- A re-evaluation of the risks and benefits of treatment for all women should be carried out every two years in those who wish to continue use [E].
- For women with significant lifestyle and/or medical risk factors for osteoporosis, other methods of contraception should be considered.

## Drug interactions

Enzyme-inducing drugs do not reduce the contraceptive efficacy of DMPA. Therefore, the injection intervals do not need to be reduced [C].

## Non-contraceptive benefits

There is improvement in dysmenorrhoea and in the symptoms of endometriosis.

---

**POIC - UKMEC Category 3 - Risks generally outweigh benefits**

- **Cardiovascular disease** – multiple risk factors for arterial cardiovascular disease
- **Hypertension** – vascular disease
- **Current and history of ischaemic heart disease and stroke**
- **Unexplained vaginal bleeding**
- **Breast cancer** – past and no evidence of disease for five years
- **Diabetes** – nephropathy, retinopathy, neuropathy and other vascular disease
- **Cirrhosis** – severe (decompensated)
- **Liver tumours** – hepatocellular adenoma and malignant hepatoma
- **SLE** – positive or unknown antiphospholipid antibodies

---

**POIC – UKMEC Category 4 – Unacceptable health risk and should not be used**

- **Breast cancer** – current

---

**KEY POINTS**

**Progestogen-only injectable contraception**
- The main reasons for discontinuation are bleeding problems and weight gain.
- Fertility can be delayed for up to 12 months on discontinuation of Depo Provera.
- DMPA is associated with a small loss of BMD, which mostly recovers after discontinuation. However, there is no increased fracture risk in past and present users.
- Enzyme-inducing drugs do not decrease the contraceptive efficacy of Depo Provera. There is no need to decrease the time intervals between injections for women on enzyme inducing drugs.

---

# PROGESTOGEN-ONLY IMPLANT

Implanon is the only POI available in the UK. It is a single rod which contains 68 mg of etonogestrel (ENG) in a membrane of ethylene vinyl acetate. It is licensed for three years [C] and is available in a preloaded disposable introducer.

Other POIs are Norplant, a six rod LNG implant, and Jadelle, a two rod LNG implant. These implants are licensed for five years' use. They are not available in the UK but UK healthcare professionals may see women who have had them inserted in other countries.

## Mode of action

The main mode of action is inhibition of ovulation [B]. Thickening of the cervical mucus prevents sperm penetration into the upper reproductive tract. It also brings about changes in the endometrium making the environment unfavourable for implantation.

## Effectiveness

The overall pregnancy rate is <1 in 1000 over three years' use [B].

The interaction of any enzyme-inducing medication, for example certain anticonvulsants, antiretroviral therapy, rifampicin or rifabutin, is likely to reduce the effectiveness of the implant, therefore consistent use of condoms is recommended. Use of other contraceptives should be encouraged for women who are long-term users of any of these drugs.

## Side effects

### Bleeding problems
Bleeding irregularities are common with POIs. They include prolonged bleeding, irregular bleeding, oligomenorrhoea and amenorrhoea. Up to 20 per cent of women using implants will be amenorrhoeic [C].

Management
Women who experience problematic bleeding while using a POI should have a sexual history taken to establish STI risk and/or be investigated for gynaecological pathology if clinically indicated. When these have been excluded, bleeding problems can be treated with mefenamic acid or ethinylestradiol (alone or as an oral contraceptive), provided there are no contraindications to oestrogen therapy [C].

### Weight gain
Weight gain has been reported in various studies ranging from 3 to 12 per cent.

### Other changes
Mood changes and loss of libido can occur. Acne can improve, occur or worsen while using the implant. There is no evidence of a causal association between the use of an implant and headache [C].

## Discontinuation

Discontinuation rates of up to 43 per cent within three years have been reported [C]. A third of the women discontinue because of bleeding irregularities. Less than 10 per cent discontinue the method because of other side effects.

## Complications with removal

Complications with removal are low, in the region of 1 per cent. They include deeply sited, non-palpable, broken or migration of implants. Ultrasound and magnetic resonance imaging can be used to locate the implants.

Complicated implants should be referred to specialized centres for removal.

## Health concerns

### Venous thrombo-embolism

There is little or no increase in the risk of VTE with the use of POIs [C].

### Bone marrow density

There is no evidence to suggest that POIs have any clinically significant effect on BMD [C].

### Endocarditis

Prophylactic antibiotics to prevent endocarditis are not needed for insertion and removal of implants [E].

---

**POI – UKMEC Category 3 – Risks generally outweigh benefits**

- Current and history of ischaemic heart disease and stroke - continuation of the method
- Unexplained vaginal bleeding
- Breast cancer - past and no evidence of disease for five years
- Cirrhosis - severe (decompensated)
- Liver tumours - hepatocellular adenoma and malignant hepatoma
- SLE - positive or unknown antiphospholipid antibodies

---

**POI – UKMEC Category 4 – Unacceptable health risk and should not be used**

- Breast cancer - current

---

**KEY POINTS**

**Progestogen-only implant**

- Single rod - lasts for three years.
- Common side effects - bleeding irregularities and weight gain.
- Interaction with enzyme inducing medication decreases the contraceptive effectiveness of the implant.
- There is no evidence to suggest that POIs decrease BMD.

---

# EMERGENCY CONTRACEPTION

In 2002, a judicial review ruled that pregnancy begins at implantation and not at fertilization, thus emergency contraception (EC) is not considered an abortifacient.

A sexual history should be taken from all women attending for EC to assess the risk of STIs. Effectiveness for various methods of EC is shown in Figure 50.3.

## Hormonal method

### Progestogen-only emergency contraception – Levonorgestrel – Levonelle1500, Levonelle one step

#### Mode of action

It is probably multifocal depending when it is given during the cycle. It alters cervical mucus, impairs sperm transport, inhibits ovulation and implantation.

Levonorgestrel is given as a single dose as soon as possible after unprotected sexual intercourse (UPSI) and within 72 hours [A]. However, it can also be given between 73 and 120 hours outside product licence, but there is limited evidence of efficacy [E].

It can be used more than once in a cycle. The WHOMEC for contraceptive use advises that there are no medical contraindications to the use of hormonal EC.

Women who are on liver enzyme-inducing drugs should be advised to take double the dose, i.e. 3 mg of LNG [C]. This use is outside product licence.

## Intrauterine device

A copper IUD can be inserted up to 5 days after the first episode of UPSI. If the timing of ovulation can be estimated, insertion can be beyond 5 days of UPSI, as long as it does not occur beyond 5 days after ovulation [C]. It is effective immediately after insertion. IUDs with banded copper on the arms and containing at least 380 mm$^2$ of copper have the lowest failure rates and should be the first-line choice, particularly if the woman intends to continue the IUD as long-term contraception [A]. Failure rate is 1 per cent.

## Prerequisites

Prior to emergency IUD insertion, women at higher risk of STIs (age <25 years, change in sexual partner, or more than one partner in the last year) should be offered screening for *Chlamydia trachomatis* (as a minimum) [C]. For women assessed as being at higher risk of STIs, if results of screening are not available at the time of emergency IUD insertion, the use of prophylactic antibiotics, at least to cover Chlamydia, should be considered (good practice point).

Reproductive medicine

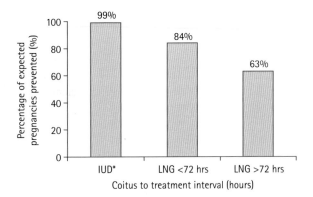

**Figure 50.3** Efficacy of emergency contraception and time since unprotected sexual intercourse. *Within 5 days. IUD, intrauterine device; LNG, levonorgestrel. Reproduced from FFPRHC/FSRH Emergency Contraception Guidance, April 2006

## Mode of action

The same as for IUD.

## Contraindications

The same contraindications apply as for routine IUD insertions.

## Ulipristal acetate – ellaOne

ellaOne® consists of one 30 mg tablet containing ulipristal acetate. It is a selective progesterone receptor modulator. The introduction of ulipristal to the UK market marks an important development in EC. It will be the first oral emergency contraceptive to be licensed for use between 72 and 120 hours of UPSI.[20] Its place in UK contraceptive practice will become clearer as new data are published and clinical experience increases.

### Mechanism of action

Its primary mode of action is thought to be inhibition or delay of ovulation. Endometrial changes also play a role which may inhibit implantation.

How should it be used? One tablet should be taken orally as soon as possible, but no later than 120 hours after UPSI or contraceptive failure. If vomiting occurs within 3 hours, another tablet should be taken. Ulipristal is not recommended to be used more than once per cycle as the safety and efficacy of repeated exposure has not been assessed. If hormonal contraception is continued after administering ulipristal, barrier contraception should be used until the next period or withdrawal bleed.

### Effectiveness

Individual studies suggest that ulipristal is as effective as levonorgestrel for EC. There have been no studies comparing the efficacy of ulipristal to the IUD for the purpose of emergency contraception.

A meta-analysis suggests that regardless of the type of EC drug used, the risk of pregnancy is significantly increased with increasing body mass index (BMI) (8 per cent per point increase in BMI). However, ulipristal acetate appears to be more efficacious compared to levonorgestrel in women who are categorized as overweight or obese.[21]

Ulipristal is contraindicated in pregnancy or suspected pregnancy, as well as in those with a hypersensitivity to any of the excipients. Ulipristal is not recommended in those with severe hepatic impairment, nor in women with severe asthma. As it is not known whether ulipristal is excreted in breast milk, breastfeeding women are advised not to breastfeed for 36 hours after treatment.

### Side effects

The most commonly reported side effects are abdominal pain and menstrual disorders, for example irregular vaginal bleeding, premenstrual syndrome and uterine cramps.

### Does ulipristal interact with other drugs?

Liver enzyme inducers, for example rifampicin, phenytoin, carbamazepine, ritonavir and St John's wort, may reduce plasma concentrations of ulipristal and may reduce efficacy. Use of ulipristal with antacids, proton pump inhibitors and $H_2$ receptor antagonists, or any other drugs that increase gastric pH, may reduce absorption of ulipristal and decrease efficacy.

Ulipristal binds to progesterone receptors and so may reduce the efficacy of progestogen-containing contraceptives.

> **KEY POINTS**
>
> **Emergency contraception**
> - IUD 99 per cent effective as an EC.
> - Levonelle 1500 – licensed up to 72 hours of UPSI, but can be given up to 120 hours as an unlicensed prescription.
> - ellaOne – licensed up to 120 hours of UPSI. It is as effective as Levonelle for EC. Repeat dose not advised in the same cycle.

## STERILIZATION

Sterilization is a permanent and usually an irreversible method of contraception. In the UK, about 50 per cent of the couples over the age of 40 use this method.

Counselling and written information regarding the procedure, its risks, benefits and failure rates should be provided to the client. Discussion and information should also be given regarding other methods, especially the long-acting reversible methods of contraception.

Both men and women should be informed that reversal operations are rarely provided by the National Health Service.

## Female sterilization – tubal occlusion

### Methods

Female sterilization usually involves blocking both the Fallopian tubes during laparotomy, minilaparotomy, laparoscopy or via hysteroscopy.

The Pomeroy technique is the most widely used ligation technique. It involves using absorbable sutures to tie the base of a loop of the Fallopian tube near the mid-portion and cutting off the top of the loop. This procedure destroys 3–4 cm of the tube, making reversal more difficult. A modified Pomeroy procedure rather than Filshie clip application may be preferable for postpartum sterilization performed by mini-laparotomy or at the time of caesarean section, as this leads to lower failure rates [B]. Mechanical occlusion of the tubes by either Filshie clips or rings should be the method of choice for laparoscopic tubal occlusion [A]. Diathermy should not be used as the primary method of tubal occlusion because it increases the risk of subsequent ectopic pregnancy and is less easy to reverse than mechanical occlusive methods [C].

### Essure method

Micro-inserts made from nickel-titanium and stainless steel are inserted hysteroscopically through the cornual ends of both tubes. These generate fibrosis around the devices and the tubes are occluded by three months of the procedures. Some departments carry out a hysterosalpingogram at three months to confirm full occlusion of the tubes. It is an irreversible procedure and the failure rates quoted are the same as for the other methods of tubal occlusion.

#### Failure rate

The failure rate for female sterilization is one in 200. Women should be informed that with tubal occlusion, pregnancy can occur several years after the procedure.

#### Bleeding problems

There is no evidence to suggest that there is an increased incidence of bleeding problems and consequently an increased hysterectomy rate after tubal occlusion.

### Adiana method

The Adiana sterilization method is a combination of controlled thermal damage to the lining of the Fallopian tube followed by insertion of a non-absorbable silicone elastomer matrix within the tubal lumen. Failure rates are less than 2 per cent after two years and the procedure is safe and well tolerated.

## Male sterilization – vasectomy

### Methods

The technique of vasectomy involves division of the vas with fascial interposition or diathermy. The RCOG advise that a no scalpel technique should be used to identify the vas as there is a lower rate of early complications [A]. The procedure can be carried out under a local anaesthetic and is safer than female sterilization. Following the procedure, men should be advised to use effective contraception until two consecutive semen samples 4 weeks apart confirm azoospermia. (The first sample should be taken at least 8 weeks after surgery).

### Risks

#### Failure rate

The failure rate for vasectomy is one in 2000. Both early and late failures can occur. Therefore, men should be informed that pregnancies can occur several years after vasectomy.

Early failures can occur because the wrong structure has been occluded (leaving one or both vasa intact) or because the vas is partially occluded (if ligatures or clips are applied too loosely). There could be congenital duplication of one or both vas. Although the vasa may have been occluded bilaterally, if there are any more vasa, spermatozoa can still be released.

Recanalization of the vas can occur at an early or late stage. Early recanalization is recognized by post-vasectomy sperm counts which may at first be azoospermic or reduced, but then rapidly increase again. Late recanalization presents with a pregnancy several months or years after two consecutive azoospermic samples.

#### Chronic testicular pain

This is probably due to distension and granuloma formation in the epididymis and vas deferens following the operation [B]. Men should be informed of this and reassured that there is no sinister association.

#### Cancer

There is no increase in testicular or prostatic cancers following the vasectomy operation [B].

#### Heart disease

There is no increased incidence of heart disease associated with vasectomy.

---

### KEY POINTS

#### Sterilization

- 50 per cent of the couples over the age of 40 use this method.
- It is irreversible.
- Female sterilization: Involves various occlusive methods performed via the transabdominal or transcervical routes. Failure rate is 1 in 200.
- Male sterilization: Vasectomy. Failure rate 1 in 2000.

# INDUCED ABORTION

The 1967 Abortion Act came into effect on 27 April 1968. The Human Fertilisation and Embryology Authority made changes to the Abortion Act in 1990 which came into effect on 1st April 1991.

Section 4 of the Abortion Act 1967 states that no person is under any obligation to participate in any treatment authorized by the act. This does not apply in an emergency, where the woman's life is in immediate danger or there is immediate risk of grave or permanent injury.

The Abortion Act 1967 states that:

- the abortion is performed within an NHS hospital or approved clinic;
- the chief medical officer is informed of the abortion that has taken place;
- two registered medical practitioners must certify in good faith that the operation is being performed for grounds specified within the act.

The 1967 Abortion Act amended by the Human Fertilization and Embryology Authority in 1990 has five categories. They are:

1 the continuance of the pregnancy would involve risk to the life of the pregnant woman;
2 the termination is necessary to prevent grave permanent injury to the physical or mental health of the pregnant woman;
3 the pregnancy has not exceeded its 24th week and that the continuance of the pregnancy would involve risk, greater than if the pregnancy were terminated or injury to the physical or mental health of the pregnant woman;
4 the pregnancy has not exceeded its 24th week and that the continuance of the pregnancy would involve risk, greater than if the pregnancy were terminated, or injury to the physical or mental health of any existing child(ren) of the family of the pregnant woman;
5 there is substantial risk that if the child were born it would suffer from such physical or mental abnormalities as to be seriously handicapped.

Ninety-eight per cent of the abortions are carried out under the terms of 'C' of the Abortion Act. Abortion under clause 'E' of the abortion act is legal beyond 24 weeks. Common reasons are chromosomal abnormalities and congenital malformations. Down's syndrome is the most commonly reported chromosomal abnormality.

## Pre-abortion management

Pre-abortion management should include non-directive counselling to address alternatives to abortion, i.e. continuing with the pregnancy, adoption or fostering.

Most women will come to a decision quickly but there will be others who will require additional support. Care pathways for additional support, including access to social services, should be available.

A full medical history is taken. An ultrasound scan is usually carried out prior to the procedure to confirm an intrauterine pregnancy and its gestation. Blood tests include haemoglobin measurement, a full blood count and ABO and Rhesus grouping. Other tests are carried out if indicated, depending on clinical grounds. Chlamydia screening should be offered to all. Details of the abortion methods, the procedures and their risks should be discussed with the woman. In order to prevent repeat terminations, discussion of future contraception is vital at this stage. Prophylactic antibiotics should be prescribed during and after the procedure to prevent infective complications.

The following regimens are suitable for periabortion prophylaxis [C]:

Metronidazole 1 g rectally at the time of abortion plus doxycycline 100 mg orally twice daily for 7 days, commencing on the day of abortion

or

Metronidazole 1 g rectally at the time of abortion plus azithromycin 1 g orally on the day of abortion.

All chlamydia-positive women should have a full STI screening and contact tracing and treatment of partners.

## Methods

Methods of abortion and when they can be used are shown in Figure 50.4.

First trimester:
    up to 9 weeks – Early Medical Abortion (EMA)
    up to 10–11 weeks – Manual Vacuum Aspiration (MVA)
    6–15 weeks – Suction TOP under local or general anaesthesia

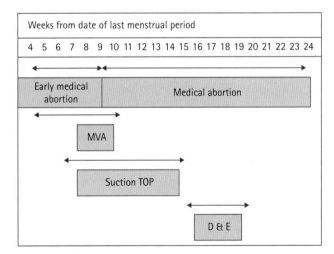

**Figure 50.4** Methods of abortion and when they can be used. Adapted from RCOG Guidelines on care of women requesting induced abortion, September 2004. D&E Dilatation and Evacuation; MVA, manual vacuum aspiration.

Second trimester:

15–20 weeks – Dilatation and Evacuation (D&E) (cervical preparation)

9+ to 24 weeks – Medical Abortion.

## Surgical procedures

Suction termination should be avoided at gestations below 7 weeks as the failure rate is higher. Conventional suction termination is an appropriate method at gestations of 7–15 weeks and can be carried out either under local or general anaesthesia [B]. For first-trimester suction termination, either electric or manual aspiration devices may be used as both are effective and acceptable to women and clinicians. For gestations above 15 weeks, surgical abortion by dilatation and evacuation (D&E), preceded by cervical preparation, is safe and effective and should be undertaken by specialist practitioners who have a reasonable caseload to maintain their skills. Cervical preparation is beneficial prior to surgical abortion and should be routine if the woman is aged under 18 [B].

## Medical abortion

Medical abortion using mifepristone plus prostaglandin is the most effective method of abortion at gestations of less than 9 weeks [A].

The following regime is safe and effective:

- Mifepristone 200 µg orally followed 36–48 hours later by misoprostol 800 µg vaginally. A second dose of 400 µg of misoprostol may have to be given, especially for gestations between 7 and 9 weeks.

For gestations between 9–24 weeks, the regimen is as follows:

- Mifepristone 200 mg orally followed 36–48 hours later by misoprostol 800 µg vaginally. A maximum of four further doses of misoprostol 400 µg may be administered at 3-hourly intervals, vaginally or orally (depending on the amount of bleeding).
- This regimen is unlicensed.

## Complications

### Retained products of conception
This is the most common complication following abortion, more so following a medical abortion. An ultrasound scan is helpful in diagnosing retained products, but the decision to intervene and perform a surgical evacuation should be made on clinical grounds.

### Haemorrhage
The risk of haemorrhage is one in 1000 abortions. The risk is lower for early abortions (0.88 in 1000 at less than 13 weeks; 4.0 in 1000 at more than 20 weeks) [B].

### Uterine perforation
The incidence is 1–4 in 1000. The risk is lower for abortions performed early in pregnancy and those performed by experienced clinicians.

Uterine rupture has been reported in association with mid-trimester medical abortion. However, the risk is under one in 1000 [B].

### Cervical trauma
The risk of damage to the external cervical os at the time of surgical abortion is moderate (no greater than one in 100) [B]. The risk is lower when abortion is performed early in pregnancy and when it is performed by an experienced clinician. Cervical preparation prior to the procedure decreases the risk of cervical trauma.

### Failed abortion and continuing pregnancy
All methods of first-trimester abortion carry a small risk of failure to terminate the pregnancy. The risk for surgical abortion is around 2.3 in 1000 and for medical abortion between one and 14 in 1000 (depending on the regimen used and the experience of the centre) [B].

### Post-abortion infection
Genital tract infection, including pelvic inflammatory disease of varying degrees of severity, occurs in up to 10 per cent of cases. The risk is reduced when prophylactic antibiotics are given or when lower genital tract infection has been excluded by bacteriological screening [B].

### Breast cancer
Induced abortion is not associated with an increase in breast cancer risk [B].

### Future reproductive outcome
There is no evidence to suggest that induced abortion has any effect on subsequent ectopic pregnancy, placenta previa or fertility. However, it may be associated with a small increase in the risk of subsequent miscarriage or preterm delivery [B].

### Psychological sequelae
Some studies suggest that rates of psychiatric illness or self-harm are higher among women who have had an abortion [B].

## Aftercare

### Rhesus prophylaxis
Anti-D immunoglobulin G (250 IU before 20 weeks of gestation and 500 IU thereafter) should be given to all non-sensitized Rh negative women within 72 hours following abortion, whether by surgical or medical methods [B].

## Contraception

This should have been discussed at the pre-abortion assessment. The chosen method of contraception can be initiated immediately following the abortion. Oral contraceptives can be commenced on the following day of the procedure. Injectables can be administered on the same day, while the subdermal implant and intrauterine contraception can be inserted immediately following a first or second trimester termination of pregnancy. Sterilization can also be safely performed at the time of induced abortion. However, this is associated with higher rates of failure and regret on the part of the woman [B].

## Follow up

Women should be given written information about the symptoms they may experience following the abortion. They should be given a 24-hour telephone helpline number to contact in case of any problems. They should be offered a follow-up appointment within 2 weeks of the procedure. A minority of women can experience long-term post-abortion distress and they should be referred for further counselling.

### KEY POINTS

#### Induced abortion

- There are five categories of the Abortion Act.
- Two registered medical practitioners must certify in good faith that the operation is being performed for grounds specified within the Act.
- Medical abortion is safer than the surgical method. It can be carried out from 4+ till 24 weeks.
- Cervical preparation should be carried out for women under 18 years of age and for gestations more than 10 weeks.
- Prophylactic antibiotics should be prescribed during and after the procedure to prevent infective complications.

## Published Guidelines

In addition to the Key References the following guildelines are essesntial reading and were used in the writing of this chapter:

**FFPRHC guidelines - All guidelines are available on the Faculty's website www.ffprhc.org.uk or www.fsrh.org**

Condoms – Male and Female
Combined Oral Contraceptive – First Prescription of COC
Combined Oral Contraception – Missed Pills
Emergency Contraception Guidance
Female Barrier Methods
Intrauterine Contraception
Management of Unscheduled Bleeding in Women Using Hormonal Contraception
Progestogen-only Implants
Progestogen-only Injectable Contraception
Progestogen-only Pills

UK Medical Eligibility Criteria for Contraceptive Use (2009)
UK Selected Practice Recommendations for Contraceptive Use (2002)

**RCOG Guidelines – Available on the RCOG website www.rcog.org.uk**

Male and female sterilization
The care of women requesting induced abortion

**NICE Guideline – the following guideline is available on the NICE website www.nice.org.uk**

Long Acting Reversible Contraception

## Key References

1. WHO. Medical eligibility criteria for contraceptive use 3rd edn. Geneva: World Health Organization 2008.
2. UK Medical Eligibility Criteria for Contraceptive Use. *Faculty of Sexual and Reproductive Healthcare*. London: Royal College of Obstetrics and Gynaecology, 2009.
3. World Health Organization. Task Force a Methods for the Determination of the Fertile Period, Special Programme of Research and Training in Human Reproduction. *Am J Obstet Gynecol* 1980; **138**: 383.
4. Glasier A, Gebbie A. *Handbook of Family Planning and Reproductive Healthcare*, 5th edn. Edinburgh: Churchill Livingstone Elsevier, 2008.
5. Marshall J. A prospective trial of mucothermic method of natural family planning. *Int Rev Nat Fam Plann* 1985; **9**:139–43.
6. World Health Organization. A prospective multi-centre trial of the ovulation method of natural family planning II. The effectiveness phase. *Fertil Steril* 1981; **36**: 591–8.
7. Kennedy KI, Rivera R, McNeilly AS. Consensus statement on the use of breast feeding as a family planning method. *Contraception* 1989; **39**: 477–96.
8. Guillebaud J. *Contraception, Your Questions Answered*, 5th edn. Edinburgh: Churchill Livingstone Elsevier, 2009.
9. Lidegaard Ø, Løkkegaard E, Svendsen AL, Agger C. Hormonal contraception and risk of venous thromboembolism: national follow-up study. *BMJ* 2009; **339**: b2890.
10. Van Hylckama Vlieg A, Helmerhorst FM, Vandenbroucke JP *et al.* Effects of oestrogen dose and progestogen type on venous thrombotic risk associated with oral contraceptives: results of the MEGA case-control study. *BMJ* 2009; **339**: b2921.
11. Khader YS, Rice J, John L, Abueita O. Oral contraceptive use and the risk of myocardial infarction: a meta-analysis. *Contraception* 2003; **68**: 11–17.
12. Szarewski A, Guillebaud J. *Contraception – A User's Guide*, revised 3rd edn. Oxford: Oxford University Press, 2002.

13. Mansour D. Qlaira: A 'natural' change of direction. *J Fam Plann Reprod Health Care* 2009; **35**: 139–42.

14. Shimoni N, Westhoff C. Review of the vaginal contraceptive ring (Nuva Ring). *J Fam Plann Reprod Health Care* 2008; **34**: 247–50.

15. Faculty of Sexual and Reproductive Healthcare Clinical Effectiveness Unit. Recommendation: Antibiotic prophylaxis for intrauterine contraceptive use in women at risk of bacterial endocarditis, July 2008.

16. Kulier R, O'Brien P, Helmerhorst F *et al.* Copper containing, framed intra-uterine devices for contraception. *Cochrane Database Syst Rev* 2007; (**4**): CD005347.

17. Robinson GE, Bounds W, Kubba AA *et al.* Functional ovarian cysts associated with the levonorgestrel releasing intrauterine device. *Br J Fam Plann* 1989; **14**: 132.

18. Canto De Cetina TE, Canto P, Ordoñez Luna M. Effect of counseling to improve compliance in Mexican women receiving depot-medroxyprogesterone acetate. *Contraception* 2001; **63**: 143–6.

19. Medicines and Healthcare Products Regulatory Agency. *Updated Guidance on the Use of DepoProvera-Contraception*, 8 November 2004. Available from: www.mhra.gov.uk/Safetyinformation/Safetywarning salertsandrecalls/Safetywarningsandmessagesform edicines/CON1004262.

20. Faculty of Sexual and Reproductive Healthcare. New Product Review, Ulipristal Acetate (ellaOne). Clinical Effectiveness Unit, October 2009.

21. Ulmann A, Scherrer B, Mathe H *et al.* Meta-analysis demonstrating superiority of the selective progesterone receptor modulator ulipristal acetate versus levonorgestrel for emergency contraception. Abstract and Poster Presentation presented at the 8th Congress of the European Society of Gynecology, Rome, Italy, 10–13 September 2009.

# 51.1 Endometrial function

*Hilary OD Critchley and Christine P West*

---

### MRCOG standards

- Understand the physiology of normal menstruation.

## INTRODUCTION

The main function of the endometrium is to receive a fertilized ovum (blastocyst) during implantation. As this occurs relatively infrequently, cyclical breakdown and regeneration of the endometrium during the menstrual cycle are pivotal reproductive events. These changes are under the control of the hypothalamo–pituitary–ovarian axis, with ovarian steroids acting directly within the endometrium via local intracellular receptors. Many other local mediators are involved in the complex and dynamic processes that take place within this metabolically highly active organ.

## ENDOCRINE REGULATION OF ENDOMETRIAL FUNCTION

The uterine endometrium is a target organ for sex steroids and is exposed to an orchestrated sequence of circulating oestrogen, progesterone and progesterone withdrawal (result of regression of the corpus luteum in the absence of pregnancy). Sequential exposure to oestrogen and progesterone, as a consequence of cyclical ovarian activity, results in repeated episodes of cellular proliferation and differentiation with regular menstrual bleeding.[1] The proliferative phase of the endometrial cycle corresponds to the ovarian follicular phase. The secretory phase of endometrial differentiation is under progesterone domination and corresponds to the ovarian luteal phase. In the follicular phase, oestrogen secreted from the dominant follicle promotes regeneration and proliferation of the endometrium with upregulation of both oestrogen receptors (ER) and progesterone receptors (PR). The mid-secretory phase is a period of peak exposure to circulating

progesterone and is often referred to as the 'implantation window' (day 19–24). Endometrial expression of sex steroid receptors permits the endometrium to respond to ovarian oestradiol and progesterone. Exposure of the endometrium to sex steroids, acting via their nuclear receptors (ER and PR), results in a cascade of gene expression that is essential for preparation of the endometrium (receptive) in anticipation of successful implantation. In the absence of a pregnancy, the corpus luteum regresses, progesterone levels fall and progesterone withdrawal is the trigger for the cascade of events that culminate in shedding of the upper functional layer of the endometrium. Menstruation is a fundamental reproductive process in women and displays all the hallmarks of an inflammatory event. Equal in importance with the shedding of the endometrium is its regeneration, which commences 36 hours after the onset of bleeding and is normally completed by day 5–6 of the cycle.

## MORPHOLOGICAL CHANGES

The three classic phases of the menstrual cycle are the oestrogen dominated proliferative phase, the post-ovulatory and progesterone dominated secretory phase, and the menstrual phase.[2] The endometrium is composed of two layers. The upper functional layer is shed during menstruation. During the follicular phase of the cycle, the endometrium proliferates from the basal layer in response to oestradiol. The developing glands are initially straight and tubular within a compact stroma but later become more convoluted. Following ovulation, exposure to rising levels of progesterone from the corpus luteum induces secretory changes in the endometrial glands. Subnuclear vacuoles appear initially, followed by evidence of glandular secretory activity. This is accompanied in the late luteal phase by oedema and predecidual changes in the stroma and increased coiling of the spiral arterioles, which supply the endometrium.

Failure of conception results in regression of the corpus luteum and an abrupt decline in circulating levels of oestrogen and progesterone. In the endometrium, there is loss of tissue fluid, stromal infiltration of leukocytes and intense vasoconstriction of the spiral arterioles. Distal ischaemia and vasodilatation lead to tissue breakdown and bleeding from the damaged vessels. Thirty-six hours after the onset of bleeding, the process of endometrial regeneration commences in the basal layer.

## CELLULAR AND MOLECULAR EVENTS

Progesterone is the endocrine signal that is responsible for the establishment and maintenance of pregnancy. Progesterone withdrawal is the primary initiating event for the cascade of molecular and cellular events that lead to menstruation. Following shedding of the upper functional layer, the endometrium displays remarkable and immediate regenerative capacity.

The precise local mechanisms involved in the control of the highly coordinated cyclical tissue 'injury' and 'repair' that occurs in the absence of a pregnancy have still to be fully elucidated. Modern molecular technologies have permitted an expansion of knowledge of gene profiles across the menstrual cycle, including during the 'putative window' of implantation and at the time of progesterone withdrawal (menstruation). The molecular and cellular mechanisms within the uterine endometrium regulating the key reproductive events – implantation and menstruation, involve complex interactions between the endocrine, vascular and immune systems.[3]

The receptors for sex steroids are members of a large family of nuclear transcription factors that regulate the expression of numerous genes. Members of the nuclear receptor superfamily expressed by endometrial cells include progesterone (PR), oestrogen (ERα and ERβ), androgen (AR) and glucocorticoid receptors (GR). The role for these latter two steroid receptors in regulation of endometrial function has thus far received limited attention.[4] The endometrial expression of PR, ERα and ERβ varies temporally and spatially across the menstrual cycle. The expression of ERα and PR are under dual control by oestradiol and progesterone.

Two isoforms of the human PR have been described. PRA and PRB derive from a single gene and function as transcriptional regulators of progestin-responsive genes. There is a decline in PR expression in the glands of the functional layer of the endometrium with the transition from the proliferative to the secretory phase of the cycle. PR persists in the stromal cells in the upper functional layer. The basal region is regulated differently as the glands and stroma of the deeper zones express PR throughout the cycle. Differences between expression of the PR in the superficial and basal regions of the endometrium is likely to have functional importance because only the superficial layers are shed during menstruation. Progestogens have an anti-oestrogenic effect with inhibition of endometrial growth and induction of maturation and differentiation of the glandular and stromal cells.

Oestrogen action is mediated by two subtypes of oestrogen receptor referred to as ERα and ERβ. These two structurally related subtypes of ER are derived from separate genes. In the upper functional layer, ERα expression increases in both glandular and stromal cells in the proliferative phase and declines in the secretory phase due to suppression by progesterone. In the basal layer, ERα is expressed in glandular and stromal cells throughout the menstrual cycle. In endometrium, the only sex steroid receptor present in the endothelium of endometrial blood vessels is ERβ. Thus, any direct effects of oestrogen on endometrial vessels, including angiogenesis and permeability, will be mediated by ERβ. The function of ERβ in the uterus is still to be determined. The physiological role of endometrial androgen receptor (AR) has also not been established. During the normal cycle, stromal cells are the predominant cell type expressing the AR and thus androgen effects in the endometrium will likely be mediated by the stromal cells. A more detailed discussion of the mechanisms of steroid receptor function in the endometrium is outwith the scope of this brief overview.

The availability of molecular technologies, including gene microarray studies and detailed bioinformatics analysis, has contributed to the expanding literature on identification of genes that are likely to be important for endometrial function during the progesterone dominant 'receptive phase'.[5] This knowledge is important for understanding the requirements for a receptive endometrium and successful implantation and how disturbances of endometrial structure and function may play a role in subfertility. Equally important is the insight such knowledge has provided for fertility control (contraception). Valuable insight about progesterone action, progesterone withdrawal and endometrial function has come from the observations of pharmacological withdrawal of progesterone from the endometrium. Studies with pharmaceutical compounds that bind to the PR, for example the antiprogestin, mifepristone, have advanced our understanding of local mechanisms that may be targeted to modulate both endometrial receptivity and endometrial bleeding.[6]

The regenerative capacity of the endometrium is also remarkable and an essential component of regulated endometrial function. Disturbance of the tightly controlled sequence of 'injury and repair' events within the endometrium will contribute to menstrual disorders, such as heavy menstrual bleeding (HMB, menorrhagia). Early studies of menstruation identified a role for prostaglandins. Progesterone withdrawal results in increases in endometrial prostaglandin (PG) synthesis and decreases in PG metabolism. More recent research has shed light upon the complex molecular and cellular events within the endometrium at the time of menses (when progesterone levels fall).[1,3] Local mediators within the endometrium that have been implicated in the regulation of the menstrual process include the inducible enzyme responsible for synthesis of prostaglandins – COX-2 and chemokines (for example: CXCL8, neutrophil chemotactic factor, interleukin-8; and CCL-2, monocyte chemotactic peptide-1, MCP-1). Prostaglandin synthesis via COX-2 is relevant since non-steroidal anti-inflammatory agents are widely used in the treatment of menstrual complaints, including heavy and painful periods. Changes in the structure and viability of the endometrium are due to the release of mediators that degrade the extracellular matrix including matrix metalloproteinases (MMPs).[7] A phenomenon of blood vessel function at menstruation is modest platelet aggregation and fibrin deposition. It is notable that menstrual bleeding extends over 3–5 days and is not accompanied with scarring. The uterus is a rich source of prostaglandins and uterine fluid contains high fibrinolytic activity and fibrin degradation products, suggesting active fibrinolysis occurs. Indeed, agents targeting the fibrinolytic system are a first-line management for complaints of heavy menstrual bleeding. Following menses, the endometrium rapidly repairs with regeneration of all cell types (epithelial, vascular and stromal). The exposed surface is rapidly covered with fibronectin, leukocytes are removed and the epithelium regenerates. Full repair is usually complete by day 6 of the menstrual cycle. A host of local mediators are involved in regeneration including EGF, TGFa, endothelins and VEGF. These factors also play a key role in the angiogenic processes necessary for reconstitution of the endometrial vasculature.[8]

## KEY POINT

Knowledge of basic uterine physiology is necessary to understand the physiological basis of disorders of the menstrual cycle. Future research efforts should aim to delineate cellular and molecular pathways that may be targets for therapeutic intervention when implantation or menstruation is problematic.

## Key References

1. Jabbour HN, Kelly RW, Fraser HM, Critchley HO. Endocrine regulation of menstruation. *Endocr Rev* 2006; **27**: 17–46.
2. Noyes RW, Hertig AT, Rock J. Dating the endometrial biopsy. *Fertil Steril* 1950; **1**: 3–25.
3. Critchley HO, Kelly RW, Brenner RM, Baird DT. The endocrinology of menstruation – a role for the immune system. *Clin Endocrinol* 2001; **55**: 701–10.
4. Critchley HO, Saunders PT. Hormone receptor dynamics in a receptive human endometrium. *Reprod Sci* 2009; **16**: 191–9.
5. Giudice LC. Microarray expression profiling reveals candidate genes for human uterine receptivity. *Am J Pharmacogenomics* 2004; **4**: 299–312.
6. Critchley HO, Kelly RW, Baird DT, Brenner RM. Regulation of human endometrial function: mechanisms relevant to uterine bleeding. *Reprod Biol Endocrinol* 2006; **4** (Suppl. 1): S5.
7. Salamonsen LA. Tissue injury and repair in the female human reproductive tract. *Reproduction* 2003; **125**: 301–11.
8. Girling JE, Rogers PA. Recent advances in endometrial angiogenesis research. *Angiogenesis* 2005; **8**: 89–99.

# 51.2 Uterine fibroids and heavy menstrual bleeding

*Christine P West*

## INTRODUCTION

Uterine fibroids are common in women of reproductive age. They are a frequent indication for gynaecological surgery, most commonly hysterectomy, although in the past many hysterectomies were carried out for asymptomatic fibroids because of concerns about the nature and consequences of a pelvic mass. Advances in imaging have facilitated the diagnosis of fibroids and enabled more women to be managed conservatively. Fibroids may be implicated in the causation of miscarriage and subfertility, but this chapter primarily addresses the evidence base for the management of heavy menstrual bleeding (HMB) associated with the presence of fibroids.

## DEFINITIONS

Uterine fibroids, also known as myomas or leiomyomas, are benign tumours arising from the myometrium. They are composed of round whorls of smooth muscle and connective tissue and may be single, multiple or very numerous. Their site may be intramural, submucosal or subserous and their presentation and symptoms vary according to their size and site of origin. They are commonly asymptomatic and found incidentally during routine pelvic or ultrasound examination. Their most common symptomatic presentation is with heavy menstrual bleeding or pressure symptoms.

## INCIDENCE

Fibroids are present in up to 25 per cent of women of reproductive age.[1] In studies in which heavy blood loss has been subjectively confirmed by direct measurement,[2] 40 per cent of women with losses >200 mL were found to have fibroids, compared with only 10 per cent whose losses were <100 mL. In a review of risk factors,[1] fibroids were reported to be more common and to occur at a younger age in black women. They are also associated with nulliparity and are more common in women with a family history of fibroids. Smoking and the long-term use of the oral contraceptive pill and Depo-Provera are associated with a reduced risk. Fibroids regress in size and undergo degeneration after the menopause.

## AETIOLOGY

Fibroids are hormone dependent and contain increased levels of receptors for both oestrogen and progesterone compared with normal myometrium.[3] The actions of steroid hormones on the uterus are mediated by a number of growth factors and it is likely that these are involved in fibroid growth. However, it is not clear how fibroids are initiated and there is no explanation for their heterogeneity in terms of numbers, size, site and behaviour within and between individuals. Although a causal relationship with heavy menstrual bleeding has not been firmly established, it is likely that fibroids contribute to heavy bleeding if present submucosally or where intramural fibroids cause distortion of the endometrial cavity. There is little evidence that subserosal or pedunculated fibroids contribute to heavy blood loss.[4]

# MANAGEMENT

The management of uterine fibroids is covered in detail in a comprehensive evidence-based guideline.[4] Recommendations relevant to the management of heavy bleeding associated with fibroids are also made in a national evidence based clinical guideline on heavy menstrual bleeding.[5] In common with all gynaecological disorders, the age and reproductive status of the individual woman and her preferences in relation to the various options influence management.

## Investigation

History and examination are supplemented by a full blood count.[5] Suspicion of fibroids is usually based on a palpably enlarged uterus on pelvic or abdominal examination. If the uterine enlargement is no greater than a 10–12 week gestation size, medical management can be initiated within primary care without further investigation.[5] Failure to respond to medical therapy or a uterus that is palpable abdominally is an indication for further assessment [E].

Investigation of abnormal bleeding is covered elsewhere (Chapter 51.3, Heavy and irregular menstruation) and these recommendations apply to the investigation of suspected fibroids. Transvaginal ultrasound (TVS) should be the preliminary investigation [A],[4,5] combined with abdominal ultrasound where the uterine enlargement is in excess of a 12-week size. It is important to visualize the ovaries and endometrium and, where possible, to document the size, number and position of individual fibroids, as well as the overall uterine dimensions [E]. Where submucosal fibroids are suspected, hysteroscopy or transvaginal saline infusion sonography improve diagnostic accuracy [A].[4] Magnetic resonance imaging (MRI) has no advantage over ultrasound for the detection and routine imaging of fibroids[6] and is considerably more costly. However, it has greater precision and can be used if there is doubt about the nature of a fibroid mass[7] or to assess suitability for uterine artery embolization [B].[8]

Endometrial biopsy should be carried out if there is irregular or intermenstrual bleeding[5] [E] or abnormal endometrial thickening on TVS [A].

## Conservative management

First-line management of HMB in the presence of fibroids should follow national guidelines.[5] These state that medical therapies which are effective in the management of HMB can be used in women with fibroids less than 3 cm in diameter which are causing no distortion of the uterine cavity [E]. Anaemia should be treated with oral iron. Some women will wish to avoid further treatment, either medical or surgical, and this preference should be respected [E]. The evidence supporting the use of medical therapies for HMB in women with fibroids is reviewed below.

## Non-hormonal therapy

Non-steroidal anti-inflammatory drugs (NSAIDs) are not effective in the reduction of heavy bleeding secondary to the presence of fibroids [C].[4] There have been no randomized, controlled trials evaluating antifibrinolytics in the management of HMB associated with fibroids, but a non-random comparative study[9] reported a highly significant blood loss reduction of around 50 per cent in women with clinically diagnosed fibroids. This was similar to the response in women with normal-sized or slightly enlarged uteri. On the basis of this information, tranexamic acid should be used in preference to NSAIDs in the first-line management of fibroid-associated HMB [D].

## Combined oral contraceptives

There is no evidence that the oral contraceptive pill causes enlargement of fibroids; indeed, long-term use may be protective [D].[1] There have been no randomized trials of its use to control bleeding in women with fibroids, but one comparative study demonstrated a significant reduction in measured blood loss (around 50 per cent) with a high-dose combined oral contraceptive pill (COCP) in women with clinically diagnosed fibroids.[9] For women desiring contraception or for whom the use of the COCP is acceptable, this is a reasonable option [D].

## Progestogens, antiprogesterones and androgens

Progestogens, even in high doses, do not shrink fibroids[4] thus use of oral progestogens in women with fibroids should be purely symptomatic and in a regimen that is effective for HMB, i.e. for 21 days out of 28. The long-term use of depot medroxyprogesterone acetate (MPA) protects against the development of fibroids [C],[10] but its role in the symptomatic management of fibroid-associated bleeding problems is unclear.

Both the androgen danazol[4] and the androgenic antiprogesterone gestrinone[4] reduce fibroid size and blood loss during treatment. After cessation of gestrinone, fibroid regrowth is gradual, potentially increasing the usefulness of this therapy. Androgenic side effects are less with gestrinone compared with danazol and thus gestrinone is a potentially useful short-term management option [B].

The antiprogesterone mifepristone causes amenorrhoea and significant regression of fibroids at various doses[11] without having any detrimental effect on bone density. Currently it is not available for the treatment of fibroids, but antiprogesterones are likely to be an important future option.

## Levonorgestrel-releasing intrauterine system

The role of the levonorgestrel-releasing intrauterine system (LNG-IUS) has not been fully evaluated in women with fibroids. Presence of fibroids greater than 3 cm and/or cavity distortion has been generally regarded as a contraindication to inclusion in clinical trials of the LNG-IUS for heavy menstrual bleeding.[5] Rates of expulsion of between 6 and 13 per cent have been reported in women with fibroids, compared with around 3 per cent in the general population.[12–14] Users of the LNG-IUS for contraception have a lower rate of development of fibroids compared with users of copper-containing devices.[4,12] Six small prospective studies all reported reduction of menstrual loss with the LNG-IUS in women with HMB and fibroids,[12,13] although duration of follow up was limited to 12 months and effect on fibroid size was variable. A prospective cohort study comparing LNG-IUS use in women with fibroid-related and non-fibroid-related HMB[14] reported a significant decrease in uterine volume in both groups of women with HMB, but not in a control group of women using the LNG-IUS for contraception. However, reduction of fibroid volume, as distinct from overall uterine volume, was not significant. Forty per cent of the women with fibroids were amenorrhoeic after two years, compared with 50 per cent of the women with non-fibroid HMB and 57 per cent of the control group. The prevalence of spotting was 27 per cent in the fibroid group, compared with 11 and 7 per cent in the other two groups, respectively. Continuation with the LNG-IUS in the fibroid group was 67 per cent at two years and 37 per cent at three years, but reasons for discontinuation were not stated. None of the studies mentioned above related bleeding patterns or expulsion risk to fibroid size or to the degree of cavity distortion. On the basis of current limited information, the use of the LNG-IUS can be considered in women with fibroids, but they should be warned of the increased risk of expulsion [C], particularly in the presence of an enlarged or distorted uterine cavity [C].

## GnRH analogues

Treatment with gonadotrophin-releasing hormone (GnRH) agonists induces amenorrhoea and shrinkage of fibroids [A].[4] However, after cessation, regrowth is rapid. These changes are secondary to temporary ovarian suppression, and long-term treatment with GnRH agonists is contraindicated due to the risk of bone loss. Currently, the role of these agents is largely limited to pre-operative shrinkage of fibroids, although there is scope for their longer term use with the addition of hormonal add-back.

### GnRH agonists prior to hysterectomy and myomectomy

Shrinkage of fibroids prior to hysteroscopic or conventional surgery has been advocated on the basis of reduced fibroid size and vascularity. Their use prior to hysterectomy or myomectomy has been the subject of a systematic review[15] that was based on 26 randomized, controlled trials. When used together with iron therapy, they are effective in the treatment of preoperative anaemia [A]. They significantly

reduce intraoperative blood loss, particularly in women with very large uteri. With large uteri, they significantly increase the likelihood of a transverse abdominal incision or a vaginal rather than an abdominal hysterectomy [A]. However, their cost effectiveness for routine use for women who do not fall into these specific categories has been challenged.[16]

There have been no randomized trials of GnRH agonists prior to hysteroscopic myomectomy, although they are widely used in this situation. One non-randomized, controlled study[17] reported a significant reduction in operating time, blood loss, volume of distending medium and treatment failure following pre-treatment with a GnRH agonist [C].

### GnRH agonists plus hormonal add-back for longer term treatment of fibroids

In women who have contraindications to or decline surgery and in whom other medical measures have failed, long-term relief of HMB may be achieved with GnRH agonists in combination with low-dose hormone replacement therapy (HRT). The GnRH agonist should be administered alone for three months to obtain fibroid shrinkage [D][4] before addition of the HRT. Low-dose oral oestrogen–progestogen combinations, progestogens alone and tibolone have been tested in randomized, controlled trials. Oral oestrogen combined with cyclical norethisterone 0.7 mg was compared with continuous norethisterone 10 mg daily[4] in women treated with leuprolide acetate for a period of two years. Both add-back therapies prevented bone loss, but regrowth of the fibroids and a less favourable bleeding pattern occurred with norethisterone alone. In a randomized, double-blind study,[18] tibolone add-back was more effective than placebo in the relief of vasomotor symptoms and equally effective in reducing fibroid size and menstrual symptoms. Bone density was maintained in the group given tibolone, and irregular bleeding was a problem for only a minority of the patients in this group. On the basis of this limited evidence, combined HRT preparations or tibolone are effective for add-back therapy with GnRH agonists for the longer-term treatment of fibroids [B].

## HRT in menopausal women with fibroids

Conservative management is often offered to women with symptomatic fibroids who are perimenopausal on the basis that their symptoms will resolve spontaneously when they reach the menopause. It is therefore relevant to consider the effect of HRT on fibroids. Limited information from randomized trials is based on the use of continuous combined preparations or tibolone in women with pre-existing fibroids and an established menopause. Use of transdermal oestradiol (50 μg) in combination with 5 mg MPA resulted in significant uterine enlargement at one year of follow up, compared with 0.625 μg conjugated equine oestrogens (CEE) in combination with 2.5 mg MPA.[4] However, symptomatic response and bleeding patterns were no different. The same dose of CEE combined with 5 mg MPA, when compared with tibolone,[19] caused less amenorrhoea and more irregular bleeding, but neither caused uterine enlargement. Information from these studies suggest that oral continuous combined HRT preparations or tibolone can be used in postmenopausal women with fibroids [B].

## SURGICAL TREATMENT

### Hysteroscopic surgery

Small submucous fibroids can be removed hysteroscopically.[4,5] However, assessment of the effectiveness of hysteroscopic resection has been based on retrospective reports from single centres.[4,5] The procedure is normally restricted to type I fibroids that are largely intracavitary and less than 3–5 cm in diameter, although removal of larger, partly intramural, type II fibroids has also been described.[4] The complications of hysteroscopic surgery include fluid overload, uterine perforation, haemorrhage and infection. Case review and cohort studies[4,5,20] have reported relief of menstrual symptoms in 69–84 per cent of women up to 15 years of follow up. Effectiveness can be increased by concurrent endometrial ablation in women not desiring future pregnancies.[5,20] Hysteroscopic myomectomy is thus an effective approach for the relief of heavy menstrual bleeding associated with small submucous fibroids [D].

### Myomectomy

Myomectomy is a well-established alternative to hysterectomy for women wishing to preserve their fertility.[4,21] Reduction of menstrual bleeding in more than 80 per cent of women has been reported in retrospective case series [C]. Recurrence of fibroids is common, with a ten-year recurrence of 27 per cent in one large follow-up study.[4] Heavy blood loss is a potential problem at myomectomy, and techniques such as the use of occlusive clamps and tourniquets, vasopressin, adrenaline and misporostol[21,22] have been described to reduce it, although there is no clear consensus as to which is most effective.[4,22] GnRH agonists have been shown to reduce operative blood loss when used for the pre-treatment of large uteri [A].[15] Intramural fibroids smaller than 6 cm diameter may be removed successfully by laparoscopy in specialist centres [C],[4,5] but meticulous suturing is required in order to avoid the risk of uterine rupture in subsequent pregnancies.[4] Laparotomy remains the preferred route for myomectomies performed outwith specialist centres and is associated with low morbidity and a favourable outcome for subsequent pregnancies [E].[4,5,21]

### Hysterectomy

Hysterectomy offers a definitive cure for women with heavy bleeding associated with fibroids who have completed childbearing. The abdominal route is most commonly used for large fibroids, although there are reports of use of the vaginal route by experienced operators.[21] The role of the pre-operative use of GnRH agonists is discussed above. Hysterectomy is not recommended for the routine management of women with asymptomatic fibroids, even if they are very large [E].[4,5]

### Uterine artery embolization

This technique was initially performed for the control of postpartum haemorrhage but is now widely used for the treatment of fibroids. It is performed under radiological screening after selective catheterization of the uterine arteries via one or both femoral arteries. Polyvinyl alcohol particles are injected to embolize the uterine vascular bed.[4] It is carried out under local anaesthesia but requires overnight hospitalization for opiate analgesia because of severe post-procedural ischaemic uterine pain. Fibroid shrinkage is gradual, reaching a mean of around 60 per cent at six months. A 50 per cent reduction in median measured menstrual blood loss 6–9 months after uterine artery embolization (UAE) and 80 per cent reduction after 36–48 months has been reported.[23] Complications are usually minor and include local haematomas at the puncture sites, urinary retention, mild febrile reactions (post-embolization syndrome), vaginal discharge and delayed passage of infarcted submucus fibroids.[4] Severe complications have also been reported including overwhelming sepsis which has proved fatal.[24] A complication-related hysterectomy rate of around 1 per cent in the first 12 months after the procedure was reported in large prospective studies.[5,24,25]

Data from a systematic review of three RCTs[26] comparing UAE with hysterectomy (two studies) or myomectomy (one study), together with a subsequently published RCT[27] is now available. UAE is associated with shorter duration of hospital stay and faster return to work and normal activities compared with surgery. Complication rates were similar in the two groups, with major complications more frequent following hysterectomy. Satisfaction rates and quality of life scores were high in both groups although further intervention rates were higher following UAE. Long-term data from these studies are not yet available and assessment of longer term efficacy is largely based on case series.[4,5] A large retrospective UK cohort study of 1100 women comparing UAE with hysterectomy reported a lower complication rate with UAE but better symptomatic improvement with hysterectomy.[25] There was a 23 per cent chance of requiring further treatment for fibroids a mean of 4.6 years after UAE with 4.9 per cent undergoing myomectomy and 11.2 per cent hysterectomy. One RCT and three cohort studies have compared UAE with myomectomy.[5,26] All reported fewer adverse events with UAE and no significant difference in symptom or quality of life scores at various time intervals after the procedure. One showed a significantly greater reduction in menstrual blood loss after UAE [C].

In women of reproductive years, choice between myomectomy and UAE will be influenced by prospects for future pregnancy. To date, pregnancies after UAE have been limited in number[25] and, although reassuring, there is insufficient evidence upon which to base advice on this important issue. The procedure is associated with a small risk of ovarian failure which largely affects women aged 45 years and over.[28]

Although early results support the use of uterine artery embolization for symptomatic fibroids associated with heavy menstrual bleeding [B], there is a clear need for more information based on longer-term outcome from randomized trials comparing UAE with both hysterectomy and myomectomy.

## MRI-guided focused ultrasound

This technique uses a non-invasive thermal ablation device integrated with an MR imaging system for the ablation of soft tissue.[29] It has a potential role as a fertility conserving option for the management of fibroids and its use in the USA has been approved by the FDA. Although initial results from prospective cohort studies are positive, data are limited and the technique remains under evaluation in the UK.

---

### EBM

These recommendations are based on two evidence-based clinical guidelines (one specific to the management of fibroids) and three systematic reviews. Many of the recommendations regarding management are based on information from non-randomized trials, case series or prospective cohort studies.

---

### KEY POINTS

- Transvaginal ultrasound, combined with abdominal ultrasound for uteri larger than 12-week size, is the primary investigation for suspected fibroids [A].
- Both hysteroscopy and transvaginal sonohysterography (saline infusion sonography) are of value in the further investigation of suspected submucosal fibroids [A].
- MRI scanning should not be used as a primary investigation but can be used if there is doubt about the nature of a uterine mass or in assessment of suitability for uterine artery embolization [B].
- Medical therapies which are effective in the management of heavy menstrual bleeding can be used in women with fibroids less than 3 cm in diameter which are causing no distortion of the uterine cavity [E].
- Tranexamic acid should be used in preference to NSAIDs in the first-line management of HMB associated with fibroids [D].
- The COCP is not contraindicated in the presence of fibroids and may relieve HMB [D].

- Progestogens do not shrink fibroids but may relieve HMB at high doses if used continuously or for 21 days out of 28 [D].
- Progestogen-releasing intrauterine devices may be beneficial for HMB associated with fibroids but patients should be warned of the increased risk of expulsion [C].
- Gestrinone is a useful drug for the short-term symptomatic management of fibroids [B].
- GnRH agonists shrink fibroids and relieve HMB [A] and may be used in conjunction with add-back HRT for long-term treatment [B].
- GnRH agonists are useful adjuncts to surgery in cases of anaemia, very large fibroids and where uterine shrinkage may result in a transverse abdominal incision or a vaginal rather than an abdominal hysterectomy [A].
- Oral administration of HRT is preferable to the transdermal route for postmenopausal women with fibroids [B].
- Small submucous fibroids may be removed by hysteroscopic surgery [D].
- Myomectomy is an alternative to hysterectomy for women with HMB associated with fibroids who wish to retain their fertility [B].
- Hysterectomy is not recommended for the routine management of women with asymptomatic fibroids, regardless of their size [E].
- Uterine artery embolization is a promising alternative to surgery for fibroids [B], but information based on longer term follow up is required.

## Key References

1. Vollenhoven B. The epidemiology of uterine leiomyomas. *Baillière's Clin Obstet Gynaecol* 1998; **12**: 169–76.
2. Rybo G, Leman J, Tibbin R. Epidemiology of menstrual blood loss. In: Baird DT, Michie EA (eds). *Mechanisms of Menstrual Bleeding*. New York: Raven Press, 1985: 181–93.
3. Nowak RA. Fibroids: pathophysiology and current medical treatment. *Baillière's Clin Obstet Gynaecol* 1999; **13**: 223–8.
4. Farquhar C, Arroll B, Ekeroma A et al. An evidence-based guideline for the management of uterine fibroids. *Aust N Z J Obstet Gynaecol* 2001; **41**: 125–40.
5. National Collaborating Centre for Women's and Children's Health. *Heavy Menstrual Bleeding*. London: RCOG Press, 2007.
6. Dueholm M, Lundorf E, Hansen ES et al. Accuracy of magnetic resonance imaging and transvaginal ultrasonography in the diagnosis, mapping and measurement of uterine myomas. *Am J Obstet Gynecol* 2002; **186**: 409–15.
7. Schwartz LB, Zawin M, Carcangiu ML et al. Does pelvic magnetic resonance imaging differentiate among the histologic subtypes of uterine myomata? *Fertil Steril* 1998; **70**: 580–7.

8. Volkers NA, Hehenkamp WJ, Spijkerboer AM *et al.* MR reproducibility in the assessmsnt of uterine fibroids for patients scheduled for uterine artery embolization. *Cardiovasc Intervent Radiol* 2008; **31**: 260–68.

9. Nilsson L, Rybo G. Treatment of menorrhagia. *Am J Obstet Gynecol* 1971; **10**: 713–20.

10. Lumbiganon P, Rugpao S, Phandhu-fung S *et al.* Protective effect of depot-medroxyprogesterone acetate on surgically treated uterine leiomyomas: a multi-centre case-control study. *Br J Obstet Gynaecol* 1995; **103**: 909–14.

11. Murphy AA, Morales AJ, Kettel LM, Yen SSC. Regression of uterine leiomyomata to the antiprogesterone RU486: dose–response effect. *Fertil Steril* 1995; **64**: 187–90.

12. Kaunitz AM. Progestin-releasing intrauterine systems and leiomyoma. *Contraception* 2007: **75**: S130–33.

13. Varma R, Sinha D, Gupta JK. Non-contraceptive uses of levonorgestrel-releasing hormone system (LNG-IUS) – A systematic enquiry and overview. *Eur J Obstet Gynecol* 2005; **125**: 9–28.

14. Magalhaes J, Aldrighi JM, deLima GR. Uterine volume and menstrual patterns in users of the levonorgestrel-releasing intrauterine system with idiopathic menorrhagia or menorrhagia due to leiomyomas. *Contraception* 2007: **75**: 193–8.

15. Lethaby A, Vollenhoven B, Sowter M. Pre-operative GnRH analogue therapy before hysterectomy or myomectomy for uterine fibroids. *Cochrane Database Syst Rev* 2001; (**2**): CD000547.

16. Farquhar C, Brown PM, Furness S. Cost effectiveness of pre-operative gonadotrophin releasing analogues for women with uterine fibroids undergoing hysterectomy or myomectomy. *Br J Obstet Gynaecol* 2002; **109**: 1273–80.

17. Perino A, Chianchino N, Petronio M, Ciltadini E. The role of leuprolide acetate depot in hysteroscopic surgery: a controlled study. *Fertil Steril* 1993; **59**: 507–10.

18. Palomba S, Affinito P, Tommaselli GA, Nappi C. A clinical trial of the effects of tibolone administered with gonadotropin-releasing hormone analogues for the treatment of uterine leiomyomata. *Fertil Steril* 1998; **70**: 111–18.

19. de Aloysio D, Altieri P, Penacchioni P *et al.* Bleeding patterns in recent postmenopausal outpatients with uterine myomas: comparison between two regimens of HRT. *Maturitas* 1998; **29**: 261–4.

20. Derman SG, Rehnstrom J, Neuwirth RS. The long-term effectiveness of hysteroscopic treatment of menorrhagia and leiomyomas. *Obstet Gynecol* 1991; **77**: 591–4.

21. West CP. Hysterectomy and myomectomy by laparotomy. *Baillière's Clin Obstet Gynaecol* 1998; **12**: 317–35.

22. Kongnyuy EJ, Wiysonge SU. Interventions to reduce haemorrhage during myomectomy for fibroids. *Cochrane Database Syst Rev* 2007; (**1**): CD005355.

23. Khaud A, Moss JG, McMillan N, Lumsden MA. Evaluation of the effect of uterine artery embolisaation on menstrual blood loss and uterine volume. *Br J Obstet Gynaecol* 2004; **111**: 700–5.

24. Pron G, Mocarski E, Cohen M *et al.* Hysterectomy for complications after uterine artery embolization for leiomyoma: results of a Canadian multicenter clinical trial. *J Am Assoc Gynecol Laparosc* 2003; **10**: 99–106.

25. Duttton D, Hirst A, McPherson K *et al.* A UK multi-centre retrospective cohort study comparing hysterectomy and uterine artery embolisation for the treatment of uterine fibroids (HOPEFUL study): main results on medium term safety and efficacy. *Br J Obstet Gynaecol* 2007; **114**: 1340–51.

26. Gupta JK, Sinha A, Lumsden MA, Hickey M. Uterine artery embolization for symptomatic uterine fibroids. *Cochrane Database Syst Rev* 2006; (**1**): CD005073.

27. The REST Investigators. Uterine-artery embolization versus surgery for symptomatic uterine fibroids. *N Eng J Med* 2007; **356**: 360–70.

28. Spies JB, Roth AR, Gonsalves SM, Murphy-Skrzyniarz KM. Ovarian function after uterine artery embolization for leiomyomata: assessment with use of serum follicle stimulating hormone assay. *J Vasc Interv Radiol* 2001; **12**: 437–42.

29. Zowall H, Cairns JA, Brewer C *et al.* Cost-effectiveness of magnetic resonance-guided focused ultrasound surgery for treatment of uterine fibroids. *Br J Obstet Gynaecol* 2008; **115**: 653–62.

# 51.3 Heavy and irregular menstruation

*Christine P West*

## MRCOG standards

### Theoretical skills

- Understand the causes of abnormal uterine bleeding.
- Know the principles of investigation and treatment of heavy or irregular menstrual bleeding.

### Practical skills

- Be familiar with the practical skills of endometrial sampling, hysteroscopy, transvaginal ultrasound.
- Be familiar with the insertion of the levonorgestrel intrauterine system.
- Be familiar with techniques of endometrial ablation.
- Be familiar with surgical techniques of abdominal and vaginal hysterectomy.

## INTRODUCTION

Regular menstruation is a feature of contemporary society. In the past, large family size, prolonged breastfeeding and reduced life expectancy limited the number of menstrual cycles experienced by women. Currently, women may experience more than 400 menstrual periods during reproductive life, and problems related to menstruation are a common cause of referral, both to general practitioners and to gynaecologists. Abnormal bleeding can be a consequence of pelvic pathology, including malignant disease, but the majority of women who present with bleeding problems have no underlying abnormality. Indeed, a significant proportion of women who complain of heavy bleeding are found to have normal menstrual loss if this is measured objectively. Concerns about the widespread use of hysterectomy in this situation have led to a well-developed evidence base for medical management. This, together with less invasive surgical methods, has increased the range of options available for the relief of menstrual bleeding problems.

## DEFINITIONS

In its 1997 evidence-based guideline, commissioned by the National Institute for Health and Clinical Excellence (NICE),[1] the National Collaborating Centre for Women's and Children's Health, rejected the term menorrhagia in favour of heavy menstrual bleeding (HMB). HMB is defined as 'excessive menstrual blood loss which interferes with the woman's physical, emotional, social and material quality of life, and which can occur alone or in combination with other symptoms'. The former definition of heavy blood loss based on objective measurement of loss more than 60–80 mL per period[2] should be used only as a research tool. Bleeding patterns that may be associated with underlying histological or hormonal abnormalities fall into a category termed 'abnormal uterine bleeding', whereby 'a woman experiences a change in her menstrual loss or the degree of loss or menstrual bleeding pattern differs from that experienced by the age-matched general female population'.[1] This category includes intermenstrual, postcoital and post-menopausal bleeding, as well as prolonged or irregular menstruation. The guideline defines dysfunctional uterine bleeding (DUB) as abnormal bleeding that occurs during an anovulatory menstrual cycle or the occurrence of irregular or excessive bleeding in the absence of pregnancy, infection, trauma, new growth or hormone treatment.

## PREVALENCE

The reported prevalence of HMB in various studies varies between 4 and 50 per cent, depending upon the population under study and the methods used.[1] Those using objective measurement of blood loss[2] report a more consistent prevalence of around 10 per cent. Impact on healthcare resources is considerable with 5 per cent of women aged between 30 and 49 consulting their general practitioner for excessive menstrual bleeding in a year[3] and accounting for around 12 per cent of gynaecology referrals. Prior to the more widespread and recent availability of effective medical and surgical alternatives, it was estimated[4] that one in five women in the United Kingdom had undergone hysterectomy by the age of 55 years. Although the rate of hysterectomy has declined sharply with the availability of simpler and less invasive alternatives, this represents a considerable economic burden to the National Health Service, as well as a major impact on the general workforce.

# AETIOLOGY

The aetiology of heavy or abnormal menstrual bleeding depends on the pattern of the bleeding and is also influenced by the age of the patient and other factors. Postmenopausal bleeding and abnormal bleeding secondary to contraceptives, hormone replacement therapy (HRT) or tamoxifen are not considered here.

## Heavy menstrual bleeding

Fibroids are the most common structural cause of HMB with a prevalence of around 30 per cent of women with this complaint (see below and Chapter 51.2, Uterine fibroids and heavy menstrual bleeding). Heavy bleeding associated with fibroids is often painless; painful heavy periods may be secondary to adenomyosis (see Chapter 51.6, Adenomyosis). Coagulation disorders, in particular von Willebrand disease, have been reported in between 5 and 20 per cent of women with HMB.[1] These usually present in young women in whom there is likely to be a history of other bleeding problems.

The majority of women reporting HMB have no underlying structural, histological or endocrine abnormality.[1] Studies involving objective measurement of blood loss have shown that in a high proportion of women reporting heavy periods, blood loss is not abnormal.[2] However, a study of women referred to gynaecological clinics because of excessive menstrual loss showed that more than half did not perceive this as severe or as their main problem.[5] There was considerable overlap between problems related to bleeding and other menstrual problems, such as pain and cyclical symptoms. Psychosocial factors may also influence presentation.

## Abnormal uterine bleeding

Anovulatory menstrual cycles are common following the menarche and in the lead up to the menopause, and abnormal bleeding is a consequence of prolonged stimulation of the endometrium by oestrogen, unopposed by progesterone. Bleeding is painless and in teenagers is usually limited to a few cycles. In the perimenopause, various histological abnormalities may occur, ranging from simple or complex hyperplasia, reversible by progestogens, to severe atypia and malignancy. Anovulatory dysfunctional bleeding is also a well-recognized consequence of polycystic ovary syndrome. Irregular bleeding may be associated with other endocrine disorders, particularly thyroid disease, although the underlying mechanism is unclear.

Intermenstrual and postcoital bleeding frequently coexist and may have a common aetiology. While serious pathology, in particular cervical carcinoma, may be present, most cases are due to benign causes and often no cause can be found. Bleeding at mid-cycle is secondary to the mid-cycle oestradiol surge and is regarded as physiological. In young sexually active women, chlamydial infection[6] may present with intermenstrual or postcoital bleeding. On visualization of the cervix, benign cervical conditions, such as polyps or ectopy, may be present, but are more likely to be asymptomatic incidental findings. Similarly, the significance of abnormalities of the uterine cavity is uncertain. A review of 20 observational and diagnostic studies[1] showed that the majority of women investigated for menstrual bleeding disorders have no histological or structural abnormality. Fibroids are present in approximately 30 per cent and polyps in 10 per cent. It was estimated that the rate of endometrial cancer in women consulting with HMB in primary care is less than one per 10 000 below the age of 40, three per 10 000 between 40–44 and eight per 10 000 in women of 45 and over,[1] although these data do not relate to bleeding patterns or to those referred to secondary care. A retrospective review of 2500 outpatient hysteroscopies[7] reported a 16.8 per cent incidence of endometrial polyps in women presenting with intermenstrual or postcoital bleeding compared with 10 per cent of those with menorrhagia, although the incidence of submucous fibroids was lower in this group (20.4 per cent compared with 29.8 per cent in those with menorrhagia). The incidence of both polyps and fibroids is reduced in younger women,[7,8] but age alone is poorly predictive of the presence of these structural lesions.

# MANAGEMENT

Decisions regarding both investigation and treatment are influenced by a number of factors, which include the age and reproductive status of the individual woman, the pattern and severity of her symptoms and the degree of social disruption that she experiences. Many women may simply seek reassurance. A detailed and accurate history is essential in eliciting any relevant medical problems and in assessing the impact of the problem for each individual woman. While simple menstrual calendars may be helpful in clarifying the pattern of bleeding, use of objective blood loss measurement or pictorial charts[9] are not recommended in routine clinical practice [E].

## Investigation

### Heavy regular menstrual bleeding

This is covered in the national evidence-based guideline[1] and falls within the scope of primary care. History taking should define the presenting problem, determine the impact that it is having on the woman's life and detect abnormal bleeding patterns and/or symptoms that may indicate significant pathology [E]. Abdominal and bimanual pelvic examinations should be performed [E]. If examination is normal, no additional investigations are required prior to the initiation of therapy [E]. If the uterus is felt to be enlarged (>10–12-week gestation size), an ultrasound scan is the first-line investigation for delineating fibroids or excluding other causes of a pelvic mass [A]. A full blood count should be carried out in all women with HMB [C]. Additional blood tests, such as ferritin, female hormone levels or thyroid function, should not be carried out in the absence of specific indications [C]. If coagulation disorders are suspected, particularly in young women, a clotting screen should be carried out [C].[1] Where medical treatment has failed or where there are specific risk factors for endometrial cancer (obesity, tamoxifen therapy, polycystic ovary syndrome), more detailed evaluation of the endometrial cavity should be carried out[1] as described below [E].

### Abnormal uterine bleeding

Most cases will be associated with the perimenopause. Endocrine investigation is unnecessary unless there is clinical suspicion of thyroid disease or premature ovarian failure [C]. Endometrial biopsy should be taken to exclude endometrial cancer or atypical hyperplasia in cases of prolonged or persistent intermenstrual bleeding or, in women over 45 with HMB, where treatment has failed [E].[1] Various outpatient endometrial sampling techniques are available; of which the most common is the Pipelle technique which has been shown to have high sensitivity in the detection of both endometrial cancer and atypical hyperplasia.[10] However, endometrial biopsy does not detect polyps or fibroids[8,11] and if these are suspected, the first-line investigation is transvaginal ultrasound (TVS) [A].[1,11,12] Abdominal ultrasound is required if the uterus is palpable abdominally. Hysteroscopy provides accurate visualization of the uterine cavity and is more accurate than TVS in distinguishing between polyps or submucosal fibroids.[8,11,12] However, it is more costly and invasive than TVS and current guidelines[1,13] recommend that TVS should be used together with endometrial biopsy for the initial investigation of abnormal bleeding, with hysteroscopy as a back up [A]. In centres where provision for outpatient hysteroscopy is limited, the ultrasound-based technique of saline infusion sonography (transvaginal sonohysterography)[12] is useful in delineating the uterine cavity, but should not be used as a first-line investigation [A]. Dilatation and curettage has no advantage over the clinic-based techniques described above for routine investigation and should not be used alone as a diagnostic tool [B].[1,11]

### Intermenstrual and postcoital bleeding

Careful examination of the cervix is essential and any suspicious findings are an indication for colposcopy. In young sexually active women, chlamydial infection should be excluded [B].[6] Where the bleeding is confined to mid-cycle, further investigation is not required. Although the incidence of structural and histological abnormalities rises with increasing age,[8,10] fibroids and polyps can be problematic in younger women. As discussed above, TVS is the primary investigation for the detection of endometrial polyps or submucosal fibroids [A], backed up by biopsy and or hysteroscopy if additional investigations are required.

## MEDICAL MANAGEMENT

### Non-hormonal therapy

For women with HMB requiring non-hormonal treatment, antifibrinolytics (tranexamic acid)[14] or non-steroidal anti-inflammatory drugs (NSAIDs; e.g. mefenamic acid)[15] are first-line drugs [A]. Both are used only during menstruation and are generally well tolerated. Reduction of blood loss is greater with the antifibrinolytic [A],[14] but associated menstrual pain is more effectively treated with NSAIDs (see Chapter 51.4, Dysmenorrhoea). There is no evidence that the long-term use of antifibrinolytics increases the incidence of thrombosis.[14] As antifibrinolytics and NSAIDs have different mechanisms of action in menorrhagia, they may be used in combination [E]. Ethamsylate (a drug that reduces capillary fragility) was used in the past for menorrhagia, but recent evidence does not confirm its efficacy [A].[7] If effective, use of tranexamic acid and/or NSAIDs can be continued long term, but they should be stopped if they do not improve symptoms within three menstrual cycles [E].

### Combined oral contraceptive pill

For women requiring contraception or for whom hormonal agents are acceptable, combined oral contraceptive pill (COCP) preparations are effective in reducing menstrual bleeding, controlling cycle irregularities and relieving menstrual pain, although reports of efficacy have largely been based on indirect evidence from contraceptive studies and one small randomized, controlled trial.[16] A 53 per cent reduction of menstrual blood loss was reported in one non-randomized study. There is some reluctance on the part of both professionals and consumers to use the COCP for the management of menstrual disorders in older women. For non-smokers who have no risk factors for vascular disease, there is no upper age limit for the use of the COCP, and current guidelines recommend its use as a first-line therapy for HMB [B].[1]

### Progestogens

Cyclical progestogens were commonly used in the past, but current evidence does not support their use for HMB when given only during the luteal phase of the cycle [A].[17] They are effective when given at high doses between days 5 and 26 of the cycle (e.g. norethisterone 5 mg tid or medroxyprogesterone acetate 10 mg tid, both for 21 days out of 28) [A].[17] Cyclical progestogens are traditionally the drug of first choice for the control of anovulatory dysfunctional bleeding through their action in opposing the proliferative effects of oestrogen. When evaluated in two small comparative studies,[18] both norethisterone and medroxyprogesterone acetate, given cyclically, were effective in reducing blood loss [C].

Long-acting high-dose progestogens (e.g. Depo-Provera) may be used to induce amenorrhoea [A].[1] However, their usefulness is limited by side effects, including a high incidence of breakthrough bleeding. A recent randomized controlled trial (RCT) has shown the levonorgestrel-releasing intrauterine system (LNG-IUS) to be more effective than either continuous oral or depot medroxyprogesterone acetate in the control of perimenopausal heavy menstrual bleeding.[19]

## Progestogen-releasing intrauterine system

The levonorgestrel-releasing intrauterine system is a well-established treatment for HMB. The continuous exposure of the endometrium to progestogen induces progressive atrophy, with reduction of menstrual bleeding by more than 80 per cent after three to six months and more than 90 per cent at 12 months.[20,21] Spontaneous expulsion occurs in 3–6 per cent of women and there is an initial incidence of breakthrough bleeding as high as 25–55 per cent in the early months. Progestogenic side effects of bloating, breast tenderness, mood swings and acne may occur, and these together with the incidence of prolonged breakthrough bleeding adversely affect compliance. Continuation rates between 60–88 per cent have been reported in various prospective studies.[20–25] Careful counselling is therefore essential prior to insertion [E].

The LNG-IUS has been compared in randomized trials and three systematic reviews[17,20–23] with other medical therapies, with endometrial ablation and with hysterectomy. Reduction of menstrual blood loss was significantly greater than with tranexamic acid or an NSAID.[21] The side effects of breakthrough bleeding and breast tenderness were more common in women with the LNG-IUS compared with high-dose cyclical norethisterone,[17,20,21] but overall satisfaction was greater with the LNG-IUS.

In a study of women awaiting hysterectomy,[22] 64.3 per cent of those randomized to insertion of LNG-IUS cancelled their operation after six months, compared with 14.3 per cent in the control group. In a direct comparison with hysterectomy,[23] 20 per cent of the group assigned to the LNG-IUS opted for hysterectomy in the first year. However, quality of life assessment at 12 months was not significantly different in the two groups, with the exception

of lower pain scores after hysterectomy. Costs were three times higher in the hysterectomy group. The LNG-IUS has also been compared with endometrial resection[21,23] and with thermal balloon ablation.[23–25] Although reduction of blood loss was greater following resection and side effects were more common with the LNG-IUS, overall satisfaction rates were similar. Results of three RCTS included in a systematic review,[23] together with two subsequent RCTs[24,25] comparing the LNG-IUS with thermal balloon ablation (TBA) again show similar results. These results indicate that the LNG-IUS is a highly effective treatment for HMB [A] that has advantages over existing medical treatments and is a potential alternative to surgery.

## Other medical therapies

Second-line drugs are available for the control of severe bleeding when simpler measures have failed and, as they more reliably induce amenorrhoea, are useful in the management of severe anaemia or in the presence of medical disorders when surgery may be contraindicated. Androgens, such as danazol and gestrinone, induce amenorrhoea by a combination of negative feedback and direct effects on the endometrium, (see Chapter 51.5, Endometriosis and gonadotrophin-releasing hormone analogues), while gonadotrophin-releasing hormone (GnRH) agonists induce a hypogonadal state via their central action. While effective, these approaches are usually limited to short-term use because of their side effects [A]. They are also of value as endometrial-thinning agents prior to hysteroscopic surgery [A].[26] In severe cases in which simple measures have failed, long-term therapy with a GnRH agonist plus hormonal add-back can be considered if there are contraindications to surgery (see Chapter 51.5) [B].

## SURGICAL MANAGEMENT

While medical treatment should normally be used as first-line therapy for HMB [E], limitations in efficacy and side effects[23] will result in many women seeking a surgical solution for their problem. Until recently, hysterectomy has been the principal surgical management for menstrual disorders. As the majority of hysterectomies were carried out for benign conditions or, in many cases, where no pathology was demonstrable, this policy was called into question.[3] The use of the diagnostic techniques described above identifies some women with benign lesions (small submucosal fibroids or endometrial polyps) that are suitable for removal by hysteroscopic surgery [D],[1,13] although the role of such surgery in the management of menstrual disorders has not been subject to critical evaluation. Various methods of endometrial ablation are now well established as day case or outpatient procedures and recent developments include second-generation techniques that are simpler and safer than conventional methods. The availability and relative safety of the latter methods has led to the view that endometrial ablation may be offered as an initial treatment for HMB after a full discussion of the risks and benefits and of other treatment options [A].[1]

## Endometrial ablation

The objective of endometrial ablation is the complete destruction of the endometrium down to the basal layer, resulting in fibrosis of the uterine cavity and amenorrhoea. In practice, it is very difficult to achieve complete destruction, and rates of amenorrhoea vary between 10 and 40 per cent.[23–31] However, patient satisfaction rates are over 70 per cent in the short term [A]. Life-table analysis of follow up after endometrial resection[28] reported a cumulative hysterectomy rate of 27.4 per cent after four years. A desire for future fertility is an absolute contraindication to endometrial ablation and women must be counselled regarding the appropriate use of contraception [E].

Initially, ablation techniques were carried out under direct hysteroscopic vision and involved the use of fluid for distension and irrigation. They comprised laser ablation, endometrial loop resection using electrodiathermy and rollerball electrodiathermy ablation. Of these, laser ablation was limited by its costs to a very few centres. All three are operator dependent, time consuming and carry risks of systemic fluid absorption, haemorrhage and uterine perforation with heat damage to adjacent structures. The MISTLETOE study,[26] a prospective national survey of more than 10 000 procedures in the United Kingdom, reported an overall immediate complication rate of 4.4 per cent. Complications were lower with laser and rollerball techniques, and highest with loop resection. Complications were also related to the experience of the operator. Increasingly, these methods have been replaced by the techniques described below. However, they may be carried out, if appropriate, in conjunction with hysteroscopic myomectomy or fibroid resection (see Chapter 51.2, Uterine fibroids and heavy menstrual bleeding) [D].

Newer techniques, the so-called second generation methods of endometrial ablation, have been developed with the object of reducing operator dependency and minimizing risk. Several techniques are currently available, including fluid-filled TBA, microwave endometrial ablation (MEA) and impedance-controlled bipolar radiofrequency ablation.[1] Second-generation methods have been compared with each other,[30,31] with first-generation methods,[30] with abdominal and vaginal hysterectomy,[27] and with LNG-IUS,[21,23–25] in randomized trials and systematic reviews. To date, they appear to have similar efficacy when compared with the first-generation methods with the advantage of shorter operating times and fewer complications, making them safer and more cost effective [A]. They are also more suitable for use with local rather than general anaesthesia. All methods of endometrial ablation are less effective than hysterectomy in reducing blood loss and pain, but costs and complication rates are much lower, making endometrial ablation an appropriate first-line surgical approach where medical methods have failed or are deemed inappropriate. Prior assessment of the uterine cavity with TVS or hysteroscopy is recommended [E] as second-generation methods are not suitable for women with submucosal fibroids greater than 3 cm or an enlarged uterine cavity [A].[30] In contrast to first-generation methods, endometrial thinning agents are not usually required.[26] Although the risk of uterine perforation is lower than with the first-generation methods,[30] it is recommended that hysteroscopy should be performed after cervical dilatation, prior to placement of the device to reduce the risk of uterine perforation and thermal damage to adjacent structures cavity [E]. Prophylactic antibiotics are commonly used prior to endometrial ablation procedures,[26] although evidence to support their use is lacking.

Outcome and patient satisfaction with second-generation methods of endometrial ablation is similar to that with the LNG-IUS and patient preference, as well as perception or experience of side effects will largely determine selection. There are, to date, relatively few published randomized controlled trials of direct comparison between second-generation methods of ablation.[30,31] Until there is clear evidence favouring one method above others, the choice will depend on factors such as the local availability of equipment and marketing strategies by the companies concerned.

## Hysterectomy

Recent randomized trials comparing hysterectomy with endometrial ablation have highlighted the greater costs and morbidity of hysterectomy, together with its longer recovery time.[27] However, longer-term patient satisfaction rates are greater for hysterectomy and thus cost differentials tend to narrow with time. Satisfaction after hysterectomy is not universal; there may be long-term implications for bladder function. A systematic review[32] estimated a 60 per cent increase in the odds of developing urinary incontinence following hysterectomy. A large cohort study of 37 298 hysterectomies performed in the UK for benign indications reported an operative complication rate of 3.5 per cent, a post-operative complication rate of 9 per cent and an overall mortality rate of 0.38 per 1000.[33] Mortality was 0.25 per 1000 in women undergoing hysterectomy for menstrual problems.

Currently, there is interest in the optimal method of carrying out hysterectomy. This is partly motivated by short-term issues of hospital stay and recovery time, based on economic factors. This has accompanied the development of techniques, such as laparoscopically assisted vaginal hysterectomy (LAVH), laparoscopic total and subtotal hysterectomy and an increased use of the vaginal route. A systematic review[34] based on five RCTs and four large case series has concluded that laparoscopic hysterectomy is associated with a shorter hospital stay, but is more expensive, takes longer than abdominal or vaginal hysterectomy and is associated with more complications, particularly

**Table 51.3.1** Morbidity of hysterectomy

| Complication | Abdominal (%) | Vaginal (%) | Laparoscopic (%) |
|---|---|---|---|
| Bowel injury | 0.67 | 0 | 0.20 |
| Urinary tract injury (bladder or ureter) | 0.86 | 1.60 | 2.33 |
| Vascular injury | 0.77 | 0.94 | 1.81 |
| Blood transfusion | 3.33 | 3.87 | 4.23 |
| Laparotomy | – | 2.66 | 4.17 |
| Pelvic haematoma | 6.00 | 4.04 | 3.94 |
| Abdominal wound infection | 7.38 | 0.00 | 1.92 |
| Urinary tract infection | 4.87 | 1.27 | 4.77 |
| Chest infection | 4.55 | 6.67 | 0.56 |
| Other febrile morbidity | 13.15 | 7.73 | 10.01 |
| Thromboembolism | 0.00 | 0.00 | 0.59 |

- Data from 3643 women included in a systematic review of randomized controlled trials[34] comparing surgical approaches for hysterectomy.
- Adapted with permission from Heavy Menstrual Bleeding Clinical Guideline[1]

bladder and ureteric injuries (see Table 51.3.1) [A]. Vaginal hysterectomy has advantages over abdominal hysterectomy in terms of cost and speed of recovery [A], but is technically more challenging [E]. The role of subtotal hysterectomy and its laparoscopic equivalent remains unclear. Despite a lay perception that retention of the cervix may have a positive impact on sexual function, evidence from three RCTs[35] has failed to identify any difference in sexual, bladder or bowel function, although surgery is faster and blood loss and febrile morbidity is reduced with the subtotal abdominal approach [A]. No comparative data are currently available for laparoscopic subtotal hysterectomy. Women undergoing subtotal hysterectomy should be warned about the occurrence of ongoing menstrual bleeding [A]. Individual assessment is essential when deciding the method and route of hysterectomy.[1] Factors to be considered include the size and mobility of the uterus, vaginal access and other factors, such as previous surgery, and presence of other gynaecological disease, such as endometriosis, as well as the skill and experience of the individual surgeon [E]. Taking into account the need for individual assessment, current evidence supports vaginal hysterectomy in favour of abdominal hysterectomy as the first-line approach where possible [A].[1] Where vaginal hysterectomy is not possible, laparoscopic hysterectomy offers advantages over abdominal hysterectomy, although it brings a higher chance of bladder or ureteric injuries and requires special expertise. All decisions regarding hysterectomy must be accompanied by a detailed discussion with the individual woman of the benefits, risks and future implications of the procedure [E].

Removal of healthy ovaries at the time of hysterectomy for heavy menstrual bleeding should not be undertaken without detailed discussion of the potential impact on the woman's subsequent health and well-being and consideration of relevant issues including her personal and family history of breast and ovarian cancer and her attitude to the use of hormone replacement therapy [E].[1]

## EBM

These recommendations for the management of heavy and irregular menstruation are based on a national evidence-based guideline, two other evidence-based guidelines, an Effective Health Care review, a systematic review of diagnostic procedures, seven systematic reviews of medical therapy and seven systematic reviews relating to surgical management.

## KEY POINTS

- The term 'menorrhagia' is no longer appropriate and should be replaced by heavy menstrual bleeding.
- Heavy menstrual bleeding should be recognized as having a major impact on a woman's quality of life and any intervention should aim to improve this rather than focusing on menstrual blood loss [E].
- The initial management of HMB should take place within a primary care setting following abdominal and pelvic examination and measurement of full blood count [E].
- Young sexually active women presenting with intermenstrual or postcoital bleeding should be tested for chlamydia [B].
- If the history or clinical findings are suggestive of a structural abnormality, ultrasound should be the primary investigation [A], backed up by hysteroscopy or saline infusion sonography if the nature of an intracavity lesion is uncertain [A].
- Endometrial biopsy is indicated in cases of prolonged or persistent intermenstrual bleeding and in cases of treatment failure in women over 45 years [E].
- NSAIDs and anti-fibrinolytics are effective in the management of HMB [A], but ethamsylate is ineffective [A].
- The COCP is effective for HMB provided there are no contraindications [B].
- Cyclical progestogens are effective for HMB when given for 21 days out of 28 and for control of anovulatory dysfunctional bleeding [B].
- Continuous high-dose progestogens (e.g. depot preparations) may be useful if they induce amenorrhoea [B].
- The LNG-IUS device is highly effective in reducing HMB, but adequate counselling is needed prior to insertion [A].
- Drugs that induce amenorrhoea are useful for the short-term management of severe menorrhagia or for endometrial thinning prior to endometrial ablation [A].
- Endometrial polyps and small submucous fibroids should be removed by hysteroscopic surgery [D].

- Endometrial ablation is cheap, safe and effective for the relief of HMB [A] and may be offered as a first-line treatment for women who decline medical options [A].
- Newer techniques of ablation are as effective as older techniques and are safer and simpler to perform [A].
- Long-term satisfaction is high with hysterectomy, but it is associated with significant morbidity and mortality [A] and should be offered only if simpler alternatives have failed [E].
- Healthy ovaries should not be removed at hysterectomy without detailed consideration of the risks and benefits [E].
- Laparoscopic hysterectomy is more expensive than abdominal or vaginal hysterectomy and carries a greater risk of serious complications, particularly in inexperienced hands [A].
- Vaginal hysterectomy is more cost effective than the abdominal route and should be considered preferable to abdominal hysterectomy where possible [A].
- Subtotal hysterectomy offers no long-tem advantages over abdominal hysterectomy and may be associated with continued menstrual bleeding, although short-term morbidity is reduced [A].
- The route selected for hysterectomy should be determined by assessment of the individual patient, as well as by the skill and experience of the individual surgeon [E].

# Key References

1. National Collaborating Centre for Women's and Children's Health. *Heavy Menstrual Bleeding*. London: RCOG Press, 2007.
2. Hallberg L, Hogdahl AM, Nilsson L, Rybo G. Menstrual blood loss – a population study. Variation at different ages and attempts to define normality. *Acta Obstet Gynaecol Scand* 1966; **45**: 320–51.
3. Nuffield Institute for Health, University of Leeds and NHS Centre for Research and Dissemination, University of York Research Unit, Royal College of Physicians. *Effective Health Care. The Management of Menorrhagia*. Leeds: University of Leeds, 1995.
4. Vessey M, Villard-MacKintosh L, McPherson K *et al.* The epidemiology of hysterectomy: findings of a large cohort study. *Br J Obstet Gynaecol* 1992; **99**: 402–7.
5. Warner P, Critchley HOD, Lumsden MA *et al.* Referral for menstrual problems: cross sectional survey of symptoms, reasons for referral and management. *BMJ* 2001; **323**: 24–8.
6. Scottish Intercollegiate Guidelines Network. Management of Genital *Chlamydia trachomatis* Infection. A National Clinical Guideline. Edinburgh: SIGN Secretariat, Royal College of Physicians, 2000.
7. Nagele F, O'Connor H, Davies A *et al.* 2500 outpatient diagnostic hysteroscopies. *Obstet Gynecol* 1996; **88**: 87–92.
8. Critchley HO, Warner P, Lee AJ *et al.* Evaluation of abnormal uterine bleeding: comparison of three outpatient procedures within cohorts defined by age and menopausal status. *Health Technol Assess* 2004; **8**: iii–iv, 1–139.
9. Higham JM, O'Brien PM, Shaw RW. Assessment of menstrual blood loss using a pictorial chart. *Br J Obstet Gynaecol* 1990; **97**: 734–9.
10. Dijkhuizen FP, Mol BW, Brolmann HA, Heintz AP. The accuracy of endometrial sampling in the diagnosis of patients with endometrial carcinoma and hyperplasia: a meta-analysis. *Cancer* 2000; **89**: 1765–72.
11. Tahir MM, Bigrigg MA, Browning JJ *et al.* A randomised controlled trial comparing transvaginal ultrasound, outpatient hysteroscopy and endometrial biopsy with inpatient hysteroscopy and curettage. *Br J Obstet Gynaecol* 1999; **106**: 1259–64.
12. Farquhar C, Ekeroma A, Furness S, Arroll B. A systematic review of transvaginal ultrasonography, sonohysterography and hysteroscopy for the investigation of abnormal uterine bleeding in premenopausal women. *Acta Obstet Gynecol Scand* 2003; **82**: 493–504.
13. Farquhar C, Arroll B, Ekeroma A *et al.* An evidence-based guideline for the management of uterine fibroids. *Aust NZ J Obstet Gynaecol* 2001; **41**: 125–40.
14. Lethaby A, Farquhar C, Cooke I. Antifibrinolytics for heavy menstrual bleeding. *Cochrane Database Syst Rev* 2004; (**4**): CD002439.
15. Lethaby A, Augood C, Duckitt K. Nonsteroidal anti-inflammatory drugs for heavy menstrual bleeding. *Cochrane Database Syst Rev* 2007; (**4**): CD000400.
16. Iyer V, Farquhar C, Jepson R. Oral contraceptive pills for heavy menstrual bleeding. *Cochrane Database Syst Rev* 2000; (**2**): CD000154.
17. Lethaby A, Irvine G, Cameron I. Cyclical progestogens for heavy menstrual bleeding. *Cochrane Database Syst Rev* 2008; (**1**): CD001016.
18. Hickey M, Higham J, Fraser IS. Progestogens versus oestrogens and progestogens for irregular uterine bleeding associated with anovulation. *Cochrane Database Syst Rev* 2007; (**4**): CD001895.
19. Kucuk T, Ertan K. Continuous oral or intramuscular medroxyprogesterone acetate versus the levonorgestrel releasing intrauterine system in the treatment of perimenopausal menorrhagia: a randomised prospective, controlled clinical trial in female smokers. *Clin Exp Obstet Gynecol* 2008; **35**: 57–60.
20. Lethaby AE, Cooke I, Rees M. Progesterone/progestogen releasing intrauterine systems versus either placebo or any other medication for heavy menstrual bleeding. *Cochrane Database Syst Rev* 2005; (**4**): CD002126.
21. Stewart A, Cummins C, Gold L *et al.* The effectiveness of the levonorgestrel-releasing intrauterine system in menorrhagia: a systematic review. *Br J Obstet Gynaecol* 2001; **108**: 74–86.
22. Hurskainen R, Teperi J, Rissanen P *et al.* Quality of life and cost effectiveness of levonorgestrel-releasing intrauterine system versus hysterectomy for treatment of menorrhagia: a randomised trial. *Lancet* 2001; **357**: 273–7.

*Reproductive medicine*

23. Marjoribanks J, Lethaby A, Farquhar C. Surgery versus medical therapy for heavy menstrual bleeding. *Cochrane Database Syst Rev* 2003; (**2**): CD003855.

24. Busfield RA, Farquhar CM, Sowter MC *et al.* A randomised trial comparing the levonorgestrel intrauterine system and thermal balloon ablation for heavy menstrual bleeding. *Br J Obstet Gynaecol* 2006; **113**: 257–63.

25. Shaw RW, Symonds IM, Tamizian O *et al.* Randomised comparative trial of thermal balloon ablation and levonorgestrel intrauterine system in patients with idiopathic menorrhagia. *Aust NZ J Obstet Gynaecol* 2007; **47**: 335–40.

26. Sowter MC, Singka AA, Lethaby A. Pre-operative endometrial thinning agents before hysteroscopic surgery for heavy menstrual bleeding. *Cochrane Database Syst Rev* 2000; (**2**): CD001234.

27. Lethaby A, Shepperd S, Cooke I, Farquhar C. Endometrial resection and ablation versus hysterectomy for heavy menstrual bleeding. *Cochrane Database Syst Rev* 1999; (**2**): CD000329.

28. Pooley AS, Ewen P, Sutton CJ. Does transcervical resection of the endometrium for menorrhagia really avoid hysterectomy? Life table analysis of a large series. *J Am Assoc Gynecol Laparosc* 1998; **5**: 229–35.

29. Overton C, Hargreaves J, Maresh M. A national survey of the complications of endometrial destruction for menstrual disorders: the MISTLETOE study. *Br J Obstet Gynaecol* 1997; **104**: 1351–9.

30. Lethaby A, Hickey M, Garry R. Endometrial destruction techniques for heavy menstrual bleeding. *Cochrane Database Syst Rev* 2009; (**4**): CD001501.

31. Garside R, Stein K, Wyatt K *et al.* The effectiveness and cost effectiveness of microwave and thermal balloon endometrial ablation for heavy menstrual bleeding: a systematic review and economic modelling. *Health Technol Assess* 2004; **8**: iii, 1–155.

32. Brown JS, Sawaya G, Thom DH, Grady D. Hysterectomy and urinary incontinence: a systematic review. *Lancet* 2000; **356**: 535–9.

33. Maresh MHJ, Metcalfe MA, McPherson K *et al.* The VALUE national hysterectomy study: description of the patients and their surgery. *Br J Obstet Gynaecol* 2002; **109**: 302–12.

34. Nieboer T, Johnson N, Barlow D *et al.* Surgical approach to hysterectomy for benign gynaecological disease. *Cochrane Database Syst Rev* 2009; (**3**): CD003677.

35. Lethaby A, Ivanova V, Johnson N. Total versus subtotal hysterectomy for benign gynaecological conditions. *Cochrane Database Syst Rev* 2006; (**2**): CD004993.

# 51.4 Dysmenorrhoea

*Christine P West*

## INTRODUCTION

Pain during menstruation is an almost universal experience among women and, when severe, it has a significant economic impact through loss of time from work or education. Recognition of the consequences of this problem has led to several large-scale reviews of treatments for dysmenorrhoea, including alternative therapies. There is thus a well-founded evidence base for its management. Pain related to or exacer-bated during menstruation or sexual intercourse may be a consequence of underlying pelvic pathology, although not all women with pelvic pain have a gynaecological disorder. This chapter is mainly concerned with gynaecological causes of cyclical pelvic pain, but some reference is made to the multifactorial nature of the problem.

## DEFINITIONS

Dysmenorrhoea is pain that occurs during menstruation. Primary dysmenorrhoea is also known as 'primary spasmodic dysmenorrhoea'. This is a useful descriptive term for a condition of cramping lower pain that may radiate to the lower back and thighs, often associated with gastrointestinal and neurological symptoms. It typically lasts for between 8 and 72 hours, although young women almost universally experience milder manifestations.

Secondary dysmenorrhoea is menstrually related pain, which is secondary to identifiable pelvic pathology. It is characteristically associated with deep dyspareunia and the pain may precede the onset of menstrual bleeding. It is regarded as distinct from the condition of chronic pelvic pain in which pain of at least six months duration is present continuously or intermittently, not associated exclusively with menstruation or sexual intercourse.[1] However, there is considerable overlap between the two conditions, and many women who present with chronic pain describe dyspareunia and/or premenstrual exacerbation.

## INCIDENCE

In a large random sample of 19-year-old Swedish women,[2] dysmenorrhoea was experienced by 72 per cent of the women. Fifteen per cent reported limitation of daily activity and lack of relief from analgesics and 7.9 per cent reported repeated absence from work or school. Follow up of the same cohort five years later[3] found that the prevalence and severity were reduced only in those who had completed a pregnancy or were pill users. It was unchanged in those who remained nulliparous or who had a history of early pregnancy loss or abortion. A systematic review[4] of published papers on pelvic pain in women in the United Kingdom estimated a prevalence rate of between 45 and 95 per cent for dysmenorrhoea. The studies did not distinguish between primary and secondary dysmenorrhoea, but 48 per cent of middle-aged women experienced pain during at least half their menses. The reported prevalence of chronic pelvic pain among women aged 18–50 years in a large community-based US study was 15 per cent.[5]

## AETIOLOGY

Uterine myometrial hyperactivity has been demonstrated in women with primary dysmenorrhoea. This is likely to be secondary to increased uterine production of prostaglandins.[6] Other local mediators may also be involved, and increased circulating levels of vasopressin have been reported. These responses represent the extremes of the normal physiological response of the uterus to progesterone withdrawal, as primary dysmenorrhoea is not regarded as a pathological condition.

Severe dysmenorrhoea in young women is rarely due to any underlying abnormality. One exception is pain secondary to congenital abnormalities that are associated with obstruction to menstrual flow, for example cryptomenorrhoea in an accessory uterine horn.

Many of the conditions that cause secondary dysmenorrhoea may also present with chronic pelvic pain, in particular endometriosis, which occurs in around one-third of laparoscopies carried out for pelvic pain (Table 51.4.1). Adenomyosis is a cause of secondary dysmenorrhoea in older multiparous women. Uterine fibroids do not characteristically cause pain unless there is an acute complication, such as torsion or expulsion. Chronic pelvic inflammatory disease and other causes of pelvic pain that are non-cyclical, such as adhesions or ovarian cysts, are not considered in this chapter.

Around one-third of laparoscopies carried out for the investigation of pelvic pain or secondary dysmenorrhoea are negative (see Table 51.4.1).[7] This must not be interpreted as implying that the pain is psychogenic. Non-gynaecological conditions can be exacerbated or enhanced during menstruation. In particular, irritable bowel syndrome (IBS) is commonly diagnosed following negative investigations for pelvic pain.[1] In a sample of 5051 UK women on a GP database with a recorded diagnosis of chronic pelvic pain,[8] 21 per cent had gastrointestinal symptoms and 29 per cent were eventually diagnosed with IBS; this diagnosis being more common in the older age group. Interstitial cystitis

**Table 51.4.1** Causes of pelvic pain

| Cause | Percentage |
|---|---|
| Normal findings | 35 |
| Endometriosis | 33 |
| Adhesions | 24 |
| Chronic pelvic inflammatory disease | 5 |
| Ovarian cyst | 3 |
| Pelvic varicosities | 1 |
| Fibroids | 1 |
| Other | 4 |

- Results of 1524 laparoscopies for pelvic pain (13 studies reviewed by Howard[7]).

is also commonly diagnosed in women with chronic pelvic pain.[9] Pelvic pain may be musculoskeletal or, if highly localized and sharp, stabbing or aching in nature, related to nerve entrapment.[9]

A systematic review of studies of risk factors for chronic pelvic pain[10] concluded that drug or alcohol abuse, psychological comorbidity and a history of physical or sexual abuse are all associated with an increased risk of chronic pelvic pain. They also reported an association between non-cyclical pelvic pain and many gynaecological and obstetric factors including miscarriage, caesarean section, heavy menstrual flow and pelvic inflammatory disease. Factors, such as personality traits, coping strategies, health beliefs and influences of family members, may predispose an individual to the development of chronic pain.[1]

Pelvic venous congestion is a condition described in multiparous women of reproductive age.[11] Chronic dull, aching pain is characteristically exacerbated perimenstrually, by activity and by sexual intercourse, and relieved by lying down. It is attributed to the presence of dilated veins in the broad ligament and ovarian plexus. Typical appearances have been described at venography and reported with both ultrasound[12] and magnetic resonance imaging (MRI), although studies reporting accuracy, sensitivity and specificity have not been undertaken. Indirect evidence for the existence of the condition was obtained from a small therapeutic study in which the vasoconstrictor dihydroergotamine[13] was more effective than placebo in relieving symptoms. However, the existence of the condition as an entity distinct from unexplained chronic pelvic pain is disputed.

## MANAGEMENT

### Investigation

The diagnosis of primary dysmenorrhoea is based on the clinical history and does not require investigation [E]. It is normally managed by the general practitioner or primary care physician. Referral for specialist advice is required if there is a lack of response to standard therapies or if symptoms are atypical, giving rise to a suspicion of endometriosis or other pathology. Although a pelvic examination can provide reassurance, this is not indicated in a teenager who is not sexually active [E]. A transabdominal ultrasound scan will exclude congenital uterine abnormalities or significant ovarian pathology and should provide reassurance if negative.

If there are atypical features in the history, for example premenstrual pain, deep dyspareunia, abnormal bleeding or atypical bowel or urinary symptoms, further assessment is required. Abdominal and pelvic examination should be performed to assess tenderness, uterine size and the presence of any masses. Reduced uterine mobility together with tenderness and thickening or nodularity in the pouch of Douglas is suggestive of endometriosis. In cases of suspected pelvic inflammatory disease, samples should be taken to screen for sexually transmitted infection. Ultrasound should be performed if there are abnormal findings on examination. Ultrasound is sensitive in detecting uterine and ovarian pathology and has the advantage of being non-invasive [A].[14] MRI scanning is useful as an additional tool if ultrasound findings are equivocal. Laparoscopy has an established role in the diagnosis and treatment of endometriosis (see Chapter 51.5, Endometriosis and gonadotrophin-releasing hormone analogues), but is not without risk[15] and is not routinely required prior to a therapeutic trial of medical therapy [E].[9]

For women presenting with chronic pelvic pain, there is evidence that the quality of the initial consultation influences later progress.[9] Detailed history taking, together with pelvic examination is essential; not necessarily at the same visit. The initial history should include questions about the pattern of the pain and its association with other problems, such as bladder and bowel symptoms, and the effect of movement and posture on the pain. Psychosocial factors must be explored and the women given time to express her ideas, concerns and expectations [E]. Laparoscopy is commonly performed to investigate chronic pelvic pain, but in the absence of abnormal clinical or ultrasound findings the likelihood of abnormal findings at laparoscopy is also very low.[16,17] Although negative findings may provide reassurance, a study assessing the value of photographic reinforcement after a negative laparoscopy showed no additional benefit.[13]

## Management of primary dysmenorrhoea

### Non-steroidal anti-inflammatory drugs

These drugs inhibit prostaglandin synthesis via inhibition of the enzyme cyclo-oxygenase-2. A systematic review of 56 clinical trials[18] concluded that naproxen, ibuprofen, mefenamic acid and aspirin are all effective in primary dysmenorrhoea [A]. Response rate ratios generally favour naproxen and ibuprofen, aspirin having the lowest response rate ratio. The overall incidence of side effects is low and generally related to the gastrointestinal tract. Naproxen causes more side effects than ibuprofen and mefenamic acid. The reviewers conclude that ibuprofen is superior in terms of its efficacy and favourable side-effect profile [A]. NSAIDs may be use in combination with other analgesics, such as paracetamol or codeine.

### Combined oral contraceptive pill

These preparations have been widely used for many years for the relief of primary dysmenorrhoea. The theoretical basis for their action is via inhibition of ovulation. A systematic review[19] concluded that combined oral contraceptive pills (COCP) are significantly more effective than placebo for pain relief. Only four randomized, controlled trials met the criteria for inclusion in the review; all based

on higher dose formulations than those in current use. Despite these reservations about the evidence base, the COCP should be regarded as a safe and effective therapy for the relief of primary dysmenorrhoea [A].

### Other hormonal therapies

Other ovulation suppressive therapies used for the treatment of menstrual pain secondary to endometriosis, such as high-dose progestogens, androgens and GnRH analogues are highly effective [A], but have limitations for long-term use. The levonorgestrel releasing intrauterine system (LNG-IUS) can be used for treatment of menstrual pain secondary to both endometriosis and adenomyosis (see Chapters 51.5, Endometriosis and gonadotrophin-releasing hormone analogues and Chapter 51.6, Adenomyosis), although evidence of its effectiveness has largely been based on case series and small-scale randomized trials. Its use in primary dysmenorrhoea is likely to be limited to women also seeking contraception who have contraindications to the combined pill [E].

### Surgical interruption of pelvic nerve pathways

Because of the chronic and recurrent nature of pelvic pain, surgical techniques have been described for division of the nerves which innervate the uterus. Sensory fibres from the lower uterus, cervix and upper vagina exit along autonomic nervous system pathways that run along the lower margins of the uterosacral ligaments. These pass superiorly via bilateral inferior hypogastric plexuses in the pararectal spaces to the superior hypogastric plexuses that lie over the bodies of L4 and L5 and the sacral promontory.[14] Presacral neurectomy (PSN) involves removal of the nerve bundles of the hypogastric plexus, a procedure traditionally performed by laparotomy, but more recently laparoscopic methods have been described. Laparoscopic uterine nerve ablation (LUNA) is a simpler procedure that involves division of the uterosacral ligaments.

A systematic review has assessed the role of these surgical interventions in primary and secondary dysmenorrhoea.[20] There was some evidence of effectiveness in primary but not secondary dysmenorrhoea and of a greater benefit with PSN compared with LUNA. The overall conclusion was that there is insufficient evidence to support the use of either procedure in the management of dysmenorrhoea, regardless of its cause [A]. Significant morbidity has been described following both procedures, but is more common following PSN. Availability of the latter is restricted to specialized centres.

### Alternative therapies

These are popular with the lay public and are widely used. There have been four systematic reviews of alternative therapy in dysmenorrhoea. A review of five randomized, controlled trials of spinal manipulation found this to be ineffective [A].[21] Another reviewed herbal and dietary therapies comprising vitamin $B_1$ (one large trial), vitamin $B_6$ (one small trial comparing it with magnesium), vitamin E (in combination with ibuprofen), magnesium (three small trials), omega-3 fatty acids, and Japanese herbal combination.[22] Although results were generally encouraging for all except vitamin E, the reviewers concluded that both magnesium and vitamin $B_1$ are promising for the relief of dysmenorrhoea [B], but that insufficient evidence exists for the use of any of the other therapies. Reviews of 39 trials of Chinese herbal medicine[23] and five trials of behavioural interventions,[24] including relaxation and pain management training, found promising evidence of benefit, but conclusions were limited by poor methodological quality of the included trials [A].

## New therapeutic approaches in primary dysmenorrhoea

Non-steroidal anti-inflammatory drugs (NSAID) in current use inhibit two different isoforms of the enzyme cyclo-oxygenase-2, known as COX-1 and COX-2. Selective inhibitors of the enzyme COX-2 may have similar analgesic efficacy, but fewer of the side effects of the drugs in current use. However, there are concerns about cardiotoxicity which have limited clinical trials of their use for dysmenorrhoea. The smooth muscle relaxant glyceryl trinitrate,[6] vasopressin antagonists and sildafenil are all under current evaluation for management of primary dysmenorrhoea.[25]

## Secondary dysmenorrhoea and chronic pelvic pain

Management of secondary dysmenorrhoea will depend on its underlying cause. In cases of secondary dysmenorrhoea or chronic pelvic pain where a diagnosis of endometriosis is suspected, laparoscopic confirmation of the diagnosis is not required prior to a trial of medical therapy provided that there are no other indications for surgery, such as the presence of an adnexal mass [E]. Interventions for the management of chronic pelvic pain have been the subject of an RCOG Green-top guideline[9] and a systematic review.[13] Management of chronic pain attributed to IBS, chronic pelvic inflammatory disease (PID) or interstitial cystitis is not considered here.

## Multi-disciplinary approach

One study[17] randomized women with chronic pelvic pain between routine laparoscopy followed by conventional management and an integrated approach without initial laparoscopy. In the latter group, a gynaecologist, psychologist, physiotherapist and nutritionist assessed all the women and management was then directed as appropriate.

One year later, evaluation showed a significantly greater improvement in daily activities and perception of pain in the latter group, although pain scores were not significantly different. Following negative laparoscopy, another study[13] compared expectant management with intervention comprising an ultrasound scan and an educational and counselling session. Interval reassessment showed a significant improvement in mood and pain scores in the intervention group. These studies highlight the importance of a multidisciplinary approach to chronic pelvic pain [B].

## Centrally acting drugs

In the absence of pelvic pathology, there is a tendency for chronic pain to be attributed to depression. Although symptoms of depression and sleep disturbances may be more prevalent among women with chronic pain,[1] the interaction is likely to be complex and not necessarily causative. A randomized comparison of the antidepressant sertraline (a serotonin reuptake inhibitor) with placebo in chronic pelvic pain sufferers[13] failed to show any difference in pain scores [B]. Amitriptyline and gabapentin are useful for the treatment of neuropathic pain, but there are no randomized trials of their use in chronic pelvic pain.

## Ovarian suppression

Although there is some dispute about the existence of the condition, treatment with continuous medroxyprogesterone acetate (MPA) has been advocated for women with chronic pelvic pain and dyspareunia attributed to the presence of pelvic varicosities. In a large randomized trial,[26] MPA 50 mg daily for four months was compared with placebo. In addition, both were used alone or in conjunction with psychotherapy. MPA was more effective than placebo for the duration of therapy, but the benefit was not sustained after completion. Psychotherapy was no better than placebo. In a subsequent study, 47 women with chronic pelvic pain and pelvic venous congestion diagnosed by venography[12] were randomized between six months of the GnRH agonist goserelin or MPA 30 mg/day. Both groups had improved pain scores at the end of treatment, but the improvement was sustained for 12 months after the end of treatment only in the group which had received goserelin. On the basis of this evidence, as well as studies of women with endometriosis-associated pelvic pain, there seems to be a role for empirical ovarian suppression in the management of chronic pelvic pain which is cyclically exacerbated [B].

## Surgical approaches for chronic pelvic pain

Studies of conservative surgical approaches, including surgical interruption of pelvic nerve pathways and division of adhesions, have shown minimal or no improvement of pelvic pain symptoms [A], with the exception of women undergoing laparoscopic division of severe adhesions.[13,20] Hysterectomy may be beneficial for secondary dysmenorrhoea attributed to endometriosis or adenomyosis, but its role in chronic pelvic pain is unclear. A trial of therapy with a GnRH agonist should be undertaken before consideration of hysterectomy in such cases [E]. A review of five studies of women undergoing hysterectomy for chronic pain presumed to be of uterine origin[27] reported that symptoms were relieved in 83–97 per cent of women at 12-month follow up [D]. However, the results of these studies showed that failure of pain relief was greatest among women with no demonstrable pelvic pathology, once again emphasizing the importance of a multidisciplinary approach for women with unexplained pelvic pain.

## EBM

Recommendations for the management of primary dysmenorrhoea are based on eight systematic reviews. The management of chronic pelvic pain has been the subject of one systematic review and an RCOG Green-top guideline.

## KEY POINTS

- Primary dysmenorrhoea is experienced by more than two-thirds of women and a minority are severely incapacitated.
- Investigation is unnecessary, unless there are atypical symptoms or abnormal findings on pelvic examination [C].
- Ultrasound is a useful non-invasive method for the detection of pelvic abnormalities [A].
- Laparoscopy has a limited role in the investigation of chronic pelvic pain [B].
- NSAIDs are effective for the first-line management of primary dysmenorrhoea [A].
- COCPS are effective in primary dysmenorrhoea, although the evidence is largely based on higher dose formulations than those in current use [A].
- There is insufficient evidence to support the use of pelvic nerve interruption for the relief of primary or secondary dysmenorrhoea [A].
- Alternative therapies, including dietary supplements (magnesium, vitamin B$_1$), Chinese herbal medicine and behavioural interventions, may have a role in the management of primary dysmenorrhoea [A].
- Dysmenorrhoea secondary to suspected endometriosis or adenomyosis can be treated empirically with a trial of ovulation suppression [A].
- Chronic pelvic pain with cyclical exacerbation may be relieved by continuous high-dose MPA or goserelin [B].
- Antidepressants are not effective in the management of chronic pelvic pain [B].

- There is no evidence that division of adhesions relieves chronic pelvic pain, with the possible exception of severe dense avascular adhesions [B].
- The multifactorial nature of chronic pelvic pain should be discussed and explored from the start [A].
- Where possible, chronic pelvic pain should be managed in a multi-disciplinary clinic [A].

## Key References

1. Moore J, Kennedy S. Causes of chronic pelvic pain. *Baillière's Clin Obstet Gynaecol* 2000; **14**: 389–402.
2. Andersch B, Milsom I. An epidemiological study of young women with dysmenorrhoea. *Am J Obstet Gynecol* 1982; **144**: 655–60.
3. Sundell G, Milsom I, Andersch B. Factors influencing the prevalence and severity of dysmenorrhoea in young women. *Br J Obstet Gynaecol* 1990; **97**: 588–94.
4. Zondervan KT, Yudkin PL, Vessey MP *et al.* The prevalence of chronic pelvic pain in women in the United Kingdom: a systematic review. *Br J Obstet Gynaecol* 1998; **105**: 93–9.
5. Mathias SD, Kuppermann M, Liberman RF *et al.* Chronic pelvic pain: prevalence, health-related quality of life and economic correlates. *Obstet Gynecol* 1996; **87**: 321–7.
6. Facchinelti F, Sgarbi L, Piccinini F, Volpe A. A comparison of glyceryl trinitrate with diclofenac for the treatment of primary dysmenorrhoea: an open, randomized, cross-over trial. *Gynecol Endocrinol* 2002; **16**: 39–43.
7. Howard FM. The role of laparoscopy as a diagnostic tool in chronic pelvic pain. *Baillière s Clin Obstet Gynaecol* 2000; **14**: 467–94.
8. Zondervan KT, Yudkin PL, Vessey MP *et al.* Patterns of diagnosis and referral in women consulting for chronic pelvic pain in UK primary care. *Br J Obstet Gynaecol* 1999; **106**: 1156–61.
9. Royal College of Obstetricians and Gynaecologists. *The Initial Management of Chronic Pelvic Pain.* Green-top guideline No. 41. London: RCOG, 2005.
10. Latthe P, Mignini L, Gray R *et al.* Ractors predisposing women to chronic pelvic pain: systematic review. *BMJ* 2006; **332**: 749–51.
11. Beard RW, Reginald PW, Wadsworth J. Clinical features of women with lower abdominal pain and pelvic congestion. *Br J Obstet Gynaecol* 1988; **95**: 153–61.
12. Soysal ME, Soysal S, Viedan K, Ozer S, A randomized controlled trial of goserelin and medroxyprogesterone acetate in the treatment of pelvic congestion. *Hum Reprod* 2001; **5**: 931–9.
13. Stones RW, Cheong YC, Howard FM. Interventions for treating chronic pelvic pain in women. *Cochrane Database Syst Rev* 2005; (**2**): CD000387.

Reproductive medicine

14. Moore J, Copley S, Morris J *et al.* A systematic review of the accuracy of ultrasound in the diagnosis of endometriosis. *Ultrasound Obstet Gynecol* 2002; **20**: 630–4.

15. Royal College of Obstetricians and Gynaecologists. *Diagnostic Laparoscopy.* Consent Advice No. 2. London: RCOG, 2008.

16. Okaro E, Condous G, Khalid A *et al.* The use of ultrasound based 'soft markers' for the prediction of pelvic pathology in women with chronic pelvic pain – can we reduce the need for laparoscopy? *Br J Obstet Gynaecol* 2006; **113**: 251–6.

17. Peters AA, van Dorst E, Jellis B *et al.* A randomized clinical trial to compare two different approaches in women with chronic pelvic pain. *Obstet Gynecol* 1991; **77**: 740–4.

18. Zhang WY, Po ALW. Efficacy of minor analgesics in primary dysmenorrhoea: a systematic review. *Br J Obstet Gynaecol* 1998; **105**: 780–9.

19. Proctor ML, Roberts H, Farquhar CM. Combined oral contraceptive pill (OCP) as treatment for primary dysmenorrhoea. *Cochrane Database Syst Rev* 2001; (**4**): CD002120.

20. Proctor ML, Farquhar CM, Sinclair OJ, Johnson NP. Surgical interruption of pelvic nerve pathways for primary and secondary dysmenorrhoea. *Cochrane Database Syst Rev* 2005; (**4**): CD001896.

21. Proctor ML, Hing W, Johnson TC, Murphy PA. Spinal manipulation for primary and secondary dysmenorrhoea. *Cochrane Database Syst Rev* 2001; (**4**): CD002119.

22. Proctor ML, Murphy PA. Herbal and dietary therapies for primary and secondary dysmenorrhoea. *Cochrane Database Syst Rev* 2001; (**3**): CD002124.

23. Zhu X, Proctor M, Bensoussan A *et al.* Chinese herbal medicine for primary dysmenorrhoea. *Cochrane Database Syst Rev* 2009; (**4**): CD005288.

24. Proctor M, Murphy PA, Pattison HM *et al.* Behavioural interventions for primary and secondary dysmenorrhoea. *Cochrane Database Syst Rev* 2009; (**4**): CD002248.

25. Proctor M, Farquhar C. Diagnosis and management of dysmenorrhoea. *BMJ* 2006; **332**: 1134–8.

26. Farquhar CM, Rogers V, Franks S *et al.* A randomized controlled trial of medroxyprogesterone acetate and psychotherapy for the treatment of pelvic congestion. *Br J Obstet Gynaecol* 1989; **96**: 1153–62.

27. Vercellini P, De Giorgi O, Pisacreta A *et al.* Surgical management of endometriosis. *Baillière's Clin Obstet Gynaecol* 2000; **14**: 501–23.

# 51.5 Endometriosis and gonadotrophin-releasing hormone analogues

*Christine P West*

## INTRODUCTION

Endometriosis is a common condition with many diverse manifestations and a clinical course that is highly variable and unpredictable. It may be asymptomatic, but most commonly presents with pelvic pain that is usually cyclical and in severe cases there may be bowel or bladder involvement. The site of the lesions deep in the pelvis can cause dyspareunia and there is a well-recognized, but poorly understood, association with subfertility. Management is individualized and will depend on the patient's symptoms, her age and reproductive plans. This chapter deals mainly with the management of pain in endometriosis, which has attracted a large literature and for which evidence-based management is relatively well developed.

## DEFINITION

Endometriosis is the presence of ectopic endometrial tissue in extrauterine sites, usually within the pelvis, but very rarely at distant sites, such as the lung. Endometriosis may be regarded as distinct from adenomyosis, in which endometrial tissue is present within the myometrium.

Endometriomas, also known as chocolate cysts, are retention cysts that develop as a consequence of ovarian endometriosis. They commonly form when adhesions develop between endometriotic deposits on the ovary and the pelvic sidewall or may result from an inflammatory reaction to a superficial ovarian lesion, leading to adhesions developing around the lesion, producing progressive inversion of the surrounding cortex. Endometriomas may be multiple and very large, when they inevitably interfere with fertility by adhesion and distortion of the Fallopian tubes.

In some women with endometriotic lesions predominantly affecting the uterosacral ligaments, marked fibrosis and scarring may develop, with infiltration of active endometriotic tissue into the rectovaginal septum or laterally to involve the ureters. Dense adhesions involving the rectum may lead to partial or complete obliteration of the pouch of Douglas. Both processes may be associated with the development of tender nodules that are easily palpable on vaginal examination and are associated with bowel symptoms. Deep nodular lesions may also be visible as small, tender, bluish cysts in the posterior fornix. So-called deep infiltrating endometriosis may also be present on the uterovesical fold, leading to bladder involvement.

## INCIDENCE

The widespread use of laparoscopy has led to increased detection of endometriosis. Reported prevalence has varied very widely within and between different societies and according to the indications for laparoscopy. In a prospective study of 1542 Caucasian women in a single Scottish centre,[1] endometriosis was visualized in 6 per cent of women undergoing sterilization, 21 per cent being investigated for infertility and 15 per cent being investigated for pelvic pain. However, in a review of 1524 laparoscopies for pelvic pain,[2] the prevalence of endometriosis was reported to be 33 per cent.

# AETIOLOGY

It is generally accepted that endometriotic tissue reaches the pelvis by retrograde menstruation,[3] initiating a local inflammatory response. Failure of this response is believed to lead to implantation of the endometriotic tissue and its subsequent activity. Whether this failure is related to the volume of menstrual debris that reaches the pelvis or to a defect in the local peritoneal defence system remains unresolved. Retrograde menstruation occurs in the majority of women, but only a minority develop endometriosis. Factors that reduce menstruation, such as pregnancy and the use of oral contraceptives,[1,3] reduce its prevalence. Genetic factors also appear to be relevant and these may influence local response mechanisms and the subsequent course of the disease. Whatever the underlying mechanisms, it is evident that the progress of the disease differs considerably among individuals.[3] There is a suggestion that minimal or mild endometriosis is a natural condition that occurs intermittently in most women,[3] but in a minority progresses to cystic ovarian endometriosis or deeply infiltrating disease.

The mechanism of pain in endometriosis is presumably by the release of inflammatory mediators, such as prostaglandins from superficial lesions. Pain related to deep lesions may be caused by infiltration or constriction of nerves or may be secondary to adhesions.[4]

# MANAGEMENT

## Investigation

The most common presentation of endometriosis is with pelvic pain (which is usually cyclical in nature) characteristically preceding the onset of menstruation and associated with deep dyspareunia. There may be tenderness on bimanual examination, with palpable nodules in the pouch of Douglas or ovarian lesions on ultrasound suggestive of endometriomas. More often, examination is unhelpful and the decision to carry out further investigation is based largely on the history and the wishes of the patient. There is no evidence that serum CA-125 is useful as a screening test [A],[5,6] although levels are likely to be raised in severe disease. Transvaginal ultrasound is of value in detecting ovarian endometriomas [A],[5-7] but these may be confused with haemorrhagic functional cysts. Negative ultrasound findings do not exclude the disease. Magnetic resonance imaging

(MRI) has no advantage over ultrasound in the assessment of endometriomas [A],[5,6] but may assist in the evaluation of deep lesions.

The 'gold standard' investigation for diagnosis of endometriosis is by laparoscopy [B]. This is an invasive procedure and for some patients with pain symptoms suggestive of the disease, it will be preferable to undertake a therapeutic trial of hormonal suppression as initial management.[5,6] All cases require an informed discussion of the various options and, for those undergoing laparoscopy, its nature and risks must be fully discussed [E].[8] Counselling must include discussion about the possible courses of action should endometriosis be diagnosed at the primary procedure. Best practice is to carry out surgical ablative therapy at the initial laparoscopy, depending on the facilities and expertise available, providing that adequate informed consent has been obtained [E].

Laparoscopy must involve a two-port approach with careful inspection of the pouch of Douglas, the uterosacral ligaments, the pelvic sidewall and the anterior surfaces of both ovaries [E].[2,5,6] Where necessary, careful mobilization of the ovaries should be attempted in order to inspect their anterior surface, as the presence of adhesions is strongly suggestive of endometriosis. Where there is doubt about the nature of a lesion, this should be confirmed by biopsy [E], but this procedure is not without risk and is not necessary as a routine. It is recommended that endometriomas greater than 3 cm in diameter are biopsied [E].[5,6] The operator must appreciate the varied appearances of endometriosis and be familiar with the American Fertility Society (AFS) classification.[9] Photographs or DVD recordings are helpful in the documentation of disease extent and use should be made of diagrams, in particular those based on the AFS classification, which should be available in all gynaecological theatres [E]. It should be noted that although such classification systems are useful in the management of disease associated with impaired fertility, they correlate poorly with pain symptoms [C].[6]

## Medical management of pelvic pain associated with endometriosis

Endometriosis-associated pain can be managed effectively by medical therapy [A]. The majority of therapies act by ovarian suppression and induction of amenorrhoea. Since this merely inactivates and does not remove local disease, symptoms recur after cessation in a proportion of patients and, for some, treatment may potentially be long term. As all the therapies discussed below have similar efficacy, their tolerability in terms of side effects and health risks is important when selecting the most appropriate treatment for an individual woman [A].[5,6] As discussed above, medical therapy may be initiated for the relief of pain symptoms in the absence of a definitive diagnosis of endometriosis.

In contrast to the important role that medical therapy has in the symptomatic management of endometriosis, it has no role in the management of endometriosis-associated infertility, and indeed delays rather than enhances fertility

[A].[5,6] Medical suppression may be of temporary value in pain control, for example in women awaiting *in-vitro* fertilization (IVF) [E].

## Non-steroidal anti-inflammatory drugs

These offer a non-hormonal approach that is particularly useful in women trying to conceive and are widely used in clinical practice. Only one randomized controlled trial (RCT), comparing naproxen with placebo,[5] has been conducted on patients with endometriosis and this was insufficiently powered to give a conclusive result. Evidence for their efficacy is largely based on their use in the treatment of primary dysmenorrhoea [A].

## Combined oral contraceptives

Continuous use of a low-dose combined oral contraceptive pill (COCP) is a common management strategy, although evidence to support its continuous use is lacking.[10] In a randomized trial comparing cyclical administration of a low-dose COCP with a GnRH agonist,[10] both were effective in the management of non-menstrual pain and dyspareunia. This evidence, albeit limited, supports the use of the COCPs as a first-line therapy [B]. In the absence of further information, the mode of administration, whether cyclical, tricyclical, six-monthly or continuous, should be a matter for discussion between the clinician and the individual patient [E]. Because of their relative safety, COCPs are suitable for long-term use.

## Progestogens

Progestogens given continuously and at high doses inhibit ovulation and have direct anti-proliferative effects on endometriotic implants, causing decidualization and eventual atrophy. They have been widely used for the treatment of endometriosis and are the subject of two large reviews.[11,12] However, most published studies of their efficacy predated the era of evidence-based medicine and their small scale and poor design limited critical evaluation. In randomized controlled trials, both high-dose oral medroxyprogesterone acetate (MPA) (100 mg daily) and depot MPA (Depo-Provera 150 mg three-monthly) were found to be effective in the relief of pain symptoms [A]. Considerably lower daily doses of MPA (30 mg, 50 mg) were effective in non-randomized trials [C].[12]

The most commonly reported side effect of progestogens is breakthrough bleeding, with an overall incidence of around 33 per cent,[12] which is not dose related. Other side effects experienced by up to 10 per cent of women include weight gain, breast tenderness, bloating, headache and nausea. Progestogens, in particular long-acting depots, have an important role in the long-term management of endometriosis because of their low cost and good safety profile [A].

## Levonorgestrel-releasing intrauterine system

There are currently limited data on the effectiveness of the levonorgestrel-releasing intrauterine system (LNG-IUS) in the management of pain in endometriosis. The LNG-IUS does not suppress ovulation, but acts locally on the endometrium. Its effect on extra-uterine endometrial tissue is therefore locally mediated. An RCT comparing LNG-IUS with a GnRH agonist depot in 82 women with laparoscopically confirmed endometriosis[13] reported a significant reduction in pain scores over six months in both groups. Although bleeding scores were higher in the LNG-IUS group, there was no difference in pain or quality of life assessments between the two groups. A second RCT compared use of a LNG-IUS with a GnRH agonist in 40 parous women following laparoscopic surgery for endometriosis.[14] Reduction of menstrual pain was significantly better in the group treated with the LNG-IUS. On the basis of these results together with data from a longer-term cohort study,[5] the LNG-IUS seems to have a role in the management of pain associated with endometriosis [B].

## Gestrinone

Gestrinone is a 19-nortestosterone derivative that also has progestogenic and anti-progestogenic actions. It has been compared in randomized trials[11] with placebo, with danazol and with a GnRH analogue. Gestrinone was as effective as danazol and a GnRH analogue in reducing pain scores [A], but both androgenic and hypo-oestrogenic side effects were less frequent with gestrinone. Side effects of gestrinone were reduced by lowering the dose from 2.5 mg twice weekly to 1.25 mg twice weekly without a reduction in efficacy [A].[11]

No direct comparison has been made between gestrinone and progestogens, but the reported incidence of breakthrough bleeding is much lower with gestrinone, making it a potentially useful alternative to progestogens, danazol or GnRH analogues [A]. However, there is a lack of information relating to its safety for long-term use.

## Danazol

Danazol is an androgenic steroid, which acts both centrally and locally to suppress steroidogenesis and induce endometrial atrophy. It has also been the subject of a systematic review.[15] It induces amenorrhoea and significantly improves pain and AFS scores at doses of 400–600 mg daily [A]. Androgenic side effects, such as weight gain, limb tingling, acne, greasy skin, hirsutism and deepening of the voice, are common, and atherogenic effects on lipid profiles have been reported. Although there is evidence that danazol suppresses endometriosis at low doses that are insufficient to suppress menstruation [C],[16] the dose selected is usually the lowest that will achieve amenorrhoea. Thus, while effective for the treatment of symptomatic endometriosis, its side effects preclude its long-term use.

## GnRH analogues

The GnRH analogues are derived from native hypothalamic GnRH by peptide substitutions that increase their potency and duration of action. Both agonist analogues and antagonists have been developed, of which the agonists have been in established clinical practice for much longer. The antagonists act by competitive inhibition of pituitary GnRH receptors, with a rapid onset of action, whereas the agonists cause initial stimulation of gonadotrophin production followed by prolonged down-regulation. The antagonists are used for short-term pituitary suppression (e.g. during superovulation prior to IVF), but are unlikely to take over from agonists for longer-term indications, such as the management of endometriosis.

Downregulation of pituitary GnRH receptors by GnRH agonists leads to the inhibition of follicle-stimulating hormone (FSH) and luteinizing hormone (LH) production and gonadal suppression. The GnRH agonists are thus useful in the management of hormone-dependent conditions in both men and women. Administration of GnRH agonists is by nasal spray or monthly or three-monthly depot injection (Table 51.5.1). The intranasal route tends to be less costly, while depot administration improves compliance.

Results of a systematic review of 26 randomized, controlled trials of GnRH agonist therapy have demonstrated its effectiveness in the treatment of pain associated with endometriosis [A].[17] In the only trial which was placebo controlled, 27 of 31 patients randomized to placebo discontinued because of poor efficacy. Comparison with gestrinone, a COCP and danazol (15 studies) demonstrated no significant differences in clinical response, but expected differences in side-effect profiles. The side effects of GnRH agonists include hot flushes, insomnia, vaginal dryness, reduced libido and headaches – all secondary to oestrogen suppression.

Various GnRH agonists were used in these studies (see Table 51.5.1), the majority for six months duration. Comparison of different intranasal doses (600 versus 900 μg buserelin; 400 versus 800 μg nafarelin) showed no difference in symptomatic response and AFS scores, but side effects were reduced at the lower doses [A]. When three months of treatment was compared with six months, clinical response was similar, with the exception of deep dyspareunia, for which improvement was significantly greater after six months [A].

Like other medical treatments, GnRH agonists do not produce permanent disease regression. A life-table analysis of follow up of women treated with various GnRH agonists for six to nine months[18] reported a cumulative symptomatic recurrence rate of 53.4 per cent after seven years [C]. For severe disease, the recurrence rate was 74.4 per cent, while for minimal disease it was 36.9 per cent.

## Longer-term use of GnRH analogues

The side effects of the GnRH analogues are largely related to oestrogen deficiency and are often well tolerated. However, loss of bone mineral density is a major concern and for this reason GnRH analogues should not be given as single agents for longer than six months [A]. In women needing longer-term treatment, hormonal add-back therapy can be used with the object of reducing or preventing bone loss and minimizing other unwanted side effects. Several continuous combined regimens have been compared with placebo in patients treated with GnRH agonists for endometriosis.[19] These have included various progestogens in combination with transdermal oestradiol 25 μg twice weekly, oral oestradiol 2 mg daily and conjugated equine oestrogens 0.3–1.25 mg daily. All were effective in relieving pain while reducing side effects and maintaining bone density during treatment and up to 6 and 12 months after discontinuation of treatment. The longest treatment duration was two years.

Progestogens alone as add-back therapy are not effective in preventing bone loss.[19] For women who cannot tolerate hormonal add-back or for whom it is contraindicated, antiresorptive agents, such as bisphosphonates, have been used for bone protection, but evidence of their efficacy to date is currently insufficient.[19]

These results support the role of add-back therapy with GnRH agonists to suppress endometriosis-associated pain when given as continuous low-dose oestrogen–progestogen combinations for up to two years years [A]. Tibolone is

**Table 51.5.1** Gonadotrophin-releasing hormone agonists for the treatment of endometriosis

| Name | Monthly depot | Licensed indication | Three-monthly depot | Licensed indication | Intranasal | Licensed indication |
|---|---|---|---|---|---|---|
| Buserelin | | | | | 300 mg tid | Yes |
| Goserelin | 3.6 mg s.c. | yes | 10.8 mg | No | | |
| Leuprorelin acetate | 3.75 mg s.c. or i.m. | yes | 11.25 mg i.m. | Yes | | |
| Nafarelin | | | | | 200 μg bd | Yes |
| Triptorelin | 3.75 mg i.m. | yes | 11.25 mg i.m. | Yes | | |

- Data from British National Formulary indicating whether each preparation is licensed for treatment of endometrosis.
- bd, twice a day; tid, three times a day.

licensed in the United Kingdom for bone protection when used in conjunction with GnRH analogues, although there are a lack of published data to compare its effectiveness with that of other add-back therapies.

# ROLE OF SURGERY IN ENDOMETRIOSIS-ASSOCIATED PAIN

Unlike medical therapies, there have been few controlled studies of surgical approaches for the management of endometriosis-associated pain, although the latter have gained a large literature, and surgical interventions, mainly involving laparoscopy, are widely used. Because operative laparoscopy is associated with a significant risk of major complications and potential litigation [C],[8] such interventions are in urgent need of critical review.

To date, there have been only two randomized double-blind controlled trials of surgery compared with expectant management for relief of endometriosis-associated pain. In the first, active treatment comprising local laser ablation combined with adhesiolysis and laparoscopic uterine nerve ablation (LUNA) was compared with diagnostic laparoscopy.[20] Outcome was assessed in relation to the stage of the disease, but women with stage IV disease were excluded on ethical grounds. Women with mild and moderate disease (stages II–III) showed a significant improvement in pain scores at six months, with no improvement in those with minimal (stage I) disease. Overall, 62.5 per cent of those treated reported an improvement, compared with 22.6 per cent of controls. In a follow up of the original study at one year,[21] which included second-look laparoscopy in women who remained symptomatic, 90 per cent of those who initially responded remained well, but only 29 per cent of the control women showed signs of disease progression.

The second study[22] compared full excisional surgery with a diagnostic procedure, followed by a second-look laparoscopy after six months. Eighty per cent of the surgically treated group compared with 32 per cent of the control group reported symptomatic improvement. Patients with all degrees of severity of endometriosis were included. Disease progression was seen in 45 per cent of the control group, with static disease in 33 per cent and an improvement in 22 per cent.

These important but small-scale studies, carried out in nationally recognized laparoscopic surgery centres, support the use of conservative laparoscopic surgery for the relief of pain in endometriosis [A], but more data are needed from larger studies to establish the duration of benefit and how this is influenced by the severity of the disease. No serious surgical complications were reported, but these results may not be reproducible in a more general context, in terms of both efficacy and safety [E]. The studies highlight the variability of disease progression and also the placebo response associated with surgical intervention.

Several studies evaluating the role of laparoscopic uterine nerve ablation alone or as an adjunct to laparoscopic surgical treatment for pain in endometriosis have failed to show any benefit of this procedure [A].[23]

Surgical ablation of advanced disease, particularly where there are dense adhesions and deeply infiltrating lesions, is a technically difficult procedure involving a high risk of bowel and ureteric damage[5] and should only be carried out in specialist regional centres [E] if it is to be attempted laparoscopically. Where issues of safety arise, laparotomy still has a role in the conservative management of advanced disease [C],[24] both for pain management and for enhancement of fertility.

## Surgical management of endometriomas

The relationship between the presence of endometriomas and pain symptoms is unclear, but their presence in association with pain or infertility is usually regarded as an indication for laparoscopic surgical intervention. Endometriomas do not resolve during medical suppression, although, if small, they may reduce in size and become asymptomatic. Simple drainage of an endometrioma is followed by rapid recurrence, even if it is fenestrated and irrigated [A].[25] A systematic review of two randomized trials[25] has indicated a higher rate of recurrence following coagulation of the inner lining of the cyst compared with excision. Laparoscopic excision is therefore the surgical treatment of choice in endometriomas [A].

## Medical adjuncts to surgery

There is no evidence to support the use of medical adjuncts prior to conservative surgery for endometriosis [A], although they may be valuable in the control of symptoms. Drugs which suppress ovarian activity are frequently used following conservative surgery of endometriosis. Published evidence on their role are, however, conflicting. A systematic review of 11 RCTs, which included GnRH analogues, danazol, medroxyprogesterone and an oral contraceptive, concluded that there was insufficient evidence to recommend their use [A].[26] There was, however, a significant improvement in AFS scores, but a non-significant improvement in pain scores during follow up. In contrast, the authors of an evidence-based guideline[6] have stated that 'treatment with danazol or a GnRH for six months after surgery reduces endometriosis-associated pain and delays recurrence at 12 and 24 months compared with placebo and expectant management'. This was a grade A recommendation. The same authors concluded that post-operative treatment with a COCP is not effective. On the basis of this conflicting evidence, it seems that management decisions should be based on individual clinical circumstances including the patient's desire for pregnancy and severity and recurrence of symptoms [E].

The LNG-IUS can also be considered appropriate as a post-operative adjunct to surgical treatment.[14]

## Long-term follow up after surgery

Symptomatic recurrence rates of between 15 and 57 per cent two years after both laparoscopic surgery and laparotomy have been reported in multicentre studies [C].[24,27,28] Such figures are likely to be dependent on both the disease severity and the experience of the operator. There are no randomized studies comparing medical and surgical therapies, in terms of either short-term efficacy or long-term recurrence.

## Definitive surgery

In women with symptomatic endometriosis who have completed childbearing, hysterectomy offers a long-term cure, but only if combined with bilateral oophorectomy [C].[5] In advanced disease with dense adhesions and deep lesions in the recto-vaginal pouch, complete removal of the disease will require a very radical approach [C][5] with careful consideration of the risks, especially if the symptoms are well controlled with medical therapy.

## HORMONE REPLACEMENT THERAPY AND ENDOMETRIOSIS

Following hysterectomy with oophorectomy, or oophorectomy alone for severe endometriosis, there is a risk that use of HRT may activate small foci of residual endometriosis [C].[5,6] This risk is likely to be greater with unopposed oestrogen compared with combined oestrogen and progestogen therapy.[5,6] Unfortunately, there is a shortage of evidence to address this issue. A systematic review[29] identified only two RCTs. One was a very small study comparing tibolone with continuous transdermal oestradiol in combination with cyclical progestogen. The other was a larger study comparing transdermal oestradiol and cyclical progesterone with no treatment. There was a small incidence of symptom recurrence in all treatment groups, but not in the placebo group. Results did not reach statistical significance. The risk of symptom recurrence with HRT has to be balanced against the well-established sequelae of oestrogen deficiency in young women. Similarly, the theoretical benefit of using an oestrogen–progestogen combination or tibolone rather than oestrogen alone needs to be balanced against the slightly greater risk of breast cancer with combined HRT. The consensus view is that HRT should be used in young women following oophorectomy and the choice of preparation should be determined by individual risk factors [E].

---

### EBM

- Management of pain in endometriosis is supported by two evidence-based guidelines and six systematic reviews based on a large number of randomized, controlled trials.
- Surgical management of pain in endometriosis is based on two evidence-based guidelines, two small randomized, controlled trials and a systematic review of the use of pelvic denervation.
- There have been no randomized studies comparing medical with surgical management in the relief of endometriosis-associated pain.

### KEY POINTS

- Laparoscopy is the gold standard for diagnosis of endometriosis [A], but adequate counselling is essential prior to the procedure [E].
- Where appropriate, surgical ablative therapy should be carried out at the time of the initial laparoscopy [E].
- Measurement of CA-125 is not helpful as an aid to diagnosis [A].
- Transvaginal ultrasound is useful in identifying endometriomas, but lacks specificity [A].
- Hormonal suppression of ovulation is effective in the management of pain associated with endometriosis [A].
- COCPs, progestogens, danazol, gestrinone and GnRH agonists are all effective therapies and selection should be determined by the relative side-effect profiles [A].
- Because of a high risk of recurrence, medical treatment may need to be intermittent or long term [A].
- Levonorgestrel-releasing intrauterine systems may have a role in long-term pain control [B], but further evaluation is required.
- If GnRH agonists are used for longer than six months, add-back therapy with low-dose continuous combined HRT or tibolone should be given [A].
- Laparoscopic surgery is effective in the treatment of pain secondary to endometriosis in experienced hands [B].
- There is insufficient evidence to recommend surgical pelvic nerve interruption for the relief of pain associated with endometriosis [A].
- The role of post-operative medical therapy as an adjunct to surgery is uncertain [A].
- Operative laparoscopy carries a significant risk, and cases of advanced disease should be referred to specialist centres for laparoscopic surgery [E].
- Surgical treatment of endometriomas should be by laparoscopic cystectomy [A].
- If fertility is no longer an issue, hysterectomy with bilateral oophorectomy may provide a cure, but disease excision may be incomplete [C].

- Because of a risk of disease recurrence [C], low-dose continuous combined HRT or tibolone is preferable to oestrogen-only HRT following hysterectomy with oophorectomy for severe endometriosis [E].

## Key References

1. Mahmood TA, Templeton A. Prevalence and genesis of endometriosis. *Hum Reprod* 1991; **6**: 544–9.

2. Howard FM. The role of laparoscopy as a diagnostic tool in chronic pelvic pain. *Baillière's Clin Obstet Gynaecol* 2000; **14**: 467–94.

3. Wardle PG, Hull MRG. Is endometriosis a disease? *Baillière's Clin Obstet Gynecol* 1993; **7**: 673–85.

4. Moore J, Kennedy S. Causes of chronic pelvic pain. *Baillière's Clin Obstet Gynecol* 2000; **14**: 389–402.

5. Royal College of Obstetricians and Gynaecologists. *The Investigation and Management of Endometriosis*. Green-top guideline No. 24. London: RCOG, 2006.

6. Kennedy S, Bergquist A, Chapron C *et al.* ESHRE guideline for the diagnosis and treatment of endometriosis. *Hum Reprod* 2005; **20**: 2698–704.

7. Moore J, Copley S, Morris J *et al.* A systematic review of the accuracy of ultrasound in the diagnosis of endometriosis. *Ultrasound Obstet Gynecol* 2002; **20**: 630–4.

8. Royal College of Obstetricians and Gynaecologists. *Diagnostic Laparoscopy*. Consent Advice No. 2. London: RCOG, 2008.

9. American Fertility Society. Revised American Fertility Society classification of endometriosis. *Fertil Steril* 1985; **43**: 351–2.

10. Moore J, Kennedy S, Prentice A. Modern combined contraceptives for pain associated with endometriosis. *Cochrane Database Syst Rev* 2007; (**3**): CD001019.

11. Prentice A, Deary AJ, Bland E. Progestagens and antiprogestagens for pain associated with endometriosis. *Cochrane Database Syst Rev* 2000; (**2**): CD002122.

12. Vercellini P, Cortesi I, Crosignani PG. Progestins for symptomatic endometriosis – a critical analysis of the evidence. *Fertil Steril* 1997; **68**: 393–401.

13. Petta CA, Ferriani RA, Abaro MS *et al.* Randomized clinical trial of a levonorgestrel-releasing intrauterine system and a depot GnRH analogue for the treatment of chronic pelvic pain in women with endometriosis. *Hum Reprod* 2005; **20**: 1993–8.

14. Vercellini P, Frontino G, DeGiorgi O *et al.* Comparison of a levonorgestrel-releasing intrauterine system versus expectant management after conservative surgery for fendometriosis: a pilot study. *Fertil Steril* 2003; **80**: 305–9.

15. Selak V, Farquhar C, Prentice A, Singla A. Danazol for pelvic pain associated with endometriosis. *Cochrane Database Syst Rev* 2001; (**4**): CD000068.

16. Vercellini P, Trespidi L, Panazza S *et al.* Very low dose danazol for relief of endometriosis-associated pelvic pain: a pilot study. *Fertil Steril* 1994; **62**: 1136–42.

17. Prentice A, Deary AJ, Goldbeck-Wood S *et al.* Gonadotropin-releasing hormone analogues for pain associated with endometriosis. *Cochrane Database Syst Rev* 1991; (**1**): CD000346.

18. Waller KG, Shaw RW. Gonadotrophin-hormone releasing hormone analogues for the treatment of endometriosis; long term follow up. *Fertil Steril* 1993; **59**: 511–15.

19. Sagsveen M, Farmer JE, Prentice A, Breeze A. Gonadotropin-releasing hormone analogues for endometriosis: bone mineral density. *Cochrane Database Syst Rev* 2003; (**4**): CD001297.

20. Sutton CJ, Ewen SP, Whitelaw N, Haines P. Prospective randomized, double-blind, controlled trial of laser laparoscopy in the treatment of pelvic pain associated with minimal, mild and moderate endometriosis. *Fertil Steril* 1994; **62**: 696–700.

21. Sutton CJ, Pooley AS, Ewen SP, Haines P. Follow-up report on a randomized, controlled trial of laser laparoscopy in the treatment of pelvic pain associated with minimal to moderate endometriosis. *Fertil Steril* 1997; **68**: 1070–4.

22. Abbott J, Hawe J, Hunter D *et al.* Laparoscopic excision of endometriosis: a randomized, placebo-controlled trial. *Fertil Steril* 2004; **82**: 878–84.

23. Procter M, Latthe P, Farquher C *et al.* Surgical interruption of pelvic nerve pathways for primary and secondary dysmenorrhoea. *Cochrane Database Syst Rev* 2005; (**4**): CD001896.

24. Crosignani PG, Vercellini P, Biffignandi F *et al.* Laparoscopy versus laparotomy in conservative surgical management for severe endometriosis. *Fertil Steril* 1996; **66**: 706–11.

25. Hart RJ, Hickey M, Maouris P, Buckett W. Excisional surgery versus ablative surgery for ovarian endometriomata. *Cochrane Database Syst Rev* 2008; (**2**): CD004992.

26. Yap C, Furness S, Farquhar C, Rawal N. Pre- and postoperative medical therapy for endometriosis surgery. *Cochrane Database Syst Rev* 2004; (**3**): CD003678.

27. Hormstein MD, Hemmings R, Yuzpe AA, Heinrichs WL. Use of nafarelin versus placebo after reductive laparoscopic surgery for endometriosis. *Fertil Steril* 1997; **68**: 860–4.

28. Vercellini P, Crosignani PG, Fadini R *et al.* A gonadotropin-releasing hormone agonist compared with expectant management after conservative surgery for symptomatic endometriosis. *Br J Obstet Gynaecol* 1999; **106**: 672–7.

29. Al Kadri H, Hassan S, Al-Fozan HM, Hajeer A. Hormone therapy for endometriosis and surgical menopause. *Cochrane Database Syst Rev* 2009; (**1**): CD005997.

# 51.6 Adenomyosis

*Christine P West*

## INTRODUCTION

Adenomyosis is implicated as a cause of both heavy and painful menstruation, but information about its prevalence among women presenting with these problems is lacking. Similarly, its incidence in a normal population is unknown. Most published information on adenomyosis is based on studies of hysterectomy specimens. This is because, until recently, the diagnosis has only been possible in retrospect. Recent advances in imaging have facilitated its diagnosis and led to greater opportunities for clinical trials of medical and conservative management. To date, such studies have been very limited and consequently the literature on adenomyosis remains small, as is the evidence base for its management.

## DEFINITION

Histologically, adenomyosis is characterized by the presence of endometrial glands and stroma in the myometrium, with adjacent smooth muscle hyperplasia,[1] the latter often resulting in significant uterine enlargement. The lesions are seen haphazardly and at varied depths within the myometrium, and the exact diagnostic criteria may be disputed.[2] Although histologically similar, adenomyosis is traditionally regarded as distinct from endometriosis in terms of its epidemiology, being most commonly diagnosed in parous, middle-aged women who have undergone hysterectomy. However, recent studies based on imaging techniques (see below) have cast doubt on this distinction.

## INCIDENCE

Histological evidence of adenomyosis is present in 15–30 per cent of hysterectomy specimens,[2–6] but its overall contribution to menstrual disorders is unclear. Studies based on findings at hysterectomy have yielded varied conclusions about the correlation between symptomatology and the presence of adenomyosis. Some have related the severity of dysmenorrhoea to the extent of adenomyosis and its depth of invasion into the myometrium,[7,8] but others have failed to find any relationship between its presence and individual symptoms[2] or the main indication for the hysterectomy.[4] Recent small-scale studies using imaging techniques have reported appearances consistent with adenomyosis in 12 per cent of a sample of 100 healthy women[9] and in 9 per cent of 208 women following term delivery.[10] Its prevalence in a population of women attending a fertility clinic[11] was 79 per cent in 160 women with confirmed endometriosis and 28 per cent in 67 women without laparoscopic evidence of endometriosis. These limited data on prevalence have yet to be confirmed in larger studies.

## AETIOLOGY

Its cause remains speculative, but the adenomyotic tissue is presumed to be derived from the endometrium by abnormal ingrowth and invagination of its basal layer.[12] This process may be triggered by a weakness in the smooth muscle of the myometrium, by increased intrauterine pressure[1] or by surgical trauma. Among women undergoing hysterectomy, the incidence of adenomyosis is increased with increasing parity[3,4] and with a history of miscarriage[3] or induced abortion.[5,8] Some studies have reported an increased incidence following caesarean section,[5] but others have not.[2] It is decreased in smokers compared with non-smokers.[3] A relationship between the presence of adenomyosis and both endometrial hyperplasia[1,2] and uterine fibroids[1,8] has been reported, but this may be related to the age and symptomatology of the women undergoing hysterectomy.

## MANAGEMENT

### Investigation

Available evidence suggests that women with symptomatic adenomyosis are likely to present with heavy and painful menstruation.[12] Clinically, the uterus may be bulky and tender, but both the history and the clinical findings are very non-specific.

Reviews of diagnostic techniques[13,14] have concluded that transvaginal ultrasound (TVS) should be used as a primary screening modality for the diagnosis of adenomyosis [B]. Various sonographic appearances have been described[15] including:

- diffuse echogenicity,
- myometrial cysts,
- subendometrial nodules,
- subendometrial linear striations,
- poor definition of the endometrial/myometrial border,
- asymmetric myometrial thickening.

However, TVS lacks specificity, in particular in distinguishing adenomyosis from fibroids.[13,16] In such cases, magnetic resonance imaging (MRI) may be of value [B]. Both techniques, even when used in combination, may lack accuracy for the evaluation of very large uteri with a volume greater than 400 mL.[6]

Both hysteroscopic and laparoscopic myometrial biopsy techniques have been described,[17,18] but clearly have limitations when compared with non-invasive imaging.

### Medical management

The current medical management of menstrual disorders includes non-steroidal anti-inflammatory drugs (NSAIDs), combined oral contraceptives, high-dose progestogens and the levonorgestrel-releasing intrauterine system (LNG-IUS) with danazol and GnRH analogues as second-line options (see Chapter 51.2, Uterine fibroids and menorrhagia and Chapter 51.5, Endometriosis and GnRH analogues). As most of these therapies are effective in the management of heavy menstrual bleeding, dysmenorrhoea and endometriosis,

they should theoretically be beneficial for adenomyosis although evidence is lacking. A small, uncontrolled study[19] showed the LNG-IUS to reduce symptoms in 23 out of 25 women with adenomyosis diagnosed at TVS and followed up for 12 months. A prospective study of 95 women with adenomyosis treated with either LNG-IUS or expectant management following TCRE[20] reported a significantly higher rate of dysmenorrhoea and need for further treatment with expectant management. This evidence, albeit limited, supports the role of the LNG-IUS in the management of adenomyosis [C].

### Surgical management

The presence or absence of adenomyosis may influence the choice of surgical treatment for women with menstrual disorders. There is some evidence that the presence of deep lesions of adenomyosis is associated with failure of endometrial ablation,[17,21] with both regeneration of the endometrium and glandular activity within the myometrium [D]. However, further studies comparing the results of imaging before and after such procedures are needed to distinguish between pre-existing and iatrogenic lesions. It is not known whether second generation ablation techniques have any advantage over first generation methods in this regard. On the basis of current evidence, use of the LNG-IUS may be preferred to endometrial ablation where a diagnosis of adenomyosis is suspected [E]. Persistence of pain following excisional surgery for endometriosis was significantly associated with pretreatment MRI features of adenomyosis in a small prospective study.[22] Hysterectomy is well established and, for the definitive treatment of adenomyosis, should not be accompanied by oophorectomy [E] unless there are specific indications for the latter.

Where preservation of fertility is desired, management options are even less clear. There have been a few preliminary reports of laparoscopic or microsurgical excision or coagulation[12] of adenomyosis with variable results. MRI guided focused ultrasound may be applicable to adenomyosis,[23] but data are very limited. Uterine artery embolization (UAE) has an established role for conservative management of fibroids, but reports of its use for adenomyosis are less promising. Two small studies of 65 women followed up for at least two years after UAE reported symptomatic improvement in only 57 per cent.[24,25]

> **EBM**
>
> There is little supporting evidence for the management of adenomyosis, and the above text relies largely on small descriptive, non-randomized and cohort studies.

## KEY POINTS

- Adenomyosis is present in 15–30 per cent of hysterectomy specimens and is a cause of uterine enlargement.
- Its prevalence in the population is unclear and its role as a contributing factor to menstrual disorders is not well understood.
- TVS, backed up by MRI, is of value as a diagnostic tool [B].
- Medical therapies that have proven value in management of painful heavy menstruation and endometriosis have not been adequately assessed in adenomyosis but are likely to be beneficial [E].
- Limited data suggest that the LNG-IUS reduces menstrual symptoms in adenomyosis [C].
- Endometrial ablation and local excision of endometriosis may have a greater failure rate in the presence of adenomyosis [D].
- Hysterectomy is an effective treatment for menstrual symptoms attributed to adenomyosis [D].
- Preliminary data suggest that uterine artery embolization has a limited role in the management of adenomyosis [D].

## Key References

1. Ferenczy A. Pathophysiology of adenomyosis. *Hum Reprod Update* 1998; **4**: 312–22.
2. Bergholt T, Eriksen L, Berendt N *et al.* Prevalence and risk factors of adenomyosis at hysterectomy. *Hum Reprod* 2001; **16**: 2418–21.
3. Parazzini F, Vercellini P, Panazza S *et al.* Risk factors for adenomyosis. *Hum Reprod* 1997; **12**: 1275–9.
4. Vercellini P, Parazzini F, Oldani S *et al.* Adenomyosis at hysterectomy: a study on frequency distribution and patient characteristics. *Hum Reprod* 1995; **10**: 1160–62.
5. Valvis D, Agorastos T, Tzafetas J *et al.* Adenomyosis at hysterectomy: prevalence and relationship to operative findings and reproductive and menstrual factors. *Clin Exp Obstet Gynecol* 1997; **24**: 36–8.
6. Dueholm M, Lundorf E, Hansen ES *et al.* Magnetic resonance imaging and transvaginal ultrasonography for the diagnosis of adenomyosis. *Fertil Steril* 2001; **76**: 588–94.
7. Nishida M. Relationship between the degree of dysmenorrhoea and histologic findings in adenomyosis. *Am J Obstet Gynecol* 1991; **165**: 229–31.
8. Levgur M, Abadi MA, Tucker A. Adenomyosis: symptoms, histology and pregnancy terminations. *Obstet Gynecol* 2000; **95**: 688–91.
9. Hauth EA, Jaeger HJ, Libera H *et al.* MR imaging of the uterus and cervix in healthy women: determination of normal values. *Eur Radiol* 2007; **17**: 734–42.
10. Juang CM, Chou P, Yen M *et al.* Adenomyosis and risk of peterm delivery. *Br J Obstet Gynaecol* 2007; **114**: 165–9.
11. Kunz G, Beil D, Huppert P *et al.* Adenomyosis in endometriosis – prevalence and impact on fertility. Evidence from magnetic resonance imaging. *Hum Reprod* 2005; **20**: 2309–2316.
12. Mehasseb MK, Habiba MA. Adenomyosis uteri: an update. *Obstetrician Gynaecologist* 2009; **11**: 41–7.
13. Arnold LL, Ascher SM, Schruefer JJ, Simon JA. The non-surgical diagnosis of adenomyosis. *Obstet Gynecol* 1995; **86**: 461–5.
14. Meredith SM, Sanchez-Ramos L, Kaunitz AM. Diagnostic accuracy of transvaginal sonography for the diagnosis of adenomyosis: systematic review and metaanalysis. *Am J Obstet Gynecol* 2009; **201**: 107.
15. Atri M, Reinhold C, Mehio AR *et al.* Adenomyosis: US features with histologic correlation in an *in-vitro* study. *Radiology* 2000; **215**: 783–90.
16. Bazot M, Cortez A, Darai E *et al.* Ultrasonography compared with magnetic resonance imaging for the diagnosis of adenomyosis: correlation with histopathology. *Hum Reprod* 2001; **16**: 2427–33.
17. McCausland AM, McCausland VM. Depth of endometrial penetration in adenomyosis helps determine outcome of rollerball ablation. *Am J Obstet Gynecol* 1996; **174**: 1786–93.
18. Popp LW, Schwiedessen JP, Gaetje R. Myometrial biopsy in the diagnosis of adenomyosis uteri. *Am J Obstet Gynecol* 1993; **169**: 546–9.
19. Fedele L, Bianchi S, Rafaelli R *et al.* Treatment of adenomyosis-associated menorrhagia with a levonorgestrel-releasing intrauterine device. *Fertil Steril* 1997; **68**: 426–9.
20. Maia H Jr, Maltez A, Coelho G *et al.* Insertion of mirena after endometrial resection in patients with adenomyosis. *J Am Assoc Gynecol Laparosc* 2003; **10**: 512–16.
21. Tresserra F, Grases P, Ubeda A *et al.* Morphological changes in hysterectomies after endometrial ablation. *Hum Reprod* 1999; **14**: 1473–7.
22. Parker JD, Leondires M, Sinaii N *et al.* Persistence of dysmenorrhoea and nonmenstrual pain after optimal endometriosis surgery may indicate adenomyosis. *Fertil Steril* 2006; **86**: 711–15.
23. Fukunishi H, Funaki K, Sawada K *et al.* Early results of magnetic resonance-guided focused ultrasound surgery of adenomyosis: analysis of 20 cases. *J Min Invasive Gynecol* 2008; **15**: 571–9.
24. Kim MD, Kim S, Kim NK *et al.* Long term results of uterine artery embolization for symptomatic adenomyosis. *Am J Roentgenol* 2007; **188**: 176–81.
25. Bratby MJ, Walker WJ. Uterine artery embolisation for symptomatic adenomyosis – mid-term results. *Eur J Radiol* 2009; **70**: 128–32.

# 51.7 Premenstrual syndrome

*Christine P West*

## INTRODUCTION

Adverse emotional and physical symptoms are experienced by the majority of women in the lead up to menstruation, although they are usually mild and regarded as a normal physiological response to cyclical hormone changes. However, a substantial number of women are sufficiently distressed by their symptoms to seek medical help and a minority are severely incapacitated by them. Hormonal treatments were commonly used in the past, but premenstrual syndrome (PMS) is no longer regarded as an endocrine disorder and first-line management includes non-hormonal approaches. However, the symptoms are triggered by the endocrine changes of the menstrual cycle and women with PMS continue to be referred to gynaecologists for consideration of hormonal suppression when other therapies have failed. Assessment of the efficacy of treatment for PMS is complicated by the subjective nature of the diagnosis and the strong placebo effect. Prospective methods of symptom assessment are now well established and there is an expanding literature of randomized, controlled trials covering various approaches to management, including several systematic reviews.

## DEFINITIONS

Premenstrual syndrome is a cluster of menstrually related symptoms, which include:

- mood swings;
- tension, depression, anger, irritability;
- headache;
- breast discomfort;
- bloating;
- increased appetite and food cravings.

These symptoms occur during the luteal phase of the cycle and are relieved with the onset of menstruation or soon afterwards. Symptoms occur with a variable degree of severity from mild (no interference with personal or professional life) to severe in which symptoms are so disruptive that the individual is unable to function socially or professionally. PMS of this severity is classified as premenstrual dysphoric disorder (PMDD) by the American Psychiatric Association in its *Diagnostic and Statistical Manual of Mental Disorders*, 4th edition (DSM-IV), although this is a research criterion not in general use outside the United States. Because no objective tests can confirm PMS, the diagnosis is made on the basis of prospective daily symptom recording using various rating scales.[1]

Premenstrual syndrome must be distinguished from premenstrual magnification/exaggeration, in which symptoms are present throughout the cycle, but are exacerbated premenstrually. There may also be premenstrual exacerbation of underlying psychiatric or medical disorders.

## INCIDENCE

In a population-based questionnaire survey of 1083 women aged 18–46 years in Goteborg,[2] 92 per cent experienced at least one adverse symptom in the lead up to menstruation. Seventy per cent reported mental symptoms in combination with bodily swelling, and 30–40 per cent rated their symptoms as mild to moderate in intensity. Eleven per cent felt that their symptoms were severe enough to seek medical help. A study of 500 women from a UK-based general practice population[3] reported very similar findings. Such population-based studies rely on retrospective assessment and do not distinguish between PMS and premenstrual magnification, so that the true prevalence of PMS is unclear. However, it is evident that cyclical symptoms contribute significantly to menstrual cycle morbidity.

# AETIOLOGY

The frequency with which these symptoms are reported by women suggests that in their milder form they are a normal manifestation of the menstrual cycle, although it is likely that those at the more extreme end of the normal range have a pathological cause. Despite their relationship with the endocrine changes of the menstrual cycle, there is no evidence for any underlying disorder of the hypothalamo–pituitary–ovarian axis. There have been many theories of aetiology, but current evidence suggests that PMS may be a neuroendocrine disorder caused by serotonergic dysfunction,[4] which is supported by evidence that drugs that enhance serotonergic function are beneficial in its management.[5]

It is likely that there is a hormonally related trigger factor. This may be abnormal metabolism of progesterone to its metabolites allopregnenalone and pregnenalone, neuroactive steroids with differential effects on anxiety-related symptoms. Allopregnenalone has anxiolytic actions, whereas pregnenalone may promote anxiety.[4] However, the basis for any metabolic disorder remains unclear.

A study of prospective daily symptom self-assessment by women referred for specialist help because of cyclical symptoms found that PMS was confirmed in only one-third,[6] the remainder showing premenstrual magnification of ongoing psychological symptoms or symptoms exacerbated by menstruation itself. There was a significant relationship between menstrual and premenstrual magnification and previous psychiatric disorders, marital breakdown and increased parity.[6] Other studies have shown a relationship between self-reported PMS and personality disorders[3] and psychosocial stress.[7]

# MANAGEMENT

Management of PMS has been the subject of a recent RCOG Green Top guideline.[8] Women with mild degrees of PMS may respond to reassurance and general advice about exercise, diet and stress reduction [E]. Basic management lies within the scope of primary care. Referral for specialist help will depend on the severity of the problem, the experience of individual general practitioners and the expectations of the women involved. Most women referred for specialist help will be experiencing disruption of family or professional life and have a history of previous treatment failures. Ideally, women with severe PMS should be seen in a multidisciplinary specialist clinic or at least by a gynaecologist or a psychiatrist with a particular interest in the problem, preferably in a community-based setting [E].

A diagnosis of PMS based on retrospective history taking is unreliable, and prospective charting of symptoms for at least two menstrual cycles is essential in order to clarify the symptom pattern [E]. This must be preceded by a detailed medical, social and psychiatric history. Many methods of symptom assessment are available,[8,9] but as they are time consuming to analyse, most are only suitable for use in a specialist clinic or research setting. Simple pictorial charts are available for use in primary care.

All randomized, controlled trials of treatment for PMS have shown a very marked placebo response. This emphasizes the importance of critical appraisal of the evidence base before recommending specific therapies. The strength of the placebo effect in all trials of therapy for PMS may reflect the positive role of detailed history taking and a sympathetic approach.

# Complementary and alternative therapies

These approaches are popular with patients and, given the high level of placebo response, are likely to be perceived as effective without the potential disadvantage of side effects associated with conventional medications. However, interactions with conventional medicines should be considered, such as those reported with the use of St John's wort.[8] Many randomized trials have been reported using a variety of alternative therapies for PMS. There have been three systematic reviews of trials of such therapies: one covering a wide range of approaches,[10] one addressing dietary supplements[11] and one on the use of vitamin $B_6$.[12]

## Dietary supplements

Vitamin $B_6$, evening primrose oil, isoflavones, calcium, magnesium and vitamin E have all been compared with placebo in small-scale, controlled trials. Beneficial effects were reported with calcium, calcium combined with vitamin D, magnesium, vitamin E and isoflavones.[8,10–12] Only one of these, comparing calcium 1200 mg daily with placebo, was a large-scale multicentre study. Despite these positive results, the reviewers felt that weaknesses in methodology limited their recommendations of the value of such interventions [E]. Similarly, studies of nutritional supplements containing high doses of vitamins and other micronutrients have yielded inconclusive results.[8,10,11]

Dietary supplements are popular because they are perceived to have fewer side effects than conventional medicines. However, high-dose vitamin $B_6$, used for many years for the treatment of PMS, was reported to have neurotoxic effects at doses above 200 mg daily.[12] A meta-analysis of ten randomized, controlled trials comparing various doses of vitamin $B_6$ with placebo in 940 women[12] showed results significantly in favour of vitamin $B_6$ for overall symptomatic response and for depression. There was no dose–response effect. Despite their comments on the methodological weaknesses of the studies, the authors concluded that 'doses of vitamin $B_6$ up to 100 mg daily are likely to be of benefit in treating premenstrual symptoms and premenstrual depression' [A].

A meta-analysis of placebo-controlled trials of evening primrose oil[13] failed to find sufficient evidence to support its use for PMS [A], although at high dosage it is licensed for the relief of premenstrual mastalgia.

Despite the negative conclusions of the reviewers cited above, an Expert Consensus Group has endorsed the use of nutritional approaches for women with severe PMS and PMDD [E].[14]

## Herbal medicine

The fruit of the chaste tree (*Vitex agnus castus*) contains a mixture of iridoids and flavonoids and some compounds similar in structure to sex steroids. Initial controlled studies of its use were felt to be inconclusive.[10] A more recent multi-centre, randomized, controlled study[15] has shown the active treatment to be significantly more effective than placebo for the majority of the symptoms assessed (with the exception of bloating), with an overall response rate of 53 per cent for active treatment and 24 per cent for placebo. On the basis of this evidence, *Vitex agnus castus* fruit extract seems to be a potentially useful therapy for PMS [B], although there is no standard quality controlled preparation available. Similarly, reports of benefit from the use of Chinese herbal medicine[16] are limited by the lack of standard formulations. Ginko biloba and pollen extract have both been shown to be beneficial in small-scale studies, although further data would be needed to support their use.[9]

## Cognitive behavioural therapy

A randomized trial comparing cognitive behavioural therapy (CBT) with fluoxetine and with both treatments in combination, showed all three to be similarly effective for women with PMDD after six months of treatment, but the groups receiving CBT showed better maintenance of benefit after 12 months of follow up.[17] There did not appear to be any advantage of combined therapy over CBT alone. CBT has also been evaluated by comparing immediate treatment with delayed treatment, showing a substantial improvement in the immediate treatment group.[18] Although CBT is effective for severe PMS [A], such therapy is intensive, involving weekly sessions of individual cognitive therapy, and thus not available for the majority of sufferers.

## Other alternative approaches

Massage, relaxation and aromatherapy are popular therapies for which benefit is likely to outweigh any possible harm [E], although controlled studies of their use for PMS have yielded inconclusive results.[11] Chiropractic therapy and light therapy have not been found to be effective. Similarly, although advice about graded exercise is useful for general health, there is no evidence for or against a specific benefit in PMS.

Support and self-help groups are commonly used for PMS. This approach has been evaluated in a controlled study. A package of strategies including self-monitoring, personal choice, self-regulation and environmental modification was administered within a peer support group with

professional guidance. Comparison was with a control group waiting for the intervention. The active intervention was reported to be effective [B],[19] with a 75 per cent reduction in severity of PMS.

The Expert Consensus Group cited above[14] has endorsed the use of psychobehavioural approaches for women with PMDD.

## Selective serotonin reuptake inhibitors

Selective serotonin reuptake inhibitors (SSRIs) are now regarded as first-line therapy for moderate to severe PMS, particularly in women who fulfil the criteria for PMDD.[9] The use of SSRIs for PMS has been the subject of a systematic review.[5] Forty trials, which included 2294 women, compared various SSRIs with placebo. Most commonly studied were fluoxetine ($n = 14$) and sertraline ($n = 11$), followed by citalopram ($n = 3$), paroxetine ($n = 9$), clomipramine ($n = 2$) and fluvoxamine ($n = 1$). Some compared different dose levels and others included luteal-phase-only administration. The results strongly favoured active treatment over placebo for both behavioural and physical symptoms. The onset of effectiveness was rapid, and luteal-phase-only therapy seemed to be as effective as continuous treatment. Withdrawals due to side effects were twice as likely in the active treatment groups. Insomnia, gastrointestinal disturbances and fatigue were the most commonly reported side effects, reported by up to 20 per cent of subjects.

On the basis of this review, SSRIs, used continuously or cyclically, can be regarded as a first-line treatment for severe PMS [A]. They have the advantage of being suitable for long-term use. Despite this convincing evidence for their efficacy, side effects are a common reason for poor compliance, and 30–40 per cent of women with PMS fail to respond to SSRIs. Use of these medications falls outside the expertise of the average gynaecologist and should be prescribed in the context of a specialist clinic [E].

# HORMONAL MANIPULATION FOR THE MANAGEMENT OF PMS

Although the majority of women with PMS have no identifiable underlying endocrine disorder, ovulation appears to act as a trigger factor and thus various strategies that suppress ovulation or abolish the cycle altogether have a potential role in management.

## Progesterone and progestogens

Luteal-phase supplements of progesterone have been widely used, based on the unfounded assumption that PMS was secondary to a progesterone deficiency. In the United Kingdom, progesterone is available only for vaginal or rectal administration, hence the use of synthetic progestogens for

*Reproductive medicine*

this indication. However, evidence from hormone replacement therapy (HRT) studies indicate that these therapies might actually exacerbate PMS-type symptoms in susceptible individuals.[20]

A systematic review assessed 14 randomized, controlled trials of progesterone and four of progestogens in PMS.[21] Overall results of meta-analysis for progesterone showed no difference compared with placebo. Results with progestogens were difficult to interpret due to the small number of studies and differences in the treatment protocols. Overall, odds ratios were marginally but significantly in favour of progestogens for both physical and behavioural symptoms, but drop-out due to side effects was high. The response to progestogens may have been influenced by the fact that two of the four studies used progestogens in an ovulation-suppressing regimen. However, this evidence does not support the use of either progesterone or progestogens in the management of PMS when given during the luteal phase of the cycle [A]. While the continuous use of progestogens in ovulation suppressive doses (e.g. Depo-Provera or oral desogestrel) may be beneficial, there is insufficient evidence to support this approach.

## Combined oral contraceptives

The occurrence of PMS symptoms in the post-ovulatory phase of the menstrual cycle and the observation that spontaneous anovulation causes the disappearance of cyclical symptoms in women with PMS[22] strongly suggest that any therapy that suppresses ovulation should relieve PMS. The combined oral contraceptive pill (COCP) has the advantage of being cheap and suitable for long-term use. Population and contraceptive studies have yielded varied results. Some have shown a reduction in the prevalence and severity of PMS,[23,24] while others have failed to show any difference in cyclical symptoms between COCP users and non-users.[25] An oral contraceptive containing the progestogen drospirenone, which has anti-androgenic and anti-mineralocorticoid activities may have advantages over older preparations. A systematic review of five RCTs[26] including a total of 1500 women, compared a combined pill containing drospirenone with placebo (three trials) or another combined pill (two trials); one with desogestrel and the other with levonorgestrel. Pills containing drospirenone were significantly more effective than placebo over a three-month period of treatment in women with a pre-treatment diagnosis of PMDD (severe PMS). Both 30 μg (one study) and 20 μg (two studies) doses of ethinyloestradiol were included. In the other two studies, PMS or PMDD was not an inclusion criteria. Patients treated with drospirenone reported fewer premenstrual symptoms than those treated with levonorgestrel (both combined with 30 μg ethinyloestradiol) after six months. However, after two years of treatment with either desogestel or drospirenone combined with 30 μg ethinyloestradiol, PMS symptoms were similar.

Taken overall, this evidence suggests that a trial of therapy with a low-dose COCP is appropriate for women with no contraindications to its use. Pills containing third-generation progestogens may be more effective than second-generation combinations [B], in particular preparations containing drospirenone in combination with either 20 or 30 μg ethinyloestradiol [A]. Although continuous use of COCP preparations may have a theoretical advantage over cyclical use in PMS,[9] there is limited evidence to support this strategy.

## Transdermal oestradiol

Transdermal oestradiol has been used in ovulation-suppressive doses in combination with cyclical luteal-phase progestogen for the management of severe PMS. A dose of 200 mg twice weekly was found to be more effective than placebo in an initial crossover study. Subsequently, a lower dose of 100 mg twice weekly was found to be as effective in the suppression of ovulation and symptom relief as the 200 mg dosage,[27] but with fewer oestrogenic side effects. The authors did not comment on side effects related to the progestogen. Overall satisfaction at eight months was around 50 per cent. These limited data support the role of ovulation-suppressive doses of transdermal oestradiol for the relief of PMS [A], although information on its long-term safety in relation to breast and endometrial cancer and cardiovascular risk is lacking. Its use in combination with the levonorgestrel-releasing intrauterine system for endometrial protection is an approach that merits future investigation.

## Danazol

Several studies have supported the use of danazol for PMS. At a dose of 200 mg twice a day in a crossover study,[28] 44 per cent of subjects on active therapy experienced a clinically significant improvement, compared with only 8 per cent of those treated with placebo. Although effective [B], the side effects and metabolic sequelae of danazol limit its usefulness for the long-term management of PMS.

## Gonadotrophin-releasing hormone agonists

Ovarian suppression with gonadotrophin-releasing hormone (GnRH) agonists should eliminate PMS if the symptoms are triggered by ovulation. A meta-analysis[29] of five studies comparing a GnRH agonist with placebo reported a reduction in both physical and behavioural symptoms with the active therapy [A]. However, the use of hormonal add-back is necessary if treatment is to be long term. The meta-analysis[29] included three studies in which add-back HRT combined with a GnRH agonist was compared with the GnRH agonist alone. In two of these, add-back was with continuous oestrogen and cyclical progestogen HRT; the third used tibolone. Results showed no significant difference in efficacy, even with the use of cyclical hormones, although one trial reported a reduced response and a greater drop-out rate in the cyclical add-back group.

GnRH agonists are effective in the management of severe PMS [A], but the cost and potentially long-term nature of treatment when used with hormonal add-back should limit its use to women with severe symptoms that are socially disruptive and resistant to other forms of therapy [E]. Patient selection is also important. All the women included in the trials cited above had prospectively confirmed PMS. Women with premenstrual exacerbation of ongoing dysphoric symptoms do not experience symptom relief.[30] GnRH agonists therefore offer a useful means of further assessment of the pattern and nature of cyclical symptoms in situations in which the diagnosis is unclear or, in particular, when oophorectomy is being considered [E].

## Oophorectomy

Although there have been reports of its efficacy in the literature,[31,32] oophorectomy is not recommended for the management of PMS unless the problem is very severe and has been confirmed by prospective assessment and there has been genuine failure of conservative therapies [E].[31,32] It should not be considered unless supported by a trial of ovarian suppression with danazol[31] or, preferably, a GnRH agonist.[33] The latter also gives an opportunity to assess the response of the patient to add-back HRT. In the latter situation, the advantages and disadvantages of continuing medical suppression together with add-back HRT need to be considered carefully. Unless there are additional indications for hysterectomy, laparoscopic oophorectomy offers a less invasive surgical approach [E]. In women undergoing hysterectomy for other indications, a history of PMS is not a sufficient indication for concurrent oophorectomy without careful assessment [E],[33] as cyclical symptoms may improve following hysterectomy [C].[34] Indeed, improvement of PMS has been reported following endometrial ablation.[34]

## MANAGEMENT OF WOMEN WITH PREMENSTRUAL MAGNIFICATION

There is now a wide evidence base for the management of PMS. However, eligibility for treatment trials included prospective confirmation of the diagnosis by daily self-rating, so that the majority excluded the group of women whose management tends to be most problematic – those with premenstrual magnification. The presence of high baseline postmenstrual symptom scores has been identified as one factor that leads to treatment failure with SSRIs[35] and GnRH agonists[30] and to poor response to the COCP.[23] Women with premenstrual magnification are therefore likely to be over-represented among those who present because of treatment failure. It is important that this group is identified and the nature of the problem and the limitations of management appreciated by both the clinician and the patient so that these women are not subjected to inappropriate and over-aggressive interventions, such as hormonal manipulation or even surgery.

## CONCLUSION

There is a wide range of therapies that have proven efficacy for severe PMS. However, response rates to any individual therapy are rarely in excess of 60 per cent, and thus it is important that those involved in management are aware of these limitations and of different approaches to the problem. Ideally, women with severe symptoms and treatment failure should be managed in specialist multidisciplinary clinics. The importance of making a correct diagnosis based on adequate prospective daily symptom assessment cannot be over-emphasized.

### EBM

- There are many published randomized, controlled trials covering various approaches to the management of PMS, but some of those relating to alternative therapies are open to methodological criticism.
- These recommendations are based on an RCOG Green Top Guideline and seven systematic reviews or meta-analyses of PMS therapy, three of which relate to alternative or dietary approaches.

### KEY POINTS

- Diagnosis of premenstrual syndrome should be confirmed by at least two cycles of prospective daily symptom rating [E].
- Management of severe PMS should take place in a multidisciplinary clinic or by a specialist with a special interest in the condition [E].
- All treatment trials to date have demonstrated a strong placebo effect [A].
- Expert opinion is divided about the benefit of complementary therapies, such as nutritional and herbal approaches [E].
- Limited evidence supports the role of group support, lifestyle modification and physical interventions, such as acupuncture and relaxation [C].
- Cognitive behavioural therapy is effective for the treatment of severe PMS [A].
- SSRIs are effective for relieving both the physical and psychological symptoms of PMS [A].
- SSRIs are equally effective when given during the luteal phase of the cycle, and this is associated with fewer side effects [A].
- Progesterone or progestogens given during the luteal phase of the menstrual cycle are not effective for PMS [A], although ovulation-suppressive regimens may be beneficial [C].

- Suppression of ovulation with a third-generation COCP containing drospirenone is beneficial in the management of PMS [A], although other third-generation preparations may also be beneficial [B].
- Suppression of ovulation with transdermal oestradiol combined with progestogen for endometrial protection is effective in around 50 per cent of women [A], but information on its safety for long-term use is lacking [A].
- Danazol is effective for PMS, but is not suitable for long-term use [A].
- GnRH analogues are effective for severe PMS and may be used in combination with low-dose hormonal add-back therapy [A].
- Oophorectomy may be considered in severe PMS, but only when medical measures have failed, and should be preceded by a trial of GnRH agonist therapy [E].
- The presence of high baseline symptom scores (premenstrual magnification) is an important contributor to treatment failure [C].

## Key References

1. Born L, Steiner M. Current management of the premenstrual syndrome and premenstrual dysphoric disorder. *Curr Psychiatry Rep* 2001; 3: 463–9.
2. Andersch C, Wendestram L, Hahn L, Ohman R. Premenstrual complaints. 1. Prevalence of premenstrual symptoms in a Swedish urban population. *J Psychosom Obstet Gynecol* 1986; 5: 39–49.
3. Coppen A, Kessel N. Menstruation and personality. *Br J Psychiatry* 1963; 109: 711–21.
4. Berga SL. Understanding premenstrual syndrome. *Lancet* 1998; 351: 465–6.
5. Brown J, O'Brien PMS, Marjoribanks J, Wyatt KM. Selective serotonin reuptake inhibitors for premenstrual syndrome. *Cochrane Database Syst Rev* 2009; (2): CD001396.
6. West CP. The characteristics of 100 women presenting to a gynaecological clinic with premenstrual complaints. *Acta Obstet Gynaecol Scand* 1990; 68: 743–7.
7. Warner P, Bancroft J. Factors related to self reporting of the premenstrual syndrome. *Br J Psychiatry* 1990; 157: 249–60.
8. Royal College of Obstetricians and Gynaecologists. The management of premenstrual syndrome. Green-Top Guideline No. 48. London: RCOG, 2007.
9. Steiner M, Streiner DL, Steinberg S et al. The measurement of premenstrual mood symptoms. *J Affect Disord* 1999; 53: 269–73.
10. Stevinson C, Ernst E. Complementary/alternative therapies for premenstrual syndrome: A systematic review of randomized controlled trials. *Am J Obstet Gynecol* 2001; 185: 227–35.
11. Carter J, Verhoef MJ. Efficacy of self-help and alternative treatments of premenstrual syndrome. *Women's Health Issues* 1994; 4: 130–7.
12. Wyatt KM, Dimmock PW, Jones PW et al. Efficacy of vitamin B6 in the treatment of premenstrual syndrome: Systematic review. *BMJ* 1999; 318: 1375–81.
13. Budeiri D, Li Wan Po A, Dornan JC. Is evening primrose oil of value in the treatment of premenstrual syndrome? *Control Clin Trials* 1996; 17: 60–8.
14. Altshuler LL, Cohen LS, Moline ML et al. The Expert Consensus Panel for Depression in Women. The Expert Consensus Guideline Series. Treatment of depression in women. *Postgrad Med* 2001; **March**: 1–107.
15. Schellenberg R. Treatment for the premenstrual syndrome with agnus castus fruit extract: Prospective, randomised, placebo controlled study. *BMJ* 2001; 322: 134–7.
16. Jing Z, Yang X, Ismail KMK et al. Chinese herbal medicine for premenstrual syndrome. *Cochrane Database Syst Rev* 2009; (1): CD006414.
17. Hunter MS, Ussher JM, Browne SJ et al. A randomized comparison of psychological (cognitive behaviour therapy), medical (fluoxetine) and combined therapy for women with premenstrual dysphoric disorder. *J Psychom Obstet Gynecol* 2002; 23: 193–9.
18. Blake F, Salkovskis P, Gath D et al. Cognitive therapy for premenstrual syndrome: A controlled trial. *J Psychosom Res* 1998; 45: 307–18.
19. Taylor D. Effectiveness of professional-peer group treatment: Symptom management for women with PMS. *Res Nurs Health* 1999; 22: 496–511.
20. Bjorn I, Bixo M, Nojd KS et al. Negative mood changes during hormone replacement therapy: A comparison between two progestogens. *Am J Obstet Gynecol* 2000; 183: 1419–26.
21. Wyatt K, Dimmock P, Jones P et al. Efficacy of progesterone and progestogens in management of premenstrual syndrome: Systematic review. *BMJ* 2001; 323: 776–80.
22. Hammarback S, Ekholm UB, Backstrom T. Spontaneous anovulation causing disappearance of cyclical symptoms in women with the premenstrual syndrome. *Acta Endocrinol (Copenh)* 1991; 125: 132–7.
23. Backstrom T, Hansson-Malmstrom Y, Lindhe BA et al. Oral contraceptives in premenstrual syndrome: A randomized comparison of triphasic and monophasic preparations. *Contraception* 1992; 46: 253–68.
24. Serfaty D, Vree ML. A comparison of the cycle control and tolerability of two ultra low-dose oral contraceptives containing 20 micrograms ethinyloestradiol and either 150 micrograms desogestrel or 75 micrograms gestodene. *Eur J Contracep Reprod Health Care* 1998; 3: 179–89.
25. Bancroft J, Rennie D. The impact of oral contraceptives on the experience of perimenstrual mood, clumsiness, food craving and other symptoms. *J Psychosom Res* 1993; 37: 195–202.

26. Lopez LM, Kaptein AA, Helmerhorst FM. Oral contraceptives containing drospirenone for premenstrual syndrome. *Cochrane Database Syst Rev* 2009; (**2**): CD006586.

27. Smith RN, Studd JW, Zamblera D, Holland EF. A randomised comparison over 8 months of 100 micrograms and 200 micrograms twice weekly doses of transdermal oestradiol in the treatment of severe premenstrual syndrome. *Br J Obstet Gynaecol* 1995; **102**: 475–84.

28. Hahn PM, Van Vugt DA, Reid RL. A randomized, placebo-controlled, crossover trial of danazol for the treatment of premenstrual syndrome. *Psychoneuroendocrinology* 1995; **20**: 193–209.

29. Wyatt KM, Dimmock PW, Ismail KMK *et al.* The effectiveness of GnRHa with and without 'add-back' therapy in treating premenstrual syndrome: A meta analysis. *Br J Obstet Gynaecol* 2004; **111**: 585–93.

30. Freeman EW, Sondheimer SJ, Rickels K. Gonadotropin-releasing hormone agonist in the treatment of premenstrual symptoms with and without ongoing dysphoria; a controlled study. *Psychopharmacol Bull* 1997; **33**: 303–9.

31. Casson P, Hahn PM, Van Vugt DA, Reid RL. Lasting response to ovariectomy in severe intractable premenstrual syndrome. *Am J Obstet Gynecol* 1990; **162**: 99–105.

32. Casper RF, Hearn MT. The effect of hysterectomy and bilateral oophorectomy in women with severe premenstrual syndrome. *Am J Obstet Gynecol* 1990; **162**: 105–9.

33. Argent V, Woodward Z. Consent and the ovary. *Obstet Gynecol* 2001; **3**: 206–10.

34. Pinion SB, Parkin DE, Abramovich DR *et al.* Randomised trial of hysterectomy, endometrial laser ablation, and transcervical endometrial resection for dysfunctional uterine bleeding. *Lancet* 1994; **309**: 979–83.

35. Freeman EW, Sondheimer SJ, Polansky M, Garcia-Espagna B. Predictors of response to sertraline treatment of severe premenstrual syndromes. *J Clin Psychiatry* 2000; **61**: 579–84.

# 52.1 Normal conception

*Yakoub Khalaf*

## INTRODUCTION

The fusion of the male and female gametes is the core event in reproduction. The genetic material in the two haploid gametes combines to produce a diploid zygote. In mammals, the fusion of the gametes occurs within the female reproductive tract, and is followed by implantation and the development of the fetus in the uterus. Gametes are produced in the gonads, which also have endocrine functions that are essential for successful reproduction. It is important to explore the embryology, anatomy and some physiological aspects of the ovary and testis in order to understand conception and infertility.

## THE OVARY AND FEMALE GAMETE

The functions of the ovary are to engineer the periodic release of gametes (oocytes) and to produce steroid and glycoprotein hormones. Both functions are integrated in the continuous process of growth and maturation of the Gräafian follicle, containing the oocyte, followed by ovulation and formation of the corpus luteum, which then regresses if pregnancy does not occur. The ovary is a heterogeneous, ever-changing organ whose cyclicity is measured in weeks. The human ovary consists of three major components:

1 the outer cortex, the outer part of which is the tunica albugenia, and the internal part consists of primordial follicles embedded in stromal tissue;
2 the inner medulla;
3 the rete ovarii (hilum), which is attached to the mesovarium and contains nerves, blood vessels and hilar cells, which have the potential to become active in steroidogenesis. The hilar cells are similar to the testosterone-producing Leydig cells of the testes.

The embryonic development of the ovary passes through four stages.

1 *The indifferent gonadal stage.* This stage lasts about 7–10 days and starts at approximately 5 weeks gestation. It starts with the development of the gonadal ridges, which consist of consolidated coelomic projections overlying the mesonephros. At this stage, the ridges are indistinguishable as testes or ovaries. The gonadal ridge is the only site where the germ cells (the direct precursors of the sperm and oocytes) can survive. By the sixth week, the indifferent stage is completed, leaving the indifferent gonads consisting of germ cells and supporting cells derived from the coelomic epithelium and the mesenchyme of the gonadal ridge.
2 *The stage of differentiation.* This occurs at 6–9 weeks if the gonad is destined to be a testis.
3 *The stage of oogonial multiplication and maturation.* This starts at 6–8 weeks and represents the first sign of ovarian differentiation. A rapid mitotic division of the germ cells takes place, giving rise to the oogonia, and by 10–12 weeks the number of oogonia reaches 6–7 million. This is the

maximal oogonial content of the gonads. From this point onwards, the germ cell content will irretrievably decrease and will be exhausted approximately 50 years later. The germ cells undergo mitosis to produce the oogonia that enter the first meiotic division and arrest in the prophase to become oocytes. This process begins at 11–12 weeks, perhaps in response to a factor or factors produced by the rete ovarii.[1] Progression of meiotic prophase to the diplotene stage takes place throughout the rest of the intrauterine life. The completion of the first meiotic division occurs just before ovulation, and the second meiotic division takes place at sperm penetration. As a result of the two meiotic divisions, a single haploid ovum is produced and the excess genetic material is extruded as one polar body at the completion of each meiotic division.

There is a continuous loss of germ cells during all these events, as a result of several mechanisms: (1) follicular growth, atresia and regression during meiosis; (2) the follicles, which fail to become enveloped by granulosa cells, undergo atresia; (3) some germ cells migrate to the surface of the gonads and become incorporated into the surface epithelium or become eliminated into the peritoneal cavity. Once all the oocytes are incorporated into follicles (shortly after birth), the loss of oocytes will only take place as a result of follicular growth and atresia.

4  *The stage of follicular formation.* This starts at 14–20 weeks, when the entire follicle undergoes various stages of maturation leading to the production of the primary follicle before atresia takes place. However, ovulation does not occur in the fetal ovary.

At the onset of puberty, the germ cell mass, incorporated into primordial follicles, is usually reduced to approximately 300 000 follicles. These regularly undergo various stages of maturation, development and atresia. In all, less than 0.1 per cent of follicles will grow beyond the pre-antral stage and develop into a dominant follicle, which ovulates. This enormous attrition of primordial follicles forms part of the process of natural selection, by which only a tiny number of randomly selected germ cells pass through the reproductive cycle and form a new individual.

As the dominant follicle grows, it produces oestrogens, predominantly oestradiol, and inhibins, predominantly inhibin B. These hormones synchronize the development of the endometrial lining of the uterus with that of the follicle, and prepare the pituitary for eventual triggering of the luteinizing hormone (LH) surge. Once oestradiol production from the dominant follicle passes a threshold, a positive feedback is triggered at the pituitary and the LH surge occurs, leading to ovulation. Ovulation results in the physical release of the oocyte, allowing it to enter the Fallopian tube, with potential for fertilization. The follicle then becomes blood filled and develops into the corpus luteum, the source of progesterone and inhibin A in the second half (luteal phase) of the cycle. Production of the sex steroids by the corpus luteum results in preparation of the uterus and the entire woman's body for the occurrence of conception. For this regular periodic process to occur, accurate communication between the ovary and the pituitary gland is essential.

## THE TESTIS AND MALE GAMETE

The physiological responsibilities of the testis are, in principle, similar to those of the ovary, i.e. the production of gametes (spermatozoa) and sex steroids (testosterone). However, sex steroid production in the male is a continuous, non-episodic process, which is independent of the development of gametes. The early embryonic stages of testicular development also follow those of the ovary, starting from the indifferent gonad stage. However, at 6–7 weeks of embryonic life of the male fetus, the production of testes-determining factor (TDF) results in differentiation of the gonads to testes. TDF is the product of a gene located on the Y chromosome. However, the male phenotype is dependent on the production of anti-Müllerian hormone and testosterone. The absence of these two factors leads to the development of the female phenotype. Differentiation of the testis leads to the production of the spermatic cords, which include the Sertoli cells and primordial germ cells that later become the spermatogonia. The mature Sertoli cells produce androgen-binding protein and inhibin B. The former is responsible for maintaining the high local androgen environment necessary for spermatogenesis. The Leydig cells develop from the mesenchymal cells surrounding the spermatic cords. They produce testosterone, the secretion of which increases with the increase in the number of Leydig cells. The Leydig cell number reaches a peak at 15–18 weeks, after which they regress, leaving a few cells present at birth. These cells become responsive to gonadotrophins at puberty, leading to the production of testosterone and the initiation of spermatogenesis. The spermatogonia divide mitotically to produce primary spermatocytes, which then divide meiotically to produce the haploid secondary spermatocytes. Secondary spermatocytes undergo a maturation process to produce the spermatid, then the mature spermatozoon.

The Sertoli cells influence the process of spermatogenesis and are directed by genes on the Y chromosome. Approximately 74 days are required to produce a mature spermatozoon, of which about 50 days are spent in the seminiferous tubules. After leaving the testicle, the sperm takes 12–21 days to travel to the epididymis and appear in the ejaculate.

## FOLLICULAR DEVELOPMENT, MATURATION AND OVULATION

### Follicular development

This involves several stages, starting with the mobilization of the dormant primordial follicles to form a cohort of growing follicles, which progress through the pre-antral,

antral, and pre-ovulatory stages to produce (usually) one dominant follicle that reaches ovulation. The mechanism determining which primordial follicles and how many will be released into the pool of growing follicles in each menstrual cycle is not known. However, this may be regulated by an intra-ovarian mechanism. The number of primordial follicles released from quiescence to enter the pool of growing follicles each cycle seems to be proportional to the size of the residual pool. Therefore, the reduction of the primordial follicle pool by total or partial unilateral oophorectomy, or towards the end of reproductive life, may result in a smaller cohort of growing follicles. The onset and the time span of folliculogenesis have been controversial. Mais *et al.*[2] suggested that the follicle destined to ovulate is recruited in the first few days of the cycle, whereas Gougeon[3] suggested that such a process occurs over a time span of several cycles, estimated to be 85 days to achieve a pre-ovulatory status. The initiation of follicular growth in the early stages is independent of pituitary control; however, without a rise in follicle-stimulating hormone (FSH), these follicles are destined for atresia.

Soon after the initial resumption of maturation, the follicle develops FSH receptors and becomes capable of responding to circulating FSH. This is known as the pre-antral stage, which starts to occur towards the end of the luteal phase of the preceding cycle. FSH, aided by other autocrine/paracrine factors, initiates steroidogenesis and granulosa cell proliferation, and is also responsible for upregulation and downregulation of its own receptors. Therefore, the fate of each pre-antral follicle in the developing pool depends on its ability to convert an androgen microenvironment to an oestrogen microenvironment. This requires the development of aromatase within the granulosa cells that line the follicle. Once one follicle acquires sufficient aromatase to produce and secrete significant quantities of oestradiol, the remainder of the cohort stop growing and gradually become atretic.

The granulosa cell layer is separated from the stromal cells by a basement membrane called the basal lamina (lamina basalis). The surrounding stromal cells differentiate into concentric layers designated as the theca interna (closest to the basal lamina) and the theca externa (the outer portion). As the follicle develops, the theca cells develop LH receptors, leading to LH-stimulated production of androgens, which form the substrate for the production of oestrogen in the granulosa cell layer.

Under the influence of FSH and as the follicles grow, intrafollicular fluid secretion increases, to form a cavitated antral follicle. The intrafollicular fluid contains oestrogens and a variety of peptide growth factors, which provide the oocytes and the surrounding granulosa cells with an endocrine-rich environment essential for maturation and eventually ovulation.

## The selection of a dominant follicle

In primates and humans, usually one follicle proceeds to ovulation and the rest of the cohort is destined for atresia. Oestradiol and inhibin B are produced in increasing amounts by the rapidly growing lead follicle in the cohort. These hormones exert a negative feedback on the pituitary, leading to a decrease in the circulating level of FSH. This in turn withdraws gonadotrophic support from the less developed follicles, but is sufficient for the continued growth of the most advanced follicle, which contains the highest number of FSH receptors. In the antral stage, the dominant follicle maintains the production of oestradiol and inhibin B, which further reduces the FSH level and seals the fate of the other less developed follicles in the cohort. The accumulation of a greater mass of granulosa cells is accompanied by advanced development of the thecal vasculature, which facilitates preferential delivery of gonadotrophins to the follicles, allowing the dominant follicle to maintain FSH responsiveness and continue to develop and function despite the decreasing levels of FSH.

In the pre-ovulatory stage, the granulosa cells enlarge, the theca cells become vacuolated and richly vascular, the oocyte resumes meiosis, and the oestradiol level continues to rise, reaching a peak approximately 24–36 hours prior to ovulation.[4]

## Ovulation

The continuous production of oestradiol by the growing follicle leads to the surge in LH through a positive-feedback mechanism. The LH surge usually lasts 48–50 hours. Ovulation (follicular rupture and oocyte release) occurs 24–36 hours after the LH surge. The LH surge leads to several events essential for oocyte maturation and preparation of the endometrium for implantation. The oocyte resumes its first meiotic division, leading to the production and extrusion of the first polar body, and enters the second meiotic division, which will be completed on fusion of the sperm with the oocyte later on. This stage is essential for the oocyte to be fertilized by the sperm. Stimulation of the granulosa cells by LH leads to the production of progesterone necessary for converting the endometrium from the proliferative to the secretory phase. Furthermore, progesterone enhances the activity of proteolytic enzymes and prostaglandins to digest the follicular wall, leading to the rupture of the follicle and the release of the oocyte.

## Fertilization

The oocyte released at the time of ovulation is surrounded by granulosa cells known as the cumulus oophorus, which is separated from the actual oocyte by a layer of glycoprotein known as the zona pellucida. Within 2–3 minutes of ovulation, the oocyte (surrounded by the cumulus) is within the ampullary part of the Fallopian tube. The fertilizable life span of the human ovum is estimated to be 24–36 hours. Although several million sperm are deposited in the vagina, only about 200 will come in contact with the oocyte. For the sperm to bind with the zona pellucida, a receptor is required, which is species specific. The sperm has to undergo a process known as 'capacitation' in order to be able to bind with the receptor and penetrate the egg. The zona pellucida not only contains the receptors for the sperm, but also has a mechanism by which it prevents more than one sperm from entering the oocyte (polyspermy). This mechanism is known as the zona reaction.

## IMPLANTATION

This is defined as the process by which the embryo attaches itself to the endometrial side of the uterine wall and gradually penetrates the epithelium to reach the circulatory system of the mother. This process requires preparation of both the endometrium and the embryo for a successful implantation to take place.

### Embryo preparation

For the first post-fertilization week, the embryo prepares for implantation while dividing. Sufficient cell division needs to take place to produce the inner cell mass essential for the formation of the blastocyst. The embryo usually reaches the blastocyst stage by day 5 post-fertilization, with a prominent inner cell mass and trophoectoderm. The two structures expand and hatch through the zona pellucida from day 7 onwards. The hatched blastocyst is capable of producing human chorionic gonadotrophin (hCG), which acts on the corpus luteum to maintain the production of progesterone and oestradiol. This prevents the onset of menstruation and allows the early pregnancy to continue. At the time of hatching, the trophoblast cells begin to differentiate into cytotrophoblasts and syncytiotrophoblasts. The expression of adhesion molecules in the trophoblast may be responsible for the initial attachment of embryo to the uterus. The embryo gradually develops its self-regulatory paracrine system and establishes a communication system with the endometrium. This leads to interaction with the uterine epithelium and decidua during apposition and invasion by the trophoblast.

### Endometrial preparation

After ovulation, oestradiol and progesterone from the corpus luteum alter the molecular structure of the endometrium from proliferative to secretory. The individual components of the endometrium continue to grow, leading to tortuosity of the glands and coiling of the spiral arterioles. Intracytoplasmic glycogen vacuoles appear and transudation of plasma occurs, contributing to endometrial secretion. The peak secretory phase is reached by 7 days post-ovulation. At this point, the endometrial cells are rich in glycogen and

lipids. The receptivity of the endometrium is limited to days 16–19 (of a 28-day cycle), and it is essential that the hatched blastocyst impacts and adheres to the surface of the endometrium during this 'implantation window' if pregnancy is to occur.

## ACKNOWLEDGEMENT

This chapter has been revised and updated. The author and editors acknowledge the contribution of Hany AMA Lashen to the chapter on this topic in the previous edition of the book.

### KEY POINTS

- At the onset of puberty, the size of the primordial follicles pool is approximately 300 000 follicles.
- Once oestradiol production from the dominant follicle passes a threshold, a positive feedback is triggered at the pituitary and the LH surge occurs, leading to ovulation.
- The oestradiol level continues to rise, reaching a peak leading to the LH surge, which is followed 24–36 hours later by ovulation.
- The fertilization life span of the released ovum is 24–36 hours.
- The zona pellucida precludes more than one sperm entering the oocyte through a mechanism known as the zona reaction.
- The embryo usually reaches the blastocyst stage by day 5 post-fertilization with a prominent inner cell mass and trophectoderm.

### Key References

1. Gondos B, Westergaard L, Byskov A. Inhibition of oogenesis in the human fetal ovary: ultrasound structural and squash preparation study. *Am J Obstet Gynecol* 1986; **155**: 189–95.
2. Mais V, Kazer RR, Cetel NS *et al.* The dependence of folliculogenesis and corpus luteum function on pulsatile gonadotrophin secretion in cycling women using a gonadotrophin-releasing hormone antagonist as a probe. *J Clin Endocrinol Metab* 1986; **62**: 1250–55.
3. Gougeon A. Dynamics of follicular growth in the human: a model from preliminary results. *Hum Reprod* 1986; **1**: 81–7.
4. Pauerstein CJ, Eddy CA, Croxatto HD *et al.* Temporal relationships of oestrogen, progesterone, and luteinizing hormone levels to ovulation in women and infrahuman primates. *Am J Obstet Gynecol* 1978; **130**: 876–86.

# 52.2 Female infertility

*Yakoub Khalaf*

## INTRODUCTION

Infertility is defined as the inability to conceive despite regular unprotected sexual intercourse over a specific period of time, usually 1–2 years. The cumulative spontaneous pregnancy rate for a couple is approximately 57 per cent after three months, 72 per cent after six months, 85 per cent after one year and 93 per cent after two years [D].[1] Accordingly, only 50 per cent of couples failing to conceive during the first year will conceive in the second year, which justifies starting investigations for infertility after one year. However, if the physician or the patient has a reason to suspect impaired fertility, the process should be started sooner. Furthermore, if the female partner is 35 years of age or older, the investigations should not be delayed, given the rapid decline of female fecundity after this age. Over the past three decades the introduction of *in-vitro* fertilization (IVF) and the wide public interest in this aspect of infertility treatment, together with the increasing ease of obtaining information, have increased patients' expectations of infertility treatment.

## EPIDEMIOLOGY

It has been estimated that infertility affects 9 per cent of couples, of whom 70 per cent suffer from primary infertility, i.e. no previous conception, and 30 per cent secondary infertility, i.e. have achieved a previous pregnancy (regardless of the outcome of that pregnancy). Worldwide, more than 70 million couples suffer from infertility, the majority being residents of the developing countries. The recent advances in infertility treatment and the access of patients to such information have led to early presentation of these patients and their request for treatment. This may give a false impression of an increasing infertility problem.

## CAUSES OF INFERTILITY

For pregnancy to occur, there must be fertile sperm and egg, a means of bringing them together and a receptive endometrium to allow the resulting embryo to implant. A defect at any of these stages can lead to subfertility. It has been estimated that in 35 per cent of cases a male factor is the reason for infertility [C]. In the remaining 65 per cent of cases, a female factor is identified in 50 per cent of couples and no cause will be identified in the remainder [C]. The most common causes of infertility in the female are ovulatory and tubal factors. Endometriosis in its moderate to severe forms has also been linked to infertility, despite a lack of clear understanding of the connection between the two phenomena [C]. Although failure of implantation will cause infertility, it is difficult to determine whether the embryo or the endometrium is at fault in such cases. The effect of age on female fertility is not a new concept, with a gradual decline in female fertility and an increase in the miscarriage rate being observed many years before the menopause [D]. As discussed earlier, women enter the reproductive age at puberty with a pool of primordial follicles of a pre-determined number. The size of this pool and the rate of follicular depletion are the deciding factors in the timing of the menopause. Female fertility declines after the age of 35 and declines more rapidly after the age of 40 [C]. The rate of follicular loss is inversely proportional to the size of the primordial pool, i.e. the smaller the pool, the faster the rate. Delaying starting a family to the later years of reproductive life also increases the risk of developing endometriosis and the risk of miscarriage.

## Anovulatory infertility

Anovulation is a frequent cause of infertility. Negative-feedback and positive-feedback mechanisms allow the ovaries to interact successfully with the hypothalamo–pituitary axis. The causes of anovulation can be classified according to the clinical findings when the level of disruption between the hypothalamic–pituitary axis and the ovary is assessed. This divides the causes of anovulartory infertility into three main categories – ovulatory dysfunction, hypogonadotrophic hypogonadism and hypergonadotrophic hypogonadism, with other less common causes considered separately.

### Ovarian dysfunction

The most common presentation of anovulation is associated with normal gonadotrophin concentrations. Such normogonadotrophic anovulation is usually seen in polycystic ovary syndrome (PCOS). Polycystic ovary syndrome is the most common endocrine disorder in women of reproductive age. In its classic form – a combination of oligomenorrhoea/anovulation and hyperandrogenism – it is estimated to affect >5 per cent of the female population. Polycystic ovary syndrome is also associated with a metabolic disturbance, central to which is peripheral insulin resistance and compensatory hyperinsulinaemia. Significant abnormalities in the very earliest stages of folliculogenesis may be the root cause of anovulation in PCOS.

### Hypogonadotrophic hypogonadism

Failure of the pituitary gland to produce gonadotrophins will lead to lack of ovarian stimulation. There are a number of disorders of the anterior pituitary gland that lead to failure of production of FSH. These include destruction of the anterior pituitary by a tumour (e.g. a benign non-functioning adenoma or craniopharyngioma), by a pituitary inflammatory reaction as in tuberculosis or following ischaemia as in Sheehan's syndrome. Rare congenital causes include Laurence–Moon–Biedl, Kallmann's and Prader–Willi syndromes. The pituitary can also be damaged by cranial irradiation or surgically at the time of hypophysectomy for a pituitary tumour.

Hypogonadotrophic hypogonadism will also occur if pulsatile secretion of gonadotrophin-releasing hormone (GnRH) is slowed or stopped. This is seen in hypothalamic dysfunction, commonly secondary to excessive exercise, psychological stress or anorexia nervosa.

### Hypergonadotrophic hypogonadism

This occurs as a result of failure of the ovary to respond to gonadotrophic stimulation by the pituitary gland. The absence of negative feedback (by oestradiol and inhibin B) from a developing follicle results in excessive secretion of the gonadotrophic hormones, follicle-stimulating hormone (FSH) and luteinizing hormone (LH). Concentrations of these hormones reach menopausal levels. Hypergonadotrophic hypogonadism classically results from premature ovarian failure with exhaustion of the ovarian follicle pool. A variant of the condition, resistant ovary syndrome, describes the occurrence of elevated levels of serum gonadotrophins in the presence of a good reserve of follicles. Abnormalities in the FSH receptor may produce this picture. Neither premature ovarian failure nor resistant ovary syndrome is treatable by injection of FSH.

### Other discrete causes

Endocrine disorders, most commonly hyperprolactinaemia and hypothyroidism, are possible causes of anovulation and should be excluded by appropriate biochemical testing.

## Tubal infertility

Tubal damage underlies infertility in approximately 14 per cent of couples and 40 per cent of infertile women [C]. Any damage to the Fallopian tube can prevent the sperm from reaching the oocyte or the embryo from reaching the uterine cavity, leading to infertility and tubal ectopic pregnancy, respectively. The Fallopian tube is more than just a 'tube': a number of key events occur within the tube, including capacitation of the sperm, fertilization and the early development of the zygote and embryo. Therefore, the Fallopian tube may maintain its patency but lose the ability to promote these other functions. Currently accepted investigations can only test tubal patency.

The main causes of tubal damage are either pelvic inflammatory disease (PID) or iatrogenic causes. Pelvic inflammatory disease remains the major cause of tubal damage in the western world, with *Chlamydia trachomatis* infection the prime pathogen in most cases. Pelvic infection or abscess caused by appendicitis, other bowel disorders or septic abortion is responsible for a lesser proportion of cases. Fallopian tubes can be damaged iatrogenically either directly, as in tubal ligation for sterilization, or indirectly as a consequence of pelvic surgery. Other rare causes of tubal damage include tuberculosis, schistosomiasis, viral infection and abdominal inflammatory disorders, such as Crohn's disease.

## Endometriosis

It is apparent that severe endometriosis can lead to mechanical tubal damage due to adhesion formation caused by the pelvic endometrial deposits. However, it is less certain whether the lesser degrees of endometriosis can lead to infertility. Both mild endometriosis and infertility are common, and may occur together as epiphenomena [C]. Endometriosis is discussed further in Chapter 51.5, Endometriosis and gonadotrophin-releasing hormone analogues.

## Uterine factors

Submucous leiomyomata, congenital uterine abnormalities, endometrial polyps and intrauterine adhesions are all potential causes of infertility. The presence of a fibroid that occludes or distorts the Fallopian tubes will lead to tubal infertility [D]. Fertility outcomes are decreased in women with submucosal fibroids, and removal seems to confer benefit. Subserosal fibroids do not affect fertility outcomes, and removal does not confer benefit. Intramural fibroids appear to decrease fertility, but the results of therapy are unclear. Distortion of the uterine cavity, by a fibroid, a septum or in the T-shaped uterus following exposure of the female fetus to diethystilbestrol *in utero*, can lead to implantation failure and recurrent early miscarriage [D]. Such cases should be assessed individually and the likelihood of their contribution to infertility should be examined. Excessive uterine curettage after a miscarriage or abortion, especially in the presence of uterine infection, can lead to the destruction of the strata basalis endometrium. Intrauterine scarring and synechiae develop as a result, which is known as Asherman's syndrome. This condition can also result after caesarean section, uteroplasty or myomectomy.

It has been difficult to demonstrate a relationship between endometritis and subfertility, except when the cause of endometritis is tuberculosis. In the UK, tuberculous endometritis is a rare, but increasing, cause of infertility. The effect of chlamydial endometritis on implantation remains controversial, although there is evidence that patients with tubal disease undergoing IVF have significantly lower pregnancy and implantation rates.

## Unexplained infertility

Completion of standard investigation of infertility fails to reveal a cause in 15–30 per cent of cases [C]. This does not indicate absence of a cause, but rather the inability to identify it. The results of IVF have shown that there may be undiagnosed problems of oocyte or embryo quality or of implantation failure, neither of which can easily be tested unless IVF is undertaken. Unexplained infertility causes great distress to couples, who often find it harder to bear when a cause cannot be found.

# INVESTIGATION OF THE FEMALE PARTNER

Investigation of infertility will usually be initiated in general practice, frequently followed by referral to a secondary or tertiary centre, where most treatments will take place. The RCOG and NICE have recently published guidelines for the management of infertility. These define the role of the medical practitioner at each level, and outline the evidence base for investigation and treatment.

## History taking and examination

It is important to recognize that infertility is a problem that faces couples, and that both partners should be seen and investigated together whenever possible [E]. Consultations involving infertility require tact and sensitivity on behalf of the clinician, a quiet, private environment and sufficient clinical time to allow exploration of the couple's anxieties and explanation of available treatments, as well as classical history taking. A rapport must be established before more personal and sensitive details can be sought.

### Personal and social history

The couple's age, in particular that of the female partner, is important, as discussed earlier. The occupation of the couple, especially the male, can have an impact on their fertility. Exposure to high temperature, chemicals and ionizing radiation can seriously affect sperm production [D]. If either of the partners works away from home, this may affect the frequency of sexual intercourse around the time of ovulation. Smoking, alcohol and recreational drug use can also influence fertility. Appropriate advice should be given.

### Menstrual history

The age of menarche and regularity of periods are important factors. Information about the frequency and length of the menstrual cycle and any associated problems such as dysmenorrhoea or heavy menstrual loss should be sought. Irregular menstrual cycles, oligomenorrhoea and amenorrhoea are all suggestive of anovulation. If amenorrhoea is reported, enquiries should be made about any menopausal symptoms, weight loss or gain, and symptoms of hyperprolactinaemia and hypothyroidism. These patients should be investigated in specialized centres [E].

## Obstetric history

The clinician should enquire about any previous pregnancies, both in the current and any previous relationships, as well as the outcome of these pregnancies. It may be wise to ask about breastfeeding and any sustained galactorrhoea at this stage. It is also important to establish if there were any difficulties encountered or treatment required prior to achieving a previous pregnancy.

## Contraception

The use of the oral contraceptive pill and the long-acting progestogens can be followed by a period of amenorrhoea. In particular, use of long-acting progestogen-based contraceptives may be followed by delay in the resumption of ovulation [D]. The use of intrauterine contraceptive devices may increase the risk of pelvic infection, especially in young nulliparous women, leading to tubal disease [D].

## Past medical history

It is important to establish any previous medical disorders that may affect either fertility or pregnancy. Pre-conceptional counselling may be necessary if a serious medical condition is identified. The possible impact of prescription medications on ovulation should be investigated: for example, some antidepressants can increase prolactin secretion and non-steroidal anti-inflammatory drugs can interfere with ovulation.

## Sexual history

The clinician should enquire about the couple's frequency of sexual intercourse and associated problems, such as dyspareunia or ejaculatory dysfunction. Regular intercourse (two to three times a week) is sufficient for most couples to achieve a pregnancy. It is frequently the case that infertile couples restrict their sexual activity to the period around mid-cycle and some use commercially available ovulation detection kits to time intercourse. There is no evidence that such practices can increase fecundability, and the increase in psychological stress that results from such practices is unhelpful [C]. Sensitive enquiry concerning sexually transmitted diseases should be made.

## Other important points

The discussion should include advice concerning the use of folic acid and enquiry about rubella vaccination [A]. A cervical smear history should be taken and a smear offered if indicated [E]. A family history, including enquiry concerning diabetes, endometriosis and PCOS, should be taken, as this information can be useful in the diagnosis and treatment of infertility [D]. A history of familial disorder should lead to an offer of genetic counselling before starting investigation and treatment [E].

## Examination of the female partner

Unless there is an indication from the patient's history that examination would be of any value in establishing the cause of infertility, there would seem to be little to be gained from routine examination. Indications from the history, for example of cyclical pelvic pain or dyspareunia, should prompt pelvic examination. Other features of the physical examination, for example detection of an asymptomatic pelvic mass, have been supplanted by transvaginal ultrasound examination.

Assessment of body mass index is important, as both obesity and underweight can cause anovulation [C]. If the patient is found to be obese, central obesity can be assessed by measuring the waist:hip ratio [C].

## Laboratory investigations, endoscopy and imaging

The aim of these investigations is to assess ovulation, tubal patency and uterine factors (Table 52.2.1).

### Ovulation

A history of regular periods usually indicates ovulation. However, a reliable marker is useful to confirm that ovulation has occurred. After the release of the oocyte and the formation of the corpus luteum, progesterone levels rise sharply, reaching a peak level approximately 8 days after the LH surge. The detection of high levels of progesterone in serum or evidence of progesterone effect can be used as a secondary marker of ovulation. Historically, the effects of progesterone on basal body temperature, endometrial histology or cervical mucus were commonly used. Measuring serum progesterone at its peak in the mid-luteal phase is a reliable, safe and inexpensive test. Levels in excess of 30 nmol/L are diagnostic of ovulation [C]; however, lower (suboptimal) levels may be due to incorrect timing of blood sampling or may be caused by a luteinized unruptured follicle. It is important to remember that the mid-luteal phase is approximately 7 days before the next expected period, i.e. day 21 and day 28 in 28-day and 35-day cycles, respectively.

Commercially available urinary LH detection kits can detect the LH surge and can be used to time intercourse with ovulation induction or donor insemination treatments.

### Ovarian reserve tests

Another test added to the investigation of couples with infertility includes assessment of ovarian reserve. Women with advanced age or history of prior ovarian surgery are at risk for diminished ovarian function or reserve. Given the relatively non-invasive nature of the testing, several practitioners are including the evaluation of ovarian reserve as first-line work up for infertility. The testing includes a cycle day 3 serum follicle-stimulating hormone (FSH) and estradiol level, antimüllerian hormone (AMH) or an

**Table 52.2.1** Interpretation of female infertility investigations

| Test | Result | Interpretation |
| --- | --- | --- |
| Progesterone | <30 nmol/L | Anovulation |
| | | Check cycle length and timing in mid-luteal phase |
| | | Complete other endocrine tests |
| | | Scan for PCO |
| | | Advise re. weight gain/loss |
| | | May need ovulation induction |
| | | Clomiphene should not be started without test of tubal patency |
| FSH | >10 IU/L | Reduced ovarian reserve: |
| | | May respond poorly to ovulation induction |
| | | May need egg donation |
| LH | >10 IU/L | May be PCO |
| | | Ultrasound to confirm |
| Testosterone | >2.5 nmol/L | May be PCO |
| | | Need ultrasound to confirm |
| Prolactin | >1000 IU/L | May be pituitary adenoma |
| | | Repeat prolactin to confirm raised level |
| | | Exclude hypothyroidism |
| | | Arrange MRI/CT scan |
| | | If confirmed hyperprolactinaemia, start dopamine agonist |
| HSG/HyCoSy | Abnormal | May be tubal factor |
| | | Arrange laparoscopy and dye to evaluate further |
| | | May be intrauterine abnormality |
| | | Evaluate further by hysteroscopy |
| Lap and dye | Blocked tubes | Tubal factor |
| | | ? suitable for transcervical cannulation, surgery or IVF (also depends on semen quality) |
| | Endometriosis | Endometriosis |
| | | Assess severity, may benefit from diathermy laser |
| | | Medical suppression not helpful for fertility |
| | | May need IVF |
| Rubella | Non-immune | Offer immunization and one month contraception |

ultrasonographic ovarian antral follicle count. However, NICE guidelines recommend that women who have high levels of gonadotrophins should be informed that they are likely to have reduced fertility. The results of these tests are not absolute indicators of infertility but abnormal levels correlate with decreased response to ovulation induction medications and lowered live birth rates after IVF.

## Tubal patency tests

Although the Fallopian tube has functions other than as a conduit for the sperm, oocyte and embryo, it is not yet feasible to assess these functions in routine practice. Tubal patency can be assessed by three different methods: ultrasound scanning with hydrotubation, hysterosalpingography, laparoscopy and dye hydrotubation [D].

## Ultrasound scan and hydrotubation

HyCoSy (**hy**sterosalpingo **co**ntrast **so**nography) has recently been introduced as a method for studying tubal patency using ultrasonography. Ultrasonographic contrast medium is slowly injected into the uterine cavity under direct visualization, with imaging of the cavity and of flow along the Fallopian tubes. This method does not require x-ray and allows the ultrasound assessment of the pelvic organs, i.e. the uterus including the uterine cavity, tubes and ovaries. This screening method should be reserved to cases where history is not suggestive of tubal pathology. Finding a normal cavity and bilateral fill and spill of contrast is reassuring, but where there is doubt, hysterosalpingography or a laparoscopy and dye hydrotubation test should be performed.

## Hysterosalpingography

Hysterosalpingography is a simple, safe and inexpensive x-ray-based contrast study of the uterine cavity and the Fallopian tubes with a 65 per cent sensitivity and 83 per cent specificity for detecting tubal blockage. The principle of this test is to inject a radio-opaque contrast medium through the cervix into the uterus and take abdominal x-rays at intervals during and after the injection. The images should reveal the uterine outline and passage of contrast along the tubes, with free spill into the peritoneal cavity. HSG is usually carried out in the first 10 days of the menstrual cycle, to avoid disruption of an early pregnancy in the secretory phase of the cycle. It will cause period-like pain in most patients and may occasionally lead to a vasovagal attack. The main complication of hysterosalpingography is flare up of PID. The overall risk of infection from this test in the normal population is approximately 1 per cent, rising to 3 per cent in high-risk patients. Therefore, it is wise to carry out laparoscopy and dye test in high-risk patients and to use prophylactic antibiotics to cover the test. The RCOG recommends the routine screening for Chlamydia in any patient before carrying out any intrauterine instrumentation [E]. Hysterosalpingography is recommended by the RCOG as the primary screening procedure in low-risk patients [E].

## Laparoscopy and dye test

A laparoscopy and dye hydrotubation ('lap and dye') test is the most reliable, albeit expensive, tool used to diagnose tubal subfertility. The principle of this procedure is to visualize the passage of methylene blue dye through the Fallopian tubes. The procedure enables inspection of the fimbrial ends of the tubes and the pelvic structures for the presence of endometriosis or adhesions. Combining this procedure with electrocoagulation of any endometriotic spots or adhesiolysis adds therapeutic value. Hence, it is advisable that such procedures are carried out in centres where the necessary expertise is available [E].

Laparoscopy and dye test requires general anaesthetic and carries the risk of bowel or visceral injury. It is therefore not recommended as a first-line screening test [E]. However, it should be considered in patients with a history suggestive of endometriosis, previous PID or previous pelvic surgery. Furthermore, if the hysterosalpingography reports abnormal results, verification should be carried out with diagnostic laparoscopy [E]. To diagnose unexplained infertility, both peritoneal factor and endometriosis should be excluded, even in patients with normal hysterosalpingography, by carrying out laparoscopic examination. When comparing hysterosalpingography with laparoscopy, keep in mind that both procedures provide extra information in addition to the assessment of the Fallopian tubes. Hysterosalpingography provides information about the status of the uterine cavity, whereas laparoscopy allows inspection of the intra-abdominal cavity, excludes peritoneal disease and allows laparoscopic treatment of pelvic pathology.

Visualization and assessment of the uterine cavity are not possible unless hysteroscopy is performed concurrently. However, the value of routine hysteroscopy is questionable [E], as the frequency of asymptomatic intrauterine lesions that are not seen on transvaginal ultrasound is low. Hysteroscopy should probably therefore be reserved for cases where there is an indication from the history or previous investigations.

## Assessment of the uterus

Uterine anatomy can be visualized by saline hysterosonography, hysterosalpingography or hysteroscopy. Conventional transvaginal ultrasound may not always provide a good quality image of the cavity, but 3D ultrasound, when available, can provide an accurate assessment of the uterine cavity. This may outline intrauterine polyps or synechiae. Routine hysteroscopy for infertile patients has been discouraged by the RCOG [E].

## Postcoital test

The postcoital test provides information concerning the ability of the sperm to penetrate and survive in cervical mucus. However, reproducibility of the test is low and the false-positive rate is high. A diagnosis of an adverse cervical factor does not alter therapeutic decisions, as both 'cervical factor' and unexplained infertility are treated with intrauterine insemination or IVF. According to NICE guidelines on the management of infertility, the routine use of post-coital testing in the investigation of fertility problems is not recommended because it has no predictive value on pregnancy rate.

## Management of female infertility

Any discussion about the management of infertility should begin with an explanation of the physiology of the cycle, with information about the 'fertile period'. Among healthy women trying to conceive, nearly all pregnancies can be attributed to intercourse during a 6-day period ending on the day of ovulation.

Lifestyle issues, including advice on smoking, alcohol consumption and 'fitness for pregnancy', should be raised. Further planning of treatment protocols will depend on the presumed cause of the problem.

## Management of tubal infertility

Tubal infertility can be treated with tubal surgery, IVF and embryo transfer (IVF-ET) or selective salpingography.

Reproductive medicine

Although tubal surgery is no longer recommended for severe tubal disease since the introduction of IVF-ET, it still has a place in less severe forms of the disorder.

## Tubal surgery

Successful tubal surgery requires surgical skill and experience. The decline in the number of suitable cases has reduced training opportunities, and some advocate restriction of this practice to tertiary centres to allow concentration of expertise [E]. This permits audit of outcome and estimation of realistic, single-centre pregnancy rates. Comparison between tubal surgery and IVF is difficult. The cost, success rate, complications and benefits must be assessed in every case individually. Decision-making may be altered in favour of IVF by the presence of other causes of infertility, particularly male factor and anovulation. The success rate after tubal surgery depends on the underlying disease, site of damage (proximal or distal) and patient's age. NICE guidelines have suggested that for women with mild tubal disease, tubal surgery may be more effective than no treatment. In centres where appropriate expertise is available, it may be considered as a treatment option.

The cost of a single cycle of IVF has been calculated to be comparable to that of tubal surgery, and apart from patients with mild tubal disease, the cost-effectiveness argument is in favour of IVF-ET. However, tubal surgery, if successful, offers less risk of multiple pregnancy and ovarian hyperstimulation syndrome (OHSS), and avoids the ethical issues that fertilization in vitro can engender. Patients should be informed that the risk of ectopic pregnancy after tubal surgery is significantly higher than after IVF-ET [C].

Once tubal surgery is being contemplated, careful assessment of the tubes and pelvis with hysterosalpingography and laparoscopy should be carried out [E]. The route of access should then be decided, i.e. laparotomy or laparoscopy. Laparoscopic surgery is less costly and offers less morbidity, more technical advantages and a marginally better pregnancy rate. If pregnancy does not occur within 6–12 months of tubal surgery, reassessment of the tubes with hysterosalpingography should be carried out. If the tubes remain blocked, IVF-ET is indicated. If the tubes remain patent, ovulation should be assessed and perhaps a short period of ovulation induction could be tried. This decision will depend on the patient's age and whether IVF-ET is affordable to the couple. The key issues here are to present the couple with all the available facts and to involve them in the decision-making process.

## IVF-ET

Absent or irreparably damaged Fallopian tubes were the main reason for the development of IVF-ET. A lower pregnancy rate after IVF-ET in tubal infertility couples compared to other causes of infertility has been reported. The reason is not entirely clear, but it is possible that fluid from a hydrosalpinx could be hostile to embryo development and implantation. Salpingectomy of an ultrasonographically visible hydrosalpinx should therefore be considered to improve the success rate of IVF treatment [C], although careful counselling is needed before performing salpingectomy for an infertile patient, even if the tubal damage is severe [E].

## Selective salpingography and tubal cannulation

These procedures can be carried out under image intensification or at hysteroscopy. These methods were originally developed for diagnostic purposes, but were subsequently proven to be useful in treating proximal tubal damage, for which surgery yielded disappointing success rates. The outcome of these procedures in terms of regaining tubal patency is immediately known. According to NICE guidelines, for women with proximal tubal obstruction, selective salpingography plus tubal catheterization, or hysteroscopic tubal cannulation, may be treatment options because these treatments improve the chance of pregnancy.

## Management of anovulatory infertility

A number of therapeutic interventions for the induction of ovulation are available. Selecting the most appropriate method depends on the cause of anovulation. Patients with ovarian failure and resistant ovary syndrome will not respond to ovulation induction and should be offered oocyte donation [C]. Normalization of body weight in underweight and obese patients can help to regain ovulation without the need for medical intervention [B]. Medical treatment of prolactinoma can also help regain normal ovulation [A]. Ovulation induction in patients with hypogonadotrophic hypogonadism can be achieved with the pulsatile administration of GnRH or by daily injection of gonadotrophin [C]. Ovulation induction in PCOS patients (80 per cent of anovular women) can be achieved by weight normalization in obese patients [C] (40–60 per cent of PCOS patients), medical or surgical methods. The medical methods include the use of clomiphene citrate or gonadotrophins – discussed further in Chapter 52.4, Assisted reproduction. NICE has recommended that women with World Health Organization group II ovulation disorders (hypothalamic pituitary dysfunction), such as PCOS, should be offered treatment with clomifene citrate (or tamoxifen) as the first line of treatment for up to 12 months because it is likely to induce ovulation [A]. Additionally, women undergoing treatment with clomifene citrate should be offered ultrasound monitoring during at least the first cycle of treatment to ensure that they receive a dose that minimizes the risk of multiple pregnancy.

The surgical methods are either ovarian drilling or wedge resection. Stein and Leventhal suggested ovarian wedge resection in 1935. Their theory was that the thick tunica albugenia prevented the release of the ovum, hence the anovulation in PCOS patients. Although pregnancies resulted, the operation (performed by laparotomy) led to complications, including tubal damage and adhesion formation, and fell into disrepute. Ovarian drilling involves focal local destruction of the ovarian stroma with laser or diathermy, applied laparoscopically. The route of access reduces morbidity and post-operative complications. Ovarian drilling achieves equivalent ovulation and pregnancy rates to medical ovulation induction. Predictors of success have included LH level >10 IU/L, normal BMI and shorter duration of infertility. However, evidence suggests that ovarian drilling has less risk of multiple pregnancies and no risk of OHSS. Economic analyses of two RCTs suggest that treating women with CC-resistant PCOS by LOS resulted in reduced direct and indirect costs. On the other hand, the long-term advantages and risks of ovarian drilling require further assessment. Destroying ovarian tissue inevitably leads to destruction of primordial follicles and reduction of the ovarian reserve. These anxieties have partially been resolved by studies that demonstrate that a good therapeutic response can be achieved by minimal application of energy and after reduction of the number of diathermy burns to 4 per ovary.

## Management of endometriosis-related infertility

This depends on the severity of the condition and the presence of any other infertility factors. The two main lines of treating endometriosis are medical and surgical. Medical treatment of minimal and mild endometriosis does not enhance fertility in infertile women and should not be offered [A].

Women with minimal or mild endometriosis who undergo laparoscopy should be offered surgical ablation or resection of endometriosis plus laparoscopic adhesiolysis because this improves the chance of pregnancy [A].

As many infertile patients will undergo diagnostic laparoscopy, diathermy to endometriosis can be delivered at the same session, alleviating the need for a further anaesthetic. Women with moderate or severe endometriosis should be offered surgical treatment because it improves the chance of pregnancy [B]. Assisted reproduction has lent itself to treating endometriosis-related infertility. Whether medical or conservative surgical treatment of endometriosis before carrying out IVF-ET can improve the ovarian response and pregnancy rates remains unclear.

## Management of unexplained infertility

The lack of an identifiable reason for infertility in this category makes the treatment empirical. Conservative management, ovulation induction with or without intrauterine insemination, and IVF-ET are the main approaches to managing unexplained infertility. Approximately 60 per cent of couples with unexplained secondary infertility (diagnosed after one year) achieve a pregnancy within three years of conservative management [C]. Results are less good in primary infertility. However, the woman's age should be taken into consideration when advising this line of management. Ovulation induction (or, more properly, 'augmentation') with clomiphene citrate along with timed sexual intercourse has been used frequently in patients with unexplained infertility However, recent meta-analysis of studies in this area has not demonstrated benefit over theconservative approach [A], and treatment with clomiphene citrate carries a risk of multiple pregnancy.

A cumulative pregnancy rate of 40 per cent has been reported after controlled ovarian stimulation (COS) with gonadotrophins and intrauterine insemination (IUI) [C]. The pregnancy rates after IUI alone in couples with unexplained infertility have been disappointing and its use does not appear to confer any additional benefit over expectant management. However, the advantage of IUI over timed sexual intercourse after COS has been controversial, and firm evidence is lacking. For logistic reasons, IUI may provide a better timing compared to sexual intercourse. Many centres advise two or three cycles of COS–IUI before moving to IVF-ET in this group. COS-IUI may be less stressful, less physically demanding and less costly per attempt than IVF.

*In-vitro* fertilization–embryo transfer in unexplained infertility has diagnostic as well as therapeutic value, as it provides information about fertilization and egg and embryo quality. Owing to its high cost, IVF-ET is usually seen as a last resort in unexplained infertility. The cost of three cycles of COS-IUI is comparable to that of one IVF-ET cycle, with the former offering a better pregnancy rate [D].

Gamete intrafallopian transfer (GIFT) used to be the treatment of choice for patients with unexplained infertility. However, IVF-ET, with its diagnostic potential, has superseded this modality. Although GIFT offered a high pregnancy rate, the ectopic pregnancy risk was also high [C], and the treatment requires general anaesthesia and laparoscopy in order for gametes to be placed within the ampulla of the Fallopian tube. This method has largely been supplanted by IVF-ET.

## Management of uterine factor infertility

Congenital defects, leiomyomas and intrauterine adhesions and polyps are the only treatable uterine factors. However, before offering surgical treatment, the impact of such findings on the couple's fertility should be carefully assessed [E]. Myomectomy can be carried out either laparoscopically or by laparotomy with similar post-operative pregnancy rates [A]. Entry into the uterine cavity should be avoided if possible, and adhesion barriers and microsurgical technique should be used to reduce the risk of post-operative adhesions. The risk of a scar rupture during pregnancy is less if the endometrial cavity remains intact at myomectomy [D], although some fibroids cannot be removed without breach of the cavity. Post-operative adhesions can have a detrimental effect on tubal patency.

Submucous fibroids can successfully be resected hysteroscopically, depending on the size of the fibroid and its degree of protrusion into the uterine cavity. The risk of tubal damage with this procedure is minimal, but there is a risk of haemorrhage, uterine perforation and endometrial scarring leading to intrauterine adhesions. Hysteroscopic division of intrauterine adhesions and excision of polyps are usually straightforward, with low morbidity. Assisted reproductive technology is not applicable to uterine factor infertility. However, treatment of a uterine factor should be considered if failure of implantation seems to be the only cause of an unsuccessful IVF-ET treatment [E].

## EBM

- There is no evidence that ovulation detection kits and temperature charts increase the chance of conception.
- There is no evidence that thorough physical examination of every patient is necessary.
- The post-coital test is of limited value with regard to discriminating between couples achieving and not achieving a pregnancy.
- Drug treatment is ineffective in the treatment of endometriosis-related infertility.
- Ovarian stimulation and IUI is effective in the management of mild male factor and unexplained infertility.

## ACKNOWLEDGEMENT

This chapter has been revised and updated. The author and editors acknowledge the contribution of Hany AMA Lashen to the chapter on this topic in the previous edition of the book.

## KEY POINTS

- Around 9 per cent of couples are affected by infertility and half of them seek help.
- The most important determinant of a couple's fertility is the woman's age.
- Delaying starting a family until later life does not only reduce fertility, but also increases the risk of miscarriage.
- PCOS is the most common cause of anovulatory infertility.
- Ovulatory disorders are the most common cause of female infertility.
- PID and iatrogenic causes are the main reasons for tubal infertility.
- *Chlamydia trachomatis* is the most common pathogen leading to PID in the western world.
- Unexplained infertility represents approximately 15–30 per cent of cases.
- Careful history taking is a very important starting point to the investigation of infertility.
- The mid-luteal phase is approximately 7 days from the next menstrual cycle, which is important when measuring serum progesterone levels for ovulation detection.
- Combining laparoscopy and dye test with electrocoagulation of minimal and mild endometriosis adds a therapeutic dimension to a diagnostic procedure.

## Key References

1. Gutmacher AF. Factors affecting normal expectancy of conception. *J Am Med Assoc* 1956; **161**: 855–60.
2. Boivin J, Bunting L, Collins JA, Nygren KG. International estimates of infertility prevalence and treatment-seeking: potential need and demand for infertility medical care. *Hum Reprod* 2007; **22**: 1506–12.
3. Ombelet W, Cooke I, Dyer S *et al*. Infertility and the provision of infertility medical services in developing countries *Hum Reprod* 2008; **14**: 605–21.
4. Balen AH, Rutherford AJ. Management of infertility. *BMJ* 2007; **335**: 608–11.
5. Franks S, Stark J, Hardy K. Follicle dynamics and anovulation in polycystic ovary syndrome. *Hum Reprod* 2008; **14**: 367–78.
6. Goswami D, Conway GS. Premature ovarian failure. *Hum Reprod* 2005; **11**: 491–510.

# 52.3 Male infertility

*Yakoub Khalaf*

---

## MRCOG standards

### Theoretical skills

- Understand epidemiology, aetiology and pathogenesis of male infertility.
- Understand clinical treatment and prognosis of male factor infertility.
- Understand indications, limitations and interpretation of relevant investigations.
- Read and understand the RCOG and NICE guidelines on this subject.

### Practical skills

- Be able to take a history and examine the male partner with regard to infertility investigations.
- Be able to interpret and understand the seminal analysis report.

## INTRODUCTION

Other than in cases of absolute azoospermia or severe oligozoospermia/asthenzooospermia, the impact of the male factor on a couple's fertility is difficult to quantify. In other words, any man with motile normal spermatozoa in his ejaculate should be credited with some degree of fertility. Women undergoing donor insemination treatment have a higher probability of pregnancy if they are partners of azoospermic men than if they are partners of oligozoospermic men. This reflects that a degree of compensation can exist between the female and male partners. Accordingly, in most circumstances, it is easier to define male fertility than infertility. The ability to make a woman pregnant or father a child can be considered evidence of the male's fertility. There are many causes of male infertility, although primary testicular disorders are most commonly responsible.

## AETIOLOGY

### Primary testicular disease

The majority of cases of male factor infertility lie in this category. The pathogenesis of testicular dysfunction is poorly understood, with no obvious predisposing factors being identifiable in more than 50 per cent of cases. Recent studies have linked azoospermia and severe oligozoospermia to microdeletions of genes on the Y chromosome, which appear to be involved in at least some cases of 'idiopathic' male infertility [D]. Other causes of failure of spermatogenesis include testicular maldescent, particularly if left uncorrected until puberty, testicular torsion, trauma or infection, neoplasm and effects of subsequent chemotherapy, haemosiderosis and Klinefelter's syndrome [D]. Mumps orchitis and severe epididymo-orchitis are the main inflammatory causes of testicular damage [D]. Other chromosomal anomalies can also lead to male infertility; however, Klinefelter's syndrome remains the only relatively commonly seen anomaly. Azoospermic and severely oligozoospermic men should have chromosomal karyotyping before their sperm is used for intracytoplasmic sperm injection (ICSI) in order to counsel the couple adequately about the risk of transmission of a chromosomal disorder (commonly deletion or translocation) to the offspring [E].

### Obstructive male infertility

Obstruction can occur at any level of the male reproductive tract from the rete testis and the epididymis to the vas deferens. Obstruction can be due to congenital, inflammatory or iatrogenic causes. Desire for fertility following vasectomy is common. Congenital absence of the vas is also fairly common, being the cause of azoospermia in approximately 10 per cent of cases [D]. Bilateral congenital absence of the vas is seen in carriers of genes for cystic fibrosis [C], and pre-treatment screening of both partners is essential to avoid the possibility of cystic fibrosis in the offspring.

## Endocrinological causes of male infertility

Endocrinopathies are rarely identified in cases of male infertility. The more common conditions seen in this category include hypogonadotrophic hypogonadism, thyroid and adrenal disease [D]. Although rare, these conditions should be diagnosed, as their treatment is straightforward and can restore fertility. Hyperprolactinaemia in men can lead to impotence, but has little effect on sperm production [C].

## Autoimmune causes

Approximately 12 per cent of men have anti-sperm antibodies [C]. This can lead to decreased sperm motility and may impede the binding of the spermatozoon to the zona pellucida of the oocyte, hindering fertilization. Low levels of anti-sperm antibodies are not thought to have a significant impact on fertility [D]. The reason why some men develop anti-sperm antibodies is not known, although damage to the testis following trauma and surgery can be found in many cases.

## Drugs

Drugs taken for medicinal and recreational purposes can affect sperm production and/or function. Alcohol, cigarettes, opiates and marijuana can suppress spermatogenesis and affect sperm function [D]. Anabolic steroids, antifungal drugs, sulfasalazine, corticosteroids and other classes of drugs also affect spermatogenesis. The effect of most of these drugs is reversible. In contrast, chemotherapy can cause permanent damage to spermatogenesis. Other drugs, including antidepressants, sedatives and antihypertensives, can lead to male infertility by causing erectile dysfunction.

## Environmental factors

Exposure to heat, chemicals and ionizing irradiation can damage sperm production, and it is important to enquire about the male partner's occupation. Evidence for the extent of the effects of environmental toxins on male fertility is lacking. Although epidemiological studies have demonstrated a decline in sperm quality in the developed world, it is difficult to extrapolate from this population-based data to individual cases. However, it seems sensible to advise the avoidance of excessive heat and exposure to chemicals such as paints, organic solvents, lead-based products and pesticides in oligospermic/asthenospermic subfertile men.

## Varicocele

Varicocele is a dilatation of the veins along the spermatic cord in the scrotum. Dilatation occurs when valves within the veins along the spermatic cord obstruct normal blood flow, causing a back flow of blood. The mechanisms by which varicoceles would affect fertility have not yet been explained, and neither have the mechanisms by which surgical treatment of the varicoceles might restore fertility. It occurs in both fertile and infertile men, although the incidence seems to be higher among infertile men [C]. The impact of varicocele on male fertility remains controversial. Increased testicular temperature (which is unfavourable for spermatogenesis) has been suggested as a mechanism of action in these cases, but surgical or radiological correction of the disorder is not thought to improve the chances of conception [A].[1] Additionally, there is no increase in pregnancy rates following varicocele treatment compared to no treatment in subfertile couples, in whom varicoceles in the man is the only abnormal finding.

## Ejaculatory disorders

Retrograde ejaculation, in which sperm enter the bladder rather than the penile urethra at ejaculation, can follow from neurological disorders, diabetes or bladder neck or prostate surgery. Failure of ejaculation due to neurological disorders, medication or psychological difficulties is a rare cause of male infertility.

## INVESTIGATION OF THE MALE

All referrals to an infertility clinic should be seen as a couple, with concurrent investigation of the male and female partners. A routine semen analysis can be performed before seeing the couple in the clinic. A normal result can provide a degree of reassurance to the male partner, and erectile and ejaculatory problems can usually be excluded by a sensitively taken medical history. If the seminal parameters are abnormal, further investigations should be instigated. It is important to elicit from the history any of the causes of male infertility mentioned above. This should be followed by examination of genital development, the testicles, the epididymis and the vas deferens. Any of the aforementioned reversible causes can usually be corrected, and advice regarding smoking, alcohol and substance abuse should be given. Testicular cooling by wearing boxer shorts or taking cold baths is probably of little value, although occupational exposure to extreme heat should be avoided.

## Semen analysis

The value of a diagnostic test depends on its sensitivity (ability to identify disease), specificity (ability to identify normality) and reproducibility (obtaining similar results each time the test is carried out). The wide overlap of the results of the various components of a semen analysis between fertile and infertile men reduces the sensitivity and specificity of routine semen analysis as a test of infertility. Moreover, the large biological variation seen in the quality of sperm in repeated tests on the same individual limits the reproducibility of semen analysis as a diagnostic test. Routine semen analysis should be performed according to criteria established by the World Health Organization (WHO) in order to achieve standardization (Table 52.3.1). The test assesses several measures of sperm quality, some of which are more sensitive in identifying infertile men than others. The WHO-recommended method of semen analysis includes determination of the volume of ejaculate, concentration, motility and percentage of morphologically normal forms. Semen analysis can be carried out manually or using computer-assisted sperm analysis (CASA). Several population-based studies have produced statistical correlation between the different semen parameters and fertility potential in men. It is also important to remember that these values are not the minimum requirement to achieve a pregnancy; therefore they are referred to as 'reference' and not 'normal' values.

Many other tests of semen quality have been devised. These include biochemical analysis of the seminal fluid and detection of anti-sperm antibodies. Biochemical analysis of the seminal fluid can provide information about the prostate, seminal vesicles and epididymis. Zinc, fructose, carnitine and acid phosphatase have all been studied, but are not thought to impart useful diagnostic or prognostic information. The detection of anti-sperm antibodies using the immunobead or mixed antibody reaction (MAR) test may alter treatment and continues to be performed in most centres.

## Sperm function tests

The functions of the sperm *in vivo* are to negotiate the cervical mucus, reach the ampullary part of the Fallopian tube in sufficient numbers, undergo capacitation and finally fertilize the egg. However, routine semen analysis does not test these functions. Therefore several tests, known as 'sperm function tests', have been developed in tertiary centres. These tests are still of academic rather than practical value and have become less significant following the introduction of *in-vitro* fertilization (IVF) treatments, which circumvent most of the steps necessary for fertilization *in vivo*. Their role in routine infertility investigations has yet to be established. Some of these tests are listed in Table 52.3.2 and the interested reader can refer to the WHO manual for more details.

## Other tests

Unexplained severe sperm abnormality including azoospermia merits further investigation. The objectives of such tests are to identify whether azoospermia is due to a primary testicular disorder or an outflow obstruction. Obstructive azoospermia is usually associated with normal concentration of follicle-stimulating hormone (FSH) in serum, as the testes continue to function normally. In contrast, disorders of spermatogenesis result in interruption of the gonadal–pituitary feedback loop with elevation of serum FSH. Measurement of FSH can thus be useful in the investigation of azoospermia. Invasive investigation using testicular biopsy can assess the extent of damage to the spermatogenesis and identify whether it is possible to obtain testicular sperm for use in ICSI, even if the patient is azoospermic. Karyotyping and cystic fibrosis gene screening are necessary if a chromosomal abnormality is suspected or to assess the carrier status for cystic fibrosis genes in patients with congenital absence of the vas. However, the modern management of male infertility and the introduction of ICSI treatment has reduced the need for extensive investigations, especially in less severe cases of oligozoospermia or athenozoospermia. Where an endocrinol024gical reason is suspected, the diagnosis should be made, as the treatment strategy in these cases differs from the usual treatment modalities for male infertility (Figure 52.3.1).

## Examination of the male partner

In the presence of a normal semen analysis, there is little to gain from examination of the male. On the other hand, in

**Table 52.3.1** Semen analysis reference values

| Parameter | Reference value |
| --- | --- |
| Volume | 2 mL or more |
| pH | 7.2 or more |
| Sperm concentration | 20 million/mL or more |
| Total sperm number | 40 million or more per ejaculate |
| Motility | 50% or more (grade a + b) or 25% with progressive motility |
| Morphology | See note below |
| Vitality | 75% or more live |
| White cell count | Fewer than 1 million |
| Immunobead test | Less than 5% motile sperm with beads bound |
| MAR test | Less than 50% sperm with adherent particles |

Note: Multicentre population-based studies utilizing the methods of morphology assessment in the manual are now in progress. Data from assisted reproduction suggest that fertilization rates drop if sperm morphology falls below 15% of the normal forms. MAR, mixed agglutination reaction.

**Table 52.3.2** Sperm function tests

| |
| --- |
| Objective assessment of motility |
| Hypo-osmotic swelling test |
| Tests for sperm nuclear maturity |
| Measure of acrosome status |
| Acrosome reaction and acrosin activity |
| Hamster zona-free oocyte penetration |
| Human sperm zona binding and penetration |

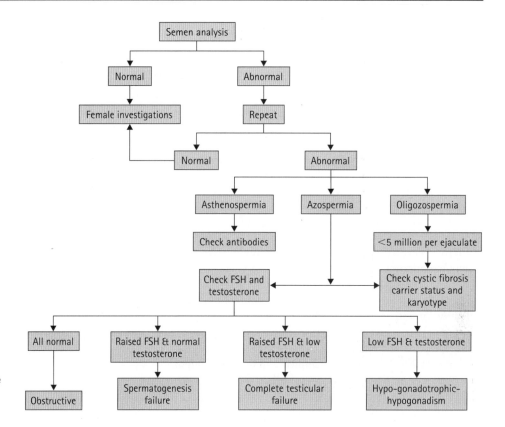

**Figure 52.3.1** Investigations of male infertility. FSH, follicule-stimulating hormone

severe male factor infertility and especially in azoospermic men, examination is warranted to help establish the cause of the problem. Both general and genital examinations should be undertaken. The objectives of the general examination are to assess the level of masculinization and to detect any stigmata of chromosomal abnormality, inguinal hernia or relevant surgical scars, gynaecomastia or evidence of systemic illnesses. The genital examination should include assessment of the testes, epididymis and vas deferens and detection of any scrotal swellings or varicocele. If the history suggests penile or prostatic problems, it is advisable to refer for a urological opinion. The examination should be carried out in standing and supine positions in a warm private room. The testicular axis, volume and consistency should be assessed with a Prader orchiometer to measure the testicular volume. It should be noted that testicular volume is related to ethnic origin, weight and height and there is normally a small difference between the left and right testicles. For Caucasian men the normal volume is above 12 mL per testis. The consistency of the testicles can also be assessed. A soft consistency is associated with impaired spermatogenesis. Examination of the epididymis should assess its position in relation to the testicle, volume, any tenderness and any nodularity or swellings. Normally, the epididymis is small and may not be palpable. The vas should have no thickenings or nodules. Careful examination for the presence of the vasa is essential in azoospermic men, especially if the testicular volume is normal. Scrotal examination for varicocele should be carried out in the standing position. If any other scrotal swelling is palpable, the patient should be referred for a urological

opinion. Testicular maldescent in infancy is associated with an increased risk of testicular cancer in later life. Such patients may present to an infertility clinic for investigation of oligospermia. They should be appraised for this risk and taught to self-examine. Similarly, tissue collected at testicular biopsy that is used to obtain sperm for ICSI in azoospermic men should also be sent for histological examination.

## MANAGEMENT OF MALE INFERTILITY

Until recently, men with primary testicular dysfunction or obstructive azoospermia were unable to reproduce. *In vitro* fertilization and micromanipulation of sperm now offer these men the opportunity to father children and has become the mainstay in the treatment of male factor infertility. The treatment of male factor infertility, including the use of donor insemination, is discussed in Chapter 52.4, Assisted reproduction. However, some more traditional methods of treatment merit consideration.

### Varicocelectomy

This procedure refers to the ligation of varicocele, which was carried out both prophylactically and therapeutically for many decades. Varicocele repair does not seem to be an effective treatment for male or unexplained subfertility [A]. The modern management of infertility has made the procedure redundant, removing the opportunity for further randomized trials to investigate its value.

## Management of endocrine disorders

Hypogonadotrophic hypogonadism, often in association with Kallmann's syndrome, has been successfully treated with pulsatile GnRH or human menopausal gonadotrophins to restore spermatogenic drive and hence fertility.Initiation of spermatogenesis can take several months and treatment can become costly.

Men with idiopathic semen abnormalities should not be offered anti-oestrogens, gonadotrophins, androgens, bromocriptine or kinin-enhancing drugs because they have not been shown to be effective [A].

## Management of anti-sperm antibodies

Many empirical therapies have been suggested for men with anti-sperm antibodies. The use of condoms and corticosteroids and intrauterine insemination of washed spermatozoa are some examples [A]. The value of all these modalities has been controversial, and IVF-ET (*in vitro* fertilization and embryo transfer) and ICSI are currently the methods of choice in these cases. Donor insemination can be an alternative for financial reasons.

## Reversal of vasectomy

Vasectomy reversal can be carried out successfully, with up to an 80 per cent chance of a subsequent pregnancy. The chance of success is inversely proportional to the length of time since the vasectomy was carried out. Although the integrity of the vas deferens can be restored in most cases, anti-sperm antibodies are common after vasectomy and reversal, and are probably the major bar to conception. In these cases and in those whose operation has failed, IVF with ICSI is the recommended treatment. A growing number of centres are offering collection and storage of sperm from the epididymis at the time of vasectomy reversal, for subsequent use in ICSI treatment if the reversal operation fails.

---

### EBM

- The use of gonadotrophin drugs in hypogonadotrophic hypogonadal men is an effective treatment [B].
- The use of bromocriptine in men with sexual dysfunction as a result of hyperprolactinaemia is effective [B].
- Testicular biopsy should only be undertaken in tertiary centres [E].

---

- Vasectomy reversal is an effective treatment [A].
- Anti-oestrogens, androgens and bromocriptine are not effective in improving sperm quality [C].
- The use of steroids in the treatment of anti-sperm antibodies is ineffective and further validation is required [B].
- Surgery on the male genital tract should be undertaken only in centres where expertise is available [E].
- Men found to have abnormal chromosomal analysis (14 per cent in azoospermia and 7 per cent in severe oligotertatoastheonzoospermia) should receive genetic counselling.

---

## ACKNOWLEDGEMENT

This chapter has been revised and updated. The author and editors acknowledge the contribution of Hany AMA Lashen to the chapter on this topic in the previous edition of the book.

---

### KEY POINTS

- Semen analysis is an appropriate starting point in the investigation of the male partner.
- If a severe sperm abnormality is found, clinical examination and bacteriological and endocrinological tests should be undertaken.
- Tact and sensitivity are important when obtaining a history, examining patients and discussing abnormal results with them.
- If reversal of vasectomy is to be undertaken, efforts should be made to obtain epididymal sperm for freezing and future use in case of operation failure.
- There is a considerable variability in sperm quality when assessed in the same individual over time.
- Semen analysis, unlike many modern investigative tests, is operator dependent. Adequate training of the operator is therefore essential to minimize both intraobserver and interobserver variations.
- The andrology laboratory should be subject to external and internal quality control.

---

## Key Reference

1. Evers JLH, Collins JA. Assessment of efficacy of varicocele repair for male subfertility: A systematic review. *Lancet* 2003; **361**: 1849–52.

# 52.4 Assisted reproduction

*Yakoub Khalaf*

## INTRODUCTION

The term 'assisted reproductive technology' (ART) includes all methods of infertility treatment that require laboratory handling of gamete(s). Assisted reproduction originated from the practices of donor insemination and intrauterine insemination (IUI) by the male partner, which were practised long before *in vitro* fertilization (IVF). The introduction of IVF and the later introduction of sperm micromanipulation were major developments in the management of infertility. Assisted reproduction technologies have opened many avenues for infertile couples, although not without financial cost and ethical considerations. The first 'IVF child', Louise Brown, was the result of IVF of an oocyte obtained in a natural cycle, which was carried out by Patrick Steptoe and Robert Edwards in 1977. Advances in pharmaceuticals, vaginal ultrasound and laboratory practice have significantly improved the success rates of assisted reproduction since that time.

A typical cycle of ART passes through several steps: initial assessment and counselling, ovarian stimulation and monitoring, oocyte retrieval, IVF, embryo transfer (ET), luteal support, pregnancy test and confirmation of viability with ultrasound. Variations on this theme may take place, depending on the modality of assisted reproduction. However, counselling is a common denominator in all ART modalities and is discussed first. The indications for the different forms of assisted reproduction have already been discussed under the individual causes of infertility.

## COUNSELLING

Counselling in the context of IVF treatment refers either to information counselling, i.e. providing sufficient information to patients to allow them to take informed and considered decisions regarding treatment, or to therapeutic and implication counselling. The former falls within the duties of the medical professional, while the latter should be carried out by trained counsellors and has different objectives. To avoid confusion, the roles of both the clinician and the counsellor are considered separately.

### Counselling and the clinician

It is imperative for the clinician who deals with infertile couples to understand their feelings and any psychological and/or social stresses imposed on them. Infertile couples frequently report feelings of inadequacy, with low self-esteem, blame and social exclusion [C]. This significantly affects their social abilities, their marital relations and frequently their work performance [D]. The clinician should be able to assess these impacts, give the couple the opportunity to discuss their anxieties and direct them towards therapeutic counselling, if appropriate. Establishing a rapport with the infertile couple is usually not difficult, as they are willing to put their hope in the clinician, who may help them overcome their childlessness. Seeing the couple together is essential [E]. They should be made to feel at ease and feel that the doctor is sympathetic to their problem, and should be given ample opportunity to address all their points of concern. A clear plan of action should be agreed from the outset, along with a discussion of the reasons for undertaking all the proposed investigations. Providing the couple with written information and useful addresses is very important. The doctor should be prepared to discuss at length all aspects of the modalities of treatment available to them. It is not unusual to find that the couple have studied the literature and searched the internet looking for evidence, and that they are aware of the latest advances and the relevant statistics. Consequently, they may lose confidence if they sense any lack of knowledge on behalf of their doctor.

## The counsellor

The counsellor plays a pivotal role in the success of assisted conception treatment. The adequate provision of counselling is a key HFEA licensing requirement for any unit that proposes to provide assisted conception treatment. The diversity and versatility of the counsellor role requires specific training and experience, as well as a great deal of understanding and compassion. The counsellor should be able to provide therapeutic and implication counselling. The objective of the former is to alleviate the stresses imposed on the couple by infertility and to help them through the grieving process after a failed cycle or pregnancy loss. The latter modality should provide the couple with a means of dealing with potential stresses or ethical dilemmas that they may encounter during a particular form of treatment. Couples intending to undergo treatments involving gamete donation are particularly vulnerable and should spend time in discussion with the counsellor before starting the treatment cycle.

## MODALITIES OF ASSISTED REPRODUCTION

The major forms of ART are IVF-ET, possibly including intracytoplasmic sperm injection (ICSI), gamete intrafallopian transfer (GIFT), zygote intrafallopian transfer (ZIFT), IUI, donor insemination (DI) and egg donation.

Legal issues dominate practice in this area, and in the United Kingdom some of these treatments are regulated by the HFEA. Until recently, the provision of GIFT and IUI treatment did not require a licence from HFEA. This has now changed and a HFEA licence is required for these two procedures. Micromanipulation of gametes for ICSI or assisted hatching is additional to basic IVF treatment. Micromanipulation refers to any technique that involves working with gametes or embryos microscopically. Currently, the most commonly used technique of micromanipulation is ICSI, which has revolutionized the management of male infertility and helped overcome fertilization difficulties. ICSI supplanted other, now obsolete, methods of improving sperm penetration into the oocyte, such as zona drilling (ZD) and subzonal sperm injection (SUZI). Assisted hatching as a micromanipulation technique refers to partial drilling or dissection of the zona pellucida to aid implantation of the embryo. The embryo has to 'hatch' by breaking through the zona pellucida before it can implant. Embryos resulting from IVF were thought to have a hardened zona, resulting in a low implantation rate. Weakening the zona mechanically or chemically was therefore thought to enhance embryo hatching and potentially aid implantation. Since the risk of damage to the embryo is increased, routine assisted hatching is not recommended, and this procedure is reserved for older patients and those with multiple cycle failures [E].

Pre-implantation genetic diagnosis (PGD) involves embryo micromanipulation for diagnostic rather than therapeutic purposes. The technique was developed initially to allow identification of the sex of the embryo and sex selection to prevent transmission of X chromosome-linked genetic disorders. However, in theory, any heritable disease for which the gene or chromosome defect is known can be identified in the embryo by PGD, with avoidance of transmission. Several single gene disorders are currently diagnosed using PGD, and the list is growing rapidly. The applicability of this technique for infertility treatment is limited and its real value is for patients who are carriers of genetic disorders [E]. However, it is being applied as a means of aneuploidy screening (pre-implantation genetic screening (PGS)), in an attempt to avoid the replacement of chromosomally abnormal embryos that may result in implantation failure or miscarriage. This application has failed to improve live birth rates or reduce miscarriage rates in several randomized controlled trials and therefore is no longer recommended.

## OVARIAN STIMULATION AND MONITORING

Although the first attempt of IVF was carried out in a natural ovulatory cycle, ovarian stimulation soon became the cornerstone of assisted conception treatment.

Controlled ovarian stimulation (COS) is now universally used in IVF in order to produce multiple mature oocytes capable of fertilization, implantation and pregnancy. A dazzling number of protocols have been developed using a combination of several agents to achieve this goal. The lack of uniformity amongst different centres in the regimens used reflects the lack of properly randomized studies and the shortage of knowledge regarding the regulation of ovarian function and folliculogenesis. This section reviews the available techniques of COS, as well as the stimulating agents and ovarian monitoring.

## Ovarian stimulatory agents

Several agents have been used individually and in combination to stimulate folliculogenesis and ovulation, with various degrees of success, as judged by the individual woman's response and the pregnancy rates achieved.

### Human gonadotrophins

The use of gonadotrophins to stimulate ovulation was first described by Cole and Hart in 1930,[1] using pregnant mare serum gonadotrophins (PMSG) that could stimulate ovulation in hypophysectomized animals. In 1938 and 1939, two groups induced ovulation in humans using intravenous injection of purified gonadotrophic substance from pregnant mare serum.[2,3] In the 1950s, a variety of gonadotrophins of both human and animal origin was developed for the use of ovulation induction. However, these preparations lacked consistency, and monitoring of ovarian response was extremely basic, using basal body temperature, endometrial biopsy and daily vaginal smears, which were inaccurate and tedious. Others used human pituitary gonadotrophin to avoid the problem of antibody formation to animal proteins, but the availability of this preparation was limited by the difficulty in obtaining human pituitaries. A commercially available preparation of human gonadotrophin extracted from the urine of postmenopausal women was first described by Gemzel et al. in 1958.[4]

Human menopausal gonadotrophins (hMG) were used initially for ovulation induction in anovulatory women until the introduction of IVF led to their use to induce multiple ovulation so that a large number of follicles and oocytes could be obtained. Jones et al.[5] and Garcia et al.[6] used a low hMG dose (150 IU follicle-stimulating hormone (FSH)/day), and the ovarian response was monitored using ultrasound and serum oestradiol (E2) assay. Purified human urinary FSH preparations were later made available and successfully used to induce ovulation. The first IVF pregnancy using purified urinary human FSH was reported by Shaw et al. in 1985.[7] Several studies on the use of FSH alone, or in combination with hMG, have been reported and suggest that pure urinary FSH and hMG are equally effective in ovulation induction for assisted reproduction procedures [A].

### Recombinant FSH

The production of urinary gonadotrophins requires the collection of vast amounts of urine from post-menopausal women. The difficulties associated with this collection and anxieties about the contamination of urinary FSH with other urinary excreted proteins led to the development of recombinant FSH (rFSH), which is 99 per cent pure FSH. Recombinant human FSH is produced from a Chinese hamster ovary cell line transfected with genes for the alpha and beta subunits of FSH. The polypeptide chain of rFSH is identical to the native molecule, although there are subtle differences in glycosylation and sialation. Several randomized controlled trials have reported that ovarian stimulation with rFSH and urinary FSH resulted in significantly more oocytes and embryos in favour of rFSH.[8] However, the clinical pregnancy and live birth rates were similar in the two groups of patients.

### Clomiphene citrate

Clomiphene citrate was first synthesized in 1956 and introduced for clinical trial use in 1960. It was first used successfully to induce ovulation in 1961 and continues to be the most commonly used drug for this purpose, as well as in the empirical treatment of unexplained infertility. After early failure with the use of hMGs in COS for the purpose of IVF, attention turned to clomiphene citrate. Clomiphene citrate is a non-steroidal oestrogen designed as triphenylchloroethylene derivative and administered as a racemic mixture of cis and trans isomers. These isomers were relabelled as enclomiphene (E) and zuclophene (Z) isomers. The racemic mixture used to induce ovulation comprises 38 per cent Z and 62 per cent E.

The exact mechanism of action of clomiphene citrate is not known. However, it has been suggested that it reacts with oestrogen receptors at the level of the hypothalamus and pituitary and its anti-oestrogenic action results in an increase in gonadotrophin secretion. The rise in FSH and luteinizing hormone (LH) results in the stimulation of follicular growth, and the subsequent ovulation results from the positive feedback of oestrogen produced by the growing follicles on the hypothalamus and pituitary. However, the cycle cancellation rate with clomiphene citrate or with combined clomiphene citrate and hMG was significant, mainly due to abnormal or poor ovarian response, poor follicular growth, or premature LH surge [C]. Consequently, most ART centres have moved away from this approach to COS.

### Gonadotrophin-releasing hormone analogues

Native GnRH was first isolated from hypothalamic extracts and sequenced as a decapeptide by Schally et al.[9] Pharmaceutical modification of the amino acid sequence of the GnRH molecule resulted in the development of a large number of GnRH agonists, which are now widely used clinically. The administration of a GnRH agonist results in an initial agonistic effect, leading to the production of both FSH and LH, followed by a sustained decline in both pituitary response and gonadotrophin production, a process known as pituitary down-regulation. GnRH agonists are used with COS to improve the outcome of ovarian stimulation by allowing synchronous folliculogenesis and later to prevent premature luteinization by suppressing the endogenous LH surge. Suppression of the LH surge allows prolonged stimulation with FSH, producing a cohort of large ovarian follicles with mature oocytes.

## Downregulation protocols

Different protocols have been used to induce pituitary downregulation, based on the timing of administration of the agonist.

- Most commonly, GnRH agonist treatment is begun in the mid-luteal phase of the preceding cycle. The woman will then experience a withdrawal bleed, after which FSH injection is started. This is known as the 'long protocol'.
- The 'short or flare-up protocol' involves agonist treatment being started 2–3 days before or concurrently with ovarian gonadotrophin stimulation. This protocol takes advantage of the initial endogenous release of stored pituitary gonadotrophin as a result of the agonistic effect of the GnRH agonist, followed by the direct stimulatory effect of the exogenous gonadotrophin.
- In the 'ultra-short follicular phase protocol', GnRH agonist is administered for the first 3 days of the cycle only. This protocol has proved less popular and is rarely used in practice.

Although numerous reports have been published on different agonist regimes, there are few randomized studies that prospectively compare the efficacy of the various GnRH agonist protocols. Hughes et al.[10] carried out a meta-analysis of ten prospective, randomized trials on the use of GnRH agonists in IVF and concluded that the routine use of GnRH agonists in IVF was associated with a better ovarian response (higher number of oocytes and lower cycle cancellation rate) and greater clinical pregnancy rates [A]. They also commented that the available studies comparing the long and the short protocols did not demonstrate any significant difference in terms of cycle cancellation rate or clinical pregnancy rates. However, some concern about the possibility of adverse effects of increased follicular phase LH and progesterone levels seen in the flare-up protocol was later expressed.

## Gonadotrophin-releasing hormone antagonists

The GnRH antagonists are synthesized from the native GnRH molecule by multiple amino acid substitutions. They are capable of immediate inhibition of pituitary gonadotrophin secretion and are likely to offer advantages over the currently available agonists due to the absence of the flare-up effect. The early development of these compounds was hampered by the side effects of histamine release and problems in developing a depot formation, with variable levels of absorption. However, these problems have been overcome and the results of large randomized clinical trials have been published. These suggest that pregnancy and live birth rates from GnRH antagonist-controlled IVF are equivalent to those seen in the 'traditional' long protocol [B]. The use of an antagonist avoids the prolonged prestimulation period of pituitary downregulation, speeding up the cycle and removing the experience of menopausal side effects. There is also a suggestion that the incidence of OHSS is lower with this approach, although that has yet to be demonstrated in an adequately powered trial.

## Monitoring of response to ovarian stimulation

Monitoring the ovarian response to FSH stimulation is a critical part of good ART practice. Under-response may prompt cycle cancellation or an increase in FSH dosage, while over-response can lead to OHSS, with serious consequences. Both hormonal and ultrasonographic criteria have been used to monitor ovarian response to controlled stimulation and to manage the cycle. Serum concentrations of E2 reflect the growth and maturity of the follicle. The antral follicle produces increasing amounts of oestrogen while maturing. However, improvement in image quality of transvaginal ultrasound has resulted in a growing reliance on direct measurement of follicle growth, follicles of ≥17 mm mean diameter being regarded as 'mature'.

The aims of cycle monitoring are:

- to determine the optimum time to administer human chorionic gonadotrophin (hCG) to induce final oocyte maturation before egg collection;
- to predict and therefore prevent the severe forms of OHSS;
- to identify poor responders with a view to improving their response or cancelling the cycle.

## In vitro fertilization–embryo transfer

In vitro fertilization refers to extracorporeal fertilization of an oocyte. However, the term has been more loosely applied to the whole treatment cycle in which fertilization in vitro is utilized. A typical IVF cycle begins with ovarian stimulation and final maturation of oocytes with a single hCG injection, followed by transvaginal ultrasound-guided oocyte collection, fertilization in vitro, incubation of embryos and ET.

Reproductive medicine

## Oocyte maturation *in vivo*

The oocyte will only become fertile if exposed to an LH surge, causing it to re-enter meiosis and extrude the first polar body. In an IVF cycle in which the endogenous LH surge is prevented by GnRH antagonist or agonist treatment, hCG is used to mimic the natural surge. Human chorionic gonadotrophin is usually given when three or more follicles are larger than 16 mm in mean diameter. Oocyte retrieval is then carried out 34–36 hours later – delay can lead to loss of oocytes due to ovulation.

## Oocyte collection

Historically, oocyte collection was carried out laparoscopically, but this has been supplanted by transvaginal ultrasound-guided oocyte retrieval, an approach that offers simplicity and safety and yields more oocytes. Under ultrasound guidance, a 16–17-gauge needle is passed through the lateral vaginal fornix into the ovary to pierce the follicle and aspirate the intrafollicular fluid using a suction apparatus. The oocyte is then microscopically retrieved from the follicular fluid. The potential risks of transvaginal oocyte collection include ovarian infection (estimated at less than 1 per cent) and excessive vaginal bleeding, which can usually be controlled with pressure. Oocyte retrieval can be carried out under general anaesthesia or with local anaesthetic and sedation.

## Laboratory procedures

The embryologist retrieves the oocyte from the follicular fluid, grades it for maturity and pre-incubates each oocyte before mechanically stripping the outer cumulus cells from the oocyte itself by repeated aspiration into a glass pipette. The sperm sample is prepared by washing and isolation of motile sperm, and a number of spermatozoa are added to each egg. Following incubation, the oocytes are examined microscopically for the presence of two pronuclei, confirming fertilization. The presence of more than two pronuclei indicates polyspermy, and the eggs are discarded as they contain excessive genetic material.

The fertilized eggs (zygotes) are then incubated for a further 1–2 days to allow for the development of the embryos. Embryos are then graded according to the size and number of their cells (blastomeres) and the presence of any fragmentation. The embryologist will select embryos for transfer, and 'spare' embryos can be cryopreserved at this stage, if deemed suitable to withstand the freezing process.

## Embryo transfer

The number of embryos routinely transferred varies in different countries. In the UK, a maximum of three embryos can be legally transferred. However, the HFEA and the British Fertility Society recommend transfer of a maximum of two embryos in patients under 40 years of age. In order to reduce the risk of multiple pregnancy, serious consideration should be given to identifying good prognosis patients (younger than 35 years and have more than one good quality embryo) where only an elective single embryo transfer is recommended. Several reports have shown that the transfer of a single embryo and freezing additional embryos with a view to replacing them subsequently does not affect the pregnancy rate but significantly reduces the multiple pregnancy rate, which in turn considerably reduces neonatal morbidity and mortality [B].

The embryos are transferred transcervically into the uterine cavity using a soft polyethylene catheter. The procedure is usually painless and straightforward. Manipulation of the cervix by distending the urinary bladder or using ultrasound guidance is helpful to facilitate a difficult ET, although its impact on pregnancy rate is controversial.

## Luteal phase support

The luteal phase is 'supported' until the pituitary gland recovers from pituitary suppression and produces the required LH to maintain the corpus luteum. This can be achieved by administering hCG to maintain the corpus luteum directly, or indirectly by administering progesterone to the patient. In earlier reports, the administration of hCG was held to have a marginal advantage over progesterone administration in terms of pregnancy rates, but with increasesd risk of OHSS [A]. Recent evidence has not shown any difference in pregnancy rates between the two treatments [A]. Progesterone can be administered in several forms; however, the intramuscular and transvaginal routes are most commonly used.

## Pregnancy test and confirmation of a clinical pregnancy

If a pregnancy occurs, a positive urinary pregnancy test will be obtained approximately 14 days post-ET. Elevated serum levels of hCG can be detected earlier. The risk of ectopic pregnancy should be considered in all cases until an intrauterine pregnancy is later confirmed by ultrasound scan. If necessary, b-hCG levels should be serially measured to exclude ectopic pregnancy.

The definition of clinical pregnancy varies in different countries. The presence of fetal cardiac activity on ultrasound scan is important to make the diagnosis in most European countries, whereas in the United States the presence of a gestational sac is sufficient to diagnose a clinical pregnancy. A positive pregnancy test that is followed by a decline in the hCG levels without evidence of a clinical pregnancy is referred to as biochemical pregnancy.

# ALTERNATIVES TO IVF

## Intrauterine insemination

Washed partner or donor sperm can be inseminated into the uterine cavity using a polyethylene catheter. Intrauterine insemination of the partner's sperm without ovarian stimulation has been used to treat unexplained and cervical factor infertility, but with poor results. With the introduction of COS, this approach was revived and has yielded good success rates in treating mild male factor and unexplained infertility. The presence of patent Fallopian tubes is essential for this treatment. The majority of clinicians do not consider patients with a history of ectopic pregnancy to be suitable for this treatment, as tubal disease is the precipitating factor in most of these patients. Intrauterine insemination can be used in conjunction with ovarian stimulation with either clomiphene citrate or gonadotrophin. However, the results with gonadotrophins are generally better than with clomiphene citrate [C]. The success rates with this line of treatment have been discussed above under Clomiphene citrate.

## Use of donor gametes

Sperm from anonymous or known donors has been used to treat infertile couples for centuries. More recently, legislation has regulated this practice and recognized the need for careful counselling before treatment, particularly considering the welfare of the potential child. As IVF has grown, oocyte donation has also become feasible and is now widely practised. There are similarities between sperm and egg donation with regard to the screening of donors. Any potential donor should be interviewed and a thorough medical, social and family history taken. Donors have a legal obligation to divulge any previous history of medical illnesses and particularly any family history of congenital or hereditary diseases. Screening for human immunodeficiency virus (HIV), hepatitis (B and C), syphilis, cytomegalovirus, gonorrhoea and chlamydia should be conducted on every prospective donor. A negative HIV test should be repeated six months later. Donor insemination is now only carried out using quarantined frozen sperm, to reduce the risk of HIV transmission.

## Counselling

The counsellor's role is also to make sure that the couple have carefully considered the implications of their decision to undergo treatment, and to support them through a stressful time of their lives. Matching the physical characteristics of the donor with the recipient should also be discussed. This is usually straightforward if donor sperm is to be used, but more difficult given the smaller number of oocyte donors. The couple should also be informed that, despite careful screening of donors, the normal population risk of congenital anomalies still exists. Their plans to discuss the method of conception with the child should also be explored, as this can lead to conflict later.

## Donor recruitment

It has been much easier to recruit male than female donors. An oocyte donor has to undergo ovarian stimulation and oocyte retrieval as described for IVF. Such risks and inconveniences do not apply to the male. Previous fertility, although desirable, is not always a prerequisite for accepting a donor. Some couples may choose to receive gametes from a known donor. However, the majority of couples prefer an anonymous donor, which is usually encouraged to avoid emotional and ethical complications. In 2004, the government in the United Kingdom announced that people who donate eggs, sperm or embryos in the UK are to lose their right to anonymity. The change to the existing law – which did not allow children conceived using donor sperm to discover the identity of donors, but only to find out small amounts of non-identifying information when they reach the age of 18 – came into effect from April 1, 2005. This means that for the first time, people will be able to receive identifying information about donors in 2023. This has, at least initially, resulted in a significant shortage of gamete donors. Given the rarity of volunteer female donors, the HFEA has recently allowed 'egg sharing', in which patients undergoing IVF for their own benefit donate a proportion of their oocytes in exchange for reduced treatment costs.

### Indications for use of donated sperm

The uptake of donor insemination (DI) has fallen since the introduction of ICSI, which can be used for severely oligospermic males or for azoospermic males if sperm can be retrieved from a testicular biopsy. However, this is not always possible, and ICSI will fail to result in pregnancy in some couples. Testicular failure with complete absence of spermatogenesis, typically after chemotherapy, and the high cost of ICSI treatment are now the main indications for DI. DI is also used to remove the risk of transmission of inherited disorders and in the treatment of single women. It can be carried out intracervically or by IUI. Cumulative pregnancy rates of up to 80 per cent after 6–12 treatment cycles have been reported, much depending on the fertility and age of the female. IVF using donor sperm can be resorted to if the female partner has tubal disease or if insemination treatments fail.

### Changes in the legal parenthood legislation that affect users of donor sperm

The HFEA has released guidance in accordance with the HFE Act 2008, that as long as an individual is willing to take on the legal rights and responsibilities of parenthood, they may be named on the birth certificate of a child born through fertility treatment. In addition, as of April 6, 2009, the third party parent will be able to sign IVF clinic consent forms. This will primarily affect couples receiving treatment with donor sperm or embryos created with donor sperm.

### Use of donor oocytes

Oocyte donation can be offered to women with ovarian failure or oocyte abnormalities, and also for the prevention of some hereditary disorders. Although initially used in cases of premature ovarian failure, the technique has now been controversially applied to women beyond natural menopause, and pregnancies with donated oocytes have been reported for women in their 60s and 70s.

Egg donation treatment is effectively carried out in an IVF cycle. The donor undergoes ovarian stimulation and oocyte collection, while the recipient undergoes the ET. The success rates from this treatment are similar to, if not slightly higher than, the average success rate expected from IVF treatment.

---

> ## KEY POINTS
>
> ### Alternatives to IVF
> - Donor insemination is useful in cases of severe male factor infertility and genetic diseases in the male partner or rhesus iso-immunization.
> - Unless the male partner is azoospermic and testicular sperm retrieval fails, the role of DI is becoming less evident in severe male factor infertility. However, financial constraints may force some couples to accept this form of treatment over ICSI.
> - Intrauterine insemination using donor sperm with or without superovulation offers better pregnancy rates compared to intracervical insemination.
> - Unless the female partner is anovulatory, DI treatment should be carried out in a natural cycle in the first place to avoid multiple pregnancies. The timing of introduction of ovarian stimulation in DI programmes is debatable. However, three to six natural treatment cycles need to be considered prior to starting ovarian stimulation.

## COMPLICATIONS OF ASSISTED REPRODUCTION

### Multiple pregnancy

Multiple birth is the single biggest risk to the health and welfare of children born after *in vitro* fertilization. *In vitro* fertilization pregnancy rates are improved by the transfer of more than one embryo. However, the incidence of multiple pregnancy increases with the number of embryos transferred. Approaches to this problem vary around the world, but UK legislation and guidance restrict the number of embryos transferred to two, except in patients who are >40 years old where a maximum of three embryos can be transferred. This policy has been effective in reducing triplets and high order multiple pregnancies but failed to address the increased incidence of twin births. Multiple pregnancy is a major cause of stillbirth, neonatal death and disability. Compared with singletons, twins are four times more likely to die in pregnancy, seven times more likely to die shortly after birth, ten times more likely to be admitted to a neonatal special care unit, and have six times the risk of cerebral palsy. Maternal morbidity and mortality is also increased due to late miscarriage, high blood pressure, pre-eclampsia and haemorrhage, amongst others.

Therefore, efforts should be made to reduce such risks and to counsel patients accordingly. Elective single embryo transfer for selected good prognosis patients has been recommended by the HFEA and each licensed clinic has to follow a multiple birth minimization strategy so that multiple births can be reduced in the next 3 years to 10 per cent.

## Ovarian hyperstimulation syndrome

This is a serious and potentially life-threatening complication of COS. The incidence of significant OHSS complicating assisted conception is variably quoted as between 0.6 and 14 per cent [D]. The underlying cause of OHSS is not known, but release of a vasoactive ovarian factor is likely to be involved. Several studies have reported that women with ultrasonographic or biochemical features of polycystic ovary syndrome are at higher risk of developing OHSS compared to those with normal ovaries. A link between lean habitus and OHSS has also been suggested.

The best approach to the management of OHSS is avoidance [C], as the syndrome only develops after the administration of hCG, and identifying those at high risk of developing OHSS can lead to prevention by cycle cancellation. This is costly and disappointing to patients and clinicians alike. The features used to identify 'high-risk' patients include a rapid rise in E2 in response to ovarian stimulation, high peak E2 level on the day of hCG administration, and the presence of large numbers of follicles on ultrasound. However, the predictive value of these commonly used criteria is low, and cases continue to occur in 'low-risk' women. Cessation of exogenous FSH or hMG administration (coasting) and withholding hCG administration until E2 levels have fallen to what is considered to be a safe level (<13 000 pmol/L) is another strategy that has been reported to reduce the incidence of OHSS. If the risk is deemed excessive after hCG has been given, abandoning the embryo transfer, with elective cryopreservation of all embryos and later frozen embryo transfer, is effective in reducing the severity, but not the incidence, of symptomatic OHSS.

The clinical picture and the management of the syndrome depend on its degree of severity. It may present 3–7 days post-hCG injection (early presentation) or 12–17 days post-hCG (late presentation). The early presentation is an acute effect of the pre-ovulatory dose of hCG, whereas the late presentation is induced by the rising serum concentration of hCG produced by the pregnancy. A classification of OHSS based on the clinical signs is widely used to guide diagnosis and treatment. Golan et al.[11] described several degrees of severity of the syndrome. In the mild form, the clinical picture of OHSS includes abdominal distension, nausea and vomiting, diarrhoea and moderate ovarian enlargement (<12 cm in average diameter). The moderate form is similar to the mild, but includes the presence of ascites on ultrasound scan. The severe form includes clinical evidence of ascites and/or hydrothorax, haemoconcentration and significant ovarian enlargement (>12 cm in average diameter).

In women with a mild/moderate form of OHSS (haematocrit value <44 per cent), bed rest and fluid replacement, together with monitoring of the biochemical profile, are all that is needed for their management. However, in the severe form of the syndrome (haematocrit, >44 per cent) hospitalization is always mandatory. Paracentesis under direct ultrasound guidance is indicated in severely compromised patients and when respiration becomes difficult due to severe abdominal distension. It has also been reported that reinfusion of the ascitic fluid with or without ultrafiltration can be useful in some severe cases. Some reports suggest that albumin infusion can prevent severe OHSS. Owing to the potential risk of human albumin infusion, many units restrict its use to cases of biochemically proven hypoalbuminaemia.

## Risk of ovarian cancer

Case reports of ovarian tumours in women undergoing infertility treatment led to concern about the potential neoplastic effect of ovarian stimulatory agents, such as clomiphene citrate and gonadotrophins. Such an effect was hypothesized to occur because ovulation induction results in the development of a higher number of ovulatory follicles per cycle than occur naturally. Ovarian epithelial cells proliferate after ovulation to cover the exposed surface of the ovary. In some instances, epithelium may be incorporated into the ovarian stroma to form epithelial inclusion cysts. These inclusion cysts have been suspected to be the areas most likely to undergo malignant transformation. Anxiety concerning a possible effect of ovulation induction on the development of ovarian cancer was raised following publication of an analysis of pooled data from case–control studies in this area.[12] Recently, however, a study including 54 362 women with infertility problems referred to Danish fertility clinics from 1963 to 1998,[13] found that use of four groups of fertility drugs (gonadotrophins, clomifenes, human chorionic gonadotrophin and gonadotrophin-releasing hormone) was not associated with an overall increase in the risk of ovarian cancer.

> **KEY POINTS**
>
> **Complications of assisted reproduction**
> - The surest way of avoiding OHSS is to withhold the hCG injection.
> - The use of clomiphene citrate should be restricted to six months to avoid the risk of ovarian epithelial neoplasia.
> - More evidence is needed to establish any potential risk of ovarian neoplasia caused by externally administered gonadotrophins.

## ETHICAL ISSUES

From the outset, human use of assisted conception technology brought with it numerous ethical concerns. A detailed review of this aspect of ART practice is beyond the scope of this chapter, but certain controversial areas stand out as frequently encountered ethical problems in clinical practice. These include problems of funding and access to treatment, payment for donors and the use of donated gametes, fetal reduction and human embryo research. These aspects are discussed here as examples of the ethical dilemmas that can occur.

## Funding issues

In the UK, the limited resources of the National Health Service have dictated the government position on funding infertility treatment. In some parts of the country, patients have limited access to NHS funding for IVF. Such funds are rationed by restrictive eligibility criteria, usually a mixture of factors relating to the chance of success (female age, normal body mass) and social criteria (neither partner should have a child already, no funding if either partner has been sterilized). The absence of a national policy on funding infertility treatment, coupled with overt rationing of access where some funds are available, has led to a protracted public debate. The National Institute for Health and Clinical Excellence (NICE) has now produced guidance in this area, which may help to resolve some of the discrepancies between regions.

### Payment for donors

The HFEA Act (1990) stipulates that no money or other benefits should be given or received for supplying gametes or embryos, other than expenses and nominal fees. This has little effect on the number of volunteers offering to donate sperm, a procedure that is free of risk to the health of the donor. In contrast, oocyte donation carries significant risks of side effects of ovarian stimulation and oocyte recovery. Some have argued that oocyte donors should be allowed to receive payment to compensate them for the risk they encounter. To overcome the shortage of egg donors, egg sharing has also been allowed by the HFEA.

## Fetal reduction

Assisted conception has increased the risk of multiple pregnancies, with the attendant increase in perinatal mortality and morbidity and cost to the health service. Even with strict embryo transfer policy, the risk of triplet pregnancy, although significantly reduced, cannot be completely eliminated. If a higher order multiple pregnancy does occur, this can be reduced by selective fetal reduction. This is a difficult decision, made harder by the many years of unsuccessful treatment that may have led up to the pregnancy. The objective of fetal reduction is to reduce the perinatal mortality and morbidity associated with high-order multiple pregnancies. In most cases, triplets and quadruplet pregnancies are reduced to twins, but occasionally some couples request the reduction of twins to a singleton pregnancy. Selective fetal reduction is usually carried out at the beginning of the second trimester to allow for spontaneous reduction in some cases to take place. However, this is too early to screen for congenital anomaly. The procedure is not without risk and complete miscarriage can be a very distressing consequence in about 15 per cent of cases. Careful, sympathetic counselling is obviously vital before selective reduction is undertaken.

## Embryo cryopreservation

Cryopreservation of extra embryos allows more cycles of embryo transfer from one IVF cycle. Although the success rate for frozen embryo transfer may be inferior to that for fresh cycles, such practice increases the potential success rate obtained from a single IVF cycle. So far, no risk has been linked to embryo freezing. The couple's consent should be obtained prior to freezing any embryos. Furthermore, the potential ethical issues that may arise should be carefully discussed with the couple, especially the fate of the embryos if either partner were to die or become mentally incapacitated.

## Embryo research

Research on human embryos has been licensed by the HFEA since its inception in 1990. Study protocols are only approved if they ask questions that cannot be answered using other methods. Until recently, most human embryo research was directly linked to improving the outcomes of infertility treatment, for example in the development of PGD or the study of embryo and blastocyst culture conditions. The recent surge of interest in the therapeutic use of human embryonic stem cells has stimulated a heated debate on the ethics of using 'spare' IVF embryos for the creation of stem cell lines, resulting in a House of Lords' ruling that such research can be carried out within the UK within strict guidelines and governance.

## Human Fertilisation and Embryology Authority

The UK HFEA replaced the Voluntary Licensing Authority established by the Warnock Committee following passage of the Human Fertilisation and Embryology Act in 1990. The role of the HFEA is to monitor and licence centres that offer IVF treatment or deal with human gametes or embryos. The licence given to centres by the HFEA is subject to renewal after the inspection of the relevant centre. The HFEA also regulates research on human embryos and gametes. The organization is largely funded by fees paid by couples undergoing treatment. The HFEA has a code of practice that guides licensed centres, and publishes on its website the results of all centres that offer IVF and gamete donation along with a patient guide (‹www.hfea.gov.uk›).

## ACKNOWLEDGEMENT

This chapter has been revised and updated. The author and editors acknowledge the contribution of Hany AMA Lashen to the chapter on this topic in the previous edition of the book.

### KEY POINTS

- Counselling is at the heart of ART treatment.
- IVF is effective in treating all types of infertility, with similar success rates.
- It is clear from the available evidence that eSET can be offered to a significant subgroup of patients without jeopardising live-birth rates.
- OHSS can be prevented by withholding hCG injection. However, its severity could be reduced by freezing all the embryos and not proceeding with fresh ET.
- OHSS is a potentially life-threatening condition. Anticipation of its occurrence, early diagnosis and appropriate management are essential to avoid any fatalities.
- Clomiphene citrate should be given for a total period of no longer than 12 months.
- Every clinician should be aware of all the ethical issues surrounding ART, as it represents a key issue when counselling patients for such treatment modalities.

## Key References

1. Cole HH, Hart GH. The potency of blood serum of mares in progressive stages of pregnancy in effecting the sexual maturity of the immature rat. *Am J Physiol* 1930; **93**: 57–68.
2. Davis ME, Koff AK. The experimental production of ovulation in the human subject. *Am J Obstet Gynecol* 1938; **36**: 183–99.
3. Siegler SL, Fein MJ. Studies in artificial ovulation with the hormone of pregnant mares' serum. *Am J Obstet Gynecol* 1939; **38**: 1021–36.
4. Gemzel CA, Diczfalusi E, Tillinger G. Clinical effect of human pituitary follicle stimulating hormone (FSH). *J Clin Endocrinol Metab* 1958; **18**: 1333–48.
5. Jones HW Jr, Jones SG, Andrews MC *et al.* The programme for *in vitro* fertilisation at Norfolk. *Fertil Steril* 1982; **38**: 14–21.
6. Garcia J, Jones G, Acosta A *et al.* Human menopausal gonadotrophin–human chorionic gonadotrophin follicular maturation for oocyte aspiration: phase II 1981. *Fertil Steril* 1983; **39**: 174–9.
7. Shaw RW, Ndukwe G, Imoedemhe DA *et al.* Twin pregnancy after pituitary desensitisation with LHRH agonist and pure FSH. *Lancet* 1985; **2**: 506.
8. Out HJ, Mannaerts B, Driessen S *et al.* Recombinant follicle stimulating hormone (rFSH: Puregon) in assisted reproduction: more oocytes, more pregnancies. Results from five comparative studies. *Hum Reprod Update* 1996; **2**: 162–71.
9. Schally AV, Kastin AJ, Arimura A. Hypothalamic FSH and LH-regulating hormone: structure, physiology and clinical studies. *Fertil Steril* 1971; **22**: 703–21.
10. Hughes EG, Sagle MA, Fedorkow DM *et al.* The routine use of gonadotropin-releasing hormone agonists prior to *in vitro* fertilization and gamete intrafallopian transfer: a meta-analysis of randomized controlled trials. *Fertil Steril* 1992; **58**: 888–95.
11. Golan A, Ron-El R, Herman A *et al.* Ovarian hyperstimulation syndrome: an update review. *Obstet Gynaecol Survey* 1989; **6**: 430–40.
12. Thurin Kjellberg A, Carlsson P, Bergh C. Randomized single versus double embryo transfer: obstetric and paediatric outcome and a cost-effectiveness analysis. *Hum Reprod* 2006; **21**: 210–16.
13. Jensen A, Sharif H, Frederiksen K, Kjaer SK. Use of fertility drugs and risk of ovarian cancer: Danish population based cohort study. *BMJ* 2009; **338**: b249.

# Polycystic ovarian syndrome

*Mostafa Metwally and William Ledger*

## MRCOG standards

### Theoretical skills

- Revise the normal physiology of ovulation and steroid formation.
- Understand the difficulty in defining polycystic ovarian syndrome (PCOS).
- Be able to discuss the importance of lifestyle/ environmental factors on the progress of PCOS.
- Understand how androgens are formed in the female, and their mode of action.

### Practical skills

- Be able to describe the classical ultrasound appearance of polycystic ovaries.
- Know the different types of drugs used in the management of PCOS, the indications for use and their mode of action.

## INTRODUCTION

Polycystic ovarian syndrome (PCOS) is a common endocrine disorder, affecting women of reproductive age. The syndrome is characterized by chronic oligo/anovulation and a variable combination of symptoms, including menstrual disturbances, obesity and hyperandrogenism. Stein and Leventhal first described the syndrome in 1935 and since then our understanding of the spectrum of disorders involved in this condition has evolved dramatically. However, many aspects of this common condition remain obscure.

## DEFINITIONS

Over the years, the definition of PCOS has evolved considerably. This is due to the fact that the syndrome encompasses a wide spectrum of clinical and biochemical findings making it difficult to define a 'core' condition. Following an international conference on PCOS sponsored by the US National Institute of Health (NIH), a consensus statement defined PCOS by the presence of the following criteria and after exclusion of other possible causes:

- Hyperandrogenism and/or hyperandrogenaemia
- Menstrual dysfunction

It has since been recognized that the spectrum of disorders was larger than encompassed by the previous definition. The most recent definition was set out during a consensus meeting by the American Society of Reproductive Medicine (ASRM) and the European Society of Human Reproduction and Embryology (ESHRE) in Rotterdam in May 2003.[1] Based on the modified criteria defined at this meeting, the diagnosis of PCOS is made when two out of three of the following criteria are found:

1. Clinical or biochemical evidence of androgen excess after the exclusion of other related disorders.
2. Oligo and/or anovulation.
3. Ultrasound appearance of the ovaries: presence of >12 follicles in each ovary measuring 2–9 mm and/or increased ovarian volume (>10 mL).

It is important to note that these ultrasound findings do not apply in women taking the oral contraceptive pill. Also, if a dominant follicle is found, then the scan needs to be repeated in the next cycle (Figure 53.1).

It is important to note that certain previous diagnostic criteria, such as increased luteinizing hormone (LH) concentrations, increased LH/FSH ratio and the peripheral distribution of the follicles on ultrasound scan, are no longer necessary to make the diagnosis.

The overlap in ultrasound, biochemical and clinical features of the syndrome and the realization that the condition is a continuum or spectrum can confuse diagnosis in 'non-classical' cases, and it is likely that the condition is often over-diagnosed.

## PREVALENCE

Based on the earlier NIH definition, PCOS is thought to occur in about 6–8 per cent of women worldwide, making

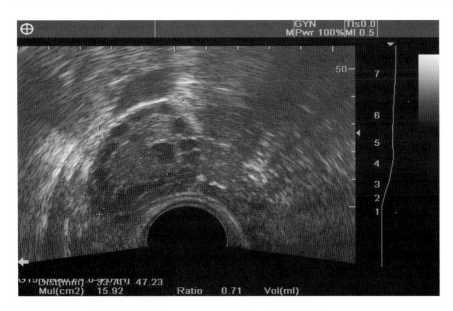

**Figure 53.1** Ultrasound appearance of a polycystic ovary

it the most common reproductive disorder. However, when applying the new Rotterdam/ESHRE criteria, it is likely that the prevalence is even higher. The prevalence is also higher in certain ethnic groups, such as South Asians, who may also suffer from more severe symptoms.

## AETIOLOGY AND PATHOPHYSIOLOGY

The aetiology of PCOS is largely unknown, but seems to involve a complex interaction between environmental (e.g. diet and exercise) and multiple genetic factors. The mode of inheritance appears akin to an autosomal dominant pattern.

Several factors have been implicated in the pathogenesis of PCOS, including a dysfunction of ovarian function characterized by increased production of ovarian androgens, a dysfunction in hypothalamic function resulting in increased LH secretion which in turn stimulates androgen production by the theca cells (Figure 53.2) and insulin resistance which is a characteristic of both obese and non-obese PCOS patients.

The exact mechanism of insulin resistance is not entirely understood. In obese patients, it may be a consequence of alteration in some of the adipokines; a range of diverse proteins produced by the adipose tissue. One particular adipokine, resistin, has been related to insulin resistance.

In non-obese PCOS patients, the mechanism is less clear, although it is possible that some form of adipose cell dysfunction still exists.[2] Other possible causes include β-cell dysfunction, increased insulin secretion in response to dietary stimuli, decreased hepatic clearance of insulin and deficient insulin action.[3–7]

Hyperinsulinaemia then leads to hyperandrogenism by inhibition of the hepatic production of sex hormone-binding globulin and insulin-like growth factor binding protein-I and stimulation of ovarian P450c17α activity.[8]

Hyperandrogenism can then lead to anovulation by inducing granulosa cell apoptosis. An increase in the peripheral conversion of androgens to oestrogen will also lead to an increase in the negative feedback on gonadotropin secretion.

## OTHER MANIFESTATIONS OF POLYCYSTIC OVARIAN SYNDROME

### Obesity

Obesity and PCOS are closely related conditions, and 50 per cent or more of patients with PCOS are obese. The onset of obesity around puberty may be related to the occurrence of PCOS later in life. It is not known which of these two conditions is the precursor of the other. Obesity may be a result of hyperinsulinaemia or problems with energy balance.

### The metabolic syndrome

Women suffering from insulin resistance are at an increased risk of developing the metabolic syndrome characterized by type 2 diabetes, hypertension, dyslipidaemia, atherosclerosis and ischaemic heart disease.

### Dermatological manifestations

PCOS can be associated with a number of dermatological manifestations that are a reflection of the metabolic and biochemical disturbances. The most common of these is hirsutism (Chapter 54, Virilism and hirsutism). Other changes include oily skin, seborrhoea, alopecia, acne and acanthosis nigricans. Hirsutism, acne, alopecia and oily skin are all manifestations of hyperandrogenism. The

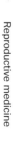

Reproductive medicine

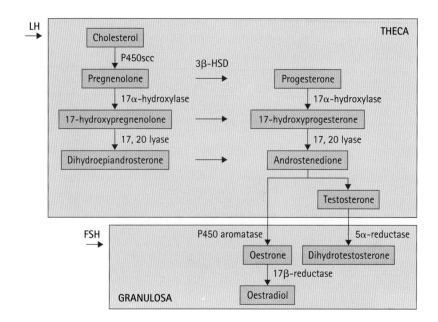

**Figure 53.2** Steroid production in the ovary. FSH, follicle-stimulating hormone; HSD, hydroxysteroid dehydrogenase; LH, luteinizing hormone

'SAHA' syndrome is a combination of seborrhoea, acne, hirsutism and alopecia and is associated with PCOS, cystic mastitis, obesity and infertility. On the other hand, acanthosis nigricans, which is characterized by pigmented, velvety skin patches in the axilla, nape of the neck, antecubital fossa and groin, is a marker of insulin resistance. Its presence also helps differentiate hirsutism due to PCOS from that due to androgenic secreting ovarian tumours in which it is absent.[9]

## MANAGEMENT

The treatment of PCOS depends on whether or not fertility is desired. If fertility were required then the aim would be to induce ovulation using oral anti-oestrogens, gonadotropins or more recently aromatase inhibitors. Insulin-sensitizing agents are also now commonly used to reduce insulin resistance and consequent hyperandrogenism. Induction of ovulation may also be induced surgically using laparoscopic ovarian drilling. Even if normalization of ovulation is not required, then it is still important to protect the endometrium against the long-term effects of prolonged unopposed oestrogen using, for example, progestagens or the oral contraceptive pill. The presence of obesity further compounds the problem and should be addressed in all cases.

### Treatment of obesity

#### Lifestyle changes

In obese PCOS patients, weight loss is the cornerstone of treatment, where even a small amount of weight loss can lead to the spontaneous resumption of ovulation.[10] Weight loss is also important prior to conception to minimize the associated risks of maternal and fetal morbidities that can occur during pregnancy and delivery.

Weight loss is best achieved through a combination of diet and exercise. Various diets have been investigated in different studies, but so far there is no substantive evidence to favour one diet over the other. A summary of some studies investigating different diets is seen in Table 53.1. Similarly, there is no evidence to prescribe a particular programme of physical activity; however, as little as 1 hour per week of rigorous activity can lead to a 5 per cent drop in the risk of anovulatory infertility.[11]

### Pharmacological agents

Some obese PCOS patients, however, will find it difficult to achieve adequate weight loss with diet and exercise alone in which case the use of weight-losing drugs may be indicated. There are two weight-losing drugs currently licensed in the United Kingdom, the centrally acting serotonin and norepinephrine uptake inhibitor, sibutramine, and the peripherally acting lipase inhibitor, orlistat. Both medications have been shown to be effective at producing a modest weight loss together with a well-balanced diet. However, in PCOS patients, it needs to be remembered that fertility treatment is often the main target and therefore the safety of these drugs in the presence of an early pregnancy needs to be considered. Although there is no definitive evidence, it seems that the pharmacokinetics of orlistat make it a favourable option since only about 1 per cent of the drug is absorbed into the systemic circulation. The main side effect of orlistat is gastrointestinal disturbance that can be limited with the use of a low fat diet.

Recently, another centrally acting anti-obesity agent, rimonabant, has been withdrawn from the EU market due to reports of serious side effects, including psychiatric disorders.

**Table 53.1** Summary of some studies investigating the effect of different diets in women with polycystic ovarian syndrome

| Study | Type of diet | Study design | Main finding(s) |
|---|---|---|---|
| Mavropoulos et al.[28] | LCKD | Cohort study | Significant improvement in: Weight  Free testosterone  LH/FSH ratio  Fasting insulin |
| Stamets et al.[29] | Low energy high protein diet vs low energy high carbohydrate diet | RCT | No evidence for a difference between the two diets |
| Moran et al.[30] | High protein vs low protein diet | RCT | Minor endocrine and metabolic advantages for the high protein diet |
| Douglas et al.[8] | Eucaloric MUFA vs eucaloric low carbohydrate diet | Cross-over study | Lower fasting insulin concentrations after the low carbohydrate diet |
| Kasim-Karakas et al.[31] | PUFA diet | Cohort | Higher fasting glucose concentrations |
|  |  |  | No change in sex steroid hormone profile |

- FSH, follicle stimulating hormone; LCKD, low-carbohydrate ketogenic diet; LH, luteinizing hormone; MUFA, monounsaturated fatty acids; PUFA, polyunsaturated fatty acids; RCT, randomized controlled trials.

## Bariatric surgery

The guidelines of the National Institute for Health and Clinical Excellence (NICE) state that, 'Surgery is recommended as a treatment option for people with morbid obesity (body mass index equal to or greater than 40 kg/m²) or with a body mass index (BMI) equal to or greater than 35 kg/m² in the presence of significant co-morbid conditions that could be improved by weight loss'. Laparoscopic adjustable gastric banding (LAGB) is a technique particularly suitable for women with fertility problems, since the band tightness can be varied to accommodate the increased demands of pregnancy when it occurs.

There is still controversy regarding the outcome of this technique should pregnancy occur during the period of weight loss. Since weight loss after banding is often rapid, it seems prudent to suggest that the couple delay trying to conceive for a few months after banding, even if regular menses resume, since the obstetric consequences of morbid obesity will be avoided if weight is normalized before conception.

## Ovulation induction

### Anti-oestrogens

Clomifene citrate has been used for ovulation induction in women with anovulatory infertility for over 40 years. On the hypothalamus, clomifene binds to and blocks oestrogen receptors leading to a release of the pituitary gland from the negative feedback by circulating oestrogen. This results in an increase in GnRH pulse amplitude and consequent increase in follicle stimulating hormone (FSH)

secretion leading to follicular growth. Clomifene citrate can be offered for 6–12 months provided there is evidence for ovulation. The main side effect is that of multiple pregnancies, which may occur in 6–8 per cent of cases; hence, the rationale of offering ultrasound cycle monitoring at least in the first cycle to ensure monofollicular development.

A potential problem in obese PCOS patients is that of clomifene resistance and hence again the importance of weight loss in these patients prior to starting ovulation induction. Tamoxifen is another anti-oestrogen similar to clomifene. Available evidence suggests that both tamoxifen and clomifene are equally effective [A].[12,13]

### Gonadotropins

Ovulation induction using FSH is mainly indicated in cases of clomifene resistance and in those who fail to conceive or have intolerable side effects with clomifene. Gonadotropin therapy is associated with an increased risk of multiple follicular development and multiple pregnancies. Furthermore, PCOS patients are particularly prone to ovarian hyperstimulation syndrome (OHSS), a serious complication of ovarian stimulation. This condition can vary in severity from mild to severe and is caused by the release of vasoactive substances that lead to third space fluid loss and multi-organ dysfunction. The risk of severe OHSS is about 5–8 per cent and is a life-threatening condition, unless appropriate measures such as fluid control and anti-coagulant measures are taken.[14] The tendency of PCOS patients to over-respond to gonadotropin treatment is mainly due to the altered FSH threshold, which is the FSH concentration that needs to be reached before follicular development occurs. Patients with PCOS have an increased threshold that may lead to multifollicular rather than monofollicular development. Furthermore, polycystic ovaries may also have an increased sensitivity to gonadotropins partially due to the larger size of the FSH sensitive cohort of small antral follicles. Careful monitoring of treatment and dosage manipulation is therefore necessary.

## GnRH agonists

The pulsatile use of GnRH agonists using a subcutaneous pump can lead to monofollicular growth, while minimizing the risks of multiple pregnancies and OHSS. Its main use is in women with hypogonadoptropic hypogonadism; however, in women with PCOS, there is no clear evidence that GnRH treatment is associated with better pregnancy rates compared to gonadotropins alone or in combination. The use of the pump can be uncomfortable and the response to treatment unpredictable. For these reasons, its use in PCOS patients cannot currently be recommended [A].[15]

## Aromatase inhibitors

The use of the third-generation aromatase inhibitors, anastrozole and letrozole, is a novel approach to ovulation induction. These drugs inhibit ovarian aromatase activity leading to a decrease in circulating oestradiol concentrations and a consequent increase in FSH release, leading to follicular growth. Central negative feedback on FSH secretion is maintained, thus limiting multifollicular development. It follows that the risk of OHSS and multiple pregnancies is also much lower than with clomifene. Unlike clomifene, these drugs do not have an anti-oestrogenic effect on the endometrium or cervical mucus. The evidence so far suggests that letrozole is as effective as clomifene for inducing ovulation, although further randomized controlled trials (RCT) are needed before a definitive conclusion can be drawn [A].[13,16] Aromatase inhibitors are not licensed for use in the treatment of anovulation.

## Insulin sensitizing agents

Metformin, a biguanide, is the most common sensitizing agent used for ovulation induction in PCOS patients. Metformin has been used for ovulation induction either as a first-line therapy, a second-line therapy or in combination with clomifene. However, recent evidence has cast doubt on the benefit gained from using metformin as a first-line therapy or in combination with clomifene [B].[17] With the exception of patients with clomifene resistance where there is some evidence that a combination of clomifene with metformin may be beneficial,[18,19] the current evidence does not support using metformin as a first-line single agent or combination therapy with clomifene and supports the use of metformin only as a second-line therapy.

It is also controversial whether obese or non-obese PCOS patients would benefit more from metformin. Some studies have shown that non-obese patients respond better,[20] while others have shown an opposite effect.[21]

The exact mechanism of action of metformin in PCOS patients is not clearly defined, although there is a clear advantage from the insulin-sensitizing effect of this drug. Although controversial, metformin may also assist weight loss. A recent randomized controlled study has compared metformin to orlistat in the management of obese anovulatory women, most of them suffering from PCOS, and has shown that both drugs have a similar effect on ovulation rates, as well as producing a similar reduction in weight and testosterone concentrations.[22] Other studies, however, have not shown any effect for metformin on BMI.[23]

Current evidence also suggests that metformin is safe if taken while trying to conceive and if continued into the first trimester, may decrease the risk of miscarriage in obese patients [D].[24,25] However, more studies are needed to clarify its effect on pregnancy outcomes.

A second insulin sensitizing agent, rosiglitazone, is not recommended for use due to concerns regarding an increased risk of myocardial infarction.

## Laparoscopic ovarian drilling

Laparoscopic ovarian drilling (LOD) is mainly indicated in clomifene-resistant patients where it has been shown to have a similar efficacy to gonadotropins with the advantage of a lower multiple pregnancy rate [A].[26] LOD can result in ovulation in approximately 80 per cent and a clinical pregnancy in 60 per cent of cases. Apart from inducing ovulation, LOD can also lead to correction of the biochemical abnormalities in PCOS, such as high LH and androgen concentrations.

The exact mechanism by which LOD may stimulate ovulation is not entirely known, but it is possible that the thermal damage associated with the procedure may lead to release of inflammatory intra-ovarian cytokines, with a paracrine effect on androgen production and eventual normalization of pituitary LH secretion. Patients with high LH are more likely to respond to LOD, while those with marked obesity, marked hyperandrogenism and/or long duration of infertility are more likely to be resistant.[27]

## KEY POINTS

- PCOS involves a wide spectrum of biochemical and clinical disorders.
- PCOS can result from an interaction between multiple environmental and genetic factors.
- Insulin resistance is a key factor in the pathogenesis of PCOS.
- Long-term consequences are related to the effects of prolonged unopposed oestrogen and effects of the metabolic syndrome.

- Management depends on whether or not fertility is desired.
- Clomifene citrate and tamoxifen remain the first option for first-line ovulation induction.
- In patients with clomifene resistance, options for ovulation induction include metformin or LOD.
- Weight loss remains the cornerstone for improving the ovulatory status and minimizing the long-term effects of PCOS in obese patients.

# Key References

1. Rotterdam ESHRE/ASRM-Sponsored PCOS consensus workshop group. Revised 2003 consensus on diagnostic criteria and long-term health risks related to polycystic ovary syndrome (PCOS). *Hum Reprod* 2004; **19**: 41–7.
2. Carmina E, Orio F, Palomba S *et al.* Evidence for altered adipocyte function in polycystic ovary syndrome. *Eur J Endocrinol* 2005; **152**: 389–94.
3. Wang JX, Warnes GW, Davies MJ, Norman RJ. Overweight infertile patients have a higher fecundity than normal-weight women undergoing controlled ovarian hyperstimulation with intrauterine insemination. *Fertil Steril* 2004; **81**: 1710–12.
4. Ehrmann DA, Liljenquist DR, Kasza K *et al.* Prevalence and predictors of the metabolic syndrome in women with polycystic ovary syndrome. *J Clin Endocrinol Metab* 2006; **91**: 48–53.
5. Hirschberg AL, Naessen S, Stridsberg M *et al.* Impaired cholecystokinin secretion and disturbed appetite regulation in women with polycystic ovary syndrome. *Gynecol Endocrinol* 2004; **19**: 79–87.
6. Ciampelli M, Fulghesu AM, Cucinelli F *et al.* Heterogeneity in beta cell activity, hepatic insulin clearance and peripheral insulin sensitivity in women with polycystic ovary syndrome. *Hum Reprod* 1997; **12**: 1897–901.
7. Dunaif A, Xia J, Book CB *et al.* Excessive insulin receptor serine phosphorylation in cultured fibroblasts and in skeletal muscle. A potential mechanism for insulin resistance in the polycystic ovary syndrome. *J Clin Invest* 1995; **96**: 801–10.
8. Douglas CC, Gower BA, Darnell BE *et al.* Role of diet in the treatment of polycystic ovary syndrome. *Fertil Steril* 2006; **85**: 679–88.
9. Lowenstein EJ. Diagnosis and management of the dermatologic manifestations of the polycystic ovary syndrome. *Dermatol Ther* 2006; **19**: 210–23.
10. Clark AM, Ledger W, Galletly C *et al.* Weight loss results in significant improvement in pregnancy and ovulation rates in anovulatory obese women. *Hum Reprod* 1995; **10**: 2705–12.
11. Rich-Edwards JW, Spiegelman D, Garland M *et al.* Physical activity, body mass index, and ovulatory disorder infertility. *Epidemiology* 2002; **13**: 184–90.
12. Steiner AZ, Terplan M, Paulson RJ. Comparison of tamoxifen and clomiphene citrate for ovulation induction: a meta-analysis. *Hum Reprod* 2005; **20**: 1511–15.
13. Beck JI, Boothroyd C, Proctor M *et al.* Oral anti-oestrogens and medical adjuncts for subfertility associated with anovulation. *Cochrane Database Syst Rev* 2005; (**4**): CD002249.
14. Royal College of Obstetricians and Gynaecologists. The management of ovarian hyperstimulation syndrome. Green Top Guideline No. 5. London: RCOG, 2006.
15. Bayram N, van Wely M, van der Veen F. Pulsatile gonadotrophin releasing hormone for ovulation induction in subfertility associated with polycystic ovary syndrome. *Cochrane Database Syst Rev* 2004; (**2**): CD000412.
16. Requena A, Herrero J, Landeras J *et al.* Use of letrozole in assisted reproduction: a systematic review and meta-analysis. *Hum Reprod Update* 2008; **14**: 571–82.
17. Legro RS, Barnhart HX, Schlaff WD *et al.* Clomiphene, metformin, or both for infertility in the polycystic ovary syndrome. *N Engl J Med* 2007; **356**: 551–66.
18. Khorram O, Helliwell JP, Katz S *et al.* Two weeks of metformin improves clomiphene citrate-induced ovulation and metabolic profiles in women with polycystic ovary syndrome. *Fertil Steril* 2006; **85**: 1448–51.
19. Moll E, Bossuyt PM, Korevaar JC *et al.* Effect of clomifene citrate plus metformin and clomifene citrate plus placebo on induction of ovulation in women with newly diagnosed polycystic ovary syndrome: randomised double blind clinical trial. *BMJ* 2006; **332**: 1485.
20. Maciel GA, Soares Jr JM, Alves da Motta EL *et al.* Nonobese women with polycystic ovary syndrome respond better than obese women to treatment with metformin. *Fertil Steril* 2004; **81**: 355–60.
21. Moghetti P, Castello R, Negri C *et al.* Metformin effects on clinical features, endocrine and metabolic profiles, and insulin sensitivity in polycystic ovary syndrome: a randomized, double-blind, placebo-controlled 6-month trial, followed by open, long-term clinical evaluation. *J Clin Endocrinol Metab* 2000; **85**: 139–46.
22. Metwally M, Amer S, Li TC *et al.* An RCT of metformin versus orlistat for the management of obese anovulatory women. *Hum Reprod* 2009; **24**: 966–75.
23. Lord JM, Flight IH, Norman RJ. Metformin in polycystic ovary syndrome: systematic review and meta-analysis. *BMJ* 2003; **327**: 951–3.
24. Turner MJ, Walsh J, Byrne KM *et al.* Outcome of clinical pregnancies after ovulation induction using metformin. *J Obstet Gynaecol* 2006; **26**: 233–5.
25. Thatcher SS, Jackson EM. Pregnancy outcome in infertile patients with polycystic ovary syndrome who were treated with metformin. *Fertil Steril* 2006; **85**: 1002–9.
26. Farquhar C, Lilford RJ, Marjoribanks J, Vandekerckhove P. Laparoscopic 'drilling' by diathermy or laser for ovulation induction in anovulatory polycystic ovary syndrome. *Cochrane Database Syst Rev* 2007; (**3**): CD001122.

Reproductive medicine

27. Amer SA, Li TC, Ledger WL. Ovulation induction using laparoscopic ovarian drilling in women with polycystic ovarian syndrome: predictors of success. *Hum Reprod* 2004; **19**: 1719–24.

28. Mavropoulos JC, Yancy WS, Hepburn J, Westman EC. The effects of a low-carbohydrate, ketogenic diet on the polycystic ovary syndrome: A pilot study. *Nutr Metab (Lond)* 2005; **2**: 35.

29. Stamets K, Taylor DS, Kunselman A *et al*. A randomized trial of the effects of two types of short-term hypocaloric diets on weight loss in women with polycystic ovary syndrome. *Fertil Steril* 2004; **81**: 630–7.

30. Moran LJ, Noakes M, Clifton PM *et al*. Dietary composition in restoring reproductive and metabolic physiology in overweight women with polycystic ovary syndrome. *J Clin Endocrinol Metab* 2003; **88**: 812–19.

31. Kasim-Karakas SE, Almario RU, Gregory L *et al*. Metabolic and endocrine effects of a polyunsaturated fatty acid-rich diet in polycystic ovary syndrome. *J Clin Endocrinol Metab* 2004; **89**: 615–20.

# Hirsutism and virilism

*Mostafa Metwally and William Ledger*

---

# HIRSUTISM

## Definition

Hirsutism is defined as male pattern hair growth in a female as a result of increased androgen production or increased skin sensitivity to circulating androgens. Hirsutism must be differentiated from hypertrichosis, which is a generalized non-sexual (vellus) hair growth that may be hereditary, a result of various medications or malignancies. It is important to recognize that hirsutism in itself is not a diagnosis but rather a manifestation of a large spectrum of abnormalities; so careful searching for the underlying cause is essential.

## The physiology of hair growth

Adults have two types of hair, vellus and terminal. Vellus hair is the fine lightly pigmented hair that covers most areas of the body during the prepubertal years, while terminal hair, that is referred to by the term 'hirsutism', is the thick pigmented hair normally present on the face, limbs, axilla and pubic area. Terminal hair is androgen dependent and is influenced by genetic and racial factors.

Hair growth is a dynamic process and can be divided into three distinct phases. The relative duration of these different stages influences the length and appearance of hair in different parts of the body:

1 *Anagen*: This is the growing phase during which active mitotic division occurs in the basal matrix. This stage is relatively long in areas such as the scalp where hair appears to be continuously growing. Similarly, facial hair also has a long growth phase, which is why the effects of therapy require six to nine months before becoming apparent.[1] Consequently, the focus of hirsutism treatment is to shorten this phase.[2]
2 *Catagen*: During this phase, hair growth ceases and the hair follicle prepares to enter the resting (telogen) phase.
3 *Telogen*: During this resting phase, the hair is short and loosely attached to be ultimately expelled as the follicle again enters the anagen phase and a new hair starts growing.

## Incidence

It is difficult to state exactly the prevalence of hirsutism since it is highly variable depending on the studied ethnic group, being higher in those of African or Mediterranean origin. The condition, however, is believed to affect 5–10 per cent of women of reproductive age.[3]

## Female androgens and hair growth

Pivotal to the understanding of hirsutism is an understanding of the metabolism of androgens in the female and how they can affect hair growth. Female androgens are produced by two sources, namely the ovaries and adrenal glands. The ovaries produce testosterone and androstendione, whilst the adrenals produce androstendione and dehydroepiandrosterone (DHEA). Testosterone in the ovary is produced by the theca cells under the control of luteinizing hormone (LH) and insulin acting through insulin-like growth factor

1 (IGF-1). Testosterone is then converted by the granulosa cells to oestradiol. This transition of the ovarian environment from androgen dominant to oestrogen dominant is vital to normal ovulation and ovarian function. In conditions such as polycystic ovarian syndrome (PCOS) where this process is disturbed, there is a relative increase in ovarian androgen production. Adrenal androgens are also peripherally converted to testosterone, which then circulates in two forms, an inactive form bound to sex hormone binding globulin (SHBG) and a metabolically active free form. To stimulate hair growth, free testosterone needs to be further metabolized at the level of the hair follicle into a more active form, dihydrotestosterone (DHT) by the enzyme, 5α reductase. Consequently, hirsutism can be caused by any of the following disturbances:

- Increased production of adrenal or ovarian androgens: Adrenal androgens can increase in Cushing's syndrome, delayed onset congenital adrenal hyperplasia (CAH) and androgen producing adrenal tumours. However, the most common cause in clinical practice is an increased production of ovarian and to a lesser extent adrenal androgens as a result of PCOS.
- An increase in the free fraction of testosterone due to a decreased concentration of SHBG despite normal testosterone production. Decreased SHBG can occur due to increased insulin concentrations in women with insulin resistance, which again is a common finding in women with PCOS.[4]
- An increased local activity of 5α reductase. Two forms of this enzyme exist, type 1 and type 2. Type 1 is mainly present in the sebaceous gland, while type 2 is found mainly in the hair follicle. Relative activity of these isoenzymes can lead to a discrepancy between the severity of hirsutism and acne in women with hyperandrogenism.[5] In PCOS, women – especially those who are obese or are insulin resistant – insulin and insulin-like growth factor (IGF) act to stimulate this enzyme.
- Iatrogenic hirsutism can be caused by the administration of certain medications, such as danazol, androgen therapy, sodium valporate and anabolic steroids.

## Clinical assessment of hirsutism

### History

A detailed history should include the following:

- The severity and duration of hirsutism, as well as the presence of any other symptoms of virilization. Rapidly progressive virilization or severe hirsutism point to the possibility of a more ominous cause, such as an ovarian or adrenal tumour.
- Associated menstrual disturbances or history of infertility may point to chronic anovulation as a result of PCOS.
- History suggestive of other related medical conditions, such as Cushing's syndrome or hypothyroidism.
- Medications such as steroids, androgen therapy or danazol.

## Examination

- Evaluation of the severity of hirsutism is commonly performed using the Ferriman–Gallwey scoring system. The score includes an evaluation of nine androgen-sensitive body areas. Each area is assigned a score from 0 to 4 and the scores are then added. A minimal score of 8 is required for the diagnosis of hirsutism. The disadvantages of this method are that it does not account for focal hirsutism. In addition, it ignores some androgen sensitive areas, such as the buttocks and side burns.[1]
- General examination may show other manifestations of androgen excess, such as acne or even signs of virilization (e.g. clitoromegaly).
- The presence of velvety, pigmented skin patches (acanthosis nigricans) in the groin, neck or axillae may point to associated insulin resistance. The combination of hirsutism together with acanthosis nigricans and insulin resistance is a hereditary condition known as HAIR-AN syndrome. It is possibly due to an insulin receptor defect and can be associated with severe hirsutism.[6]
- Pelvic examination in severe cases may reveal the presence of a pelvic mass (androgen producing ovarian tumour).

## Investigations

- Testosterone concentrations: The need to measure testosterone concentrations in patients with mild isolated hirsutism is debatable, since over half of these women will have normal concentrations and results are unlikely to influence treatment.[1] Testosterone concentrations also correlate poorly with the severity of hirsutism due to individual variations in hair follicle response. Testosterone measurements are however indicated in women with other symptoms, such as menstrual irregularities, infertility, severe hirsutism or in the presence of virilism. Measurement of the free androgen index (FAI) is particularly useful since it reflects changes in SHBG as well as testosterone. Obese and PCOS patients may have an elevated FAI when the testosterone concentrations are normal due to a decrease in SHBG. High testosterone concentrations (>5 mmol/L) may suggest an androgen-producing tumour. DHEA concentrations may also be measured and if markedly elevated may suggest an adrenal cause.
- Baseline 17-OH progesterone measurements should be performed to screen for suspected cases of late onset CAH. Equivocal results will need a short Synacthen test to confirm the diagnosis. After measurement of baseline 17-OH progesterone concentrations, the patient is given an intramuscular injection of 250 mg of Synacthen and measurements are taken again after 1 hour. A significant rise in 17-OH progesterone concentrations is diagnostic of CAH.

- Tests for insulin resistance (75 g GTT and insulin concentrations) are particularly important in PCOS and obese patients.
- Dexamethasone suppression test or 24 hour urinary free cortisol for suspected cases of Cushing's syndrome.
- Pelvic imaging may show the presence of polycystic ovaries or an androgen producing ovarian tumour. More detailed imaging (computed tomography (CT) and magnetic resonance imaging (MRI)) may be required in cases with suspected androgen producing ovarian or adrenal tumours. In cases where imaging is negative, selective venous sampling from the ovarian and adrenal veins may be performed.

## VIRILISM

Hirsutism may occur together with other symptoms of defeminization in a condition known as 'virilism'. Other signs and symptoms include secondary amenorrhoea, male pattern baldness, clitoromegaly and deepening of voice. The condition is far more ominous than hirsutism and usually indicates significant pathology, including the following:

- Androgen producing ovarian and adrenal tumours: This should be suspected in the presence of progressive severe virilization.
- Adult onset CAH: This is most commonly due to 21-hydroxylase deficiency, leading to a blockage of the production of 11-deoxycortisol from 17-OH progesterone with a consequent diversion of steroidogenesis to the androgen pathway.
- XY females with functioning testicles will usually present around the time of puberty with primary amenorrhoea and signs of virilization. The diagnosis can be confirmed with karyotyping.
- Iatrogenic, due to androgen therapy or the use of danazol to treat endometriosis.
- Cushing's syndrome and acromegaly.

## Treatment

In addition to treatment of the excessive hair growth, treatment should be directed to any possible cause. For example, weight loss in obese PCOS patients may improve hirsutism through a decrease in ovarian androgen production, an improvement in insulin resistance and an increase in SHBG (see Chapter 53, Polycystic ovarian syndrome). Treatment of hirsutism can prevent or slow further hair growth but will not treat the already existent hair growth, which will need to be physically removed using a variety of methods, including electrolysis, plucking, waxing, shaving and laser removal. Targeting the hair follicles in the anagen stage can lead to permanent hair removal.[5]

## Pharmacological agents

### Oral contraceptive pill

The oral contraceptive pill (OCP) is usually the first line of therapy, particularly for those requiring contraception or for those with period irregularities.[1] The OCP acts by increasing sex hormone binding globulin thus decreasing the free testosterone fraction. Other actions include antagonising LH stimulated androgen production by the theca cells, a mild decrease in adrenal androgen production and a mild blockage of the androgen receptors.[1] Pills with an oestrogen dominant effect, such as those containing desogesterel, gestodene or norgestimate should be used. Levenorgestrel can oppose the oestrogen-driven increase in SHBG, while norethisterone is an androgen derivative. Pills containing these two progestagens should therefore be avoided. Dianette® is an OCP that contains the progestagen, cyproterone acetate (2 mg) that also has an anti-androgenic effect through gonadotropin inhibition and increased hepatic clearance of androgens. Cyproterone acetate in higher doses (50–100 mg/day) can also be used, but needs to be combined with an effective contraceptive due to the risk of feminization of a male fetus should pregnancy occur. Cyproterone acetate has a long half-life and therefore can be combined with ethinyl oestradiol in a reverse sequential regimen which involves the administration of ethinyl oestradiol 25–50 μg/day from day 5 to day 25 and cyproterone acetate in the first ten days (days 5–15). After improvement, the dose of cyproterone acetate can be decreased (5 mg/day).[1] The efficacy of cyproterone acetate combined with ethinyl oestradiol compared to placebo has been demonstrated in a Cochrane review.[7]

Similar to Dianette is Yasmin®, which contains the progestagen, drosperinone that has an anti-androgen effect through inhibition of ovarian androgen production, as well as blockage of androgen receptors similar to the effect of spironolactone from which it is derived.[5] A recent randomized controlled trial compared two OCPs containing either drosperinone or cyproterone acetate and showed them to be similarly effective.[8]

### Androgen antagonists

These medications are usually used as second-line monotherapy or in combination with the OCP in severe cases. They should be used in combination with an effective contraceptive to avoid feminization of a male fetus. They include the following:

- Spironolactone: This is the most common used antiandrogen due to its relative safety and demonstrated effectiveness.[9] Spironolactone acts by blockage of the androgen receptors and by inhibition of 5α reductase. The effect of spironolactone is dose-dependent[1] and side effects include diuresis and postural hypotension in early stages, as well as menstrual irregularities and rarely hyperkalaemia.[1]
- Flutamide: This is a potent androgen receptor antagonist that can result in hepatotoxicity. Hence, it should only be

Reproductive medicine

used with caution and under tertiary care supervision. The dose varies from 250 to 500 mg/day.[1] Flutamide alone has shown to have similar efficacy to a combination of spironolactone and Dianette.[10,11]

- Finasteride: This is an inhibitor of 5α reductase that is used at dose of 5 mg/day. It can result in mild gastrointestinal disturbances, as well as dry skin and decreased libido.[5] The most important concern, however, is its teratogenicity and hence the importance of effective contraception.

### Eflornithine

Eflornithine (Vaniqa®) is a topical antiprotozoal drug that acts locally to inhibit hair follicle ornithine decarboxylase enzyme that is essential for hair growth and can result in visible improvement within a few weeks. However, on discontinuation of treatment, hair growth returns. It can also result in obstruction of the sebaceous glands and hence worsening of acne. Vaniqa has been shown to enhance the effect of laser treatment for hair removal.[12,13]

### Insulin sensitizing agents

Metformin has been shown to improve ovulation rates in women with PCOS (Chapter 53, Polycystic ovarian syndrome) and may also improve hirsutism through an improvement in insulin resistance. A recent meta-analysis has shown that metformin has similar efficacy to an OCP containing 2 mg cyproterone acetate and 35 μg of ethinyl oestradiol.[14] On the other hand, other studies have shown little or no benefit from the use of metformin.[15]

### GnRH agonists

GnRH agonists can be used to suppress pituitary gonadotropins and ovarian activity in severe resistant cases. However, treatment is associated with significant menopause-like symptoms and prolonged treatment can lead to loss of bone mineral density.

## Surgical treatments

Surgical approaches include the treatment of identifiable causes, such as hypophysectomy for Cushing's syndrome, adrenal suppression for CAH and surgical removal of ovarian and adrenal tumours.

A therapeutic approach to hirsutism is summarized in Figure 54.1.

### KEY POINTS

- Polycystic ovarian syndrome is one of the most common causes of hirsutism.
- Weight loss in obese patients may improve hirsutism.
- Virilism usually indicates significant pathology.
- The oral contraceptive pill is the most commonly used single therapy for hirsutism.

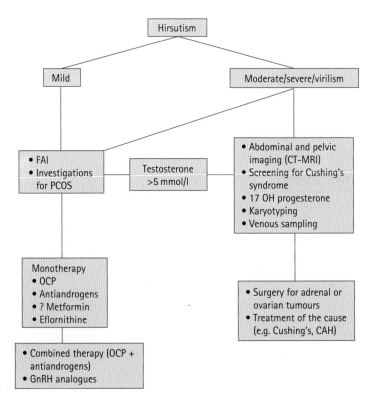

**Figure 54.1** A simplified algorithm for the management of hirsutism

# Key References

1. Martin KA, Chang RJ, Ehrmann DA *et al.* Evaluation and treatment of hirsutism in premenopausal women: an endocrine society clinical practice guideline. *J Clin Endocrinol Metab* 2008; **93**: 1105–20.

2. Randall VA. Androgens and hair growth. *Dermatol Ther* 2008; **21**: 314–28.

3. Olsen EA. Evaluation and treatment of hirsutism. Introduction. *Dermatol Ther* 2008; **21**: 313.

4. Hunter MH, Carek PJ. Evaluation and treatment of women with hirsutism. *Am Fam Physician* 2003; **67**: 2565–72.

5. Archer JS, Chang RJ. Hirsutism and acne in polycystic ovary syndrome. *Best Pract Res Clin Obstet Gynaecol* 2004; **18**: 737–54.

6. Somani N, Harrison S, Bergfeld WF. The clinical evaluation of hirsutism. *Dermatol Ther* 2008; **21**: 376–91.

7. Van der Spuy ZM, le Roux PA. Cyproterone acetate for hirsutism. *Cochrane Database Syst Rev* 2003; (**4**): CD001125.

8. van Vloten WA, van Haselen CW, van Zuuren EJ *et al.* The effect of 2 combined oral contraceptives containing either drospirenone or cyproterone acetate on acne and seborrhea. *Cutis* 2002; **69**: 2–15.

9. Brown J, Farquhar C, Lee O *et al.* Spironolactone versus placebo or in combination with steroids for hirsutism and/or acne. *Cochrane Database Syst Rev* 2009; (**2**): CD000194.

10. Inal MM, Yildirim Y, Taner CE. Comparison of the clinical efficacy of flutamide and spironolactone plus Diane 35 in the treatment of idiopathic hirsutism: a randomized controlled study. *Fertil Steril* 2005; **84**: 1693–7.

11. Karakurt F, Sahin I, Guler S *et al.* Comparison of the clinical efficacy of flutamide and spironolactone plus ethinyloestradiol/cyproterone acetate in the treatment of hirsutism: a randomised controlled study. *Adv Ther* 2008; **25**: 321–8.

12. Hamzavi I, Tan E, Shapiro J, Lui H. A randomized bilateral vehicle-controlled study of eflornithine cream combined with laser treatment versus laser treatment alone for facial hirsutism in women. *J Am Acad Dermatol* 2007; **57**: 54–9.

13. Smith SR, Piacquadio DJ, Beger B, Littler C. Eflornithine cream combined with laser therapy in the management of unwanted facial hair growth in women: a randomized trial. *Dermatol Surg* 2006; **32**: 1237–43.

14. Jing Z, Liang-Zhi X, Tai-Xiang W *et al.* The effects of Diane-35 and metformin in treatment of polycystic ovary syndrome: an updated systematic review. *Gynecol Endocrinol* 2008; **24**: 590–600.

15. Cosma M, Swiglo BA, Flynn DN *et al.* Clinical review: Insulin sensitizers for the treatment of hirsutism: a systematic review and metaanalyses of randomized controlled trials. *J Clin Endocrinol Metab* 2008; **93**: 1135–42.

# Amenorrhoea and oligomenorrhoea

*Mostafa Metwally and William Ledger*

---

# DEFINITIONS

## Amenorrhoea

Amenorrhoea is the absence of menses. Based on the previous occurrence of menstruation, amenorrhoea is divided into primary and secondary.

- **Primary amenorrhoea**: Menstruation has not occurred by the age of 14 in the absence of secondary sexual characters or by the age of 16, even if secondary sexual characters are present.
- **Secondary amenorrhoea**: Periods have not occurred for a time equivalent to the length of three previous cycles (or six months).

## Oligomenorrhoea

This is defined as infrequent menstruation, where the duration between periods is more than 35 days.

# CAUSES OF AMENORRHOEA

It is important to remember that amenorrhoea and oligomenorrhoea are symptoms and not a final diagnosis. The occurrence of regular menses requires a co-ordinated interaction between the hypothalamus, pituitary, ovaries and the outflow tract (uterus and vagina). A disturbance at any of these levels can lead to amenorrhoea (Figure 55.1).

## Hypothalamus (normal or low gonadotropins)

- **Congenital**: Kallman syndrome is a condition associated with congenital absence of GnRH secretion from the arcuate nucleus. Since GnRH-producing cells develop in the olfactory area, Kallman syndrome can be associated with defective olfactory development manifesting with anosmia.
- **Trauma**: This may be physical trauma, such as in the case of head injuries, or psychological trauma, such as in cases of severe emotional stress.
- **Inflammation**: For example, encephalitis and meningitis.
- **Neoplastic**: Hypothalamic and other brain tumours.
- **Weight related**: Leptin is one of the adipokines (a range of proteins secreted by white adipose tissue) that can influence the hypothalamus and is involved in various aspects of female reproductive function. Leptin has a stimulatory effect on the hypothalamus and may be responsible for signalling information to the brain on the critical amount of fat stores that are necessary for GnRH secretion and activation of the hypothalamic–pituitary–gonadal axis.[1] Rising levels of leptin have also been associated with the initiation of puberty in animals and humans, possibly acting in concert with gonadotropins and the growth hormone axis.[2] This is further supported by the occurrence of amenorrhoea associated with a drop in body fat seen in eating disorders, such as anorexia nervosa, which can affect about 0.7 per cent of teenage girls[3] and in strenuously exercising athletes.[4] Exogenous recombinant leptin replacement has been shown to improve reproductive and neuroendocrine function in women with hypothalamic amenorrhoea.[5]

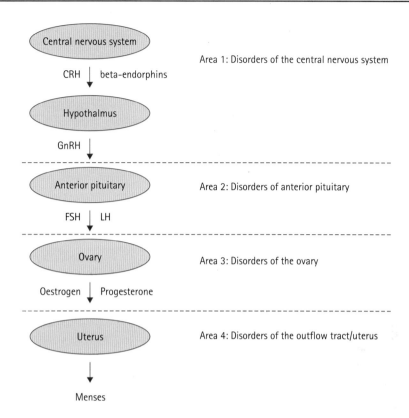

**Figure 55.1** Different compartments that may be involved in occurrence of amenorrhoea

In contrast, obesity is often associated with elevated serum or follicular fluid leptin levels, raising the possibility of relative leptin deficiency or resistance which may explain the poor reproductive performance in such conditions.[2]

## Pituitary: (normal or low gonadotropins)

- **Congenital**: Mutation of the β-subunit of FSH.[6]
- **Trauma**: After surgical removal of pituitary tumours.
- **Neoplastic**: Microadenomas producing prolactin, macroadenomas or an extra pituitary tumour compressing the pituitary stalk and hence leading to hyperprolactinaemia due to interference with dopamine (prolactin inhibitory factor).
- **Sheehan syndrome** is a condition of hypopituitrism due to ischaemic necrosis of the pituitary after massive postpartum haemorrhage. The first hormones to be affected are the gonadotropins and growth hormone followed by ACTH and finally TSH.

## Ovarian: (normal or raised gonadotropins)

- **Congenital**:
  - Complete androgen insensitivity in an XY female.
  - Turner's syndrome (XO) presents with primary amenorrhoea, while women with mosaic Turner (XX/XO) may present with secondary amenorrhoea.

  - Other forms of abnormal gonadal development may also present with primary or secondary amenorrhoea, such as cases of gonadal dysgenesis (pure or mixed).
  - Resistant ovary syndrome is a condition that can present with premature menopause. The condition is characterized by a normal cohort of primordial follicles and absence of autoimmune disease. The condition can be due to a defect in the gonadotropin receptors.[7]
- **Trauma**: Radiotherapy, chemotherapy and surgical removal.
- **Inflammation**: Rarely severe genital tuberculosis causing ovarian damage.
- **Neoplastic**: A variety of benign or malignant ovarian tumours.
- **Polycystic ovarian syndrome (PCOS)**: This is discussed in more detail in Chapter 53.
- **Premature ovarian failure (POF)**: This is characterized by cessation of ovarian function due to depletion of the follicular cohort before the age of 40 years. Gonadotropins are raised in the menopausal range. The cause is usually idiopathic in 74–90 per cent of cases,[8] but may be associated with a variety of autoimmune conditions, chromosomal abnormalities (such as mosaic Turner), galactosaemia and carriers of fragile X pre-mutation. The occurrence of premature menopause should prompt the search for chromosomal abnormalities associated with the presence of a Y chromosome due to the high risk of malignant tumours in these gonads.

## Outflow tract (normal gonadotropins)

- **Congenital**: Congenital absence of the uterus is due to faulty development of the Müllerian ducts (Meyer–Rokitansky–Kuster–Hauser syndrome). Since the Müllerian and Wolffian ducts are closely related, this condition is often associated with developmental abnormalities in the urinary tract. Other developmental abnormalities that present with primary amenorrhoea include imperforate hymen and transverse vaginal septum. These two conditions lead to cryptomenorrhoea, where cyclic bleeding and pain occur every month, but the bleeding is not revealed. Eventually haematocolpos and haematometra occur and commonly present with acute urinary retention due to stretching of the urethra.
- **Trauma**: Surgical removal (hysterectomy) or over curettage of the endometrium.
- **Inflammation**: Post-partum or post-abortive infection. Surgical or inflammatory destruction of the basal endometrial layer will lead to the formation of intrauterine adhesions (Asherman syndrome).

## INVESTIGATIONS

Clinical examination particularly in cases of primary amenorrhoea may reveal physical characteristics of Turner's syndrome, outflow obstruction and allow for examination of secondary sexual character development. According to the findings, investigations may be required at this stage including karyotyping or gonadotropin measurement.

Other preliminary tests include exclusion of pregnancy, which is a must in all cases of secondary amenorrhoea. Thyroid function tests will exclude thyroid disorders, although it is a rare cause of amenorrhoea. Prolactin measurement is needed to exclude hyperprolactinaemia as the cause.

## Progesterone challenge test

An oral progestagen given for 5–10 days will usually induce a withdrawal bleed if the endometrium has been primed by endogenous oestrogen. A positive withdrawal bleed therefore establishes the cause as anovulation (e.g. PCOS), while a negative withdrawal bleed is an indication for addition of oestrogen to the progestagen. A positive bleed means that the ovary is not producing adequate oestrogen (hypogonadism). This may be due to ovarian (hypergonadotropic hypogonadism) or central deficiency of FSH/LH (hypogonadoptropic hypogonadism). The two conditions can be differentiated by measurement of gonadotropin concentrations. On the other hand, a negative withdrawal bleed is an indication for investigation of the outflow tract (e.g. hysteroscopy to diagnose and treat Asherman syndrome,

ultrasonography or magnetic resonance imaging (MRI) to investigate obstructive outflow lesions or Müllerian abnormalities).

## Pituitary imaging

Imaging of the sella turcica using computed tomography (CT) scans or MRI is indicated in women with exceedingly high prolactin concentrations.

## Investigations for women with premature ovarian failure

The diagnosis is usually established by finding a raised FSH concentration in the menopausal range. The test should be repeated since fluctuations in FSH concentrations can occur and are associated with intermittent episodes of ovarian activity. However, other tests of ovarian reserve may be more accurate and include measuring AMH (anti-Müllerian hormone) and inhibin B concentrations. Both these hormones are produced by the existing cohort of follicles and decrease with diminished ovarian reserve. However, AMH has the advantage of not fluctuating with the different phases of the cycle and therefore can be measured at any time. Other tests that may be indicated after the diagnosis is established include karyotyping, screening for autoantibodies, galactosaemia and fragile X syndrome permutations.

## TREATMENT

This should be directed to the cause and depends on the patient's current desire for fertility.

Specific pathologies that will require intervention include:

- Hysteroscopic resection of intrauterine adhesions in cases with Asherman syndrome. In one series, the conception rate after treatment ranged from 33 to 58 per cent, depending on the severity of adhesions.[9]
- Removal of space-occupying pituitary or brain tumours. The majority of pituitary microadenomas, however, can be managed conservatively with a dopamine agonist. For women with hyperprolactinaemia, not due to a pituitary adenoma, dopamine agonists can lead to resumption of ovulation and menstruation.
- Treatment of feeding disorders and normalization of body weight.
- Surgical correction of outflow tract obstruction, e.g. incision of an imperforate hymen.
- Correction of thyroid disorders.

Treatment depends on whether fertility is required. Where fertility is not required, regular withdrawal bleeds may be induced using cyclic oestrogen/progestagen therapy (e.g. oral contraceptive pill (OCP)). Women who suffer from chronic anovulation should be treated with a cyclic oestrogen/progestagen or a progestagen alone to protect the endometrium against the effects of prolonged unopposed oestrogen stimulation. The OCP or another form of combined HRT should also be used for women with POF to protect the bone density and avoid the unpleasant side effects of oestrogen deficiency.

Where fertility is required in anovulatory women, the primary method of ovulation induction depends on the level of the defect:

- Polycystic ovarian syndrome (see Chapter 53).
- Oocyte donation and *in vitro* fertilization (IVF) offer the best chance for conception in women with premature ovarian failure. Spontaneous conception, although very rare (5–10 per cent),[10] can still occur due to bouts of ovarian activity. There are also some reports of successful ovulation induction after suppression of FSH using ethinyl oestradiol.[11–13]
- Women with pituitary or hypothalamic causes of amenorrhoea (hypogonadoptropic hypogonadism) are treated with gonadotropins (FSH and LH) or less commonly with pulsatile GnRH administration using a subcutaneous pump.

## KEY POINTS

- Amenorrhoea and oligomenorrhoea can arise from a disturbance at the level of any of the key structures controlling the menstrual cycle.
- Pregnancy should always be excluded in a patient presenting with secondary amenorrhoea.
- Premature ovarian failure should prompt the search for underlying pathologies, although the most common cause remains idiopathic.
- In women with premature ovarian failure not requiring fertility, treatment should be directed to the prevention of the long-term health consequences of oestrogen deficiency.
- Contraception should still be advised for women with premature ovarian failure not desiring pregnancy, since spontaneous pregnancy can still occur, albeit rarely.
- Measurement of anti-Müllerian hormone is a better ovarian reserve test than follicle-stimulating hormone.

- Investigations for amenorrhoea should follow a systematic approach that methodically addresses all the potential levels at which the cause may occur.
- Fertility treatment depends on the anatomical level of the pathology.

## Key References

1. Mantzoros CS. Role of leptin in reproduction. *Ann NY Acad Sci* 2000; **900**: 174–83.
2. Moschos S, Chan JL, Mantzoros CS. Leptin and reproduction: a review. *Fertil Steril* 2002; **77**: 433–44.
3. Lock J, Fitzpatrick KK. Anorexia nervosa. *Clin Evid (Online)* 2009; 2009.
4. Thong FS, Graham TE. Leptin and reproduction: is it a critical link between adipose tissue, nutrition, and reproduction? *Can J Appl Physiol* 1999; **24**: 317–36.
5. Welt CK, Chan JL, Bullen J et al. Recombinant human leptin in women with hypothalamic amenorrhea. *N Engl J Med* 2004; **351**: 987–97.
6. Layman LC, McDonough PG. Mutations of follicle stimulating hormone-beta and its receptor in human and mouse: genotype/phenotype. *Mol Cell Endocrinol* 2000; **161**: 9–17.
7. Huhtaniemi I, Alevizaki M. Gonadotrophin resistance. *Best Pract Res Clin Endocrinol Metab* 2006; **20**: 561–76.
8. Vujovic S. Aetiology of premature ovarian failure. *Menopause Int* 2009; **15**: 72–5.
9. Roy KK, Baruah J, Sharma JB et al. Reproductive outcome following hysteroscopic adhesiolysis in patients with infertility due to Asherman's syndrome. Arch Gynecol Obstet 2009 [Epub ahead of print].
10. Rebar RW. Premature ovarian failure. *Obstet Gynecol* 2009; **113**: 1355–63.
11. Check JH. Pharmacological options in resistent ovary syndrome and premature ovarian failure. *Clin Exp Obstet Gynecol* 2006; **33**: 71–7.
12. Blumenfeld Z. Pregnancies in patients with POF gonadotropin stimulation and pretreatment with ethinyl estradiol (author's reply). *Fertil Steril* 2007; **88**: 763.
13. Tartagni M, Cicinelli E, De Pergola G et al. Effects of pretreatment with estrogens on ovarian stimulation with gonadotropins in women with premature ovarian failure: a randomized, placebo-controlled trial. *Fertil Steril* 2007; **87**: 858–61.

Reproductive medicine

# Menopause and hormone replacement therapy

*Michael Paterson*

## MRCOG standards

There are no MRCOG standards for this topic. We would suggest the following guidelines:

### Theoretical skills

- Understand the pathophysiology of the menopause.
- Understand the medication available.
- Be aware of the complications and contraindications.
- Be able to advise regarding the advantages and disadvantages of the different treatment modalities.

## INTRODUCTION

The term 'menopause' is derived from the Greek *menos* (month) and *pauses* (cessation), but the term has come to be used to describe the climacteric, which is again derived from the Greek *klimakter* (rung of a ladder). The dictionary definition of the climacteric is the period of life when fertility and sexual activity decline. The definition may be accurate, but does not describe the profound changes that occur when the ovaries cease to function.

The average age of the menopause has not changed for centuries, but life expectancy has improved enormously, particularly in the last century. The life expectancy of women in Roman times was 29 years and, even by the late nineteenth century only 30 per cent of women survived to experience the menopause. Life expectancy among women is now almost 80 years and it has been estimated that there are 10 million post-menopausal women in the United Kingdom. The vast majority of women will reach the menopause and will spend one-third of their lives in this state. The long-term metabolic problems of the menopause are therefore becoming increasingly important.

## PATHOPHYSIOLOGY

The number of primordial follicles declines even before birth and although the decline is dramatic just before the menopause, there are still a significant number present at the onset of the menopause. Hypothalamic–pituitary activity increases from about ten years before the menopause. This is shown by the rising plasma levels of luteinizing hormone (LH) and, particularly, follicle-stimulating hormone (FSH). Closer to the menopause, anovulation occurs and luteal inadequacy becomes more frequent. There is a reduction in the production of progesterone and, as oestrogen levels do not decline as quickly, this may result in dysfunctional uterine bleeding and endometrial hyperplasia. Oestrogen levels decline dramatically at the menopause and menstruation ceases. The ovarian stroma still produces small quantities of androstenedione and testosterone, but the main post-menopausal oestrogen is estrone, which is produced in the peripheral fat from adrenal androgens. It is the lack of oestrogen that causes the majority of symptoms and pathology of the menopause.

## SYMPTOMS

The characteristic symptoms of the menopause include hot flushes, night sweats, headaches, depression and lack of concentration and energy. The most obvious symptom is the hot flush. This is very different from a blush, which characteristically occurs over the face and chest. The hot flush, although it may start in the head or neck area, involves the whole body and is often followed by intense sweating and then by shivering. There is a rise in skin temperature of 1°C [B],[1] and although women may feel embarrassment, there are no obvious signs that they are having a hot flush. Hot flushes and sweats occur in 75 per cent of women and tend to be more severe following a surgical menopause. They will usually continue for more than a year, and 25 per cent will continue with hot sweats for more than five years [D].

The diagnosis is straightforward when the patient is a year post-menopausal and has significant hot flushes and sweats, but if the patient is peri-menopausal, the diagnosis may be much more difficult, particularly if her only symptom is that of depression. Depression is more common in the decade before the menopause than after it, and if the patient has a long history of depression, it is unlikely that her symptoms are due to a lack of oestrogen. Many women request oestrogens in the hope that other causes of depression may be helped. There are many other causes of depression at the time of the menopause, including loss of reproductive potential, lack of femininity, marital problems and the 'empty nest' syndrome. There have been studies to show the beneficial effects of oestrogen in the treatment of depression, but the main benefit seems to be among pre-menopausal women.

Many of the symptoms that can be related to ovarian failure are shown in Box 56.1, but it can be difficult to determine whether a particular symptom is caused by the menopause. If the diagnosis is uncertain, the only way of determining whether the symptom is oestrogen related is to prescribe a short course of hormone replacement therapy (HRT).

## Cardiovascular disease

Coronary heart disease (CHD) is uncommon among pre-menopausal women, particularly if they do not smoke. There is a rapid increase in risk following the menopause and cardiovascular disease is now a leading cause of death among post-menopausal women. Even though the post-menopausal incidence increases, it does not reach the incidence in men at any age.

Why are pre-menopausal women given this protection? The mechanism is not clear, but the lipoprotein profile, with a higher high-density lipoprotein (HDL) and lower low-density lipoprotein (LDL) cholesterol concentration when compared with men, may in part be the answer. In post-menopausal women, the HDL:LDL ratio becomes much closer to the male ratio, but this may not explain all the differences, and oestrogen may well have a more direct effect on the vessel wall.

Oral oestrogens when given to post-menopausal women cause an increase in HDL and a lowering of LDL cholesterol concentrations, which should be beneficial. They also increase triglyceride levels, which are associated with an increased risk of cardiovascular disease. There have been a huge number of studies to try to find a drug with the ideal lipid profile, but none has been conclusive.

Early observational studies suggested that women taking or who have taken HRT have a lower CHD incidence and mortality by around 30 per cent, but there has been only one small randomized study [C], the Heart and Estrogen/Progestin Replacement Study (HERS). This showed no CHD benefit of taking HRT among women with stable CHD, but a significant increased risk of thromboembolic events [B].[2] The study was surprising in view of all the previous epidemiological evidence, but the epidemiological studies could be criticized for possible selection bias and, on the other hand, there were a large number of drop-outs in the HERS. However, the picture has changed, owing to the publication of the Women's Health Initiative (WHI) trial in the United States, which has led to a reappraisal of the long-term use of HRT.[3] This was the largest trial ever undertaken in the field, with more than 16 000 women. The main aim of the study were to test whether post-menopausal use of HRT protected women against heart disease. The trial randomized women to receive continuous combined HRT in the form of 0.625 mg conjugated equine oestrogen (Premarin® in United Kingdom) and 2.5 mg medroxyprogesterone acetate daily, or placebo. After five years of follow up, the women taking HRT were found to have a higher incidence of breast cancer, myocardial infarction, stroke and pulmonary embolus, although there were reductions in the numbers of hip fractures and colorectal cancers. Part of the trial was then stopped early because of these events.

## Osteoporosis

Osteoporosis is a major cause of morbidity and mortality in women in the UK. Bone mass reaches a peak in women towards the end of their third decade. It then remains relatively constant until the menopause, after which the loss is lifelong. Seventy per cent of women over the age of 80 will have measurable osteoporosis. It is estimated that there are 60 000 hip fractures, 50 000 Colles fractures and 40 000 clinically apparent vertebral fractures a year in the UK. The clinical consequences are enormous, and women who have a fracture of the neck of femur have a 25 per cent of dying within a year and a 50 per cent chance of not being able to resume their social independence. The other fractures also cause significant morbidity, particularly as they often occur in elderly women who live alone and are just able to maintain their independence.

---

### Box 56.1 Menopausal symptoms

- Hot flushes
- Night sweats
- Palpitations
- Globus hystericus
- Formication
- Depression
- Anxiety
- Insomnia
- Headaches
- Loss of libido
- Loss of concentration
- Skin atrophy
- Joint pains
- Urge incontinence
- Myalgia

Reproductive medicine

A minimum of 2 mg of oestradiol or equivalent is needed to increase rather than maintain bone mass. The combined oestrogen/progestogen preparations are effective, as is tibolone, a synthetic hormone preparation. There are plenty of randomized studies to show that HRT maintains bone mass, but no long-term study has shown a significant reduction in fractures. The major problem in running such a study is that there is a 30-year gap between the menopause and most of the fractures, and to sustain any such trial for that length of time is almost impossible. However, it does appear that bone density is maintained following treatment with combined preparations and that it will fall following cessation of treatment at the same rate as it does after the menopause [B].[4]

There are other treatments that may be useful in the treatment of osteoporosis. Calcium supplementation is of little value in younger, active patients but has been shown to be beneficial in elderly post-menopausal patients living in care. Bisphosphonates are also effective in the treatment of relatively elderly patients with established osteoporosis. Fluoride is not thought to be effective, but physical exercise is thought to be important in the prevention of osteoporotic fractures, mainly through improvement in posture, mobility and muscle function.

## Urogenital system

Embryologically, the female genital tract and lower urinary system develop in close proximity, both developing from the primitive urogenital sinus. Vaginal discomfort, dyspareunia, dysuria, recurrent lower tract infections and urinary incontinence are all more common after the menopause. The urethra and vagina have a high concentration of oestrogen receptors and there is now significant evidence to support the use of oestrogens in the treatment of urogenital symptoms. Evidence exists that oestrogens relieve urogenital atrophic symptoms, induce an increase in lactobacilli in the vagina, prevent recurrent urinary tract infections, and alleviate urge incontinence, frequency and nocturia. In combination with alpha-adrenergic agonists, oestrogens improve stress incontinence [C].

## DIAGNOSIS AND INVESTIGATION

The triad of hot flushes, amenorrhoea for a year and a raised serum FSH level of >15 IU/L makes the diagnosis easy and in the majority of cases it can be made on the history alone. The differential diagnosis includes depression, premenstrual syndrome, migraine and, very rarely, carcinoid syndrome. It can sometimes be more difficult when the patient has had a hysterectomy because this is associated with an earlier menopause, and a serum FSH level will often help to establish the diagnosis.

There are no essential investigations that must be carried out before commencing HRT, but it is a screening opportunity that should not be missed. This would include, if appropriate, breast self-examination, mammography, pelvic examination and cervical cytology. The patient should be weighed and her blood pressure checked before commencing treatment. Perceived weight gain is a common reason for discontinuing HRT, but randomized studies have not shown any significant gain in weight on HRT [B].

There is no indication to perform routine bone density measurements or endometrial biopsies. However, any erratic bleeding should be investigated before commencing HRT.

## TREATMENT

### Oestrogens

Oestrogens are effective at relieving menopausal symptoms and this has been confirmed by several randomized, double-blind studies [B].[5] For all women who have not had a hysterectomy, a progestogen should be added for at least 10 days each month to reduce risk of endometrial hyperplasia and carcinoma [C]. This will result in a regular withdrawal bleed and, as many women find this unacceptable, continuous regimens of oestrogen and a progestogen have been introduced to reduce its incidence. The routes of administration are shown in Box 56.2. All these regimens are effective, but have different side effects. This is important when prescribing HRT, because if the initial drug is ineffective, it is unlikely that changing to another route of administration will improve the symptoms. However, if the drug is effective but has unacceptable side effects, a different route of administration may well be more acceptable.

Oral preparations are by far the most common and they have the advantage of flexibility, a short half-life, ease of administration and lower cost. However, they do deliver a relatively high level of oestrogen to the liver, with an increased risk of gallstone formation and a tendency to increase triglyceride levels. The so-called sequential regimens that have oestrogen in the first half of the 28-day pack and oestrogen and a progestogen in the second half are particularly useful in treating patients close to the menopause, as they give better cycle control.

> **Box 56.2 Routes of administration of hormone replacement therapy**
> - Oral
> - Patches
> - Implants
> - Vaginal ring
> - Gel

Combined continuous therapy, which has progestogen every day, is useful for those women who are a few years past the menopause and who do not wish to have vaginal bleeding. There is now evidence that there is an increased risk of endometrial carcinoma if sequential regimens are taken for more than five years [C].[6] This is not seen with combined continuous regimens, and there may be a reduced risk of endometrial carcinoma [C]. Women should therefore consider changing after a few years from a sequential regimen to continuous combined therapy for long-term treatment.

Patches offer an alternative to oral preparations for those women who do not wish to take tablets or who have side effects. The matrix patch has removed most of the skin irritation problems, but there is a huge range of alternative routes of administration that are beneficial, including gels, vaginal rings and implants. Implants are useful in that as well as lasting for six months, they can also be used in combination with testosterone in those women who have loss of libido [C].[7] Implants may continue to release oestrogen for up to two years and if they are given too frequently, supraphysiological levels may occur [C].[8]

## Side effects and complications

The main side effect is vaginal bleeding in patients with a uterus. This may be acceptable in women aged 50, but not ten years later. The combined continuous preparations are associated with few bleeding problems in women over the age of 55, but erratic vaginal bleeding may be a problem close to the menopause. The addition of a progestogen may well cause many of the side effects, including bloating, fluid retention and mastalgia. Progestogens can be administered vaginally as a gel or pessary or as an intrauterine device to try to reduce the severity of any side effects.

## Breast disease

Hormone replacement therapy increases the rate of benign breast disease and increases the incidence of benign mastalgia and mammographic density. With the use of mammography to detect early breast cancer, HRT leads to an increase in the psychological and surgical morbidity because of the increased numbers of mammographically guided or open breast biopsies that have to be performed.

There has been a large number of studies showing that HRT is associated with an increased risk of breast cancer. An analysis of 51 epidemiological studies [A][9] showed that the cumulative excess risk for women starting HRT at the age of 50 was two cases/1000 women after five years, 6/1000 after ten years, and 12/1000 after 15 years. The background risk was 45/1000. This risk fell on discontinuing HRT, with no excess risk after five years. HRT does not increase mortality, and some studies have shown an improvement in prognosis [C]. A more recent report from the WHI study suggests that women who have had a hysterectomy and are

### Box 56.3 The evidence against prescribing hormone replacement therapy (HRT) to women with breast cancer

- Oestradiol stimulates some breast cancer cells in culture
- Oophorectomy reduces rate of recurrence
- Breast cancer risk relates to age at menarche and menopause
- Stopping HRT may cause some breast cancers to regress
- Long-term HRT increases the risk of breast cancer

taking oestrogen only do not have an increased risk and may have a slight benefit.

Breast cancer has been regarded as an absolute contraindication to HRT and for that reason very few patients with breast cancer have been prescribed it. A study from Australia [D][10] involving more than 100 women with breast cancer was unable to find a significant increased risk of recurrence, but this was only 10 per cent of the total number with breast cancer treated in that institution. The case against prescribing HRT in women with breast cancer is still strong (Box 56.3). Great care needs to be taken before prescribing HRT to women with breast cancer, but the risks to women who have good-prognosis disease are probably small and the risks may be justified in women who have severe symptoms.

## Venous thrombosis

There are marked haematological changes that occur secondary to the menopause, and users of HRT have further favourable and unfavourable changes. In the past, it has been difficult to determine whether or not these changes indicate that women on HRT are at an increased risk. In 1996 and 1997, there was a total of five epidemiological studies of various study design showing that there was a very small increased risk for HRT users. The absolute risk years was 2/10 000 treatment-years for venous thrombosis, 0.6/10 000 treatment-years for pulmonary embolus and 2/million treatment-years for death. The first 12 months of treatment were associated with the highest risk [C].[11]

The risk of the occurrence of a venous thrombosis for any one individual is very small, but care needs to be taken before prescribing HRT for a patient with a history of deep vein thrombosis. HRT should be avoided in those patients who have had a serious proven event and in those who have ongoing risk factors. HRT should be considered a risk factor for venous thrombosis in women undergoing surgery but does not require to be routinely stopped prior to surgery provided that appropriate thromboprophylaxis is used.

## Acceptability

Hormone replacement therapy is effective in relieving menopausal symptoms and is likely to reduce deaths from osteoporosis. One might expect a high uptake of the drug, but most studies have shown poor continuation rates on HRT. One study[12] showed that 31 per cent of women had discontinued HRT within six months, 51 per cent within six months and 75 per cent within three years, which is typical of the published data.

The reasons for stopping HRT are numerous and the reasons given in the study cited above are again fairly typical of many reported studies [D]: 36 per cent discontinued because of side effects, 24 per cent because of lack of efficacy, 18 per cent because the side effects were worse than the menopausal symptoms, 9 per cent because their symptoms had ceased, 9 per cent because of bleeding problems, and 18 per cent because of long-term risks.

Oestrogenic side effects are shown in Box 56.4 and progestogenic side effects in Box 56.5. The oestrogenic effects can be reduced by prescribing the lowest effective dose or by changing the route of administration. The progestogenic effects are often more troublesome, and may be improved by changing the progestogen, changing to a three-monthly regimen or changing the route of administration.

The levonorgestrel intrauterine system has been used in combination with an oestrogen, and may be particularly useful in the peri-menopausal woman with dysfunctional bleeding.

If the drug is not effective, the diagnosis should be reconsidered and perhaps one further type of HRT prescribed. If bleeding is the main problem, the progestogen can be changed and, for the older patient, combined continuous therapy or tibolone is available.

---

### Box 56.4 Oestrogenic side effects

- Leg cramps
- Headaches
- Bloating
- Nipple sensitivity
- Nausea

---

### Box 56.5 Progestogenic side effects

- Premenstrual syndrome
- Depression
- Poor concentration
- Acne
- Headaches
- Breast tenderness
- Fluid retention
- Dysmenorrhoea

---

## Duration of treatment

Prior to the publication of the WHI study the long-term advantages of HRT were deemed to outweigh the disadvantages.

A second 'landmark' publication, the Million Women Study, provided further high-quality evidence concerning the risks and benefits of HRT in women aged 50–64. This UK-based study collected data from women attending for breast screening as part of the National Health Service breast screening programme. Women were classified according to their reported use of HRT, menopausal status, etc. Combined oestrogen/gestagen HRT use was associated with an increased number of breast cancers when compared with non-users. Users of oestrogen-only HRT (usually reserved for hysterectomized women) were at lower risk, and the risks to users of combined oestrogen/gestagen HRT only applied to current, not past, users.[13]

Following publication of these findings, the UK Committee on Safety of Medicines issued advice to prescribers of HRT, which can be summarized as follows.

- For short-term (e.g. two to three years) use of HRT for the relief of menopausal symptoms, the benefits outweigh the risks for most women.
- Longer-term use of HRT is licensed for the prevention of osteoporosis. However, patients should be aware of the increased incidence of some conditions with long-term HRT use and of alternative options for the prevention of osteoporosis.
- The decision to use HRT should be discussed with each women on an individual basis, taking into consideration her history, risk factors and personal preferences.
- Individual risks and benefits should be regularly reappraised (e.g. at least annually) while using HRT.
- HRT should not be used for the prevention of CHD.

The results of these trials had a major impact on patterns of HRT used throughout the Western world. Other than the lack of a protective effect against heart disease, there was little new in the findings, but the study did re-emphasize the cautionary notes raised by earlier, smaller studies. Clearly, alternative strategies exist for protection against post-menopausal osteoporosis, including the use of selective oestrogen receptor modulators (SERMS) or bisphosphonates. The control of peri-menopausal symptoms without resort to HRT is more problematic and it may be that many women will continue to use HRT for a few years during their early fifties. However, it seems likely that long-term use will decline over time.

The majority of women will require HRT for a few years until their symptoms cease, but there will be a small number whose symptoms continue for more than five years and the risk and benefit of continuing on HRT should be made on an annual basis.

## Alternative treatments

Norethisterone 5 mg daily has been shown to be effective in reducing hot flushes and sweats, but it has little effect on other menopausal symptoms [B].[14] Medroxyprogesterone acetate and megestrol acetate 40 mg daily are also effective and these drugs may be useful in women who have relative contraindications to HRT. The WHI study[3,15] suggested that is was the combination of oestrogen and progestogen rather than oestrogen alone that led to the increase in the risk of breast cancer and therefore we should urge caution when treating women who have an increased risk of breast cancer with progestogens.

Propranolol and clonidine have been used in the treatment of hot flushes, but the effect is probably no better than placebo.

Selective serotonin and noradrenaline reuptake inhibitors may help with vasomotor symptoms, but nausea can be a significant side effect and long-term studies are awaited.

Vaginal oestrogen preparations can be used to treat patients with symptoms of urogenital atrophy and recurrent urinary tract infections after underlying pathology has been excluded.

Selective oestrogen receptor modulators are effective in the prevention of bone loss and are likely to have a cardiovascular benefit and reduce the incidence of breast cancer. They may increase hot flushes slightly and therefore are useful in those women whose hot flushes have settled, but who are concerned about long-term osteoporosis.

Naturally occurring oestrogens, such as phytoestrogens, occur in cereals, legumes and vegetables. Women living in countries that have a diet rich in phytoestrogens have fewer menopausal symptoms, but although a lifetime's use may be beneficial, these drugs have not yet been shown to be effective in randomized studies. Therefore, although these drugs are widely used, particularly in the United States, their efficacy needs to be established. Red clover has been shown to reduce the incidence of hot flushes in five placebo controlled trials, but the differences reached statistical significance in only two of the five studies.

There are many herbal remedies available but there is no good evidence to show that they are effective in relieving menopausal symptoms.

---

### KEY POINTS

- Oestrogens are effective at relieving climacteric symptoms.
- Progestogens must be given if the patient has a uterus.
- There are few absolute contraindications.
- The long-term benefits, particularly in the prevention of osteoporosis, may be reduced because of the problems of compliance.

## Published Guidelines

Royal College of Obstetricians and Gynaecologists. Hormone replacement therapy and venous thromboembolism. Guideline No. 19 (revised). London: RCOG, January 2004.

## Key References

1. Sturdee DW, Wilson KA, Pipili E, Crocker AD. Physiological aspects of menopausal hot flush. *BMJ* 1978; **2**: 79–80.

2. Hulley S, Grady D, Bush T *et al*. Randomized trial of estrogen plus progestogen for secondary prevention of coronary heart disease in postmenopausal women. *JAMA* 1998; **280**: 605–13.

3. Writing Group for the Women's Health Initiative Investigators. Risks and benefits of estrogen plus progestin in healthy postmenopausal women: principal results from the Women's Health Initiative randomized controlled trial. *JAMA* 2002; **288**: 321–33.

4. Christiansen C, Christensen MS, Transbol I. Bone mass in postmenopausal women after withdrawal of oestrogen/gestagen replacement therapy. *Lancet* 1981; **I**: 459–61.

5. Campbell S, Whitehead M. Oestrogen therapy in the menopausal syndrome. *Clin Obstet Gynaecol* 1977; **4**: 31–7.

6. Beresford SAA, Weiss NS, Voigt LF, McKnight B. Risk of endometrial cancer in relation to use of oestrogen combined with cyclic progestogen therapy in postmenopausal women. *Lancet* 1997; **349**: 458–61.

7. Studd JWW, Chakravarti S, Collins WP *et al*. Oestradiol and testosterone implants in the treatment of psychosexual problems in postmenopausal women. *Br J Obstet Gynaecol* 1977; **84**: 314–15.

8. Ganger KF, Cust MP, Whitehead MI. Symptoms of oestrogen deficiency associated with supraphysiological plasma oestradiol concentrations in women with oestradiol implants. *BMJ* 1989; **299**: 601–2.

9. Collaborative Group on Hormonal Factors in Breast Cancer. Breast cancer and hormone replacement therapy: collaborative reanalysis of data from 51 epidemiological studies of 52,705 women with breast cancer and 108,411 women with breast cancer. *Lancet* 1997; **350**: 1047–59.

10. Dew J, Eden J, Beller E *et al*. A cohort study of hormone replacement therapy given to women previously treated for breast cancer. *Climacteric* 1998; **1**: 137–42.

11. Daly E, Vessey MP, Hawkins MM *et al*. Case–control study of venous thromboembolism risk in users of hormone replacement therapy. *Lancet* 1996; **348**: 977–80.

12. Hope S, Wager E, Rees M. Survey of British women's views on the menopause and HRT. *J Br Menopause Soc* 1998; **4**: 33–6.

13. Million Women Study Collaborators. Breast cancer and hormone-replacement therapy in the Million Women Study. *Lancet* 2003; **362**: 419–28.

14. Paterson MEL. A randomised double blind cross-over trial into the effect of norethisterone on climacteric symptoms and biochemical profiles. *Br J Obstet Gynaecol* 1982; **89**: 464–72.

15. Anderson GL, Limacher M, Assaf AR *et al.* Effects of conjugated equine estrogen in post-menopausal women with hysterectomy: the Women's Health Initiative randomised trial. *JAMA* 2004; **291**: 1701–12.

# Chapter 57

# Problems in early pregnancy

*Ying Cheong and Aarti Umranikar*

## COMMON PROBLEMS ENCOUNTERED IN AN EARLY PREGNANCY UNIT/ EMERGENCY GYNAECOLOGY UNIT

### Pregnancy related

- Miscarriage associated with bleeding and or pain
- Suspected ectopic with severe abdominal pain or signs of intra-abdominal bleeding (fainting, shoulder tip pain, cervical excitation, signs of peritonitis)
- Haemodynamic instability due to ruptured ectopic
- Hyperemesis gravidarum
- Complications from a medical or surgical abortion.

### Differential diagnosis of abdominal pain in a non-pregnant patient

- Acute pelvic inflammatory disease
- Endometriosis
- Complications of ovarian cyst (haemorrhage, rupture, torsion)
- Fibroid torsion or degeneration
- Acute appendicitis
- Irritable bowel syndrome
- Cholecystitis
- Pancreatitis
- Diverticulitis
- Urinary tract infection
- Acute urinary retention
- Urinary calculus.

## INTRODUCTION AND DEFINITION

Miscarriage and ectopic pregnancy are two large groups of problems in early pregnancy. Both are life-threatening conditions that are commonly seen in our emergency departments.

Miscarriage is defined as spontaneous loss of pregnancy at or before 24 weeks gestation.

Ectopic pregnancy is defined as implantation of a conceptus outside the normal uterine cavity. Common sites of implantation are Fallopian tubes (95 per cent), ovaries (3 per cent) and peritoneal cavity (1 per cent). In the Fallopian tubes, common sites are the ampulla (74 per cent), isthmus (12 per cent), fimbrial end of the tube (12 per cent) and interstitium (2 per cent).

Miscarriage and ectopic pregnancy are both important causes of maternal morbidity and mortality. The CEMACH report highlights the number of maternal deaths due to miscarriage and ectopic pregnancy. There were 11 deaths/100 000 maternities due to ectopic pregnancy in 1985–87; 9/100 000 in 1991–93, which increased to 10/100 000 in 2003–05.

The mortality rates from miscarriage have reduced over the past decade. CEMACH has reported a mortality rate of 4/100 000 maternities due to miscarriage in 1985–87, which fell to 1/100 000 in 2003–05.

## ECTOPIC PREGNANCY

### Incidence and aetiology

The incidence of ectopic pregnancy in the UK is 11.1/1000 pregnancies. Approximately 11 000 cases of ectopic pregnancies are diagnosed each year in the UK. The incidence has been reported to be rising and this is in part due to better and earlier diagnosis and also an increase in the use of assisted conception techniques. IVF and related treatments increase the likelihood of ectopic pregnancy. The incidence of ectopic pregnancy after IVF is 1–3 per cent, which is twice the normal rate.

Heterotopic pregnancy is simultaneous development of a conceptus within and outside the uterine cavity. The incidence in the general population is 1:25000–30000. The incidence is around 1 per cent after IVF treatment.

Known aetiological factors contributing to the risk of ectopic pregnancy are:

- tubal disease due to previous pelvic infection: Chlamydia infection has been estimated to account for 40 per cent of all ectopic pregnancies;
- previous ectopic pregnancy;
- previous tubal surgery;
- subfertility;
- use of assisted reproductive techniques.

## Diagnosis

Any patient presenting to the emergency unit in early pregnancy with pain and bleeding should be investigated with a view to rule out an ectopic pregnancy.

Transvaginal ultrasound (TVS), in conjunction with serial βhCG, has facilitated the diagnosis of ectopic pregnancy. It allows clear visualization of normal and abnormal pregnancies at an early stage of pregnancy. Identification of an intrauterine pregnancy (gestation sac, yolk sac along with fetal pole) on TVS effectively excludes the possibility of an ectopic pregnancy in most patients. The exceptions are those pregnancies conceived as a result of IVF in whom the incidence of heterotopic pregnancy can be as high as 1 per cent.

Ultrasonographic features suggestive of ectopic pregnancy can be variable. The presence of an extra uterine sac with a live embryo is diagnostic of an ectopic pregnancy, whereas visualization of an adnexal mass is suggestive of an ectopic pregnancy in 65–70 per cent of cases with a positive predictive value between 63–100 per cent.[1] Other features that should raise the suspicion of an ectopic pregnancy are an empty uterus or a pseudo sac at a βhCG level greater than 1500 IU/L or the presence of free fluid in the pelvis in the absence of an intrauterine pregnancy. Transvaginal ultrasonography should therefore be the initial investigation for pregnant patients presenting with first trimester bleeding and/or pain.

The concept of a discriminatory threshold of βhCG level (i.e. visualization of an intrauterine gestation sac above that βhCG level) has been known since the 1980s. Advances in the ultrasound imaging technology have enabled visualization of an intrauterine sac at a βhCG level greater than 1500 IU (TVS). However, this threshold is user-and machine-dependent and therefore varies between different units.

Serum βhCG can be detected as early as 1 week before an expected menstrual period. In a viable intrauterine pregnancy (IUP), βhCG concentration rapidly increases, doubling every 2 days. An increase of at least 66 per cent over 48 hours has been used as a cut-off point for viability. This optimum rise is noted in around 85 per cent of IUP. The βhCG level increases more slowly in a non-viable IUP or an ectopic pregnancy (suboptimal rise). However, 10–15 per cent of viable IUP may also show a suboptimal rise in βhCG. Hence the interpretation of βhCG must be done in context with the clinical picture and ultrasound findings. Ideally, the assays should be performed in the same laboratory to maintain consistency in the results.

## Management

Ectopic pregnancy can be managed using the expectant, medical or the surgical approach.

## Expectant

Expectant management is based on the assumption that a significant proportion of all tubal pregnancies will resolve through regression or a tubal abortion without any treatment. This option is suitable for patients who are haemodynamically stable and asymptomatic [C].

Data from observational studies suggest a subsequent pregnancy rate of around 80–85 per cent.[2,3]

The METEX study[4] (methotrexate versus expectant management), an ongoing randomized controlled trial of methotrexate versus expectant management, will hopefully throw some light on this topic.

> ### The RCOG criteria for expectant management of ectopic pregnancy are:
> - βhCG at initial presentation <1000 IU/L
> - Adnexal mass <4 cm on transvaginal (TV) scan
> - Less than 100 mL free fluid in the pelvis
> - Dedicated unit with facilities available for TV scan and βhCG monitoring.

## Medical

Systemic methotrexate is an option of treatment in a carefully selected subgroup of patients. Methotrexate, a folic acid antagonist, inhibits DNA synthesis in trophoblastic cells. It can be administered as a single intramuscular injection or in a multiple fixed dose regimen. The dose is calculated from the patient's body surface area as 50 mg/m².

The following are some indications for the use of methotrexate: (1) cornual pregnancy; (2) persistent trophoblastic disease; (3) patient with one Fallopian tube and fertility desired; (4) patient who refuses surgery or in whom risks of surgery is too high; and (5) treatment of ectopic pregnancy where trophoblast is adherent to bowel or blood vessel.

Medical treatment should be offered only if facilities are present for regular outpatient follow-up visits.

The few contraindications to medical treatment include: (1) chronic liver, renal or haematological disorder; (2) active infection; (3) immunodeficiency; and (4) breastfeeding. There are also known side effects such as nausea, vomiting, stomatitis, conjunctivitis, gastrointestinal upset, photosensitive skin reaction and about two-thirds of patients suffer nonspecific abdominal pain. It is important to advise women to avoid sexual intercourse during treatment and take some form of contraception for three months after methotrexate treatment. It is also important to give advice regarding the avoidance of alcohol and exposure to sunlight during treatment.

---

### Criteria for medical treatment are [B]:

- Haemodynamically stable patient with no evidence of haemoperitoneum on ultrasound scan with minimal or no pain or bleeding.
- βhCG <3000 (although some centres have used multiple dose methotrexate successfully with βhCGs between 5000 and 10 000 IU/L)
- No contraindications to the use of methotrexate
- Adnexal mass <4 cm size on ultrasound
- No fetal cardiac activity in the ectopic sac
- Patient compliance with follow-up visits to the hospital.

---

Patients treated with methotrexate should be followed up closely. A suggested follow-up regime will be as follows: serum βhCG is monitored on day 4 and 7 after methotrexate. The level of βhCG can rise slightly before it starts to fall and is therefore not done earlier than 4 days after the methotrexate treatment. If the fall in βhCG is greater than 15 per cent, a repeat βhCG is performed on day 7. If the fall is satisfactory, weekly blood tests are performed until βhCG is under 25 IU/L. This may usually take 4–5 weeks. If the βhCG has not fallen by >25 per cent by day 7, a repeat dose is administered.

Most hospitals use single-dose methotrexate treatment with additional doses administered based on subsequent βhCG levels during follow-up visits. Single-dose methotrexate treatment is effective in around 65–85 per cent of patients. Medical treatment in appropriately selected patients is as effective as laparoscopic treatment.

Mol et al.[5] concluded from a meta-analysis and systematic review of 15 RCTs that there is no statistical difference in the treatment success of systemic methotrexate (intramuscular) in a fixed multiple dose compared to laparoscopic salpingostomy (RR 1.15, 95 per cent CI 0.93–1.43). Systemic fixed multiple dose methotrexate was only cost effective if βhCG was less than 3000 IU/L and single dose regimen was cost effective if βhCG was <1500 IU/L. Also, the addition of mifepristone to methotrexate does not appear to improve the success rate of treatment.

## Surgical management

### Is surgery necessary?

Surgery offers many significant advantages in the management of ectopic pregnancy as compared to medical treatment. First, in the vast majority of cases, a firm diagnosis of the presence or absence of an ectopic pregnancy can be made. Second, follow-up arrangements are generally less prolonged and less demanding. Third, after surgery, patients can attempt to conceive as soon as they recover from the operation whereas if a chemotherapeutic agent such as methotrexate is used, patients will have to wait at least three months because of the potential teratogenic effects of methotrexate.

### Laparoscopy or laparotomy

The laparoscopic approach offers significant advantage when compared to laparotomy as it results in less blood loss, a shorter hospital stay, shorter operating time, less analgesia requirement and a shorter convalescence than laparotomy [A]. One would expect in this day and age that there remains a very little role for laparotomy in the management of ectopic pregnancies. However, we would like to emphasize that many around the world would still justifiably be performing a laparotomy on patients with ectopic pregnancies due to the lack of endoscopic facilities. There have been three randomized controlled trials published in the early 1990s examining the effectiveness of laparotomy versus laparoscopy in the treatment of ectopic pregnancy. Combining the results of these three studies, a Cochrane review[6] reported that laparoscopic salpingostomy is less successful than salpingotomy performed at laparotomy in the elimination of the tubal pregnancy (RR 0.90, 95 per cent CI 0.83–0.97). This mainly resulted from the higher persistent trophoblastic rate in the laparoscopic group (RR 3.6, 95 per cent CI 0.63–21). There was, however, no difference in the number of future IUPs (RR 1.2, 95 per cent CI 0.88–1.5) or in the repeat ectopic pregnancy rate (RR 0.43, 95 per cent CI 0.15–1.2) between the two groups.

The higher persistent trophoblastic rate in the laparoscopic salpingotomy group suggests that there is a trade off for the various advantages of laparoscopic conservative surgery (salpingotomy) in the management of ectopic pregnancy. The likely explanation is that surgeons were better able to remove the ectopic tissue completely from the tube during laparotomy than at laparoscopy. This is not at all surprising given that all the RCTs were conducted in the 1990s, when laparoscopic skills were not as well established and instruments were not as refined. Many surgeons were in the 'learning phase' of laparoscopic surgery. The results would have been quite different if the RCTs were conducted more recently. Nevertheless, it does highlight the need to pay meticulous attention to the complete removal of the ectopic tissue during laparoscopic salpingotomy and to ensure that our trainees acquire the proper skills in this respect. Furthermore, it is important to highlight that there were no RCTs comparing laparoscopic salpingectomy with salpingectomy by laparotomy. On balance, we feel that there is little place for open surgery as a routine management of women with ectopic pregnancy, except for the rare incidences of a severely compromised patient. This view is no doubt reciprocated by many other gynaecologists.[7-9] Most gynaecologists will resort to a route that will stop the bleeding quickly when patients are in hypovolaemic shock with a large amount of haemoperitoneum and, in most centres, this will be via laparotomy.

## Salpingostomy or salpingectomy

Laparoscopic salpingotomy should be considered as primary treatment in the presence of contralateral tubal disease and the desire for future fertility [B]. In the pre-sence of a healthy contralateral tube, there is no clear evidence that salpingotomy is preferable to salpingectomy [B]. The subsequent IUP rates are similar for both the procedures. The rate of persistence of trophoblastic activity and chance of repeat ectopic are higher with salpingotomy than salpingectomy. However, one needs to appreciate that except for the macroscopic inspection of the Fallopian tubes during laparoscopy, there is currently no effective way of assessing function of the Fallopian tube. Tubal patency tests check for mechanical patency rather than tubal function. The ESEP study[10] is an ongoing international multicentre randomized controlled trial of salpingo(s)tomy versus salpingectomy for tubal pregnancy with a primary outcome measure being the occurrence of spontaneous viable intrauterine pregnancy, with the secondary outcome measure being the persistence of trophoblasts and repeat ectopic pregnancy ESEP will hopefully provide us with more conclusive data in the near future.

## Ovarian function

One possible complication of salpingectomy is the impairment of blood supply to the ovary and thus ovarian reserve. In attempting to minimize the complication of salpingectomy, i.e. compromise of ovarian blood supply, some surgeons advocate partial salpingectomy, i.e. removing only the distal part of the tube, leaving the proximal stump. However, this is not advisable because of two concerns. First, it increases the likelihood of ectopic pregnancy following IVF and second, leaving a long stump behind may have a similar effect to that of a hydrosalpinx, adversely affecting pregnancy rates and increasing the miscarriage rate following IVF. If we consider the anatomical relationship between the ovary and the Fallopian tube (Figure 57.1), it becomes apparent that the infundibulopelvic ligament is in close proximity to the suspensory ligament of the ovary; the latter carries the ovarian artery which together with the collaterals from the uterine artery, form the main blood supply to the ovaries. Hence, while performing a salpingectomy, one must keep close to the Fallopian tube and away from the suspensory ligament, thereby resulting in minimal compromise of the blood supply to the ovary. The use of non-traumatic forceps to help elevate the Fallopian tube away from the suspensory ligament of the ovary will allow the surgeon to divide the infundibulo-pelvic ligament without significantly compromising the blood supply from the ovarian artery (Figure 57.2). There have been several studies reporting a decrease in ovarian function in women who have had salpingectomy compared to those who have had salpingotomy.[11-13] Most of these studies have performed ovarian function assessment by measuring antral follicular count, ovarian volume and ovarian stromal flow by power Doppler ultrasonography (2D or 3D). Although Meng and Zhu[13] and Lass et al.[12] found no difference in the pregnancy rates between women who have had previous salpingectomy and the control group, they showed that the salpingectomy group had significantly fewer follicles and number of oocytes retrieved. The findings of these studies imply that surgery may have an impact on the functional physiology of the ovaries. Hence, while carrying out a salpingectomy, a complete salpingectomy is preferable to a partial salpingectomy with precautionary measures taken to preserve the ovarian blood supply.

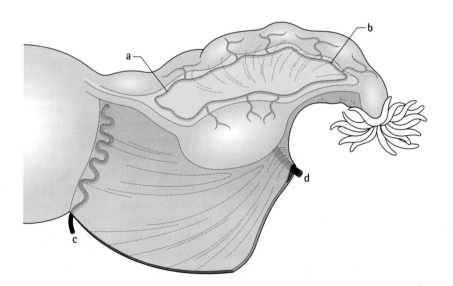

**Figure 57.1** Anatomical relationship of the ovary and F allopian tube: (a) medial tubal artery; (b) lateral tubal artery; (c) uterine artery; (d) ovarian artery.

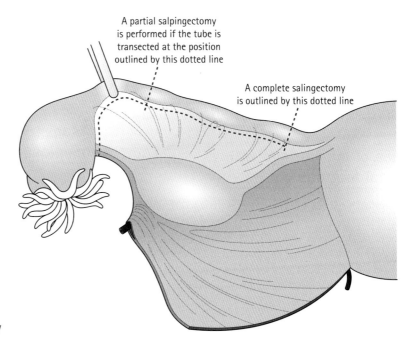

A partial salpingectomy
is performed if the tube is
transected at the position
outlined by this dotted line

A complete salingectomy
is outlined by this dotted line

**Figure 57.2** Fallopian tube with ectopic pregnancy

## Technical aspects

Many surgeons regard salpingectomy as an easier procedure to perform in comparison to salpingotomy. Laparoscopic salpingectomy can be performed by using pre-tied ligatures, coagulation of the mesosalpinx with monopolar or bipolar diathermy forceps and cutting with scissors or the use of laser or staplers. Bipolar diathermy and laparoscopic scissors are simple and safe and, with appropriate training, the necessary surgical skill may be easily acquired.

On the other hand, salpingotomy is usually performed by making an incision on the anti-mesenteric border of the Fallopian tube. This can be achieved either with diathermy scissors, monopolar needle diathermy or laser. None of these methods has been shown to be better than the other. Fujishita et al.[14] showed that the cumulative pregnancy rate, the adhesion formation/reformation rate and the tubal patency rate were similar whether the opening of the tubes was sutured or not. Bleeding from the diathermy site can be a troublesome problem. If extensive diathermy was applied to these bleeding sites, the tubal mucosa may be damaged. It has been suggested that local injection of vasopressin during the operation into the ectopic pregnancy might decrease bleeding; however, this has only been supported by a very small trial in 1996. Furthermore, vasopressin may rarely be associated with serious cardiovascular side effects. The use of hydro-dissection is a useful method for 'teasing' out the trophoblastic tissue without the need to use the grasping forceps. If the entire gestational sac were expelled rather than being removed 'piece-meal', the risk of persistent bleeding from the trophoblastic bed is less likely. The use of micro-diathermy can reduce the amount of tubal damage caused by diathermy as bleeding sites can be better tackled with pin-point accuracy. Gentle tissue handling is also vital in the prevention of future peritubal adhesions, and this can be achieved by using

non-traumatic instruments (e.g. forceps). At the end of the operation, adequate use of suction and irrigation to remove all residual blood in the pelvis is important to reduce the chances of fibrin deposition and adhesion formation/ reformation. Some surgeons advocate the use of adhesion prevention solution, such as 4 per cent Icodextrin (Adept, Baxter Healthcare, USA), which utilizes the hydroflotation theory to prevent adhesion formation/reformation.

## Conclusions

Management of an ectopic pregnancy should be based on the clinical presentation, βhCG and ultrasound findings. Methotrexate is an option for a selected group of patients with βhCG <5000 IU/L who are haemodynamically stable and compliant. Units offering this treatment must be well equipped to deal with out-of-hour emergencies and must be able to offer follow-up visits. Surgical treatment will remain the mainstay treatment modality for ectopic pregnancy in most units. It is important for every surgeon to understand the limitations of each procedure (salpingectomy versus salpingostomy) and to provide appropriate counselling. Laparotomy should be considered in the absence of adequate laparoscopic expertise and/or the presence of haemodynamic instability.

## MISCARRIAGE

Miscarriage is a pregnancy that ends spontaneously before the fetus has reached a viable gestational age. At present, the legal definition of miscarriage in the UK is spontaneous loss of pregnancy at or before 24 weeks gestation.

Reproductive medicine

## Risk of miscarriage

Sporadic miscarriage is the most common complication of pregnancy. The incidence in a clinical recognizable pregnancy is 10–20 per cent. The incidence decreases after the 8th week of pregnancy to about 10 per cent and drops to 3 per cent if a viable fetus has been recognized on ultrasound scan.

## Types of miscarriage with clinical features

The clinical features of types of miscarriage are shown in Table 57.1.

Maternal age is an independent risk factor for miscarriage. Advanced maternal age leads to a decreased number of good quality oocytes, resulting in chromosomally abnormal conceptus leading to a miscarriage.

## Recurrent miscarriage

It is defined as spontaneous loss of three or more consecutive pregnancies. It affects 1 per cent of all women. However, it is not in the remit of this chapter to discuss this entity in detail.

## Management

There is currently no evidence to support the use of the following in the management of miscarriage:

- progesterone supplement for prevention of miscarriage;
- progesterone supplement for treatment of threatened miscarriage;
- uterine muscle relaxant for prevention of miscarriage;
- bed rest;
- oestrogen supplementation – avoid especially diethyl-stilbestrol;
- multivitamins.

## Management – expectant, medical or surgical

Patients with miscarriage can have expectant, medical or surgical management.

### Expectant

The natural course of an early pregnancy loss is unknown, and it is questionable if all women with a miscarriage should have any intervention at all. Expectant management allows for the avoidance of surgery and general anaesthesia; patients also potentially feel more in control. In a survey of women attending a family planning clinic, respondents indicated a strong preference for expectant treatment as a future preferred therapy, but the physician's recommendation would clearly influence their decision. Patients undergoing expectant care are more likely to have retained products of conception or incomplete miscarriage, with a complete evacuation rate of around 30 per cent. This is more likely in the presence of an intact gestational sac on ultrasound. Comparatively, expectant management is relatively effective in women with incomplete miscarriage, with a complete success rate of around 95 per cent.

Thong et al.[15] observed a complete miscarriage rate of 81 per cent over an observation period of 2 weeks and 93 per cent over 7 weeks. Clearly, studies conducted over a shorter

| Type of miscarriage | Ultrasound findings | Clinical presentation | Action |
|---|---|---|---|
| Threatened miscarriage | Intrauterine pregnancy, i.e. gestation sac with yolk sac ± fetal pole and cardiac activity | Bleeding ± pain | Reassure. Follow up depending on symptoms |
| | | Speculum/pelvic examination - Os closed | |
| Inevitable miscarriage | Intrauterine pregnancy i.e. gestation sac with yolk sac ± fetal pole and cardiac activity | Bleeding ± pain | Loss of pregnancy inevitable. Admit and discuss options |
| | | Speculum/pelvic examination - Os open | |
| Incomplete miscarriage | Retained products of conception | Bleeding ± pain | Admit and discuss options |
| | | Speculum/pelvic examination - Os open, ± products at the Os | |
| Complete miscarriage | Empty uterus or ultrasound appearances showing less than 15 mm in diameter of retained tissue | Minimal bleeding ± pain | Reassure and GP follow. βhCG monitoring if ectopic not ruled out |
| | | Speculum/pelvic examination - Os closed | |
| Missed/early fetal demise/ anembryonic pregnancy | RCOG/RCR criteria | Bleeding ± pain | Expectant/medical/surgical |
| | CRL >6 mm, no FHM Empty gestation sac with mean diameter >20 mm | | |

follow up period will potentially report a higher incidence of failure of treatment. The use of ultrasound assessment versus clinical assessment will also affect the success rate of any treatment of miscarriage, although an ultrasound assessment of the uterine cavity with shadows identified as AP diameter less than 15 mm is unlikely to contain any retained products on histology. However, it is important to appreciate that if an ultrasound cut-off of greater than 15 mm is used, the proportion of women classed as failure of treatment will increase.

Women undergoing expectant care are more likely to require unplanned surgery due to unacceptable pain and bleeding compared to those who have had surgical evacuation,[16] although pelvic infection is less common in women managed with expectant care compared to those who had surgery due to the lack of instrumentation of the uterus.

## Surgical

Some clinicians recommend surgical intervention to avoid the uncertainty regarding passage of tissue with expectant management, since this may be upsetting to some women. Surgical management or evacuation of products of conception (ERPC) has a high success rate of 95–100 per cent. A Cochrane review in 2001[17] concluded that vacuum (suction) aspiration was associated with significantly decreased blood loss (mean difference 17 mL, CI –24 to –10 mL), less pain and shorter duration of procedure than sharp curettage [A]. Sharp curettage is therefore only routinely recommended at the end of the surgical procedure.

However, surgical evacuation has its drawbacks, including risks such as cervical trauma and subsequent cervical incompetence, uterine perforation, intrauterine adhesions or post-operative pelvic infection. The incidence of serious morbidity is about 2 per cent with a mortality of 0.5/100 000. The use of prostaglandin vaginally prior to the surgical evacuation can help prime the cervix, make dilatation of the cervix easier and potentially reduce some of the risks and morbidity. Hysteroscopic assessment of the uterine cavity following ERPCs has demonstrated that intrauterine adhesions form in up to 8 per cent of patients, although mostly these adhesions do not result in long-term fertility issues or menstrual problems. Very occasionally, moderate to severe adhesions can result from ERPCs and these adhesions can be a challenge to treat.

## Medical management

Approximately 20 per cent of women with miscarriage will opt for medical management. Prostaglandins are used in single or divided doses administered orally (misoprostol) or vaginally (Gemeprost). Misoprostol is cheap and effective in both oral and vaginal forms. Several studies have been conducted comparing oral and vaginal misoprostol. Most RCTs have shown similar success rates with either routes of administration of misoprostol.

In delayed miscarriage, addition of a progesterone antagonist to the prostaglandin regime is often used to promote cervical ripening and placenta separation. Overall, medical management is successful in 70–95 per cent of incomplete miscarriage and in about 50–90 per cent of delayed miscarriage. It has been shown to be most successful in pregnancies under 10 weeks or with a mean gestational sac diameter under 24 mm.

A meta-analysis in 2004[18] identified 13 trials comparing expectant management to medical management in patients with missed and incomplete miscarriage and showed that in women with missed miscarriage, the success rate with expectant management was 21 per cent as against 81 per cent patients who were managed using medical treatment. In women with incomplete miscarriage, the success rate with expectant management was 94 per cent and it was 99 per cent in the group that underwent medical management. Thus, medical management has a higher success rate than expectant management in women with missed miscarriage. Both these methods have similar success rates for incomplete miscarriage. Both the expectant and medical management regimes are good alternatives to surgical treatment in appropriately selected patients [A].

Few randomized controlled trials[19-21] have compared the efficacy of one or two doses of 600–800 μg of misoprostol with surgical evacuation. The efficacy with misoprostol was reported to be 85 per cent at the end of 1 week and it was 93 per cent with the surgical group. Thus, medical management is clinically useful since it reduces the need for surgical curettage and has a lower complication rate.

Surgical uterine evacuation has been the standard treatment offered to patients for many years.

Several randomized controlled trials[22,23] have compared medical versus surgical treatments in women with missed or incomplete miscarriage. Overall, the success rate of surgical treatment is superior to that of medical treatment (95–99 per cent versus 50–90 per cent, respectively).

A meta-analysis in 2005[24] compared expectant, medical and surgical management of first trimester miscarriage. They concluded that expectant management had a markedly variable success rate (39 per cent) depending upon the type of miscarriage. The overall efficacy with the medical and surgical management was 62 and 95 per cent, respectively.

## Conclusion

Surgical treatment has a higher success rate than expectant or medical treatment in missed or incomplete miscarriage. Both expectant and medical treatments have an equal success rate in incomplete miscarriage. Medical treatment is more successful than expectant management in women with missed miscarriage.

Expectant and medical management are effective alternatives to surgical management. They should be offered to women with easy access to the hospital. Patients need to be counselled appropriately regarding the efficacy and side effects of medication used, along with the potential risks involved with each treatment. Finally, patients preference (after appropriate counselling) plays an important role in the decision making process regarding the treatment options.

---

## KEY POINTS

- Miscarriages and ectopic pregnancies are two large groups of life-threatening emergencies.
- Diagnosis is based on correlation of ultrasound scan findings with βhCG levels.
- Expectant, medical and surgical management options are all well known and are based on haemodynamic stability.
- Ultrasound findings, βhCG levels and patient preference.

---

## Key References

1. Jauniaux ERM, Jurkovic D. The role of ultrasound in abnormal early pregnancy. In: Grudzinkas TG, O'Brien PMS (eds). *Textbook of Problems in Early Pregnancy. Advances in Diagnosis and Management.* London: RCOG Press, 1997.

2. Elson J, Tailor A, Banerjee S *et al.* Expectant management of tubal ectopic: prediction of successful outcome using decision tree analysis. *Ultrasound Obstet Gynecol* 2004; **23**: 552–6.

3. Helmy S, Sawyer E, Ofili-Yebovi D *et al.* Fertility outcomes following expectant management of tubal ectopic pregnancy. *Ultrasound Obstet Gynecol* 2007; **30**: 988–93.

4. Van Mello NM, Mol F, Adriaanse AH *et al.* The METEX Study: methotrexate versus expectant management in women with ectopic pregnancy: a randomised controlled trial. *BMC Women's Health* 2008; **8**: 10.

5. Mol F, Mol W, Ankum WM *et al.* Current evidence on surgery, systemic methotrexate and expectant management in the treatment of tubal pregnancy: a systematic review and meta-analysis. *Human Reprod Update* 2008; **14**: 309–19.

6. Hajenius PJ, Mol F, Mol BWJ *et al.* Interventions for tubal ectopic pregnancy. *Cochrane Database Syst Rev* 2007; (**1**): CD000324.

7. Garry R. Laparoscopic surgery. *Best Pract Res Clin Obstet Gynaecol* 2006; **20**: 89–104.

8. Orazi G, Cosson M. Surgical treatment of ectopic pregnancy. *J Gynecol Obstet Biol Reprod* 2003; **32** (7 Suppl): S75–82.

9. Takacs P, Chakhtoura N. Laparotomy to laparoscopy: changing trends in the surgical management of ectopic pregnancy in a tertiary care teaching hospital. *J Minim Invasive Gynecol* 2006; **13**: 175–7.

10. Mol F, Strandell A, Jurkovic D *et al.* The ESEP study: salpingostomy versus salpingectomy for tubal ectopic pregnancy, the impact on future fertility: a randomised controlled trial. *BMC Women's Health* 2008; **8**: 11.

11. Chan CC, Ng EH, Li CF, Ho PC. Impaired ovarian blood flow and reduced antral follicle count following laparoscopic salpingectomy for ectopic pregnancy. *Hum Reprod* 2003; **18**: 2175–80.

12. Lass A, Ellenbogen A, Croucher C *et al.* Effect of salpingectomy on ovarian response to super ovulation in an *in vitro* fertilisation–embryo transfer program. *Fertil Steril* 1998; **70**: 1035–8.

13. Meng XH, Zhu U. Effect of salpingectomy on ovarian function. *Zhejiang Da Xue Xue Bao Yi Xue Ban* 2006; **35**: 555–9.

14. Fujishita A, Masuzaki H, Khan KN *et al.* Laparoscopic salpingotomy for tubal pregnancy: comparison of linear salpingotomy with and without suturing. *Hum Reprod* 2004: **19**: 1195–200.

15. Thong KJ, Mahmood TA, Shehata KI. A randomized trial comparing conservative management versus surgical uterine evacuation for first trimester miscarriage with retained products of conception. Available from: www.show.scot.nhs.uk/cso/Publications/ExecSumms/Oct_Nov02.htm.

16. Nanda K, Peloggia A, Grimes D. Expectant care versus surgical treatment for miscarriage. *Cochrane Database Syst Rev* 2006; (**2**): CD003518.

17. Forna F, Gulmezoglu AM. *Cochrane Database Syst Rev* 2001; (**1**): CD001993.

18. Graziosi GC, Mol BW, Ankum WM, Bruinse HW. Management of early pregnancy loss. *Int J Gynaecol Obstet* 2004; **86**: 337–46.

19. Graziosi GC, Mol BW, Reuwer PJ *et al.* Misoprostol versus curettage in women with early pregnancy failure after initial expectant management: a randomised controlled trial. *Hum Reprod* 2004; **19**: 1894–9.

20. Dempsey, AMD. Early pregnancy disorders: An update and eye to the future. *Semin Reprod Med* 2008; **26**: 401–10.

21. Bagratee JS, Khullar V, Regan L *et al.* A randomised controlled trial comparing medical and expectant management of first trimester miscarriage. *Hum Reprod* 2004; **19**: 266–71.

22. Hinshaw K, Cooper K, Henshaw R *et al.* Management of uncomplicated miscarriage. *BMJ* 1993; **307**: 259.

23. Chung TK, Lee DT, Cheung LP *et al.* Spontaneous abortion: a randomised controlled trial comparing surgical evacuation with conservative management using misoprostol. *Fertil Steril* 1999; **71**: 1054–9.

24. Sotiriadis A, Makrydimas G, Papatheoudorou S, Ioannidis JP. Expectant, medical or surgical management of first trimester miscarriage: a meta analysis. *Obstet Gynecol* 2005; **105**: 1104–13.

# Chapter 58

# Reproductive ageing and ovarian reserve

*Dimitrios Nikolaou*

## INTRODUCTION

The 'biological clock' is emerging as one of the most agonising issues for women in their late thirties and forties in developed countries. Women are anxious to know particularly if they can assess and safely postpone their fertility potential. In order to address these issues properly one needs to have not only training in assisted reproduction technology (ART), but also a good understanding of the biology, epidemiology and demography of ageing in general and reproductive ageing in particular, as well as the basic principles of 'screening' and evidence-based medicine. The advice to patients will be individualized, based on their circumstances. The aim of this chapter is to provide an overview of the key facts and hypotheses currently surrounding the issue of reproductive ageing and ovarian reserve assessment, both in the management of infertility and in the general population.

## OVARIAN AGEING AND THE POPULATION OF HUMAN FOLLICLES

Although there has been some controversy in recent years, it is generally accepted that women are born with a finite supply of eggs which is not renewed after birth. The primordial germ cells originate from the endoderm of the yolk sac, near the caudal end of the embryo, where they have been identified by the end of the third week. Some 1000–2000 migrate to the gonadal ridge, where they multiply until about the 20th week of gestation, when a maximum of seven million has been reached. Follicles begin to form during the fourth month of fetal life. Although some of these newly formed follicles start to grow almost immediately, most of them remain in the resting phase until they either degenerate or some signals(s) activate them to enter the growth phase. After growth has started, most follicles will become atretic with apoptosis. Only one million follicles remain at birth and by the time of menarche their number is reduced to about 300 000. During the entire reproductive life, only about 400 follicles will reach full maturation and ovulation.

## GRANULOSA CELLS OR OOCYTES?

Where exactly in the follicle does the atresia start? One theory is that it is caused by the failing of the granulosa cell compartment. According to this theory, the 'pacemaker' for the onset and progression of reproductive senescence in women is granulosa cell competence: within the ageing follicles there are fewer granulosa cells. These granulosa cells demonstrate decreased mitosis and increased apoptosis. As a result of compromised endocrine, paracrine and autocrine signals, there is altered communication between the granulosa cells and the oocyte. This causes abnormal nuclear and cytoplasmic maturation within the oocyte. These authors believe that timely interventions, directed at improving or replacing granulosa cell function, may help delay reproductive ageing.

Although there is no doubt that the granulosa cells have an important contribution, the most recent evidence suggests that the oocyte drives its own development and is responsible for the proliferation, development and function of the granulosa cells. It seems that there are oocyte-derived growth factors that are obligatory for normal foliculogenesis and female fertility. Furthermore, there is evidence to suggest that the target cells for the action of these growth factors are the granulosa cells. In the ovaries of all mammals examined to date, the oocyte is the only cell type that expresses these genes. One example of these factors is GDF-9. Studies of GDF-deficient mice have provided strong evidence that GDF-9 has a critical physiological role in stimulating granulosa-cell proliferation during the gonadotropin-independent period. Importantly, GDF-9 acts directly on granulosa cells from pre-antral, as well as developing follicles, to stimulate DNA synthesis.

## EPIDEMIOLOGY OF MENOPAUSE AND VARIABILITY OF MENOPAUSAL AGE

The obvious end-point of reproductive ageing, the menopause, has enormous variation between individuals. The median age of menopause in the western world is around 50–51 years, although there is a wide range between 35 and 60 years. As with every human characteristic, it depends on a number of genetic and environmental factors, including the fetal environment. Genetic and epidemiological studies, including twin studies, have shown that the age of menopause has high inheritability.[1] This means that it is mostly genetically determined, and the effect of the various environmental factors is very limited. Smoking seems to be one factor that has a statistically significant effect on the age of menopause, albeit a reduction by 1–2 years. Long-term use of the combined oral contraceptive seems to have a very small protective effect and can prolong reproductive life by one year or so [C].

It was proposed in the early 1990s, on the basis of mathematical modeling on previously collected pathological datasets, that the rate of atresia of follicles follows a biphasic pattern, with an accelerated loss starting at an average age of 37.5 years.[2] This model was nicknamed the 'broken stick' model, because of the break-point at 37.5 years. In fact, it seems unlikely that something very sudden happens at the exact level of 25 000 remaining follicles, but it is certain that there is an accelerated loss of follicles in the late thirties.

At the same time, Faddy et al. put forward this important hypothesis: the rate of follicular atresia in the ovary depends not on age per se but on the number of remaining follicles.[2] At the age of 37.5, an estimated 25 000 follicles remain in the ovaries. They hypothesized that an accelerated decline of follicles will always start when there are fewer than 25 000 follicles in the ovary, regardless of age. On this basis, they speculated that the age at menopause could be predicted using mathematical models, on the basis of total follicle counts at different ages. For example, a unilateral oophorectomy before the age of 30 years would not lower follicle numbers below 25 000 and so the rate of disappearance would continue at the lower rate for some years before a more rapid depletion began. The threshold number of 1000 remaining follicles (menopause) would then be reached at around the age of 44. When the same operation was performed between the ages of 30 and 37.5 years, the remaining follicles would abruptly fall below 25 000 and the phase of rapid loss would be entered immediately, resulting in the age by which menopausal threshold was reached increasing (from 44 years) by $0.6 \pm 0.06$ years for each year after the age of 30 years.

## DECLINE OF NATURAL FERTILITY WITH AGE

Natural fertility is known to decline with maternal age.[3] Women normally experience their peak fertility in the early twenties. There is a small decline of fertility until the age of 30, followed by a slightly accelerated decline until the age of 35–37, and a very rapid decline thereafter. This is true for both the natural fertility rates and the assisted conception rates [C]. Some of the evidence had been recorded in the Hutterites, a sect of anabaptist refugees from Europe who settled in North America over a century ago. This community forbade any form of fertility control while enjoying a high standard of living and health care. In the 1950s, women in this community were delivering an average of 11 babies each, and the peak age of fertility was 30 years of age. Half of the women had delivered the last child by 40, when only 1 per cent was postmenopausal.

Even the most sensitive pregnancy assays cannot detect a rise in hCG until about 6 or 7 days after conception. The risk of fetal loss appears to be highest very early in pregnancy. As a result, most population studies of fertility report the monthly probability of conception that survives long enough to produce a detectable pregnancy.[3] In a nine month prospective endocrinological study in a natural fertility population in rural Bangladesh, O'Connor et al. used a model to estimate fecundability and fetal loss, that was based on previous work by Wood and Boklage.[3] The results indicated that much of the decline in fertility could be attributed to an increasing risk of fetal loss with maternal age. The probability of fetal loss showed a steady increase from about 45 per cent at age 18 to 92 per cent at age 38. In contrast, total probability of conception per month was high and nearly constant until age 40, when it dropped rapidly to nearly zero by age 46. These results suggested that the observed decline in fertility from the early twenties to the early forties was not caused by a decline in the monthly probability of conception; rather, it was a result of an increasing risk of fetal loss with maternal age.

## ASSISTED CONCEPTION SUCCESS RATES DECLINE WITH AGE

In assisted conception, live-birth rates have been shown in many studies to depend on the woman's age and decline sharply after the age of 35.[4] After adjustment for age, other important factors are the duration of infertility and history of previous pregnancy and live-birth [C]. Although there has been an improvement of IVF success rates among younger women in the last ten years, data from the Human Fertilization and Embryology Authority show that the success rates have remained almost unchanged, less than 10 per cent live-birth rate per attempt, for women over 40 and less than 5 per cent for women over 42.[4] In other words, ART is not a good treatment for the age-related decline of fertility, other than offering egg-donation [C].

## THE FIXED INTERVALS HYPOTHESIS

The only reproductive event that is clearly recognizable is the menopause. This occurs when the remaining number of resting follicles in the ovaries falls below a critical number, which has been estimated at 1000 follicles. It was proposed by te Velde and colleagues that the time-differences between all the major reproductive milestones and the menopause are more or less fixed.[5] Furthermore, that the same factors that affect age at menopause – which are mainly genetic – affect all major reproductive milestones that depend on number of resting follicles in the ovary. These milestones are the beginning of subfertility, the loss of fertility and the loss of menstrual regularity (Figure 58.1).

Support for this hypothesis came from epidemiological and laboratory observations. It was found that the time interval between the loss of menstrual regularity and menopause was 6–7 years, regardless of age at menopause.[6] Richardson et al. had previously shown that women with regular periods had ten times more follicles than women with irregular periods. Also, te Velde et al. quoted data that the age of last delivery for Canadian women in the nineteenth century showed the same variation as the age of menopause, but ten years earlier.

However, as we will see later, epidemiological and clinical observations in assisted conception suggest that the time-interval between loss of fertility and menopause is not stable; it is shorter in cases of very early menopause and much

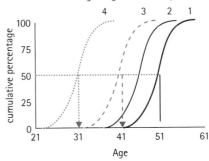

**Figure 58.1** Fixed intervals theory. Reproduced with permission from ref. 6

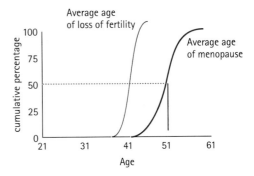

**Figure 58.2** Age of infertility and age of menopause

longer in cases of very late menopause [E].[7] In other words, the variation of age of menopause is much greater and not exactly parallel with the age of infertility. This has important implications in the management of infertility in women of different ages (Figure 58.2).

## OVARIAN RESERVE

The term 'ovarian reserve' is used to describe the number and quality of oocytes in a woman's ovary. Direct measurement of the resting follicle pool of each individual woman is not possible. Ovarian biopsies combined with computerized calculations have been evaluated and there is an ongoing debate, but there are problems caused by the uneven distribution of the follicles within the ovary. A further contribution of ART has been the development of the so-called 'ovarian reserve tests'. The main focus has been the prediction of IVF outcome. There is an ever-growing literature on this subject and numerous possible markers and combinations of them have been assessed. In general, these tests fall into one of the following categories: 'Basal' endocrine markers, such as the day 2 FSH, LH, oestradiol and inhibin B; dynamic biochemical tests, such as the clomiphene citrate challenge test, the exogenous FSH stimulation test and the GnRH stimulation test; Basal biophysical tests, including Doppler studies of the blood-flow in the ovaries, ovarian volume and follicular counts.

Most of the known baseline ovarian reserve tests, apart from the antral follicle counts, provide an indirect reflection of the size of cohort of antral follicles, which is thought to be associated with the size of the large pool of resting follicles. Anti-müllerian hormone (AMH) is involved in folliculogenesis and shows good correlation with chronological age, antral follicle counts and IVF outcome. Because it is related to a much earlier stage of follicle development than all other common markers of the ovarian reserve, AMH measurement is the closest we can get, so far, to measuring the actual primordial follicle pool.

## BASIC ENDOCRINOLOGY OF OVARIAN AGEING

In considering a hormone as a possible marker for ovarian ageing in general, it is important to study the way the serum levels of this hormone change over the course of the reproductive life of healthy fertile woman. It has been known for some time that the early follicular phase FSH of normally cycling women starts to rise considerably in the late thirties. However, there seems to be a large overlap between FSH levels of older and younger women. Schipper et al. found no correlation between age and maximum FSH levels in the early follicular phase in 38 volunteers, and there were important differences in the FSH level between these individuals.[8] Faced with similar observations, Brown et al. had proposed the 'threshold' concept: women have different FSH levels above which follicles are stimulated for further growth.[9] It is difficult to be sure, therefore, whether a moderately elevated FSH in a relatively younger woman reflects early ovarian ageing (EOA) or not. In terms of IVF, the early follicular FSH can predict poor response only if the cut-off level is set quite high. Interestingly, it has been proposed that the duration, rather than the magnitude, of elevated FSH plays the crucial role in determining the number of follicles that will undergo further development. This is the concept of the 'FSH window', which has been substantiated by the finding that elevating FSH levels high above the 'threshold' level for a short period of time in the early follicular phase does not increase the number of dominant follicles. It has been suggested that individual differences in ovarian sensitivity for FSH are determined by the balance between ovarian factors that enhance or attenuate the FSH signal. It has also been hypothesized that measuring changes in early follicular phase FSH over a time in a given individual could provide a more sensitive test of ovarian ageing.[9]

LH levels are also known to rise with age, but 5–10 years later than the rise of FSH. Oestradiol and progesterone levels tend to vary in the various studies, but the general impression is that oestradiol and progesterone levels do not show important changes with increasing age. Oestradiol, progesterone and inhibin A levels reflect the function of the dominant follicle, whereas inhibin B in the early follicular phase reflects the cohort of follicles recruited for further development. The dominant follicle itself in women of advanced reproductive age still manages to produce an almost normal hormonal output, whereas the cohort of antral follicles declines both quantitatively and qualitatively.

With regards to inhibin B, our whole understanding has changed since the introduction of the specific inhibin B assay. There appears to be an inverse relationship between inhibin B and FSH in the early follicular phase. It has been shown that early follicular phase secretion of inhibin B is decreased in older women who demonstrate a monotropic FSH rise. In IVF studies, a decrease in day 3 serum inhibin B has been observed before a rise in day 3 FSH in women with poor ovarian responsiveness. Inhibin B is the dominant circulating form of inhibin in the early and mid-follicular phase, while inhibin A is the dominant form of circulating inhibin in the late follicular and luteal phases.

## SELECTABLE FOLLICLES, OVARIAN AGEING AND THE ROLE OF ULTRASOUND

One of the most widely accepted models of follicular development and depletion is the one proposed by Gougeon.[11] According to this model, at any time a proportion of follicles are moving through various stages of follicular maturation. Eight classes were proposed to describe follicular development from the pre-antral stage to ovulation. It takes several months for a primordial follicle to reach the pre-antral stage. The subsequent period of development required for a follicle to pass through all eight classes is approximately 85 days. During the basal growth (classes 1–4), the development of human follicles requires only small levels of gonadotrophins. These follicles are faintly responsive to cyclic gonadotropin changes. From a size of 2 mm, the follicles enter the 'rapid' growth phase and become more dependent on FSH.[10] Follicles 2–5 mm in diameter are present throughout the menstrual cycle. During the late luteal phase, the 2–5 mm follicles, which have entered the preantral stage 70 days earlier, become selectable follicles (class 5) and constitute the pool of follicles from which the one destined to ovulate in the subsequent cycle is selected. Their number in the late luteal phase is 3–11 per ovary in 24–33-year-old women and rapidly decrease with advancing age, with an abrupt drop in women over the age of 40. This evolution parallels that observed for non-growing follicles, suggesting that the number of selectable follicles (2–5 mm) at the late luteal and early follicular phase of the menstrual cycle reflects the size of the stock of non-growing follicles. The size of the antral follicle cohort may be a reflection of the actual ovarian reserve of a woman and can easily be assessed using transvaginal ultrasound. This assessment has been shown to be accurate and reproducible.

# POOR RESPONSE TO OVARIAN STIMULATION AS A MODEL OF OVARIAN AGEING

Women of the same age respond differently to gonadotropin stimulation in ART. Some have fewer oocytes collected and lower peak oestradiol levels than others who receive the same amount of FSH. Generally, these women are called 'poor responders', although there is still no universally accepted definition of 'poor response'. It has been observed that increasing the exogenous FSH dose beyond a certain limit does not usually improve the outcome in terms of live-birth rate. This limit has been estimated at around 300 IU FSH/day. Various stimulation protocols have been tried to improve the success rate of poor responders and these generally involve a higher dose of FSH, lower dose and duration of GnRHa and various adjuvant treatments, such as aspirin, dexamethasone, etc. None of these treatments, however, has so far been very successful. Poor responders generally have a poorer prognosis for future IVF cycles.

## Poor responders go into menopause earlier

Another significant contribution of ART was to shed light on the time-interval between subfertility, infertility and menopause. These would otherwise be difficult to study epidemiologically, as the transition between fertility and infertility is asymptomatic. It was found that regularly menstruating women aged 35–40, with normal baseline FSH, who did not respond to high-dose ovarian stimulation, went into their menopause significantly earlier than age-matched controls with a good response.[11] If we accept that non-response corresponds to the end of fertility, the above observation would suggest that there is a similar (if not parallel) variation between loss of fertility and menopause. This would be in keeping with the fixed intervals hypothesis. Further studies have confirmed the above findings. Furthermore, it was found that women who had a relatively poor response to ovarian stimulation (not just the absolute non-responders) also went into the menopause earlier than age-matched controls. In addition, it was found that the relative poor responders had poorer future fertility prognosis with lower cumulative success rates. If we accept that a relative poor response to stimulation represents a stage between optimal fertility and infertility, these findings from ART would suggest that women with earlier decline of their fertility also go into the menopause earlier [C].

# 'EARLY OVARIAN AGEING'

The average woman will go into the menopause at the age of 51, having started an accelerated decline of the ovarian follicles at the age of 38, some 13 years earlier. On the basis of a fixed interval of around 13 years between onset of accelerated decline of the ovarian reserve and the menopause, women who go into the menopause before the age of 46 (early menopause) will have started an accelerated decline of their ovarian reserve before the age of 32. It has been proposed that this process, which represents a shift to the left of the normal ageing process, should be called 'early ovarian ageing'.[12,13] On the basis of epidemiological data, that 10 per cent of women go into 'early menopause' before the age of 46, it was estimated that 10 per cent of women in the general population might be at risk of 'early ovarian ageing' [E]. While they are still young, these women are still fertile and completely asymptomatic. It was suggested that EOA has a long latent phase (some 13 years before the menopause) and a predictable natural history, in accordance with the model of Faddy et al.[2] It is associated with a number of predictable sequelae, in terms of fertility prognosis, reproductive and general health. For these reasons, it was also proposed that EOA might be suitable for screening among asymptomatic young women in the general population or in high risk groups, using tests that were initially developed to predict the outcome of IVF, especially the AMH and antral follicular counts (AFC).[12,13] A significant role for ART would be to provide a model for the initial development and validation of these tests. On the basis of the fixed intervals theory, it was suggested that the same epidemiological factors that determine the age of menopause are likely to determine the risk of EOA. The main factors are genetic, but there are also acquired factors. On this basis, it is possible to describe high-risk groups for EOA in the general population.[12,13]

## 'Early ovarian ageing' versus 'premature ovarian failure'

Premature ovarian failure (POF) is the end-point of an extreme form of EOA and affects 1 per cent of the general population [C]. It is associated with irregular periods or secondary amenorrhea and menopausal symptoms, as well as very abnormally high baseline FSH. There is no effective fertility treatment for POF other than egg-donation. On the contrary, EOA is much more common (10 per cent). It refers to asymptomatic young women in the general population. Women with EOA have regular periods and their baseline FSH may be within normal limits. They are fertile and will remain fertile for a few years following the diagnosis. Therefore, unlike POF, EOA is a public health issue.[7] It may be amenable to primary prevention, screening, secondary prevention of childlessness through early intervention.

# What is the cause of the age-related deterioration of oocyte quality?

The rapid decline of pregnancy rates in the late thirties, both naturally and with IVF, is accompanied by an increasing rate of spontaneous miscarriage, chromosomal abnormalities in the embryos and is mainly attributed to a deterioration of oocyte quality. The cause of age-related deterioration of oocyte quality has been an issue of scientific debate for some time. It is generally accepted that the main mechanism is meiotic non-disjunction. Generally, one approach has been that it is caused by an accumulation of damage in the DNA of the oocyte as a woman grows older. Another, that differentiation of oocyte quality is already established, to some degree, in fetal life and the best oocytes are simply recruited and selected first, so that oocytes of inferior quality remain at a more advanced age. The 'two-hit' model of non-disjunction appears to combine all the previous theories of oocyte-ageing.[6] The overall impact of the second 'hit', which is the effect of the environment on the quality of the pool of oocytes, depends on the duration of the exposure and therefore age.[14]

## Fertility in early ovarian ageing

On the basis of the 'two hit' theory, in cases of EOA, caused by unilateral oophorectomy for example, the quantitative decline of the ovarian reserve (number of remaining follicles) is faster than the qualitative decline (proportion of good quality oocytes) (Figure 58.3). Hence, young women with EOA are not infertile.[14] Women who are undergoing an EOA process are fertile in their early thirties. They are also asymptomatic, with regular periods. There are two reasons: first that they still have enough follicles. Second, and most important,

that the quality of their oocytes is still good, as it mainly depends on their chronological age; hence, the scope for early diagnosis.[7,12,13] This is reflected in the better IVF success rates of 'poor responders' who are chronologically young, compared to the extremely poor IVF outcome of older 'poor responders' [C].[14] Hence, the scope for screening: an early indication may help women with EOA make informed decisions about having their own families before it is too late. Eventually, of course, as the best oocytes are recruited and selected first, fertility will be lost earlier than expected by age alone.

Do young women with EOA have the exactly the same or less fertility than women of the same age with 'normal' ovarian biological age? Data from IVF suggest that young true poor responders (who have received at least 300 IU of FSH a day for ovarian stimulation and had fewer than four eggs collected) have lower live-birth rates than women of the same age with normal response. This would suggest that young women with EOA have reduced fertility potential. This would be in keeping with laboratory observations: Brook et al., working on ovariectomized mice, reported that mice that had undergone unilateral oophorectomy started to produce aneuploid embryos at a much younger age than expected.[15] They suggested that there was a continuum of age-related aneuploidy in women, governed by biological age, and that any factor, which depleted the oocyte population, could also advance the maternal age for aneuploidy [C].

## Sequelae of early ovarian ageing

The sequelae of EOA are predictable on the basis of the above [E]. When they are still in their early thirties, most women with EOA will be completely asymptomatic with regular menstrual cycles and normal baseline endocrine markers. They will be fertile for a few more years following the early diagnosis. However, their fertility will be less than the fertility of their peers with normal ovarian ageing and will reach extremely low levels much earlier than expected on age alone.[13] They will eventually go into the menopause before the age of 46. In the years following the diagnosis, they may take longer to conceive or present with 'unexplained infertility'. During an IVF cycle, they may behave as 'poor responders' to ovarian stimulation in IVF and need higher doses of gonadotrophins. Apart from reduced likelihood of conception, both natural and with IVF, they will have a higher incidence of fetal aneuploidy, miscarriage and dizygotic twinning. They will have a tendency towards shorter menstrual cycles, although menstrual irregularity will not appear for 3–4 more years on average after the total loss of fertility. They may also have a tendency towards adverse lipid profiles and an increased cardiovascular risk.

There is evidence to support the above: the link between unexplained subfertility and poor ovarian reserve has been a finding of many studies. There have been studies linking

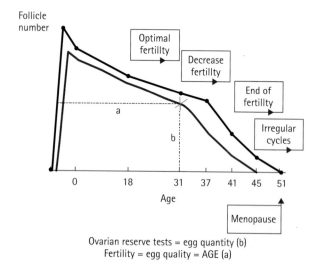

Ovarian reserve tests = egg quantity (b)
Fertility = egg quality = AGE (a)

**Figure 58.3** Fertility in early ovarian ageing

unexplained subfertility and a poorer obstetric outcome. Elevated FSH concentrations in the early follicular phase of the menstrual cycle have been shown to be associated with trisomy-21 and other aneuploidies.[17,18] In order to clarify whether this rise of FSH was due to diminished ovarian reserve, van Montfrans et al. measured inhibin B and E2 in women with a history of a Down's syndrome baby and in controls. They found that basal FSH concentrations were significantly elevated in Down's syndrome mothers and that there was a statistically significant negative correlation between basal FSH and inhibin B concentrations.[16,17] Trout and Seifer[18,19] showed that women with unexplained recurrent pregnancy loss had a greater incidence of elevated day 3 serum FSH and E2 levels than women with a known cause for recurrent miscarriage. Epidemiological studies have long shown a link between dizygotic twinning and an earlier menopause.[20,21] The association between increased pituitary FSH and dizygotic twinning has also been observed for many years. Martin et al. concluded that being a mother of DZ twins was a significant risk factor for premature ovarian failure.[20] In an interesting report, pre-menopausal women with serum FSH >7 mIU/L had significantly elevated total serum cholesterol and LDL levels compared with premenopausal women of the same age with FSH levels <7 mIU/L.

The findings of the last study would be in agreement with some very interesting research linking early reproductive ageing to early general ageing. Some of the evidence comes from observations on accelerated ageing syndromes, such as Werner's syndrome, ataxia telangiectasia, Hutchison-Gilford progeria and Down's syndrome: patients suffering from these syndromes are either infertile or have an early menopause. Other studies have shown an association between early menopause and shorter life-expectancy. It has also been reported that women who delivered a child beyond the age of 45 tended to live longer and women who had a child with Down's syndrome before the age of 36 had a higher chance of developing Alzheimer's disease relatively early in life.

## Causes of early ovarian ageing and possibility for primary prevention

On the basis of te-Velde's hypothesis, that the time-interval between major reproductive events is fixed and that factors determining the age at menopause also affect the age of all reproductive events that depend on ovarian reserve, it can be speculated that the main causes of EOA are genetic.[12] A family history of early menopause is a high risk factor for EOA but is obviously not preventable. From epidemiological studies and from data produced on the IVF model, we can identify several acquired factors that play some role in the pathogenesis of early ovarian ageing. Smoking has long been identified as a preventable environmental factor that can cause an earlier menopause and a poor ovarian response to exogenous stimulation. Pelvic inflammatory disease has

been linked to poor ovarian response and is also potentially preventable. In an analysis of factors affecting IVF outcome, tubal disease appeared to have the worst prognosis. However, this has not been confirmed by others and the issue is still controversial. A meta-analysis showed a very good link between poor response and endometriosis,[22] which is not a preventable disease, although its progress may be modified with drugs. Chemotherapy and pelvic surgery – not just ovarian surgery – are obvious important causes of EOA in some women. Surgeons should consider carefully the possible impact on the ovarian reserve of any procedure they are contemplating.[7]

All the above factors can theoretically result in a poor response to ovarian stimulation. An analysis of our own database (Chelsea and Westminster Hospital) has shown that the absolute numbers of cases of either endometriosis or PID were too small to explain the observed variability of ovarian response between poor and good responders. Just like the variability of the age of menopause, the variability of ovarian response among women of the same age cannot be fully explained by medical or environmental factors. The poor responders had significantly poor overall outcome and future fertility prognosis than women with normal response. These data seem to confirm that the main reasons for EOA are indeed genetic.

## Possibility for secondary prevention

In recent years, the tendency to postpone childbearing has spread throughout the developed countries. This trend started mainly with the introduction of the oral contraceptive pill, which provided reliable contraception. However, it leads to more attempts to become pregnant at a more advanced age and this contributes considerably to the increase of the incidence of infertility. In terms of avoiding subfertility associated with EOA, this trend is definitely avoidable. There have been many reports in the press, illustrating the fact that women are unaware of the way fertility declines after the early thirties [E].[23] It seems that the significant achievements of assisted reproduction technologies have created the false impression that fertility can be safely postponed, which is clearly misleading. Screening for EOA in the early thirties, if an effective strategy could be developed, would provide information to women on which to base rational decisions about their fertility without risking involuntary childlessness [E].

It is possible that the management of certain antenatal conditions, such as growth retardation, could influence the size of the ovarian reserve at birth. It may be possible to use drugs that will limit the extent of ovarian reserve damage during chemotherapy, radiotherapy or illness. There is ongoing research into the possibilities for altering the rate of decline of the ovarian reserve, but there is currently very little that can be offered in routine clinical practice.[23] Embryo – not egg – freezing is currently the only reliable option for preserving fertility, providing that there are enough good-quality embryos to freeze.[23] Improvement of oocyte cryopreservation techniques and research in the area of 'stem cells' may open new possibilities in the future [E].

# SYSTEMATIC REVIEWS OF THE VARIOUS OVARIAN RESERVE TESTS

In the last few years, there have been systematic reviews of the literature on ovarian reserve tests. The conclusion is that some, especially FSH, AMH and antral follicule count, are reasonable in predicting the number of eggs that are collected in an IVF cycle. The correlation with live-birth rates is rather disappointing. One of the reasons is that most of the currently known ovarian reserve markers reflect the size of the cohort of antral follicles, with the exception of AMH which reflects the number of pre-antral follicles. A woman's current fertility depends mainly on the quality of her eggs. Quantity and quality normally co-variate, as fewer eggs remain in older age. However, in cases of a sudden reduction of the ovarian reserve, following unilateral oophorectomy for example, the quality of the ovarian reserve (percentage of good eggs) is better than the quantity (total number of eggs) (Figure 58.4).[7] Apart from this, it is well known that the IVF outcome for younger women varies significantly between clinics, and even within the same clinic in different years, for a number of reasons. However, it seems that in women over 40 the outcome is almost invariably low, as advanced age alone has such a major effect on egg quality (Figure 58.3).[23]

## Baseline FSH

Pregnancy rates decline significantly as day 3 FSH rises above 15 mIU/mL. Very few pregnancies were reported when FSH exceeded 25 mIU/mL. The meta-analysis of

Broekmans *et al.* showed that in women with an increased FSH level, the probability of poor response only increases substantially (3-fold or more) in studies applying a high threshold level for FSH, resulting in a very limited number of patients with an abnormal test result.[24]

The authors concluded that the use of basal FSH in regularly cycling women had little clinical utility as the threshold whereby sufficient accuracy would be achieved would result in very few positive results. The test would not be suitable as a diagnostic test to exclude patients from treatment, but only as screening test for counselling purposes and further diagnostic steps, in which a first IVF attempt may be the step of choice.

## Clomiphene challenge test

Twelve studies were included in the meta-analysis.[24] They were based on either day-10 FSH alone or on both basal FSH and day-10 FSH results. The CCCT performed no better than other tests such as the AFC or basal FSH, again largely because of poor specificity.

## Inhibin B

A total of nine studies were included in the meta-analysis.[24] The authors concluded that with the use of basal inhibin B in regularly cycling women, the accuracy in the prediction of poor response and non-pregnancy was only modest at a very low threshold level. At best, the test may be used to screen for counselling purposes or to direct further diagnostic steps, like a first IVF attempt.

## Antral follicle count

In the meta-analysis of Broekmans *et al.*, 15 studies were included. They concluded that the accuracy of the AFC for predicting poor response in regularly cycling women was adequate at a low threshold level, but because of the very limited numbers of abnormal tests had hardly any clinical value for pregnancy prediction.

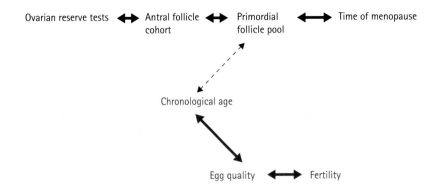

**Figure 58.4** Ovarian reserve tests. No text predicts egg quality directly. IVF offers some information on the quality of embryos and eggs

The test would not be suitable as a diagnostic test to exclude patients on the basis of the presumed diagnosis of AOE. It might be used as a screening test for possible poor responders and for directing further diagnostic strategies.

## Anti-müllerian hormone

Anti-müllerian hormone is a member of the transformin growth factor-B (TGF-B) family synthesized exclusively by the gonads of both sexes.

Two studies report on the predictive capacity of AMH. The meta-analysis revealed a sensitivity of 75 per cent and specificity of 85 per cent in the prediction of poor response, so the test performed only moderately, especially in terms of sensitivity. Additional studies are awaited. Overall, AMH has a number of advantages as a screening test. Its level corresponds well with AFC, it remains constant throughout the menstrual cycle and it has superior intercycle reproducibility compared with FSH and AFC.

The summary ROC curve for prediction of non-pregnancy runs close to the line of equality, indicating that the test has little predictive value for pregnancy. Comparison with AFC indicates that AMH behaves in a very similar manner in terms of prediction of poor response, as well as non-pregnancy [A].[25,26]

The overall performance in an IVF cycle can give more information about a woman's current reproductive potential, as it permits direct access to oocytes, embryos, as well as implantation and early pregnancy loss rates [E].[7,24]

## PREGNANCY AND INFERTILITY IN OLDER WOMEN

The risks associated with pregnancy increase steadily over the age of 35 [C]. Current best advice is that the safest age to have a baby is before 30.[23] It should be recognized that pregnancy in women over 40 in particular, especially following IVF, especially if it is a multiple pregnancy, poses increased risks. In terms of current management of these pregnancies, one of the challenges is to make the necessary resources available in order to minimize the adverse outcomes.[23]

As the live-birth rates of IVF have remained particularly low for women in their forties, almost invariably less than 10 per cent per attempt, the management of women in this age group presenting with infertility cannot be solely focused on achieving a live-birth. Rather, it needs to be much more holistic and aim at the improvement of the overall quality of their life through education, support and counseling. This includes protecting them from non-evidence-based treatments or treatments that evidence has shown to be ineffective and may be very costly and potentially dangerous.

## CONCLUSIONS

The sexual revolution that followed the introduction of reliable hormonal contraception in the 1960s did not lead to the true emancipation of women, as the biological clock stubbornly refused to adjust to the new time. Women can opt to avoid pregnancy when they are young. However, there is no guarantee that they will be able to have children later. There is no reliable way to assess, predict or preserve fertility. For now, chronological age remains the most reliable marker of current fertility potential. Women should be informed that the assisted reproduction technology cannot overcome the problem of the ageing ovary if it presents too late. Thus, postponing childbearing to the late thirties remains a gamble. The medical profession may have some responsibility for not highlighting the misconception earlier. In addition, it is important to raise awareness of the possibility of EOA, especially if there is a significant family history or other risk factors. There is some room for primary prevention, with lifestyle adjustment.

We are fortunate to live in an era when there are large amounts of data which are easily accessible. Making sense of these data is a challenge for all. The description of EOA was based on a synthesis of clinical, laboratory and epidemiological observations. The development of screening strategies will need global collaboration, just as we did with antenatal screening. This collaboration is more feasible than ever before.

## KEY POINTS

- Fertility declines with female age. This decline accelerates in the late thirties and a woman's fertility is almost invariably very low in the forties.
- The underlying mechanism is the progressive loss of follicles from the ovary by apoptosis, and the deterioration of the quality of the remaining oocytes.
- With the exception of egg donation, assisted reproduction technology (ART) cannot overcome the problem of declining oocyte quality caused by advanced maternal age.
- 'Ovarian reserve' is a term used to describe the quantity and quality of the remaining oocytes in a woman's ovaries.
- Various tests have been developed to assess the ovarian reserve. With the exception of the IVF process itself, ovarian reserve tests mainly assess the number, not the quality of the remaining oocytes. However, a woman's current fertility depends mainly on the quality, not the number of the oocytes in her ovary.
- 'Ovarian reserve' tests are reasonably good at predicting poor response in an IVF cycle, but are poor at predicting live-births. They might better be called 'ovarian response' tests.

Reproductive medicine

- 'Early ovarian ageing' is a term introduced in 2003 to describe women who undergo an accelerated decline of their ovarian reserve, which is normally seen in the late thirties, much earlier (before the age of 32). It was estimated that it affects 10 per cent of women in the general population.
- Women with 'early ovarian ageing' are fertile and totally asymptomatic in the early thirties but their fertility declines much sooner than expected by age alone.
- It may be possible to use 'ovarian response' tests to screen for 'early ovarian ageing' in the general population, however further work is required before this can be offered to women.

## Key References

1. Cramer DW, Huijuan XMPH, Harlow BL. Family history as a predictor of early menopause. *Fertil Steril* 1995; **64**: 740–5.
2. Faddy MJ, Gosden RG, Gougeon A *et al.* Accelerated disappearance of ovarian follicles in mid-life: implications for forecasting menopause. *Hum Reprod* 1992; **7**: 1342–6.
3. O'Connor KA, Holman DJ, Wood JW. Declining fecundity and ovarian ageing in natural fertility populations. *Maturitas* 1998; **30**: 127–36.
4. Human Fertilisation and Embryology Authority. www.hfea.gov.uk
5. te Velde ER, Dorland M, Broekmans FJ. Age at menopause as a marker of reproductive ageing. *Maturitas* 1998; **30**: 119–25.
6. te Velde ER, Pearson PL. The variability of female reproductive ageing. *Hum Reprod* 2002; **8**: 141–54.
7. Nikolaou D. How old are your eggs? *Curr Opin Obstet Gynaecol* 2008; **20**: 540–44.
8. Schipper I, de Jong FH, Fauser BCJM. Lack of correlation between maximum early follicular phase serum follicle-stimulating hormone levels and menstrual cycle characteristics in women under the age of 35 years. *Hum Reprod* 1998; **13**: 1442–8.
9. te Velde ER, Scheffer GJ, Dorland M *et al.* Age dependent changes in serum FSH levels. In: Fauser BCJM (ed.). *FSH Action and Intraovarian Regulation.* Studies in Profertility Series, vol. 6. New York: Parthenon, 1997: 145–55.
10. Gougeon A. Regulation of ovarian follicular development in primates: facts and hypotheses. *Endocr Rev* 1996; **17**: 121–55.
11. Nikolaou D, Lavery S, Turner C *et al.* Is there a link between an extremely poor response to ovarian hyperstimulation and early ovarian failure? *Hum Reprod* 2002; **17**: 1106–11.
12. Nikolaou D, Templeton A. Early ovarian aging: a hypothesis. Detection and clinical relevance. *Hum Reprod* 2003; **18**: 1137–9.
13. Nikolaou D, Templeton A. Early ovarian ageing. *Eur J Obs Gynecol* 2004; **113**: 126–33.
14. Nikolaou D, Gilling-Smith C. Early ovarian ageing: are women with polycystic ovaries protected? *Hum Reprod* 2004; **19**: 2175–9.
15. Brook JD, Gosden RG, Chandley AC. Maternal ageing and aneuploid embryos: evidence from the mouse that biological and not chronological age is the important influence. *Hum Genet* 1984; **66**: 41–5.
16. van Montfrans JM, Dorland M, Oosterhuis G *et al.* Increased concentrations of follicle-stimulating hormone in mothers with Down's syndrome. *Lancet* 1999; **353**: 1853–4.
17. van Montfrans JM, van Hooff MH, Martens F *et al.* Estradiol and inhibin B concentrations in women with a previous Down's syndrome affected pregnancy. *Hum Reprod* 2002; **17**: 44–7.
18. Trout S, Seifer D. Do women with unexplained recurrent pregnancy loss have higher day 3 serum FSH and estradiol values? *Fertil Steril* 2000; **74**: 335–7.
19. Scott RT, Leonardi MR, Hofman GE *et al.* A prospective evaluation of clomiphene citrate challenge test screening of the general infertility population. *Obstet Gynaecol* 1993; **82**: 539–44.
20. Martin NG, Heath AC, Turner G. Do mothers of dizygotic twins have earlier menopause? *Am J Med Genet* 1997; **69**: 114–16.
21. Lambalk CB, Koning CH, Braat DD. The endocrinology of dizygotic twinning in the human. *Mol Cel Endocrinol* 1998; **145**: 97–102.
22. Barnhart K, Dunsmoor R, Coutifaris C. Effect of endometriosis on *in vitro* fertilization. *Fertil Steril* 2002; **77**: 1148–55.
23. Bewley S, Ledger W, Nikolaou D (eds). *Reproductive ageing. Recommendations for clinical practice.* London: RCOG Press, 2009.
24. Broekmans F, Kwee J, Hendriks DJ *et al.* A systematic review of tests predicting ovarian reserve and IVF outcome. *Hum Reprod Update* 2006; **12**: 685–718.
25. Maheshwari A, Fowler P, Bhattacharya S. Assessment of ovarian reserve – should we perform tests of ovarian reserve routinely? *Hum Reprod* 2006; **21**: 2729–35.

## Further Essential Reading

Nikolaou D, Trew G. Contribution of assisted reproduction technology to the understanding of early ovarian ageing. In: Studd J (ed.). *The Management of the Menopause*, 3rd edn. London: Parthenon, 2003: 185–98.

Templeton A, Morris J, Parslow W. Factors that affect outcome of *in-vitro* fertilization treatment. *Lancet* 1996; **348**: 1402–6.

te Velde ER, Scheffer GJ, Dorland M *et al.* Developmental and endocrine aspects of normal ovarian ageing. *Mol Cel Endocrinol* 1998; **145**: 67–73.

Van Rooij IA, Broekmans FJ, Hunault CC *et al.* Use of ovarian reserve tests for the prediction of ongoing pregnancy in couples with unexplained or mild male infertility. *Reprod Biomed Online* 2006; **12**: 182.

# SECTION B
## Pelvic floor and lower urinary tract dysfunction

# Assessment of lower urinary tract function

*Angie Rantell*

## INTRODUCTION

Lower urinary tract symptoms (LUTS) are common and can be due to a wide variety of underlying mechanisms. It is therefore important to approach the investigation of such symptoms in a logical and objective manner. An accurate and detailed history and examination provide a framework for diagnosis. However, it is important to recognize that different underlying conditions can cause the same urinary symptoms and that the medical history alone is a poor predictor of pathophysiology.

## HISTORY

According to the International Continence Society (2002), symptoms are the subjective indicator of a disease or change in condition as perceived by the patient, carer or partner and may lead him/her to seek help from health care professionals. Symptoms may be volunteered by the patient or described during the patient interview. In general, lower urinary tract symptoms cannot be used to make a definitive diagnosis.[1]

Although urinary symptoms alone do not lead directly to a diagnosis, this should in no way detract from the central importance of the medical history in assessing a woman who presents with urinary problems. Listening to any patient is important, and an appropriate history should be obtained in a targeted and methodical manner. Not only will this enable the woman's own words to be turned into a graduated list of symptoms, but it will also provide information about how the woman's quality of life is affected by the condition. There are a number of ways in which a woman can ameliorate her urinary symptoms through behavioural changes. When taking a history, it is important to elucidate these restrictions and adaptations in order to gain a proper impression of the morbidity of the disorder. For example, by severely restricting fluid intake and never venturing far from a toilet, it is possible that a woman could greatly reduce the number of episodes of leaking. However, these adaptations do not lessen the severity of the disorder, or the need for appropriate treatment that will reduce this social restriction.

Urinary symptoms are valuable in directing further management by guiding the investigator in his or her choice of additional tests. Investigations may produce a diagnosis that is inconsistent with the problems complained of by the woman. It is very important to establish which problems bother her most, so that management can be targeted at these problems. This can only be done by taking the time to listen to the patient's description of her urinary symptoms in her own words. To ensure that a complete picture of lower urinary tract symptoms is gained, it is often useful to question the patient about individual symptoms. This can take the form of a questionnaire or of a series of structured questions, and ensures that important features of the history

**Table 59.1** Classification of urinary symptoms into groups

| Abnormal storage | Abnormal voiding | Abnormal sensation |
|---|---|---|
| Stress incontinence | Hesitancy | Urgency |
| Urge incontinence | Incomplete emptying | Dysuria |
| Frequency | Poor stream | Painful bladder |
| Nocturia | Post-micturition dribble | Loin pain |
| Nocturnal enuresis | Straining to void | Absent sensation |

are not omitted because the woman is unable to describe a symptom or is too embarrassed to mention it.

Lower urinary tract symptoms can be grouped into three main areas. These reflect disorders of different aspects of bladder and urethral function. That is, to store urine in a low-pressure reservoir until such time as it is socially convenient to void, when the bladder should be efficiently emptied to completion. The first group of symptoms reflects abnormal storage, the second group includes symptoms associated with abnormal voiding or post-micturition symptoms and the final group relates to abnormal bladder sensations (Table 59.1).

# URINARY SYMPTOMS

All the following definitions are as defined by the ICS (2002).[1]

## Storage symptoms

### Increased daytime frequency

Increased daytime frequency is the complaint by the patient who considers that she voids too often by day. A normal frequency is around four to seven times per day but this symptom is subjective to the patient and a frequency of six voids a day may be normal for one woman, but bothersome for another.

### Nocturia

Nocturia is the complaint that the individual has to wake at night one or more times to void. It is important to establish whether the woman wakes due to the desire to pass urine or for other reasons (e.g. insomnia, breathing problems) and going to the toilet as they are awake.

### Urgency

Urgency is the complaint of a sudden compelling desire to pass urine which is difficult to defer. If this desire is not relieved it may result in urge incontinence.

## Overactive bladder syndrome

Overactive blabber syndrome (OAB) can be defined as urgency, with or without urge incontinence, usually with frequency and nocturia.

## Urinary incontinence

Urinary incontinence is the complaint of any involuntary leakage of urine. It is important to consider factors such as type, frequency, severity, precipitating factors, social impact, effect on hygiene and quality of life, the measures used to contain the leakage and whether or not the individual seeks or desires help because of urinary incontinence. Urinary leakage may need to be distinguished from sweating or vaginal discharge.

## Stress urinary incontinence

Stress urinary incontinence is the complaint of involuntary leakage on effort or exertion, or on sneezing or coughing. The leakage of urine is usually in small, discrete amounts, coinciding with the physical activity. It is important to distinguish the subjective symptom of stress incontinence from the objectively demonstrated diagnosis of urodynamic stress incontinence, which can only be made following urodynamic assessment.

## Urge urinary incontinence

Urge urinary incontinence is the complaint of involuntary leakage accompanied by or immediately preceded by urgency. It is frequently described as an inability to reach the toilet in time, and women suffering from this symptom often restrict their social activities to ensure that they are constantly near a toilet. Typical triggers for urge incontinence include hearing running water, opening the front door (latch-key incontinence) and sudden changes in temperature. Urge incontinence can present in different symptomatic forms; for example, as frequent small losses between micturitions or as a catastrophic leak with complete bladder emptying.

## Mixed urinary incontinence

Mixed urinary incontinence is the complaint of involuntary leakage associated with urgency and also with exertion, effort, sneezing or coughing. It is important to distinguish between urodynamic mixed incontinence which is the presence of urodynamic stress incontinence and detrusor overactivity based on urodynamic observations from the symptoms of OAB with stress or urge incontinence.

## Nocturnal enuresis

Enuresis means any involuntary loss of urine. Nocturnal enuresis is the complaint of loss of urine occurring during sleep. It can be primary or secondary. Primary nocturnal enuresis starts in infancy and can persist in adulthood. Secondary nocturnal enuresis occurs when the nocturnal incontinence restarts following a period of night-time continence. It is important to distinguish enuresis from night-time urge incontinence, in which the woman is awoken by urgency and leaks before making it to the toilet.

## Other types of urinary incontinence

There are several other types of urinary incontinence. These may be situational, for example the report of incontinence during sexual intercourse, or giggle incontinence. Women may also complain of continuous urinary leakage.

## Voiding symptoms

### Slow stream

Slow stream is reported by the individual as her perception of reduced urine flow, usually compared to previous performance or in comparison to others. Urinary flow rate is dependent on the total volume voided, the pressure generated by the detrusor muscle, and outflow resistance. In order to differentiate between these causes, urodynamic investigations need to be undertaken. Bladder outflow obstruction is rare in women who have not undergone previous surgery. Other causes of poor urinary stream include an underlying neurological condition and a pelvic mass.

### Intermittent stream

'Intermittent stream' (intermittency) is the term used when the individual describes urine flow which stops and starts, on one or more occasions, during micturition.

### Hesitancy

'Hesitancy' is the term used when an individual describes difficulty in initiating micturition resulting in a delay in the onset of voiding after the individual is ready to pass urine. It is not uncommon for most women to experience this occasionally. Even in those women who complain of persistent hesitancy, only a small minority are found to be obstructed. The other causes of persistent hesitancy include poor detrusor contractility and a lack of co-ordination in the normal neurological control of micturition (detrusor sphincter dyssynergia).

### Straining

Straining to void describes the muscular effort used to either initiate, maintain or improve the urinary stream. Straining to empty the bladder is suggestive of voiding difficulty. Like the other symptoms in this category, it can be the result of a number of different disorders affecting bladder contractility, as well as outflow resistance. Raising intra-abdominal pressure by a Valsalva manoeuvre exerts increased intravesical pressure to aid bladder emptying. Suprapubic pressure may be used to initiate or maintain urine flow. The Credé manoeuvre is used by some spinal cord injury patients. The urinary flow produced is characteristically intermittent and prolonged.

## Post-micturition symptoms

### Incomplete emptying

Feeling of incomplete emptying is a self-explanatory term for a feeling experienced by the individual after passing urine. It does not always correlate with the presence of a significant urinary residual. Similarly, women with large residuals are often unaware of it. This sensation can also arise as a result of an open bladder neck, abnormal bladder sensation, and a cystocele acting as a urinary sump.

### Post-micturition dribble

'Post-micturition dribble' is the term used when an individual describes the involuntary loss of urine immediately after she has finished passing urine, usually after rising from the toilet in women. This symptom is associated with a collection of fluid left in the bladder after voiding, such as is found with a cystocele. It is also seen where there is a separate reservoir of urine, such as a urethral diverticulum, which fills up during voiding and subsequently drains.

## Bladder sensations

Bladder sensation according to five categories:

1 *Normal.* The individual is aware of bladder filling and increasing sensation up to a strong desire to void.
2 *Increased.* The individual feels an early and persistent desire to void. Suprapubic bladder pain on filling is a significant symptom and, if it persists, is an indication for cystoscopy and bladder biopsy. Inflammation of the bladder, such as interstitial cystitis, as well as stones, bladder tumours, endometriosis and pelvic infections are associated with this symptom.
3 *Reduced.* The individual is aware of bladder filling, but does not feel a definite desire to void. This can lead to bladder over-distension if women are not advised to void at regular intervals.
4 *Absent.* The individual reports no sensation of bladder filling or desire to void. Bladder hyposensitivity is usually due to denervation caused by spinal cord injury or pelvic trauma. It leads to infrequent micturition and a large-capacity bladder. It is often associated with overflow incontinence.
5 *Non-specific.* The individual reports no specific bladder sensation but may perceive bladder filling as abdominal fullness, vegetative symptoms or spasticity.

Pelvic floor and lower urinary tract dysfunction

## Dysuria

Dysuria is pain experienced in the bladder or urethra on passing urine. It is most frequently associated with a urinary tract infection or urethritis, but can also be caused by inflammatory bladder conditions, such as interstitial cystitis.

## Loin pain

Loin pain is referred from the nerves innervating the kidney and urethra. If the ureter is involved, it often radiates around to the ipsilateral groin. There are many causes for this symptom and it is an indication for further assessment of the upper urinary tracts.

## Haematuria

The presence of blood in the urine is always significant and should not be ignored. It warrants investigation of the upper urinary tracts with ultrasound or an intravenous urogram (IVU) and of the lower tract with cystoscopy and urine cytology.

## PHYSICAL EXAMINATION

Abdominal and pelvic examinations form an essential part of the assessment of any woman who presents with urinary tract symptoms. Depending upon the medical history, there may be certain additional aspects of the physical examination that require particular attention. If there are any symptoms that point to a possible neurological cause, it is important to perform a screening neurological examination. The patient's mobility and mental state affect her ability to react to her symptoms and it may be appropriate to test these formally as part of the examination, as they will influence management. Similarly, an assessment of motivation and manual dexterity is important in determining the treatment most likely to prove effective.

As part of the gynaecological examination, the condition of the vulval skin should be noted. There may be signs of erythema, oedema and inflammation from chronic exposure to urine (incontinence-associated dermatitis). This can cause pain, discomfort and increase the risk of developing pressure sores. Vulval and vaginal atrophy may also be noted. Because of the close proximity of the lower urinary and genital tracts in the female, the presence of pelvic organ prolapse can have an important bearing on urinary symptoms and their management. This is best assessed in the left lateral position, using a Sims' speculum and asking the patient to cough and bear down. It is important to note that in order to demonstrate stress incontinence during examination, the bladder needs to be reasonably full, which is often not the case. Speculum examination should be complemented by performing a digital examination with the woman standing, legs abducted and performing a Valsalva manoeuvre. This gives a more accurate impression of the size and origin of any prolapse that is present. The grade of prolapse can be classified subjectively as mild, moderate or severe or graded according to the International Continence Society (ICS) Pelvic Organ Prolapse Quantification (POP-Q) score. While performing a vaginal examination in a woman who complains of leaking urine, it is important to assess the degree of anterior vaginal wall mobility and note any scarring that may be present, as this will influence the most appropriate choice of continence surgery. In addition, the anterior vaginal wall should be examined for any mass that may be a urethral diverticulum or cyst. Pelvic masses, such as ovarian cysts or uterine enlargement, can cause urinary symptoms and need to be excluded by bimanual examination. If this cannot be done with confidence, for example in the obese patient, a transvaginal ultrasound scan should be considered. For some women, a rectal examination may be indicated to further assess pelvic organ prolapse and to rule out faecal impaction.

It is important to ensure that informed consent has been gained and that all examinations are performed in line with Royal College of Obstetricians and Gynaecologists (RCOG) guidelines.[2]

## INVESTIGATIONS

The bladder has been described as an 'unreliable witness'. Although urinary symptoms provide a framework for diagnosis, they do not on their own allow an accurate impression to be formed of the underlying pathology. This may lead to inappropriate treatment being given and is especially important if surgical management is being considered, as the effects of surgery are irreversible. Investigations can be divided into basic tests, which all gynaecologists should be capable of performing and interpreting, and more complex investigations that require specialist expertise to perform (Table 59.2).

**Table 59.2** Investigations of lower urinary tract disorders

| Basic investigations | Midstream urine specimen |
| --- | --- |
| | Frequency-volume chart |
| | Pad test |
| Specialist investigations | Uroflowmetry |
| | Subtracted cystometry |
| | Videourodynamics |
| | Ambulatory urodynamics |
| | Urethral pressure profilometry |
| | Leak-point pressures |
| | Neurophysiological studies |
| | Radiological imaging |
| | Ultrasonography |
| | Endoscopy |

# Midstream urine specimen

A midstream urine specimen must be taken for microscopy, culture and sensitivity from all women presenting with urinary symptoms. Bacteriuria is considered to be significant if $>10^5$ organisms/mL of urine are reported. It is important to rule out a urinary tract infection before going on to perform more invasive investigations. The presenting lower urinary tract symptoms can be exacerbated or entirely caused by a bacterial infection, and effective treatment with appropriate antibiotics may be all that is required. If it proves necessary to proceed to urodynamic studies, it is important to ensure that there is not an infection already present, which would lead to unrepresentative findings and the risk of an ascending urinary infection of the upper tracts. In some situations, such as investigating a patient with recurrent urinary tract infections, it is necessary to request cultures for 'fastidious organisms' such as *Mycoplasma hominis*, *Ureaplasma urelyticum* and *Chlamydia trachomatis*.

## Frequency–volume chart

This is also known as a bladder diary or micturition time chart (Figure 59.1). The patient is asked to record on a standard time sheet the volume of all fluid consumed and of all urine passed, as well as indicating any episodes of urgency and incontinence. The value of this simple, non-invasive tool is often overlooked, which is unfortunate as, if filled in conscientiouoly, it provides a good indication of fluid input and a natural volumetric record of bladder function.

An accurately filled out chart provides invaluable information about the patient's voiding function in her natural environment and adds objectivity to the medical history (Table 59.3).

Frequency–volume charts can be completed prior to the initial hospital consultation to triage care and determine the urgency and complexity of the condition. They provide a useful form of feedback to the practitioner and the patient

(a)
**Bladder Diary**
IMPORTANT – PLEASE READ INSTRUCTIONS CAREFULLY

It is very important that you fill in the chart overleaf as accurately as possible over a 3 day period prior to attending your test.

It is designed to help us take a closer look at your fluid intake and output, and leakage if any. It also helps us to plan the right treatment for you.

For each day, record *how much* (mL if possible) and *what time* you drink and write it down in the *IN* column.

When you go the toilet, measure the urine you pass using a jug (mL if possible) and write it down in the *OUT* column.

If you leak urine, put an X, yes or ✓ in the *WET* column. If you experience urgency i.e a sudden desire to pass urine that is difficult to defer please score 0, 1, 2, 3 or 4 according to the urge score that is described on the next page. Then according to how severe your urgency was please enter the appropriate number in the URGE SCORE column.

FOR EXAMPLE:

| Time | DAY 1 | | | |
|---|---|---|---|---|
| | IN | OUT | WET | URGE SCORE |
| 07:10 am | | 140 mL | | |
| 08:30 am | 250 mL | | | |
| 10:40 am | | 90 | Yes | |
| 12:00 noon | | 150 | | 2 |
| 12:45 pm | 200 mL | | | |
| 02:00 pm | | 60 | | 0 |

This means that you passed 140 mL at 07:10 am and had 250 mL of a drink (maybe a cup of tea with breakfast). At 10:40 you leaked urine and passed 90 mL. At 12:00 noon you had 'moderate urgency' with a score of 2 which according to the urgency score means 'you could postpone voiding for a short while without fear of wetting yourself'.

Please write the time you got up and time you went to bed at the top and bottom of the chart for each day. This allows us to see the difference between what is happening during the day and during the night.

(b) Urogynaecology Department, King's College Hospital Bladder Diary

| TIME | DAY 1 | | | | DAY 2 | | | | DAY 3 | | | |
|---|---|---|---|---|---|---|---|---|---|---|---|---|
| | IN | OUT | WET | URGE SCORE | IN | OUT | WET | URGE SCORE | IN | OUT | WET | URGE SCORE |
| | | | | | | | | | | | | |
| | | | | | | | | | | | | |
| | | | | | | | | | | | | |
| | | | | | | | | | | | | |
| | | | | | | | | | | | | |
| | | | | | | | | | | | | |
| | | | | | | | | | | | | |
| | | | | | | | | | | | | |
| | | | | | | | | | | | | |
| | | | | | | | | | | | | |
| | | | | | | | | | | | | |
| | | | | | | | | | | | | |
| | | | | | | | | | | | | |
| | | | | | | | | | | | | |
| | | | | | | | | | | | | |
| | | | | | | | | | | | | |

Time got up: _____ Time got up: _____ Time got up: _____

Time went to bed: _____ Time went to bed: _____ Time went to bed: _____

**Urge score**

| 0 | No urgency: I felt no need to empty my bladder but did so for other reasons |
|---|---|
| 1 | Mild Urgency: I could postpone voiding for as long as necessary without fear of wetting myself |
| 2 | Moderate Urgency: I could postpone voiding for a short while without fear of wetting myself |
| 3 | Severe Urgency: I could not postpone voiding but had to rush to the toilet in order not to wet myself |
| 4 | Urge Incontinence: I leaked before arriving at the toilet |

**Figure 59.1** Bladder diary. (a) Instructions for patient (b) Three day frequency volume chart for patient to fill in

Pelvic floor and lower urinary tract dysfunction

**Table 59.3** Information that can be derived from a frequency volume chart

| |
|---|
| An idea of the normal functional bladder capacity, which should be fairly consistently around 300–500 mL. Frequent voids of variable amounts throughout the day imply bladder overactivity or behavioural adaptation to symptoms |
| A volumetric summary of diurnal urinary frequency and nocturia |
| Quantification of total fluid intake and its distribution throughout the day |
| A semi-objective evaluation of the severity of urinary incontinence and associated or provocative events |

so that they can objectively evaluate the effectiveness of any therapy, for example in women undergoing bladder training for detrusor over-activity. In addition, they can also aid diagnosis for conditions such as nocturnal polyuria. A frequency–volume chart should always be completed prior to urodynamic testing so that the patient's functional bladder capacity is known. This prevents over-distension during filling cystometry. There is no standardized format for frequency–volume charts; the duration varies between 48 hours and 7 days in different centres. In addition to the standard volumetric information, the patient may be asked to quantitate incontinent episodes, note associated or provocative activities, and state the number of pads used per day. Measures of urinary urgency (e.g. Patient Perception of Intensity of Urgency Scale (PPIUS)) can provide additional information on a bladder diary.

## Quality of life assessment

Symptom and quality of life scoring is used to give some quantification of the impact of urinary symptoms and provides a measure that can be used to assess outcomes of treatment at a later stage.[1] This employs carefully designed and validated patient-assessed health questionnaires. Traditionally, doctors have categorized the severity of a condition using objective clinical measures. However, the impact of a disease and the success of any treatment should no longer be measured purely in terms of 'doctor-centred' clinical parameters alone. It is increasingly recognized that a patient's quality of life and psychosocial adjustment to an illness are equally as important as the status of their physical disease. Two major types of QoL questionnaire are available: generic questionnaires, which can be used across a range of medical conditions, and disease-specific questionnaires, which focus on the likely impacts of a particular disorder. It is very important that any questionnaires used for this form of assessment have been subjected to rigorous reliability testing and validation in order to derive meaningful data from them. Quality of life assessment is particularly useful in determining the response of patients to treatment. It gives useful information about therapeutic effects as

seen from the patient's perspective across a range of different domains. This form of patient assessment has many applications. It is now widely used as an outcome measure in the evaluation of clinical practice and in research trials. There are many disease-specific questionnaires to assess women with urinary incontinence. These include the King's Health Questionnaire (KHQ), International Consultation on Incontinence Questionnaire (ICIQ), Bristol Female Urinary Tract Symptoms (BFLUTS), Overactive Bladder Questionnaire (OAB), Urogenital Distress Inventory (UDI) and Incontinence Impact Questionnaire (IIQ).

## Pad test

The objective demonstration of leaking is essential in reaching a diagnosis of urinary incontinence. A pad test provides a simple, non-invasive, objective method for detecting and quantifying urinary leakage. Various protocols exist for performing a pad test. To obtain a representative result, especially for those who have variable or intermittent urinary incontinence, the test should be as long as possible in circumstances that approximate those of everyday life. It should be conducted in a standardized fashion so that results are comparable and reproducible. This allows the effect of treatment to be objectively assessed in a non-invasive manner.

The ICS has produced guidelines for a standardized 1-hour pad test.[3] The patient wears a pre-weighed pad or sanitary towel, drinks 500 mL of water and rests for 15 minutes. She then performs 30 minutes of moderate exercise, such as stair climbing and walking. The remaining 15 minutes are spent performing more provocative exercises, including coughing vigorously, bending over, hand washing and running. At the end of 1 hour, the pad is removed and re-weighed. An increase of >2 g is considered a significant loss. A weight gain of >10 g is categorized as severe incontinence.

The standard 1-hour ICS pad test has been shown to have good reproducibility, and reliably differentiates normal from abnormal continence mechanisms. However, the short period of study and lack of a standardized bladder volume before starting the test mean that there is a significant false-negative rate.

Long-term protocols also exist in which the patient is given several pre-weighed pads to be worn at home for periods of 12, 24 or 48 hours. The used pads are collected in sealed plastic bags and reweighed at the end of the specified period to determine total urine loss. The extended pad test is particularly useful to confirm or refute leakage in those patients complaining of incontinence that has not been demonstrated on urodynamic studies.

Recent studies have shown that pad tests bare little relationship to the underlying urodynamic diagnosis but there is a positive relationship with symptom severity.[3] The 1-hour pad test has poor predictive value in the diagnosis of urinary incontinence.[4] However, the 24-hour pad test appears to be a more useful tool clinically that the 1-hour test, but should be used in conjunction with other investigations.[3]

## Methylene blue test

For women who are unable to differentiate urinary leakage from vaginal discharge, or in cases of possible vesico-vaginal or urethra-vaginal fistula, a methylene blue test can be performed. During this test, a solution of normal saline and methylene blue is instilled into the patient's bladder to half the cystometric capacity. Gauze swabs are then placed into the upper, mid and lower vagina and a pre-weighed pad into the patient's underwear. They are then asked to mobilize for 1 hour and perform provocative exercises. At the end of the test, patients are asked to void and then each vaginal swab is removed. Staining on the pad represents urinary leakage. Blue on the lower vaginal swab may represent urethro-vaginal reflux or contamination from the test. Blue on the mid-vaginal swab may be indicative of a urethro-vaginal fistula and on the upper vaginal swab could suggest a vesico-vaginal fistula. A heavy vaginal discharge can also be assessed from this test. During the instillation of methylene blue into the bladder, it is important to ensure that there is no contamination of dye on to the labia or vagina as this will give false-positive results from the test. Figure 59.2 demonstrates the placement of swabs during the test.

## Uroflowmetry

Uroflowmetry is the simplest and one of the most useful investigations in the assessment of voiding dysfunction. It consists simply of measuring urinary flow over time and allows a rapid and non-invasive analysis of the normality or otherwise of flow rate. When combined with the measurement of residual urine volume by ultrasound or catheterization, it provides information on the efficiency of micturition in emptying the bladder. One or more symptoms of voiding disorder are commonly described in women complaining of urinary tract disorders, and it is important to diagnose or eliminate voiding difficulty. This is particularly so when treatment is being considered for incontinence. Both surgical treatment of urodynamic stress incontinence and drug treatment for detrusor over-activity have the potential to cause voiding difficulty. Therefore

pretreatment uroflowmetry and the measurement of residual urine are essential.

### Indications

Uroflowmetry should be regarded as a screening test for voiding difficulty in all women with symptoms of lower urinary tract dysfunction. It is important to appreciate that urinary flow is dependent upon a number of factors, including detrusor contractility, neurological co-ordination of sphincter relaxation and outflow patency. Uroflowmetry on its own cannot successfully distinguish between the causes of voiding dysfunction.

### Methods

There are several different physical principles that can be utilized to provide an accurate assessment of flow. The following three methods are in common use.

1  *Gravimetric method.* The rate of change of the weight of the voided urine in the collecting jug is converted into a flow rate (Figure 59.3).
2  *Rotating disc method.* A known amount of power is required to keep a rotating disc spinning at a constant rate. Voided fluid is directed on to the disc, increasing its inertia. The flow rate is proportional to the amount of extra power that is required to keep the disc spinning at a constant rate.
3  *Capacitance dipstick.* A metal capacitor strip is attached to the side of the flowmeter. As urine accumulates in the container, the electrical capacitance of the dipstick changes and from this the rate of flow can be calculated.

It should be noted that the environment in which the woman performs the flow rate recording will have a considerable influence on the results. It is important that every effort is made to make the patient feel as comfortable and relaxed as possible, and that privacy and dignity are maintained at all times.

### Interpretation

The definitions for urine flow rate measurements have been standardized by the ICS and should be expressed in millilitres per second (Figure 59.4).

The two most useful parameters are the maximum flow rate and the voided volume. The maximum flow rate is partially dependent on the voided volume, as this determines how distended the bladder muscle fibres are. For this reason, small voided volumes of less than 150 mL are insufficient to obtain an accurate impression of flow, and the test needs to be repeated.

The third major factor to consider when interpreting flow rate is the pattern of flow, in particular whether flow is continuous or intermittent. A normal flow curve is bell-shaped and characterized by a rapid rise to maximal flow. A prolonged, intermittent flow curve is suggestive of voiding dysfunction, with the patient using abdominal straining to achieve bladder emptying. The results must always be interpreted

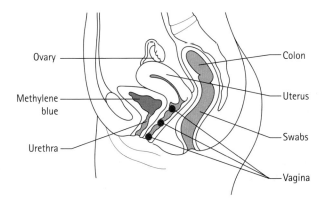

**Figure 59.2** Diagrammatic representation of methylene blue test

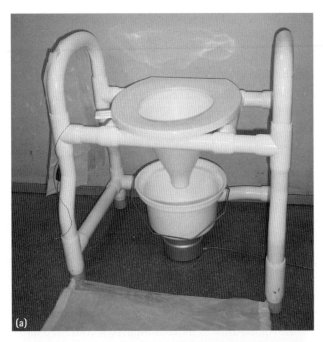

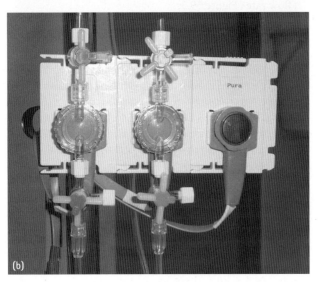

**Figure 59.3** (a) Gravimetric flow meter. (b) External pressure transducers connected to the patient via fluid-filled lines inserted into the bladder and rectum. This allows accurate measurement of intravesical and intra-abdominal pressure

within the context of the clinical situation, and the limitations of the study should be recognized. These include the reliability of the apparatus, and the ability of the staff interpreting the trace in recognizing artefact. More information concerning the cause of voiding difficulty is provided by the addition of simultaneous pressure measurements as part of cystometry (pressure flow studies).

### Factors influencing urine flow rate

The peak flow rate (PFR) is highly dependent on voided volume, as has already been discussed. Most commonly, a minimum accepted PFR of 15 mL/s is used. Urine flow

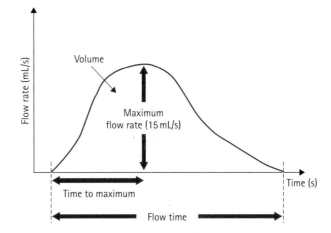

**Figure 59.4** Diagrammatic representation of urinary flow rate with standardized International Continence Society (ICS) terminology. Voided volume: total volume expelled via the urethra; the area beneath the flow–time curve. Maximum flow rate: maximum measured value of the flow rate. Flow time: the time over which measurable flow actually occurs. If flow is intermittent, the time intervals between flow episodes are not included. Average flow rate: volume voided divided by the flow time. Time to maximum flow: elapsed time from onset of flow to maximum flow

rates are higher in women than in men for a comparable voided volume. Age and parity have not been shown to have a significant effect on urine flow rates in asymptomatic women. As might be expected, there is a progressive decline in flow rate with increasing grades of pelvic floor prolapse, especially uterine prolapse and cystourethrocele.

Altered detrusor function influences flow rate by determining the contractile force with which urine is expelled. In addition, bladder neck and urethral anatomy influence urine flow by affecting outflow resistance. To distinguish between these two major causes of voiding dysfunction, more complex urodynamic tests are required in which simultaneous pressure/flow measurements are taken.

### Subtracted cystometry

Cystometry is the method by which the pressure/volume relationship of the bladder is assessed during filling and voiding. It involves the simultaneous measurement of intravesical and intra-abdominal pressures. Electronic subtraction of the intra-abdominal pressure from the intravesical pressure enables the detrusor pressure to be calculated and compared with changes in bladder volume and flow rate. Cystometry aims to characterize detrusor and urethral function during the filling and voiding phases (Table 59.4). It can be useful, when learning to interpret cystometrograms, to break down the functions of the detrusor and urethra by phases of the micturition cycle.

### Indications

When access to investigations is limited, it is reasonable to manage patients with clear-cut symptoms empirically with conservative treatment, provided that cystometry is

**Table 59.4** Cystometry

| Phases of cycle | Urethra | Detrusor |
|---|---|---|
| Filling | Should remain closed and competent but can:<br><br>be incompetent due to physical stress, but without an associated rise in detrusor pressure (stress incontinence)<br><br>be incompetent as a direct result of an involuntary rise in detrusor pressure (detrusor over-activity) | Should remain relaxed/stable throughout filling but can:<br><br>show abnormal involuntary contractions (detrusor over-activity)<br><br>show a gradual rise in pressure with filling (low compliance) |
| Voiding | Should be appropriately relaxed but can:<br><br>be constricted, leading to outflow obstruction (obstructed cause) | Should contract efficiently under voluntary instruction but can:<br><br>be under-active or acontractile (possible neuropathic cause)<br><br>show high-pressure contractors (if over-active or needing to overcome an outflow obstruction) |

subsequently performed in those in whom empirical treatment fails. Certainly surgical treatments should never be considered without urodynamic assessment, as the inappropriate selection of surgery can have disastrous and largely irreversible consequences for the patient.

If a policy of urodynamic screening on all women with lower urinary tract symptoms is not practised, selective testing should certainly be considered in the investigation of:

- symptoms that have failed to respond to empirical conservative measures;
- a patient being considered for any form of incontinence surgery if there is a clinical suspicion of detrusor over-activity;
- voiding difficulties;
- mixed symptoms (e.g. frequency, urgency and stress incontinence);
- previous unsuccessful incontinence surgery;
- suspected neuropathic bladder disorders.

The last two complex groups are better investigated by videourodynamics, as this yields valuable information about the anatomical structure of the urinary tract, as well as the dynamic function.

A good urodynamic practice comprises three main elements:[5]

1   A clear indication for and appropriate selection of relevant measurements and procedures.
2   Precise measurement with data quality control and complete documentation.
3   Accurate analysis and critical reporting of results.

## Methods

It is important that cystometric diagnoses are related to the patient's symptoms and physical findings at the time of the investigation. The aim is to reproduce the presenting symptoms that cause the woman concern, so that a diagnosis can be made and appropriate treatment planned. Terminology and standards are defined by the ICS.[2] This allows cystometric data to be compared among different centres and used in research trials.

Modern multi-channel cystometry requires two pressure transducers (to measure the intra-abdominal and intravesical pressures), an electronic subtraction unit (to derive the detrusor pressure), an amplifying unit and a display or printout (Figure 59.5). Two types of pressure transducers are available: a fluid-filled pressure line inserted into the bladder or rectum and connected to an external transducer, and a solid microtip pressure transducer placed directly inside the body. The difference between the two is largely one of cost and convenience of use. Fluid-filled lines are generally disposable, whereas microtip pressure transducers are reusable and need sterilization between patients. Local inflection control policies should be adhered to. All pressure measurements are made in centimetres of water ($cmH_2O$).

Prior to inserting the pressure catheters, the patient is asked to void on the flowmeter to allow the measurement of a free flow rate. The presence of any residual urine on subsequent urethral catheterization is noted. The pressure catheters are then inserted and calibrated. Quality control is an essential part of performing cystometry if valid conclusions are to be drawn from the investigation. The system is checked for adequate subtraction by asking the patient to cough at regular intervals. An equal pressure rise should be observed in both the intra-abdominal and intravesical pressure traces, which should cancel out to leave the detrusor pressure unchanged. Once the integrity of the pressure readings has been checked and the system zeroed to atmospheric pressure, filling can commence.

Normal saline at room temperature is instilled into the bladder at a predetermined rate under the control of a peristaltic pump. This is usually in the range of 25–100 mL/min, depending on the indication for cystometry. This rate should be reduced to a slower filling rate closer to the normal physiological range when assessing patients with neuropathic bladders. During filling, the patient is asked to indicate her first desire to void (FDV) and when she experiences an uncontrollably strong desire to void (SDV). Any rise in detrusor pressure is noted and whether this is associated with the sensation of urgency or leaking. Filling is discontinued once there is a sustained SDV. This volume is taken as cystometric bladder capacity and is usually in the range 400–600 mL. Filling can occur when the patient is in the supine, sitting or standing position.

At the end of filling, the patient is asked to stand, to assess whether there is a postural rise in detrusor pressure, and to cough several times. More strenuous stimuli, such as star jumps, can be performed if leakage is not demonstrated by coughing in women who complain of this symptom in their history. The presence of any leakage is noted and whether a stable trace or an associated rise in detrusor pressure accompanies this. Provocative tests for detrusor over-activity are performed at this stage and the patient may be asked to listen to running water, wash her hands or heel bounce to try to induce leakage. Finally, the patient transfers back on to the flowmeter, with the pressure catheters still *in situ*. She is instructed to void and the detrusor pressure and urine flow rate are measured simultaneously to provide a simultaneous pressure/flow analysis.

## Interpretation

As has been previously discussed, it is vital that the cystometric findings are evaluated in the light of the woman's symptomatology. The following are normal cystometric parameters:

- Filling cystometry:
  - residual urine <50 mL,
  - capacity (taken as SDV) >400 mL,
  - absence of uninhibited detrusor contractions during filling,
  - negligible rise in detrusor pressure on filling: this should be <15 cmH$_2$O for a filling volume of 500 mL.
- Voiding cystometry:
  - no leakage on coughing or performing exercise,
  - no provoked detrusor contractions as a result of precipitating factors, such as postural changes, hand washing or coughing,
  - a maximum voiding detrusor pressure of <50 cm H$_2$O, with a maximum flow rate >15 mL/s for a volume voided of >150 mL.

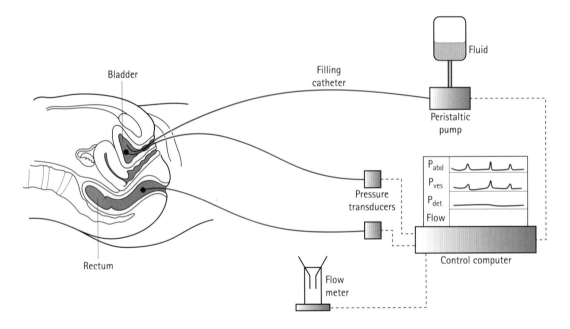

**Figure 59.5** Schematic diagram showing the position of the pressure catheters and the measurements recorded during subtracted cystometry. The following measurements are made:

- Free-flow rate and residual urine are measured at the start of the test by means of a flow meter and subsequent urethral catheterization.
- Intra-abdominal pressure ($P_{abd}$) is measured with the rectal pressure catheter. Alternatively, this could be measured with a pressure catheter in the vagina or colostomy stoma.
- Intravesical pressure ($P_{ves}$) is measured with a pressure catheter in the bladder via the urethra or suprapubic route.
- Detrusor pressure ($P_{det}$) is derived from continuous electronic subtraction of abdominal from intravesical pressure ($P_{det} = P_{ves} - P_{abd}$) and displayed concomitantly.
- Filling volume is recorded by a peristaltic pump connected to the system or calculated manually.
- Flow rate is measured by a flow meter allowing simultaneous pressure-flow analysis.
- During filling, the patient is asked to indicate her first desire to void (FDV) and when she experiences a strong desire to void (SDV). This is taken as bladder capacity.
- In addition, it is important to explain to the patient the relevance of expressing her sensations (such as urgency) during the test so that the cystometry trace can be annotated. This helps to interpret the findings

By considering urethral and detrusor function during the filling and voiding phases of cystometry, abnormalities can be systematically classified (Figure 59.6). The presence of involuntary detrusor contractions during filling or on provocation that the patient cannot suppress is diagnostic of detrusor over-activity. If there is a gradual rise in detrusor pressure during filling to >15 cmH$_2$O, but without phasic contractions, this is termed 'low compliance'. This can be artefactual owing to superphysiological or fast bladder filling. If there is a neurological condition present, such as multiple sclerosis, this is often accompanied by marked low compliance. If leakage occurs on coughing, with an associated rise in intra-abdominal pressure, but in the absence of abnormal detrusor activity, urodynamic stress incontinence is diagnosed.

## Videourodynamics

Videourodynamics offers the facility to simultaneously study the anatomical structure and the pressure/flow characteristics of the lower urinary tract. This is achieved by using contrast medium rather than saline to fill the bladder during cystometry, and radiologically screening the bladder and urethra intermittently throughout the procedure. The combination of these approaches results in the videocysto-urethrogram (VCU), which is regarded as the 'gold standard' for assessing lower urinary tract disorders. Most patients can be adequately investigated using simpler techniques, but VCU does offer several advantages over cystometry alone for the investigation of complex cases in tertiary centres. The addition of radiological screening provides valuable additional information relating to bladder morphology, the degree of bladder base support and function of the bladder neck during coughing, the presence of vesicoureteric reflux (which may be present in up to 7 per cent of incontinent patients) and the site of outflow obstruction (Figure 59.7).

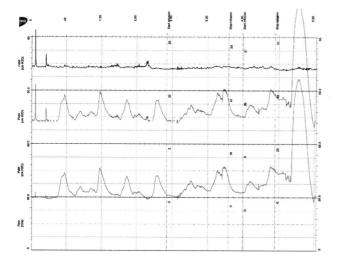

**Figure 59.6** Part of a cystometrogram trace showing detrusor overactivity. Note that intra-abdominal pressure is stable while the intravesical pressure line shows an involuntary detrusor contraction.

Clinical situations in which VCU offers significant advantages over simple cystometry include the following:

- Women in whom previous incontinence surgery has failed, as the position and mobility of the bladder neck can be assessed at rest and on straining. When combined with urethral pressure profilometry (UPP), an experienced investigator can infer information about the relative contributions of bladder neck hypermobility and sphincter deficiency as the causes of continued stress incontinence.
- Neurological lower urinary tract dysfunction. VCU is required to adequately assess the complex dysfunction seen in neuropathic bladders and to provide a framework for treatment. It is important to look for the presence of vesicoureteric reflux in this group of women.
- Assessment of voiding difficulties or symptoms suggestive of an anatomical lesion, such as a urethral diverticulum.

### Technique

The technique is identical to that used for routine subtracted cystometry, except that the investigation is performed in a room set up for radiological x-ray screening. Uroflowmetry, measurement of urinary residual and the insertion of pressure catheters are the same as for subtracted cystometry. Radio-opaque contrast is used to fill the bladder. X-ray screening takes place if the woman complains of leaking during filling and then during provocative coughing. This allows assessment of the degree of bladder neck opening, the severity of leakage and the extent of bladder-base descent. The presence of vesicoureteric reflux, bladder trabeculation and diverticulae is noted. The woman then commences voiding and, once normal flow has been established, she is asked to interrupt it. This should result in cessation of flow and urine being 'milked back' from the proximal urethra into the bladder. Finally, the presence of a post-void residual can be determined.

## Ambulatory urodynamic monitoring

Ambulatory urodynamic monitoring (AUM) is of particular use in the investigation of detrusor over-activity, where standard laboratory urodynamics have failed to replicate the symptoms that are experienced by the patient in her normal environment. Although laboratory urodynamics forms the standard method of objectively investigating bladder and urethral function, it is by design unphysiological. This is because relatively fast retrograde filling of the bladder is employed rather than slower filling from the kidneys via the ureters. In addition, the environment in which the test is performed and the focus of attention directed towards the subject are far removed from her everyday activities. In an attempt to study bladder function in circumstances that more closely approximate those in which the subject normally finds herself, ambulatory urodynamics has been developed.

Ambulatory urodynamic monitoring uses natural antero-grade bladder filling and allows the patient to reproduce

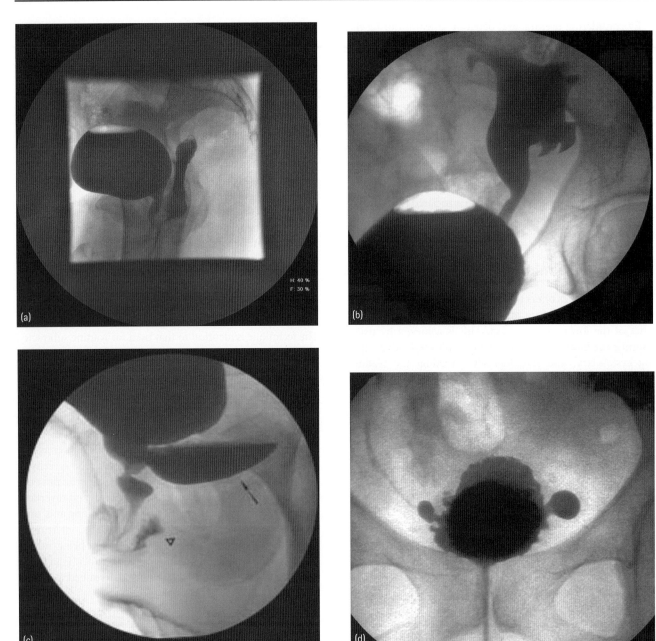

**Figure 59.7**  Urethro-vaginal reflux. a) urethro-vaginal reflux, b) vesico-uretic reflux into a transplanted kidney, c) urethral diverticulum, d) bladder diverticula and trabeculation, suggestive of a neurogenic bladder

her normal daily activities, including those that commonly provoke symptoms.

## Technique

Ambulatory systems have three main components.

1   Microtip transducers are placed in the bladder and rectum as in laboratory urodynamics.
2   A portable recording system allows several channels of data to be recorded simultaneously. This should include an event marker, to enable the patient to mark particular activities on the trace, and a method quantifying urine leakage, such as an electronic pad.
3   An analyzing system is needed to retrieve and process the data. All traces are interpreted with the patient present so that more information can be obtained about particular events.

The ICS has standardized the terminology and methodology of AUM,[6] allowing the comparison of results from different centres.

The investigation is usually carried out over a 4-hour time period. Once the transducers have been inserted into the bladder and rectum and the system has been calibrated, the patient is encouraged to drink normally and perform normal activities. During the investigation, the patient is asked to keep a careful record of symptoms and events, and the position of the catheters is checked periodically. At the conclusion of the test, provocative manoeuvres are carried out with a full bladder prior to removing the transducers and analyzing the results. Significantly more detrusor over-activity is diagnosed using AUM than with conventional laboratory urodynamics. However, it is uncertain whether this is due to a higher sensitivity or whether AUM simply has a high false-positive rate for diagnosing detrusor over-activity. Ambulatory urodynamics is subject to significant artefact, but this can be greatly reduced by rigorous methodology.

## Urethral pressure profilometry

The relationship between the intravesical pressure and the urethral pressure is the key to maintaining continence. Normally, the urethral pressure exceeds the intravesical pressure at all times, except during voluntary relaxation of the bladder neck leading to micturition. Urethral pressure profilometry can assess this ability of the urethra to exert a positive closure pressure in order to prevent leakage. This is done by simultaneously measuring the intravesical and urethral pressures using a catheter with two pressure transducers set 6 cm apart.

### Technique

The pressure catheter is inserted into the bladder with the distal pressure transducer inside the bladder and the proximal transducer near the bladder neck. It is then withdrawn at a standard speed by a mechanical retractor, allowing pressure measurements to be made along the functional length of the urethra to give a graph of pressure over distance travelled along the urethra. The ICS has also standardized the terminology and methodology of urethral pressure measurement.[7] Two types of UPP may be measured:

1 resting UPP, with the patient at rest in a supine position,
2 stress UPP, with the patient coughing throughout the test to see if the intravesical pressure exceeds the urethral pressure during increases in intra-abdominal pressure – this would result in a negative closure pressure and leakage of urine *per urethram*.

Although the closure pressures in women with urodynamic stress incontinence are generally less than in their dry counterparts, this test is not sufficiently discriminatory to be used in the diagnosis of urodynamic stress incontinence. However, it is often useful in understanding the pathophysiology of urodynamic stress incontinence and in planning the most appropriate intervention, especially in women who have had previous failed surgery for incontinence. A low maximum urethral closure pressure correlates with a poor outcome for incontinence surgery. The other group of patients in whom UPP can be useful is women with voiding difficulties. An increased maximum urethral closure pressure indicates outflow obstruction, sometimes as the result of previous surgery or a stricture. In these women, urethral dilatation or urethrotomy may be appropriate.

## NEUROPHYSIOLOGICAL INVESTIGATION

The normal co-ordinated functions of the bladder and urethra are controlled by a complex set of central and peripheral neurological reflexes. In an effort to understand these mechanisms better and to evaluate patients with lower urinary tract dysfunction, a whole range of neurophysiological tests has evolved. These techniques stimulate and record activity at different levels of the neurological pathways that control bladder and urethral function. The most commonly employed techniques in clinical neurophysiological testing are electromyography (EMG), in which recordings of bioelectrical potentials in muscles are studied, and nerve conduction studies. The latter examine the capacity of a nerve to transmit a test electrical stimulus along its length.

## Electromyography

Electromyography is the study of bioelectrical potentials generated by the depolarization of muscle fibres. It is predominantly used to study striated muscle, in particular the urethral sphincter and the pelvic floor muscles. The functional unit studied is called a motor unit and consists of the muscle fibres innervated by branches from the motor neuron of a single anterior horn cell. The potential it generates during contraction is called the motor nerve unit potential (MUP). This can be measured by means of surface electrodes or various types of needle electrode. By measuring the amplitude, duration and number of phases of the action potential, the extent of neurological denervation and subsequent reinnervation in the target muscle can be inferred. This is a highly specialist investigation and a skilled investigator is required to interpret the results. While EMG studies have greatly improved our understanding of pelvic floor, lower urinary tract and bowel function in health and disease, the results to date have had little effect on clinical management. The main clinical indication for EMG studies is as an adjunct to videourodynamics to distinguish between striated and smooth muscle in neuropathic urethral obstruction.

## Nerve conduction studies

A number of different techniques have been employed to study the conduction of central and peripheral nerve

Pelvic floor and lower urinary tract dysfunction

pathways to the bladder and urethra. These examine the capacity of a nerve to transmit a test electrical signal along its length. If the pathway being tested is damaged, there will be a delay in conduction time and thus a prolonged latency between the stimulus and the muscular response. In addition, the amplitude of the muscle response will be reduced. A wide range of neurological pathways has been investigated using variations of this technique, including the sacral reflex arc, pudendal terminal motor latencies, transcutaneous spinal stimulation and cortical evoked responses. As with EMG studies, these investigations have improved our understanding of the neurophysiological control of the normal and dysfunctional bladder, but are of limited use in the clinical investigation of most patients.

## RADIOLOGICAL IMAGING

Radiological imaging of the urinary tract is not justified as a routine investigation in all women presenting with urinary symptoms, but instead should be targeted at specific indications. The diagnostic procedures available include plain abdominal films, intravenous urography and various contrast studies of the lower urinary tracts.

### Plain x-ray

A plain abdominal film may be a useful screening investigation for a variety of conditions that affect lower urinary tract function. Foreign bodies and bladder calculi causing outflow obstruction can be diagnosed. Bladder wall calcification is rare in the United Kingdom, but is seen more frequently worldwide as a result of tuberculosis and schistosomiasis. Probably the most useful indication for plain radiographic films is to investigate spinal abnormalities, such as spina bifida or sacral agenesis, as a cause of neuropathic bladder disorder.

### Intravenous urography

This is not a routine investigation of lower urinary tract dysfunction. It provides anatomical and some functional information on the kidneys, ureters and bladder. Intravenous urography (IVU) is indicated in women with neuropathic bladders, suspected congenital or acquired abnormalities (such as uterovaginal fistulae), haematuria and suspected ureteric compromise secondary to the effects of a pelvic mass (e.g. large fibroids or a procidentia) or trauma.

### Micturating cystourethrography

This investigation requires instillation of radio-opaque contrast medium into the bladder and then screening with fluoroscopy as the patient voids. It is similar to the x-ray screening performed as part of a videocystometrogram, but without any pressure flow information. Its main value is to demonstrate bladder and urethral fistulae, vesicoureteric reflux and anatomical abnormalities of the lower tracts, such as urethral diverticulae.

## ULTRASONOGRAPHY

Ultrasound provides a relatively non-invasive method of imaging the urinary tract in real time, without exposing the patient to ionizing radiation. There is an ever-increasing range of applications for ultrasound imaging in the investigation of urinary tract dysfunction. As well as the lack of radiation exposure, ultrasound has the advantage of having significantly lower operating costs than comparable radiological investigation. The main disadvantage is that ultrasound waves do not penetrate as far and so the probe has to be held close to the target. The field of view is more limited than x-rays, so that only one part of the urinary tract can be viewed at a time. Ultrasound imaging depends on the different echogenicity of tissues to form a picture. It is especially well suited for visualizing fluid-filled and air-filled cystic structures.

### Post-micturition residual volume

Ultrasonography is widely used to estimate residual urine volumes. This obviates the need for urethral catheterization, with its concomitant risk of infection. This is particularly useful in the assessment of women with voiding difficulties. It can also be used following post-operative catheter removal or in women in labour as an alternative to repeated catheterization to ensure that the bladder is not allowed to over-distend. There are many methods of estimating bladder volume from real-time scanning, however, most portable bladder scanners presently available automatically calculate the volume of urine in the bladder.

### Assessing lower urinary tract structure

Ultrasound offers an inexpensive, non-invasive method of assessing the structure of the lower urinary tract and is advocated as an alternative to cystourethroscopy for many indications. The arguments in favour of each technique are similar to those proposed for the use of transvaginal ultrasonography and hysteroscopy for the assessment of the reproductive organs. The sensitivity of ultrasonography and endoscopy in different disorders varies, largely according to the experience of the operator and the quality of the equipment used. The majority of bladder tumours are exophytic and papillary in shape and are well visualized by ultrasound. Similarly, bladder diverticulae and calculi are easily detected.

Transabdominal ultrasound does not provide satisfactory imaging of the bladder neck and urethra, owing to their position behind the symphysis pubis. These are visualized better with the use of a transvaginal, transrectal or perineal probe. Ultrasonography is a very sensitive method of detecting urethral diverticulae and their relation to the urethral sphincter. Differentiation from para-urethral cysts may be difficult if a connection cannot be visualized. Three-dimensional ultrasound has been used as a research tool to determine urethral sphincter volumes as part of the assessment of women presenting with incontinence.

Another technique is the measurement of bladder wall thickness. This is performed using the transvaginal approach when the bladder is empty and offers a reproducible, sensitive method of screening for detrusor over-activity.[8]

## IMAGING

Computed tomography (CT) and magnetic resonance imaging (MRI) can provide confirmation of alternative pelvic pathology, by means of cross-sectional imaging. It can be used to characterize the extent and anatomical contents of a pelvic organ prolapse, especially in the standing position with MRI.[9]

## CYSTOURETHROSCOPY

Cystourethroscopy enables the inside of the bladder and urethra to be visualized (Figure 59.8). It is an invasive, but relatively low-risk, procedure that can be undertaken for women of any age as a day case. The choice between a rigid or flexible cystoscope and the anaesthetic used will depend on the individual case and the preferences of the operator. Modern cystoscopes consist of at least three elements.

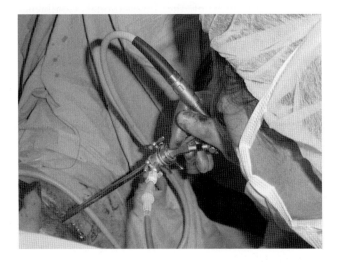

**Figure 59.8** Rigid cystometry with multiple bladder biopsies being performed under general anaesthesia in a patient with a history of recurrent urinary tract infections

1   An optical system for transmitting the image to a video monitor with maximum clarity and resolution. In a rigid endoscope this is performed by a rod-lens system, and in a flexible endoscope by a multifibre bundle of optical fibres.
2   Another system of optical fibres is needed to transmit light into the bladder.
3   An irrigating channel is needed to flush away blood and debris, and dilate the bladder under direct vision.

Most operating cystoscopes also have an outflow channel to carry debris away.

Cystourethroscopy is an invaluable tool in investigating the lower urinary tract, as it provides detailed anatomical information. It is not usually performed as part of the routine investigation of women with incontinence, but there are many indications for which direct visual inspection and targeted biopsies of the bladder and urethra are important in establishing a diagnosis.

## Indications

Cystourethroscopy is indicated:

- to investigate haematuria not related to urinary tract infection;
- when a reduced bladder capacity or painful filling is found at cystometry;
- to exclude bladder tumours and stones as a cause of recurrent or persistent urinary tract infection;
- if a lower urinary tract fistula is suspected;
- if interstitial cystitis is suspected;
- following failed incontinence surgery when the patient complains of voiding difficulty, overactive symptoms or persistent incontinence.

## Technique

The majority of cystourethroscopies undertaken by gynaecologists are performed under a general anaesthetic with a rigid scope. The advantages of a rigid cystoscope are that visualization is clearer and more magnified, and that biopsies and other manipulative procedures are relatively easily carried out through the large instrument channel. Flexible cystoscopes offer the advantage of use in the outpatient setting, with topical anaesthetic only. However, the view is more limited, as is the instrumentation that can be used, making it difficult to take histologically valid biopsy specimens. Flexible cystoscopy is more often performed by urologists.

Rigid cystoscopes are available with several viewing angles, including 0° (straight), 12°, 30° and 70°. Angled telescopes have a field marker, which appears as a notch at the edge of the field of view and helps to maintain orientation. The choice of telescope depends on the procedure being performed and the operator's preference. The cystoscope is placed into the urethral meatus and advanced towards the bladder under direct vision with the irrigation fluid running. Sterile saline is usually used as the irrigating fluid unless diathermy is planned, in which case a non-ionic solution, such as glycine, is required. Once the bladder is sufficiently distended to allow inspection of the folds of mucosa (200–400 mL), the irrigation can be switched off. The careful inspection of the urethra is a vital part of the investigation and should not be neglected. This is most commonly done while withdrawing the instrument at the end of the procedure. The trigone and the position of the ureteric orifices should be noted. Next, the mucosa is examined for colour, vascularity, trabeculation and abnormal lesions. Orientation is easily established by identifying the air bubble at the dome of the bladder. This serves as a landmark during inspection of the bladder mucosa, which is conventionally performed by going around clockwise in a series of 12 sweeps, coming back to the bubble after each one. Visualization of the bladder base can be difficult if a large cystocele is present. This is made easier by inserting a finger in the vagina to correct the prolapse.

## NATIONAL POLICIES AND GUIDANCE

In 2006, the National Institute for Health and Clinical Excellence (NICE) published guidelines on the management of urinary incontinence in women.[9] It provided recommendations and practice algorithms on assessment and investigations of LUTS. The Fourth International Consultation on Incontinence (ICI) (Paris, 2008) have recently published recommendations and guidance on the assessment of urinary incontinence.[10]

## ACKNOWLEDGEMENT

This chapter has been revised and updated. The author and editors acknowledge the contribution of James Balmforth to the chapter on this topic in the previous edition of the book.

### KEY POINTS

- Investigations of lower urinary tract dysfunction vary from simple tests that can easily be performed in an office setting, to complex investigations available in tertiary centres.
- As the correlation between lower urinary tract symptoms and underlying diagnosis is poor, early investigation is desirable so that a firm diagnosis can be established and rational treatment instigated.

- Thorough assessment, including urodynamics, is mandatory prior to considering surgical treatment.
- The choice of investigations performed should be individualized according to the patient's presenting symptoms, and past medical history.

## Key References

1. Abrams P, Cardozo L, Fall M *et al*. The standardisation of terminology of lower urinary tract function: report from the Standardisation Sub-committee of the International Continence Society. *Neurourol Urodyn* 2002; **21**: 167–78.
2. Royal College of Obstetricians and Gynecologists. *Gynaecological Examinations: Guidelines for Specialist Practice*. London: RCOG, 2002.
3. Matharu GS, Assandra RP, Williams KS *et al*. Objective assessment of urinary incontinence in women: comparison of the one hour and 24 hour pad test. *Eur Urol* 2004; **45**: 208–12.
4. Constantini E, Lazzeri M, Bini V *et al*. Sensitivity and specificity of one hour pad test as a predictive value for female urinary incontinence. *Urol Int* 2008; **81**: 153–9.
5. Schafer W, Abrams P, Lioa L. Good urodynamic practices: uroflowmetry, filling cystometry and pressure flow studies. *Neurolurol Urodyn* 2002; **21**: 261–74.
6. van Waalwijk van Doorn E, Anders K, Khullar V *et al*. Standardisation of ambulatory urodynamic monitoring: report of the Standardisation Sub-committee of the International Continence Society for ambulatory urodynamic studies. *Neurourol Urodyn* 2000; **19**: 113–25.
7. Lose G, Griffiths D, Hosker G *et al*. Standardisation of urethral measurement: report from the Standardisation Sub-Committee of the International Continence Society. *Neurourol Urodyn* 2002; **21**: 258–60.
8. Robinson D, Anders K, Cadozo L *et al*. Can ultrasound replace ambulatory urodynamics when investigating women with irritative urinary symptoms? *BJOG* 2002; **109**: 145–8.
9. National Institute for Health and Clinical Excellence. *Urinary Incontinence: The Management of Urinary Incontinence in Women*. Clinical Guideline 40. Implementation advice. London: NICE, 2006.
10. Staskin D, Kelleher C, Avery K *et al*. Initial investigations of urinary and faecal incontinence in adult male and female patients. In: Abrams P, Cardozo L, Khoury S, Wein A *(eds)*. *Incontinence*, 4th edn. Paris: Health Publication, 2009: 331–63.

# Urinary incontinence

*Dudley Robinson and Jane Rufford*

---

## MRCOG standards

### Theoretical skills

- Have good knowledge of normal pelvic anatomy, physiology and pathophysiology in relation to the functions of the pelvic floor.
- Understand the principles of all types of non-surgical and surgical interventions.

### Practical skills

- Be proficient in history taking, general and pelvic examination.
- Be able to perform the more common and basic pelvic floor surgical procedures.
- Be able to undertake non-surgical management of bladder problems, including voiding disorder and urgency.
- Be able to undertake surgery for stress incontinence under supervision.

---

## INTRODUCTION

Urinary incontinence is defined by the International Continence Society as 'the complaint of any involuntary leakage of urine'.[1] While not life-threatening, it is known to be a cause of considerable morbidity and has a considerable impact on quality of life.

## PREVALENCE

Urinary incontinence is known to be a prevalent, and often under-reported condition. A large epidemiological study of urinary incontinence has been reported in 27 936 women from Norway.[2] Overall, 25 per cent of women reported urinary incontinence, of whom 7 per cent felt it to be significant and the prevalence of incontinence was found to increase with age. When considering the type of incontinence, 50 per cent of women complained of stress, 11 per cent urge and 36 per cent mixed incontinence. Further analysis has also investigated the effect of age and parity. The prevalence of urinary incontinence among nulliparous women ranged from 8 to 32 per cent and increased with age. In general, parity was associated with incontinence and the first delivery was the most significant. When considering stress incontinence in the 20–34-year age group, the relative risk was 2.7 (95 per cent confidence interval (CI), 2.0–3.5) for primiparous women and 4.0 (95 per cent CI, 2.5–6.4) for multiparous women. There was a similar association for mixed incontinence, although not for urge incontinence.[3]

Evidence would suggest that incontinence is often under-reported. In a large study of patients assessed after tertiary referral, 60 per cent of women were found to have delayed seeking treatment for more than one year from the time their symptoms became severe. Of these women, 50 per cent claimed that this was because they were too embarrassed to discuss the problem with their doctor, and 17 per cent said that they thought the problem was normal for their age.

## EPIDEMIOLOGY

### Age

The incidence of urinary incontinence increases with increasing age. Elderly women have been found to have a reduced flow rate, increased urinary residuals, higher filling pressures, reduced bladder capacity and lower maximum voiding pressures. In a large study of 842 women aged 17–64 years, the prevalence rates of urinary incontinence increased progressively over seven birth cohorts (1900–1940) from 12 to 25 per cent. These findings agree with those of a large telephone survey in the United States which reported a prevalence of urge incontinence of 5 per cent in the 18–44 age group rising to 19 per cent in women over 65 years of age.[4] Conversely, as mobility and physical exercise decrease with advancing age, so does the prevalence of stress urinary incontinence.

# Race

Several studies have been performed examining the impact of racial differences on the prevalence of urinary incontinence in women. In general, there is evidence that there is a lower incidence of both urinary incontinence and urogenital prolapse in black women, and North American studies have found a larger proportion of white than African American women reported symptoms of stress incontinence (31 versus 7 per cent) and a larger proportion were found to have demonstrable stress incontinence on objective assessment (61 versus 27 per cent). Overall, white women had a prevalence of urodynamic stress incontinence 2.3 times higher than African American women.[5] While most studies confirm these findings, there is little evidence regarding the prevalence of urge incontinence or mixed incontinence.

# Pregnancy

Pregnancy is responsible for marked changes in the urinary tract and consequently lower urinary tract symptoms are more common and many are simply a reflection of normal physiological change. Urine production increases in pregnancy due to increasing cardiac output and a 25 per cent increase in renal perfusion and glomerular filtration rate.

Frequency of micturition is one of the earliest symptoms of pregnancy affecting approximately 60 per cent in the first trimester and mid trimester and 81 per cent in the final trimester. Nocturia is also a common symptom, although it was only thought to be a nuisance in 4 per cent of cases. Overall, frequency occurs in over 90 per cent of women in pregnancy.

Urgency and urge incontinence have also been shown to increase in pregnancy. Urge incontinence has been shown to have a peak incidence of 19 per cent in multiparous women, while other authors have reported a rate of urge incontinence of 10 per cent and urgency of 60 per cent. The incidence of detrusor overactivity and low compliance in pregnancy has been reported as 24 and 31 per cent, respectively. The cause of the former may be due to high progesterone levels, while the latter is probably a consequence of pressure from the gravid uterus.

Stress incontinence has also been reported to be more common in pregnancy, with 28 per cent of women complaining of symptoms, although only 12 per cent remained symptomatic following delivery. The long-term prognosis for this group of women remains guarded. Continent women delivered vaginally have been compared to those who had a caesarean section. While there was initially a difference in favour of caesarean section, this effect was insignificant by three months following delivery.

# Childbirth

Childbirth may result in damage to the pelvic floor musculature, as well as injury to the pudendal and pelvic nerves. The association between increasing parity and urinary incontinence has been reported in several studies. Some authorities have found this relationship to be linear, while others have demonstrated a threshold at the first delivery and some have shown that increasing age at first delivery is significant. A large Australian study has demonstrated a strong relationship between urinary incontinence and parity in young women (18–23 years), although in middle age (45–50 years) there was only a modest association and this was lost in older women (70–75 years).

Obstetric factors themselves may also have a direct effect on continence following delivery. The risk of incontinence increases by 5.7-fold in women who have had a previous vaginal delivery, although a previous caesarean section did not increase the risk.[6] In addition, an increased risk of urinary incontinence has been associated with increased exposure to oxytocic drugs, vacuum extraction, forceps delivery and fetal macrosomia.

# Menopause

The urogenital tract and lower urinary tract are sensitive to the effects of oestrogen and progesterone throughout adult life. Epidemiological studies have implicated oestrogen deficiency in the aetiology of lower urinary tract symptoms occurring following the menopause with 70 per cent of women relating the onset of urinary incontinence to their final menstrual period. Lower urinary tract symptoms have been shown to be common in postmenopausal women attending a menopause clinic, with 20 per cent complaining of severe urgency and almost 50 per cent complaining of stress incontinence. Urge incontinence in particular is more prevalent following the menopause and the prevalence would appear to rise with increasing years of oestrogen deficiency. Some studies have shown a peak incidence in perimenopausal women, while other evidence suggests that many women develop incontinence at least ten years prior to the cessation of menstruation with significantly more premenopausal women than postmenopausal women being affected.

# CAUSES OF URINARY INCONTINENCE

- Urodynamic stress incontinence (USI)
- Detrusor overactivity
- Overflow incontinence
- Fistulae (vesicovaginal, ureterovaginal, urethrovaginal)
- Congenital (e.g. ectopic ureter)
- Urethral diverticulum
- Other (e.g. urinary tract infection, faecal impaction, medication)
- Functional (e.g. immobility).

Urinary symptoms can be broadly divided into three groups. Detrusor overactivity is classically associated with frequency, urgency, urge incontinence, nocturia and nocturnal enuresis.

Urodynamic stress incontinence is classically associated with involuntary leakage on effort or on exertion or on coughing or sneezing (Table 60.1).

Continuous incontinence and/or post-micturition dribbling are more likely to be associated with neurological disorders, overflow, urethral diverticulae or a fistula. However, there are problems with making a presumptive diagnosis on the basis of symptoms alone. Many women complain of a mixture of symptoms. For instance, those women who are found to have USI often complain of frequency, as they are going to the toilet more often in order to avoid leaking. One study found that even an experienced clinician made the correct diagnosis only 65 per cent of the time when relying on symptoms alone.

# URODYNAMIC STRESS INCONTINENCE

## Definition

Urodynamic stress incontinence is noted during filling cystometry and is defined as 'the involuntary leakage of urine during increased abdominal pressure, in the absence of a detrusor contraction'.

## Incidence

Urodynamic stress incontinence is the most common cause of incontinence in women. It is difficult to assess the true incidence, as many women suffer in silence and consider it an inevitable consequence of childbirth and ageing. However, conservative estimates are that one in ten women will suffer from USI at some point in their lives.

**Table 60.1** Symptoms and definitions

| Symptom | Definition |
|---|---|
| ↑Daytime frequency | Complaint by the patient who considers that she voids too often by day |
| Urgency | Sudden and compelling desire to pass urine, which is difficult to defer |
| Urge urinary incontinence | Complaint of involuntary leakage accompanied by or immediately preceded by urgency |
| Mixed urinary incontinence | Complaint of involuntary leakage associated with urgency and also with exertion, effort, sneezing or coughing |
| Nocturnal enuresis | Complaint of loss of urine occurring during sleep |
| Continuous urinary incontinence | Complaint of continuous leakage |
| Stress urinary incontinence | Complaint of involuntary leakage on effort or exertion, or on sneezing or coughing |

## Aetiology

There are various factors that are thought to predispose to the development of USI.

- Increased intra-abdominal pressure:
  - pregnancy
  - chronic cough
  - abdominal, pelvic mass
  - constipation
  - ascites.
- Damage to the pelvic floor:
  - childbirth
  - radical pelvic surgery.
- Fixed, scarred urethra:
  - previous surgery
  - radiotherapy.

## Pathophysiology

The exact pathophysiology is unclear, but several hypotheses have been put forward.

- Failure of the supporting structures, such as the pubourethral and pubovesical ligaments.
- Failure of the intrinsic sphincter mechanism as a result of damage to the rhabdosphincter, poor collagen or reduced urethral vascularity (intrinsic sphincter deficiency (ISD)).
- Failure of the extrinsic sphincter mechanism as a result of weakness or damage to the pelvic floor musculature. This allows displacement of the bladder neck from within the intra-abdominal pressure zone.

### KEY POINTS

- Urodynamic stress incontinence is the most common cause of incontinence in women.
- The diagnosis is based on urodynamic assessment.
- Increased abdominal pressure, pelvic floor damage and urethral scarring all predispose to USI.

# MANAGEMENT OF URODYNAMIC STRESS INCONTINENCE

## Conservative management

Urodynamic stress incontinence interferes with a woman's quality of life, but it is not a life-threatening condition and therefore conservative measures should be tried in every woman prior to resorting to surgical treatment.

Conservative treatment is effective, has few complications and does not compromise further surgical procedures. It is particularly useful in those women who are medically unfit for surgery, those who have not completed their family or are breastfeeding or less than six months post-partum.

Conservative measures include:

- pelvic floor exercises
- biofeedback
- electrical stimulation
- vaginal cones
- urethral devices.

In order to maximize the benefits that can be obtained using these techniques, it is vital to ensure that the treatment is tailored to the individual and that it is properly taught.

Pelvic floor muscle training (PFMT) and pelvic floor physiotherapy remain the first-line conservative measure since their introduction in 1948. PFMT appears to work in a number of different ways:

- Women learn to consciously pre-contract the pelvic floor muscles before and during increases in abdominal pressure to prevent leakage ('the knack').
- Strength training builds up long-lasting muscle volume and thus provides structural support.
- Abdominal muscle training indirectly strengthens the pelvic floor muscles.[7]

In addition, during a contraction, the urethra may also be pressed against the posterior aspect of the symphysis pubis producing a mechanical rise in urethral pressure. Since up to 30 per cent of women with stress incontinence are unable to contract their pelvic floor correctly at presentation, some patients may simply need to be retaught the 'knack' of squeezing the appropriate muscles at the correct time. Cure rates varying between 21 and 84 per cent have been reported. Success appears to depend upon the type and severity of incontinence treated, the instruction and follow up given, the compliance of the patient and the outcome measures used. However, the evidence would suggest that PFMT is more effective if patients are given a structured programme to follow rather than simple verbal instructions.[8]

Biofeedback is used to augment the effect of pelvic floor exercises. It can range in complexity from the very simple, such as a vaginal examination measuring the strength of the squeeze, which the woman can perform herself at home, to the much more sophisticated electromyography, which is usually used in a clinic. Biofeedback has not been shown to be superior to pelvic floor exercises alone.

Electrical stimulation uses an electrical pulse to augment the ability to produce a voluntary contraction. A probe is put into the vagina near the muscles of the pelvic floor and a pulse of electricity is passed. The optimal pulse frequency is debated, but it is usually in the 35–40-Hz range. This method cannot be used in pregnancy or in those with an intrauterine contraceptive device (IUCD) *in situ*. It is not suitable for most women as it is excessively time consuming.

Vaginal cones or weights are now used infrequently, as the results are no better than those of pelvic floor exercises alone.

Many women find a tampon or an intravaginal device very helpful. These devices elevate the bladder neck and in some cases partially obstruct the flow of urine. They are particularly suitable for women who find they are incontinent only at specific times, for instance during aerobics or playing tennis. Several urethral devices are available, such as Conveen, but these are now very rarely used.

## Pharmacological management

While various agents such as $\alpha_1$-adrenoceptor agonists, oestrogens and tricyclic antidepressants have all been used anecdotally in the past for the treatment of stress incontinence, duloxetine is the first drug to be specifically developed and licensed for this indication.

Duloxetine is a potent and balanced serotonin (5-hydroxytryptamine) and noradrenaline reuptake inhibitor (SNRI) which enhances urethral striated sphincter activity via a centrally mediated pathway. The efficacy and safety of duloxetine has been evaluated in a double-blind randomized parallel group placebo controlled phase II dose-finding study in the United States involving 553 women with stress incontinence.[9] Duloxetine was associated with significant and dose-dependent decrease in incontinence episode frequency, while the most frequently reported adverse event was nausea.

A further global phase III study of 458 women has also recently been reported. There was a significant decrease in incontinence episode frequency and improvement in quality of life with duloxetine compared to placebo. Once again, nausea was the most frequently reported adverse event occurring in 25.1 per cent of women receiving duloxetine compared to a rate of 3.9 per cent in those taking placebo.

Duloxetine may also be useful in those women awaiting continence surgery. In a further double-blind, placebo-controlled study of 109 women awaiting surgery for stress incontinence,[10] there was a significant improvement in incontinence episode frequency and quality of life when compared to placebo. Furthermore, 20 per cent of women who were awaiting continence surgery changed their mind while taking duloxetine.

In addition, the role of synergistic therapy with pelvic floor muscle training and duloxetine has been examined in a prospective study of 201 women with stress incontinence. Women were randomized to one of four treatment combinations: duloxetine, PFMT, combination therapy or placebo. Overall duloxetine, with or without PFMT was found to be superior to placebo or PFMT alone, while pad test results and quality of life analysis favoured combination therapy to single treatment.[11]

## Surgical procedures

More than 200 operative procedures for the treatment of USI have been described. Many of these are modifications of similar procedures, but there is not one definitive operation.

The first operative procedure offers the best chance of cure and therefore it is very important to select the appropriate procedure for each patient.

Historically, colposuspension, originally described by Burch in 1961, has been regarded as the operation of choice in cases of primary stress incontinence. However, with the description of the 'mid-urethral theory' or 'integral theory' by Petros and Ulmsten,[12] the rationale behind surgery for stress incontinence has changed. This concept is based on earlier studies suggesting that the distal and mid-urethra play an important role in the continence mechanism and that the maximal urethral closure pressure is at the mid-urethral point. The theory proposes that damage to the pubourethral ligaments supporting the urethra, impaired support of the anterior vaginal wall to the mid-urethra, and weakened function of part of the pubococcygeal muscles which insert adjacent to the urethra are responsible for causing stress incontinence. This hypothesis has led directly to the development of both the retropubic and trans-obturator mid-urethral tape procedures and these new, minimally invasive procedures have now largely replaced retropubic suspensions and sling procedures.

For those women who may not be suitable for a mid-urethral tape procedure, urethral bulking agents may also be considered and many of these may now be performed under local anaesthesia in the ambulatory setting.

## Colposuspension

The patient is placed in the modified lithotomy position using Lloyd–Davies stirrups. A Foley catheter is inserted into the bladder and allowed to drain freely. A low transverse incision is made just above the symphysis pubis (i.e. lower than a pfannenstiel). The retropubic space is dissected until the white paravaginal tissue lateral to the bladder neck is exposed. Two to four polydioxanone sutures (PDS), Ethibond or polyglycolic acid sutures are inserted into the paravaginal fascia. Each suture is tied and the needle is then reinserted into the ipsilateral iliopectineal ligament. The first suture is placed at the level of the bladder neck and the subsequent sutures are placed 1 cm laterally and 1 cm cranially (Figure 60.1). When all the sutures have been inserted, an assistant elevates the lateral fornix on each side to allow the sutures to be tied without tension (Figure 60.2). A suction drain is left in the retropubic space, a suprapubic catheter is inserted and the urethral catheter is removed.

The suprapubic catheter is left on free drainage for at least 2 days and then a clamping regimen is initiated. This usually entails clamping the catheter at a set time and allowing the patient to void normally. Initially, the residual is checked after each void or, if the patient experiences discomfort, the clamp is released and the residual measured. If the patient is passing good volumes of urine with small residuals, the time between unclamping can be extended to 12 hours and then 24 hours. When the residuals are persistently under 100 mL, the suprapubic catheter can be removed.

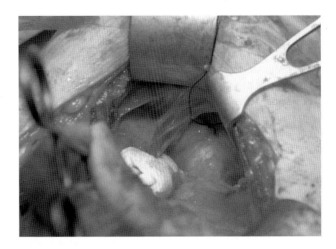

**Figure 60.1** Colposuspension: The bladder neck is mobilized medially and the first suture placed in the white paravaginal tissue

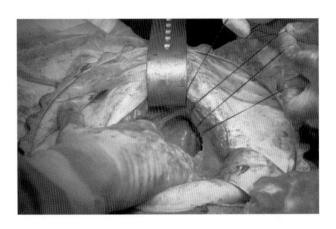

**Figure 60.2** Colposuspension: Four sutures are placed on each side to elevate the paravaginal tissue to the ipsilateral pectineal ligament

### Post-operative complications

Voiding difficulties are the main complication following a colposuspension. Overall, the incidence of voiding difficulties lasting over one month is reported as 5 per cent (confidence interval, 3–5), although other series have reported rates as high as 21 per cent.

These women are initially managed by allowing them to go home with their suprapubic catheter *in situ*, leaving it on free drainage. Two weeks later they are readmitted and a further trial of clamping is attempted. The majority of women will be able to void spontaneously at this stage. About 2 per cent will continue to complain of voiding difficulties, and these women are usually taught clean intermittent self-catheterization.

Detrusor overactivity arises *de novo* in between 12 and 18.5 per cent of women who have undergone a colposuspension. It seems to occur more commonly after previous continence surgery. It may be that a number of cases reflect pre-existing detrusor overactivity that went undetected at pre-operative cystometry. Alternatively, the autonomic nerve supply may be damaged when the bladder is medially displaced at the time of surgery.

A longer-term complication is the development of prolapse. Enterocele and rectocele formation is thought to occur as a result of elevation of the anterior vaginal wall creating a posterior defect and causing intra-abdominal pressure to be transmitted directly to the posterior vaginal wall. The incidence is estimated to be between 7 and 17 per cent. It is unclear whether these represent new defects or merely a pre-existing defect becoming symptomatic once the support of the anterior vaginal wall has been rectified.

### Outcome

Historically, there have been many prospective case series and cohort studies assessing the efficacy of colposuspension with some studies providing long-term follow-up data up to 20 years and cure rates of 80–94 per cent.

In addition, there have also been three reported meta-analyses. The first of these was reported in 1994 in a review of 1726 women with follow up of at least one year and a mean objective success rate of 84.3 per cent. Very similar results were reported from a meta-analysis of 2196 women reported by the American Urological Association in 1997. Overall mean objective cure rates were 84 per cent at 48 months (confidence interval, 79–88 per cent) with follow up to at least four years. More recently, the Cochrane group has published a meta-analysis of 39 randomized controlled trial involving 2403 women with a mean follow up of one year. Objective cure rates were found to be 85–90 per cent and there was a slow decline in cure rates to 70 per cent over five years.

## Laparoscopic colposuspension

Minimally invasive surgery is attractive and this trend has extended to surgery for stress incontinence. Although many authors have reported excellent short-term subjective results from laparoscopic colposuspension, early studies have shown inferior results to the open procedure.

More recently, two large prospective randomized controlled trials have been reported from Australia and the United Kingdom comparing laparoscopic and open colposuspension. In the Australian study, 200 women with urodynamic stress incontinence were randomized to either laparoscopic or open colposuspension. Overall, there were no significant differences in objective and subjective measures of cure or in patient satisfaction at six months, 24 months or 3–5 years. While the laparoscopic approach took longer, it was associated with less blood loss and a quicker return to normal activities.

These findings are supported by the United Kingdom multicentre randomized controlled trial of 291 women with urodynamic stress incontinence comparing laparoscopic to open colposuspension.[13] At 24 months, intention-to-treat analysis showed no significant difference in cure rates between the procedures. Objective cure rates for open and laparoscopic colposuspension were 70.1 and 79.7 per cent,

respectively, while subjective cure rates were 54.6 and 54.9 per cent, respectively.

These studies have confirmed that the clinical effectiveness of the two operations is comparable, although the cost-effectiveness of laparoscopic colposuspension remains unproven. A cost analysis comparing laparoscopic to open colposuspension was also performed alongside the UK study. Healthcare resource use over the first six-month follow-up period translated into costs of £1805 for the laparoscopic group versus £1433 for the open group.

### Post-operative complications

The incidence of urinary tract injury has been found to be higher during laparoscopic colposuspension than during the open operation. A 1–10 per cent rate of bladder injury has been reported, and although the rate of ureteric injury or kinking is less than 0.1 per cent, this is significantly higher than at the open procedure. Operative morbidity has also been extensively studied with intraoperative blood loss, febrile morbidity and length of hospital stay all higher in the open colposuspension group.

## Pubovaginal sling

Sling procedures are often performed as secondary operations where there is scarring and narrowing of the vagina. The sling material can either be organic (rectus fascia, porcine dermis) or inorganic (Prolene, Mersilene, Marlex or Silastic). The sling may be inserted either abdominally, vaginally or by a combination of both. Normally, the sling is used to elevate and support the bladder neck and proximal urethra, but not intentionally to obstruct it.

Sling procedures may be associated with a high incidence of side effects and complications. It is often difficult to decide how tight to make the sling. If it is too loose, incontinence will persist and if it is too tight, voiding difficulties may be permanent. Women who are going to undergo insertion of a sling must be prepared to perform clean intermittent self-catheterization post-operatively. In addition, there is a risk of infection, especially if inorganic material is used. The sling may erode into the urethra, bladder or vagina, in which case it must be removed and this can be exceedingly difficult.

## Mid-urethral tape procedures

### Retropubic mid-urethral tapes

#### Tension-free vaginal tape

The tension-free vaginal tape (TVT, Gynaecare), first described by Ulmsten in 1996,[14] is now the most commonly performed procedure for stress urinary incontinence in the UK and more than two million procedures have been performed worldwide.

A knitted 11 mm × 40 cm polypropylene mesh tape is inserted transvaginally at the level of the mid-urethra, using two 5-mm trochars (Figure 60.3). The procedure may be performed under local, spinal or general anaesthesia.

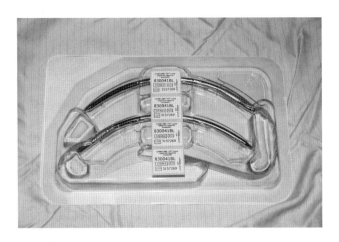

**Figure 60.3** TVT: Tension-free vaginal tape

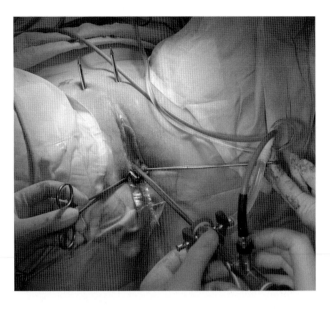

**Figure 60.4** TVT trochars inserted and check cystoscopy to exclude bladder perforation

## Technique

The procedure may be performed under local or general anaesthesia. The patient is placed in the dorsal lithotomy position and having prepared the vagina and suprapubic area an indwelling 18-Fr Foley catheter is inserted into the bladder. Once the bladder has been emptied, a rigid catheter guide is then inserted down the catheter in order to deflect the bladder away from the passage of the needle introducers. The use of local anaesthesia (20-mL bupivicaine 0.5 per cent with 1 in 200 000 adrenaline – diluted in 100-mL normal saline) allows effective hydrodissection and vasoconstriction, while at the same time providing effective intraoperative and post-operative analgesia. Dilute local anaesthetic (20 mL) is injected on each side retropubically immediately behind the pubic tubercle. In addition, a further 20 mL is injected paraurethrally on each side up to the level of the urogenital diaphragm and 5 mL suburethrally.

A 2-cm midline suburethral vaginal incision is made and paraurethral dissection performed using sharp dissection with McIndoe scissors between the vaginal mucosa and pubocervical fascia to the level of the inferior pubic ramus and the urogenital diaphragm. Two small 0.5-cm suprapubic incisions at the upper border of the pubic tubercle 2 cm lateral to the midline may be made to facilitate needle passage through the skin.

The TVT needle is then placed in the starting position within the dissected paraurethral tunnel with the tip of the needle between the index finger (in the vagina) and the lower border of the pubic ramus. Prior to the passage of the needle, the bladder is pushed away from the track of the needle using the rigid catheter guide. In a controlled movement, the needle is then pushed through the urogenital diaphragm, the retropubic space and the rectus fascia keeping in close contact to the dorsal aspect of the pubic bone. The procedure is then repeated on the contralateral side.

With the needles still in position, a cystoscopy using a 70° cystoscope is performed to check that there is no bladder injury (Figure 60.4). Should a bladder perforation be noted, the needle is withdrawn, replaced, passed once again and the cystoscopy repeated. Once the integrity of the bladder is confirmed, the bladder is again emptied completely and the tape pulled through.

In those centres which continue to use the cough stress test, the bladder is then refilled with 300-mL normal saline and the patient asked to cough vigorously. The tape may then be adjusted to a point where there is only a drop of leakage from the urethral meatus. After this final adjustment, the tape is held in position beneath the urethra using a pair of McIndoe scissors, while the plastic sheaths are removed on each side (Figure 60.5).

In those centres where a cough stress test is no longer used, the tape is positioned loosely below the mid-urethra without tension. Finally, the vaginal incision is closed using an absorbable suture and the suprapubic incisions are closed with steristrips. While an indwelling catheter is not required in all cases, a urethral catheter should be left on free drainage for 48 hours following a bladder injury.

## Outcome

The initial multicentre study carried out in six centres in Sweden reported a 90 per cent cure rate at one year in women undergoing their first operation for urodynamic stress incontinence, without any major complications. Long-term results would confirm durability of the technique with success rates of 86 per cent at three years, 84.7 per cent at five years, 81.3 per cent at seven years and 90 per cent at 11 years.[15]

The tension-free vaginal tape has also been compared to open colposuspension in a multicentre prospective randomized trial of 344 women with urodynamic stress incontinence.[16] Overall, there was no significant difference in terms of objective cure; 66 per cent in the tension-free vaginal

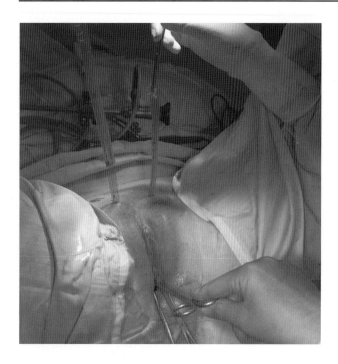

**Figure 60.5** TVT: Adjusting the tension of the tape

## Mid-urethral sling suspension system

The SPARC sling system (American Medical Systems) is a minimally invasive sling procedure using a knitted 10 mm wide polypropylene mesh which is placed at the level of the mid-urethra by passing the needle via a suprapubic to vaginal approach. The procedure may be performed under local, regional or general anaesthetic. A prospective multicentre study of 104 women with urodynamic stress incontinence has been reported from France. At a mean follow up of 11.9 months, the objective cure rate was 90.4 per cent and subjective cure 72 per cent. There was a 10.5 per cent incidence of bladder perforation and 11.5 per cent of women complained of *de novo* urgency following the procedure. More recently, SPARC has been compared to tension-free vaginal tape in a prospective randomized trial of 301 women. At short-term follow up, there were no significant differences in cure rates, bladder perforation rates and *de novo* urgency. There was, however, a higher incidence of voiding difficulties and vaginal erosions in the SPARC group.

## Transobturator sling procedures

The transobturator route for the placement of synthetic mid-urethral slings was first described in 2001.[17] As with the retropubic sling procedures, transobturator tapes may be performed under local, regional or general anaesthetic and have the theoretical advantage of eliminating some of the complications associated with the retropubic route, such as bladder and urethral perforation.

The transobturator approach may be used as an 'inside-out' (TVT-O, Gynaecare) or alternatively an 'outside-in' (Monarc, American Medical Systems) technique. To date, there have been several studies documenting the short-term efficacy of transobturator procedures.

### Technique

Transobturator 'inside-out'
The TVT-O device consists of an 11 mm wide by 40 cm long tape of polypropylene mesh, both ends of which are attached to a plastic sheath which threads over the helical needle introducer. A winged needle guide is also provided to facilitate passage of the needle through the obturator membrane (Figure 60.6).

The procedure may be performed under local or general anaesthesia. The patient is placed in the dorsal lithotomy position in 120° hyperflexion. The vagina and thighs are then prepared and an indwelling 12-Fr Foley catheter is inserted into the bladder. Next two 0.5-cm incisions are made 2 cm superior to a horizontal line level with the urethra and 2 cm lateral to the thigh folds. This marks the exit point for the helical needle introducer.

The use of local anaesthesia (20-mL bupivicaine 0.5 per cent with 1 in 200 000 adrenaline, diluted in 100-mL normal saline) allows effective hydrodissection and vasoconstriction, while at the same time providing effective intraoperative and

tape group and 57 per cent in the colposuspension group. However, operation time, post-operative stay and return to normal activity were all longer in the colposuspension arm. Analysis of the long-term results at 24 months using a pad test, quality of life assessment and symptom questionnaires showed an objective cure rate of 63 per cent in the tension-free vaginal tape arm and 51 per cent in the colposuspension arm. At five years, there were no differences in subjective cure (63 per cent in the tension-free vaginal tape group and 70 per cent in the colposuspension group), patient satisfaction and quality of life assessment. However, while there was a significant reduction in cystocele in both groups, there was a higher incidence of enterocele, rectocele and apical prolapse in the colposuspension group. Furthermore, cost–utility analysis has also shown that at six months follow up, tension-free vaginal tape resulted in a mean cost saving of £243 when compared to colposuspension.

A smaller randomized study has also compared tension-free vaginal tape to laparoscopic colposuspension in 72 women with urodynamic stress incontinence. At a mean follow up of 20 months, objective cure rates were higher in the tension-free vaginal tape group when compared to the laparoscopic colposuspension group: 96.8 versus 71.2 per cent, respectively.

### Post-operative complications

Following the procedure, most women can go home the same day, although some do require catheterization for short-term voiding difficulties (2.5–19.7 per cent). Other complications include bladder perforation (2.7–5.8 per cent), *de novo* urgency (0.2–15 per cent) and bleeding (0.9–2.3 per cent).

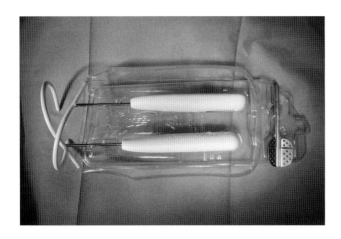

**Figure 60.6** TVTO: Tension-free vaginal tape, obturator

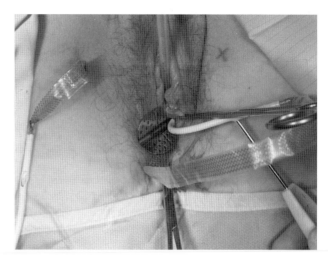

**Figure 60.7** TVTO: Insertion of TVTO using the winged guide

post-operative analgesia. Dilute local anaesthetic (20 mL) is injected paraurethrally on each side in the direction of the inferior pubic ramus.

A midline suburethral incision is then made at the level of the mid-urethra prior to paraurethral sharp dissection between the vaginal epithelium and periurethral fascia using McIndoe scissors. Dissection is continued laterally to the inferior border of the pubic ramus at the level of the mid-urethra and the medial aspect of the obturator membrane is perforated.

The winged needle guide is then passed at 45° relative to the saggital plane of the urethra until reaching the posterior aspect of the inferior pubic ramus and perforating the the obturator membrane. Having mounted the tape on to the helical introducer, the tip is then placed along the guide channel in the winged guide to pass through the obturator membrane and is then rotated so as to exit through the inner thigh incision. The tip of the tubing is then clamped and the helical introducer withdrawn. The procedure is then repeated on the contralateral side (Figure 60.7). Once both needles have been passed and the tape inserted a cystoscopy may be performed to exclude bladder or urethral injury.

The tape is then held loosely in position beneath the urethra using a pair of McIndoe scissors, while the protective plastic sheaths are removed ensuring that there is no tension on the urethra and the tape is lying flat (Figure 60.8). The vaginal incision is then closed using an absorbable suture and steristrips are used to close the two small incisions on the thighs. While an indwelling catheter is not required in all cases, a urethral catheter should be left on free drainage for 48 hours following a bladder injury.

### Transobturator 'outside-in'

The procedure may be performed under local or general anaesthesia. The patient is placed in the dorsal lithotomy position in 120° hyperflexion. The vagina and thighs are then prepared and an indwelling 12-Fr Foley catheter is inserted into the bladder. The use of local anaesthesia (20 mL

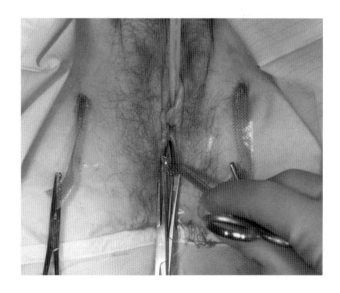

**Figure 60.8** TVTO: Adjusting the tension of the tape

bupivicaine 0.5 per cent with 1 in 200 000 adrenaline, diluted in 100-mL normal saline) allows effective hydrodissection and vasoconstriction, while at the same time providing effective intraoperative and post-operative analgesia. Dilute local anaesthetic (20 mL) is injected paraurethrally on each side in the direction of the inferior pubic ramus.

A midline suburethral incision is then made at the level of the mid-urethra prior to paraurethral sharp dissection between the vaginal epithelium and periurethral fascia using McIndoe scissors. Dissection is continued laterally to the inferior border of the pubic ramus at the level of the mid-urethra and the medial aspect of the obturator membrane is perforated. Next, a small incision is made 1.5 cm lateral to the ischiopubic ramus on each side at the level of the clitoris. The helical needle introducer is then passed 'outside-in' through the incision to perforate the medial aspect of the obturator membrane. With the index finger in the vaginal incision palpating the ischiopubic ramus and obturator internus muscle, the tip of the helical needle may then be guided through to the vaginal incision. Care should be taken to avoid perforating the lateral vaginal fornix and the urethra is guarded by the operator's finger. Once the tip of the needle has been passed through the vaginal incision, the tape may then be attached to the needle and pulled through to exit through the thigh incision. The procedure is then repeated on the contralateral side.

The tape is then held loosely in position beneath the urethra using a pair of McIndoe scissors, while the protective plastic sheaths are removed ensuring that there is no tension on the urethra and the tape is lying flat. The vaginal incision is then closed using an absorbable suture and steristrips are used to close the two small incisions on the thighs. While an indwelling catheter is not required in all cases, a urethral catheter should be left on free drainage for 48 hours following a bladder injury.

## Outcome

Initial studies have reported cure and improved rates of 80.5 and 7.5 per cent, respectively, at seven months[18] and 90.6 and 9.4 per cent, respectively, at 17 months.

More recently, the transobturator approach (TVT-O) has been compared to the retropubic approach (TVT) in an Italian prospective multicentre randomized study of 231 women with urodynamic stress incontinence. At a mean of nine months subjectively 92 per cent of women in the TVT group were cured compared to 87 per cent in the TVT-O group. Objectively, on pad test testing, cure rates were 92 and 89 per cent, respectively. There were no differences in voiding difficulties and length of stay, although there were more bladder perforations in the TVT group; 4 per cent versus none in the TVT-O group. A further multicentre prospective randomized trial comparing TVT and TVT-O has also recently been reported from Finland in 267 women complaining of stress urinary incontinence. Objective cure rates at 9 weeks were 98.5 per cent in the TVT group and 95.4 per cent in the TVT-O group. While complication rates were low and similar in both arms of the study, there was a higher incidence of groin pain in the TVT-O group.

These data are supported by a recent meta-analysis of the five randomized trials comparing TVTO with TVT and six randomized trials comparing TOT with TVT.[19] Overall, subjective cure rates were identical with the retropubic and transobturator routes. However, adverse events such as bladder injuries (odds ratio (OR) 0.12; 95 per cent CI, 0.05–0.33) and voiding difficulties (OR 0.55; 95 per cent CI, 0.31–0.98) were less common, whereas groin pain (OR 8.28; 95 per cent CI, 2.7–25.4) and vaginal erosions (OR 1.96; 95 per cent CI, 0.87–4.39) were more common after the transobturator approach. Long-term data would also seem to support the durability and efficacy of the transobturator approach. A three-year follow-up study of a prospective, observational study evaluating the use of TVT-O

has recently been reported. Of the 102 patients recruited 91 (89.2 per cent) were available for follow up at a minimum of three years. The objective cure rate was 88.4 per cent with an improvement in 9.3 per cent of cases and there was no statistical difference in outcome as compared to the results reported at one year.

### Post-operative complications

While the transobturator route may be associated with a lower risk of bladder injury, there is a risk of damage to the obturator nerve and vessels. In an anatomical dissection model, the tape passes 3.4–4.8 cm from the anterior and posterior branches of the obturator nerve, respectively, and 1.1 cm from the most medial branch of the obturator vessels. Consequently, nerve and vessel injury in addition to buttock pain, bladder injury and vaginal erosion remain a potential complication of the procedure.

## Urethral bulking agents

Urethral bulking agents are a minimally invasive surgical procedure for the treatment of urodynamic stress incontinence and may be useful in the elderly and those women who have undergone previous operations and have a fixed, scarred fibrosed urethra.

Although the actual substance which is injected may differ, the principle is the same. It is injected either periurethrally or transurethrally on either side of the bladder neck under cystoscopic control and is intended to 'bulk' the bladder neck, in order to stop premature bladder neck opening, without causing outflow obstruction. They may be performed under local, regional or general anaesthesia. There are now several different products available (Table 60.2). The use of minimally invasive implantation systems has also allowed some of these procedures to be performed in the office setting without the need for cystoscopy (Figure 60.9).

**Table 60.2** Urethral bulking agents

| Urethral bulking agent | Application technique |
|---|---|
| Gluteraldehyde crosslinked bovine collagen (Contigen) | Cystoscopic |
| Polydimethylsiloxane (Macroplastique) | Cystoscopic (MIS Implantation System) |
| Pyrolytic carbon-coated zirconium oxide beads in β-glucan gel (Durasphere) | Cystoscopic |
| Calcium hydroxylapatite in carboxymethylcellulose gel (Coaptite) | Cystoscopic |
| Polyacrylamide hydrogel (Bulkamid) | Cystoscopic |

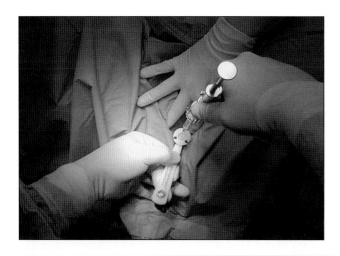

**Figure 60.9** Macroplastique: Use of the Macroplastque implantation system under local anaesthesia

### Outcome

In the first reported series, 81 per cent of 68 women were dry following two injections with collagen. There have been longer-term follow-up studies most of which give a less than 50 per cent objective cure rate at two years, but a subjective improvement rate of about 70 per cent. Macroplastique has recently been compared to Contigen in a recent North American study of 248 women with urodynamic stress incontinence. Outcome was assessed objectively using pad tests and subjectively at 12 months. Overall objective cure and improvement rates favoured Macroplastique over Contigen (74 versus 65 per cent; $p = 0.13$). While this difference was not significant, subjective cure rates were higher in the Macroplastique group (41 versus 29 per cent; $p = 0.07$).

While success rates with urethral bulking agents are generally lower than those with conventional continence surgery, they are minimally invasive and have lower complication rates meaning that they remain a useful alternative in selected women.

## Minimally invasive tape procedures

While the development of the mid-urethral retropubic and transobturator tapes has transformed the surgical approach to stress urinary incontinence by offering a minimally invasive day case procedure, there has recently been interest in developing a new type of 'mini-sling' which may offer a truly office-based approach. The TVT Secur (Gynaecare) is the first of these mini-slings to be introduced, although there are several other devices, including MiniArc (American Medical Systems) currently under investigation and development.

### Gynecare TVT Secur

#### Technique

The TVT-Secur device consists of an 11 mm wide by 8 cm long tape of polypropylene mesh both ends of which are sandwiched between a fleece pad composed of a woven polyglactin and poly-p-dioxane fibres. The pads are locked in position on the end of two stainless steel inserters allowing accurate retropubic placement. Following the release of the locking mechanism, the pads may then be released at the time of insertion.

The procedure may be performed under local or general anaesthesia. The patient is placed in the dorsal lithotomy position and having prepared the vagina and suprapubic area an indwelling 18-Fr Foley catheter is inserted into the bladder. Once the bladder has been emptied, a rigid catheter guide is then inserted down the catheter in order to deflect the bladder away from the passage of the needle introducers. The use of local anaesthesia (20 mL bupivicaine 0.5 per cent with 1 in 200 000 adrenaline, diluted in 100-mL normal saline) allows effective hydrodissection and vasoconstriction, while at the same time providing effective intraoperative and post-operative analgesia. 20 mL are injected paraurethrally on each side up to the level of the urogenital diaphragm and 5 mL suburethrally.

A 1.5-cm midline suburethral vaginal incision is made and paraurethral dissection performed using sharp dissection with McIndoe scissors between the vaginal mucosa and pubocervical fascia to a depth of 1 cm. If the placement is retropubic ('U' position) the angle of dissection is 45°, while if an obturator ('hammock') placement is planned dissection is at 90° or horizontally.

- **U position.** Once the protective cover has been removed from the tip, the introducer is then held using a needle holder making sure the inserter is in line with the handle of the instrument. The tip of the introducer is then carefully placed within the paraurethrally dissected tunnel using the index finger on the finger pad. The inserter should then be pushed at 45° towards the ipsilateral shoulder using gentle pressure. When contact is made with the posterior surface of the pubic bone, the pad is held carefully in place against the bone while the needle holder is released leaving the inserter in position (Figure 60.10). The procedure is then repeated on the contralateral side.

- **Hammock position.** Once the protective cover has been removed from the tip, the introducer is then held using a needle holder making sure the inserter is in line with the handle of the instrument. The tip of the introducer is then carefully placed within the paraurethrally dissected tunnel using the index finger on the finger pad. The inserter tip should then be orientated at 45° from the midline towards the ischiopubic ramus, while holding the needle holder parallel to the floor. Once contact is made with the posterior surface of the pubic bone, the pad is held carefully in place against the bone while the needle holder is released leaving the inserter in position. The procedure is then repeated on the contralateral side.

After both inserters have been passed, final tape positioning may be performed by adjusting the depth of

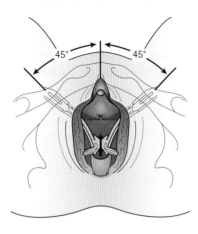

**Figure 60.10** TVT-Secur: U placement

insertion on each side. Care should be taken to ensure that the inserter tip remains in contact with the posterior surface of the pubic bone on each side and that the tape is flat and lies immediately beneath the urethra. Prior to removal of the inserters, cystourethroscopy should be performed to exclude injury to the bladder or urethra. Should a bladder perforation be noted, the inserter should be removed and replaced.

Once the tape is properly positioned, the first inserter is released by gently pulling on the release wire and then sliding the inserter out from the incision. Care should be taken not to dislodge the anchoring pad from the posterior surface of the pubic bone. The procedure should then be completed on the opposite side.

The vaginal incision is then closed using an absorbable suture. While an indwelling catheter is not required in all cases, a urethral catheter should be left on free drainage for 48 hours following a bladder injury.

### Outcome

The TVT-Secur was launched in 2006 and currently there are few long-term data supporting its use, although several short-term studies have been reported. A multicentre prospective trial has been reported from Italy in 95 women with primary stress incontinence who had a TVT-Secur. Follow up at one year reported a subjective and objective cure rate of 78 and 81 per cent, respectively, while 8 per cent of women complained of voiding difficulties. In addition, there were two cases of mesh erosion. These data are supported by a multicentre prospective observational study in France of 150 patients with one year follow up. Cure and improvement rates were 76.9 per cent in those women with pure stress incontinence, although this fell to 60 per cent in a smaller group with intrinsic sphincter deficiency.

The current evidence would appear to suggest that TVT-Secur efficacy rates may be slightly inferior to those of the retropubic mid-urethral tapes and current experience would suggest that the procedure is technically

different from a retropubic or obturator approach. Initial success rates have been disappointing in some series and the effect of the 'learning curve' has been clearly documented with objective success rates increasing from 76.2 to 94.7 per cent, depending on the experience of the operating surgeon.

From the clinical evidence available to date, it would appear that TVT-Secur offers an alternative, minimally invasive approach for the treatment of stress urinary incontinence, although more data are required to document the long-term efficacy and safety.

### KEY POINTS

- Conservative measures should be offered prior to surgical intervention.
- Duloxetine may be used in conjunction with conservative measures.
- Mid-urethral tape procedures have largely replaced colposuspension as the operation of choice in primary continence surgery.
- Laparoscopic colposuspension has a comparable outcome to open colposuspension and TVT.
- Retropubic mid-urethral tape procedures and retropubic procedures have similar success rates.
- Urethral bulking agents offer an alternative minimally invasive approach to continence surgery.

## NICE guidelines

The management of stress urinary incontinence has recently been reviewed by the National Institute for Health and Clinical Excellence (NICE). A trial of supervised pelvic floor muscle training of at least three months' duration should be offered as first-line treatment to all women with stress or mixed urinary incontinence.

Retropubic mid-urethral tape procedures using a 'bottom-up' approach with macroporous (type 1) polypropylene meshes are recommended as treatment options for stress urinary incontinence where conservative management has failed.

Open colposuspension and autologous rectus fascial sling procedures are recommended alternatives, where clinically appropriate.

Synthetic slings using materials other than polypropylene that are not of a macroporous (type 1) construction are not recommended for the treatment of stress urinary incontinence.

Intramural bulking agents (GAX collagen, Silcone, carbon-coated zirconium beads) should be considered for the management of stress urinary incontinence if conservative management has failed, although women should be made aware that repeat injections may be required, the efficacy diminishes with time and is inferior to that of a retropubic suspension or sling.

Laparoscopic colposuspension is not recommended as a routine procedure for the treatment of stress urinary incontinence in women and should only be performed by an experienced laparoscopic surgeon.

Anterior colporrhaphy, needle suspension procedures, paravaginal defect repair and the Marshall–Marchetti–Krantz procedure are not recommended.

## OVERACTIVE BLADDER

'Overactive bladder' (OAB) is the term used to describe the symptom complex of urgency with or without urge incontinence, usually with frequency and nocturia.[1]

The symptoms of OAB are due to involuntary contractions of the detrusor muscle during the filling phase of the micturition cycle. These involuntary contractions are termed detrusor overactivity[1] and are mediated by acetylcholine-induced stimulation of bladder muscarinic receptors. It has been estimated that 64 per cent of patients with OAB have urodynamically proven detrusor overactivity and that 83 per cent of patients with detrusor overactivity have symptoms suggestive of OAB.[20]

## Detrusor overactivity

Detrusor overactivity is defined as 'a urodynamic observation characterized by involuntary detrusor contractions during the filling phase which may be spontaneous or provoked' (Figure 60.11). The detrusor is shown objectively to contract (either spontaneously or with provocation) during bladder filling, while the subject is attempting to inhibit micturition.[1] Detrusor overactivity is a urodynamic diagnosis and usually presents with symptoms of frequency, urgency, urge incontinence, nocturia, nocturnal enuresis and sometimes incontinence at orgasm.

### Prevalence

Epidemiological studies have reported the overall prevalence of OAB in women to be 16.9 per cent suggesting that there could be 17.5 million women in the United States who suffer from the condition. The prevalence increases with age, being 4.8 per cent in women under 25 years to 30.9 per cent in those over the age of 65 years. This is supported by recent prevalence data from Europe in which 16 776 interviews were conducted in a population-based survey.[21] The overall prevalence of overactive bladder in individuals 40 years and above was 16.6 per cent and increased with age. Frequency was the most commonly reported symptom (85 per cent), while 54 per cent complained of urgency and 36 per cent urge incontinence. When considering management, 60 per cent had consulted a physician, although only 27 per cent were currently receiving treatment.

More recently, a further population-based survey of lower urinary tract symptoms in Canada, Germany, Italy, Sweden and the United Kingdom has reported on 19 165 men and women over the age of 18 years.[22] Overall, 11.8 per cent were found to complain of symptoms suggestive of OAB and 64.3 per cent reported at least one urinary symptom. Nocturia was the most prevalent lower urinary tract symptom being reported by 48.6 per cent of men and 54.5 per cent of women.

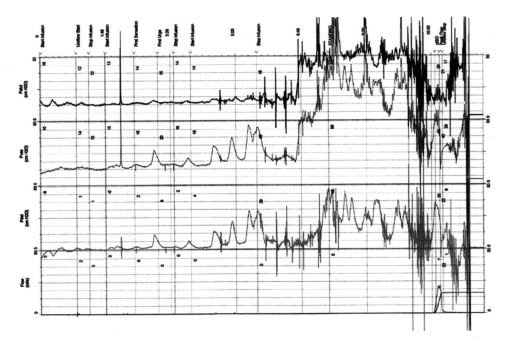

**Figure 60.11** Urodynamic trace showing detrusor overactivity

Pelvic floor and lower urinary tract dysfunction

## Muscarinic receptors

Molecular cloning studies have revealed five distinct genes for muscarinic acetylcholine receptors in rats and humans and it has been shown that there are five receptor subtypes ($M_1$–$M_5$). In the human bladder, there are $M_2$ and $M_3$ receptors and the latter is thought to cause a direct smooth muscle contraction. While the role of the $M_2$ receptor has not yet been clarified, it may oppose sympathetically mediated smooth muscle relaxation. In general, it is thought that the $M_3$ receptor is responsible for the normal micturition contraction, although in certain disease states, such as neurogenic bladder dysfunction, the $M_2$ receptors may become more important in mediating detrusor contractions.

### Pathophysiology

The pathophysiology of detrusor overactivity remains elusive. *In-vitro* studies have shown that the detrusor muscle in cases of idiopathic detrusor overactivity contracts more than normal detrusor muscle. These detrusor contractions are not nerve mediated and can be inhibited by the neuropeptide vasoactive intestinal polypeptide. Other studies have shown that increased α-adrenergic activity causes increased detrusor contractility. There is evidence to suggest that the pathophysiology of idiopathic and obstructive detrusor overactivity is different. From animal and human studies on obstructive overactivity, it would seem that the detrusor develops post-junctional supersensitivity possibly due to partial denervation, with reduced sensitivity to electrical stimulation of its nerve supply, but a greater sensitivity to stimulation with acetylcholine. If outflow obstruction is relieved, the detrusor can return to normal behaviour and reinnervation may occur.

Relaxation of the urethra is known to precede contraction of the detrusor in a proportion of women with detrusor overactivity. This may represent primary pathology in the urethra which triggers a detrusor contraction, or may merely be part of a complex sequence of events which originate elsewhere. It has been postulated that incompetence of the bladder neck, allowing passage of urine into the proximal urethra, may result in an uninhibited contraction of the detrusor. However, one study was unable to report a detrusor contraction provoked in 50 women by rapidly infusing saline into the posterior urethra using modified urodynamic equipment.

More recently, another study has suggested that the common feature in all cases of detrusor overactivity is a change in the properties of the smooth muscle of the detrusor which predisposes it to overactive contractions. They hypothesize that partial denervation of the detrusor may be responsible for altering the properties of the smooth muscle leading to increased excitability and increased ability of activity to spread between cells, resulting in coordinated myogenic contractions of the whole detrusor. They dispute the concept of neurogenic detrusor overactivity, that is, increased motor activity to the detrusor, as the underlying mechanism in detrusor overactivity proposing that there is a fundamental abnormality at the level of the bladder wall with evidence of altered spontaneous contractile activity consistent with increased electrical coupling of cells, a patchy denervation of the detrusor and a supersensitivity to potassium. Other authorities suggest that the primary defect in idiopathic and neurogenic bladders is a loss of nerves accompanied by hypertrophy of the cells and an increased production of elastin and collagen within the muscle fascicles.

## MANAGEMENT OF DETRUSOR OVERACTIVITY

The treatment options for detrusor overactivity can be divided into conservative, pharmacological, neuromodulation and surgical options.

## Conservative management

Conservative measures include advice regarding fluid intake. It may be that simply cutting down on the volume of fluid consumed throughout the day or altering the times at which drinks are taken will be enough to reduce the symptoms and improve quality of life. Women should be advised to consume between 1 and 1.5 litres in any 24-hour period. It is not advisable to restrict fluid intake severely, as a low urine output together with frequent voiding can lead to a reduction in the bladder's functional capacity. The best guide to ideal fluid intake is the colour of the urine. Caffeine and alcohol are well known to irritate the bladder, and women should be advised to try to avoid caffeine-based drinks or substitute them with decaffeinated drinks.

### Bladder retraining

The principles of bladder retraining are based on the ability to suppress urinary urge and to extend the intervals between voiding. The regimen is generally initiated at set voiding intervals and the patient is not allowed to void between these predetermined times, even if she is incontinent. When she remains dry, the time interval is lengthened. This continues until a suitable time span is achieved, usually around 3–4 hours. Cure rates using bladder retraining alone and no pharmacological agents have been reported between 44 and 90 per cent. Many professionals advise the combined use of pelvic floor exercises with bladder retraining, as this can help suppress the symptom of urinary urgency.

# Pharmacology

Drug therapy has an important role in the management of women with urinary symptoms caused by overactive bladder, although there are none which specifically act on the bladder and urethra which do not have systemic effects. The large number of drugs available is indicative of the fact that none is ideal and it is often their systemic adverse effects which limit their use in terms of efficacy and compliance. The pharmacology of drugs and recommendations for usage has recently been reviewed by the Fourth International Consultation on Incontinence (ICI) (Table 60.3).[23]

## Antimuscarinic drugs

The detrusor is innervated by the parasympathetic nervous system (pelvic nerve), the sympathetic nervous system (hypogastric nerve) and by non-cholinergic, non-adrenergic neurones. The motor supply arises from S2, 3 and 4 and is conveyed by the pelvic nerve. The neurotransmitter at the neuromuscular junction is acetylcholine, which acts upon muscarinic receptors. Antimuscarinic drugs should therefore be of use in the treatment of detrusor overactivity. Atropine is the classic non-selective anticholinergic drug with antimuscarinic activity; however, its non-specific mode of action makes it unacceptable for clinical use because of the high incidence of side effects. All antimuscarinic agents produce competitive blockade of acetylcholine receptors at postganglionic parasympathetic receptor sites. They all, to a lesser or greater extent, have the typical side effects of dry mouth, blurred vision, tachycardia, drowsiness and constipation. Unfortunately, virtually all the drugs which are truly beneficial in the management of overactive bladder produce these unwanted systemic side effects.

### Tolterodine

Tolterodine is a competitive muscarinic receptor antagonist with relative functional selectivity for bladder muscarinic receptors. While it shows no specificity for receptor subtypes, it does target the bladder muscarinic receptors rather than those in the salivary glands. Several randomized, double-blind, placebo-controlled trials have demonstrated a significant reduction in incontinent episodes and micturition frequency, while the incidence of adverse effects has been shown to be no different to placebo. When compared to oxybutynin in a randomized, double-blind, placebo-controlled parallel group study, it was found to be equally efficacious and to have a lower incidence of side effects, notably dry mouth.

Tolterodine has also been developed as an extended-release (ER) once daily preparation. A double blind multi-centre trial of 1235 women has compared extended-release tolterodine to immediate-release tolterodine and placebo. While both formulations were found to reduce the mean

**Table 60.3** Drugs used in the treatment of overactive bladder[23]

| | Level of evidence | Grade of recommendation |
|---|---|---|
| **Antimuscarinic drugs** | | |
| Tolterodine | 1 | A |
| Trospium | 1 | A |
| Solifenacin | 1 | A |
| Darifenacin | 1 | A |
| Fesoterodine | 1 | A |
| Propantheline | 2 | B |
| Atropine, hyoscamine | 3 | C |
| **Drugs acting on membrane channels** | | |
| Calcium channel antagonists | 2 | D |
| Potassium channel openers | 2 | D |
| **Drugs with mixed actions** | | |
| Oxybutynin | 1 | A |
| Propiverine | 1 | A |
| Flavoxate | 2 | D |
| **Alpha-antagonists** | | |
| Alfuzosin | 3 | C |
| Doxazosin | 3 | C |
| Prazosin | 3 | C |
| Terazosin | 3 | C |
| Tamsulosin | 3 | C |
| **Beta agonists** | | |
| Terbutaline | 3 | C |
| Salbutamol | 3 | C |
| Antidepressants | 3 | C |
| Imipramine | 3 | C |
| Duloxetine | 2 | C |
| **Prostaglandin synthesis inhibitors** | | |
| Indomethacin | 2 | C |
| Flurbiprofen | 2 | C |
| **Vasopressin analogues** | | |
| Desmopressin | 1 | A |
| **Other drugs** | | |
| Baclofen | 3 | C (Intrathecal) |
| Capsaicin | 2 | C (Intravesical) |
| Resiniferatoxin | 2 | C (Intravesical) |
| Botulinum Toxin (idiopathic) | 3 | B (Intravesical) |
| Botulinum Toxin (neurogenic) | 2 | A (Intravesical) |

Pelvic floor and lower urinary tract dysfunction

number of urge incontinence episodes per week, the extended-release preparation was found to be significantly more effective.

Extended-release oxybutynin and extended-release tolterodine have also been compared. In the OPERA (overactive bladder: performance of extended release agents) study, which involved 71 centres in the United States, improvements in episodes of urge incontinence were similar for the two drugs, although oxybutynin ER was significantly more effective than tolterodine ER in reducing frequency of micturition.[24]

In summary, the available evidence would suggest that tolterodine is as effective as oxybutynin, although since it has fewer adverse effects, patient tolerability and compliance are improved.

## Trospium chloride

Trospium chloride is a quaternary ammonium compound which is non-selective for muscarinic receptor subtypes and shows low biological availability. It crosses the blood–brain barrier to a limited extent and hence would appear to have few cognitive effects.[25] A placebo-controlled, randomized, double-blind multicentre trial has shown trospium to increase cystometric capacity and bladder volume at first unstable contraction, leading to significant clinical improvement without an increase in adverse effects over placebo. When compared to oxybutynin, it has been found to have comparable efficacy, although it was associated with a lower incidence of dry mouth and patient withdrawal. At present, trospium chloride would appear to be equally effective as oxybutynin, although it may be associated with fewer adverse effects.

## Solifenacin

Solifenacin is a potent $M_3$ receptor antagonist that has selectivity for the $M_3$ receptors over $M_2$ receptors and has much higher potency against $M_3$ receptors in smooth muscle than it does against $M_3$ receptors in salivary glands.

The clinical efficacy of solifenacin has been assessed in a multicentre, randomized, double-blind, parallel group, placebo-controlled study of solifenacin 5 mg and 10 mg once daily in patients with overactive bladder. The primary efficacy analysis showed a statistically significant reduction of the micturition frequency following treatment with both 5- and 10-mg doses when compared with placebo, although the largest effect was with the higher dose. The most frequently reported adverse events leading to discontinuation were dry mouth and constipation. These were also found to be dose related.

In order to assess the long-term safety and efficacy of solifenacin, a multicentre, open label, long-term follow-up study has been reported. This was essentially an extension of two previous double-blind, placebo-controlled studies in 1637 patients. Overall, the efficacy of solifenacin was maintained in the extension study with a sustained improvement in symptoms of urgency, urge incontinence, frequency

and nocturia over the 12-month study period. The most commonly reported adverse events were dry mouth (20.5 per cent), constipation (9.2 per cent) and blurred vision (6.6 per cent) and were the primary reason for discontinuation in 4.7 per cent of patients.

Solifenacin has also been compared with tolterodine ER in the solifenacin (flexible dosing) once daily and tolterodine ER as an active comparator in a randomized trial (STAR).[26] This was a prospective double-blind, double-dummy, two-arm, parallel-group, 12-week study of 1200 patients with the primary aim of demonstrating non-inferiority of solifenacin to tolterodine ER. Solifenacin was non-inferior to tolterodine ER with respect to change from baseline in the mean number of micturitions per 24 hours. In addition, solifenacin resulted in a statistically significant improvement in urgency, urge incontinence and overall incontinence when compared with tolterodine ER. The most commonly reported adverse events were dry mouth, constipation and blurred vision, and were mostly mild to moderate in severity. The number of patients discontinuing medication was similar in both treatment arms (3.5 per cent in the solifenacin arm versus 3.0 per cent in the tolterodine arm).

## Darifenacin

Darifenacin is a tertiary amine with moderate lipophilicity and is a highly selective $M_3$ receptor antagonist which has been found to have a five-fold higher affinity for the human $M_3$ receptor relative to the $M_1$ receptor.

A review of the pooled darifenacin data from the three phase III, multicentre, double-blind clinical trials in patients with overactive bladder has been reported in 1059 patients. Darifenacin resulted in a dose-related significant reduction in median number of incontinence episodes per week. Significant decreases in the frequency and severity of urgency, micturition frequency and number of incontinence episodes resulting in a change of clothing or pads were also apparent, along with an increase in bladder capacity. Darifenacin was well tolerated. The most common treatment-related adverse events were dry mouth and constipation, although together these resulted in few discontinuations. The incidence of central nervous system (CNS) and cardiovascular adverse events were comparable to placebo.

## Fesoterodine

Fesoterodine is a new and novel derivative of 3,3-diphenyl-propyl-amine which is a potent antimuscarinic agent that has recently been developed for the management of OAB. A phase II, dose-finding study was conducted in 728 patients in Europe and South Africa. Fesoterodine 4, 8 and 12 mg were all found to show significantly greater decreases in micturition frequency than placebo. The most commonly reported side effect was dry mouth with an incidence of 25 per cent in the 4-mg group rising to 34 per cent in the 12-mg group. Discontinuation rates were 6 and 12 per cent, respectively. Subsequently, a phase III, randomized, placebo-controlled trial has been reported comparing fesoterodine 4 and 8 mg with tolterodine ER 4 mg in patients complaining of OAB in 1135 patients at 150 sites throughout Australia, New Zealand, South Africa and Europe.[27] Both doses of fesoterodine demonstrated significant improvements over placebo in reduction of daytime frequency and number of urge incontinence episodes per day and were found to be superior to tolterodine. The current evidence would suggest that fesoterodine may offer some advantages over tolterodine in terms of efficacy and flexible dosing regimens.

## Drugs that have a mixed action

### Oxybutynin

Oxybutynin is a tertiary amine that undergoes extensive first-pass metabolism to an active metabolite, N-desmethyl oxybutynin which occurs in high concentrations and is thought to be responsible for a significant part of the action of the parent drug. It has a mixed action consisting of both an antimuscarinic and a direct muscle relaxant effect in addition to local anaesthetic properties. Oxybutynin has been shown to have a high affinity for muscarinic receptors in the bladder and has a higher affinity for $M_1$ and $M_3$ receptors over $M_2$.

The effectiveness of oxybutynin in the management of patients with detrusor overactivity is well documented. A double-blind, placebo-controlled trial found oxybutynin to be significantly better than placebo in improving lower urinary tract symptoms, although 80 per cent of patients complained of significant adverse effects, principally dry mouth or dry skin.

The antimuscarinic adverse effects of oxybutynin are well documented and are often dose limiting, with 10–23 per cent of women discontinuing medication. Using an intravesical route of administration, higher local levels of oxybutynin can be achieved while limiting the systemic adverse effects. Intravesical administration of oxybutynin is an effective and useful alternative for patients with neurogenic detrusor overactivity who need to self-catheterize or who suffer from 'bypassing' an indwelling catheter.

In order to improve tolerability, a controlled release oxybutynin preparation using an osmotic system (OROS) has been developed which has been shown to have comparable efficacy when compared with immediate-release oxybutynin, although are associated with fewer adverse effects. In order to maximize efficacy and minimize adverse effects, alternative delivery systems are currently under evaluation. An oxybutynin transdermal delivery system has recently been developed and compared with extended-release tolterodine in 361 patients with mixed urinary incontinence. Both agents significantly reduced incontinence episodes, increased volume voided and lead to an improvement in quality of life when compared to placebo. The most common adverse event in the oxybutynin patch arm was application site pruritis in 14 per cent, although the incidence of dry mouth

was reduced to 4.1 per cent compared to 7.3 per cent in the tolterodine arm.

More recently, a large prospective multicentre, randomized, double-blind placebo-controlled study has been reported investigating the use of oxybutynin gel in the management of overactive bladder in 704 patients.[28] Overall, there was a significant reduction in urge incontinence episodes in the gel arm compared to placebo, a significant reduction in daytime frequency and increase in volume voided. When considering adverse events, dry mouth was more common in the treatment arm when compared to placebo (6.9 versus 2.8 per cent) and skin site reactions were infrequent in both arms – 5.4 and 1.0 per cent, respectively. Consequently, oxybutynin gel may represent an important development over the oxybutynin patch in terms of patient acceptability.

In summary, the efficacy of oxybutynin is well documented, although very often its clinical usefulness is limited by adverse effects. Alternative routes and methods of administration may produce better patient acceptability and compliance.

### Propiverine

Propiverine has both antimuscarinic and calcium channel-blocking actions. Open studies have demonstrated a beneficial effect in patients with overactive bladder and neurogenic detrusor overactivity. Dry mouth was experienced by 37 per cent in the treatment group as opposed to 8 per cent in those taking placebo, with dropout rates being 7 and 4.5 per cent, respectively. Overall propiverine was found to have comparable efficacy to oxybutynin, but was better tolerated in terms of adverse effects.

More recently, propiverine extended release has been introduced and been shown to be as effective as the immediate-release preparation in the management of overactive bladder.

## Tricyclic antidepressants

These drugs have a complex pharmacological action. Imipramine has antimuscarinic, antihistamine and local anaesthetic properties. It may increase outlet resistance by peripheral blockage of noradrenaline uptake and it also acts as a sedative. The side effects are antimuscarinic, together with tremor and fatigue. Imipramine is particularly useful for the treatment of nocturia and nocturnal enuresis. In light of relatively poor evidence and the serious adverse effects associated with tricyclic antidepressants, their role in detrusor overactivity remains of uncertain benefit, although they are often useful in patients complaining of nocturia or bladder pain.

## Anti-diuretic agents

### Desmopressin

Desmopressin (1-desamino-8-D-arginine vasopressin; synthetic vasopressin (DDAVP)) has been shown to reduce

*Pelvic floor and lower urinary tract dysfunction*

nocturnal urine production by up to 50 per cent. It can be used for children or adults with nocturia or nocturnal enuresis, but must be avoided in patients with hypertension, ischaemic heart disease or congestive cardiac failure. There is good evidence to show that it is safe to use in the long term and it may be given orally or as buccal preparation. Desmopressin has also been used as a 'designer drug' for daytime incontinence and also in the treatment of overactive bladder.

Desmopressin is safe for long-term use; however, the drug should be used with care in the elderly due to the risk of hyponatraemia and the current recommendations are that serum sodium should be checked in the first week following the start of treatment.

## Oestrogens in the management of overactive bladder

Oestrogens have been used in the treatment of urinary urgency and urge incontinence for many years, although there have been few controlled trials to confirm their efficacy.

To try and clarify the role of oestrogen therapy in the management of women with urge incontinence, a meta-analysis of the use of oestrogen in women with symptoms of 'overactive bladder' has been reported by the HUT (hormones and uorgenital therapy) Committee. In a review of ten randomized, placebo-controlled trials, oestrogen was found to be superior to placebo when considering symptoms of urge incontinence, frequency and nocturia, although vaginal oestrogen administration was found to be superior for symptoms of urgency. In those taking oestrogens, there was also a significant increase in first sensation and bladder capacity as compared to placebo.

## Intravesical therapy

### Capsaicin

This is the pungent ingredient found in red chillies and is a neurotoxin of substance P-containing (C) nerve fibres. Patients with neurogenic detrusor overactivity secondary to multiple sclerosis appear to have abnormal C fibre sensory innervation of the detrusor, which leads to premature activation of the holding reflex arc during bladder filling. Intravesical application of capsaicin dissolved in 30 per cent alcohol solution can be effective for up to six months. The effects are variable and the long-term safety of this treatment has not yet been evaluated.

### Resiniferatoxin

This is a phorbol-related diterpene isolated from the cactus and is a potent analogue of capsaicin that appears to have similar efficacy, but with fewer side effects of pain and burning during intravesical instillation. It is 1000 times more potent than capsaicin at stimulating bladder activity. As with capsaicin, the currently available evidence does not support the routine clinical use of the agents, although they may prove to have a role as an intravesical preparation in neurological patients with neurogenic detrusor overactivity.

### Botulinum toxin

In 1817, an illness caused by *Clostridium botulinum* toxin was first recorded, when Justinus Kerner described a link between a sausage and a paralytic illness that affected 230 people. He was a district health officer and made botulism (Latin *botulus* meaning sausage) a notifiable disease. In 1897, the microbiologist Emile-Pierre van Ermengen identified a Gram-positive, spore-forming, anaerobic bacterium in a ham that caused 23 cases of botulism in a Belgian nightclub. He termed the bacterium *Bacillus botulinus*; it was later re-termed *Clostridium botulinum*.

The bacterium produces its effect by production of a neurotoxin – different strains produce seven distinct serotypes, designated A–G. They interfere with neural transmission by blocking the calcium-dependent release of neurotransmitter, acetylcholine, causing the affected muscle to become weak and atrophic. The affected nerves do not degenerate, but as the blockage is irreversible, only the development of new nerve terminals and synaptic contacts allows recovery of function.

The use of intravesical botulinum toxin was first described in the treatment of intractable neurogenic detrusor overactivity in 31 patients with traumatic spinal cord injury. Subsequently, a larger European study has reported on 231 patients with neurogenic detrusor overactivity. All were treated with 300 units of botulinum-A toxin which was injected cystoscopically into the detrusor muscle at 30 different sites sparing the trigone. At 12- and 36-week follow up, there was a significant increase in cystometric capacity and bladder compliance. Patient satisfaction was high, the majority stopped taking antimuscarinic medication and there were no significant complications. More recently, the first randomized placebo-controlled trial has been reported in 59 patients with neurogenic detrusor overactivity.[29] At six months, there was a significant reduction in incontinence episodes in the botox group compared to placebo and a corresponding improvement in quality of life evaluation.

While the role of botulinum toxin has been established in the treatment of neurogenic detrusor overactivity, the data regarding its use in intractable idiopathic detrusor overactivity is less robust. A prospective, open label study has recently been reported assessing the use of botulinum-A toxin in both neurogenic (300 units) and idiopathic (200 units) detrusor overactivity in 75 patients. When considering urodynamic outcome parameters in both groups, there was a significant increase in cystometric capacity and decrease in maximum detrusor pressure during filling in both groups. Clinically, there was also a significant reduction in frequency and episodes of urge incontinence. Interestingly, however, 69 per cent of patients with neurogenic detrusor overactivity required self-catheterization following treatment compared to 19.3 per cent of those with idiopathic detrusor overactivity.

At present, the evidence would suggest that intravesical administration of botulinum toxin may offer an alternative to surgery in those women with intractable detrusor overactivity, although the effect is only temporary and there are few long-term data regarding the efficacy and complications associated with repeat injections.

## Neuromodulation

### Sacral neuromodulation

Stimulation of the dorsal sacral nerve root using a permanent implantable device in the S3 sacral foramen has been developed for use in patients with overactive bladder and neurogenic detrusor overactivity. The sacral nerves contain nerve fibres of the parasympathetic and sympathetic system providing innervation to the bladder, as well as somatic fibres providing innervation to the muscles of the pelvic floor. The latter are larger in diameter and hence have a lower threshold of activation, meaning that the pelvic floor may be stimulated selectively without causing bladder activity.

Before implantation, temporary cutaneous sacral nerve stimulation is performed to check for a response and, if successful, a permanent implant is inserted under general anaesthesia. Initial studies in patients with overactive bladder refractory to medical and behavioural therapy have demonstrated that after three years, 59 per cent of 41 urinary urge incontinent patients showed greater than 50 per cent reduction in incontinence episodes, with 46 per cent of patients being completely dry.

While neuromodulation remains an invasive and expensive procedure, it does offer a useful alternative to medical and surgical therapies in patients with severe, intractable overactive bladder prior to considering reconstructive surgery, although technical failure may often necessitate surgical revisions.

### Peripheral neuromodulation

Stimulation of the posterior tibial nerve in patients with urge incontinence was first reported in 1983 and has also been proposed for pelvic floor dysfunction. The tibial nerve is a mixed nerve containing L4-S3 fibres and originates from the same spinal cord segments as the innervation to the bladder and pelvic floor. Consequently, peripheral neural modulation may have a role in the management of urinary symptoms.

In a prospective multicentre study, 35 patients with urge incontinence underwent 12 weekly sessions of posterior tibial nerve stimulation (PTNS) with 70 per cent of patients reporting a greater than 50 per cent reduction in urinary symptoms and 46 per cent being completely cured. More recently, a prospective randomized multicentre North American study has been reported comparing

PTNS with tolterodine 4 mg ER in 100 patients. Overall, there was an improvement in 75 per cent of patients with PTNS compared to 55.8 per cent with tolterodine ER and there was a significant improvement in quality of life in both groups.

Consequently, peripheral neuromodulation may offer an alternative therapeutic option for those patients with intractable overactive bladder who have failed to respond to medical therapy.

## Surgery

Approximately 10 per cent of women with overactive bladder remain refractory to medical and behavioural therapy and may be considered for surgery. Various different surgical techniques have been developed, although currently augmentation is the most commonly performed technique using a clam cystoplasty or auto-augmentation using detrusor myectomy.

### Clam cystoplasty

In clam cystoplasty, the bladder is bisected almost completely and a patch of gut (usually ileum) equal in length to the circumference of the bisected bladder (about 25 cm) is sewn in place. This often cures the symptoms of overactive bladder by converting a high-pressure system into a low-pressure system, although inefficient voiding may result. Patients have to learn to strain to void or may have to resort to clean intermittent self-catheterization, sometimes permanently. In addition, mucus retention in the bladder may be a problem and chronic exposure of the ileal mucosa to urine may lead to malignant change.

### Detrusor myectomy

Detrusor myectomy offers an alternative to clam cystoplasty by increasing functional bladder capacity without the complications of bowel interposition. In this procedure, the whole thickness of the detrusor muscle is excised from the dome of the bladder, thereby creating a large bladder diverticulum with no intrinsic contractility. While there is a reduction in episodes of incontinence, there is little improvement in functional capacity and thus frequency remains problematic.

### Urinary diversion

As a last resort, for those women with severe overactive bladder or neurogenic detrusor overactivity who cannot manage clean intermittent catheterization, it may be more appropriate to perform a urinary diversion. Usually this will utilize an ileal conduit to create an incontinent abdominal stoma for urinary diversion. An alternative is to form a continent diversion using the appendix (Mitrofanoff) or ileum (Koch pouch) which may then be drained using self-catheterization.

Pelvic floor and lower urinary tract dysfunction

## KEY POINTS

- Bladder retraining should be considered as first-line therapy, although it has high recurrence rates.
- There is a marked placebo effect associated with all pharmacological interventions.
- Oxybutinin is effective, although it may have significant adverse side effects.
- More specific antimuscarinic agents may have similar efficacy to oxybutynin, but with fewer side effects.
- Oestrogens are frequently prescribed, although there is little objective evidence to support their use.
- Botulinum toxin may offer a useful therapeutic option in patients with intractable detrusor overactivity.
- Neuromodulation may be an alternative to reconstructive surgery.
- Surgical interventions, such as diversion, are reserved for cases for which no other treatment has succeeded and quality of life is poor.

## NICE guidelines

The medical management of OAB has recently been reviewed by the National Institute for Health and Clinical Excellence. In the first instance, bladder retraining lasting for a minimum of 6 weeks should be offered to all women with mixed or urge incontinence. In those women who do not achieve satisfactory benefit from bladder retraining alone, the combination of an antimuscarinic agent, in addition to bladder retraining should be considered.

When considering drug therapy, immediate-release non-propriety oxybutynin should be offered to women with OAB or mixed urinary incontinence as first-line drug treatment if bladder retraining has been ineffective. If immediate-release oxybutynin is not well tolerated darifenacin, solifenacin, tolterodine, trospium or an extended-release or transdermal formulation of oxybutynin should be considered as alternatives. In addition, women should be counselled regarding the adverse effects of antimuscarinic drugs.

Propiverine should be considered as an option to treat frequency of micturition, but is not recommended for the treatment of urinary incontinence. Flavoxate, propantheline and imipramine should not be used for the treatment of OAB. While desmopressin may be considered specifically to reduce nocturia in women, this is currently outside the marketing authorization and hence informed consent must be obtained.

When considering the role of oestrogens, the recommendations are that systemic hormone replacement therapy should not be recommended, although intravaginal oestrogens are recommended for the treatment of OAB in postmenopausal women with urogenital atrophy.

# URINARY FISTULAE

The development of a genitourinary fistula has profound effects on both the physical and psychological health of the woman. The most common simple genitourinary fistulae are (Figure 60.12):

- vesicovaginal (42 per cent)
- ureterovaginal (34 per cent)
- urethrovaginal (11 per cent)
- vesicocervical (3 per cent).

The development of a fistula following surgery has considerable legal implications. While most gynaecologists accept that the development of a fistula is deeply regrettable, it was generally thought that this was, on occasion, unavoidable. However, more recent legal cases involving ureteric injury would seem to refute that. There is a body of opinion that holds the view that ureteric damage can always be avoided and that not to do so constitutes negligence.

## Vesicovaginal fistulae

### Aetiology

The most common cause of vesicovaginal fistulae in the developed world is gynaecological surgery. The procedure with the highest incidence of post-operative fistula formation is a hysterectomy, either abdominal or vaginal. This accounts for about 75 per cent of cases. Particular risk factors include distorted anatomy, for example previous surgery, fibroids or endometriosis. Other procedures associated with fistula formation include anterior colporrhaphy, laparoscopic pelvic surgery and urological surgery. Fistula formation has also been associated with pelvic malignancy, pelvic trauma and radiotherapy.

In the developing world, the most common cause remains obstetric trauma. It is estimated that the incidence is 1–3/1000 deliveries in West Africa.

### Presentation

The majority of women with a vesicovaginal fistula present with continuous leakage of urine, both day and night. This leads to discomfort and excoriation in the genital region as the urine irritates the skin of the vulva and thighs. However, if the fistula is relatively small, a woman may just complain of increased vaginal discharge. The timing of presentation is variable, although the most common time to present is 5–10 days following surgery.

### Diagnosis

A large fistula is usually obvious and may easily be seen by examining the woman in the left lateral position using a Simms' speculum. Urine may be seen pooling in the vagina.

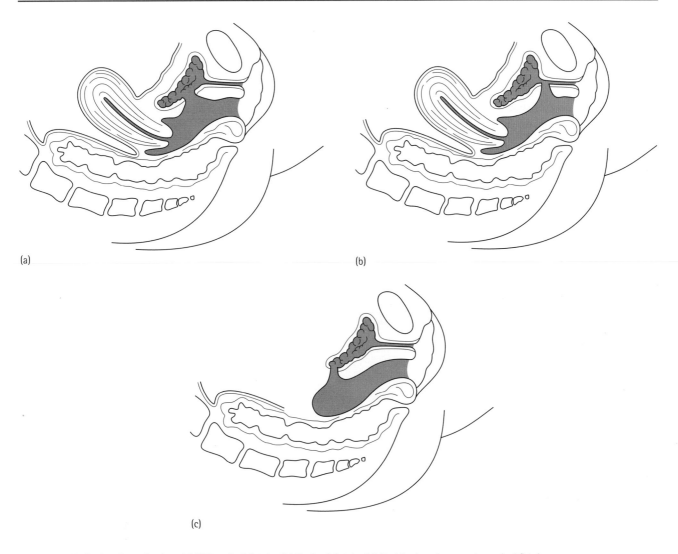

**Figure 60.12** Genitourinary fistulae. (a) Mid-vaginal fistula. (b) Urethral fistula. (c) Post-hysterectomy vesicovaginal fistula

If no fistula can be seen, useful diagnostic tests include the introduction of methylene blue into the bladder, via a urethral catheter. The blue dye may then be seen draining into the vagina. Alternatively, Bonney's 'three swab test', in which three swabs are placed in the vagina prior to instilling the dye, may help to locate the site of the fistula, which is indicated by the swab that emerges with the most dye. However, this may mask the presence of multiple fistulae. Intravenous urogram (IVU) is not usually helpful in the diagnosis of a vesicovaginal fistula, but it is mandatory to rule out a ureterovaginal fistula or ureteric obstruction, which is seen concurrently in as many as 12 per cent of cases and is obviously very important when planning future treatment. If an IVU has failed to elucidate the ureteric anatomy, retrograde ureteropyelography should be undertaken at the same time as a cystoscopy and examination under general anaesthesia.

When the woman is anaesthetized, it is often possible to palpate the vaginal opening of the fistula tract. The vesical opening may be seen at cystoscopy, usually on the posterior wall or at the bladder base. If the fistula is not related to recent gynaecological surgery for a benign condition, both the vaginal and the vesical openings should be biopsied to exclude the possibility of malignancy.

### Treatment

Treatment options range from simple conservative measures to more complex surgical procedures using either an abdominal or vaginal approach. In addition, it is important to give general advice regarding the management of symptoms experienced as a result of the fistula. Barrier creams may help prevent the skin becoming sore and excoriated. Advice about incontinence pads, the increased risk of urinary tract infection and the need in some cases for prophylactic antibiotics may be required.

### Urethrovaginal fistulae

In the developed world, these occur most commonly following an anterior repair with or without a vaginal hysterectomy. However, they may develop as a result of a urethral diverticulum or its repair or following bladder neck suspension procedures. In the developing world, the overwhelming majority are again caused by childbirth.

Symptoms vary depending on the site of the fistula. With a fistula higher up in the urethra, there may be continuous incontinence; a fistula nearer the bladder neck may present with stress incontinence and recurrent urinary tract infections; and one lower down may cause symptoms of spraying of urine at micturition or post-micturition dribble.

Women should initially be managed using a conservative approach with a urethral catheter, although almost all patients will need surgical repair. Due to the complex nature of such procedures, this should be performed in a specialist centre.

## KEY POINTS

- In the developed world, gynaecological surgery is the most common cause, with 75 per cent being attributable to hysterectomy.
- Obstetric trauma is the most common cause in the developing world.
- Most present between 5 and 10 days after surgery.
- Presentation varies from a mild discharge with small fistulae to continuous urine loss with larger fistulae.
- IVU is mandatory as part of the assessment because of high ureteric co-morbidity.

# OVERFLOW INCONTINENCE AND VOIDING DYSFUNCTION

## Symptoms

These may be a result of the voiding difficulty, such as:

- poor stream
- prolonged voiding time
- double void
- incomplete emptying
- hesitancy
- frequency
- nocturia
- urgency
- pain
- abdominal distension

or may reflect the underlying disease:

- abdominal distension, due to a mass such as fibroids or an ovarian cyst
- pregnancy

- peri-anal pain
- peripheral paraesthesia
- herpetic rash

or a consequence of the voiding difficulties:

- recurrent urinary tract infections.

## Aetiology

### Neurological

The aetiology depends on the underlying neurological condition and the level at which the anatomy is affected. Central nervous system conditions that commonly cause voiding difficulties include multiple sclerosis, spinal injuries, cerebrovascular accidents and brain tumours. Peripheral lesions include lesions at the sacral outflow, for instance a prolapsed intervertebral disc, cauda equina syndrome or herpes zoster.

### Myogenic

This usually results from ischaemia due to acute retention, for example after an epidural block or spinal shock.

### Iatrogenic

Post-operative retention is relatively common and may be associated with long operation times, epidural anaesthesia, patient-controlled analgesia, high doses of opiates and large volumes of intravenous fluids. It may also be associated with obstructive outflow procedures, such as continence procedures.

### Obstructive

This may be extrinsic, for example pregnancy or a large fibroid uterus, or intrinsic, such as a urethral stricture or foreign body. Alternatively, it may be as a result of kinking of the urethra, as can occur with a large prolapse.

### Inflammatory

Any lesion may be sufficiently painful to inhibit the voiding reflex. This is seen, for instance, with vulval abscess or acute herpetic infections.

## Diagnosis

Voiding difficulties should be suspected if a pelvic mass that is dull to percussion is palpable on clinical examination. The diagnosis can be confirmed using ultrasound. The patient is asked to empty her bladder and then an abdominal ultrasound scan can easily be performed to assess the residual urine. Alternatively, a urethral catheter can be inserted to assess the residual urine. In either case, it is very important that the residual volume is measured and accurately recorded.

## MANAGEMENT

It is vital that all clinicians are aware of the complications associated with an episode of acute retention and that all possible steps are taken to avoid it happening. If it does occur, catheterization should be undertaken as soon as possible and the catheter should be left in for at least 2 days, after which it is reasonable to undertake a trial without catheter, but only under strict supervision. If there is a further episode of retention, this should be managed with a suprapubic catheter and the bladder allowed to rest for a period of 2–6 weeks.

### Medical therapy

Bethanechol, 25 mg three times a day, has been shown to enhance bladder emptying, providing there is no evidence of outflow obstruction, although is seldom useful clinically.

### Surgery

If the voiding difficulties are a result of extrinsic compression, this is usually best treated by removing the underlying cause, for example a hysterectomy or myomectomy in the case of fibroids. However, in the case of pregnancy causing obstruction, supportive measures are usually used in the form of a urethral catheter until the uterus has grown a little more and the obstruction relieves itself.

If the obstruction is intrinsic, this may be treated by the removal of a foreign body or offending material. Alternatively, if a urethral stricture is suspected, a cystoscopy and an Otis urethrotomy may be required, in which case the patient would need to be counselled about having a urethral catheter on free drainage for 2 weeks on discharge from hospital and the possibility of post-operative urinary incontinence.

In the long term, intractable voiding difficulties may need to be treated with clean intermittent self-catheterization. The patient needs to be able to perform the technique and this usually requires a degree of manual dexterity, in addition to willingness to undertake it.

## CONCLUSIONS

Urinary incontinence is common and, while not life threatening, is known to have a significant effect on quality of life. Appropriate investigation and management allows an accurate diagnosis and avoids inappropriate treatment. While many forms of conservative therapy may be initiated in primary care continence surgery, the investigation of more complex and recurrent cases of incontinence,

should be performed in specialist secondary and tertiary referral units. Ultimately, an integrated pathway utilizing a multidisciplinary team approach, including specialist nurses, continence advisors, physiotherapists, urologists and colorectal surgeons, will ensure the best possible outcomes in terms of 'cure' and patient satisfaction.

## Key References

1. Abrams P, Cardozo L, Fall M et al. The standardisation of terminology of lower urinary tract function. Report from the standardisation committee of the International Continence Society. Neurourol Urodynam 2002; **21**: 167–78.
2. Hannestad YS, Rortveit G, Sandvik H, Hunskar S. A community-based epidemiological survey of female urinary incontinence: The Norwegian EPINCONT Study. J Clin Epidemiol 2000; **53**: 1150–7.
3. Rortveit G, Hannnestad YS, Daltveit AK, Hunskaar S. Age and type dependent effects of parity on urinary incontinence: The Norwegian EPINCONT study. Obstet Gynaecol 2001; **98**: 1004–10.
4. Stewart WF, Corey R, Herzog AR et al. Prevalence of overactive bladder in women: Results from the NOBLE program. Int Urogynaecol J 2001; **12**: S66.
5. Bump RC. Racial comparisons and contrasts in urinary incontinence and pelvic organ prolapse. Obstet Gynaecol 1993; **81**: 421.
6. Hojerberg KE, Salvig JD, Winslow NA et al. Urinary incontinence; prevalence and risk factors at 16 weeks of gestation. Br J Obstet Gynaecol 1999; **106**: 842.
7. Bo K. Pelvic floor muscle training is effective in treatment of female stress urinary incontinence, but how does it work? Int Urogynaecol J Pelvic Floor Dysfunct 2004; **15**: 76–84.
8. Bo K, Hagen RH, Kvarstein B et al. Pelvic floor muscle exercise for the treatment of female stress urinary incontinence. III: Effects of two different degrees of pelvic floor muscle exercise. Neurourol Urodyn 1990; **9**: 489–502.
9. Norton PA, Zinner NR, Yalcin I, Bump RC and the Duloxetine Urinary Incontinence Study Group. Duloxetine versus placebo in the treatment of stress urinary incontinence. Am J Obstet Gynaecol 2002; **187**: 40–8.
10. Cardozo L, Drutz HP, Baygani SK, Bump RC. Pharmacological treatment of women awaiting surgery for stress urinary incontinence. Obstet Gynaecol 2004; **104**: 511–19.
11. Ghoniem GM, Van Leeuwen JS, Elser DM et al. and the Duloxetine/Pelvic Floor Muscle Training Clinical Trial Group. A randomised controlled trial of duloxetine alone, pelvic floor muscle training alone, combined treatment and no active treatment in women with stress urinary incontinence. J Urol 2005; **173**: 1453–4.

12. Petros P, Ulmsten U. An integral theory of female urinary incontinence. Experimental and clinical considerations. *Acta Obstet Gynaecol Scand* 1990; **153** (Suppl.): 7–31.

13. Kitchener HC, Dunn G, Lawton V *et al.* on behalf of the COLPO study group. Laparoscopic versus open colposuspension – results of a prospective randomised controlled trial. *Br J Obstet Gynaecol* 2006; **113**: 1007–13.

14. Ulmsten U, Henriksson L, Johnson P, Varhos G. An ambulatory surgical procedure under local anesthetic for treatment of female urinary incontinence. *Int Urogynaecol J* 1996; **7**: 81–6.

15. Nilsson CG, Palva K, Rezapour M, Falconer C. Eleven years prospective follow up of the tension free vaginal tape procedure for the treatment of stress urinary incontinence. *Int Urogynaecol J Pelvic Floor Dysfunct* 2008; **19**: 1043–7.

16. Ward K, Hilton P, United Kingdom and Ireland Tension Free Vaginal Tape Trial Group. Prospective multicentre randomised trial of tension free vaginal tape and colposuspension as primary treatment for stress incontinence. *BMJ* 2002; **325**: 67.

17. Delorme E. [Transobturator urethral suspension: Mini-invasive procedure in the treatment of stress urinary incontinence in women.] *Prog Urol* 2001; **11**: 1306–13.

18. Costa P, Grise P, Droupy S *et al.* Surgical treatment of female stress urinary incontinence with a transobturator tape (TOT). Uratape: Short term results of a prospective multicentric study. *Eur Urol* 2004; **46**: 102–6.

19. Latthe PM, Foon R, Toozs-Hobson P. Transobturator and retropubic tape procedures in stress urinary incontinence: A systematic review and meta-analysis of effectiveness and complications. *Br J Obstet Gynaecol* 2007; **114**: 522–31.

20. Hashim H, Abrams P. Do symptoms of overactive bladder predict urodynamic detrusor overactivity? *Neurorol Urodyn* 2004; **23**: 484.

21. Milsom I, Abrams P, Cardozo L *et al.* How widespread are the symptoms of overactive bladder and how are they managed? A population-based prevalence study. *BJU Int* 2001; **87**: 760–6.

22. Irwin DE, Milsom I, Hunskaar S *et al.* Population-based survey of urinary incontinence, overactive bladder and other lower urinary tract symptoms in five countries; results of the EPIC study. *Eur Urol* 2006; **50**: 1306–15.

23. Andersson KE, Chapple CR, Cardozo L *et al.* Pharmacological treatment of urinary incontinence. In: Abrams P, Cardozo L, Khoury S, Wein A (eds). *Incontinence*, 4th edn. Paris: Health Publication Ltd, Editions 21, 2009: 631–700.

24. Diokno AC, Appell RA, Sand PK *et al.* and the OPERA Stuy Group. Prospective, randomised, double blind study of the efficacy and tolerability of the extended-release formulations of oxybutynin and tolterodine for overactive bladder: Results of the OPERA trial. *Mayo Clin Proc* 2003; **78**: 687–95.

25. Fusgen I, Hauri D. Trospium chloride: An effective option for medical treatment of bladder overactivity. *Int J Clin Pharmacol Ther* 2000; **38**: 223–34.

26. Chapple CR, Martinez-Garcia R, Selvaggi L *et al.* for the STAR study group. A comparison of the efficacy and tolerability of solifenacin succinate and extended release tolterodine at treating overactive bladder syndrome: Results of the STAR trial. *Eur Urol* 2005; **48**: 464–70.

27. Chapple CR, Van Kerrebroeck PE, Junemann KP *et al.* Comparison of fesoterodine and tolterodine in patients with overactive bladder. *BJU Int* 2008; **102**: 1128–32.

28. Staskin DR, Dmochowski RR, Sand PK *et al.* Efficacy and safety of oxybutynin chloride topical gel for overactive bladder: A randomised double-blind, placebo controlled, multicentre study. *J Urol* 2009; **181**: 1764–72.

29. Schurch B, de Seze M, Denys P *et al.* Botox Detrusor Hyperreflexia Study Team. Botulinum toxin type A is a safe and effective treatment for neurogenic urinary incontinence: Results of a single treatment, randomized, placebo controlled 6-month study. *J Urol* 2005; **174**: 196–200.

# Chapter 61

# Other lower urinary tract disorders

*Arasee Renganathan*

## INTRODUCTION

In the preceding chapters, the common urogynaecological disorders have been discussed together with the evidence-base that exists to guide clinicians in the management of these conditions. This chapter includes some less frequently seen disorders of the lower urinary tract. There is far less supporting evidence for the efficacy of different clinical interventions for these disorders, and the established management is based largely on non-randomized, observational data and expert opinion.

## BLADDER PAIN SYNDROME

Bladder pain syndrome (BPS) is defined as chronic pelvic pain, pressure or discomfort of greater than six months duration, perceived to be related to the urinary bladder. This is usually accompanied by at least one other urinary symptom, such as persistent urge to void or urinary frequency. BPS has a strong relationship to other pain syndromes, such as irritable bowel syndrome, fibromyalgia and chronic fatigue syndrome. Therefore, confusable diseases as the cause of the symptoms of BPS must be excluded. Based on this, a comprehensive article has been published by the European Society for the Study of Bladder Pain Syndrome/Interstitial Cystitis (ESSIC).[1] Other diseases that can cause similar symptoms must be excluded before the diagnosis is made. The presence of other cognitive, behavioural, emotional and sexual symptoms should also be addressed. The diagnosis may change after findings at cystoscopy or bladder biopsies. Historically, interstitial cystitis has been defined as a chronic severe inflammatory disease of the bladder that is difficult to diagnose and treat. It has been agreed by the members of the International Consultation on Incontinence that the term 'bladder pain syndrome' complies with the current knowledge and understanding of the pain syndrome.[2] However, BPS/IC is being used in parallel for the time being, until the term becomes better known.

### Incidence

The prevalence of chronic pain in the general population due to benign conditions is at least 10 per cent.[3] The lack of a clear definition and valid diagnostic criteria have been deterrents to epidemiological studies of BPS. There is also an overlap of lower urinary tract symptoms in conditions like overactive bladder and BPS[4] which makes it difficult to estimate the true incidence. The prevalence of painful bladder syndrome symptoms is 0.83–2.71 per cent in women depending on the definition used. Painful bladder symptoms are more common than suggested by coded physician diagnoses and show a female preponderance of 5:1 or more.[5]

The presence of BPS is associated with a significant adverse impact on quality of life. There is a higher incidence of comorbidities like anxiety, depression and overall mental health problems in BPS sufferers. Consequently, there is a six-fold increase in absenteeism due to sickness than the general population.[6]

## Aetiology

Due to the lack of consensus relating to the definition and classification of BPS, the aetiology still remains obscure. However, there are several hypotheses with little evidence to support them. Inflammation and mast cell activation have been put forward as factors in ulcerative BPS. A defect in the glycosaminoglycan (GAG) layer has been proposed by some[7] and bladder epithelial dysfunction by others.[8] Although certain histopathological characteristics present in BPS patients are similar to autoimmune diseases, only a portion of BPS patients have auto-antibodies. Infection, autonomic nerve changes, disorders of nitric oxide metabolism, toxic agents, hypoxia and genetic susceptibility are other factors that are considered as aetiological factors. Numerous propositions without solid evidence show that the aetiology of BPS is more complex than previously believed.

## Management

### History

Patients presenting with frequency and urgency need to be carefully questioned about associated urinary symptoms. Associated urgency incontinence and its severity are important, as is any associated dysuria or suprapubic pain. If haematuria is reported, this must be investigated further. The presence of a urinary tract infection, a bladder carcinoma, a calculus or a lesion of the upper urinary tracts needs to be excluded. A thorough history should be undertaken with special emphasis on previous pelvic surgeries, urinary tract infections and urological diseases. Characteristics of pain including onset, correlation with events, description, location, relation to bladder filling and emptying, must be sought. History of previous pelvic radiation treatment and autoimmune diseases are also important.

### Examination

Examination should be undertaken in the standing position for kyphosis, scars, hernia and in the supine position to assess abduction/adduction of the hips and hyperaesthetic areas. An abdominal examination will rule out a mass or large distended bladder. Vaginal examination should be performed with pain mapping of vulvar region and vaginal palpation for tenderness of the bladder, urethra, levator and adductor muscles of the pelvic floor. Tenderness might be graded as mild, moderate or severe. A neurological assessment is important to exclude

an upper motor neuron lesion. The S2, S3, S4 nerve roots innervate the bladder and particular regard should be paid to these dermatomes.

## Investigation

Initial investigation should always include a midstream urine sample for culture and sensitivity, and urine for cytology. Appropriate cultures for 'fastidious organisms' (*Mycoplasma hominis*, *Ureaplasma urealyticum* and *Chlamydia trachomatis*), tuberculosis and schistosomiasis may be indicated. A completed frequency–volume chart is an invaluable tool, providing useful information on fluid input and output, drinking habits, voided volumes and the episodes of urgency and incontinence. Where the cause for the symptoms is not revealed by such assessment, the more specialist investigations should be considered. Ultrasound scan can be used to assess urinary residual volumes accurately and to give more information on any masses detected on pelvic examination. Once a urinary tract infection has been ruled out, uroflowmetry, post-void residual urine volume and pressure-flow study may be performed.

In 1914, Hunner described the classic cystoscopic picture of a bladder ulcer with a corresponding appearance of patches of red mucosa exhibiting small vessels radiating to a central pale scar[9] in patients with BPS. Glomerulations, described as punctuate petechial haemorrhages observed after hydrodistention, have become the primary cystoscopic feature of BPS. However, these findings are not always present and do not correlate with the severity of the disease. There is also a considerable variation in the procedure of cystoscopy and hydrodistension. The ESSIC has recently recommended a standardized procedure using a rigid cystoscope to enable biopsies to be performed at the same time.[10] The bladder is filled using a dripping chamber at 80 cm above the symphysis pubis and filling is stopped after fluid dribbling stops. Continuous inspection is necessary to inspect the mucosa for radiating vessels, hyperaemia, oedema, cracks, scars or any other mucosal changes. When maximum capacity is reached, the distension should be maintained for 3 minutes. The bladder is then emptied and the degree of bleeding if any is noted. The total volume drained is the measured maximum bladder capacity. The bladder is then refilled to a third or two-thirds of the capacity to look for changes and perform biopsies. It has to be borne in mind that the absence of the initial findings of glomerulations or haematuria does not preclude further developments of these features in subsequent evaluation. At least three biopsies including detrusor muscle should be taken and used for mast cell counting in addition to biopsies taken from abnormal areas. Only the biopsy with the highest number of mast cells/mm$^2$ should be reported and 27 mast cells/mm2 is considered indicative of mastocytosis.[11]

Confusable diseases can be mistaken for BPS or BPS may coexist together with confusable diseases,[12] such as chronic

**Table 61.1** Confusable diseases

| Confusable disease | Exclude or confirm by |
|---|---|
| Carcinoma | Cystoscopy and biopsy, MRI |
| Common intestinal bacteria | Routine bacterial culture |
| *Chlamydia trachomatis, Ureaplasma urealyticum* | Special cultures |
| *Mycoplasma hominis, Mycoplasma genitalium* | |
| *Corynebacterium urealyticum, Candida* sp. | |
| *Mycobacterium tuberculosis* | If dipstick shows sterile pyuria culture |
| Herpes simplex virus and human papilloma virus | Physical examination |
| Radiation | Medical history |
| Chemotherapy | Medical history |
| Bladder neck obstruction | Uroflowmetry and ultrasound |
| Bladder stone | Imaging or cystoscopy |
| Urethral diverticulum | History and examination |
| Urogenital prolapse | History and examination |
| Endometriosis | History and examination |
| Cervical, uterine and ovarian cancer | History and examination |
| Incomplete bladder emptying | History and ultrasound |
| Overactive bladder | Urodynamics |
| Pudendal nerve entrapment | History and examination |
| Pelvic floor muscle-related pain | History and examination |

or remitting urinary infections or endometriosis. The diagnosis of BPS is usually made on the basis of exclusion of these confusable diseases. If the main urinary symptoms are not explained by a single diagnosis, the presence of a second diagnosis should be considered. Table 61.1 lists some of these confusable diseases related to BPS and the diagnostic procedures to exclude them.

# Treatment

## Conservative treatment

In motivated patients, behavioural therapy has been noted to be efficacious in treating urinary frequency and urgency without any side effects. Behavioural therapy includes timed voiding, controlled fluid intake, pelvic floor muscle training[13] and bladder training. Physical therapy for the pelvic floor is effective for genitourinary and anorectal disorders. Biofeedback and soft tissue massage may help in the relaxation of the pelvic floor muscles. Stress reduction and dietary manipulation are other methods of conservative management.

## Oral medications

Several groups of drugs have been used in the management of BPS. These include non-opioid analgesics, like acetaminophen and the nonsteroidal anti-inflammatory drugs

(NSAIDs), gabapentin and pregabalin. Opioid analgesics are used as a last resort and better administered in a pain clinic to reduce the incidence of addiction. Amitriptyline is a tricyclic anti-depressant with the property of blocking H1-histaminergic receptors. It stabilizes mast cells, inhibits painful nociception from the bladder and facilitates urine storage.

The most widely used antihistamine for BPS is hydroxyzine. It also inhibits bladder mast cell activation and has anticholinergic and anxiolytic properties.[14] In addition, it has a good safety profile which makes it desirable. Sodium pentosanpolysulphate (PPS) is the most intensively studied treatment for BPS and is the only medication approved by the Food and Drug Administration for the pain of interstitial cystitis. A defective glycosaminoglycan layer is hypothesized to be one important cause for BPS and PPS may replenish it.[15]

## Intravesical medications

Intravesical therapies have always been the next line of treatment in patients in whom oral medications have failed. DMSO (dimethyl sulphoxide) has been used as a therapy for BPS for a long time. It is believed to reduce inflammation, degranulate mast cells, relax muscles and eliminate pain.[16] The exact mechanism of action, however, is not known. The instillation is performed weekly for 6–8 weeks and treatment is suspended after an initial course until symptoms recur. A further 6-week course with monthly maintenance can be initiated if the results are good. Heparin, hyaluronic acid, chondroitin sulphate, pentosan polysufate, capsaicin, resiniferatoxin, BCG, oxybutynin, lidocaine and botulinum toxin are other agents used.

## Surgical treatment

Although BPS is a chronic and debilitating disease, surgical management should only be considered when other conservative and medical therapies have been unsuccessful. Bladder augmentation-cystoplasty has been used for refractory BPS for 50 years.[17] Urinary diversion with or without total cystectomy and urethrectomy is the ultimate, final and most invasive option. It should be used as a last therapeutic resort in selected patients. Simple urinary diversion with formation of an ileal conduit is the most common surgical treatment for BPS/IC. Initially, diversion can be performed without cystectomy, and only when bladder pain is persistent, cystectomy may be considered. To avoid further bowel resection, a bowel segment used for cystoplasty can often be converted to a conduit.

---

## KEY POINTS

- BPS is defined as chronic pelvic pain, pressure or discomfort, related to the urinary bladder accompanied by urgency or urinary frequency.
- Confusable diseases as the cause of the symptoms must be excluded.
- The initial assessment should consist of a frequency/volume chart, focused physical examination, urinalysis and urine culture.
- Urine cytology and cystoscopy are recommended if clinically indicated.
- Patient education, dietary manipulation and pelvic floor relaxation techniques comprise the initial treatment of BPS.
- When conservative therapy fails oral medication, intravesical treatment or physical therapy can be prescribed.
- If medical therapy fails, further evaluation should include urodynamics, pelvic imaging and cystoscopy with distension, and biopsy under anaesthesia.
- Urinary diversion with and without cystectomy may be the ultimate option for refractory patients.

---

# URETHRAL CARUNCLES

Urethral caruncles are found only in females, typically in post-menopausal women, and they usually represent ectropion of the urethral wall secondary to post-menopausal regression of the vaginal mucosa. It is thought that oestrogen deficiency plays a role in their aetiology. Urethral prolapse is often mistakenly diagnosed as a caruncle in a child. On physical examination, a urethral caruncle is seen as a solitary red polypoid lesion protruding from one segment of the urethral meatus, usually the posterior aspect. Most caruncles measure only a few millimetres in diameter. The caruncle consists of well-vascularized transitional epithelium and is sometimes uncomfortable during voiding, but more often does not give rise to any urinary symptoms. The patient may alternatively present with post-menopausal 'spotting'. Initial treatment is with topical oestrogen therapy. If the lesion does not respond to oestrogen, it is important to biopsy it to exclude more serious pathology. Once malignancy is ruled out, it can be treated by either excision or cautery. There is a high rate of recurrence.

# Urethral problems

The female urethra is a complex muscular tube, approximately 40 mm in length. It is composed of several layers of muscle, the richly vascular submucosa and the mucosa. There is considerable debate as to the relative roles of different components of the muscles, both within the wall of the urethra and surrounding it, in maintaining continence. A number of changes occur to the urethra with age. The strength and the amount of urethral connective tissue fall as a result of oestrogen deficiency. This causes the support of the urethrovesical junction to weaken. In addition, urethral vascular pulsations in the submucosal plexus gradually decrease with age.

## Urethritis

Urethritis is inflammation of the urethra leading to symptoms of frequency, urgency, dysuria and localized urethral pain. It is caused either by an infectious pathogen or by chemical irritation. Evidence of the use of causative chemical agents, such as bubble baths, vaginal deodorants and perfumed cosmetics, should be sought as part of the medical history in women with such symptoms. Responsible infectious agents include many of the microorganisms associated with sexually transmitted infections, such as herpes simplex virus, *Neisseria gonorrhoeae* and *Chlamydia*. The group of organisms that typically cause acute bacterial cystitis, such as *Escherichia coli*, may also cause urethritis. Where urethritis is suspected, appropriate cultures should be taken from the urethra and vagina, as well as a midstream urine culture. Urine microscopy typically shows evidence of pyuria and bacteria.

Acute urinary retention can occur secondary to urethritis and needs to be considered. Prompt treatment with an indwelling catheter until symptoms have resolved is important in order to prevent overdistension of the bladder. The initiation of treatment with the appropriate antibiotic usually results in a rapid recovery, but scarring of the urethra can result in strictures and subsequent voiding difficulties. Referral to a genitourinary medicine clinic for contact tracing and treatment of partners is important if sexually transmitted organisms are responsible. Cessation of the use of the offending chemical agent results in fairly rapid resolution of symptoms without the need for further treatment.

## Urethral diverticulae

Urethral diverticulae are usually found on the anterior vaginal wall along the distal two-thirds of the urethra bulging into the vagina. They are occasionally found congenitally, but thought to arise more often from repeated inflammation of the paraurethral glands and are found mainly in parous women. Urethral diverticulae are formed as a consequence of infected periurethral glands or cysts rupturing into the urethral lumen. Common organisms include *Escherichia coli*, *Gonococcus* and *Chlamydia*. The presenting symptoms vary, but usually include frequency, dysuria, dyspareunia, voiding difficulties and recurrent urinary tract infection. The classical symptom associated with this condition is post-micturition dribble, caused by the delay in the diverticulum draining after voiding. On vaginal examination, it is sometimes possible to palpate a suburethral mass or even a calculus that has formed in the diverticulum. An infected urethral diverticulum is tender on examination and clear urine or purulent material can be expressed from the urethral meatus on compression. Alternatively, there may be no physical signs. However, Neitlich *et al.* demonstrated that high resolution, fast spin echo magnetic resonance imaging (MRI) has a higher sensitivity for detecting diverticula and has a higher negative predictive rate than double balloon urethrography.[18]

Often, urethral diverticulae are found incidentally as part of x-ray screening during videourodynamics (Figure 61.1). Similarly, they may be seen on transvaginal ultrasound examination. Urethral pressure profilometry shows a characteristic 'dip' in urethral closure pressure and gives useful information about the position of the opening of the diverticulum relative to the urethral sphincter and bladder neck. If a patient has symptoms suggestive of a diverticulum and a diagnosis is required, a voiding cystourethrogram or a positive-pressure double-balloon urethrography using a Trattner catheter will give useful information about the size and position of the defect prior to surgery. These lesions are not always easy to see on cystourethroscopy unless the opening into the diverticulum is large.

Surgical repair is usually undertaken if the patient displays related symptoms, such as suffering from recurrent urinary infections. Endoscopic incision has been described, but transvaginal excision is the preferred treatment.[19] The techniques described include marsupialization and vaginal diverticulectomy. There are no good long-term studies to guide clinicians as to the best surgical techniques for treating urethral diverticulae. Recurrence is fairly common, especially if there has been failure to remove the whole sac. If the diverticulum is small and not causing any problems, it is better left alone.

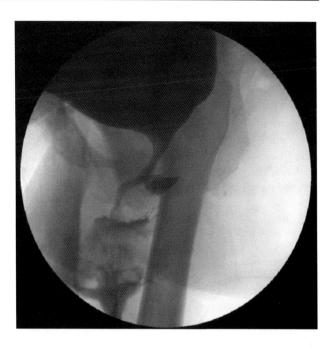

**Figure 61.1** A urethral diverticulum is clearly seen during the voiding phase of videourodynamic assessment

## Iatrogenic urinary tract injury

Damage to the urinary tract at the time of pelvic surgery is an important consideration for all gynaecological surgeons. It is estimated to occur in 0.5–2.5 per cent of routine pelvic operations and in as many as 30 per cent of radical pelvic procedures for malignancy.[20] Although relatively uncommon, when it does occur, it presents a difficult challenge both to identify the injury and then to repair the damage. A good understanding of female pelvic anatomy and how this may be altered as the result of previous surgery or pelvic pathology is essential in order to minimize the risk of inadvertently damaging the urinary tract. Prompt recognition of the injury and the early involvement of an experienced urologist are important in ensuring a good outcome.

### Aetiology

There are three common sites of ureteric injury during gynaecological surgery:

1 at the point where the ureters cross over the pelvic brim and enter the pelvis in close proximity to the ovarian vessels;
2 as the ureters course medially in the base of the broad ligament with the uterine artery crossing directly over the top of them; this is the site at which the ureters may be crushed by a clamp or divided while taking the uterine pedicle at hysterectomy;
3 at the ureterovesical junction as the ureters sweep medially to enter the bladder.

Any disease process that alters the normal anatomical course of the ureters or that makes their intraoperative identification more difficult increases the risk of injury. Malignant disease, advanced stage endometriosis and previous abdominal surgery or radiotherapy all make it more difficult to predict the path of the ureters. Similarly, the normal anatomical relations of the bladder are often distorted in these circumstances. It is often wise to consider the use of a pre-operative intravenous urogram or the placement of ureteric stents at cystoscopy before proceeding to pelvic surgery. The path of the ureters should always be identified prior to any extensive pelvic dissection.

## Management

A keen awareness of the proximity of the lower urinary tract during gynaecological surgery is the key to preventing these injuries. Such damage is largely preventable and forms an ever-increasing source of medical litigation. The success of managing these problems once they occur is largely dependent on whether the injury was detected at the time of operation and on close liaison with urological colleagues. Most bladder injuries are relatively straightforward to repair, provided they are identified intraoperatively. Methylene blue dye instilled into the bladder via a urethral catheter can aid in the identification of bladder injuries. If damage is found, associated ureteric injury should also be borne in mind. The bladder can be satisfactorily repaired with two layers of absorbable suture and left to drain freely with an indwelling catheter for at least 7 days. The bladder heals well and the prognosis for such repairs is extremely good.

If ureteric injury is suspected intraoperatively, the advice of a urologist should be sought. The course of the ureter above and below the area of concern needs to be demonstrated. Indigo carmine dye can be given intravenously to aid in checking the integrity of the ureters. The most appropriate method of repairing damage to the ureters depends largely on the site of the injury and should only ever be undertaken by an experienced surgeon with appropriate urological training. It is not appropriate for a gynaecologist who has not received such training to embark on these procedures. The most commonly employed techniques are summarized in Table 61.2.

In those cases in which injury to the lower urinary tract goes unnoticed at the time of operation, the patient is likely to develop symptoms and signs within a few days post-operatively. These may include fever, abdominal or loin pain, abdominal distension, sepsis, decreased urine output and rising serum creatinine. These result from the extravasation of urine into the peritoneal cavity or from ureteric obstruction. However, the presentation may be delayed and the patient subsequently complains of persistent discharge from a fistula or abdominal wound. Sometimes,

**Table 61.2** Repair of ureteric injuries

| Position of ureteric injury | Possible methods of repair |
| --- | --- |
| Mid-ureter | Boari flap |
| | Primary ureteric anastomosis (uretero-ureterostomy) |
| | Ureteric anastomosis to the contralateral ureter (transuretero-ureterostomy) |
| Lower ureter (distal 4 cm of the ureter) | Primary ureteric anastomosis (uretero-ureterostomy) |
| | Psoas hitch |
| | Ureteric reimplantation into the bladder |

ureteric obstruction is only discovered many years later as an incidental finding.

If damage to the bladder or ureters is suspected post-operatively, an intravenous urogram is the diagnostic study of choice.[21] Repair of the damaged bladder is dependent upon the extent of urinary leakage. Extraperitoneal injuries and small leaks in women who are still voiding spontaneously can be managed with a trial of catheter drainage for 7–10 days in order to rest the bladder. In patients with more extensive bladder damage, intraperitoneal injuries with physical signs and in those in whom conservative management has failed, surgical exploration and repair of the defect are required. In cases where ureteric injury is recognized post-operatively, it is important to identify the site of damage in order to plan the most appropriate course of action. A retrograde pyelogram can give more information regarding the precise location of the injury. If the patient is septic or not well enough to undergo immediate surgical re-exploration, a nephrostomy tube can be inserted to improve renal function to the point at which surgery is a more realistic alternative. In a small minority of cases where ureteric obstruction is caused by suture entrapment, nephrostomy drainage alone may resolve the damage. More often, surgical intervention is required. The techniques available are the same as those discussed previously for performing an intraoperative repair at the time of the initial injury.

## ACKNOWLEDGMENT

This chapter has been revised and updated. The author and editors acknowledge the contribution of James Balmforth to the chapter on this topic in the previous edition of the book.

## KEY POINTS

- The ureters and bladder should always be respected by gynaecologists operating in the pelvis.
- A thorough knowledge of their anatomical relationships and of how these may be modified by pathological processes is important in order to minimize the risk of inadvertently damaging the lower urinary tract.
- The possibility of such an injury should always be borne in mind, both at the time of surgery and in the post-operative period.

## Key References

1. Van De Merwe J, Nordling J, Bouchelouche K et al. Diagnostic criteria, classification, and nomenclature for painful bladder syndrome/interstitial cystitis: an essic proposal. *Eur Urol* 2008; **53**: 60–7.

2. Hanno P, Lin A, Nordlin J et al. Bladder pain syndrome international consultation on incontinence. In: Abrams P, Cardozo L, Khoury S, Wein A (eds). *Incontinence.* France: Health Publications, 2009: 1458–518.

3. Verhaak PFM, Kerssens JJ, Dekker J et al. Prevalence of chronic benign pain disorder among adults: a review of the literature. *Pain* 1998; **77**: 231–9.

4. Abrams P, Hanno P, Wein A. Overactive bladder and painful bladder syndrome: there need not be confusion. *Neurourol Urodyn* 2005; **24**: 149–50.

5. Clemens JQ, Link CL, Eggers PW et al. Prevalence of painful bladder symptoms and effect on quality of life in black, Hispanic and white men and women. *J Urol* 2007; **177**: 1390–4.

6. Michael YL, Kawachi I, Stampfer MJ et al. Quality of life among women with interstitial cystitis. *J Urol* 2000; **164**: 423–7.

7. Parsons CL, Lilly JD, Stein P. Epithelial dysfunction in nonbacterial cystitis (interstitial cystitis). *J Urol* 1991; **145**: 732–5.

8. Keay S, Kleinberg M, Zhang CO et al. Bladder epithelial cells from patients with interstitial cystitis produce an inhibitor of heparin-binding epidermal growth factor-like growth factor production. *J Urol* 2000; **164**: 2112–18.

9. Hunner GL. A rare type of bladder ulcer in women; report of cases. *Boston Med Surg J* 1915; **172**: 660–4.

10. Nordling J, Anjum FH, Bade JJ et al. Primary evaluation of patients suspected of having interstitial cystitis (IC). *Eur Urol* 2004; **45**: 662–9.

11. Larsen MS, Mortensen S, Nordling J, Horn T. Quantifying mast cells in bladder pain syndrome by immunohistochemical analysis. *BJU Int* 2008; **102**: 204–7.

12. Fries J, Hochberg M, Medsger T, Hunder G. Criteria for rheumatic disease. Different types and different functions. *Arthr Rheum* 1994; **37**: 454–62.

13. Lukban JC, Whitmore K. Pelvic floor muscle reeducation treatment of the overactive bladder and painful bladder syndrome. *Clin Obst Gynecol* 2002; **45**: 273–85.

14. Minogiannis P, El Mansoury M, Betances JA et al. Hydroxyzine inhibits neurogenic bladder mast cell activation. *Int J Immunopharmacol* 1998; **20**: 553–63.

15. Parsons CL, Schmidt JD, Pollen JJ. Successful treatment of interstitial cystitis with sodium pentosanpolysulfate. *J Urol* 1983; **130**: 51–7.

16. Peeker R, Haghsheno MA, Holmang S, Fall M. Intravesical bacillus Calmette-Guerin and dimethyl sulfoxide for treatment of classic and nonulcer interstitial cystitis: a prospective, randomized double-blind study. *J Urol* 2000; **164**: 1912–15.

17. Dounis A, Gow JG. Bladder augmentation – a long-term review. *Br J Urol* 1979; **51**: 264–8.

18. Neitlich JD, Foster HE Jr, Glickman MG, Smith RC. Detection of urethral diverticula in women: comparison of a high resolution fast spin echo technique with double balloon urethrography. *J Urol* 1998; **159**: 408–10.

19. Ockrim JL, Allen DJ, Shah PJ, Greenwell TJ. A tertiary experience of urethral diverticulectomy: diagnosis, imaging and surgical outcomes. *BJU Int* 2009; **103**: 1550–4.

20. Mariotti G, Natale F, Trucchi A et al. Ureteral injuries during gynecologic procedures. *Minerva Urol Nefrol* 1997; **49**: 95–8.

21. Mann WJ. Intentional and unintentional ureteral surgical treatment in gynaecologic procedures. *Surg Gynecol Obstet* 1991; **17**: 453–6.

# Lower urinary tract infections

*Ismaiel A Mahfouz and Dudley Robinson*

---

## MRCOG standards

- Have comprehensive knowledge of lower urinary tract infections (UTI) affecting pregnant and non-pregnant women.
- Appreciate the pathogenesis of lower UTI.
- Identify those at risk of developing UTI and those at risk of recurrence.
- Collect appropriate specimens, use the laboratory appropriately and order additional investigations when necessary.
- Make accurate diagnoses and appreciate definition of different terms.
- Successfully manage uncomplicated and complicated UTI and its recurrence.
- Make recommendations for follow-up care.

## INTRODUCTION

'Urinary tract infection' is a term that is used to describe various infections involving the urinary tract. The spectrum ranges from asymptomatic bacteriuria to severe pyelonephritis.

There are different classifications for UTI and these could be divided into lower urinary tract infection, i.e infection involving the urethra and bladder, or upper urinary tract infection, mainly involving the kidneys. UTI may also be classified as uncomplicated, when the infection happens without underlying structural or functional abnormalities, or complicated UTI, where several anatomical abnormalities predispose to UTI. The classification system is important in patient management, as it provides a guide to investigation, treatment and prophylaxis.

## DEFINITIONS

### Bacteriuria

This is used to describe the presence of small numbers of bacteria in the urine. In a clean-catch freshly voided sample, this represents 10 000 colony-forming units (CFU)/mL.

### Significant bacteriuria

This term is used to describe the presence of at least 100 000 CFU/mL of urine in a voided midstream clean-catch specimen, or at least 100 CFU/mL of urine from a catheterized specimen.[1]

While 20–40 per cent of women with symptomatic UTIs may present with bacterial counts of 100 000 CFU/mL,[2] bacterial counts of 100–10 000 CFU/mL have also been associated with symptoms of cystitis. This may represent the early stages of infection.

### Asymptomatic bacteriuria

This is used to describe the presence of bacteria in the urine of an asymptomatic woman. Asymptomatic bacteriuria is common, the prevalence depends on age, sex, sexual activity and the presence of urological abnormalities. In women it is only diagnosed if the same species is present in quantities of at least 100 000 CFU/mL of urine in at least two consecutive voided specimens.

Whilst the organisms causing asymptomatic bacteriuria and symptomatic UTI are the same, it is not fully understood why patients with asymptomatic bacteriuria do not develop symptoms. This is probably related to organism virulence, where organisms with decreased virulence may only colonize the urine without causing symptoms.

### Complicated lower urinary tract infection

This term is used to describe UTIs that may be related to other pathology (Table 62.1) One of the most common forms of complicated urinary tract infection is related to the use of urinary catheters. The incidence of bacteriuria associated with an indwelling urinary catheter is 3–10 per cent per day, and the duration of catheterization is the most important risk factor for developing UTI. They represent a huge reservoir of resistant bacteria in the hospital environment.

**Table 62.1** Conditions associated with complicated lower urinary tract infection

| Type | Condition |
| --- | --- |
| Structural | Urolithiasis |
| | Malignancy |
| | Ureteric stricture |
| | Urethral stricture |
| | Bladder diverticulae |
| | Renal cysts |
| | Fistulae |
| | Urinary diversions |
| Functional | Neurogenic bladder |
| | Vesicoureteric reflux |
| | Voiding difficulties (incomplete bladder emptying) |
| Foreign bodies | Indwelling catheter |
| | Ureteric stent |
| | Nephrostomy tube |
| | Suburethral tapes for urinary surgery |
| Other | Diabetes mellitus |
| | Pregnancy |
| | Renal failure |
| | Renal transplant |
| | Immunosuppression |
| | Multi-drug resistance |
| | Hospital-acquired (nosocomial) infection |

## Recurrent lower urinary tract infection

This is defined as three or more episodes of UTI during a 12-month period,[3] or two infections in a six-month period. It is symptomatic infection that follows clinical resolution of an earlier UTI. In a study involving college students with their first UTI, Foxman et al.[4] have shown that 27 per cent had at least one culture-confirmed recurrence within the six months following the initial infection, and 2.7 per cent had a second recurrence over the same period of time. The risk of recurrence of UTI is age related. In a study of women with age range between 17 and 82 years with E. coli cystitis, 44 per cent had a recurrence within one year, and recurrence is more common in older than younger women.[5]

## EPIDEMIOLOGY

UTIs are common medical conditions. In the United States, they account for 7–8 million clinic visits, and more than 100 000 hospital admissions mainly due to pyelonephritis.[6] They are more common in females than males with a female to male ratio of 14:1. The reasons are probably related to anatomical and functional differences; the female urethra is shorter with the distal third contaminated by bacteria from the vagina and rectum. In addition, during intercourse, bacteria are introduced into the urethra and bladder, and also female bladder emptying may be incomplete compared with males.

The woman's lifetime risk of at least one UTI is around 20 per cent, with a prevalence that is age related, and increases by 1 per cent per decade of life.

## RISK FACTORS FOR LOWER URINARY TRACT INFECTION

Risk factors for UTI seem to vary according to age. Data regarding recurrent UTI are scarce. Tables 62.2 and 62.3 summarize congenital and acquired risk factors for urinary tract infection.

### Pre-menopausal women

Behavioural factors are thought to increase the risk of UTI. In a large case–control study of women with and without a history of recurrent UTI, the strongest risk factor for recurrent UTI was the frequency of sexual intercourse. Other risk factors include spermicidal use during the past year, having a new sexual partner during the past year, having a first UTI at or before 15 years of age, and having a mother with a history of UTIs.[7]

### Post-menopausal women

Anatomical and functional factors are thought to increase the risk of UTI. Raz et al.[8] have shown that in healthy postmenopausal women with a history of recurrent UTI, when compared with a control group, three factors were found to be strongly associated with recurrent UTI, namely urinary incontinence, cystocele and post-void residual urine.

**Table 62.2** Congenital risk factors for urinary tract infection

| | Risk factor |
| --- | --- |
| Urethra | Hypospadias |
| | Epispadias |
| Bladder | Vesico-ureteric reflux |
| | Ectopic ureters |
| | Obstructive mega-ureter |
| Pelvis | Pelvic–ureteric junction obstruction |
| Central nervous system | Meningomyelocele |
| | Tethered cord syndrome |

**Table 62.3** Acquired causes of urinary tract infection

|  | Cause |
|---|---|
| Traumatic | Surgery (urinary diversion, clam cystoplasty) |
|  | Sexual intercourse |
|  | Sexual abuse |
|  | Foreign bodies (catheters, stents) |
|  | Contraceptive diaphragm |
| Inflammatory | Vulvo-urethritis |
|  | Chronic inflammation (tuberculosis, syphilis, schistosomiasis) |
|  | Interstitial cystitis |
|  | Radiotherapy |
|  | Fistulae |
| Metabolic | Calculi |
|  | Diabetes mellitus |
| Drugs | Cyclophosphamide |
|  | Tioprofenic acid |
| Anatomical | Cystocele |
|  | Urethral diverticulae |
| Functional | Detrusor hypotonia |
|  | Detrusor dyssynergia |
|  | Constipation |
| Malignancy | Bladder tumours |
|  | Other pelvic tumours (cervix, uterus, ovary) |

# PATHOGENESIS

Urinary tract infections are the result of a complex interaction between several factors related to both the host and the uropathogens.

## Host factors

The main route of bacterial entry into the urethra and bladder is ascending from the bowel to the vaginal vestibule, and then to the urethra and bladder. In support of that, it has been shown that the vaginal vestibule of women with recurrent UTI had higher enterobacterial colonization than women with no recurrent UTI. Changes in the vaginal microflora are important in the aetiology. These changes may be caused by the use of spermicides, antibiotics and lack of oestrogen.

## Host defence

There are several protective mechanisms against UTI; the main function is to prevent colonization with uropathogens.[9] These mechanisms include:

- Urinary hydrodynamics: urine production and micturition provide a washout mechanism to prevent uropathogens from colonizing the urinary tract, if this mechanisms is impaired, a significant post-void residual urine may result in increased risk of UTI.
- Urine biochemical characteristics, namely high osmolality and low pH prevent bacterial multiplication.
- Urinary tract epithelium has bactericidal activities.
- Inhibitors of bacterial adherence: several protective mechanisms work to prevent bacterial adherence to the urinary tract epithelium which is a prerequisite for infection. The factors that prevent bacterial adherence include Tamm–Horsfall protein, bladder mucopolusaccarides and oligosaccharides and lactoferrin.
- Inflammatory response will take effect when bacteria adhere to epithelium. The inflammatory response includes polymorph nuclear leukocytes and cytokines.
- Both humoral and cell-mediated arms of the immune system play an important part in the resistance against bacterial infection of the urinary tract.

## Virulence factor

Microorganisms have the ability to survive and multiply in the bladder and are able to adhere to the bladder epithelium.[10] E. coli is responsible for 80 per cent of UTIs, and this is why most virulence studies focused on it. The virulence factors that are thought to play a role in the pathogenesis of UTI include:

- *Adherence factors:* The two most important fimberiae thought to play a role in the *E. coli* UTI are type P and type 1. These fimberiae will bind to specific receptors on the urinary tract epithelium, and eventually provoke an inflammatory reaction. It seems that they are site specific, where type 1 is present in the majority of *E. coli* causing lower UTI, and type P is mostly found in *E. coli*-causing pyelonephritis.
- *Invasion factors:* Uropathogens produce substances that aid in the direct invasion of the urinary tract mucosa with subsequent systemic dissemination. The most important bacterial toxins are lipopolysaccarides and haemolysins.
- *Bacterial resistance:* This represents a microorganism defence mechanism against anti-microbials.

# ORGANISMS OF LOWER URINARY TRACT INFECTION

The organisms responsible for UTI are well-established and consistent. *Escherichia coli* is responsible for almost 80 per cent of acute community-acquired uncomplicated infections, followed by *Staphylococcus saprophyticus* (10–15 per cent). *Klebsiella, Enterobacter, Proteus* and enterococci are infrequent causes of uncomplicated UTI. The commonly

**Table 62.4** Common uropathogens in general practice and hospital

| Organism | Community (%) | Hospital (%) |
|---|---|---|
| *Escherichia coli* | 77.5 | 62.9 |
| *Proteus mirabilis* | 4.5 | 4.5 |
| *Klebsiella–Enterobacter* spp. | 4.7 | 9.3 |
| *Enterococcus* spp. | 4.9 | 9.2 |
| *Staphylococcus* spp. | 1 | 2.7 |
| Others (*Ureoplasma, Mycoplasma, Chlamydia*) | 7.4 | 7.6 |
| *Pseudomonas aeruginosa* | | 3.8 |

**Table 62.6** Common antibiotic sensitivities

| Gram-negative bacilli | Norfloxacin |
|---|---|
| Staphylococci | Ciprofloxacin |
| Streptococci | Gentamycin |
| | Sulphonamides |
| | Co-trimoxazole |
| | Trimethoprim |
| | Nitrofurantoin |
| *Pseudomonas* | Norfloxacin |
| | Ciprofloxacin |
| | Gentamycin |

occurring organisms in community practice differ when compared to those found within the hospital environment (Table 62.4).[11]

## Viral urinary tract infections

Lower UTIs are most often caused by bacteria; however, in the immunocompromised host, viruses are being increasingly recognized as a cause, especially in haemorrhagic cystitis, predominent viruses include the BK virus (a type of polyomavirus that infects most people, but generally causes no symptoms) adenovirus and cytomegalovirus. The diagnosis is based on molecular techniques. Cidofovir is becoming a drug of choice in viral UTIs.[12]

## ANTIBIOTIC SENSITIVITIES

The antibiotic sensitivities of uropathogens in the community (Table 62.5) differ from the sensitivities of the same organisms within the hospital.[11] Common antibiotic sensitivities are shown in (Table 62.6).

**Table 62.5** Comparison of the sensitivities to antibiotics in the community and in hospital

| Antibiotic | Community (%) | Hospital (%) |
|---|---|---|
| Amoxycillin/ampicillin | 56.9 | 48.8 |
| Cephaloradine | 86.9 | 73.1 |
| Ciprofloxacin | 90.3 | 83.3 |
| Co-trimoxazole | 86.8 | 74.1 |
| Nalidixic acid | 85.7 | 73.5 |
| Nitrofurantoin | 88.4 | 79.3 |
| Sulphonamide | 64.5 | 55.5 |
| Tetracycline | 65.0 | 57.9 |
| Trimethoprim | 74.0 | 64.9 |

## MANAGEMENT

The management of lower urinary tract infection is aimed at treating the current infection and preventing further recurrences. The aims of treatment may be summarized as follows:

- symptomatic relief,
- microbiological cure,
- detection of predisposing factors,
- prevention of upper urinary tract involvement,
- management of recurrence.

## DIAGNOSIS

### Symptoms and signs

Women with lower urinary tract infections typically complain of symptoms of cystitis, i.e. dysuria, suprapubic discomfort, frequency, urgency and nocturia. While the diagnostic accuracy of clinical assessment of UTI is uncertain, the presence of both dysuria and frequency increases the probability of UTI by 90 per cent. Of these women, approximately 30 per cent will also have an upper urinary tract infection, which may present as loin pain and tenderness. Whilst young children may present with general malaise and pyrexia, in the elderly, urinary tract infections may present with atypical symptoms, such as confusion and falls. History is also important in the differentiation between uncomplicated and complicated UTI.

Physical examination is usually unremarkable; however, suprapubic or loin tenderness may be the only physical signs.

## INVESTIGATIONS

In the majority of women with simple acute lower UTI, there is no need for further investigation. However, some cases do warrant further investigation in order to exclude an underlying cause.

Indications for investigation include:

- children,
- proven recurrent urinary tract infection,
- adults with a childhood history of urinary tract infection,
- haematuria,
- atypical infection,
- atypical organism,
- persistent infection,
- failure to respond to antibiotic therapy.

## Basic investigations

- *Urine appearance.* Whilst urine turbidity has been shown to have a specificity of 66.4 per cent and sensitivity of 90.4 per cent for predicting symptomatic UTI, it is prone to observer error.[13]
- *Urine microscopy* has a sensitivity of 60–100 per cent and specificity of 49–100 per cent of predicting significant bacteriuria in women.[14]
- *Urine dipstick for nitrites and leukocytes.* If the test is positive for both, then the probability of UTI is higher that each alone; however if both are negative, the likelihood of UTI is less than 20 per cent.[15]
- *Urine culture* will isolate the causative organism and provide antibiotic sensitivities that should guide antimicrobial treatment.

## Other investigations

- In women who have recurrent or complicated urinary infections, renal function should be assessed with serum creatinine, urea and electrolytes. In addition, urine should be sent for culture of fastidious organisms (*Mycoplasma hominis*, *Ureaplasma urealyticum* and *Chlamydia trachomatis*) to rule out the more unusual causes of infection.
- Ultrasound of the upper urinary tract will exclude renal causes, such as hydronephrosis or calculi, a postmicturition ultrasound scan will rule out a significant urinary residual.
- An alternative is radiological imaging using an intravenous urogram, although this involves exposure to ionizing radiation and has not been shown to influence treatment in the majority of cases.
- A transvaginal ultrasound should be performed to exclude the possibility of a pelvic mass.
- Cystourethroscopy and bladder biopsy will exclude an intravesical lesion, such as a bladder tumour, and anomalies, such as diverticulae and calculi, and also synthetic tapes eroded through bladder wall. A bladder biopsy may show evidence of chronic follicular or interstitial cystitis.

## TREATMENT

### General measures

Patients with cystitis should be encouraged to increase their fluid intake in order to achieve a short voiding interval and a high flow rate, which will help to dilute and flush out the infecting organism. Using potassium citrate preparations may provide symptomatic relief; it is thought to act by reducing urinary pH.

### Antimicrobials

When treating UTI, an antimicrobial should be selected that has the appropriate sensitivity and is also able to achieve a high concentration within the urinary tract. Drugs should be safe and efficacious, have a broad spectrum of activity and few side effects. Ideally, the drugs should be rapidly absorbed and not induce bacterial resistance.

### Duration

Compliance with therapy may be improved by using shorter courses of antimicrobial therapy or, ideally, by using a single-dose regimen, which also has the advantage of reducing the effect on faecal and vaginal flora and may help in reducing the emergence of resistant organisms. Several studies have documented the dosing and effectiveness of single-dose antimicrobial regimens for uncomplicated UTI. With success rates of 80–100 per cent, trimethoprim/sulfamethoxazole, fluoroquinolones and fosfomycin trometamol are highly effective as single-dose therapy in uncomplicated cystitis.[16] A recent Cochrane review concluded that a 3-day course of antimicrobial is as effective as longer courses for clinical outcome, but less effective for microbial outcome.[17]

### Antimicrobial sensitivities

Antimicrobial therapy should ideally be based upon culture and sensitivity results from a midstream specimen of urine, although initially treatment often needs to be on a 'best guess' basis.

Community-acquired infections often have a different range of sensitivities from those found in the hospital setting (Tables 62.5 and 62.6). Some antimicrobials are particularly useful when treating urinary infections. Nitrofurantoin is specific to the urinary tract and therefore has little effect on bowel and vaginal flora. It is bactericidal to most common uropathogens and is particularly useful as a prophylactic measure; it is contraindicated in cases of renal failure. Trimethoprim, primarily bacteriostatic, is also useful in the treatment of urinary tract infection.

# PREVENTION OF RECURRENT URINARY TRACT INFECTION

Women with recurrent UTI, who use spermicides mainly in conjunction with diaphragms, should be advised about their association with recurrent UTI, and hence a reduction in use or elimination would be expected to reduce recurrence. Early post-coital voiding and increased fluid intake might be helpful.

Methenamine hippurate may be effective for preventing UTI in patients without renal tract abnormalities, particularly when used for short-term prophylaxis. It does not appear to work in patients with a neuropathic bladder or in patients who have renal tract abnormalities.[18]

Cranberry juice has been used for many years for the prevention and treatment of UTI. It is thought to act by preventing bacterial adherence to bladder epithelium, although there is no good quality evidence to suggest that it is effective for the treatment of UTIs. Some reports have shown that the incidence of bacteriuria in those taking cranberry juice was 42 per cent of those in the control group and they were also found to be four times more likely to clear bacteria spontaneously.[19]

In post-menopausal women, the prevalence rate for having one episode of UTI in a given year varies from 8 to 10 per cent. This increased risk is associated with a decrease in oestrogen levels. Vaginal oestrogens have been shown to reduce the number of UTIs in post-menopausal women with recurrent UTI.[20]

When compared to placebo, continuous antibiotic prophylaxis for 6–12 months reduces the rate of UTI; however, this is associated with more side effects. In women with recurrent UTI related to intercourse, antibiotic prophylaxis has been shown to reduce the recurrence rate, with no difference between continuous daily therapy and postcoital treatment.[3]

# URINARY TRACT INFECTION IN PREGNANCY

Urinary tract infections are the most common medical complication of pregnancy.

The incidence of asymptomatic bacteriuria in pregnancy is 2–5 per cent.[21] If not treated, up to 20 per cent will develop lower UTI. The overall incidence of UTI in pregnancy is 8 per cent and the incidence of acute pyelonephritis is 2 per cent.

## Aetiology

The increased susceptibility in pregnancy is due to a number of physiological changes that make asymptomatic bacteriuria progress to symptomatic UTI. These include changes in bladder volume, decreased bladder tone and ureteric dilatation secondary to an increased level of progesterone. This will lead to urinary stasis and chronic residual urine with subsequent UTI.

A review of randomized, controlled studies has found good evidence that urine culture and dipstick testing for leukocytes and nitrites reduced the risk of pyelonephritis and was cost effective, thus offering a rationale for screening.[22]

Uropathogens responsible for UTI in pregnancy are similar to non-pregnant women, with *E. coli* responsible for over 80 per cent of the cases.

## Maternal/fetal complication

Urinary tract infections in pregnancy have been associated with increased risks of chorioamnionitis and endometritis. With regards to the fetus, it has been shown that UTI is associated with fetal growth restriction, stillbirth, preterm labour and delivery, increased perinatal mortality, mental retardation and developmental delay.[23]

## Treatment

### Asymptomatic bacteriuria
Treatment of asymptomatic bacteriuria reduces the risk of pyelonephritis and, consequently, the risks of preterm delivery and low birth weight.

### Symptomatic UTI
Treatment is directed by urine culture and sensitivity. A Cochrane review has shown that antibiotic treatment is effective for the cure of UTIs, and there are insufficient data to recommend any specific treatment regimen. An antibiotic course for 5–7 days would be appropriate, although in an attempt to increase patient compliance and reduce side effects; some studies suggested single dose treatment.[24]

Penicillins and cephalosporins have been shown to be safe in the first and second trimesters. As it is a folate antagonist, trimethoprim should be avoided in the first trimester, although it may be used safely in late pregnancy. Conversely, nitrofurantoin and sulphonamides are safe in early pregnancy, although they should be avoided in the third trimester when the former may cause a haemolytic anaemia and the latter hyperbilirubinaemia and kernicterus. Tetracyclines should be avoided because of their chelating action, which will lead to hypoplasia and staining of the teeth. While in general erythromycin is considered safe, the estolate salt may be associated with cholestatic jaundice. Finally, fluoroquinolones may affect fetal cartilage formation, and chloramphenicol may be associated with neonatal cardiovascular collapse.

### Recurrent UTI in pregnancy
The risk of recurrence in pregnancy is 4–5 per cent. While the exact aetiology of recurrence is uncertain, it is believed

Pelvic floor and lower urinary tract dysfunction

that the causes of the first infection are likely to cause recurrence. Postpartum urological investigation to exclude urinary anomalies should be considered. Long-term, low-dose antimicrobial cover and single-dose antimicrobial in intercourse-related UTI are suggested as prophylactic measures.[25]

## KEY POINTS

- Lower urinary tract infections are a common cause of morbidity.
- Risks of lower UTI are related to behavioural, anatomical and functional factors.
- Community-acquired infections may be caused by different organisms from those acquired in hospital.
- In the majority of women with uncomplicated cystitis, there is no indication for further investigation.
- Antimicrobial therapy should be based upon culture and sensitivity results, although often initial treatment is on a 'best guess' basis.
- Short and low-dose antibiotics may be used as prophylaxis and reduce infection rates by 95 per cent, compared with placebo.
- Urinary tract infection in pregnancy may be associated with pyelonephritis, preterm delivery and low birth weight.

## Key References

1. Saint S, Chenoweth CE. Biofilms and catheter-associated urinary tract infections. *Infect Dis Clin North Am* 2003; **17**: 411–32.
2. Hanson LA. Prognostic indicators in childhood urinary infection. *Kidney Int* 1982; **21**: 659–67.
3. Albert X, Huertas I, Pereiro I *et al.* Antibiotics for preventing recurrent urinary tract infection in non-pregnant women. *Cochrane Database Syst Rev* 2004; (**3**): CD001209.
4. Foxman B. Recurring urinary tract infection: incidence and risk factors. *Am J Public Health* 1990; **80**: 331–3.
5. Ikaheimo R, Sutonen A, Heiskanen T *et al.* Recurrence of urinary tract infection in a primary care setting: analysis of a 1-year follow-up of 179 women. *Clin Infect Dis* 1996; **22**: 91–9.
6. Stamm WE, Hooton TM. Management of urinary tract infections in adults. *N Engl J Med* 1993; **329**: 1328–34.
7. Scholes D, Hooton TM, Roberts PL *et al.* Risk factors for recurrent UTI in young women. *J Infect Dis* 2000; **182**: 1177–82.
8. Raz R, Stamm WE. A controlled trial of intravaginal estriol in postmenopausal women with recurrent urinary tract infections. *N Engl J Med* 1993; **329**: 753–6.
9. Sobel JD. Pathogenesis of UTI. Role of host defences. *Infect Dis North Am* 1997; **11**: 531–49.
10. Svanborg C, Godaly G. Bacterial virulence in urinary tract infection. *Infect Dis Clin N Am* 1997; **11**: 513–29.
11. Gruneberg R. Pathogenesis and microbiology. In: Stanton SL, Dwyer PL (eds). *Urinary Tract Infection in the Female*. London: Martin Dunitz, 2000: 19–33.
12. Paduch DA. Viral lower urinary tract infections. *Curr Urol Rep* 2007; **8**: 324–35.
13. Flanagan PG, Rooney PG, Davies EA, Stout RW. Evaluation of four screening tests for bacteriuria in elderly people. *Lancet* 1989; **1**: 1117–19.
14. Jenkins RD, Fenn JP, Matsen JM. Review of urine microscopy for bacteriuria. *JAMA* 1986; **255**: 3397–403.
15. Hurlbut TA 3rd, Littenberg B. The diagnostic accuracy of rapid dipstick tests to predict urinary tract infection. *Am J Clin Pathol* 1991; **96**: 582–8.
16. Nicolle LE. Short-term therapy for urinary tract infection: success and failure. *Int J Antimicrob Agents* 2008; **31** (Suppl. 1): S40–5.
17. Katchman EA, Milo G, Paul M *et al.* Three-day vs. longer duration of antibiotic treatment for cystitis in women: systematic review and meta-analysis. *Am J Med* 2005; **118**: 1196–207.
18. Lee BB, Simpson JM, Craig JC, Bhuta T. Methenamine hippurate for preventing urinary tract infections. *Cochrane Database Syst Rev* 2007; (**4**): CD003265.
19. Foxman B, Geiger AM, Palin K *et al.* First time urinary tract infection and sexual behaviour. *Epidemiology* 1995; **6**: 162–8.
20. Perrotta C, Aznar M, Mejia R *et al.* Oestrogens for preventing recurrent urinary tract infection in post-menopausal women. *Cochrane Database Syst Rev* 2008; (**2**): CD005131.
21. Foley ME, Farquharson R, Stronge JM. Is screening for bacteriuria in pregnancy worthwhile? *BMJ* 1987; **295**: 270.
22. Villar J, Bergsjo P. Scientific basis for the content of routine antenatal care. *Acta Obstet Gynaecol Scand* 1997; **76**: 1–14.
23. McCormick T, Ashe RG, Kearney PM. Urinary tract infection in pregnancy. *Obstet Gynaecol* 2008; **10**: 156–62.
24. Harris RE, Gilstrap LC 3rd, Pretty A. Single-dose antimicrobial therapy for asymptomatic bacteriuria during pregnancy. *Obstet Gynecol* 1982; **59**: 546–9.
25. Romero R, Oyarzun E, Mazor M *et al.* Meta-analysis of the relationship between asymptomatic bacteriuria and preterm delivery/low birth weight. *Obstet Gynecol* 1989; **73**: 576–82.

# Chapter 63

# Urogenital prolapse

*Sushma Srikrishna and Dudley Robinson*

## MRCOG standards

### Theoretical skills

- Have comprehensive knowledge of the functional pelvic anatomy as applied to gynaecological surgery.
- Understand the aetiology of urogenital prolapse.
- Understand preventative measures.

### Practical skills

- Know how to clinically assess women presenting with urogenital prolapse.
- Be able to undertake conservative management of prolapse.
- Be able to undertake surgical management of urogenital prolapse.

### STRAT OG: Learning objectives

To achieve a better understanding of:

- the incidence and epidemiology of urogenital prolapse;
- the classification and grading scales to indicate the severity of the prolapse;
- means of preventing urogenital prolapse;
- management procedures;
- non-surgical;
- surgical.

## INTRODUCTION

Urogenital prolapse occurs when there is a weakness in the supporting structures of the pelvic floor allowing the pelvic viscera to descend and ultimately fall through the anatomical defect.

While usually not life-threatening, prolapse is often symptomatic and is associated with a deterioration in quality of life and may be the cause of bladder and bowel dysfunction.

Increased life expectancy and an expanding elderly population mean that prolapse remains an important condition, especially since the majority of women may now spend a third of their lives in the post-menopausal state. Surgery for urogenital prolapse accounts for approximately 20 per cent of elective major gynaecological surgery and this increases to 59 per cent in elderly women. The lifetime risk of having surgery for prolapse is 11 per cent; a third of these procedures are operations for recurrent prolapse.

The economic cost of urogenital prolapse is considerable, with figures from the United States revealing a total expenditure of $1012 million in 1997: vaginal hysterectomy accounted for 49 per cent, pelvic floor repairs for 28 per cent and abdominal hysterectomy for 13 per cent of costs.[1]

## EPIDEMIOLOGY

### Age

The incidence of urogenital prolapse increases with increasing age, with approximately 60 per cent of elderly women having some degree of prolapse and up to half of all women over the age of 50 years complaining of symptomatic prolapse. In a study of women with severe vaginal vault prolapse following hysterectomy, 60 per cent were over the age of 60 years.

### Parity

Urogenital prolapse is more common following childbirth, although it may be asymptomatic. Studies have estimated that 50 per cent of parous women have some degree of urogenital prolapse and, of these, 10–20 per cent are symptomatic. Only 2 per cent of nulliparous women are reported to have prolapse.

### Race

Prolapse is generally thought to be more common in Caucasian women and less common in women of Afro-Caribbean origin. However, a study examining racial differences in North

America has shown that this may not be the case, as there was little racial variation noted, although this may simply reflect cultural differences in reporting.

## CLASSIFICATION

Urogenital prolapse is classified anatomically depending on the site of the defect and the pelvic viscera that are involved.

- *Urethrocele:* prolapse of the lower anterior vaginal wall involving the urethra only.
- *Cystocele:* prolapse of the upper anterior vaginal wall involving the bladder. Generally, there is also associated prolapse of the urethra and hence the term cystourethrocele is used.
- *Uterovaginal prolapse:* this term is used to describe prolapse of the uterus, cervix and upper vagina.
- *Enterocele:* prolapse of the upper posterior wall of the vagina, usually containing loops of small bowel. A traction enterocele is secondary to uterovaginal prolapse, a pulsion enterocele is secondary to chronically raised intra-abdominal pressure, and an iatrogenic enterocele is caused by previous pelvic surgery. An anterior enterocele may be used to describe prolapse of the upper anterior vaginal wall following hysterectomy.
- *Rectocele:* prolapse of the lower posterior wall of the vagina involving the anterior wall of the rectum.

## GRADING OF UROGENITAL PROLAPSE

- *First degree:* The lowest part of the prolapse descends halfway down the vaginal axis to the introitus.
- *Second degree:* The lowest part of the prolapse extends to the level of the introitus and through the introitus on straining.
- *Third degree:* The lowest part of the prolapse extends through the introitus and lies outside the vagina. Procidentia describes a third-degree uterine prolapse.

## PROLAPSE SCORING SYSTEM

Recently, the International Continence Society (ICS) produced a standardization document in order to assess urogenital prolapse more objectively.[2] The ICS Prolapse Scoring System (POPQ) allows the measurement of fixed points on the anterior and posterior vaginal walls, cervix and perineal body against a fixed reference point, the genital hiatus (Figure 63.1). Measurements are performed in the left lateral position at rest and at maximal valsalva, thus providing an accurate and reproducible method of quantifying urogenital prolapse.

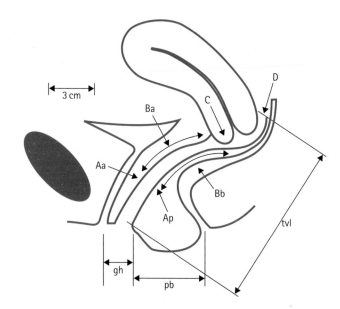

**Figure 63.1** International Continence Society (ICS) Prolapse Scoring System (POPQ)

## ANATOMY OF THE PELVIC FLOOR

The pelvic floor provides support to the pelvic viscera and consists of the levator ani muscles, urogenital diaphragm, endopelvic fascia and perineal body. The levator ani, when considered with its associated fascia, is termed the 'pelvic diaphragm'.

The muscle fibres of the pelvic diaphragm are arranged to form a broad U-shaped layer of muscle with a defect anteriorly. This physiological defect is the urogenital hiatus and allows the passage of the urethra, vagina and rectum through the pelvic floor.

### Pelvic floor musculature

The muscles of the pelvic floor are composed of the levator ani and coccygeus, which form a cradle within the bony pelvis supporting the pelvic organs. The levator ani originate on each side from the pelvic sidewall, arising anteriorly just above the arcus tendineus fasciae pelvis (the white line) and inserting posteriorly into the arcus tendineus levator ani. The arcus tendineus fasciae pelvis and arcus tendineus levator ani fuse near the ischial spine; the levator ani unite in the midline to form the anococcygeal raphe (Figure 63.2).

The levator ani has three divisions: the pubococcygeus, iliococcygeus and puborectalis muscles (Figure 63.3). The iliococcygeus and pubococcygeus arise from the arcus tendineus levator ani fascia overlying the obturator internus and insert into the midline anococcygeal raphe and the coccyx, while the latter forms the inner fibres of the pelvic floor musculature inserting into the rectum and

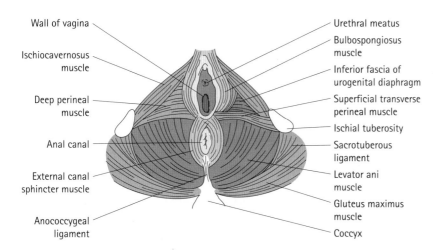

**Figure 63.2** Anatomy of the pelvic floor

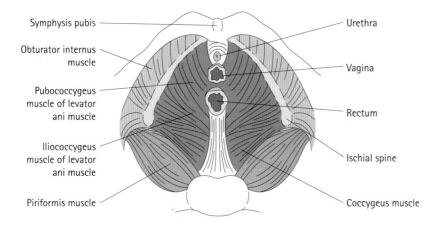

**Figure 63.3** Anatomy of the pelvic floor showing the divisions of levator ani

perineal body. Posteriorly, the coccygeus arises from the ischial spine and sacrospinous ligament and inserts into the coccyx and sacrum.

The striated muscle of the pelvic floor is composed of both slow and fast twitch muscle fibres. The slow twitch fibres provide muscle tone over a long period of time, thus supporting the pelvic viscera, while the fast twitch fibres react to sudden increases in intra-abdominal pressure.

## Urogenital diaphragm

The urogenital diaphragm (perineal membrane) is a triangular sheet of dense fibrous tissue spanning the anterior half of the pelvic outlet, which is pierced by the vagina and urethra. It arises from the inferior ischiopubic rami and attaches medially to the urethra, vagina and perineal body, thus supporting the pelvic floor.

## Perineal body

The perineal body lies between the vagina and the rectum and provides a point of insertion for the muscles of the pelvic floor. It is attached to the inferior pubic rami and ischial tuberosities through the urogenital diaphragm and superficial transverse perineal muscles. Laterally, it is attached

to the fibres of the pelvic diaphragm; posteriorly, it inserts into the external anal sphincter and coccyx.

## Pelvic fascia

The endopelvic fascia is a meshwork of collagen and elastin that represents the fused adventitial layers of the visceral structures and pelvic wall musculature. Condensations of the pelvic fascia are termed 'ligaments' and these have an important part in the supportive role of the pelvic floor.

## Uterine support

The parametrium, composed of the uterosacral and cardinal ligaments, attaches the cervix and upper vagina to the pelvic sidewall. The uterosacral ligament forms the medial margin bordering the pouch of Douglas; the cardinal ligaments attach the lateral aspects of the cervix and vagina to the pelvic sidewall over the sacrum. The former is composed mostly of smooth muscle, whereas the cardinal ligaments contain mostly connective tissue and the pelvic blood vessels. The round ligaments are not thought to have a role in supporting the uterus, although they may help to maintain anteversion and anteflexion; the broad ligaments are simply folds of peritoneum and provide no support.

## Vaginal support

Support to the upper third of the vagina is provided principally by the downward extension of the cardinal ligaments; the middle third is supported by lateral attachments to the arcus tendineus fasciae pelvis, a condensation of the obturator and levator fasciae. These supports suspend the anterior vaginal wall across the pelvis, the layer of fascia anterior to the vagina being called the 'pubocervical fascia'. Posterolaterally, the vagina is attached to the endopelvic fascia over the pelvic diaphragm and sacrum by the rectovaginal septum (fascia of Denonvilliers), which extends caudally into the perineal body and cranially into the peritoneum of the pouch of Douglas. The lower third is attached anteriorly to the pubic arch by the perineal membrane, posteriorly to the perineal body and laterally to the medial aspect of levator ani.

## Urethral support

The proximal urethra is supported by a sling of endopelvic fascia and the anterior vaginal wall, which is stabilized by lateral attachments to the arcus tendineus fasciae pelvis, and medial border of the levator ani. Contraction and relaxation of the levator muscles allows elevation or descent of the urethra, respectively, which is important in the control of voiding. In addition, an increase in intra-abdominal pressure causes compression of the urethra against the fixed anterior vaginal wall, thus maintaining continence. Bladder neck mobility and the stress continence mechanism are thus dependent on fascial integrity and connective tissue elasticity.

## AETIOLOGY

## Pregnancy and childbirth

The increased incidence of prolapse in multiparous women would suggest that pregnancy and childbirth have an important impact on the supporting function of the pelvic floor. Damage to the muscular and fascial supports of the pelvic floor and changes in innervation contribute to the development of prolapse.

The pelvic floor may be damaged during childbirth, causing the axis of the levator muscles to become more oblique and creating a funnel that allows the uterus, vagina and rectum to fall through the urogenital hiatus. In addition, the proportion of fascia to muscle within the pelvic floor tends to increase with increasing age, and thus once damaged by childbirth, muscle may never regain its full strength. This is supported by studies showing decreased cellularity and increased collagen content in 70 per cent of women with urogenital prolapse, compared to 20 per cent of normal controls.

Mechanical changes within the pelvic fascia have also been implicated in the causation of urogenital prolapse. During pregnancy, the fascia becomes more elastic and thus more likely to fail. This may explain the increased incidence of stress incontinence observed in pregnancy and the increased incidence of prolapse with multiparity.

Denervation of the pelvic musculature has been shown to occur following childbirth, although gradual denervation has also been demonstrated in nulliparous women with increasing age. However, the effects were greatest in those women who had documented stress incontinence or prolapse.[3] Furthermore, histological studies have revealed changes in muscle fibre type and distribution, suggesting denervation injury associated with ageing and also following childbirth. In conclusion, it would appear that partial denervation of the pelvic floor is part of the normal ageing process, although pregnancy and childbirth accelerate these changes.

The biochemical properties of connective tissue may also play an important role in the development of prolapse. Changes in collagen content have been identified, the hydroxyproline content in connective tissue from women with stress incontinence being 40 per cent lower than in continent controls. In addition, changes in collagen metabolism may be associated with the development of urogenital prolapse, increased levels of collagenases being associated with weakened pelvic support and stress incontinence.

## Hormonal factors

The effects of ageing and those of oestrogen withdrawal at the time of the menopause are often difficult to separate. Rectus muscle fascia has been shown to become less elastic with increasing age, and less energy is required to produce irreversible damage. Furthermore, there is also a reduction in skin collagen content following the menopause. Both of these factors lead to a reduction in the strength of the pelvic connective tissue.

More recently, oestrogen receptors, alpha and beta, have been demonstrated in the vaginal walls and the uterosacral ligaments of pre-menopausal women, although the beta receptor was absent from the vaginal walls in postmenopausal women. However, a further study was unable to identify oestrogen receptors in biopsies from the levator ani muscles in urinary incontinent women participating in pelvic floor exercises. In conclusion, it would appear that oestrogens and oestrogen withdrawal have a role in the development of urogenital prolapse, although the precise mechanism has yet to be established.

## Smoking

Chronic chest disease resulting in a chronic cough leads to an increase in the intra-abdominal pressure and thus exposes the pelvic floor to greater strain. Over a period of time this will exacerbate any defects in the pelvic floor musculature and fascia, leading to prolapse.

## Constipation

Chronically increased intra-abdominal pressure caused by repetitive straining will exacerbate any potential weaknesses in the pelvic floor and is also associated with an increased risk of prolapse.

## Obesity

Although obesity has been linked to urogenital prolapse due to a potential increase in intra-abdominal pressure, there has been no good evidence to support this theory.

## Exercise

Increased stress placed on the musculature of the pelvic floor will exacerbate pelvic floor defects and weakness, thus increasing the incidence of prolapse. Consequently, heavy lifting and exercise, as well as sports such as weight lifting, high-impact aerobics and long-distance running, increase the risk of urogenital prolapse.

## Surgery

Pelvic surgery may also have an effect on the occurrence of urogenital prolapse. Continence procedures, while elevating the bladder neck, may lead to defects in other pelvic compartments. At Burch colposuspension, the fixing of the lateral vaginal fornices to the ipsilateral ileopectineal ligaments leaves a potential defect in the posterior vaginal wall that predisposes to rectocele and enterocele formation. In a five-year follow-up study of women, 36 per cent had cystoceles, 66 per cent rectocele, 32 per cent enterocele and 38 per cent uterine prolapse. A further study of 109 women with vaginal vault prolapse reported that 43 per cent had previously undergone Burch colposuspension. Overall, 25 per cent of the women who had had Burch colposuspension required further surgery for prolapse.

Needle suspension procedures, such as the Pereyra or Stamey endoscopically guided bladder neck suspension, are also associated with an increased incidence of recurrent cystocele, although this is not the case following sling procedures. In addition, there is an increased incidence of posterior compartment defects, such as enterocele and rectocele, after Manchester repair, caused by the anterior plication of the uterosacral and cardinal ligaments, which leaves a large posterior hiatus.

The association between prolapse and prior hysterectomy is not as clear. One large study reported that 37 per cent of women had the onset of symptoms more than 37 years following hysterectomy, although 39 per cent of these women became symptomatic within two years. However, other factors, such as the ageing process and oestrogen withdrawal following the menopause, may also have an important role. Prolapse of the vaginal vault may present following either vaginal or abdominal hysterectomy, although the incidence is low, with only 0.5 per cent of women who have had a hysterectomy requiring further surgical intervention for vaginal vault prolapse.

## CLINICAL SYMPTOMS

Most women complain of a feeling of discomfort or heaviness within the pelvis in addition to a 'lump coming down'. Symptoms tend to become worse with prolonged standing and towards the end of the day. Women may also complain of dyspareunia, difficulty in inserting tampons and chronic lower backache. In cases of third-degree prolapse, there may be mucosal ulceration and lichenification, which results in a symptomatic vaginal discharge or bleeding.

A cystocele may be associated with lower urinary tract symptoms of urgency and frequency of micturition in addition to a sensation of incomplete emptying, which may be relieved by digitally reducing the prolapse. Recurrent urinary tract infections may also be associated with a chronic urinary residual. While less than 2 per cent of mild cystoceles are associated with ureteric obstruction, severe prolapse may lead to hydronephrosis and chronic renal damage. Between 33 and 92 per cent of cases of complete procidentia are associated with some degree of ureteric obstruction.

A rectocele may be associated with difficulty in opening the bowels, some women complaining of tenesmus and having to digitate to defaecate.

## CLINICAL SIGNS

Women are generally examined in the left lateral position using a Simms' speculum, although digital examination when standing allows more accurate assessment of the degree of urogenital prolapse and, in particular, vaginal vault support. An abdominal examination should also be performed to exclude the presence of an abdominal or pelvic tumour that may be responsible for the vaginal findings.

Differential diagnosis includes:

- vaginal cysts,
- pendunculated fibroid polyp,
- urethral diverticulum,
- chronic uterine inversion.

## INVESTIGATION

In women who also complain of concomitant lower urinary tract symptoms, urodynamic studies or a post-micturition bladder ultrasound should be performed in order to exclude a chronic residual due to associated voiding difficulties.

In such cases, a midstream specimen of urine should be sent for culture and sensitivity.

Subtracted cystometry, with or without videocystoure-thrography, will allow the identification of underlying detrusor overactivity, which is important to exclude prior to surgical repair. In cases of significant cystocele, stress testing should be carried out by asking the patient to cough while standing. Since occult urodynamic stress incontinence may be unmasked by straightening the urethra following anterior colporrhaphy, this should be simulated by the insertion of a ring pessary or tampon to reduce the cystocele. If stress incontinence is demonstrated, a continence procedure such as colposuspension or insertion of tension-free vaginal tape (TVT) may be a more appropriate procedure.

In cases of severe prolapse in which there may be a degree of ureteric obstruction, it is important to evaluate the upper urinary tract with either a renal tract ultrasound or an intravenous urogram.

Although a cystocele itself may be responsible for irritative urinary symptoms, if these are unusually severe cystoscopy should be performed to exclude a chronic follicular or interstitial cystitis.

## MANAGEMENT

### Prevention

In general, any factor that leads to chronic increases in intra-abdominal pressure should be avoided. Consequently, care should be taken to avoid constipation, which has been implicated as a major contributing factor to urogenital prolapse in Western society. In addition, the risk of prolapse in patients with chronic chest pathology, such as obstructive airways disease and asthma, should be reduced by effective management of these conditions. Hormone replacement therapy may also decrease the incidence of prolapse, although to date there are no studies that have tested this effect.

Smaller family size and improvements in antenatal and intrapartum care have also been implicated in the primary prevention of urogenital prolapse. The role of caesarean section may also be important, although studies examining the outcome in terms of incontinence and symptomatic prolapse have had mixed results. Equally, antenatal and postnatal pelvic floor exercises have not yet been shown conclusively to reduce the incidence of prolapse, although they may be protective.

### Physiotherapy

Pelvic floor exercises may have a role in the treatment of women with symptomatic prolapse, although there are no objective evidence-based studies to support this. Education about pelvic floor exercises may be supplemented with the use of a perineometer and biofeedback, allowing quantification of pelvic floor contractions. In addition, vaginal cones and electrical stimulation may also be used, although again, while they have been shown to be effective in the treatment of urodynamic stress incontinence, there are no data to support their use in the management of urogenital prolapse.

In summary, physiotherapy probably has a role in cases of mild prolapse in younger women who find an intravaginal device unacceptable and are not yet willing to consider definitive surgical treatment, especially if they have not yet completed their family.

### Intravaginal devices

The use of intravaginal devices offers a further conservative line of therapy for those women who are not candidates for surgery. Consequently, they may be used in younger women who have not yet completed their family, during pregnancy and the puerperium, and also for those women who may be unfit for surgery. Clearly, this last group of women may include the elderly, although age alone should not be seen as a contraindication to surgery. In addition, a pessary may offer symptomatic relief while awaiting surgery.

Ring pessaries made of silicone or polythene are currently most frequently used. They are available in a number of different sizes (52–120 mm) and are designed to lie horizontally in the pelvis with one side in the posterior fornix and the other just behind the pubis, hence providing support to the uterus and upper vagina. Pessaries should be changed every six months; long-term use may be complicated by vaginal ulceration and therefore a low-dose topical oestrogen may be helpful in post-menopausal women.

Ring pessaries may be useful in the management of minor degrees of urogenital prolapse, although in severe cases, and for vaginal vault prolapse, a shelf pessary may be more appropriate. These may be difficult to insert and remove and their use is becoming less common, especially as they preclude coitus.

## SURGERY

Surgery offers definitive treatment of urogenital prolapse. As in other forms of pelvic surgery, patients should receive prophylactic antibiotics to cover both Gram-negative and Gram-positive organisms, as well as thromboembolic prophylaxis in the form of low-dose heparin, and thromboembolic deterrent (TED) stockings.

All patients should also have a urethral catheter inserted at the time of the procedure unless there is a particular history of voiding dysfunction, in which case a suprapubic catheter may be more appropriate. This allows the residual urine volume to be checked following a void without the need for recatheterization.

Patients having pelvic surgery are positioned in lithotomy with the hips abducted and flexed. To minimize blood loss, local infiltration of the vaginal epithelium is performed using 0.5 per cent xylocaine and 1/200 000 adrenaline, although care should be taken in patients with coexistent cardiac disease. A vaginal pack may be inserted at the end of the procedure, and removed on the first post-operative day.

# Anterior compartment defects

## Anterior colporrhaphy

### Indication
Anterior coporrhaphy is indicated for the correction of cystourethrocele.

### Procedure
A midline incision is made in the vaginal epithelium from 1 cm below the urethral meatus to the cervix or vaginal vault. The cystocele is dissected off the overlying epithelium using sharp and blunt dissection and is secured using two polyglycolic (Vicryl, Ethicon) or polydioxanone (PDS, Ethicon) purse-string sutures. The redundant skin edges are then trimmed and the epithelium and fascia closed using interrupted polyglycolic (Vicryl, Ethicon) sutures.

In patients who have mild concurrent stress incontinence, a 'Kelly' mattress suture[4] may be placed under the urethrovesical junction, although colposuspension is preferable in cases of severe stress incontinence and will also cure a mild to moderate cystocele.

Lower urinary tract injury is uncommon. However, should a bladder or urethral injury occur, the defect can be repaired in layers using absorbable sutures and the bladder left on free drainage for ten days.

## Paravaginal repair

### Indication
Paravaginal repair is indicated for correction of cystourethrocele.

### Procedure
First described in 1909, this offers an abdominal approach to correct an anterior compartment defect. The retropubic space (cave of Retzius) is opened through a Pfannenstiel incision and the bladder swept medially, exposing the pelvic sidewall. The lateral sulcus of the vagina is elevated with the overlying pubocervical fascia and reattached to the pelvic sidewall using interrupted polydioxanone (PDS, Ethicon) sutures from the pubis to just anterior to the ischial spine. Long-term follow up in a series of 800 patients reported a cure rate of more than 95 per cent.[5]

# Posterior compartment defects

## Posterior colporrhaphy

### Indication
Posterior coporrhaphy is indicated for the correction of rectocele and deficient perineum.

### Procedure
Two Allis forceps are first placed on the perineum at the level of the hymenal remnants, allowing the calibre of the introitus to be estimated. Following infiltration, the perineal scarring is excised and the posterior vaginal wall opened using a longitudinal incision. The rectocele is mobilized from the vaginal epithelium by blunt and sharp dissection and secured using two or more polyglycolic (Vicryl, Ethicon) or polydioxanone (PDS, Ethicon) purse-string sutures. The redundant skin edges are then trimmed, taking care not to remove too much tissue and thus narrow the vagina. The pararectal and rectovaginal fasciae from each side are approximated using interrupted polyglycolic (Vicryl, Ethicon) sutures incorporating the vaginal epithelium, and the posterior wall is closed with a continuous polyglycolic (Vicryl, Ethicon) suture. Care should be taken not to create a constriction ring in the vagina, which will result in dyspareunia. Finally, a perineoplasty is performed by placing deeper absorbable sutures into the perineal muscles and fascia, thus building up the perineal body to provide additional support to the posterior vaginal wall and lengthening the vagina.

Injury to the rectum is unusual, but should be identified at the time of the procedure so that the defect can be closed in layers using an absorbable suture and the patient managed with prophylactic antibiotics, low-residue diet and faecal softening agents to avoid constipation.

Pelvic floor surgery may also have an adverse effect on sexual function. Following pelvic floor repairs with or without vaginal hysterectomy, 50 per cent of women reported sexual dysfunction, nearly half of the cases being due to shortening of the vagina, dyspareunia or fear of injury.[6] These findings have been confirmed more recently in a follow-up study of women undergoing posterior repair.[7] This series reported an increase in sexual dysfunction from 11 per cent pre-operatively to 27 per cent following surgery. In addition, 22 per cent of women complained of vaginal pain, 11 per cent had incontinence of faeces and 33 per cent had constipation.

## Enterocele repair

### Indication
Enterocele repair is indicated for the correction of enterocele.

### Procedure
An enterocele repair is normally performed using a vaginal approach similar to that of posterior colporrhaphy. The vaginal epithelium is dissected off the

enterocele sac, which is then secured using two or more polyglycolic (Vicryl, Ethicon) or polydioxanone (PDS, Ethicon) purse-string sutures. It is not essential to open the enterocele sac, although care should be taken not to damage any loops of small bowel that it may contain. The posterior vaginal wall is then closed as described for posterior colporrhaphy.

An abdominal approach may also be used, although this is much less common. The Moschowitz procedure[8] is performed by inserting concentric purse-string sutures around the peritoneum in the pouch of Douglas, thus preventing enterocele formation.

## Uterovaginal prolapse

### Vaginal hysterectomy

#### Indication
Vaginal hysterectomy is indicated for uterovaginal prolapse. This procedure may be combined with anterior and posterior colporrhaphy.

#### Contraindications (relative)
- Uterine size >14 weeks gestation, although morcellation[9] or uterine bisection may be used.
- Two or more caesarean sections.
- Endometriosis.
- Pelvic inflammatory disease.
- Suspected malignancy (uterine or ovarian).

#### Procedure
A cervical incision is performed and the uterovesical fold and pouch of Douglas opened. The uterosacral and cardinal ligaments are divided and ligated first, followed by the uterine pedicles and finally the tubo-ovarian and round ligament pedicles. In cases of procidentia, care should be taken to avoid kinking of the ureters, which are often dragged into a lower position than normal. After closure of the pelvic peritoneum, the upper pedicles are tied in the midline to provide support for the vaginal vault, while the uterosacral ligaments are tied posteriorly to obliterate the potential enterocele space. In addition, a McCall suture[10] may be performed, bringing the two uterosacral ligaments together in the midline as a further precaution against enterocele formation. Inclusion of the upper posterior vaginal wall also provides additional vault support. The vaginal epithelium is then closed with interrupted sutures.

### Uterine preserving surgery
Uterine prolapse can also be treated with 'uterus sparing' procedures where an attempt is made to suspend the uterus rather than remove it through a hysterectomy. The evidence base for such procedures is very limited and largely anecdotal. The indications to preserve the uterus may be as follows:

- preservation of fertility,
- role of uterus in orgasm and female sexuality,
- influence on female sexual identity,
- lack of uterine pathology.

#### Routes
- *Abdominal*: Sacrospinous hysteropexy, Shirodkar's sling, pectineal ligament suspension.
- *Vaginal*: Manchester repair, sacrospinous hysteropexy and uterosacral ligament plication have been described.
- *Laparoscopic*: Round ligament plication, sacrohysteropexy, uterosacral plication.

## Manchester repair (Fothergill repair)

#### Procedure
This procedure is only rarely performed nowadays. Cervical amputation is followed by approximating and shortening the cardinal ligaments anterior to the cervical stump and elevating the uterus. This is combined with an anterior and posterior colporrhaphy. The operation has fallen from favour, as the long-term complications include fertility problems in addition to recurrent uterovaginal prolapse and enterocele formation.

## Vaginal vault prolapse

Vaginal vault prolapse occurs equally commonly following vaginal or abdominal hysterectomy, with an incidence of approximately 5 per cent, although only 0.5 per cent of women require further surgery.

### Sacrospinous ligament fixation

#### Indication
Sacrospinous ligament fixation is indicated for vaginal vault prolapse.

#### Procedure
A longitudinal posterior vaginal wall incision is performed to expose the rectovaginal space. The right ischial spine is then identified and exposed using sharp and blunt dissection. The sacrospinous ligament may then be palpated running from the ischial spine to the lower aspect of the sacrum. An absorbable braided polyglycolic suture (Dexon, Davies + Geck) is passed through the ligament using a Miya hook ligature carrier and then through the vaginal vault. Care must be taken to avoid the sacral plexus and sciatic nerve, which are superior, and the pudendal vessels and nerve, which are lateral to the ischial spine. Once the enterocele has been secured using two purse-string sutures, the upper third of the vagina is closed as previously described. The sacrospinous sutures are then tied to support the vaginal vault from the sacrospinous ligament, following which a perineorrhaphy is performed.

Success rates of 98 per cent have been reported,[11] although posterior fixation of the posterior vaginal wall increases the incidence of anterior compartment defects.

For this reason, it should not be performed routinely at vaginal hysterectomy. As the vaginal axis is changed by the procedure, there is a risk of post-operative dyspareunia and development of stress incontinence.

## Abdominal sacrocolpopexy

### Indication

Abdominal sacrocolpopexy is indicated for vaginal vault prolapse.

### Procedure

This procedure may be performed through a lower midline or Pfannenstiel incision after packing the vagina. The apex of the vagina and sacral promontory are identified and a retroperitoneal tunnel is created between the two just to the right of the midline and medial to the right ureter. A strip of Mersilene tape is then passed through the peritoneal tunnel and sutured to the vaginal vault and posterior vaginal wall using interrupted, non-absorbable ethylene sutures (Ethibond, Ethicon). Once the other end of the tape has been secured to the periosteum overlying the sacral promontory, the sutures are tied, allowing gentle elevation of the vaginal vault towards the sacrum, but without tension. The peritoneum is then closed over the vaginal vault and sacral promontory. Complications include bleeding from the presacral venous plexus and sacral artery and damage to the right ureter and sigmoid colon.

A 93 per cent success rate has been reported,[12] although associated cystocele or rectocele may still require a vaginal colporrhaphy. In addition, since the vaginal axis is changed, there is also the risk of developing dyspareunia and stress incontinence following the procedure. Mesh erosion into the vagina, and rarely into the bladder or bowel, is a possible late complication.

A recent Cochrane review into surgical management of prolapse showed that abdominal sacrocolpopexy is associated with a lower rate of recurrent vault prolapse and dyspareunia than the vaginal sacrospinous colpopexy. These benefits must be balanced against a longer operating time, longer time to return to activities of daily living and increased cost of the abdominal approach.[13]

## Posterior intravaginal slingplasty

### Indication

Posterior intravaginal slingplasty (IVS) is indicated for vaginal vault prolapse.

### Procedure

The posterior intravaginal slingplasty, using an 8-mm polypropylene tape, has been described as a minimally invasive procedure for the treatment of vaginal vault prolapse. Under tension, a 5-cm transverse full thickness incision is made in the posterior vaginal wall 1.5 cm below the scar line at the vaginal vault. Adjacent rectocele and

enterocele are than dissected out so as to avoid accidental damage while passing the IVS tunneller (Tyco Healthcare, Mansfield, MA, USA) needle. Bilateral 1-cm perineal skin incisions are then made 2 cm lateral and below the external anal sphincter at the 4 and 8 o'clock positions.

Next, the IVS tunneller is advanced 4 cm into the ischirectal fossa before being turned inwards and guided using a finger through the rectovaginal fascia so as to exit through the transverse vaginal incision. The procedure is then repeated on the contralateral side and a rectal examination performed to exclude bowel injury. The tape is then secured to the vaginal vault using polydioxanone (PDS, Ethicon) and the vagina closed with interupted polyglycolic (Vicryl, Ethicon) sutures. A posterior colpoperineorrhaphy is then performed as previously described. Finally, the polypropylene tape is pulled posteriorly through the bilateral buttock incisions pulling the vaginal vault in a posterosuperior direction. The tape is then cut flush with the skin and incisions closed using interrupted sutures.

To date, only one retrospective series of posterior intravaginal slingplast has been reported[14] with symptomatic cure rates of 91 per cent. However, there were five cases of tape rejection, one rectal tape erosion and one rectal perforation. Consequently, while early data would appear to be encouraging, more studies are required to determine its role in the management of vaginal vault prolapse.

## Recurrent urogenital prolapse

Approximately one-third of operations for urogenital prolapse are for recurrent defects. Recurrent prolapse may occur following both abdominal and vaginal hysterectomy, previous vaginal repairs and continence surgery. In addition, women with intrinsically weak connective tissue, such as patients with Elhers Danlos syndrome, are at increased risk.

In such cases, the vaginal epithelium may be scarred and atrophic, making surgical correction technically more difficult and increasing the risk of damage to the bladder and bowel. The risk of post-operative complications, such as dyspareunia secondary to vaginal shortening and stenosis, is also increased. In those women who have had a previous continence operation, such as colposuspension, there is an increased risk of recurrent incontinence that may require further surgical correction.

## Mesh repair

The use of synthetic mesh is becoming increasingly common in patients with prolapse, and may offer further support in cases in which the endopelvic fascia and vaginal epithelium are felt to be deficient. The ideal mesh should be strong and flexible, allowing ease of use. In addition, woven meshes should have an adequate pore size to allow the ingrowth of fibroblasts so as to minimize the risks of erosion and rejection.

Vaginal mesh kits are being used to surgically treat apical vaginal prolapse; however, their safety and efficacy are currently unknown. Several companies now market these 'mesh kits' despite lack of robust evidence regarding their safety and efficacy. A recent systematic review of these kits suggests that although they are associated with high objective cure rates between 87 and 95 per cent, they have a high risk of mesh erosion (4.6–10.7 per cent) and re-operation rates of up to 6 per cent.[15]

Dyspareunia is a common complication associated with the use of synthetic mesh and may be associated with erosion into the vagina, lower urinary tract and rectum. Although the use of mesh is becoming more common, it should be reserved for those patients with recurrent defects in specialist pelvic floor reconstructive surgery units.

## CONCLUSION

Although not life-threatening, urogenital prolapse is responsible for a significant degree of morbidity and impairment of quality of life. With approximately half of elective gynaecological operations being performed for correction of urogenital prolapse, the economic considerations are also considerable. In common with continence procedures, the initial procedure offers the greatest probability of success, and therefore patients should be carefully assessed with regard to their symptoms and investigations prior to surgery.

Although conservative measures may be useful in the management of mild symptomatic prolapse, surgery offers the definitive treatment. The number of surgical procedures described is indicative of the fact that there is no perfect solution, and this is reflected in the number of patients who complain of recurrent prolapse. Such women should be managed in tertiary units by surgeons with a specialist interest in pelvic floor reconstructive surgery.

### KEY POINTS

- Urogenital prolapse is a common condition associated with a high degree of morbidity.
- Incidence increases with increasing age and parity.
- Lifetime risk of surgery for urogenital prolapse is 11 per cent.
- Urogenital prolapse may be associated with concomitant urinary and faecal incontinence.
- Conservative management involves pelvic floor exercises and the use of vaginal pessaries.
- Surgery should be tailored to the needs of the individual patient.
- The use of synthetic mesh should be reserved for repeat procedures only.
- There is a high risk of recurrence following surgery, with a third of women requiring a further procedure.
- Complicated or recurrent cases are best managed using a multi-disciplinary approach.

## Key References

1. Subak LL, Waetjen E, van den Eeden S *et al.* Cost of pelvic organ prolapse surgery in the United States. *Obstet Gynecol* 2001; **98**: 646–51.
2. Abrams P, Blaivas JG, Stanton SL, Andersen JT. The International Continence Society Committee on Standardization of Terminology. The standardization of terminology of lower urinary tract function. *Scand J Urol Nephrol* 1988; **114S**: 5–19.
3. Smith ARB, Hosker GL, Warrell DW. The role of partial denervation of the pelvic floor in the aetiology of genitourinary prolapse and stress incontinence. A neurophysiological study. *Br J Obstet Gynaecol* 1989; **96**: 24–8.
4. Kelly HA. Incontinence of urine in women. *Urol Cutan Rev* 1913; **17**: 291–7.
5. Richardson AC. Paravaginal repair. In: Benson JT (ed.). *Female Pelvic Floor Disorders*. New York: Norton, 1992: 280–7.
6. Francis WJA, Jeffcoate TNA. Dyspareunia following vaginal operations. *Br J Obstet Gynaecol* 1961; **68**: 1.
7. Kahn MA, Stanton SL. Posterior colporrhaphy: its effects on bowel and sexual function. *Br J Obstet Gynaecol* 1997; **104**: 82–6.
8. Muschovitz AV. The pathogenesis, anatomy and cure of prolapse of the rectum. *Surg Gynecol Obstet* 1912; **15**: 7.
9. Magos A, Bournas N, Sinha R *et al.* Vaginal hysterectomy for the large uterus. *Br J Obstet Gynaecol* 1996; **103**: 246–51.
10. McCall ML. Posterior culdoplasty. *Obstet Gynecol* 1957; **10**: 595.
11. Shull BL, Capen CV, Riggs MW, Kuehl TJ. Pre-operative and post-operative analysis of site-specific pelvic support defects in 81 women treated with sacrospinous ligament suspension and pelvic reconstruction. *Am J Obstet Gynecol* 1992; **166**: 1764–71.
12. Addison WA, Livergood CH, Parker RT. Post hysterectomy vaginal vault prolapse with emphasis on management by transabdominal sacral colpopexy. *Post Grad Obstet Gynaecol* 1988; **81**.
13. Maher C, Baessler K, Glazener CM *et al.* Surgical management of pelvic organ prolapse in women: a short version Cochrane review. *Neurourol Urodyn* 2008; **27**: 3–12.
14. Farnsworth BN. Posterior intravaginal slingplasty (infracoccygeal sacrocolpopexy) for severe posthysterectomy vaginal vault prolapse – a preliminary report on efficacy and safety. *Int Urogynecol J* 2002; **13**: 4–8.
15. Feiner B, Jelovsek JE, Maher C. Efficacy and safety of transvaginal mesh kits in the treatment of prolapse of the vaginal apex: a systematic review. *BJOG.* 2009; **116**: 15–24.

# 64.1 Infection and sexual health

*Melanie Mann*

---

## MRCOG standards

### Theoretical competencies
- Know the evidence for diagnosing, treating and following up pelvic inflammatory disease (PID).
- Know which infections of the genital tract are transmitted sexually.
- Understand the pathological course of sexually transmitted infections (STIs).
- Understand how to investigate and manage STIs when encountered in the gynaecological setting.
- Know the law related to STIs.
- Recognize the sexual healthcare needs of vulnerable groups: young people, commercial sex workers, asylum seekers, drug users and prisoners.
- Understand the National Chlamydia Screening programme and local implementation.
- Understand local care pathways for multi-agency working and cross-referrals for individuals with sexual health needs.

### Clinical competencies
- Take a history in relation to sexual health needs: counsel women sensitively, display tact, empathy and concern.
- Respect confidentiality.
- Explain clearly and openly treatments, complications and adverse effects of drug treatment.
- Demonstrate effective liaison with colleagues in other disciplines, such as genitourinary medicine, counsellors.
- Respect cultural and sexual diversity.
- Recognize and manage common clinical presentations of STIs in the female patient, e.g. dysuria, discharge, genital ulceration (including performing appropriate investigations, treating and arranging follow up, according to local protocols).
- Revise the causes of pelvic pain.

- Recognize presentations of complications of common STIs, e.g. acute pelvic inflammatory disease.
- Recognize and manage clinical presentations of non-STI genital infections, e.g. bacterial vaginosis.
- Explain the principles of partner notification and epidemiological treatment for sexual contacts.
- Perform an HIV risk assessment and discuss HIV transmission with women, including pre-test discussion and appropriate management of results, both positive and negative.
- Give appropriate advice to an HIV-positive woman about available interventions to prevent vertical transmission in pregnancy.
- Assess risk for hepatitis A/B/C infections and arrange appropriate vaccination for at-risk groups according to local protocol.
- Understand the psychological and psychosocial aspects of living with HIV/AIDS and STIs.
- Demonstrate the ability to promote healthy lifestyles, including safer sex.

---

## PELVIC INFLAMMATORY DISEASE

This section covers the diagnosis, treatment and follow up of PID. PID is important because it can have serious long-term sequelae, such as pelvic pain, ectopic pregnancy and infertility. It is the result of post-infection scarring that is normally associated with healing. The virulence of the infection and the host–immune factors both determine the extent of the damage caused. There may be complete tubal closure, extensive peritubal adhesions, intra-tubal adhesions, mucosal and cilial damage, all of which can cause ectopic pregnancy and infertility (including interference with ovum transport and sperm migration). In a large, multicentre World Health Organization (WHO) study of more than 8000 couples in 25 countries investigated for infertility, approximately 32 per cent of diagnoses were tubal factor infertility in the female.

## Incidence

The incidence of PID is unknown, as many cases go unnoticed until investigations for infertility are performed. There is no record of cases of PID held nationally apart from diagnosed records of all attendances at genitourinary (GUM) clinics (KC60 returns). Approximately 1 in 60 consultations in general practice is for women less than 45 years for suspected PID.

## Aetiology

*Neisseria gonorrhoeae* and *Chlamydia trachomatis* are the most important organisms, although *Gardnerella vaginalis*, anaerobes and other organisms, such as mycoplasmas commonly found in the vagina may also be implicated.

Other factors associated with PID include:

- young age (<25 years),
- multiple sexual partners,
- past history of STI (in the patient or her partners),
- termination of pregnancy,
- insertion of an intrauterine contraceptive device in the previous 6 weeks,
- hysterosalpingography,
- *in-vitro* fertilization procedure,
- postpartum endometritis,
- bacterial vaginosis,
- a recent new sexual partner (within the previous three months).

## Diagnosis

Pelvic inflammatory disease can be symptomatic or asymptomatic. Even in symptomatic patients, clinical symptoms and signs lack sensitivity and specificity. The positive predictive value of a clinical diagnosis is 65–90 per cent compared to laparoscopic diagnosis in experienced hands. The symptoms suggestive of PID include:

- lower abdominal pain,
- fever >38°C,
- dyspareunia,
- unscheduled vaginal bleeding,
- abnormal vaginal discharge.

The signs associated with PID are usually also non-specific. Pyrexia may be present, but not exclusively. Lower abdominal and adnexal tenderness on bimanual examination, as well as cervical excitation (cervical motion tenderness) on bimanual examination, are indicative of acute inflammation affecting the pelvic peritoneum. However, they are not specific for PID. Other conditions that should be considered when assessing lower abdominal pain in a young woman include:

- ectopic pregnancy,
- acute appendicitis,
- urinary tract infection,
- endometriosis,
- complications of an ovarian cyst (torsion or rupture),
- constipation,
- functional pain (pain of unknown origin).

## Investigation of suspected pelvic inflammatory disease

Testing for gonorrhoea and chlamydia in the lower genital tract is recommended, as positive results support a diagnosis (see p. 739–741 for details on testing for gonorrhoea and chlamydia). Taking an additional test from the urethra in suspected PID is only recommended if nucleic acid amplification tests (NAAT) are not available.

However, the absence of infection at this site does not exclude PID. Absence of cultured organisms may be due to poor sampling technique, inadequate storage and/or transportation of swabs or the presence of organisms that cannot easily be cultured in the laboratory, such as mycoplasmas. An elevated erythrocyte sedimentation rate (ESR) or C-reactive protein (CRP) can support the diagnosis.

Laparoscopy may strongly support the diagnosis of PID, but is not justified routinely on the basis of cost and invasiveness. Furthermore, even laparoscopy lacks the sensitivity to identify mild intratubal inflammation or endometritis reliably.

Endometrial biopsy and ultrasound scanning may also be helpful when there is diagnostic difficulty, but there is insufficient evidence to support their routine use at present.

## Management

It is likely that delay in treatment increases the risk of the development of long-term sequelae of PID, such as ectopic pregnancy, pelvic pain and infertility. Owing to this, and to the lack of definitive diagnostic criteria, it is recommended that clinicians have a low threshold for treating empirically. It is also important that women are not labelled with the wrong diagnosis just because they appear to be in a high-risk group for having PID. Effort must be made to confirm the correct diagnosis, particularly in difficult or recurrent episodes of lower abdominal pain. It is also important in the gynaecological setting not to forget to investigate and treat the sexual partner(s), in order to prevent reinfection.

## General measures

- Rest is advised for severe disease (preferably as an inpatient for observation to check that there is resolution of symptoms and signs) [C].
- A pregnancy test should be performed [C].
- Appropriate analgesia is advised [C].
- Parenteral therapy as an inpatient is advised for those with severe disease [C].
- Patients should avoid sexual intercourse until they and their partners have been fully treated and contact traced [C].

A full explanation should be given to the patient regarding the short- and long-term issues associated with PID. Leaflets to clarify and back up verbal explanation should be given to the client and her partner, if present.

All patients should be offered full STI screening and human immunodeficiency virus (HIV) testing at some point in the management [C]. Good links with local genitourinary medicine (GUM) clinics are essential.

## Antibiotic treatment

Broad-spectrum antibiotics are needed that will cover gonorrhoea and chlamydia. This treatment should be commenced as soon as possible. Information on recent and current medications should be obtained and appropriate advice given regarding any interactions, e.g. with hormonal contraception. There is a lack of evidence regarding antibiotic use and the prevention of long-term complications and fewer data on oral than parenteral regimens. There are important factors to be considered when choosing a regimen:

- local antimicrobial sensitivities (especially gonorrhoea),
- local epidemiology of infections (knowing where there are high-prevalence areas for gonorrhoea),
- cost,
- patient preference and likelihood of compliance,
- severity of disease.

When considering selection for inpatient treatment, the uncertainty of the diagnosis and severity of the disease will usually be sufficient to identify those who require inpatient observation. Other cases for which inpatient supervision is advised include women who have failed to respond to orally administered outpatient therapy, those who are suspected of having a tubo-ovarian mass and those who are unable to tolerate oral therapy. Two special subgroups might also be considered for inpatient treatment: those known to have an immunodeficiency problem (where a much more severe disease situation can develop quickly) and those who are pregnant – PID can occur up to about 12 weeks of pregnancy.

### Recommended regimens

The following are evidence based. Intravenous therapy should be continued until 24 hours after clinical improvement and then switched to oral treatment [B].

Outpatient regimens
- Oral ofloxacin 400 mg twice daily plus oral metronidazole 400 mg twice daily for 14 days.
- Intramuscular (i.m.) ceftriaxone 250 mg single dose or i.m. cefoxitin 2 g single dose with oral probenecid 1 g followed by oral doxycycline 100 mg daily plus metronidazole 400 mg twice daily for 14 days.
- Ofloxacin should be avoided in women at high risk of gonococcal PID due to increased quinolone resistance in the United Kingdom.

There is no evidence of one antibiotic regime listed above being superior to the others.

Inpatient regimens
Inpatient antibiotic treatment should be based on intravenous therapy which should be continued until 24 hours after clinical improvement and followed by oral therapy. Recommended regimens are:

- ceftriaxone 2 g by intravenous infusion daily plus intravenous doxycycline 100 mg twice daily, followed by oral doxycycline 100 mg twice daily plus oral metronidazole 400 mg twice daily for a total of 14 days;
- oral doxycycline may be used, if tolerated, while on intravenous ceftriaxone.

or

- intravenous clindamycin 900 mg three times daily plus intravenous gentamicin, followed by either
  - oral clindamycin 450 mg four times daily to complete 14 days.

or

  - oral doxycycline 100 mg twice daily plus oral metronidazole 400 mg twice daily to complete 14 days.
- Gentamicin should be given as a 2 mg/kg loading dose followed by 1.5 mg/kg three times daily (or a single daily dose of 7 mg/kg may be substituted).
- Intravenous ofloxacin 400 mg twice daily plus intravenous metronidazole 500 mg three times daily for 14 days.

The clinical trial data support the use of cefoxitin for the treatment of PID, but this agent is not easily available in the UK so ceftriaxone, which has a similar spectrum of activity, is recommended. An alternative third-generation cephalosporin would also be acceptable.

If parenteral gentamicin is used, then serum drug levels and renal function should be monitored.

The choice of an appropriate treatment regimen will be influenced by robust evidence on local antimicrobial sensitivity patterns, robust evidence on the local epidemiology of specific infections, cost, the woman's preference and compliance, and severity of disease.

Evidence of the efficacy of antibiotic therapy in preventing the long-term complications of PID is currently limited.

If the above regimens are not available, 14 days therapy to cover *N. gonorrhoeae* (quinolones, cephalosporins, penicillin – bearing in mind sensitivities locally), *C. trachomatis* (tetracyclines, macrolides) and anaerobic bacteria (metronidazole) should be used. Metronidazole may be discontinued in those women with mild or moderate PID who are unable to tolerate it, since its addition provides uncertain additional efficacy in this patient group.

## Other important situations

Women with PID who are also infected with HIV should be treated with the same antibiotic regimens as women who are HIV-negative. Hospital admission and parenteral treatment is only required for those with clinically severe disease. Potential interactions between antibiotics and antiretroviral drugs should be considered.

The risk of giving any of the recommended antibiotic regimens in very early pregnancy (before a positive pregnancy test) is low, since significant drug toxicity results in failed implantation.

Pregnant women should ideally receive i.v. therapy, as PID is associated with higher maternal and fetal morbidity. (However, PID in pregnancy is rare except for septic abortion.) None of the regimens above is of proven safety in this group. There is insufficient evidence in pregnant women to suggest one treatment over another as long as the appropriate organisms are covered for 14 days treatment and this is parenteral, if possible.

Consideration should be given to removing an intrauterine contraceptive device (IUD) in women presenting with PID, especially if symptoms have not resolved within 72 hours [A].

The randomized controlled trial evidence for whether an IUD should be left in place or removed in women presenting with PID is limited. Removal of the IUD should be considered and may be associated with better short-term clinical outcomes, but the decision to remove it needs to be balanced against the risk of pregnancy in those who have had otherwise unprotected intercourse in the preceding 7 days. Hormonal emergency contraception may be appropriate for some women in this situation.

Fitz–Hugh–Curtis syndrome comprises right upper quadrant pain associated with perihepatitis, which occurs in up to 10–20 per cent of women with PID and may be the most obvious symptom. There is insufficient evidence to recommend laparoscopic adhesiolysis in this situation.

Management of partners should be by testing and treatment, ideally in a GUM clinic. Empirical treatment should be given anyway, if testing cannot be done. Contact tracing of all partners in the previous six months is recommended.

## Follow up

All patients should be followed up at 3 days to check improvement and exclude the need for parenteral or surgical treatment. Further review at 4 weeks is recommended to check resolution of symptoms, pregnancy test where appropriate and to discuss long-term issues. It is also an ideal time to check up on partner notification and treatment.

## SEXUALLY TRANSMITTED INFECTIONS

This section focuses generally on the management of women, but one should not forget to consider partners and to think about them when talking about this aspect of gynaecology. Talking about these very personal aspects

of a woman's life is very important and all gynaecologists need to be able to talk about sex sensitively and non-judgementally in order to do the best for the patient. It is therefore important that clinicians practise taking a sexual history to achieve this (see below).

Sexually transmitted infections are an important part of the everyday work of a gynaecologist and these conditions can have long-term sequelae for the patient if not managed promptly and thoroughly. The majority of large towns and cities in the UK have a department of GUM with at least one specialist employed. It is good practice to develop strong links with this local department to improve the overall management of STIs within each gynaecology unit. This will ensure that patients receive optimum evidence-based treatment and that contact tracing and partner notification are performed according to approved guidelines.

### Taking a sexual history to assess the risk of STI

Preface by warning the patient that you need to ask some personal questions to do with her relationships with partners.

*I need to ask you some personal questions now.*
*Are you in a sexual relationship?*

You need to find out if this is a heterosexual or homosexual relationship. This is one of the most difficult questions. You can ask the first name of the partner and then clarify whether male or female if the first name is equivocal, e.g. Nicky or Chris. Or you can say,

*Can I just check, is your partner male or female?*
*How long have you been with your partner?*

Avoid the term 'steady' or 'long term' as these have different meanings for different people.

*Do you or your partner have any other partners, as far as you are aware?*

In some situations, it is important to ask about different sexual practices, such as oral or anal sex. Sometimes patients may volunteer the information that sex in a particular position causes discomfort, so it is important to be able to discuss this openly.

## Basic tenets of GUM

- The patient's confidentiality is paramount and patient details are not given to other patients or other healthcare professionals without the patient's informed consent (see below). Sexual history taking should take place in a private environment.
- If a patient has an STI, at least one other person is also carrying it and needs to be sought, treated and contact traced.

- If a patient has one STI, she must be at risk of all other STIs. She should therefore be offered screening for all other infections. This will often be carried out in a GUM clinic.
- When swabs for STI are taken, it is important to obtain informed consent about the nature of the tests and explain what the follow-up procedure will be if the test is positive for a STI.
- Patients diagnosed with an STI should be advised not to have sexual intercourse until they and their partners have completed treatment and follow up. This is to minimize further spread or reinfection.
- Patients should be given a detailed account of their condition, with particular emphasis on the long-term implications for themselves and their partner(s). This should be reinforced with clear and accurate written information.

## Law relating to STIs

All National Health Service employees are required to adhere to the Caldicott principles for confidentiality and there is also explicit guidance from the General Medical Council to emphasize the importance. Confidentiality is a common law duty and is absolute except in special circumstances such as when breaking confidentiality would be in the patient's or the public's best interests, e.g. child protection cases.

The Venereal Diseases Act 1917 applies to GUM clinics and makes the rules of confidentiality even stricter: patient records are locked away and are not accessible to other clinicians outside the department, including the GP, without the express consent of the patient.

## Terms used in GUM clinics

### Partner notification

Contact slips, with a nationally agreed code for each STI, are given to patients to pass on to their sexual contacts. Contacts can then present the slip at any GUM clinic in the UK, where the infection will be managed appropriately. This is because there is communication between GUM clinics regarding partner notification.

### Contact tracing

This involves finding the sexual contacts of the index patient carrying an infection and managing them appropriately, including ongoing partner notification if possible.

### Health advisors

These are specially trained professionals whose job is to educate patients in the GUM clinics about STIs, including pretest counselling for HIV. They are also responsible for most partner notification and contact tracing.

## Gonorrhoea

Gonorrhoea is a sexually transmitted infection caused by the Gram-negative diplococcus *N. gonorrhoeae*. The primary sites of infection are the mucous membranes of the urethra, endocervix, rectum, pharynx and conjunctiva. Transmission occurs as a result of direct inoculation of secretions from one mucous membrane to another. Vertical transmission from mother to fetus may also occur during labour.

### Clinical features

Up to 50 per cent of women are asymptomatic. In those who do have symptoms, the most common are an increased or altered vaginal discharge (up to 50 per cent) and lower abdominal pain (up to 25 per cent). Urethral infection may cause dysuria (12 per cent), but not usually frequency. Gonorrhoea is a rare cause of intermenstrual bleeding or menorrhagia and this is due to infection of the endometrium (endometritis). Infection in the pharynx is usually asymptomatic.

In men, the infection may also be asymptomatic (10 per cent), but generally causes urethral discharge (80 per cent) or dysuria (50 per cent).

### Clinical signs

Less than 50 per cent of women will present with muco-purulent endocervical discharge and easily induced endocervical bleeding, and less than 5 per cent will present with pelvic or lower abdominal tenderness. Commonly, no abnormal findings are present on clinical examination. In men, there is usually a purulent urethral discharge present. Epididymal tenderness or balanitis, although reported, is rare.

Gonorrhoea is also transmitted vertically to the fetus. It can cause severe conjunctivitis (ophthalmia neonatorum) and this is a notifiable disease in the UK. Neonatal infections can be severe and should be managed systemically by a paediatrician/ophthalmologist.

### Complications

Transluminal spread of *N. gonorrhoeae* may occur, causing PID (<10 per cent) and epididymo-orchitis (<1 per cent) in men. Haematogenous dissemination can also occur, causing skin lesions, arthralgia, arthritis and tenosynovitis. Disseminated gonococcal infection is rare (<1 per cent).

### Diagnosis

The most reliable diagnosis is achieved by identification by culture of the organism from an infected site. Specimen collection in women should be from the endocervix and urethra, with the swab being rotated to obtain purulent secretions, if present. Infection of the cervix is present in 90 per cent of women with gonorrhoea, and the use of cervical culture as a single screening test for gonorrhoea has a sensitivity of 85 per cent. Ideally, culture should be directly

Pelvic floor and lower urinary tract dysfunction

onto selective medium which has been impregnated with antibiotics to prevent overgrowth of unwanted organisms. Gonorrhoea, under different circumstances, may not be cultured easily and so refrigeration of swabs prior to transport to the laboratory is recommended.

Nucleic acid amplification tests can also be used. NAATs are more sensitive than culture and can also be used as diagnostic/screening tests on non-invasively collected specimens (urine and self-taken vaginal swabs). Comparisons between NAATs and culture suggest the sensitivity of NAATs exceeds 90 per cent for genital sites, while the sensitivity of culture may be less than 75 per cent for endocervical swabs. This probably indicates that NAATs are less affected than culture by inadequacies in collection and transport of specimens. NAAT-positive tests should be confirmed by culture and sensitivities to antibiotics checked.

It is important to follow local guidance and liaise with the laboratory.

## Management

All patients should be treated if they have a positive test result or if a recent partner has confirmed gonococcal disease and testing of the patient is not possible. Referral to GUM is highly recommended [B].

Recommended treatments:

Uncomplicated anogenital infection in adults:

- Ceftriaxone 250 mg IM as a single dose. (Grade A recommendation)

or

- Cefixime 400 mg oral as a single dose. (Grade A recommendation)

or

- Spectinomycin* 2 g IM as a single dose. (Grade A recommendation)
- Surveillance data for 2004 shows significant levels of N. gonorrhoeae resistance to penicillin ( 11.2%), tetracyclines (44.5%) and ciprofloxacin (14.1%) in the UK. Most resistant infections are acquired in the UK.
- Antimicrobial therapy should take account of local patterns of antimicrobial sensitivity to N. gonorrhoeae. The chosen regimen should eliminate infection in at least 95% of those presenting in the local community

This issue of local resistance patterns is another reason why all cases should be referred to GUM in the UK.

## Treatment of gonorrhoea when pregnant or breastfeeding

Pregnant women should not be treated with quinolone or tetracycline antibiotics.

Recommended regimes
- Ceftriaxone 250 mg i.m. as a single dose [A], or
- Cefotaxime 500 mg i.m. as a single dose [A], or

- Spectinomycin 2 mg i.m. as a single dose [A], or
- Ampicillin 2 or 3 g plus probenecid 1 g orally as a single dose where regional prevalence of penicillin-resistant N. gonorrhoeae is <5 per cent [A].

In the case of allergy, the above regimes can be used.

Co-infection with C. trachomatis is common (up to 40 per cent of women) and therefore screening and, if positive, treatment should always be performed. In many departments, epidemiological treatment for chlamydia is given at the same time as gonococcal disease is treated. Partner notification and contact tracing should be performed as described previously [B].

## Follow up

At least one follow-up visit is recommended to confirm compliance with therapy, resolution of symptoms and partner notification. A test of cure is not usually performed in UK practice, if the above regimes are used for treatment.

All cases of gonorrhoea should be seen by a trained person (ideally a health advisor in genitourinary medicine) for partner notification and contact tracing.

# Chlamydia trachomatis

## National Chlamydia Screening Programme

The National Chlamydia Screening Programme (NCSP) is a control and prevention programme targeted at sexually active young people under 25 years. Chlamydia is the most common bacterial sexually transmitted infection in the UK, affecting both men and women. Most people with chlamydia have no symptoms, but left untreated, chlamydia, can lead, in women, to infertility, ectopic pregnancy and chronic pelvic pain. In men, it may cause urethritis and epydidimitis. In both sexes, it can cause arthritis.

The Chief Medical Officer's Expert Advisory Group on Chlamydia trachomatis (1998) considered the evidence base associated with screening for genital chlamydial infection. This group concluded that chlamydia screening met the criteria for a screening programme and recommended that one be established. Since then, the evidence base for chlamydial screening has continued to develop. Mathematical modelling data show that the prevalence of chlamydial infection will be reduced by 30 per cent after one year and 70 per cent after five years, if there is 30 per cent coverage and 20 per cent partner notification in both men and women. Continuous opportunistic screening at 50 per cent coverage (20 per cent partner notification) would reduce prevalence by 40 per cent after one year and 80 per cent after seven years. The National Chlamydia Screening Programme facilitates the provision of screening in core sexual health services (community contraceptive services, general practice, abortion services and community pharmacies).

Prevalence of chlamydial infection depends on age and the setting where the test is taken. Prevalence is highest in the under 20 year olds, especially those who are pregnant (antenatal and those seeking abortion) and those attending GUM, varying between 5 and 16 per cent. Infection is sustained by unrecognized and untreated, symptomless chlamydial infection. It is now thought that overall the complication of this infection costs at least £50 million annually in the UK.

## Clinical features

Eighty per cent of infected women are asymptomatic. When symptoms are present, they include postcoital or intermenstrual bleeding, lower abdominal pain, purulent vaginal discharge, mucopurulent cervicitis and/or contact bleeding. Fifty per cent of men are asymptomatic, with urethral discharge and dysuria being the most common symptoms. The risk factors associated with chlamydial infection include young age (<25 years), new sexual partner or more than one sexual partner in recent years. There is also an association with contraceptive practice, with infection being less common in barrier contraception users and more common in those using combined oral contraception. Women undergoing termination of pregnancy also appear to have a higher association with chlamydial infection.

## Complications

One of the immediate complications is developing PID. In chlamydial PID, perihepatitis can also occur; this is known as Fitz–Hugh–Curtis syndrome. As with other types of PID, the long-term sequelae include tubal damage resulting in an increased risk of infertility and ectopic pregnancy and chronic pelvic pain. Chlamydia can be transmitted to the neonate at the time of delivery, causing neonatal conjunctivitis and pneumonia. Less common outcomes include adult conjunctivitis and sexually acquired reactive arthritis or Reiter's syndrome. This is more common in men who have chronic chlamydial infection.

## Specimen collection

Chlamydia is an obligate intracellular parasite; it is therefore imperative that samples contain cellular material. Cervical swabs are ideally the best; these should be inserted inside the cervical os and firmly rotated against the endocervix. Pus on the swab is not useful for chlamydial tests, and inadequate specimens reduce the sensitivity of all diagnostic tests. There is no consensus on how to take a urethral swab in women. It is now also possible to test first-pass urine specimens and vulvovaginal swabs.

## Laboratory tests for *C. trachomatis*

This is a rapidly developing field. The current standard is to use NAAT testing which is highly sensitive for all cases including medicolegal cases. Enzyme immunoassay is now not recommended and culture is now not available.

In general, NAATs are 90–95 per cent sensitive with the majority of studies indicating that as either the number of sites sampled increases, or the number of different NAAT used increases, the greater the detection of *C. trachomatis* in any given population.

Both first-catch urine (65–100 per cent sensitivity) and self-taken vulvovaginal swabs (90–95 per cent sensitivity) are suitable for testing and for screening.

## General management

Women should be advised to take the treatment (see below under Treatment) and avoid sexual intercourse for the duration of the treatment, or for 1 week after taking the stat dose of azithromycin. Appropriate advice should be given to women also using combined hormonal contraception.

Men and women with a positive chlamydia test should be offered a full STI screen and possibly this will require a visit to the local GUM department. All contacts of positive chlamydia tests should be tested and treated epidemiologically and also offered a full STI screen. Uncomplicated chlamydia is not an indication to remove an IUD or IUS. All patients with a positive test for chlamydia should be given written information regarding the infection.

## Treatment

The recommended treatment of uncomplicated chlamydial infection is with azithromycin 1 g stat as a single dose or doxycycline 100 mg twice a day for 7 days. In both cases, there should be no sexual intercourse advised for 7 days after commencing treatment and until all other partners have also completed treatment and abstained from intercourse. Alternative regimens include erythromycin 500 mg four times a day for 7 days or erythromycin 500 mg twice a day for 14 days. Ofloxacin 400 mg once a day for 1 week can also be used. The majority of studies are flawed in design, small and give no details regarding the treatment of sexual partners. Doxycycline and azithromycin have been the most rigorously tested. Quinolones and tetracyclines should not be used in pregnancy. Azithromycin is recommended for treatment by WHO, but is not licensed in the UK for use in pregnancy. The British National Formulary (BNF) says it can be used if no other alternative is available.

Follow up of chlamydial infection is recommended to check partner notification, reinforce health education, assess treatment efficacy and exclude reinfection [B].

### Test of cure

A test of cure is not routinely recommended but should be performed in pregnancy or if non-compliance or re-exposure is suspected. It should be deferred for 5 weeks (6 weeks if azithromycin has been given) after treatment is completed.

Pelvic floor and lower urinary tract dysfunction

# Trichomonal infection

The causative organism is *Trichomonas vaginalis*. This is a flagellated protozoon, which is found in the vagina, urethra and paraurethral glands. Transmission is almost exclusively sexual in adults. It can be acquired perinatally and occurs in 5 per cent of babies born to infected mothers. If infection is found after the first year, sexual contact is implied, although other modes of transmission are postulated.

## Clinical features

Between 10 and 50 per cent of women are asymptomatic [B]; among the remainder, the most common symptoms are vaginal discharge, vulval itching, dysuria and offensive odour. Occasionally, lower abdominal pain may be present. Seventy per cent of infected women have a vaginal discharge, which can vary in consistency from thin and scanty to profuse and thick. The classical frothy yellow discharge occurs in 10–30 per cent. Vulvitis, vaginitis and cervicitis are associated with trichomonal infection. A 'strawberry cervix' appearance is visible to the naked eye in approximately 2 per cent of cases and in more women on colposcopy. No abnormalities are found in 10–15 per cent of women.

## Complications

There is increasing evidence that trichomonal infection can have a detrimental effect on pregnancy and is associated with preterm delivery and low birth-weight infants [B].

## Diagnosis

Direct observation of a wet smear from the posterior fornix will diagnose 40–80 per cent of cases, whereas culture of the organism will correctly diagnose 95 per cent of infected women. Trichomonads are sometimes reported on cervical cytology, the sensitivity being about 60–80 per cent, but the false-positive rate is about 30 per cent, so that if a cervical smear report suggests trichomonad infection, it is worth confirming the diagnosis by the above two methods. Diagnostic tests based on the polymerase chain reaction (PCR) are not available in the UK.

## Treatment

Systemic chemotherapy is recommended, as urethral and paraurethral glands are frequently infected. Most strains of *T. vaginalis* are highly sensitive to metronidazole and related drugs (approximately 95 per cent cure rate). There is a spontaneous cure rate in 20–25 per cent.

The recommended regimens for treating trichomonal infection include metronidazole 2 g orally in a single dose or metronidazole 400–500 mg twice daily for 5–7 days [A]. The single dose is cheaper with better compliance, but there

is evidence that there may be a higher failure rate, especially if partners are not treated concurrently. Patients should be advised not to drink alcohol for the duration of, and for 48 hours after completion of, treatment due to the disulfiram-like effect (severe sickness).

Treatment failures should be referred to GUM to assess the possible reasons, such as poor compliance, reinfection, co-infection and/or resistance.

There is no evidence that metronidazole is teratogenic in the first trimester of pregnancy [A], although the BNF warns against high-dose regimens. In breastfeeding women, metronidazole may change the taste of breast milk. High doses should be avoided.

# Genital herpes

Genital herpes is acquired by sexually transmitted infection with either herpes simplex type 1 virus (HSV-1) – which is the usual cause of orolabial herpes – or herpes simplex type 2 virus (HSV-2). The infection may be primary or non-primary and disease episodes may be initial or recurrent and symptomatic or asymptomatic. Severe primary attacks of herpes constitute a genitourinary emergency and patients should be dealt with quickly and referred to a department of GUM for ongoing support and partner notification.

After childhood, symptomatic primary infection with HSV-1 is equally likely to be acquired in the genital or oral areas.

After primary infection, the virus becomes latent in local sensory ganglia, periodically reactivating to cause symptomatic lesions or asymptomatic but infectious viral shedding. This may be important in the acquisition of infection in long-term relationships where there has been primary infection with no history of a new partner.

New diagnoses of genital herpes are equally likely to be caused by HSV-1 or HSV-2; however, HSV-2 is more likely to recur than HSV-1. Median recurrence rates per month after a first episode are 0.34 for HSV-2 and 0.08 for HSV-1. Recurrence rates generally reduce over time.

## Clinical features of genital herpes in women

The most common symptoms are those of vulval pain, which is usually associated with ulcers that are preceded by blisters (Table 64.1.1). In a primary attack, this can be quite severe and the whole vulva can become swollen, ulcerated and infected. This, in turn, can cause discharge and dysuria and in severe cases urinary retention. The cervix may also become ulcerated. Tender inguinal lymphadenopathy is also a feature of the primary infection, although this may be the result of secondary infection.

More generalized features of a viral illness may also be present, particularly in primary infections. These include fever and myalgia. Herpetic infection can be asymptomatic; this is more likely in recurrent episodes.

**Table 64.1.1** Clinical features of acute herpes infections in women

| Symptoms | Signs |
|---|---|
| Painful ulceration, dysuria, vaginal discharge | Blistering and ulceration of vulva ± cervix, preceded by vesicles |
| Fever, myalgia (flu-like symptoms) – more common in primary infections | Inguinal lymphadenopathy |
| May be asymptomatic | |

## Complications

Urinary retention can occur as a result of autonomic neuropathy, or because of the severe pain caused by the local reaction around the urethra and vulva. It has also been postulated that chronic vulval pain may also be a result of post-herpetic neuralgia.

## Diagnosis

Herpes simplex virus confirmation and typing are important for diagnosis, prognosis and counselling [C].

Swabs must be taken from the base of a lesion, kept cold and transported directly to the laboratory in the viral culture medium. Serology is not commonly used to make the diagnosis. Given the implications of the diagnosis and potential for recurrent infections, it is vital that an accurate diagnosis be made at the outset. It cannot be assumed that vulval ulceration is herpetic until so proven by viral culture.

PCR (polymerase chain reaction for HSV DNA) for herpes diagnosis has a higher sensitivity than virus culture, but is not universally available.

## Management

### Primary genital herpes

General advice includes drinking large quantities of fluids to make the urine less concentrated and therefore reduce the pain on micturition, saline bathing and analgesia with a combination of non-steroidal anti-inflammatory agents and topical anaesthetic gels. Antiviral drugs are indicated if commenced within 5 days of the start of the episode and if lesions are still developing. Aciclovir (200 mg five times daily), valaciclovir (500 mg twice daily) and famciclovir (250 mg three times daily) all reduce the severity and duration of episodes [A], but they do not alter the natural history of the infection. Topical agents are less effective than oral agents, and intravenous therapy is only indicated when the patient cannot tolerate oral medication.

### Management of complications

Hospitalization may be required because of urinary retention, meningism and severe constitutional symptoms. If catheterization is required, it is recommended that the suprapubic approach be used [C] to prevent the theoretical risk of ascending infection, reduce the painfulness of the

procedure and allow normal micturition to take place without multiple attempts at recatheterization.

### Recurrent genital herpes

Recurrent attacks of genital herpes are generally less severe than primary attacks and are self-limiting. It is important to make management decisions together with the patient, and advice should be given with regard to sexual activity while potentially infective. However, not all patients will be aware of their potential infective state, particularly those who do not have symptoms or a prodrome (disordered local vulval sensations prior to the onset of a recurrent attack). Supportive and episodic antiviral therapy may be given [A], but if individuals suffer more than six attacks each year, suppressive therapy using antiviral agents and under the supervision of a genitourinary physician should be considered. Counselling may be required for those with problems adapting to the diagnosis.

## Management in pregnancy

Referral of a woman with suspected herpes in pregnancy to a GU physician is recommended.

### First-episode genital herpes

#### First and second trimester acquisition

Diagnosis in pregnancy is as described above. Serological testing of HSV 1 and 2 (immunoglobulin G) has not been fully evaluated.

First trimester herpes has been associated with miscarriage, but there is no evidence of increased risk of fetal abnormality if the pregnancy continues. It is not an indication for termination of pregnancy.

Management should be as above, with oral or intravenous aciclovir in standard doses. Aciclovir is not licensed in pregnancy, but there is substantial clinical evidence supporting its safety. Unless there are other complications, vaginal delivery can be anticipated. Continuous aciclovir in the last 4 weeks of pregnancy (aciclovir 200 mg tds) reduces the risk of both clinical recurrences at term and the need for caesarean section [A]. However, this point is contentious as other RCOG guidance quotes a study which did not demonstrate that aciclovir in the last 4 weeks of pregnancy gave any further protection.

#### Third trimester acquisition

Caesarean section should be considered for those developing symptoms after 34 weeks, as the risk of viral shedding during labour is very high, and thus also the risk of vertical transmission to the neonate (risk of neonatal herpes 41 per cent). If it is difficult to differentiate between a primary or recurrent attack, it may be helpful to take viral swabs as well as serum (IgG) and if the HSV is the same type then caesarean section may be avoided. If membranes have been ruptured for more than 4 hours, then caesarean section may not prevent vertical transmission. The paediatricians should be informed. Neonatal herpes carries a mortality of 30 per cent for disseminated herpes infection and 17 per cent have long-term neurological sequelae. Caesarean section for the prevention of neonatal herpes has not been evaluated in randomized, controlled trials (RCT) and may not be completely protective against neonatal herpes. If caesarean section does not take place, prolonged rupture of membranes and invasive monitoring should be avoided, intrapartum antivirals should be given and the baby treated postnatally.

### Recurrent genital herpes

Sequential cultures in late pregnancy do not predict viral shedding at term. If there are no lesions at delivery, caesarean section should not be performed, even if there has been a brief recurrence during the third trimester. Continuous aciclovir in the last 4 weeks of pregnancy may be cost effective compared with no therapy or caesarean section. It may not reduce the risk of caesarean section, as it does not eliminate viral shedding completely. There is no proven benefit of taking swabs for viral cultures at delivery to assess asymptomatic shedding.

### Genital lesions (recurrent herpes) at delivery

The current British Association for Sexual Health and HIV (BASHH) consensus is that a caesarean section should be performed, despite lack of evidence for its effectiveness. The current RCOG consensus is that mode of delivery and pros and cons should be discussed with the mother, but that caesarean section is not necessary as recurrent lesions are associated with a much lower risk of neonatal herpes (1–3 per cent). Therefore, the risks for the fetus at vaginal delivery may be small and need to be compared to the risks to the mother of caesarean section.

## Prevention of acquisition of infection

All women should be asked about genital herpes in themselves or in their partners. The asymptomatic female partners of men known to have genital herpes should be advised to avoid sexual contact during recurrences [C]. Conscientious use of condoms during pregnancy may reduce the risk of acquisition, but this is unproven. Pregnant women should be advised about the risk of orogenital contact for acquiring HSV-1.

The identification of susceptible women by means of type-specific antibody testing has not been shown to be cost effective.

All women, not just those with a history of genital herpes, should undergo careful inspection of the vulva at the onset of labour to look for clinical signs of herpes infection.

Mothers, staff and other relatives and friends with active oral lesions should be advised about the risk of postnatal transmission.

## Bacterial vaginosis

Bacterial vaginosis is characterized by an overgrowth of predominantly anaerobic organisms (*Gardnerella vaginalis*, *Prevotella* sp., *Mycoplasma hominis*, *Mobiluncus* sp.) in the vagina. This leads to replacement of lactobacilli and an increase in pH from a normal of 4.5 to 7. Bacterial vaginosis can arise and remit spontaneously in sexually active and non-sexually active women. It is more common in black than in white women, in those with an intrauterine device and in those who smoke cigarettes.

Bacterial vaginosis is not regarded as a sexually transmitted infection and its aetiology is unknown. It is the most common cause of vaginal discharge in women of childbearing age. The reported prevalence varies from 5 per cent in a group of asymptomatic college students to 50 per cent of women in Uganda. It has been reported in 12 per cent of pregnant women and in 30 per cent of women undergoing termination of pregnancy in the UK.

### Clinical features

In approximately 50 per cent of confirmed cases, there are no volunteered symptoms. Those with symptoms usually complain of an offensive, fishy-smelling vaginal discharge, not usually associated with vulvo-vaginitis. There is also a thin, white, homogeneous discharge coating the walls of the vagina and vestibule.

### Complications

Although the incidence of bacterial vaginosis is high in women with PID, there are no prospective studies investigating whether treating asymptomatic women for bacterial vaginosis reduces their risk of developing it subsequently. The condition is common in some populations of women undergoing elective termination of pregnancy and is associated with post-termination endometritis and PID [A]. In pregnancy, bacterial vaginosis is associated with late miscarriage, preterm birth, preterm premature rupture of the membranes and postpartum endometritis [A]. It has been associated with an increased incidence of vaginal cuff cellulitis and abscess formation following transvaginal hysterectomy [B]. It is unclear how important this is in the UK, where antibiotic prophylaxis is routine practice. There are no studies investigating the role of bacterial vaginosis in the development of PID following intrauterine device insertion.

### Diagnosis

#### Amsel's criteria for diagnosing bacterial vaginosis

At least three out of the four should be present for the diagnosis to be confirmed:

- thin, white, homogeneous discharge,
- clue cells on microscopy,
- pH of vaginal fluid >4.5,
- release of a fishy odour on adding alkali (10 per cent potassium hydroxide). (This test is rarely performed these days.)

Routine use of a high vaginal swab may not be useful, as culture of *G. vaginalis* can be possible in more than 50 per cent of normal women [B]. However, criteria can be used to judge whether a vaginal smear that has been Gram-stained shows features consistent with a diagnosis of bacterial vaginosis. Realistically, if a woman has typical symptoms, history and signs together with a raised pH (>4.5), a presumptive diagnosis can be made and the woman treated.

## Management

Initially, simple advice should be offered; this includes advice against the practice of vaginal douching, use of shower gels and antiseptic bath agents [C].

Antibiotic treatment is recommended for symptomatic women [A], women undergoing surgical procedures [A] and some pregnant women [A]. Using the oral route of administration, recommended regimens for treating bacterial vaginosis include metronidazole 400–500 mg twice daily for 5–7 days [A] or metronidazole 2 g as a single dose [A]. An alternative approach is to use the vaginal route, with intravaginal metronidazole gel (0.75 per cent) once daily for 5 days [A] or intravaginal clindamycin cream (2 per cent) once daily for 7 days [A]. All these treatments have been shown to achieve cure rates of 70–80 per cent after 4 weeks in controlled trials using placebo or comparing with oral metronidazole.

No reduction in relapse rates has been reported in studies in which the male partners were treated, and therefore there is no indication to treat the male partners of women with bacterial vaginosis.

Follow up is only required if symptoms recur, although a more cautious approach should be employed in pregnancy where recurrent infection may be associated with adverse outcomes.

The optimal management of those who have recurrent episodes of bacterial vaginosis remains unresolved.

---

### EBM: Pregnancy and bacterial vaginosis

- Meta-analyses have concluded that there is no evidence for teratogenicity from the use of metronidazole in pregnancy [A].
- The results of clinical trials investigating the value of screening for and treating bacterial vaginosis in pregnancy are conflicting, and it is therefore difficult to make firm recommendations. In summary, symptomatic pregnant women should be treated in the normal way and there is insufficient evidence to treat asymptomatic women. Breastfeeding women might be better treated intravaginally as metronidazole affects the taste of the milk.

---

## Anogenital warts

### Aetiology

Warts are benign epithelial skin tumours that are caused by the human papillomavirus (HPV), of which there are

more than 100 genotypes. The mode of transmission is most often sexual, but it may be transmitted perinatally and also from digital lesions (more commonly in children). Although the majority are benign and caused by HPV subtypes 6 and 11, others may contain oncogenic subtypes that are associated with genital tract dysplasia and cancer. Warts are just one manifestation of HPV infection of the genital tract, as there may also be subclinical and latent infection. Anogenital warts are the most common sexually transmitted infection in the UK (80 000 new diagnoses in GUM clinics in the UK in 2005). Men and women with warts are best treated in a GUM department and also screened for other sexually transmitted infections.

### Clinical features

Anogenital warts may cause irritation, but generally present as 'lumps' which women find disfiguring and psychologically distressing. They can occur at any site in the genital area including peri-anally, which does not imply anal intercourse.

Occult lesions may also occur in the vagina and cervix. Extragenital lesions may occur on the oral mucosa, larynx, conjunctiva and nasal cavity. Warts may be exophytic, single or multiple, keratinized and non-keratinized, broad based or pedunculated, and some are pigmented.

Diagnosis is mainly by naked-eye examination, although any doubt about the diagnosis should prompt biopsy under local anaesthetic. Speculum examination should be performed to look for cervical and vaginal lesions.

### Management

#### General advice

Condom usage with regular partners has not been shown to affect the treatment outcome of anogenital warts. However, using condoms may result in both partners feeling more comfortable and may prevent the transmission of HPV to uninfected partners and therefore should be encouraged.

#### Treatment

Treatment is generally uncomfortable and can be painful, and patients should be made aware that all treatments have significant failure and relapse rates. The choice of treatment depends on the morphology, number and distribution of the warts. First- and second-line treatments are not based upon robust evidence.

Soft, poorly keratinized warts respond well to podophyllin, podophyllotoxin and trichloroacetic acid, whereas keratinized lesions are better treated with physical ablative therapies, such as cryotherapy, excision and electrocautery. Imiquimod, an immune modulating agent, may be suitable for both types. Podophyllotoxin is usually administered over a 4-week cycle and imiquimod for up to 16 weeks, and both are suitable for self-application at home after appropriate instruction and screening for other sexually transmitted diseases. This is best supervised from a GUM clinic, as are most anogenital wart treatments. Adequate contraception must be ensured prior to the use of podophyllin-type chemicals because of the known teratogenic effect in animals.

Cervical warts can be removed by a variety of methods. Colposcopy is recommended if there is any doubt as to the diagnosis, but otherwise warts on the cervix are not an indication for colposcopy, in themselves.

## Anogenital warts in pregnancy

Podophyllin and podophyllotoxin should be avoided because of their possible teratogenic effects, and currently imiquimod does not have approval for use in pregnancy. The objectives of treatment in pregnancy are to minimize the number of lesions present at delivery and to reduce neonatal exposure to the virus. Potential problems in the neonate are the development of laryngeal papillomatosis and anogenital warts. Very rarely, a caesarean section is indicated due to blockage of the vaginal outlet.

## Cervical cytology

The National Health Service Cervical Screening Programme (NHSCSP) recommends no changes to the screening intervals for women with anogenital warts. Furthermore, developing anogenital warts prior to the age when screening would normally start is not an indication to commence cervical screening.

## Immunosuppressed women

This category includes women with impaired cell-mediated immunity (renal transplant patients and those infected with HIV), who are likely to have poor treatment responses, increased relapse rates and dysplasia. Careful follow up is required.

### HPV vaccination for genital wart protection

There is now a licensed vaccine to prevent a large percentage of up to 99 per cent of genital warts,[1] Gardasil, in women not yet exposed to HPV. It is also licensed to protect against cervical cancer. It is non-infectious and protects against four subtypes of HPV, 6, 11, 16 and 18. It is a quadrivalent vaccine protecting against genital warts and cervical cancer. Subtypes 6 and 11 are responsible for the majority of genital warts. For a variety of reasons, including cost effectiveness, this vaccine was not taken up for the vaccination programme in the UK. The alternative bivalent vaccine, Cervarix, was chosen to protect against cervical cancer.

## Syphilis

### Aetiology

*Treponema pallidum*, the spirochaete responsible for sexually acquired syphilis, causes one type of treponemal disease. The pathological strains also cause non-sexually transmitted tropical diseases, such as yaws, endemic syphilis, bejel and pinta. These organisms are serologically and morphologically similar and cannot be grown on artificial media. Occasionally, saprophytic strains, found in the mouth in dental sepsis, can cause diagnostic confusion.

Syphilis is transmitted sexually and vertically in pregnancy; therefore, the condition can be acquired and congenital.

### Epidemiology

Syphilis first became widespread and epidemic at the end of the fifteenth century in Europe. Syphilis and gonorrhoea were recognized as STIs in the eighteenth century, but were thought to be the same disease, until they were finally shown to be separate infections in the mid-nineteenth century. Until recently, syphilis was in a steady decline in the west, but over the last 15 years the incidence has begun to increase together with HIV infection.

### Classification

Acquired syphilis can be divided into early and late infections. Early syphilis is further subdivided into primary, secondary and early latent (less than two years of infection). The subdivisions of late infection include late latent (greater than two years of infection) and tertiary, which includes gummatous, cardiovascular and neurological involvement. Cardiovascular and neurological involvement is sometimes classified as quaternary syphilis.

Congenital syphilis is divided into early (first two years) and late, which includes the classical stigmata of congenital syphilis.

### Clinical features

Primary syphilis is characterized by an ulcer (the chancre) and regional lymphadenopathy. The chancre is classically a single, painless and indurated ulcer with a clean base discharging clear serum and is usually found in the anogenital region. However, it may also be atypical, multiple, painful, purulent, destructive and occur at extragenital sites. The ulcer(s) of primary syphilis should not be confused with other genital ulcerative disorders.

### Aetiology of anogenital ulceration

- Herpes simplex
- Syphilis
- Chancroid
- Lymphogranuloma venereum
- Donovanosis
- Candidiasis (severe)
- Behçet's disease
- Scabies-excoriated.

Secondary syphilis is characterized by multisystem involvement occurring within the first two years of infection. The features include a generalized polymorphic rash, often affecting the palms and soles, condylomata lata, mucocutaneous lesions, generalized lymphadenopathy and other rare multisystem manifestations. Early latent syphilis is characterized by positive serological tests for syphilis with no clinical evidence of treponemal infection, again within the first two years of infection.

In cases testing positive serologically for treponemal infection in the absence of clinical signs, it is important to exclude other infections such as yaws, particularly in those of Caribbean origin.

All women with positive treponemal serology should be investigated and treated in a GUM department.

## Diagnosis

The diagnosis can be made by direct demonstration of *Treponema pallidum* from lesions or infected lymph nodes in early syphilis by dark field microscopy, direct fluorescent antibody testing and tests based upon the PCR.

Serological tests include:

- cardiolipin (reaginic) tests: Venereal Diseases Research Laboratory (VDRL),
- carbon antigen test/rapid plasma reagin (RPR) test,
- specific tests: treponemal EIA to detect IgG, IgG and IgM, T. pallidum haemagglutination assay (TPHA) and others.

## Treatment

All treatment should be managed in a GUM clinic.

The mainstay of treatment is parenteral penicillin, as it is given under supervision, therefore ensuring compliance, and has bioavailability guaranteed.

Early syphilis is treated with benzathine penicillin G with a single dose, which is unlicensed in the UK. Azithromycin single dose can be used as second line.

Late syphilis is treated with benzathine penicillin G at three weekly doses, except for neurosyphilis where procaine penicillin G with concomitant oral probenicid is used as first line. All patients should be offered screening for other STIs, including HIV.

## Pregnancy

All pregnant women should be screened for syphilis at the initial antenatal visit. Syphilis may be transmitted transplacentally at any stage of pregnancy and may lead to polyhydramnios, miscarriage, preterm labour, still birth, hydrops and congenital syphilis.

Seventy to 100 per cent of the infants of pregnant women with untreated early syphilis will be infected and one-third will be stillborn.

Patients should be jointly managed with GUM physicians and treated as above, but in the third trimester a second dose of benzathine penicillin G 1 week after the first dose. Ceftriaxone 500 mg i.m. for 10 days should be added to alternatives. When pregnant women are treated for syphilis after 26 weeks, the fetus should be investigated for infection and distress during treatment in a department of fetal medicine. All neonates should be treated at birth.

## Congenital syphilis

Babies of mothers with positive serology for syphilis and treated antenatally should be managed jointly by a GUM physician and a paediatrician. Laboratory blood tests should be performed on the infant's (not cord) blood. In view of the highly treatable nature of the disease and the high perinatal morbidity and mortality of congenital syphilis, it is extremely important to continue with antenatal testing.

## Human immunodeficiency virus

There are two strains of HIV, types 1 and 2, of which HIV-1 is responsible for most HIV infections. The human immunodeficiency virus carries its genetic code as RNA; this is translated by an enzyme present in the virus (reverse transcriptase) into DNA, which then integrates into the host's target cells, including CD4 T-cell lymphocytes, and other cells of the immune system. This results in a decline in CD4 cells and progression to acquired immunodeficiency syndrome (AIDS). HIV infection can cause a decline in CD4 counts from a normal level of about $1000/\mu L$ to $<200/\mu L$. The infected person then becomes susceptible to the opportunistic infections and malignancies characteristic of AIDS.

Human immunodeficiency virus disease is an extremely important, fatal disease worldwide. It is currently estimated that approximately 40 million people are infected. HIV infection increases the susceptibility to other infectious diseases, such as tuberculosis, with a huge impact on morbidity and mortality. HIV is most prevalent in economically deprived areas in the developing world where people are less likely to be able to afford the expensive anti-retroviral drugs that can limit disease progression and spread. HIV is transmitted sexually, in blood products and to the fetus vertically and through breastfeeding. In developed countries such as the UK, infected people have access to the latest evidence-based treatments and are managed by GUM physicians.

With the currently available anti-retroviral agents, eradication of HIV infection is not likely to be possible. The aims of treatment are to prolong life and improve quality of life by maintaining suppression of virus replication for as long as possible. Antiretroviral therapy is monitored by measurements of viral load together with CD4 counts. The aim of therapy is to decrease the viral load to less than 50 copies per mL within four to six months of commencing therapy. Treatment is recommended for patients with primary HIV

Pelvic floor and lower urinary tract dysfunction

infection, asymptomatic HIV infection and symptomatic HIV infection or AIDS. However, treatment should be commenced in patients when their CD4 count is <350 cells mL. There is overwhelming evidence from cohort studies to show that the dramatic fall in AIDS-related mortality seen in the developed world coincided with the introduction of highly active anti-retroviral therapy (HAART). HAART regimens should be individualized to achieve the best potency, minimize toxicity and avoid drug interactions. Prior to commencing therapy, individuals should have full tests for HIV drug resistance, and be screened for hepatitis B and C infections.

HAART consists of three drugs, which can be from a variety of types: protease inhibitors, non-nucleoside reverse transcriptase inhibitors or nucleoside reverse transcriptase inhibitors. Issues to be considered during therapy are adherence, toxicity, resistance, long-term safety, clinical trial data and stage of disease. Change of therapy is advocated for virological failure diagnosed by viral load testing. Up to date guidance should be sought on which drugs are suitable for which group of people based on evidence.

## HIV testing

A significant number of people are unaware of their HIV infection and they are at risk from HIV-related infections leading to an increase in morbidity and mortality. They are also at risk of transmitting the infection both sexually and vertically (to a fetus). HIV testing should be encouraged in a variety of settings and healthcare professionals should obtain consent for testing in the same way as for any other investigation. Lengthy pretest counselling is not necessary, simply discussion of the benefits of early diagnosis and how the results will be given. Concerns about insurance applications should be discussed: insurance companies are not allowed to ask if an individual has been tested for HIV. However, applicants should declare HIV positivity in the same way as any other medical condition.

## Post-exposure prophylaxis for HIV following sexual exposure

There is evidence that HIV infection can be aborted after sexual exposure if anti-retrovirals are given as soon as possible after exposure. This works by inhibiting viral replication once the virus has crossed the mucosal barrier. It then takes 5 days before HIV can be detected in the blood. Post-exposure prophylaxis for HIV following sexual exposure (PEPSE) drugs need to be given as soon as possible and only up to 72 hours after initial exposure. The risk of acquisition needs to be assessed depending on the HIV risk or status of the contact and the type of sexual contact that has taken place. Informed consent must be taken following full discussion including the possible side effects (mainly gastrointestinal) and the need for blood tests at the time, and at three and six months after the event. Hepatitis B screening,

immunoglobulin and accelerated vaccination should also be considered. Twenty-four hour access to starter packs for treatment (in Accident and Emergency and GUM departments) should be available, following GUM advice and arrangement for at least 4 weeks of ongoing treatment.

## Risk assessment for HIV testing/other blood-borne viruses (for women)

Several questions can be asked which enable some assessment of the risks of HIV/other blood-borne viruses, and these questions are asked routinely in GUM:

- Have you or any of your partners ever injected (recreational) drugs?
- Have you ever had any partners who come from another country? If yes, ask where and assess whether this may pose an extra risk, e.g sub-Saharan Africa.
- Have any of your partners also had sex with men?
- Do you have any tattoos, which were done in unlicensed premises without adequate precautions for sterility?

### HIV and sexual and reproductive health

- There can be huge psychosocial issues for women with HIV, especially around conception and pregnancy.
- All women with HIV should be offered an annual sexual health check to include screening for STIs and contraceptive advice, where appropriate. The majority of STIs can be treated in the same way as in the non-HIV-positive woman. If considering conception, preconception counselling should be given especially carefully and possibly should include written consent in non sero-same couples, regarding the small risk of HIV transmission. This guidance should be led by an HIV expert.
- Women with HIV on HAART have a decreased risk of HIV sexual transmission. Those whose viral loads are very low for long periods of time may have almost negligible risks of transmission, especially in the absence of any STIs. Counselling and advice to continue to use condoms should take place. In those who wish to have unprotected sex, detailed counselling by experts should be offered.

## HIV and contraception

It is important that HIV-positive women are open about their infection so that they receive the best advice. Safer sex is to be encouraged, with the concomitant use of condoms, as well as a reliable hormonal method to prevent pregnancy. For HIV-positive women not on HAART, all methods of contraception can be used.

Methods of contraception adversely affected by antiretroviral therapy are combined hormonal contraception and progestagen only pills, if on ritonavir-boosted protease inhibitors. However, depot medroxyprogesterone acetate, implants, the levonorgestrel intrauterine system and intrauterine device can all be used by HIV-positive women on HAART without increased failure rates.

Where emergency contraception is required for a woman on HAART or other liver enzyme inducing drugs, then an emergency IUD is preferable. If progesterone-only emergency contraception is requested, then a 3 mg (double stat dose) is recommended.

## HIV and cervical screening, colposcopy and cervical cancer

Cervical cancer is an AIDS-defining illness. Women with HIV need to have regular cervical cytology and all women with cervical cancer should be offered an HIV test. The current NHSCSP guidelines on screening suggest that HIV-positive women should have an annual smear. Any cytological abnormality, however minor, should be taken as an indication for colposcopy. As there is a higher incidence of inflammatory vaginocervical disorders in HIV-positive women, the accuracy of both cytology and colposcopy is less than in non-HIV-infected women.

Women with proven cervical intraepithelial neoplasia (CIN) require treatment, although the results of treatment of CIN are significantly worse than in non-HIV women. Data also suggest that HIV-positive women with normal CD4 counts have better outcomes than those who have low CD4 counts. This observation supports the concept that the host cell-mediated immune system is implicated in the eradication of CIN following local treatments.

## HIV infection and pregnancy

The prevalence of HIV in pregnancy varies over the UK. For example, in 2006, the prevalence in London was 1 in 238 live births, whereas elsewhere in the country it was 1 in 705. The majority of these women are from sub-Saharan Africa. The risk of transmission is related to maternal health, obstetric factors and infant prematurity. There appears to be a linear correlation between maternal viral load and risk of transmission. Antenatal testing is carried out in all units in the UK, and there is a recommendation to repeat test women at increased risk of acquisition during the pregnancy. Near patient testing is also recommended in untested women in labour. Checking documentation of HIV testing is important, as well as communicating results to labour ward staff. Uptake of antenatal screening for HIV was >80 per cent in over two-thirds of maternity units, in 2003. There is a greater diversity of clinical situations for women with HIV and each scenario may need individual clinical guidance.

Pregnant women with HIV should be screened for all STIs, including syphilis (and again in the third trimester or if clinically indicated) and hepatitis B. There should be social assessment of all women with HIV in pregnancy by the multi-disciplinary team.

Viral load is important in terms of transmission and should be measured every three months, at 36 weeks or 2 weeks after changing therapy, and at delivery. Any opportunistic infections suspected should be investigated and managed as in non-pregnant women.

Obstetric factors in untested women that consistently show an association with risk of transmission are mode of delivery and duration of membrane rupture. It is suggested that invasive monitoring of babies and artificial rupture of membranes is avoided in HIV-positive women. Delivery should be expedited for term pre-labour rupture of membranes. Delivery before 34 weeks has been shown to be associated with an increased risk of transmission. There is an untreated vertical transmission risk of 25 per cent. The findings of the first RCT in 1994 showed that the use of zidovudine (AZT) could reduce transmission from 25 to 8 per cent. This has since been confirmed by multiple smaller observational studies. There is more support now for elective trial of vaginal delivery if a woman has undetectable HIV virus on HAART. In 2006, for women on HAART, transmission rates were not significantly different according to mode of delivery.

Exclusive formula feeding is still recommended in all HIV-positive women in the UK. Elsewhere in the world, where formula feeding poses extra risks to the infant because of unsafe water, breastfeeding is recommended. HAART started before pregnancy can be continued throughout pregnancy. There is no evidence for teratogenicity of any retroviral drugs, but there is an increased risk of preterm delivery. Zidovudine monotherapy should commence by 28 weeks and remains a valid option in women who do not wish to use HAART in pregnancy, or do not need to.

There should be clear local referral pathways for HIV pregnant women, including specialist nurses and social workers where available. Information for the woman concerning follow up for the baby needs to be given.

## Preconception and fertility management in men and women with HIV

There are three groups to consider:

1 HIV-positive men and negative female partners;
2 HIV-negative men and positive female partners;
3 HIV-infected couples.

All three groups may have fertility problems, but for the first two groups there is also the risk of HIV transmission.

### Positive man, negative woman

The risk of transmission to the woman is approximately 1:500 per sexual encounter and until recently this was the only way couples could conceive. Limiting exposure to the most fertile period only has been shown to reduce the risk of transmission. In one study, four of 103 women seroconverted using this method. In 1992, Semprini et al.[2] invented the technique of 'sperm washing' – a process whereby spermatozoa are removed from the surrounding seminal plasma. (HIV is found in the seminal plasma, but not bound to the spermatozoa themselves.) There have not so far been any seroconversions of women after they have been inseminated with washed sperm. The technique of sperm washing is only available in a few centres in the UK and is funded by the couple in more than 50 per cent of cases.

### Negative man, positive woman

Couples are advised to use condoms and then to practise self-insemination around ovulation to minimize the risk of transmission to the man.

### Positive couples

These couples are recommended to practise safer sex (condoms) in order to reduce the risk of transmission of viral variants. They are advised to have unprotected sex around ovulation. There has been considerable debate concerning HIV-infected couples and *in-vitro* fertilization (IVF): it is now ethically acceptable as the vertical transmission rate is less than 1 per cent and there is an increased life expectancy for parents on treatment.

# HEPATITIS

## Hepatitis A

Hepatitis A is caused by a picorna virus (RNA) and is common in areas of the world where there is poor sanitation and mainly affects children in those areas. There were only 784 cases in England and Wales in 2004 in all age groups. (Hepatitis A is a notifiable disease.) Transmission is by the faeco-oral route or close personal contact and there have been outbreaks in men who have sex with men (MSM), those who have multiple partners and group sex. There are also increased risks among injecting drug users (IDU) and haemophiliacs (cases of contamination of Factor VIII) and vaccination may be important in these groups. The incubation period is 15–45 days and people are most infectious 2 weeks before the jaundice when they are asymptomatic or not yet been diagnosed. Many people have no symptoms at all, but the typical illness is characterized by a prodromal flu-like illness with possible right upper quadrant pain, followed by an icteric illness with jaundice (mixed hepatic and cholestatic, with symptoms of pale stools and dark urine) associated with nausea, anorexia and fatigue which can go on for 1–3 weeks or even longer. Hepatitis A is rarely complicated by acute liver failure (ALF, 0.4 per cent). This is more common in those with chronic other liver disease, including hepatitis B and C. Mortality rates are very low (0.1 per cent), except those complicated by ALF.

There is no evidence that hepatitis A is teratogenic, but there is an increased risk of miscarriage and premature labour.

There have been cases of possible vertical transmission. Breastfeeding can be continued and most children will have mild or asymptomatic infection.

The diagnosis can be confirmed by positive serum hepatitis A-specific IgM and can remain positive for six months or more. If the hepatitis A was acquired sexually, then tests for other STIs should be undertaken.

General advice for women should include avoiding food handling, as well as unprotected sex. Rest and fluids are advised together with advice to seek medical help if there is a deterioration in health. A full explanation including a patient information leaflet should be given.

Vaccination is recommended to travellers to developing countries, haemophiliacs and for people at risk in an outbreak.

## Hepatitis B

Hepatitis B is a hepadna virus (DNA). It is endemic worldwide with high carriage rates of up to 20 per cent in high risk areas, such as South and East Asia, Central and South America, Africa and Eastern Europe. In the UK, 0.01–0.04 per cent of blood donors have evidence of hepatitis B infection. In 2003, there were 1151 cases notified in England and Wales. Transmission is sexual, parenteral and vertical. The incubation is 40–160 days. It is mainly asymptomatic in children and in 10–50 per cent adults and is especially likely in coexistent HIV infection. The prodrome and icteric phases are similar to hepatitis A. Fulminant hepatitis can occur in <1 per cent. Chronic infection (greater than six months) occurs in 5–10 per cent and is more likely in HIV patients. Chronic active hepatitis can proceed to cirrhosis and liver cancer. Concurrent infection with HIV or hepatitis C worsens the disease. It is important to screen for other STIs, to check liver function and to advise to avoid sexual intercourse.

In pregnancy, there is an increased risk of miscarriage and premature labour in acute infection and there is a risk of vertical transmission in >90 per cent. Infants born to infected mothers are vaccinated at birth, usually in conjunction with hep B-specific antigen, which decreases transmission by 90 per cent. Women can continue to breastfeed as there is no additional risk of transmission. Partner notification should take place and all children not vaccinated at birth should be screened.

Specific hepatitis B Ig (HBIG) can be administered to a non-immune contact after sexual exposure from a known infective contact. This needs to be done before 48 hours, but works up to 7 days and should be followed up by an accelerated course of hep B vaccine (0, 7 and 21 days). Hep B vaccine should be given to MSM, sex workers, injecting drug users, victims of sexual assault and needle stick injury and sex partners of high risk patients.

All those with active infection should be referred to a hepatologist (HbsAg-positive). All should also have an HIV test, as well as a full STI screen. The screening test for hepatitis B is antiHBc. Those who have been vaccinated will have anti-HBs detectable in the blood.

All hepatitis B patients should be considered for hepatitis D testing which can coincide and make patients worse. Hepatitis D occurs in IDU and sex workers.

# Hepatitis C

Hepatitis C is an RNA virus and is prevalent (1–4.5 per cent) in Europe, Africa, the Pacific and the Eastern Mediterranean. The UK prevalence is 0.53 per cent in adults, but is >40 in IDU. There were 8346 cases in England in 2006. Transmission is parenteral via shared needles, transfusion pre-1990s and in renal dialysis. There are low rates of sexual transmission (<1 per cent per year in relationships). There are also increased levels in MSM female sex workers and tattoo recipients. Vertical transmission takes place in only 5 per cent, but is increased in HIV co-infection. Incubation is 7–140 days and serology may take three months to show.

More than 60 per cent will be asymptomatic with occasional icteric phase. There can also be chronic infections in hepatitis B. Acute fulminant hepatitis is rare. Of these, 50–85 per cent become chronic carriers and 30 per cent of these will develop severe liver disease after long periods up to 30 years with an increased risk of liver cancer. Pregnant patients should be treated as for hepatitis A.

Screening of blood is by enzyme immunoassay (EIA) then confirmed with PCR.

General advice would be to not donate blood, semen or organs. All HCV-positive patients should be referred to a liver specialist. In both the acute and chronic phases, they may respond to interferon. Interferon is also used in some hepatitis B patients. All hepatitis C patients should be vaccinated against hepatitis A and B to decrease the chances of fulminant hepatitis coinfection.

There is no firm evidence that breastfeeding increases the risk of transmission, except if the woman is very ill. Sexual contacts and children should be tested. There is no vaccine or immunoglobulin preparation that will prevent transmission.

All IDU, haemophiliacs and people receiving blood pre-1990 should be tested, as well as sex workers and tattoo recipients.

## KEY POINTS

- Pelvic inflammatory disease is most commonly caused by *Chlamydia trachomatis* and *Neisseria gonorrhoeae*; the long-term sequelae include infertility, ectopic pregnancy and chronic pelvic pain.
- The symptoms and signs of PID can be non-specific and treatment may have to be initiated empirically.
- PID should be considered as a sexually transmitted disease and therefore contact tracing, treating partners and liaison with GUM departments are important features of management.
- Gynaecologists should take sexual histories where indicated and apply the basic tenets of GUM practice.
- Many patients will have concurrent sexually transmitted diseases; therefore genitourinary screening is recommended.
- For better patient care, it is recommended that each clinician should have a thorough understanding of the chlamydia

test used in his/her clinical setting, and encourage women under 25 years to take part in the National Chlamydia Screening Programme (NCSP).
- Testing for chlamydial infection should be considered when undertaking any procedure that entails instrumentation of the upper genital tract, such as hysteroscopy and IUD insertion, because of the serious possible complications.
- The only way to assess the risk of infection is to take a sexual history, as outlined above.
- The vulva should be carefully examined in all women – not just those at high risk of genital herpes – at the onset of labour.
- The aetiology of bacterial vaginosis is unknown; it is not sexually transmitted.
- Anogenital warts are the most common STI in the UK; they do not indicate the need for cervical screening outwith the NHSCSP.
- All women with positive tests for syphilis should be referred to GUM departments to confirm or exclude neurological, cardiovascular and ophthalmic involvement.
- There has been a significant improvement in survival and quality of life for HIV-infected women treated with HAART.

## EBM

Evidence in this chapter is taken from peer-reviewed national guidance as shown below under Published guidelines and is accessible to all on the internet.

## Published Guidelines

British HIV Association Guidelines for the Treatment of HIV1-infected Adults with Antiretroviral Therapy. Gazzard B on behalf of BHIVA Guidelines Writing Group. London: BHIVA, 2008.

Emergency Contraception. Faculty of Sexual and Reproductive Health Clinical Effectiveness Unit. London: RCOG, 2006.

Guidelines for the Management of HIV Infection in Pregnant Women. De Ruiter A *et al.* for British HIV Association and Childrens HIV Association, 2008.

Guidelines for the Management of the Sexual and Reproductive Health of People Living with HIV Infection. Fakoya A on behalf of British HIV Association, BASHH and FSRH, 2008.

Intrauterine Contraception. Faculty of Sexual and Reproductive Health Clinical Effectiveness Unit. London: RCOG, November 2007.

National Guideline for the Diagnosis and Treatment of Gonorrhoea in Adults. Bignell C for the Clinical Effectiveness Group. London: British Association for Sexual Health and HIV (BASHH), 2005.

National Guideline for the Management of Bacterial Vaginosis. Hay P for the Clinical Effectiveness Group. London: BASHH, 2006.

National Guideline for the Management of Chlamydia trachomatis Genital Tract Infection. Horner PJ and Boag F for the Clinical Effectiveness Group. London: BASHH, 2006.

National Guideline for the Management of Genital Herpes. Herpes Simplex Advisory Panel for the Clinical Effectiveness Group. London: BASHH, 2007.

National Guideline for the Management of Trichomonas vaginalis. Sherrard J for the Clinical Effectiveness Group. London: BASHH, 2007.

National Guidelines – Consultations Requiring Sexual History-taking. French P on behalf of Sexual History-Taking Working Party and the Clinical Effectiveness Group of the British Association for Sexual Health and HIV. London: BASHH, 2006.

RCOG Green Top Guideline No. 30. Management of Genital Herpes in Pregnancy. London: RCOG, 2007.

RCOG Green Top Guideline No. 32. Management of Acute Pelvic Inflammatory Disease. London: RCOG, 2008.

UKMEC, 2009. Available from ‹www.fsrh.org/guidelines›.

UK National Guideline for the Management of PID. Ross J for the Clinical Effectiveness Group. London: BASHH, 2005.

UK National Guideline for the Management of Syphilis. Kingston M for the Clinical Effectiveness Group. London: BASHH, 2008.

UK National Guideline for the Management of Viral Hepatides. Brook G et al. for the Clinical Effectiveness Group. London: BASHH, 2008.

UK National Guideline for the Use of Post-exposure Prophylaxis for HIV Following Sexual Exposure. Fisher M et al. for the Clinical Effectiveness Group. London: BASHH, 2006.

UK National Guideline on the Management of Anogenital Warts. Sonnex C et al. for the Clinical Effectiveness Group. London: BASHH, 2007.

UK National Guidelines for HIV testing. BHIVA and BASHH. London BASHH, 2008.

All the BASHH guidelines are available at ‹www.bashh.org.uk›.

All HIV guidance is available at ‹www.bhiva.org.uk›.

All Faculty of Sexual and Reproductive Health guidelines are available at ‹www.fsrh.org.uk›.

All RCOG guidelines are available at ‹www.rcog.org.uk›.

Information and references regarding Chlamydia screening and prevalence are available at ‹www.chlamydiascreening.nhs.uk›.

## Key References

1. Villa LL. Overview of the clinical development and results of a quadrivalent vaccine against HPV (types 6, 11, 16 and 18). *Int J Infect Dis* 2007; **11** (Suppl. 2): S17–25.

2. Semprini AE, Levi-Setti P, Bozzo M et al. Insemination of HIV-negative women with processed semen of HIV-positive partners. *Lancet* 1992; **340**: 1317–19.

# 64.2 Dyspareunia and other psychosexual problems

*Melanie Mann*

## MRCOG standards

### Theoretical skills

- Understand the classification and causes of dyspareunia.
- Be able to manage the individual causes of dyspareunia.
- Know the anatomy and physiology of the human sexual response.
- Understand the epidemiology, aetiology, pathogenesis, clinical features and prognosis of psychosexual and sexual problems and the links with gynaecological disease.

### Practical skills

- Be able to take an appropriate sexual history with regard to dyspareunia and psychosexual problems.
- Be able to perform a clinical examination to diagnose the cause of dyspareunia.
- Be able to ask about sexual relationship problems related to the dyspareunia, either as a result of the dyspareunia or causing the dyspareunia, i.e. be able to take a related psychosexual history.
- Be able to recognize, counsel and plan initial management of psychosexual problems.

## DYSPAREUNIA

This is recurrent genital pain associated with sexual activity, usually penetration, although it can refer to any genital stimulation. Dyspareunia can be primary, where pain has always occurred, or secondary, where it occurs after a period of pain-free sexual activity. It is important to classify it further in terms of the site of pain: i.e. superficial or deep.

Dyspareunia can itself lead to relationship difficulties due to the cycle of fear. Pain at intercourse can lead to problems of sexual arousal, causing further sexual pain and then avoidance of sexual activity.

Talking to patients about the exact site, nature and other features of the pain is important. It is also important to be comfortable talking about aspects of the sexual act, especially as some dyspareunia may be position related. Remember that patients are usually more embarrassed mentioning these aspects to us and may expect us to bring up the subject.

Most of these causes are dealt with in more detail in other sections of this book.

## Main causes of superficial dyspareunia (superficial vulval and vaginal pain at intercourse)

- Vulvitis and vulvovaginitis (infection, hypo-oestrogenic)
- Vestibulodynia (provoked vulval pain)
- Vulvodynia (unprovoked vulval pain)
- Topical irritants/dermatitis
- Urethral disorders and cystitis
- Vaginismus
- Lack of vaginal lubrication (arousal problems)
- Obstetric perineal trauma, mainly episiotomy
- Radiation vaginitis.

## Main causes of deep dyspareunia

- Pelvic inflammatory disease
- Endometriosis
- Genital or pelvic masses, e.g. ovarian cyst
- Pelvic congestion syndrome
- Urinary tract infection
- Retroverted uterus in some women
- Irritable bowel syndrome
- Psychosexual issues.

It is important to confirm diagnoses as far as possible with diagnostic tests, such as pelvic ultrasonography, microbiological swabs, laparoscopy or vulval biopsy where appropriate. Some diagnoses or problems are best dealt with by general practitioners or other specialists, such as gastroenterologists.

If an organic cause for dyspareunia is found, it does not necessarily exclude emotional and/or psychological sequelae for the woman. The aetiology of dyspareunia should be viewed on a continuum from primarily physical to primarily psychological, with many women exhibiting components of both.

## HUMAN SEXUAL RESPONSE

According to Masters and Johnson,[1] there are classically four phases in the human sexual response:

1  *Excitement:* This is the first part of arousal and is caused by physical stimulation especially clitoral stimulation, thoughts of sex and emotions. It leads to vasodilatation in the genitals causing swelling of the labia and the tissues surrounding the vagina resulting in heightened labial colouring and increased vaginal lubrication. Excitement can be enhanced or inhibited by signals from the brain, which are in turn influenced by previous experience. Oestrogen affects vaginal lubrication by enhancing the vascular bed beneath the epithelium. The clitoris becomes swollen and erect, the skin flushed and the nipples erect.
2  *Plateau:* There is intensification of the above changes with increased blood flow to the genitals accompanied by increases in heart rate, blood pressure and breathing rates. The vagina lengthens and balloons with engorgement.
3  *Orgasm:* This is a genital reflex controlled by spinal neural centres (spinal injuries to vertebrae T11 to L2 can lead to orgasmic problems). There is reflex contraction of pelvic muscles located around the vaginal introitus together with release of vaginal fluids. Orgasm is the highest point of pleasure. Orgasm can last longer in women and be multiple.
4  *Resolution:* There is a feeling of satisfaction and well-being together with a return to the pre-arousal state. Men experience a refractory phase during which they cannot have another orgasm, but women do not.

There is also another phase which is necessary before the classic phases described above and this is known as desire or libido. This varies from one person to another and during the life cycle. It is also subject to changes in oestrogen and testosterone. A newer model, 'the sexual response cycle', describes physical, emotional and cognitive feedback. A variety of biological, social and psychological factors can affect the cycle.[2]

Educating patients regarding the phases above is really important. The most important of these is giving sufficient time spent for foreplay and relaxation to be sufficiently aroused and lubricated prior to penetration, together with the importance of stimulating the clitoris to achieve orgasm. Women often feel they are failing in some way if they cannot achieve orgasm with vaginal intercourse alone and may need to be reassured.

## PSYCHOSEXUAL PROBLEMS

Physiological events, such as pregnancy, childbirth, menopause and ageing, as well as gynaecological conditions, such as infertility, prolapse, urinary incontinence and gynaecological cancers, can have an impact on sexual well-being. Sexual activity in later life remains taboo, but a large number of women remain sexually active beyond 70 years. It must also be remembered that intercourse is only one way for couples to be sexual and there are other ways that sexual intimacy can be maintained at different times of the life cycle.

Psychosexual problems may present to the gynaecologist as part of general history taking for a variety of presenting complaints, and it is sometimes difficult to disentangle how much of the gynaecological complaint is due to the psychosexual problem, or whether the gynaecological problem has caused the psychosexual issue. It is therefore extremely important that the clinician feels comfortable asking about sexual problems, especially in relation to gynaecological problems, for which there is a good chance of concomitant psychosexual issues, such as vulval disorders and dyspareunia. However, there may also be circumstances in which it is important to establish sexual habits and issues, for example prior to gynaecological surgery when any interference with sexual function can cause problems within a sexual relationship. It is also very important to have an open and non-judgemental attitude to people's sexual practices (as long as they are not causing or suffering harm) and this includes those in same sex relationships.

### Psychosexual history taking

Each clinician needs to find his/her own words that feel comfortable to use when talking about sex with the patient. There is no substitute for practice, and the more you use the words and ask the difficult questions, the more comfortable you will feel. Open-ended questions are useful in order to encourage the patient to talk, for example: 'Tell me a little bit about …'. The clinician's body language is also extremely influential to the way the patient will feel about opening up in this very intimate part of history taking. For example, sitting back in the chair, putting down your pen and not having a large expanse of desk between you and the patient will go a long way towards making her feel more comfortable.

#### Typical questions for use in psychosexual history taking

Not all the questions need to be asked or are appropriate to ask every time.

- 'Are you in a sexual relationship?'
- 'Is sex comfortable for you?'
- 'Are there any problems with sex?'
- 'Do you get any pain with sex?'

- 'Where exactly does it hurt during sex – on the outside or the inside?'
- 'Is there anything that makes the pain worse, any position, for example?'
- 'Are you able to have an orgasm during sex?'
- 'Have you ever masturbated? Do you get an orgasm during masturbation?'
- 'Tell me a little bit about your relationship with your partner.'
- 'Tell me a little bit about what happens when you try to have sex with your partner.'

Most gynaecologists would refer a patient on to an expert in psychosexual medicine for further treatment. There will be local variation in availability and waiting time.

# SEXUAL PAIN DISORDERS

## Dyspareunia

This is the only sexual disorder in which physical factors are thought to play a major aetiological role. However, the psychological and interpersonal factors are significant.[3] The organic causes for this condition are discussed above. In addition to gynaecological treatment approaches, most women require an adjunctive course of cognitive–behavioural sex therapy to ensure good outcomes.[4]

## Vaginismus

Vaginismus is the involuntary spasm of the pubococcygeal and associated muscles causing painful and difficult penetration of the vagina, during sex, tampon insertion or clinical examination. Primary vaginismus occurs when a woman has never experienced vaginal penetration; secondary vaginismus is diagnosed when the problem occurs after previous successful vaginal penetration.

The patient may present with a painful vulva at intercourse. The differential diagnosis is then of organic vulval disorders, such as vulval vestibulitis. However, there is likely to be some degree of vaginismus in all women with organic vulval disease. The skill is in trying to work out whether the vaginismus is the primary problem or is a result of organic disease. The 'Q-tip' test can be helpful to elucidate the exact site of pain and whether it is in the contracted muscles or in the tender epithelium of the vestibule. (The 'Q-tip' test involves the use of a moistened cotton bud to elicit the exact site and degree of discomfort of vulval pain.) The other main form of presentation is admission of non-consummation of a relationship in the fertility clinic setting.

### Aetiology

Vaginismus is a conditioned (learned) response that often results from associating sexual activity with pain

and fear. It can occur together with a phobia of all sexual contact or as the only problem within an otherwise normal sexual relationship. Typical phrases used by the patient include: 'There's a block', 'He just can't seem to get it (his penis) in', 'It's as if it is too small (her vaginal opening)'.

Sometimes the doctor may be able to feed back to the patient that she appears to be disassociated from that area of her body, and further questioning often confirms that she does not touch that area much herself due to concerns with cleanliness, smell or religious beliefs.

### Causes of vaginismus

- Sexual abuse
- Physical abuse
- Painful medical procedure in the perineal area
- Painful first intercourse
- Relationship problems/anger between couples ('I won't let him in' – subconsciously)
- Fear of pregnancy/labour
- Religious orthodoxy
- Poor sexual education
- Sexual inhibition.

### Treatment

There needs to be discussion around the main issues in the relationship and how the woman feels about touching her own genitalia. Behavioural therapy comprising systematic desensitization, pubococcygeal muscle training and the use of vaginal trainers works well. The response to this therapy for this group is good, with complete resolution for most couples, especially if the origin is uncomplicated in nature.[5] The phobia of penetration needs to be explored so that the woman reaches a situation in which she feels in control of her vagina and can enjoy sex when and how she wishes.

- Discussion and education about sex and the condition.
- Teaching the location and control of the vaginal (pubococcygeal) muscles.
- Self-examination of the vulva and vagina when alone and relaxed, e.g. in the bath (beginning of systematic desensitization).
- Insertion of her own finger, then fingers or plastic vaginal trainers.
- Doing the above in a sexual situation with her partner present.
- The woman inserting her partner's finger, then penis with her in control.
- Insertion of the penis with her partner in control, but with the woman on top so that it is less threatening.
- Sexual intercourse as the couple would wish.

**EBM**

There have been no randomized, controlled trials. Observational studies indicate that treatment is generally very successful for women with vaginismus.

## SEXUAL DESIRE DISORDERS

This is now often referred to as hypoactive sexual desire disorder (HSDD).

This usually presents as loss of libido (loss of interest in sex). It should also be remembered that there is huge variability between individuals and within the normal range. Sometimes it is the disparity between partners that leads a woman or couple to seek help. Testosterone deficiency can be considered among the underlying causes of desire disorders in post-menopausal women. Testosterone should be replaced together with oestrogens.

Specific pathways for sexual arousal, desire, reward and inhibition exist in the brain and are altered by hormones and experience. Hypothalamic, limbic and dopamine systems are important for desire as are certain neuropeptic systems.[6]

There is also controversy about what comes first in women, arousal or desire.

The prognosis is variable, but is better when it is the female with the initial problem. One study examined 60 couples presenting with the female partner's loss of interest as the major problem. There was only modest success, with 56 per cent experiencing a relatively good outcome at the end of treatment.[7] These problems are usually the symptom of a generally poor relationship overall, and the sexual disorder is only part of the whole problem.

## SEXUAL AROUSAL DISORDER

It is difficult to separate sexual arousal disorder from sexual desire disorder and female orgasm disorder due to the close relationship of the three conditions in women. Causes of lack of arousal are numerous. They can be psychological (distractions, childhood loss, low self-esteem), endocrine (lack of oestrogen), neurological (e.g. multiple sclerosis) or drug induced (e.g. antihistamines). Additionally, the widespread use of vaginal lubricants/vaginal oestrogens may mask or alleviate the disorder.

There have been cases of persistent sexual arousal syndrome, where women with no conscious desire for sexual expression are overwhelmed by continual sensations in the genitals. This is differentiated from hypersexuality, a syndrome which does involve a high level of desire for sexual activity. Little is known about these disorders, but psychological/cognitive–behavioural treatment does seem to confer some benefit.[8]

## FEMALE ORGASMIC DISORDER (ANORGASMIA)

### Definition

This is the term used for failure to achieve orgasm due to inhibition of the orgasmic reflex or poor sexual technique/ignorance.

### Aetiology

There may be fear of losing control, holding back. It may be situational, in that the woman can achieve orgasm by masturbation or with the aid of sex toys, but not during sexual intercourse. Sometimes, realistic ideas and the discussion of what most women achieve are necessary. For example, many women do not experience orgasm by penetration alone and do need other clitoral stimulation at the same time. Education regarding sexual positions to enhance clitoral stimulation and education about the clitoris itself may be required. There may be unrealistic expectations on the part of the partner, who may equate the female orgasm with his own and will not be happy unless his female partner also has one during penetration. This pressure on the female can lead to faking of orgasm to keep the partner happy and a premature end to the sexual act and frustration on the part of the female, who has not actually achieved orgasm. Drugs, such as anti-psychotics, can also cause orgasm problems.[9]

### Treatment of anorgasmia

- Encourage self-exploration and what is pleasurable when she is alone.
- Sensate focus–concentration on the sensual pleasure of touching her partner, but avoiding the genitals.
- Masturbation.
- Use of sex toys such as vibrators, if helpful; use of DVDs to help arousal and provide ideas (e.g. *The Lovers' Guide* series by Dr Andrew Stanway).
- Discussion and resolution of unconscious fears of orgasm, if present.
- Heightening sexual arousal so that the woman is close to orgasm before penetration.

### Hysterectomy and sexual function

There has been debate in the literature about the role of hysterectomy in sexual function. This has become more important now that women are more involved in their own treatment choices and feel more able to demand a good outcome from surgery. It has also become more pertinent since there have been more non-surgical (e.g. the levonorgestrel intrauterine system) and less-complicated procedures (e.g. endometrial destruction methods) to treat one of the most common reasons for hysterectomy, namely menorrhagia. There has been a steady rise in the number of supracervical hysterectomies performed for benign conditions, in some countries. The ratio of sub-total to total hysterectomies in Scandinavia is high at 0.56 compared to the United Kingdom where in 2005 it was reported as 0.04.[10] This may reflect the changing attitudes of surgeons and women towards a less invasive procedure, which was believed to have a reduced operative morbidity and reduced the risk of urinary and sexual dysfunction. Various mechanisms have been proposed to explain why cervical conservation may have a less detrimental effect on sexual function than total abdominal hysterectomy. Early pioneering work[1] described elevation of both the cervix and uterus during excitement and the plateau phase, followed by fundal uterine contractions progressively involving the lower uterine segment as orgasm developed. Cervical os dilatation occurred immediately afterwards, implicating a role for the cervix in the female sexual response. Another theory postulates that the ability to achieve orgasm depends on the nerve endings of the uterovaginal (cervical) plexus of Frankenhauser.[11] This plexus is a matrix of nerve fibres intimately surrounding the cervix. Stimulation of the cervix may contribute to a pleasurable sensation ultimately experienced as orgasm. However, the most recent evidence does not support superiority of subtotal over total hysterectomy and instead the most rigorous studies show that the majority of women experience no negative impact on sexual satisfaction, whatever the method and whether subtotal or not [A]. Most of the studies demonstrate improvement in sexual function in general after hysterectomy, because there is relief from dyspareunia and menstrual bleeding.[12]

## OESTROGEN REPLACEMENT THERAPY AND SEXUAL FUNCTION

Women often complain about changes in sexual function after a natural or iatrogenic menopause (bilateral salpingo-oopherectomy). Oestrogens appear to be an important part of the sexual response and loss of libido is a recognized symptom of the menopause.[13] Systemic oestrogens (e.g. oral, transdermal, subcutaneous) can be used following full discussion of the pros and cons. Testosterone may also be used, but should always be used in conjunction with systemic oestrogens.

If the main problem with sex is due to vaginal dryness causing dyspareunia and diminishing sexual pleasure and desire, it may also be useful to use local oestrogens in the form of cream or pessaries (let the woman try both to see what suits her best). Even if a woman is using systemic oestrogens she may also require local therapy, especially if she has ongoing symptoms of hypo-oestrogenism (soreness, dryness, dyspareunia). Care with the type of vaginal oestrogens should be taken with longer-term use to prevent endometrial hyperplasia in the woman with an intact uterus (only use estriol cream or oestrodiol pessaries).

## TESTOSTERONE THERAPY AND SEXUAL FUNCTION

Testosterone is produced in the ovaries and in the adrenal glands in women. Testosterone has been used in women with various sexual disorders and testosterone deficiency disorders since the 1930s. Despite this, the use of testosterone therapy is still controversial. Circulating testosterone declines in the late reproductive years so that healthy women in their forties have half the level compared to women in their twenties. A direct link between sexual dysfunction and endogenous testosterone levels has not been clearly found in premenopausal women. Research on testosterone levels is mainly confined to post-menopausal women so the place of testosterone therapy in pre-menopausal women with low libido is not currently known.

Decreased levels of testosterone in post-menopausal women lead to decreased libido, sexual activity and decreased levels of physical well-being. Bilateral salpingo-oopherectomy (BSO) causes a decrease in sex drive by 50 per cent, by removing ovarian contribution of testosterone. Many gynaecologists have used subcutaneous implants for testosterone replacement, after BSO, for many years. There is also another form of hormone replacement therapy used in post-menopausal women which is licensed for libido problems, called tibolone. It has some androgen-like properties.

More recently, transdermal testosterone therapy has been shown to increase sexual activity and satisfaction in at least 51 per cent of women in randomized double-blind trials compared to placebo. The patches are well tolerated with the main side effect being atopic site reactions. Testosterone therapy overdose can also cause acne, hirsutism and lowered voice.[14]

## PLACES TO REFER WOMEN/COUPLES WITH PSYCHOSEXUAL PROBLEMS

- Relate – provides counselling for all relationship and psychosexual problems (there may be a fee).
- Local contraceptive/reproductive healthcare services may have a psychosexual service (contact your local consultant).
- Local hospital-based psychosexual services – may be within urology, gynaecology, genitourinary medicine or psychiatry departments.
- Private sex therapists (contacted via the British Association for Sexual and Relationship Therapists or the British Association for Counselling).
- Doctors trained by the Institute of Psychosexual Medicine (contact the institute directly).

Pelvic floor and lower urinary tract dysfunction

## KEY POINTS

- It is important to classify further into the site of pain: superficial or deep.
- Pain at intercourse can lead to problems of sexual arousal causing further sexual pain and then avoidance of sexual activity.
- If an organic cause for dyspareunia is found, it does not necessarily exclude emotional and/or psychological sequelae for the woman.
- In assessing gynaecological problems, where there is a good chance of concomitant psychosexual issues, such as vulval disorders and dyspareunia, it is extremely important that the clinician feels comfortable to ask about sexual problems.
- Dyspareunia is the only sexual disorder in which physical factors are thought to play a major aetiological role. However, the psychological and interpersonal factors are significant.
- Observational studies indicate that treatment is generally very successful for women with vaginismus.

## Key References

1. Masters WH, Johnson VE. *Human Sexual Response*. Boston, MA: Little, Brown, 1966.
2. Mokate T, Wright C, Mander T. Hysterectomy and sexual function. *J Br Menopause Soc* 2006; **12**: 153–7.
3. Rosen RC, Leiblum SR. The treatment of sexual disorders in the 1990s: an integrated approach. *J Consul Clin Psychol* 1995; **65**: 877–90.
4. Schover LP, Youngs DD, Cannata R. Psychosexual aspects of the evaluation and management of vulvar vestibulitis. *Am J Obstet Gynecol* 1992; **167**: 630–6.
5. Hawton K, Catalan J, Martin P, Fagg J. Long term outcome of sex therapy. *Behav Res Ther* 1986; **24**: 665–75.
6. Basson R. Biopsychosocial models of women's sexual response: applications to management of 'desire disorders'. *Sex Relations Ther* 2003; **18**: 107–15.
7. Hawton K, Catalan J, Fagg J. Low sexual desire: sex therapy results and prognostic factors. *Behav Res Ther* 1991; **47**: 832–8.
8. Hiller J, Hekster B. Couple therapy with cognitive behavioural techniques for persistent sexual arousal syndrome. *Sex Relations Ther* 2007; **22**: 91–6.
9. Murthy S, Wylie K. Sexual problems in patients on antipsychotic medication. *Sex Relations Ther* 2007; **22**: 97–107.
10. Garry R. The place of subtotal/supracervical hysterectomy in current practice. *BJOG* 2008; **115**: 1597–600.
11. Hanson HM. Cervical removal at hysterectomy for benign disease, risks and benefits. *J Reprod Med* 1993; **38**: 781–90.
12. Kupperman M, Summitt RL Jr, Varner RE *et al.*, Total or Supracervical Hysterectomy Research Group. Sexual functioning after total compared to supracervical hysterectomy: a randomised trial. *Obstet Gynecol* 2005; **105**: 1309–18.
13. Wylie KR. Sexuality and the menopause. *J Br Menopause Soc* 2006; **12**: 149–52.
14. Kingsberg S. Testosterone treatment for HSDD in postmenopausal women. *J Sex Med* 2007; **4** (Suppl. 3): 227–34.

# 64.3 Child sex abuse

*Melanie Mann*

---

## MRCOG standards

### Knowledge criteria

- The laws related to child protection, consent and the Sexual Offences Act 2003.
- Recognize the sexual health needs of vulnerable groups, e.g. young people.
- Understand local care pathways for multi-agency working for individuals with sexual health needs.

### Clinical competency

- Network with other providers in multi-disciplinary teams, e.g. social workers, counsellors.

## INTRODUCTION

The management of these problems requires special skill and sensitivity. It also requires knowledge of the legal issues surrounding allegations of child sexual abuse and the proper procedures that need to be followed. The skills required have a wide overlap with those necessary to deal with paediatric gynaecological problems and adult psychosexual problems.

The Children's Act 1989 defines a child as 'a person who has not yet reached 18 years of age'. In England and Wales, the present age of consent for sexual intercourse is 16 years.

The Sexual Offences Act 2003 made further changes to the way that prosecutions can be made against people committing sexual offences with particular emphasis on defining any sexual activity with under 13 year olds as an offence, consent being completely irrelevant. In terms of a child aged 13–16 years, the Act describes sexual offences in a wider sense, such as any kind of penetration of any orifice, intentional touching, via a third person, arranging or facilitating and incitement of any kind of sexual act. An important factor here is the 'reasonable belief that the child is over 16' (this does apply to under 13 year olds). It is intended to include all sorts of internet crime, trafficking of people and grooming. It makes provision for anyone who has any kind

of part in these sorts of crimes to be prosecuted. It also includes crimes performed by people abusing a position of trust, such as teachers or carers including vulnerable groups, such as 'looked after' children (e.g. in care homes, foster care). The Act does also make it possible to prosecute young people under 18 who also commit these crimes, particularly if it is within the public interest or there has been a breach of duty of care of trust. The important exclusion to the Act is that those who are trying to protect children, for example from sexually transmitted infections (STI) or pregnancy, are not able to be prosecuted, such as medical staff.

All health professionals play a part in ensuring that young people receive the care, support and services they require to promote their development. Sexual abuse is one form of child abuse. The others are emotional abuse, physical abuse and neglect.

## Nature of sexual acts in child sex abuse

- Exposure: the viewing of sexual acts, pornography and exhibitionism. Forcing a child to watch sex acts, exposing oneself in front of a child with the intent of one's own sexual gratification, including via a webcam on the internet.
- Molestation: fondling the genitals of the child or asking the child to fondle or masturbate the adult's genitals. Includes rubbing oneself up against a child.
- Sexual intercourse: vaginal, oral or anal intercourse without excessive force, often chronic.
- Rape: vaginal sexual intercourse without consent, often with threats or the use of violence, which may occur on an acute basis. This includes with any child under 13 years, consent being irrelevant.

## DEFINITION

Child sex abuse is the involvement of dependent, developmentally immature children and adolescents in sexual activities that they do not fully comprehend, are unable to give informed consent to, and that violate the social taboos of family roles. It may occur over a wide range of ages and can involve single incidents perpetrated by strangers or frequent contacts by a family member or friend.

## DETECTION OF CHILD SEX ABUSE

Occasionally, a child may present to a gynaecologist for investigation of symptoms and there may be a query about sexual abuse. It is important that the gynaecologist is able to bear the risk of child sex abuse in mind during the history and examination without causing mental or physical harm to the child.

The recognition of penile or digital penetration is very difficult in certain age groups and should always be referred to a paediatrician. Ideally, all children should be examined in a child-friendly environment with a paediatric-trained nurse present. All trusts in the United Kingdom have a child protection policy and it is the duty of all healthcare professionals working with children to be aware of the local referral pathways. Each trust has a named doctor and nurse who take a professional lead for child protection matters within the trust. This will ensure that each suspected case is treated promptly in the best interests of the child.

## DETECTION OF A SEXUALLY TRANSMITTED INFECTION IN A CHILD

In children under three years of age, the possibility of vertical transmission must always be considered and investigated.

In children aged 13 years or older, the possibility of consensual sexual intercourse should be considered. The proportion of young people who are sexually active before the age of 16 is increasing. The coexistence of drug or alcohol misuse and the increased vulnerability of those living away from home/accommodated by the local authority ('looked after children') must be considered and addressed. The possibility of the young person being a commercial sex worker must also be considered. Even if a child is between 16 and 18, if there is suspected abuse taking place, it should be discussed with the local child protection officer.

Liaison with local social workers, paediatricians and genitourinary physicians is mandatory. There are specific medicolegal methods for the investigation of sexually transmitted infections that need to be followed (see 'chain of evidence', as described under Genital and internal examination in Chapter 64.4).

The confidentiality of young people attending for advice is very important. In practice, a clinician must take into account both the need of the young person for a confidential sexual health service and the need to protect that young person from sexual abuse and sexual exploitation. The clinician also has a duty to consider the possibility that other young people may be at risk of abuse. This means that the clinician must work with the young person to obtain her confidence and inform her if and when confidentiality may have to be broken.

Children under the age of 16 should be assessed at the time of prescribing contraception according to Fraser guidelines (sometimes referred to as 'Gillick competence', but this term should no longer be used). The Fraser guidelines came out of a seminal case (Wisbech v Gillick, 1985) which looked at the case of confidentiality and assessing competence to consent to contraception. The points within the guidance are that the healthcare practitioner should:

- ensure the young woman understands the potential risks of the treatment/advice given;
- discuss the value of parental support, yet confidentiality is assured whether or not this is given (unless there is concern about abuse);
- assess whether the young woman will have sexual intercourse without contraception;
- assess whether the young person will suffer physical or mental harm if not given contraceptive advice or supplies;
- consider if it is in the patient's best interests to give contraception without parental consent;
- respect the duty of confidentiality given to a person under 16 years, which should be as good as that given to someone over 16.

### KEY POINTS

- Liaison with local Child Protection Team is mandatory.
- Junior clinicians should discuss all suspected cases of child abuse with their line manager as a matter of urgency.

## ADULT SEQUELAE OF CHILD SEX ABUSE

Recent prevalence studies show that about one in three adult women have had sexual contact with an older person as a child.[1] Sexual abuse is a serious mental health problem and often results in impairment as adults, but less than 20 per cent of affected women show serious psychopathology. Surprisingly, the description and literature around child sex abuse is only found for the first time over the last 20 years.[2]

There can be many manifestations of child sex abuse that has taken place in the past, and these can be mild or can cause havoc in the adult's life and can be revealed during history taking or examination. Sensitivity and care must be exercised in all consultations to ensure that the woman is enabled to reveal the intimate secret and can be directed to appropriate help as required. Occasionally, just a sympathetic attitude and 'believing her' are all that is required. The adult sequelae of child sex abuse include the following:

- Depression: the most common symptom, coinciding with low self-esteem, anxiety and sleep disorders.
- Pelvic pain: several studies have shown an association with pelvic pain and other gynaecological complaints.
- Sexual adjustment problems: these vary from retreat to apparent preoccupation with sexual matters and promiscuity.
- Interpersonal relationship problems: victims are more likely to have physically violent partners – 'continuing victims'.
- Social functioning: there is a link between child sex abuse and later prostitution; there is also evidence for increased alcohol and drug abuse in this group.

There is no clear-cut evidence as to which factors lead to a negative outcome for child sex abuse survivors, but there are trends. It would appear that the worse-case scenario is regular abuse, with force, by a close, older member of the family, such as father to daughter.

Adult survivors should be referred to an appropriately trained counsellor. The referral pathways differ locally.

## KEY POINTS

- Sensitivity during history taking and examination will aid the diagnosis of previous child sex abuse.
- The patient can then be referred to an appropriate counsellor.
- Child sex abuse is a serious mental health problem often resulting in impairment in adulthood.

## Published Guidelines

British Association for Sexual Health and HIV. *Sexually Transmitted Infections in Children*. Clinical Effectiveness Group, BASHH, 2009. Available from: ‹www.bashh.org.uk›.

## Key References

1. Sheldrick C. Adult sequelae of child sexual abuse. *Br J Psych* 1991; **158** (Suppl. 10): 55–62.
2. Ahmad S. Adult psychosexual dysfunction as a sequel of child sexual abuse. *Sex Relation Ther* 2006; **21**: 405–18.

# 64.4 Rape and rape counselling

*Susan J Houghton*

## INTRODUCTION

It is estimated that between one in four and one in six women will be raped during their lifetimes [C][1,2] and that two years following the rape, 50 per cent of victims regularly require medical review. Drug-facilitated assault is not uncommon, usually involving the use of central nervous system depressants with alcohol. Rape and sexual assault can be associated with physical harm, infection, unwanted pregnancy and severe psychological damage. The aim of this chapter is to highlight the role of the examining doctor in the assessment of victims of sexual assault (the complainants). It defines rape, details the forensic medical examination and what forensic evidence should be obtained, and what is required in the witness statement. Ideally, all victims of sexual assault should be examined by a fully qualified forensic medical examiner (FME, previously known as a police surgeon), who has received specific training in forensic gynaecology. In England and Wales, there are currently 22 sexual assault referral centres (SARC)

providing specialist multi-disciplinary care to complainants in a sensitive and secure environment [E].[3]

## DEFINITIONS

The Sexual Offences Act, 2003, in England and Wales, redefined rape as 'non-consensual penetration of the vagina, anus or mouth with the penis' [E].[4] Ejaculation is not required for a rape to have taken place and the law now includes complainants who have undergone gender reassignment surgery. The offence of 'indecent assault' was also reclassified, with 'assault by penetration' defined as 'penetration of the vagina or anus with a part of the body including the penis or with anything else'. This may result in a custodial sentence similar to those handed down for rape, i.e. a maximum penalty of life imprisonment. 'Sexual assault' defines non-penetrative acts, including touching and 'causing a person to engage in sexual activity without consent' and includes forced masturbation and forcing acts with third parties or animals.

The age of consent in the United Kingdom is 16 years; below this age, sexual intercourse is always unlawful. Proof of absence of consent is central where offences against adults are concerned. A person consents if he/she agrees by choice and has the capacity to make that choice. Absence of consent will be presumed where: violence is used or immediate violence threatened to the victim or third party; the victim is detained against their will; the victim is unable to communicate consent through physical disability or a substance has been administered without the victim's consent which was capable of stupefying or overpowering them.

In 1994, it was determined that a man could be charged with raping his wife (R v RIAC 599 House of Lords).

## MANAGEMENT

The examination of an alleged rape victim should take place as soon as possible after the alleged assault and in an appropriate environment, ideally in a SARC or a specialized 'rape suite' in a police station or hospital. A trained female police officer should be present if the complainant requests police involvement, and the complainant should choose the gender of the examining doctor. The Faculty of Forensic and Legal Medicine (‹www.fflm.ac.uk›) has guidelines on the collection and labelling of forensic specimens (updated every six months), the management of injuries and specific consent forms for the examination of rape victims.

## Management of the immediate medical needs of the complainant

The management of injuries requiring immediate medical attention takes priority over forensic sampling. Up to 80 per cent of rape victims have some form of physical injury [D],[5] with up to 5 per cent having major non-genital injuries [C].[6] A minority of rape victims sustain genital injury, with 30 per cent of pre-menopausal and 50 per cent of post-menopausal victims having demonstrable genital injury [D].[7] Injury is much more likely if forced anal intercourse has occurred.

It is extremely important that the on-call obstetrician or gynaecologist, if asked to treat a rape victim, is aware of the forensic, legal and health issues related to such cases [E].[8,9]

## Accurate history taking of the alleged incident to determine which forensic samples should be taken

Prior to the medical examination, the police officer should obtain a detailed investigative history, or 'first account', from the complainant to establish if an offence has been committed. The FME should ask direct questions based upon the first account (Table 64.4.1) and the questions and answers should be recorded in the medical records. This will determine which forensic samples should be taken. The complainant's name, age and date of birth; the date, time and place of the examination; people present at the examination and their relationship to the victim; and details of the victim's general practitioner should be clearly documented.

## Relevant medical and sexual history

This is necessary to assist with the interpretation of the medical findings and to identify any medical problems that may be attributable to the assault (Table 64.4.2).

## Informed consent for the forensic medical examination

Consent must be obtained for a medical examination (non-genital and genital), the collection of forensic evidence, the retention of relevant items of clothing for forensic examination and the disclosure of details of medical records to the police and/or Crown Prosecution Service (CPS). Consent forms may be downloaded from the following websites: ‹www.fflm.ac.uk› or ‹www.careand evidence.org›.

## Thorough medical examination

The examination should be performed with the use of a sexual offences kit, which contains modular kits with all the necessary equipment to undertake forensic sampling, including swabs, gloves, disposable speculums, specimen and blood bottles, tamper evident bags, labels, scissors, combs, a gown and a sheet of white paper. It should also contain an information sheet, medical examination record and consent form. The first response police officer may have already collected forensic samples with an early evidence kit, which may include urine for toxicology, a mouth swab or rinse if oral intercourse occurred, sanitary dressings and/or toilet tissue and a stool sample, if vaginal or anal penetrative intercourse occurred.

### External examination

The general appearance and emotional state of the complainant are assessed for evidence of alcohol/drug intoxication, damage or staining of clothes, hair, face, hands and fingernails, and evidence of the acute phase of rape trauma syndrome. Clothing should be removed by the complainant while standing on a 'sterile' white paper sheet to catch any falling debris. Each item is inspected and described in detail before the police officer places it into a labelled paper bag and submits it for forensic examination. Any debris is sent separately. The complainant is carefully examined for any injuries, and an estimate made of the timing of these injuries. All injuries should be described according to the Crane classification [E][10] and documented on a body chart. Complex injuries should be photographed. Bite marks should be swabbed to obtain samples of the assailant's saliva and photographed by a forensic odontologist. Guidance on the management of injuries caused by teeth, body charts and a consent form for photographs can be downloaded from ‹www.fflm.ac.uk›.

### Genital and internal examination

The forensic samples taken are listed in Table 64.4.3 p. 766. The samples must be clearly labelled, documented on the forensic medical examination form or in the medical notes and sealed in tamper evident bags before transport to the forensic science laboratory, to maintain the continuity or 'chain of evidence'. The identification/exhibit number and/or timings must reflect the order of sampling. Where two swabs have been taken from the same site, the first sample should be labelled 'A' and the

**Table 64.4.1** Assault history to be taken by forensic medical examiner

| Details of the assault | Date and time of assault | |
|---|---|---|
| | Time lapse from assault | |
| | Name of assailant (if known) | |
| | Relationship of assailant to victim | |
| History of assault | Source of history | |
| | Events preceding this assault | |
| | Place of assault | |
| | Drugs or alcohol consumed by the victim | |
| | Details of the assault – to direct forensic sampling | |
| | Damage or disruption to clothing | |
| | Site and mechanism of injuries – to include details of any weapons or implements used | |
| | Defence used by victim | |
| | Relative position of parties | |
| | Any loss of consciousness | |
| Exact nature of assault | Digital/vaginal | Yes/no |
| | Oral/vaginal | Yes/no |
| | Oral/penile | Yes/no |
| | Penile/vaginal | Yes/no (If yes, did ejaculation occur?) |
| | Penile/anal | Yes/no (If yes, did ejaculation occur?) |
| | Digital/anal | Yes/no |
| | Lubricant used? | |
| | Condom used? | |
| Events following assault | Description of what occurred following the assault, to include details of: | |
| | Changing of clothes | |
| | Washing the genital area | |
| | Taking a shower or bath | |
| | Washing of hair | |
| | Cleaning of teeth | |
| | Micturition or defaecation | |
| | Vomiting | |
| | Ingestion of food or drink | |
| | Any medical treatment received since assault | |

second as sample 'B'. Anonymous samples may be sent, with consent, in cases where the complainant does not want to report the assault to the police. Complainants often change their mind and wish to report an assault to the police at a later date. A photographer of the same gender as the victim should take any genital photographs. Colposcopy may be, but is not routinely, used in the United Kingdom for the assessment of rape victims.

# Management of the sexual and mental health of the victim

## Preventing and treating sexually transmitted infections

Sexually transmitted infections occur in between 4 and 56 per cent of women following sexual assault [D].[11] Screening

**Table 64.4.2** Relevant medical and sexual history

| Gynaecological history | Age at menarche | |
|---|---|---|
| | Last menstrual period – forensic analysis cannot distinguish between menstrual blood and that related to injury | |
| | Menstrual cycle | |
| | Any gynaecological problems: | Current |
| | | Past history |
| | Obstetric history: | Pregnant – presently/previously/never |
| | | Outcome of previous pregnancies |
| Sexual history | Sexually active | Presently/previously/never? |
| | Last coitus: | |
| |    Date | |
| |    Time | |
| |    Use of lubricant | Yes/no |
| | Genital problems | Past/present |
| | Sexually transmitted diseases | Yes/no |
| General medical history | History of serious illness | Past/present |
| | Psychiatric problems | Yes/no |
| | Previous operations | Yes/no |
| | Bruising tendency | Yes/no |
| | Skin problems | Yes/no |
| Social history | Current occupation | |

for gonorrhoea, chlamydia, trichomoniasis and syphilis may be performed at initial presentation or empirical antibiotic prophylaxis can be offered, depending upon patient preference:

- ciprofloxacin 500 mg plus doxycycline 100 mg twice daily for 7 days, or
- ciprofloxacin 500 mg plus azithromycin 1 g or, if pregnant or breastfeeding,
- amoxycillin 3 g plus probenecid 1 g or erythromycin 500 mg twice daily for 14 days.

Hepatitis B vaccination should be offered up to 3 weeks after sexual assault to all victims who are not known to be immune. The risk of contracting human immunodeficiency virus (HIV) infection as a result of rape is unknown, but is thought to be very low in areas of low prevalence, such as the UK. The risk may be higher in cases involving genital trauma [E],[12] forced anal intercourse, defloration and multiple assailants. Individual risk is assessed and post-exposure prophylaxis (PEP) with Truvada one tablet once a day (tenofovir disoproxil 245 mg + emtricitabine 200 mg) and Kaletra two tablets once a day (lopinavir 1333.3 mg + ritonavir 33.3 mg) is offered to those with a negative baseline HIV ELISA test. PEP should be continued for 28 days and involves pre-HIV test counselling, informed consent and monitoring by an HIV specialist. Guidance on

the management of sexual assault and HIV PEP can be downloaded from ‹www.careandevidnce.org›.

A repeat bacterial infection screen should be performed at 2 weeks follow up if antibiotic prophylaxis was not given initially. At three to six months, HIV, hepatitis B and syphilis tests should be repeated with hepatitis C testing, if there is thought to be a risk.

## Pregnancy

Rape-related pregnancy occurs in up to 5 per cent of women [C].[13] Postcoital contraception with Levonelle 2 (within 72 hours) or an intrauterine contraceptive device (within 5 days) should be offered and a pre-existing pregnancy excluded. Counselling and support, with referral to specialist agencies, should be offered to those who become pregnant.

## Psychological support

It is estimated that over half of all women who are raped suffer from post-traumatic stress disorder (PTSD). Following the rape, symptoms of anxiety, depression, tearfulness, flashbacks, humiliation, self-blame, disbelief, anger, fear, powerlessness and physical revulsion are common [D].[14] Long-term problems with social adjustment, sexual relationships, physical health and substance abuse can occur [C].[15] Verbal and written advice concerning support and counselling agencies should be given.

Pelvic floor and lower urinary tract dysfunction

**Table 64.4.3** Forensic samples to be taken at forensic medical examination

| Non-intimate samples | Unopened control swabs |
|---|---|
| | Urine sample – for alcohol and toxicology testing |
| | Blood samples – for DNA analysis, blood typing, alcohol estimation, toxicology screen |
| | Buccal scrapes (×2) – for DNA profiling if venesection refused |
| | Mouth swab (×2 dry) – if oral assault |
| | Skin swabs (×2, 1 wet and 1 dry) – at each site of kissing/sucking/ejaculation/bite, e.g. right and left breast, upper thigh, other – to be specified |
| | Head hair visible debris (collect using forceps) |
| | Head hair swabs (×2, 1 wet and 1 dry) |
| | Head hair combings |
| | Head hair cuttings (minimum 25) – collect only in stranger rape |
| | Right and left nail scrapings – if visible debris or if victim scratched assailant |
| | Right and left fingernail cuttings – if broken nails or if victim scratched assailant |
| | Right and left fingernail swabs (×2, 1 wet and 1 dry) |
| | Right and left hand swabs |
| | Couch cover |
| | Patient gown and groundsheet |
| | Gloves – should be changed at each stage of the examination and all pairs sent for analysis |
| Intimate samples | Unopened control swabs |
| | Pubic hair visible debris (collect using forceps) |
| | Pubic hair swabs (×2, 1 wet and 1 dry) |
| | Pubic hair combings |
| | Pubic hair cuttings (minimum 25) – collect only in stranger rape |
| | Vulval/perineal swabs (×1, wet or dry, as appropriate) |
| | Low vaginal swabs (×2, dry) |
| | High vaginal swabs (×2, dry) |
| | Endocervical swabs – should be taken if vaginal intercourse has taken place >48 hours ago |
| | Perianal/anal and rectal swabs (×2, dry or wet, as appropriate) – a proctoscope may need to be used in cases of anal penetration |
| | Sanitary wear – tampon/sanitary towel/toilet tissue used before and/or after offence |
| | Condom |
| | Vaginal speculum – document if and what lubricant used |
| | Proctoscope |

- Victim Support, Victim Support National Centre, Hallam House, 56–60 Hallam Street, London, W1W 6JL. Tel. 020 7268 0200; Fax. 020 7268 0210. ‹www.victimsupport.com›.
- Survivors UK Ltd, 2, Leathermarket Street, London, SE1 3HN. Helpline: 0845 1221201. e-mail: info@survivorsuk. org, ‹www.survivorsuk.org›.
- National Rape Crisis England and Wales, Rape Crisis (England and Wales), c/o WRSAC, Box 39, Bodmin, Cornwall, PL31 1XF. Tel. 0115 934 8474; ‹www.rapecrisis.co.uk›.

## Completion of a witness statement

The 'professional' witness statement should include details of the history of the assault and relevant medical, surgical and psychiatric history, document all of the normal and abnormal findings of the examination, list the forensic specimens taken, and give details about any medical treatment given and post-examination arrangements. The FME should give an opinion as to the degree of certainty about the likely cause of the injuries.

The statement should have a professional appearance, must be carefully checked for errors, and must include a statutory declaration, with the date and signature at the bottom of each page and at the end of the declaration. A witness should also sign each page. The FME should state his or her qualifications, appointment and relevant experience and it is advisable for new examining doctors to discuss the case and statement preparation with an experienced FME. Many police forces have standard statement forms for the FME to complete.

## SUMMARY

Any doctor involved in the care of a rape victim must be sensitive, sympathetic and highly professional. With advances in forensic science, it is essential that forensic samples are taken in an attempt to identify DNA for profiling. A meticulous examination, detailed medical records and an accurate and detailed statement are essential in the management of victims of sexual assault.

## EBM

The supporting evidence for the advocated management plan (and the above text) relies on observational data, cohort studies, retrospective descriptive studies and 'expert opinion'. Given the nature of the condition, it is unlikely that evidence based upon more robust methodologies will be forthcoming.

## KEY POINTS

- Be sympathetic and professional.
- Attend to immediate medical needs.
- Examine in an appropriate and comfortable environment.
- Obtain consent for examination.
- Take an accurate history.
- Clearly document findings and carefully label samples.
- Give appropriate medical, prophylactic and psychological treatment.
- Advise on counselling and support agencies.

## Key References

1. Walch AG, Broadhead WE. Prevalance of lifetime sexual victimisation among female patients. *J Fam Practice* 1992; **35**: 511–16.
2. Roberts R. Rape crisis management. *Diplomate* 1994; **1**: 6–11.
3. Sexual assault referral centre locations. Last accessed June 11, 2009. Available from: ‹www.homeoffice.gov.uk/crime-victims/reducing-crime/sexual-offences/sexual-assault-referral-centres/referral-centre-locations/?version=4›.
4. The Sexual Offences Act 2003. Last accessed June 11, 2009. Available from: ‹www.opsi.gov.uk/acts/acts2003/ukpga_20030042_en_1›.
5. Bowyer L, Dalton ME. Female victims of rape and their genital findings. *Br J Obstet Gynaecol* 1997; **104**: 617–20.
6. Marchbanks PA, Liu KJ, Mercy JA. Risk of injury from resisting rape. *Am J Epidemiol* 1990; **132**: 540–9.
7. Cartwright PS, Sexual Assault Study Group. Factors that correlate with injury sustained by survivors of sexual assault. *Obstet Gynecol* 1987; **70**: 44–6.
8. Butler B, Welch J. Dealing with sexual assault. *Br J Sex Med* 2008; **31**: 4–7.
9. Eddy JW, James HE. Forensic gynaecological examination for beginners: management of women presenting at A & E. *Obstet Gynaecol* 2005; **7**: 82–8.
10. Crane J. Injury. In: McClay WDS (ed.). *Clinical Forensic Medicine*. London: Greenwich Medical Media, 1996: 143–62.
11. Lamba H, Murphy SM. Sexual assault and sexually transmitted infections: an updated review. *Int J STD AIDS* 2000; **11**: 487–91.
12. Claydon E. Rape and HIV. *Int J STD AIDS* 1991; **2**: 200–1.
13. Holmes MM, Resnick HS, Kilpatrick DG, Best CL. Rape-related pregnancy: estimates and descriptive characteristics from a national sample of women. *Am J Obstet Gynecol* 1996; **175**: 320–5.
14. Hampton HL. Care of the woman who has been raped. *N Engl J Med* 1995; **332**: 234–7.
15. Mezey GC, Taylor PJ. Psychological reactions of women who have been raped: a descriptive and comparative study. *Br J Psych* 1988; **152**: 330–9.

# SECTION C
## Lower genital tract

# Chapter 65

# Benign vulval problems

*Elias Tzakas and Charles Redman*

## INTRODUCTION

Many women have vulval symptoms, but only a fraction will seek medical advice. Of these, only a selected few will be referred for a specialist opinion. Some may be advised to attend a genitourinary medicine (GUM) clinic, while others will be referred for a gynaecological opinion. This chapter primarily relates to women attending gynaecological or vulval clinics.

## ANATOMICAL CONSIDERATIONS

Vulval skin comprises stratified squamous epithelium as in other parts of the body. The mons pubis and labia majora contain fat, sebaceous, apocrine and eccrine sweat glands and blood vessels, which can develop varicosities. However, whereas the labia minora are rich in sebaceous glands, there are few sweat glands and no hair follicles. The epithelium of the vestibule is neither pigmented nor keratinized, but contains eccrine glands. These glands and epithelial appendages are a source of vulval lumps.

Deep to the posterior parts of the labia majora are the Bartholin's or greater vestibular glands, whose ducts open into the posterior part of the vagina, just behind the mid-point and superficial to the hymenal ring. The glands and ducts can be the site of infection or cyst formation.

## ASSESSMENT

### Extrinsic and intrinsic causes

Whereas benign vulval disease has relatively few symptoms (pruritus, burning, pain, lumps), there are a myriad of causes. It is helpful when assessing a case to consider whether the problem arises from the skin itself or from the variety of factors that it comes into contact with, such as moisture (sweat, urine, vaginal discharge, infection, allergens and irritants). The key to making a diagnosis is clinical assessment from a careful history and, in particular, examination.

### History

It is important to accurately ascertain the nature of the presenting problem and the pattern of the symptoms in terms of periodicity and aggravating and relieving factors. It is vital to ask about what treatments have been used in the past, as well as about current and previous medications and general health.

### Examination

This should include a survey of the whole of the skin and other systems as indicated. An examination of the rest of the lower genital tract should always be considered, although it is by no means always necessary.

### Vulval biopsy

Biopsy is frequently necessary to confirm the diagnosis, if not clear, and to assess or confirm whether or not a lesion is pre-invasive or malignant. It is important to biopsy chronic dermatoses that do not respond to medical treatment. By and large, vulval biopsies can be performed in the clinic using disposable biopsy punches with local anaesthesia.

## NON-NEOPLASTIC EPITHELIAL DISORDERS

The group of conditions once referred to as 'vulval dystrophies' is now termed 'non-neoplastic epithelial disorders', classified by the ISSVD in 1987 (Table 65.1).

## Lichen sclerosus

### Definition

Lichen sclerosus (LS) is a chronic lymphocyte mediated dermatosis characterized by epithelial thinning, inflammation and distinctive histological changes in the dermis. It can affect both sexes and can occur at any age, but it is typically found in the anogenital region of postmenopausal women.

Lichen sclerosus can be asymptomatic in at least one-third of patients, but the most common presentation is intractable itching (pruritus vulvae) and vaginal soreness with dyspareunia. Burning and pain are uncommon symptoms and should arouse suspicion of alternative or concomitant conditions, such as vulvodynia.

The clinical findings are distinctive but variable. The typical lesions of porcelain white papules and plaques may be characterized by a crinkled or parchment-like appearance that usually extends around the anal area in a figure-of-eight configuration. There is often loss of the normal vulval architecture, with atrophy of the labia minora, loss of clitoral hood, constriction of the vaginal orifice, and the development of adhesions, ecchymoses, telangiectasia and fissures. LS may affect the labia minora and inner portion

**Table 65.1** International Society for the Study of Vulvar Diseases (ISSVD) classification of non-neoplastic epithelial disorders of the vulva

| |
|---|
| Lichen sclerosus |
| Squamous cell hyperplasia |
| Other dermatoses |
| Primary irritant dermatitis |
| Allergic dermatitis |
| Seborrhoeic dermatitis |
| Psoriasis |
| Lichen planus |
| Hidradenitis suppuritiva |
| Behçet's syndrome |

of labia majora, interlabial sulci, clitoris, perineum and perianal area, but almost never involves the vagina and cervix (unlike lichen planus (LP)). Extragenital lesions occur in 10–20 per cent of cases, most commonly involving the lateral thighs, submammary area, neck, shoulders and wrists. Extragenital lesions rarely itch and are not associated with malignant change.

Some cases of LS may represent an overlap syndrome, sharing clinicopathological features of both LS and LP, making diagnosis difficult. These are often associated histologically with squamous cell hyperplasia and are categorized as 'complicated' LS, as response to topical corticosteroids is often poorer and they are more at risk of long-term malignant change.[1]

In a recent clinical opinion by Jones et al., it was suggested that nearly all cases of LS can be classified into one of three histologic diagnostic categories with prognostic significance: atrophic (classic) LS, LS with histologic evidence of epidermal thickening and LS with differentiated vulval intraepithelial neoplasia (VIN).[2]

### Incidence

The prevalence of lichen sclerosus is unknown, but this group of patients usually constitutes the largest single diagnostic group in a hospital-based vulval clinic.

### Aetiology/risk factors

The cause is unknown. An autoimmune origin is most likely in view of its association with other autoimmune diseases (alopecia areata, vitiligo and thyroid disease being the most common) with a seemingly genetic predisposition.

### Prognosis

Lichen sclerosus can occur in children and in about two-thirds of cases the lesions will clear at puberty.[3] In adults, lichen sclerosus is a chronic condition that can be considered to be pre-malignant, with a reported incidence of progression to squamous vulval cancer ranging from 0 to 9 per cent.[4,5] Histopathological examination indicates that approximately 60 per cent of vulval cancers arise in a background of non-HPV-related LS (occasionally LP) and/or differentiated VIN and 30 per cent in HPV-related usual type (previously undifferentiated) VIN.[6]

### Management

The aims of management are to control the symptoms, minimize any or further architectural changes and to detect changes suggestive of malignant change. It is not yet clear whether successful control of the condition influences its long-term risk of malignant progression although a protective effect is suggested.[7]

Some clinicians believe that treatment only when symptomatic is not sufficient, as there can be active disease with minimal or no symptoms, thus requiring lifelong therapy. According to the current recommendations by the British Association of Dermatologists (BAD), asymptomatic patients with evidence of clinically active LS, i.e. ecchymosis, hyperkeratosis, erosions and progressing atrophy, should receive treatment [E].[8]

### General measures

It is important to reassure patients that lichen sclerosus is a well-recognized condition, which, although unlikely to disappear, can almost always be satisfactorily controlled with simple measures.

General vulval care and hygiene measures are especially important, such as wearing cotton underwear, avoidance of panty liners, strong soaps, bubble baths, biological washing powders, perfumed products and scratching. Lubrication to facilitate intercourse is advisable [E].

Bland emollients should be used liberally and can provide significant relief [C]. The high response rates noted when these are used as the placebo arm in randomized, controlled trials (RCTs) are thought to be more than a placebo effect.[9]

### Topical steroids

Ultrapotent topical corticosteroids are currently the accepted first-line initial management of LS.

Three RCTs have found that potent topical steroids (e.g. clobetasol propionate) provided significant symptom control, particularly in the short term [A], and that they are more effective than topical testosterone or petroleum jelly. While scarring, atrophy and pallor are irreversible, plaques, ecchymoses, erosions, hyperkeratosis and fissuring should resolve with successful treatment. The regimen recommended by the 'BAD' guidelines for a newly diagnosed case is clobetasol propionate (dermovate) initially once a night for 4 weeks, then alternate nights for 4 weeks and for the final third month, twice weekly with review at two to three months. Some patients will go into complete remission requiring no further treatment, while others will continue to have flares and remissions and will require maintenance treatment, either as weaker steroid preparations or less frequent use of very potent steroids. A 30-g tube of clobetasol propionate should last at least three months, with most maintained on 30–60 g annually.[8] Some clinicians argue that maintenance therapy should be uninterrupted to ensure better clinical control. Few, if any, adverse effects have been noted in association with the use of clobetasol propionate, even when used on an 'as-required basis' for maintenance therapy for one to three years [C].[9]

Thickened hypertrophic plaques may respond better to intralesional steroids which can be combined with local anaesthetic agent (e.g. bupivacaine 0.25–0.5 per cent). A regimen reserved for patients with intractable debilitating pruritus unresponsive to topical agents is injections every 4 weeks with up to 40 mg of triamcinolone per injection for up to three injections [C].[10]

Testosterone is no more effective than petroleum jelly [B], but can be associated with virilization, hypertrichosis, pruritus and pain.

### Retinoids

Retinoids appear to reduce connective tissue degeneration in LS.[11] One small RCT has found acitretin to be more effective that placebo [B]. Acitretin is associated with severe peeling of palms and soles and with hair loss [B], as well as with congenital abnormalities in women exposed during the first trimester of pregnancy. It is therefore contraindicated in the reproductive age group. Its use may be considered in those with severe complicated disease who are intolerant of, or resistant to, standard corticosteroid treatment after consultation with a dermatologist.[8,11] Topical retinoids, such as 0.025 per cent tretinoin cream, normalize hyperkeratinization and have significant anti-inflammatory properties and thus can be especially good for hyperkeratotic lesions, but skin irritation is a major factor limiting their use [C].

### Topical calcineurin inhibitors

Tacrolimus 0.1 per cent has been shown to be effective when used for 16–24 weeks, with one multicentre trial including men and women with genital and extragenital LS showing a 77 per cent response rate with up to 43 per cent having a complete response (absence of symptoms and skin findings excepting induration and atrophy) at 24 weeks [C].[12] A study of a related topical agent, pimecrolimus 1 per cent, showed that 42 per cent of patients were in complete remission after six months of treatment [C].[13] Local irritancy was the most common side effect with both, but improved with ongoing use. Therapy with topical calcineurin inhibitors is still experimental and ideally should only be considered in a research setting as long-term safety needs to be established, in view of concern about the possibility of topical immunosuppression and increased susceptibility to cancer.

## Surgery

In general, surgery should be limited for the treatment of coexistent vulval intraepithelial neoplasia or squamous cell carcinoma (SCC) and correction of scarring complications (labial fusion and narrowed introitus) [E]. Before any corrective surgery, LS should be clinically well controlled. There is no systematic review, RCTs or good-quality observational studies demonstrating the benefits of surgery for symptomatic relief in lichen sclerosus. Three studies reported reoperation rates after vulvectomy of 23–50 per cent for recurrence of symptoms, malignant change or introital stenosis [D].[4]

## Follow up

Long-term follow up with a specialist clinic should be reserved for 'complicated' LS unresponsive to treatment and where difficulty exists with symptomatic control, i.e. those who use topical steroids three or more times a week or greater than 30 g for six months.[8] It is also recommended for those with previously treated squamous cell carcinoma of the vulva arising in LS or VIN or where the pathologist expresses concern and is unable to make a definitive diagnosis of differentiated VIN. Vulval cancer can arise surprisingly rapidly in women with LS, especially those with associated differentiated VIN. Areas of persistent localized skin thickening/hyperkeratosis, ulcers and erosions resistant to medical therapy, require biopsy to exclude intraepithelial neoplasia or malignant change. Where there is a risk of cancer, follow up should be at least every three to six months.[2] For patients with 'uncomplicated' LS that is well controlled clinically with small amounts of topical corticosteroid, annual GP follow up and examination is recommended.[8]

## Squamous cell hyperplasia

### Definition

This is not a distinct entity, but merely a description of the altered morphology of vulval skin and a diagnosis of exclusion. Histologically, there is hyperkeratosis (greater than is seen in lichen sclerosus) and lengthening and distortion of the rete pegs (acanthosis). Cellular elements of the epithelium proliferate, but maturation is normal. An inflammatory response in the dermis usually occurs, consisting of lymphocytic and plasma cell infiltration.

The skin is thickened with white hyperkeratotic, dry, elevated epithelial patches, excoriation and fissures.

### Incidence

The incidence is unknown, but squamous cell hyperplasia is less commonly seen than lichen sclerosus in vulval clinics.

### Aetiology/risk factors

Squamous cell hyperplasia may be the result of chronic, repetitive surface irritation and trauma from chemical irritants, eczema and recurrent mycotic infection, that cause scratching and rubbing.

### Prognosis

The risk of developing vulval cancer has been estimated to be 1–5 per cent.

### Management

In general terms, the management of squamous cell hyperplasia is the same as for lichen sclerosus, with withdrawal of the possible irritant, treatment of mycotic infection, emollients and steroids, although the long-term use of potent topical steroids has more adverse sequelae [C].[1]

> ## EBM: Lichen sclerosus/squamous cell hyperplasia symptom control
>
> - Bland emollients are more effective than placebo.
> - Three RCTs suggest that potent steroids are safe and effective in controlling symptoms and that testosterone is no more effective than placebo.
> - No evidence supports the use of surgery.

## Lichen planus

### Definition

This can be an acute or chronic condition affecting the skin or mucous membranes or both. Vulval LP may be part of a wide spectrum of disease involving the skin, oral mucosa (most common), scalp (scarring alopecia), nails, conjunctivae, bladder, nose, larynx, oesophagus and anus. There are three clinical variants. The erosive form (most common), affects the vulva (and vagina in up to 70 per cent of cases). The classic type affects mainly the vulva and the hypertrophic type (least common), which involves the perineum and perianal area.[14]

On keratinized skin, lichen planus is characterized by flat-topped, violaceous, shiny papules that often show reticulated white striae (Wickham's striae). On the vulva, the appearance ranges from delicate, white reticulated papules to an erosive, desquamating process. Large denuded areas may lead to profuse discharge and scarring with partial or complete obliteration of the vagina.

It may be asymptomatic or typically cause pruritus, burning, dyspareunia or apareunia, post-coital bleeding, copious malodorous sero-purulent discharge and destruction of vulvovaginal architecture.

Differential diagnosis includes other causes of erosive vulval disease, such as the immunobullous disorders (e.g. cicatricial pemphigoid), lupus erythematosus, LS, VIN, extra-mammary Paget's disease and plasma cell vulvitis.

### Incidence

Lichen planus is uncommon.

### Aetiology

The aetiology is unknown, but the evidence suggests that it is an immunologically mediated disease in a genetically predisposed individual, possibly induced by exogenous irritants and antigens (e.g. thiazides, NSAIDS, beta blockers and anti-malarials), resulting in targeting of the epidermis with immune destruction. Any irritation from chemicals, irritants, scratching and even friction with intercourse can flare LP.[15]

## Prognosis

Vulval lesions tend to disappear after weeks or months. Erosive lesions heal poorly and may be pre-malignant in up to 3 per cent of cases.[16]

## Management

The diagnosis is confirmed by biopsy and immunofluorescence may be needed to differentiate it from immunobullous disease. Histological findings are variable and nonspecific, leading to frequent delay and difficulty in diagnosis.

Therapy is challenging. It is important to stop irritation and trauma, control symptoms of itching and pain and treat any superimposed infection. Bland emollients help reduce irritation and restore barrier function. Initial treatment consists of topical high-potency corticosteroid ointments [C]. A warm sitz bath before application may allow better penetration through keratinized lesions. Hydrocortisone acetate suppositories 25 mg or foam, nightly for two to three months and then once or twice weekly, can be effective for vaginal lesions and may prevent synechiae [D].[17] Short courses of systemic corticosteroids, such as prednisone, may be needed for severe symptoms or cases refractory to topical treatments [D]. For limited areas, intralesional triamcinolone can be effective [D].

Topical calcineurin inhibitors, such as tacrolimus 0.1 per cent or pimecrolimus, have been shown to give good short-term relief [C] and can be used as a steroid sparer in areas already under control with topical steroids, but long-term safety and efficacy need to be evaluated in large randomized trials.

Other potentially useful therapies include cyclosporin, azathioprine, methotrexate and hydroxychloroquine [D]. Because no single treatment is universally effective, treatments may have to be combined to find an effective regimen.[15]

Surgery may be necessary in cases of vaginal synechiae and obliteration where blunt dissection can be used to break down the adhesions with potent topical steroids post-operatively to prevent recurrence.

## Inflammatory dermatoses

### Definition

Inflammatory dermatoses can be classified as either contact or primary irritant dermatitis or allergic dermatitis. It can be difficult to differentiate between the two.

Typical findings are diffuse reddening of the involved skin with excoriation and ulceration. Secondary infection may occur. The main differential diagnosis is vulval candidiasis.

### Aetiology

Irritants such as perfumed soaps, feminine hygiene deodorants, bubble baths, urine and tight clothing [D] cause irritant dermatitis, a common cause of vulval irritation.

In atopic individuals, non-irritant substances that include iatrogenic factors, such as local anaesthetic creams, cause allergic dermatitis.

### Incidence

The population-based incidence is unknown, but inflammatory dermatoses account for about 25 per cent of new vulval clinic patients [D].[18]

### Management

Once the causative factor has been identified and exposure to it avoided, symptomatic control can be instigated using either oral antihistamines or a topical corticosteroid. Fluorinated steroid creams may be used, but for short periods only, as atrophy can be associated with their long-term use [C].

## Seborrhoeic dermatitis

### Definition

This occurs in areas of the skin where sebaceous glands are active, such as the face, scalp, body folds and, less commonly, the genitalia. When the vulva is involved, the labia majora and mons pubis are affected. The lesions are scaly, orange-pink in colour and can be secondarily infected.

### Incidence

Seborrhoeic dermatitis is an uncommon vulval problem which may be asymptomatic or cause just mild irritation. Diagnosis is mainly clinical because histopathology is either non-specific or psoriasiform and differentiating this from psoriasis can be difficult.

### Aetiology

It is associated with *Malassezia ovalis* infection, a yeast that plays a central role in the pathogenesis of seborrhoeic dermatitis, where a change in the epidermal environment occurs with sebum accumulation, often with impaired hygiene.

### Management

The treatment of choice is an antifungal agent, such as 2 per cent miconazole or 2 per cent ketoconazole cream or shampoo, often combined with a low-dose mild to mid-potency topical steroid twice daily for 1–2 weeks and then a low dose of topical steroid and imidazole cream for maintenance.[13] Antifungal treatment is more effective than hydrocortisone creams or placebo [B].[19,20] Local hygiene is always important to keep the area cool, ventilated and non-irritated.

Lower genital tract

## Psoriasis

### Aetiology

Psoriasis is a hereditary skin disorder that affects 1–2 per cent of the general population. A defective or altered immune response in a genetically predisposed individual, results in an inflammatory mechanism that induces epidermal proliferation and sustains inflammation.[15]

### Incidence

Genetic and environmental factors are both important. About a third of people with psoriasis have a family history, but physical/chemical trauma, stress, acute infection and selected medications, such as antimalarials, lithium and beta blockers, are commonly viewed as triggers [D].

### Definition

Clinically, there is a variable degree of itching or irritation made worse by stress, heat, humidity and topical irritants. A well-defined, smooth erythematous area with a fine silvery-white scale and a sharp outline is characteristic. Secondary changes, such as excoriation, crusting and lichenification plus bacterial and yeast infections, may further confuse the presentation. Only rarely is psoriasis limited to the vulva with most often being part of a generalized condition. The diagnosis is clinical and a biopsy is seldom necessary.

### Prognosis

There are no long-term prognostic studies and at present there is no cure for psoriasis.

### Management

There are no systematic reviews or publications on the specific management of vulval psoriasis. In general terms, the aim of management is to achieve short-term suppression of symptoms with minimal adverse effects. Treatment largely depends on severity and extent of disease. Efforts should be directed towards stopping inflammation, itching and secondary lesions. It is essential that scratching must stop as it spreads the condition, irritant exposure is avoided and infection (both bacterial and yeast) is controlled.

As several trigger and perpetuating factors for psoriasis have been recognized, management of lifestyle might have been thought to be helpful. However, there is no good evidence to support this view or the use of non-drug treatments.

Emollients and keratolytics have no proven benefit [A] and tar preparations should be avoided, as they are irritating [D]. Sitz baths will help restore the epithelial barrier function [E].

In psoriasis in general, topical steroids are beneficial in the short term [A], but prolonged use should be avoided.

Vitamin D derivatives may be as effective as steroids, but without the risk of skin atrophy, although irritation may be a problem [A].[21] For mild to moderate disease, mild to mid-potency topical steroid, e.g. budesonide 0.05 per cent or triamcinolone 0.1 per cent ointment twice daily, can be used for 2–4 weeks and then tapered to intermittent use. For severe disease, superpotent topical steroids may be necessary. Steroids can then be alternated with a topical vitamin D derivative, such as calcipotriol (calcipotriene) ointment, applied twice daily.[15] Tacrolimus 0.1 per cent ointment twice daily can also be very effective [B].

With very extensive recalcitrant psoriasis, systemic therapy may be necessary, including treatments such as methotrexate, acitretin, hydroxyurea or cyclosporine.[22,23]

## Hidradenitis suppurativa

### Definition

This is a chronic, suppurative, inflammatory disorder of the apocrine glands. It is characterized by deep, painful subcutaneous nodules that may ulcerate and drain, leading to open sinuses and extensive scarring. On the vulva, the disease primarily affects the labia majora and intercrural folds, but may also involve the mons pubis, labia minora and clitoris.

### Incidence

Hidradenitis suppurativa is a common condition, particularly in black women. It is rare before puberty and less common after the climateric.

### Aetiology

The aetiology is unknown.

### Management

Multiple therapies, including topical and systemic antibiotics and oral contraceptives, steroids and isotretinoin, have been used with limited success [C]. Surgery remains a mainstay in the treatment of this disorder, and wide excision of the involved areas may be necessary [C].

## Ulcerative dermatoses

### Definition

Ulcerating lesions of the vulva may be solitary or multiple, painful or non-tender.

### Incidence

The lesions are uncommon in a standard vulval clinic, but are seen more often in a GUM clinic.

## Aetiology

The ulcers that arise from vesicles are typical of herpes simplex virus (HSV). The ulcers arising from papules are characteristic of syphilis, chancroid, granuloma inguinale and lymphogranuloma venereum. Solitary, non-tender ulcers are characteristic of syphilis, lymphogranuloma venereum and neoplasia. Multiple painful ulcers occur in HSV, Behçet's disease and Crohn's disease.

## Management

Laboratory evaluation, including serological testing and culture, is often necessary, and there should be a low threshold for seeking the opinion of the GUM team. When a single ulcer is present, biopsy is important [E].

Treatment is dependent on the diagnosis. The vulval manifestations of Behçet's disease can be treated by topical fluorinated corticosteroid creams [D].

### EBM: Vulval dermatoses other than lichen sclerosus and cell hyperplasia

The evidence relating to the management of this group of conditions is limited. A number of non-randomized studies indicate that topical steroids are useful in certain conditions, but the following points should be noted.

- *Seborrhoeic dermatitis.* A number of uncontrolled studies have confirmed the effectiveness of antifungal treatment and one small RCT indicates that it is more effective than hydrocortisone creams.
- *Psoriasis.* No vulva-specific evidence has been found. More than 30 RCTs have shown that topical steroids are beneficial in the short term, but prolonged use should be avoided. One systematic review has demonstrated that vitamin D derivatives may be as effective as steroids.

### KEY POINTS

#### Benign vulval skin conditions
- Comprehensive clinical assessment is essential.
- Multidisciplinary assessment can be useful.
- Biopsy when symptoms are refractory or there is suspicion of atypia (stop any topical steroid for 1–2 weeks prior to taking a biopsy).
- Simple measures, such as the use of emollient creams, are often effective.
- In lichen sclerosus, potent corticosteroids are effective and safe.
- In general, the prolonged use of potent corticosteroids is to be avoided.
- With the exception of hidradenitis suppurativa, surgery is best avoided.

# VAGINAL DISCHARGE

A vaginal discharge resulting from cervical and vaginal secretion is normal in women in the reproductive age group. Vulval soreness and irritation can be secondary to excessive vaginal discharge, the causes of which are listed in Table 65.2. Vaginal discharge arising as a result of a sexually transmitted infection is covered in Chapter 64.1, Infection and sexual health.

Management is based on diagnosis, which is reached by systemic clinical enquiry and examination, supplemented by appropriate investigation.

Physiological discharge can be increased in pregnancy and in oral contraception users. Heavy vaginal loss can be associated with a large cervical ectropion. Although bacterial vaginosis is at least twice as common as vulvovaginal candidiasis,[24] it does not usually cause vulvitis, although it may coexist with thrush. In the context of a vulval clinic, recurrent vulvovaginal candidiasis is an important condition.

## Candidal vulvovaginosis

### Definition

Vulvovaginal candidiasis (VVC) is a mycotic disease, which is usually caused by the dimorphic yeast *Candida albicans*, a commensal of the genital and digestive tracts. A minority of cases are caused by the non-albicans species, such as *Candida glabrata* and *Candida tropicalis*. The clinical features caused by albicans and non-albicans species are indistinguishable.

The condition is characterized by vulval itching, although burning and soreness may occur with superficial dyspareunia; however, none of these symptoms are specific.

**Table 65.2** Causes of excessive vaginal discharge

| Physiological |
| --- |
| **Infective** |
| Bacterial vaginosis |
| Monilial vaginosis |
| Trichomonal vaginosis |
| **Malignant** |
| Endometrial cancer |
| Cervical cancer |
| Vaginal cancer |
| **Miscellaneous** |
| Foreign body, e.g. retained or 'lost' tampon, vaginal ring |

Typically, the vulva is red, dry, swollen and fissured. A white, curdish discharge that adheres to the vaginal walls and cervix is classically described.

Acute infection is confirmed by the presence of candidal pseudohyphae or budding yeast forms, but this is a relatively insensitive test. Culture of a vaginal swab is the most sensitive test; the presence of more than ten yeast colonies supports the diagnosis.

The diagnosis can be further subclassified into 'uncomplicated' or 'complicated' VVC. This has treatment implications, as complicated VVC is more likely to fail standard antifungal therapy and requires more aggressive treatment.

Recurrent vulvovaginal candidiasis (RVVC) is defined as four or more episodes of symptomatic candidiasis annually.

### Classification
Uncomplicated:
    sporadic or infrequent episodes;
    mild to moderate symptoms or findings;
    suspected candida albicans infection;
    non-pregnant women without medical complications.
Complicated:
    recurrent episodes (four or more per year);
    severe symptoms or findings;
    suspected or proven non-albicans candida infection;
    women with uncontrolled diabetes, severe medical illness, immunosuppression, or those who are pregnant.

Modified from Sexually transmitted diseases treatment guidelines. Centers for Disease Control and Prevention. *MMWR Recomm Rep* 2006; **15** (RR-11):1-94.

## Incidence
The prevalence of *Candida albicans* in healthy young women is 20–25 per cent. Uncomplicated vulvovaginal candidiasis affects about 75 per cent of women at least once in their lifetime. Recurrence is said to occur in 5 per cent of cases.

## Aetiology
Most episodes occur without an obvious cause. A relatively small proportion of women treated with broad-spectrum antibiotics subsequently develop vulvovaginal candidiasis, usually as a result of prior colonization. There is a strong association with sexual activity. There are a number of other well-recognized risk factors, including:

- diabetes mellitus,
- immunosuppression,
- pregnancy,
- oral contraceptive pill,
- cunnilingus.

The aetiopathogenesis of RVVC is complex, and can be divided into genetic, behavioural and host biologic factors that predispose to both enhanced colonization and increased risk of transformation from asymptomatic carrier state to the symptomatic vaginitis phase.[25]

## Prognosis
Uncomplicated vulvovaginal candidiasis is usually self-limiting.

## Management
Patients should avoid local irritants and tightly fitting synthetic garments [C].

Topically applied azoles (clotrimazole, econazole, miconazole) are effective in treating symptoms; they should always be used with vaginal pessaries. There is no evidence to suggest that asymptomatic women need treatment [A].[26] Four-day courses will cure just over half of infections, whereas a 7-day course cures more than 90 per cent. Pregnant women should be offered longer courses of treatment than non-pregnant women [A].[26] There is no evidence that any one imidazole is more effective than another. There are no reliable studies concerning the safety or efficacy of any complimentary therapies for prevention or cure (e.g. live yoghurt), and such treatments cannot therefore be recommended.

No differences exist in terms of the relative effectiveness (measured as clinical and mycological cure) of antifungals administered by the oral and intravaginal routes for the treatment of uncomplicated vaginal candidiasis, and no definitive conclusion can be made regarding their relative safety, although pregnant women should not be given oral treatment [B]. The oral route of administration is the preferred route for antifungals for the treatment of vulvovaginal candidiasis [A] in women who are not pregnant.[27]

In women with recurrent symptoms, it is important to exclude diabetes and assess for underlying risk factors (e.g. immunodeficiency, corticosteroid use and frequent antibiotic use), although one-third to one-half of those with RVVC have no identifiable risk factors. An induction regimen of oral fluconazole 150 mg repeated every 3 days for a total of three doses to induce clinical remission, followed by maintenance suppressive fluconazole prophylaxis (150 mg once a week × six months), has become the standard of care and will effectively prevent symptomatic episodes in more than 90 per cent at six months and 40 per cent at one year[B].[28] Most recurrences are due to relapse with the same strain responsible for previous episodes rather than new strains or species, suggesting reinfection. Progressive azole resistance and selection for non-albicans candida species, are possible concerns with long-term maintenance therapy, albeit rare in immunocompetent individuals.[29]

More recently, an individualized decreasing-dose maintenance fluconazole regimen for RVVC (ReCiDiF trial), has shown excellent prevention of long-term recurrences with a relapse free period of 90 per cent at six months and 70 per cent at one year [C].[30]

The optimal treatment for non-albicans VVC is unknown. A 2-week treatment course with a non-fluconazole azole agent (oral or topical) is recommended[31] and nystatin pessaries 100 000 units daily is the usual first-line therapy [D].[28] Chronic or recurrent vaginitis due to *C. glabrata* can also be treated with 14 days of topical boric acid 600-mg capsules or intravaginal flucytosine daily either alone or in combination with amphotericin B 50 mg daily with referral to a specialist [D].[32]

---

## EBM: Vulvovaginal candidiasis

Summary of Cochrane database systematic review.

- Asymptomatic infection does not warrant treatment.
- Topical and oral antifungal azoles are both highly effective.
- The treatment of partners is ineffective.

---

## KEY POINTS

### Vaginal discharge
- Excessive vaginal discharge is a common gynaecological complaint and can cause vulval symptoms.
- Comprehensive clinical assessment is essential.
- Vulvovaginal candidiasis is highly responsive to antifungal treatment. The persistence of symptoms throws doubt on the diagnosis.
- Recurrent vulvovaginal candidiasis, which can occur in 5 per cent of cases, can be palliated by prolonged antifungal maintenance therapy.

---

# Vulval lumps

## Definition

Cysts are either congenital or arise from obstructed glands (Table 65.3). Mucous cysts arise from mesonephric duct

**Table 65.3** Types of benign vulval lumps

| Cystic | Solid | Anatomic |
|---|---|---|
| Bartholin's cyst | Lentigo | Varicosities |
| Congenital mucous cysts | Seborrhoeic keratosis | Herniae |
| Skene's duct cyst | Fibroepithelial polyp | |
| Cyst of the canal of Nuck | Papillomatosis | |
| Epidermal inclusion cyst | Fibroma | |
| Furunculosis | Dermatofibroma | |
| Sebaceous cysts | Lipoma | |
| | Condylomata | |
| | Hidradenoma | |

remnants and may be found at the introitus or labia minora. A cyst of the canal of Nuck (processus vaginalis peritonei) that fills with fluid can give rise to a hydrocoele within the labia majora (associated with a concurrent inguinal hernia in 30 per cent of cases). The clinical manifestations are either due to the cyst itself or to infection, as in a Bartholin's abscess.

Vulval skin is subject to the same range of lesions that can occur on skin in other parts of the body. Most cause no symptoms other than compromising cosmesis.

## Incidence

Vulval lumps of one sort or another are common and usually benign. Bartholin's cysts are the most common cystic lesions. Vulval varicosities are more common during pregnancy. Pigmented vulval skin lesions occur in 10 per cent of women, of which lentigo is the most common. Fibromata and fibromyomata are the most common of the benign solid tumours, usually developing along the insertion of the round ligament into the labia majora, and lipomata are the second most common solid tumours.[33]

## Prognosis

By and large, benign vulval neoplasms behave like similar lesions elsewhere. It has been suggested that vulval naevi may be more likely to undergo malignant transformation than elsewhere, but the likelihood of this occurring is small.

## Management

Most vulval lumps are benign and can be treated conservatively. Cysts can be drained and/or marsupialized, particularly if symptomatic. Solid tumours are better excised for histological assessment [E].

---

## KEY POINTS

### Benign vulval lumps
- Most vulval lumps are benign and can be treated conservatively.
- Excisional biopsy is indicated in solid lesions or when the diagnosis is uncertain.
- Cysts can be drained without risk to vulval cosmesis.

---

## Key References

1. Clark TJ, Etherington IJ, Luesley DM. Response of vulvar lichen sclerosus and squamous cell hyperplasia to graduated topical steroids. *J Reprod Med* 1999; **44**: 958–62.
2. Jones RW, Scurry J, Neill S, MacLean AB. Guidelines for the follow-up of women with vulvar lichen sclerosus in specialist clinics. *Am J Obstet Gynecol* 2008; **198**: 496.e1–496.e3.

3. Wallace HJ. Lichen sclerosus et atrophicus. *Trans St John's Hosp Dermatol Soc* 1971; **57**: 9–30.

4. Abramov Y, Elchalal U, Abramov D *et al*. Surgical treatment of vulval lichen sclerosus: a review. *Obstet Gynecol Surv* 1996; **51**: 193–9.

5. Tidy JA, Soutter WP, Luesley DM *et al*. Management of lichen sclerosus and intraepithelial neoplasia of the vulva in the UK. *J R Soc Med* 1996; **89**: 699–701.

6. Leibowitch M, Neill S, Pelisse M *et al*. The epithelial changes associated with squamous cell carcinoma of the vulva: a review of the clinical, histological and viral findings in 78 women. *BJOG* 1990; **97**: 1135–9.

7. Renaud-Vilmer C, Cavelier-Balloy B, Porcher R, Dubertret L. Vulvar lichen sclerosus: effect of long-term topical application of a potentsteroid on the course of the disease. *Arch Dermatol* 2004; **140**: 709–12.

8. Neill SM, Tatnall FM, Cox NH. Guidelines for the management of lichen sclerosus. *Br J Dermatol* 2002; **147**: 640–9.

9. Thomas E, Murphy D, Redman C. Premalignant vulval disorders. *Clin Evid* 2002; **7**: 1733–8.

10. Mazdisnian F, Degregorio F, Mazdisnian F *et al*. Intralesional injection of triamcinolone in the treatment of lichen sclerosus. *J Reprod Med* 1999; **44**: 332–4.

11. Van de Nieuwenhof HP, van der Avoort IAM, de Hullu JA. Review of squamous premalignant vular lesions. *Crit Rev Oncol/Hematol* 2008; **68**: 131–56.

12. Hengge UR, Krause W, Hofmann H *et al*. Multicentre, phase II trial on the safety and efficacy of topical tacrolimus ointment for the treatment of lichen sclerosus. *Br J Dermatol* 2006; **155**: 1021–8.

13. Nissi R, Risteli J, Niemimaa M. Pimecrolimus cream 1% in the treatment of lichen sclerosus. *Gynecol Obstet Invest* 2006; **63**: 151–4.

14. Burrows LJ, Shaw HA, Goldstein AT. The vulvar dermatoses. *J Sex Med* 2008; **5**: 276–83.

15. Margesson L. Non-neoplastic epithelial lesions of the vulva. In: Apgar BS, Brotzman GL, Spitzer M (eds). *Colposcopy Principles and Practice, An Integrated Textbook and Atlas*. Philadelphia: WB Saunders, 2002: 343–55.

16. Cooper SM, Wojnarwowska F. Influence of treatment of erosive lichen planus of the vulva on its prognosis. *Arch Dermatol* 2006; **142**: 362–4.

17. Lewis FM, Pelisse M. Vulvar lichen planus: clinical aspects and guideline to management. *J Gynecol Oncol* 2005; **10**: 188–92.

18. Ball SB, Wojnarowska F. Vulvar dermatoses: lichen sclerosus, lichen planus, and vulvar dermatitis/lichen simplex chronicus. *Semin Cutan Med Surg* 1998; **17**: 182–8.

19. Faergemann J. Seborrhoeic dermatitis and *Pityrosporum orbiculare*: treatment of seborrhoeic dermatitis of the scalp with miconazole-hydrocortisone (Daktacort), miconazole and hydrocortisone. *Br J Dermatol* 1986; **114**: 695–700.

20. Skinner RB, Noah PW, Taylor RM *et al*. Double-blind treatment of seborrheic dermatitis with 2% ketoconazole cream. *J Am Acad Dermatol* 1985; **2**: 52–6.

21. Ashcroft DM, Li Wan Po A, Williams HC, Griffiths CEM. Systematic review of comparative efficacy and tolerability of calcipotriol in treating chronic plaque psoriasis. *Clin Evid* 2001; **6**: 963–7.

22. Ashcroft DM, Liwan PO, Griffiths CE. Therapeutic strategies for psoriasis. *J Clin Pharm Ther* 2000; **25**: 1.

23. Koo JY. Current consensus and update on psoriasis therapy: A perspective from the US. *J Dermatol Clin* 1999; **26**: 723.

24. Barbone F, Austin H, Lou WC, Alexander WJ. A follow-up study of methods of contraception, sexual activity and rate of trichomiasis, candidiasis and bacterial vaginosis. *Am J Obstet Gynecol* 1990; **163**: 510–14.

25. Sobel JD. Pathogenesis of recurrent vulvovaginal candidiasis. *Curr Infect Dis Rep* 2002; **4**: 514–19.

26. Young GL, Jewell D. Topical treatment for vaginal candidiasis (thrush) in pregnancy. *Cochrane Database Syst Rev* 2001; (**4**): CD000225.

27. Watson MC, Grimshaw JM, Bond CM *et al*. Oral versus intra-vaginal imidazole and triazole anti-fungal treatment of uncomplicated vulvovaginal candidiasis (thrush). *Cochrane Database Syst Rev* 2001; (**4**): CD002845.

28. Clinical Effectiveness Group, British Association of Sexual Health and HIV. United Kingdom National Guideline on the Management of Vulvovaginal Candidiasis. London: British Association of Sexual Health and HIV, 2007.

29. Sobel JD. Management of recurrent vulvovaginal candidiasis: unresolved issues. *Curr Infect Dis Rep* 2006; **8**: 481–6.

30. Donders G, Bellen G, Byttebier G *et al*. Individualized decreasing-dose maintenance fluconazole regimen for recurrent vulvovaginal candidiasis (ReCiDiF trial). *Am J Obstet Gynecol* 2008; **199**: 613.e1–9.

31. Centers for Disease Control and Prevention. Sexually transmitted diseases treatment guidelines. *MMWR Recomm Rep* 2006; **15** (RR-11): 1–94.

32. Sobel JD, Chaim W, Nagappan V, Leaman D. Treatment of vaginitis acused by *Candida glabrata*: use of topical boric acid and flucytosine. *Am J Obstet Gynecol* 2003; **189**: 1297–300.

33. Hopkins MP, Snyder MK. Benign disorders of vulval and vagina. In: Curtis MG, Hopkins MP (eds). *Glass's Office Gynecology*, 5th edn. Baltimore: Wilkins & Wilkins, 1999, 417–26.

# Vulval pain syndromes

*David Nunns*

## INTRODUCTION

Vulvodynia has been defined by the International Society for the Study of Vulval diseases as vulval discomfort, most often described as a burning pain, occurring in the absence of relevant visible findings or a specific, clinically identifiable, neurologic disorder. Patients can be further classified by the anatomical site of the pain (e.g. generalized vulvodynia, hemivulvodynia, clitorodynia) and also by whether pain is provoked or unprovoked. Patients previously given a diagnosis of vestibulitis should now be called vestibulodynia (localized provoked vulvodynia) (see Table 66.1). Some patients may have a combination of vulvodynia with another vulval problem, e.g. herpes or thrush, and both conditions may require treatment.[1] Before a diagnosis of vulval pain syndrome can be made, infections and vulval dermatoses should be excluded (see Chapter 65, Benign vulval problems).

## PAIN PATHOPHYSIOLOGY

Clinical pain can either be inflammatory or neuropathic in origin. Inflammatory pain is associated with tissue damage or injury and clinically exhibits sensory hypersensitivity, which is characterized by hyperalgesia and allodynia. Hyperalgesia is the exaggerated response to noxious substances through a general increase in the responsiveness of tissues. Allodynia is the production of pain by stimuli that do not usually cause pain by a reduction in the sensory threshold of neurons. Hence, inflammatory pain seen with vestibulodynia is associated with pain on light touch and is usually localized. Neuropathic pain is usually caused by damage to either the central or peripheral nervous system and produces a diffuse burning, aching pain with intermittent flare-ups. Hyperalgesia and allodynia may not necessarily be present.

## ASSESSMENT

### History

An accurate pain history is essential to differentiate between the different subtypes. In addition to the nature of the pain, one should record any aggravating and relieving factors, with particular reference to sexual intercourse. Any past treatments should also be recorded to avoid duplication. A psychosexual history is essential, as many women have significant dysfunction and may require a psychosexual referral [C].[2]

### Examination

Identifying sites of vulval tenderness and discomfort can help in making a diagnosis. Clinical examination should also exclude other vulval conditions that can produce similar symptoms. Inflammatory vulval diseases, such as lichen sclerosus and seborrhoeic dermatitis, can cause vulval pain and soreness through excoriation, splitting and fissuring of the vulval skin, as well as itching. Some conditions may not be manifest at the time of examination, such as a tight posterior fourchette and the fragile fissured vulval syndrome.[3] Symptomatic dermographism is a rare cause of vulval pain, but this may be suggested by dermographism evident at other body sites.[4] Other

**Table 66.1** ISSVD classification of vulval pain

| Classification | | |
|---|---|---|
| A. Vulval pain related to a specific disorder | 1. Infectious (e.g. candidiasis, herpes, etc.) | |
| | 2. Inflammatory (e.g. lichen planus, lichen sclerosus, immunobullous disorders, etc.) | |
| | 3. Neoplastic (e.g. Paget's disease, squamous cell carcinoma, etc.) | |
| | 4. Neurologic (e.g. herpes neuralgia, spinal nerve compression, etc.) | |
| B. Vulvodynia | 1. Generalized | 1. Provoked (sexual, nonsexual, or both) |
| | | 2. Unprovoked |
| | | 3. Mixed (provoked and unprovoked) |
| | 2. Localized (vestibulodynia – previously known as vulval vestibulitis, clitorodynia, hemivulvodynia, etc.) | 1. Provoked (sexual, nonsexual, or both) |
| | | 2. Unprovoked |
| | | 3. Mixed (provoked and unprovoked) |

- ISSVD, International Society for the Study of Vulvovaginal Disease.

less common causes of vulval pain are worth considering, including aphthous ulceration, erosive lichen planus and herpes simplex infections.

# VESTIBULODYNIA

## Definition

Vestibulodynia (localized provoked vulvodynia, formerly vulval vestibulitis) is a cause of superficial dyspareunia and is characterized by vestibular tenderness on light touch.[5] This hyperaesthesia can be generalized throughout the vestibule or can be more focal, involving the opening of the ducts of the major vestibular glands or the posterior fourchette.[6]

## Clinical features

Affected women are usually Caucasian, aged between 20 and 40 years, and present with a history of provoked pain, such as superficial dyspareunia, tampon intolerance and pain during gynaecological examinations.[5,7] There is often a delay between the onset of symptoms and receiving a diagnosis, which varies from months to years. A six-month period of time has been arbitrarily suggested from the onset of symptoms to making a diagnosis of vestibulodynia so as to exclude women recovering from acute vulval inflammation from other causes.[6]

As the condition is frequently chronic, a high level of psychological morbidity is common. Some patients are prone to stress and anxiety, which may play a role in developing symptoms [D].[2] Sexual dysfunction is common and frequently reported.[8] Reduced sexual arousal, more negative sexual feelings and less spontaneous interest in sex (not elicited by a partner) have all been described in vestibulodynia. These are all risk factors for significant psychosexual dysfunction, such as vaginismus and anorgasmia, the management of which usually requires psychosexual input [D] (see Chapter 64.2, Dyspareunia and other psychosexual problems).

Clinically, simply using a Q-tip applicator can identify vestibular tenderness. A defining feature of vestibulodynia is that the labial skin is non-tender. Vestibular erythema is a subjective finding that is often present on normal examination and is usually not helpful in making the diagnosis of vestibulodynia or in planning management.[9] The application of diluted acetic acid to the vulva does not assist in making a diagnosis [C].

## Incidence

The incidence within gynaecology clinics in the United Kingdom remains unknown. However, the prevalence of vestibulodynia was 1.3 per cent of women attending a Central London genitourinary medicine clinic.[10] Misdiagnosis is common.

## Aetiology/risk factors

This remains unknown, but is likely to be multifactorial. It is often difficult to identify a cause, as symptoms usually develop insidiously. Recurrent attacks of vaginal candidiasis are frequently cited, but this may be due to initial misdiagnosis.

## Prognosis

Up to 30 per cent of women with vestibulodynia may experience resolution of their symptoms without treatment and in 50 per cent of these, resolution can occur within 12 months [C].[6]

## Management

The aims of management are to reduce vestibular tenderness and to identify the potential need for input from other disciplines, for example psychosexual counsellors.

### General measures

Reassurance and an explanation of the condition are essential, and providing written information is helpful [C].[11] Strict vulval hygiene measures should be practised to reduce the chance of contact sensitivity [D].

Only one randomized controlled trial (RCT) exists which addresses surgery, group therapy and biofeedback.[12] Good evidence for effective treatment is lacking. Many studies are methodologically flawed, for example low study numbers, short follow-up times.

### Topical agents and vaginal dilators

No RCTs have compared topical agents. Local anaesthetic gel/ointment prior to sex and emollients are worthy of mention as first-line treatment [D]. Lignocaine gel, together with the use of vaginal dilators, can help desensitize the pelvic floor for patients who are fearful of sex and where secondary vaginismus may exist [C].[13]

Other topical agents include steroids and antifungal creams, which have been used with variable results, but no control arm existed in these studies.[14] Long-term empirical prescribing of topical medicaments should be discouraged, as it places the woman at unnecessary risk of irritancy and contact allergy.

### Pain management and psychosexual counselling

A cognitive–behavioural assessment has been suggested to complement the physical treatments [B].[12] Over a series of sessions, a clinical psychologist can teach patients coping mechanisms and pain management strategies such as the pain-gate theory, and can address the patient's expectations of treatment, which might not necessarily be a cure for pain, but rather the ability to have penetrative sex. For many women with vestibulodynia, sexual rehabilitation may be required and this can be structured over several sessions with a psychosexual counsellor, preferably with the woman's partner. Improving physical non-coital sexual contact, helping to overcome pelvic floor muscle hypertonia using sensate focus therapy, and addressing secondary psychosexual dysfunction, such as low libido and anorgasmia, will be of help to many.[8]

## Surgery

The modified vestibulectomy is the procedure of choice, involving excision of a horseshoe-shaped area of the vestibule and inner labial fold followed by dissection of the posterior vaginal wall [C]. The vaginal tissue is then advanced to cover the skin defect. The complete response rate is 59 per cent. Women who respond to lignocaine gel prior to sex have a more successful outcome.[15] The response rate can be further improved with post-operative psychosexual counselling, which is likely to help overcome the fear of sex after surgery [C].[13]

In an RCT, 78 women with vestibulodynia were randomized to one of three arms: (1) group cognitive–behavioural therapy (12 weeks duration), (2) pelvic floor biofeedback therapy (12 weeks duration), and (3) vestibulectomy.[12] At follow up at six months, all patients reported significant improvements in pain scoring. Sexual functioning with surgery had the highest success rates; however, one concern was the high number of participants randomized to surgery who declined to be included in the study. The study did support both non-surgical treatments for vestibulodynia and suggested that patients prefer a behavioural approach to treatment than a surgical one.

## Other treatments

Biofeedback therapy using surface electromyographic (sEMG) signals from the pelvic floor has been used successfully to help overcome pelvic floor muscle dysfunction in women with vestibulodynia [C].[16] Using portable home machines with a special vaginal skin sensor, 78 per cent of patients with apareunia had resumed penetrative sex and there was an objective improvement in the sEMG reading of the pelvic floor; however, many of these patients were also treated with amitryptyline. The system is not routinely available and experience in the UK is lacking. It is likely that patients may benefit from desensitizing the vulval area using a variety of techniques, but the optimal technique is not clear. Biofeedback or vaginal trainers may all work in a similar way.

No evidence exists that dietary manipulations can improve outcome in vestibulodynia.

---

### EBM: Vestibulodynia

- Topical agents are commonly used, but the evidence supporting a specific application is lacking.
- Surgery is of benefit in well-selected patients.
- One RCT showed a benefit of vestibulectomy above biofeedback therapy and group cognitive-behavioural therapy.
- Biofeedback is effective, but UK experience is limited.

## UNPROVOKED VULVODYNIA

### Definition

Unprovoked vulvodynia is a cutaneous dysaesthesia causing non-localized vulval pain. Unlike women with provoked pain, those with unprovoked vulvodynia have more constant neuropathic-type pain in the vulva and occasionally the peri-anal area.[17]

### Clinical features

The affected women are typically peri-menopausal or post-menopausal and, like women with vestibulodynia, can present with a long history of multiple, inappropriate use of topical agents prior to a diagnosis.[18] Superficial dyspareunia is not consistently reported, as many women are less sexually active.[5] In addition, many experience rectal, perineal and urethral discomfort and there may be an overlap with other perineal pain syndromes.[17] Psychological morbidity is likely to be high as a consequence of chronic pain.

Clinical examination of the vulva is normal.

### Incidence

The incidence is unknown, but, as with vestibulodynia, misdiagnosis is likely.

### Aetiology/risk factors

These remain unknown.

### Prognosis

The prognosis also remains unknown.

### Management

The aims of treatment are pain relief and identification of the potential need for input from other disciplines.

#### General measures

Reassurance and an explanation of the condition are essential, and providing written information is helpful.[11] Strict vulval hygiene measures should be practised to reduce the chance of contact sensitivity.

No RCTs have been carried out to assess the management of this group of patients, and only case-controlled studies exist, which frequently contain small numbers of women.

#### Tricyclic antidepressants and neuroleptics

Amitryptyline (a tricyclic antidepressant) is of benefit and addresses the central and peripheral components of neuropathic pain seen in unprovoked vulvodynia [C].[16] A dose of 10 mg/day, increasing every week until the pain is controlled, has been suggested. The average dosage is 60 mg/day, although up to 150 mg/day can be used. Side effects may affect compliance. The duration of treatment is debatable, but three to six months has been suggested. Patients intolerant of the side effects can try dothiepin or nortryptyline. The neuroleptic gabapentin can be used as a second-line agent. In the only series to date of 17 patients with unprovoked vulvodynia, the complete response rate was 41 per cent with a follow-up period of 26 months [C].[19]

#### Surgery

Surgery is contraindicated in this group.

#### Other treatments

Acupuncture has shown limited promise in cases refractory to standard medical treatments. In one study including only 12 patients with unprovoked vulvodynia, two were completely cured [C].[20]

### EBM: Unprovoked vulvodynia

- Tricyclic antidepressants and gabapentin are of benefit.
- Surgery is contraindicated.

## CONCLUSIONS

Women with vulvodynia form a heterogeneous group, with the clinical presentation reflecting physical, psychological and psychosexual factors. As with other chronic pain syndromes, a specific cause remains elusive and is probably multifactorial. A multidisciplinary approach to the symptoms is likely to be of benefit to address the many complex issues surrounding vulval pain (Table 66.2). For some women who fail to respond to treatment, living and coping with pain become key issues in management.

### KEY POINTS

- A good history and clinical examination are essential to distinguish between different vulvodynia subgroups.
- Surgery is only suitable for well-selected patients with vestibulodynia.
- Amitryptyline/gabapentin are treatments for unprovoked vulvodynia.
- A multidisciplinary approach can be helpful.
- Good evidence for effectiveness is lacking.

**Table 66.2** The multidisciplinary approach to vulval pain syndromes

| Health professional | Treatments offered |
|---|---|
| Clinician | Topical agents |
| | Tricyclic antidepressants/ neuroleptics |
| | Modified vestibulectomy |
| Clinical psychologist | Cognitive-behavioural therapy |
| | Pain management |
| | Coping strategies |
| Psychosexual counsellors | Treatment of secondary sexual dysfunction |
| | Sensate focus therapy |
| | Increasing non-coital sexual activity |
| Physiotherapist | Biofeedback |
| | Pelvic floor muscle rehabilitation and desensitization |

# Key References

1. Haefner HK. Report of the International Society for the Study of Vulvovaginal Disease terminology and classification of vulvodynia. *J Low Genit Tract Dis* 2007; **11**: 48–9.

2. Nunns D, Mandal D. Psychological and psychosexual aspects of vulval vestibulitis. *Genitourinary Med* 1997; **73**: 541–4.

3. Harrington C. Presidential address. In: Proceedings of the British Society for the Study of Vulval Disease Biennial Meeting, Oxford, UK, 1999.

4. Lambiris A, Greaves MW. Urticaria: increasingly recognised but not adequately highlighted cause of dyspareunia and vulvodynia. *Acta Derm Venereol* 1996; **77**: 160–1.

5. Friedrich EG. Vulvar vestibulitis syndrome. *J Reprod Med* 1987; **32**: 110–14.

6. Peckham BM, Mak DG, Patterson JJ. Focal vulvitis: a characteristic syndrome and a cause of dyspareunia. *Am J Obstet Gynecol* 1986; **154**: 855–64.

7. Marinnoff SC, Turner MLC. Vulvar vestibulitis syndrome: an overview. *Am J Obstet Gynecol* 1991; **165**: 1228–33.

8. Schover LR, Youngs DD, Cannata RN. Psychosexual aspects of the evaluation and management of vulval vestibulitis. *Am J Obstet Gynecol* 1991; **167**: 630–6.

9. Van Beurden W, van der Vange N, de Craen AJM *et al.* Normal findings in vulvar examination and vulvoscopy. *Br J Obstet Gynaecol* 1997; **104**: 320–4.

10. Denbow ML, Byrne MA. Prevalence, causes and outcome of vulval pain in a genitourinary medicine clinic population. *Int J STD AIDS* 1998; **9**: 88–91.

11. The Vulval Pain Society, PO Box 7804, Nottingham, NG3 5ZQ (send a s.a.e.).

12. Bergeron S, Binik YM, Khalife S *et al.* A randomised comparison of group cognitive–behavioural therapy, surface electromyographic biofeedback and vestibulectomy in the treatment of dyspareunia resulting from vulvar vestibulitis. *Pain* 2001; **91**: 297–306.

13. Abramov L, Wolman I, David MP. Vaginismus: an important factor in the evaluation and management of vulvar vestibulitis syndrome. *Gynaecol Obstet Inv* 1994; **38**: 194–7.

14. Friedrich EG. Therapeutic studies on vulval vestibulitis. *J Reprod Med* 1988; **33**: 515–18.

15. Kehoe S, Leusley D. An evaluation of modified vestibulectomy in the treatment of vulvar vestibulitis: preliminary results. *Acta Obstet Gynecol Scand* 1996; **75**: 676–7.

16. Glazer HI. Treatment of vulval vestibulitis syndrome with electromyographic biofeedback of pelvic floor musculature. *J Reprod Med* 1995; **40**: 283–90.

17. McKay M. Dysaesthetic vulvodynia. *J Reprod Med* 1993; **38**: 9–13.

18. McKay M. Subsets of vulvodynia. *J Reprod Med* 1987; **32**: 110–14.

19. Ben-David B, Friedman M. Gabapentin therapy for vulvodynia. *Anesth Analg* 1999; **89**: 1459–60.

20. Powell J, Wojnarowska F. Acupuncture for vulvodynia. *J R Soc Med* 1999; **92**: 579–81.

# Pre-invasive disease

*Gabrielle Downey*

## INTRODUCTION

Worldwide, cervical cancer is the second most common cancer affecting women. Of the estimated 371 000 new cases in 1990, around 77 per cent were in developing countries, where about 200 000 women die each year from the disease. In developed nations, the figures for invasive cervical cancer are much lower. The disease has a relatively long natural history, and intervention and treatment in the premalignant phase is highly effective. The accessibility of the cervix and the availability of a simple test for the presence of pre-malignancy make it suitable for mass screening. Other malignancies and pre-malignancies of the lower genital tract are much less common and therefore most of this chapter focuses on the cervix.

## CERVICAL INTRAEPITHELIAL NEOPLASIA, ITS PATHOGENESIS AND THE ROLE OF HUMAN PAPILLOMAVIRUS INFECTION

### Definitions

Pre-cancer of the cervix was first described at the end of the nineteenth century. Histologically, areas were described where the whole thickness of the epithelium was replaced by neoplastic cells that had not breached the basement membrane. This was referred to as carcinoma-*in-situ* (CIS). Retrospective studies found CIS lesions in women who subsequently went on to develop cervical cancer, and so the precursor nature of CIS came to be established. Subsequent prospective studies have confirmed these findings.[1,2] After exfoliative cytology was introduced, lesser degrees of change, not amounting to CIS, were recognized and termed 'dysplasia'. In order to rationalize the classification to encompass all degrees of change, the term cervical intraepithelial neoplasia (CIN) was introduced.[3] Pre-invasive changes were divided into grades 1, 2 and 3. Grades 1 and 2 corresponded to mild and moderate dysplasia respectively, and grade 3 combined severe dysplasia and CIS into one category. The definition implied a continuum of change from CIN1 through to CIN3 and invasive cancer. As knowledge of the natural history of pre-malignancy has grown, the concept of a continuum of change has been challenged. For practical purposes, there is now a two-stage grading, with CIN1 becoming low-grade CIN (in which there is a significant chance of regression), and CIN2 and CIN3 being grouped together as high-grade CIN (Table 67.1). In North American and some European countries, this grouping has been formalized as The Bethesda Classification, consisting of low-grade

**Table 67.1** Glossary of terms

| Term | Explanation |
| --- | --- |
| CIN | Cervical intraepithelial neoplasia, graded 1–3 depending on severity |
| VaIN | Vaginal intraepithelial neoplasia, graded 1–3 depending on severity |
| VIN | Vulval intraepithelial neoplasia, graded 1–3 depending on severity |
| AIS | Adenocarcinoma-*in-situ,* pre-invasive disease of glandular tissue |
| CIGN | Cervical intraepithelial glandular neoplasia, pre-invasive disease of glandular tissue graded low- and high-grade; high-grade CIGN = AIS |
| Pap smear | Cervical smear – cytological test described by Papanicolaou |
| ASCUS | A typical squamous cells of uncertain significance – Bethesda system grade equating to borderline nuclear abnormalities |
| LSIL | Low-grade squamous intraepithelial lesion – Bethesda system grade equating to mild dyskaryosis/CIN1 |
| HSIL | High-grade squamous intraepithelial lesion – Bethesda system grade equating to moderate and severe dyskaryosis/CIN2 and CIN3 |
| Dyskaryosis | A cytological term describing the nuclear abnormalities – not synonymous with dysplasia |
| Squamo-columnar junction (SCJ) | Where squamous and columnar tissue meet; this is not fixed, but is affected by metaplasia |
| Metaplasia | A physiological process whereby columnar epithelium is replaced by squamous tissue in response to the acid environment of the vagina |
| Transformation zone | That area on the cervix that has undergone metaplasia; it is bounded by the original SCJ and the present SCJ |
| Dysplasia | A histological term describing architectural abnormalities within tissue |
| LLETZ | Large loop excision of the transformation zone |
| LEEP | Loop electrosurgical excision procedure |
| DLE | Diathermy loop excision: taking a cone biopsy with an electrosurgical loop |

squamous intraepithelial lesions (LSIL) and high-grade squamous intraepithelial lesions (HSIL).

## Incidence

The United Kingdom has the second highest recorded incidence of CIN in the European Community. In 2004, there were around 2800 new cases of invasive cervical cancer in England and Wales, which remains the same as the previous five years with just over 1000 women dying per year which equates to 20 women per week.[4,5] There had previously been a 26 per cent fall in incidence but the static incidence figures do not reflect a failure of the screening programme, rather an increasing number of migrants from countries that do not have a screening programme being diagnosed after arrival in the UK. Statistical modelling performed by the Imperial Cancer Research Fund (now a part of Cancer Research UK) has extrapolated that the current screening programme prevents around 3900–4500 deaths from cervical cancer per annum.[6,7]

It is difficult to estimate the total numbers of cases of CIN, as cancer registries only record cases of CIN3, but there are around 21 000 cases of CIN3 in England and Wales with 21 000 cases of CIN 3 in 2005–2006, with the peak incidence being between 25 and 29 years of age.[8]

## Aetiology

Human papillomavirus (HPV) infection is the essential prerequisite for the development of cervical malignancy. The most recent data on Dutch archived cervical cancer specimens, using sensitive methods of detecting HPV DNA, call into question whether HPV-negative cervical cancers actually exist: the estimated prevalence of HPV in cervical cancers is 99.7 per cent.[9] On the other hand, population-based studies have shown that genital HPV infection is extremely common with up to 80 per cent of sexually active women being HPV positive at some point during their lifetime. Using the incidence of genital warts as a marker, the incidence appears to be rising five-fold in the female population and eight-fold in the male population, with approximately 15 per cent prevalence of the oncogenic HPV types 16 and 18.

Lower genital tract

While the likelihood of acquiring the infection is high, most infections are usually transient with 90 per cent of women clearing the infection within two years. Thus, the overwhelming majority of HPV infections will not lead to the development of cancer. Progression or regression depends on several factors that interfere with the host's ability to clear the virus.

The cell-mediated arm of the adaptive immune response is responsible for clearing HPV. If cell-mediated immunity is impaired, such as in transplant patients or in HIV-positive women, the virus will not be cleared and abnormalities may develop. How the virus results in cancer has now largely been defined. The virus lives in epithelial cells and is species specific. Genital infection with HPV can only be acquired through sexual contact. It is thought that the virus enters the epithelium through a breach in the skin integrity caused by microtrauma. The virus can remain and replicate within the cytoplasm (episomal) of the cell and is often cleared by the host immune system. Occasionally, the virus enters the cell's nucleus and this step towards oncogenesis is termed 'integration'. The cell no longer undergoes programmed cell death after 40–60 cycles but now becomes immortalized. The E6 and E7 oncoproteins are necessary for this, but vary in their ability to do so according to HPV type; E6 binds to the p53 cellular protein and E7 to the RB cellular protein, both of which are cell cycle regulators.[10,11] Interfering with the cell cycle allows DNA damage to accumulate, which may result in genetic instability and transformation of the cell into a malignant cell line. This process may be accelerated by cofactors.

Why persistent infection happens in what appears to be a healthy individual is largely unknown. Smoking is a recognized cofactor for the development of disease: local immunity within the cervix appears to be suppressed in women who smoke. The major histocompatibility complex is responsible for presenting viral antigen to the host's immune system and there is limited evidence to suggest that women with particular human leukocyte antigen (HLA) types may have increased susceptibility to disease. The majority of HPV infections result in CIN 1 and 60 per cent of these will regress without the need for treatment, while approximately 10 per cent will progress to high-grade lesions. However, it should be noted that women with mild dykaryosis have a 16–47 times increased incidence of invasive disease compared with the general female population.[12,13]

Cervical pre-cancer has a long natural history, which is one of the reasons why it is a suitable condition for screening. If a cancer is going to develop at all, it will take several years to do so, even from a CIN3 lesion. It is unclear why some CIN3 lesions become invasive, while others stay as intraepithelial disease, and it is not known how many CIN3 lesions will become invasive, as prospective studies are unethical. However, the best prospective data suggest that at least 36 per cent of women with CIN3 would develop invasive cancer if left untreated.[2]

# Screening for cervical intraepithelial neoplasia

## The test

The traditional Papanicolaou (Pap) smear test is used worldwide to screen for pre-cancerous cellular changes from the cervix. Although the test has been a significant factor in the reduction of the incidence of cervical cancer by the detection of pre-malignant cells, the drive to improve the screening test has led to the development of liquid-based cytology. Traditionally, the cytology sample from the cervix was spread on a glass slide at the time of collection. Each slide would therefore have only a proportion of the cells collected from the cervix (around 20 per cent). Liquid-based cytology collects the whole sample from the sampling device in a liquid medium that is sent to a laboratory for processing. Cells are transferred from the transport liquid to a slide as a monolayer for examination. This technique reduces the proportion of inadequate smears and increases the detection of true dyskaryosis. Liquid-based cytology is now the standard test used for the NHS cervical screening programme. There are two main types in use, Surepath™ and Thinprep®, the latter allowing for HPV and sexually transmitted disease (STD) screening if required.

More than 90 per cent of cervical cancers develop within the transformation zone, the upper limit of which is the squamo-columnar junction. It is therefore important that this area is adequately sampled by direct visualization of the cervix. In order to quality assure the screening programme, all cytology samplers have a unique identification code.

## Test performance

Cervical cytology is not a perfect test: there are false-positive results (i.e. no disease is actually present) and false-negative results (i.e. genuine disease is missed). False-positive rates vary from 7 to 27 per cent and false-negative rates from 20 to 50 per cent. About 98 per cent of the smears taken are adequate for diagnosis, and just under 10 per cent of adequate smears are 'not normal'. Most smear abnormalities are at the minor end of the spectrum.

According to the NHS cervical screening programme, cervical smear abormalities can be broken down as follows:

| Type | Per cent |
| --- | --- |
| Borderline nuclear abnormalities | 3.3 |
| Mild dyskaryosis | 1.7 |
| Moderate dyskaryosis | 0.5 |
| Severe dyskaryosis | 0.5 |
| Invasion or glandular abnormalities | <0.1 |

In general, the proportion of normal smears increases in older women, but so does the proportion of abnormalities representing invasive cancer. Borderline changes and mild dyskaryosis are very common in young women; the proportion of moderate dyskaryosis is highest for women aged 20–29 years; and the proportion of severe dyskaryosis is highest in women aged 25–34 years.[13]

## The programme

By definition, a screening test is not diagnostic, but identifies a subgroup of the reference population at increased risk of the disease for which further tests should be carried out. Screening is always a trade-off between sensitivity and specificity. In this case, the reference population being screened comprises healthy, asymptomatic women.

No randomized trials have been undertaken to establish whether screening actually reduces mortality from cervical cancer. Evidence in support of screening has been extrapolated from reducing trends in incidence and mortality in those areas where screening has been introduced. This is most strikingly illustrated by considering data from Scandinavia: Iceland, Finland, Sweden and Denmark noted reductions in incidence and mortality soon after their screening programmes achieved target coverage of the population in the 1960s. Norway, on the other hand, with no organized programme in the 1960s, continued to show increasing incidence rates into the 1970s.[14]

A nationwide, organized (as opposed to opportunistic) cervical screening programme was introduced in England and Wales in 1988 with a national computerized call-and-recall system. The regions still have a degree of autonomy in planning their screening programme, but there is now a national co-ordinating network to ensure the adoption of common standards and working practices. The whole NHS cervical screening programme was rewritten in 2004.[15] This new programme differed from those that preceded it in that it incorporated all the available evidence and used this information to define a minimum standard and what was 'best practice'. There were significant changes to (1) the age to commence screening, (2) the screening interval, (3) actions to be taken following a mildly abnormal smear and (4) follow up of both treated and untreated women. There were also guidelines dealing with the immune suppressed and HIV-positive women. In general, the principle of management was to keep 'low risk' women in the community and 'high risk' women in the colposcopy service. There were regional variations in the commencement and cessation of screening which will be dealt with later in this chapter.

## Main changes to the programme

### The screening interval
The screening interval changed from three to five yearly to be defined as:

- three yearly to 49 years and
- five yearly thereafter to 64 years.

Evidence shows that a three-yearly screening programme could prevent substantially more cancers than a five-yearly programme in the younger woman with little extra cost.[16,17]

If maximum coverage for a three-yearly programme is 91 per cent and the incremental gains become less and less thereafter with increasing screening frequency, therefore, in terms of cost–benefit, there is little justification for reducing the screening interval to less than three years in the younger age group. The exit age of 65 years has been questioned, particularly on reducing the age of screening to 50 in women who have been well screened with a satisfactory negative history. The effectiveness of cervical screening in reducing invasive cancer varies with age, being greatest in younger age groups and least in women aged over 70 years. Age-specific declines in cervical cancer were confined to women aged 30 to 70 years with a nadir around ages 45–50 years.

### The age to commence and stop screening
In England and Northern Ireland, screening begins at 25 years while it is 20 years in Scotland and Wales. The incidence of cervical cancer in the under 25 year group is low and the incidence of transient infection and CIN is high. A recent review of the age to commence screening in England was undertaken as a result of media pressure following the death of a high profile TV personality. The group concluded there was no new evidence to justify lowering the age of screening and good evidence to support the current policy. Cervical screening in this age group may detect an abnormality that would resolve spontaneously, thus screening such young women could result in both physical and psychological morbidity with little evidence of benefit. There is now evidence that treatment of CIN with loop excision can result in premature labour and delivery.[18]

The reduction in mortality from cervical cancer in women over the age of 50 years is thought to be unrelated to the cervical screening process. Cervical screening is less effective in detecting CIN 3 in older women and the incidence of both CIN and cervical cancer over the age of 50 is low: 11/100 000 in well-screened women compared to 59/100 000 women in the population as a whole.[19] Women over the age of 50 who are diagnosed with cervical cancer usually have not fully participated in the cervical screening programme. Women with a history of abnormal smears before the age of 50 should continue on the screening programme, while those with a complete and negative smear history can opt out of the programme.

### Referral for colposcopy
In the main, referral remains unchanged except for a mildly abnormal smear report. Evidence suggests that best practice would be to refer all women with a mildly abnormal smear to colposcopy.[15,20] The main reasons are:

- A significant proportion have high-grade disease.
- There are psychological benefits associated with assessment and diagnosis.

Lower genital tract

- If the cervix is normal, they can be removed from the colposcopy service.
- Cost–benefit analysis demonstrates this is more cost efficient.
- The relative risk of developing cervical cancer is greater if left in the community.

There are no reported randomized trials triaging women to immediate colposcopy or community-based cytological follow up. Other case series have shown the percentage of women found with high-grade CIN after a mild dyskaryotic smear is about 40 per cent. A randomized trial in the hospital-based management of mild dyskaryosis comparing four periods of surveillance, which included immediate colposcopy, found 68 per cent of women with high-grade CIN after a single mild or moderately dyskaryotic smear.[21] Retrospective case series of women followed in the community report varying rates of referral to colposcopy (14–64 per cent) and these women are at increased risk of developing invasive cancer.[20] There is a high non-attendance rate for women who are followed up for more than 24 months.[21] An economic model suggested that immediate colposcopy was cheaper than cytological follow up. In two studies, only 25 per cent of women with a smear showing mild dyskaryosis achieved regression to a normal smear.[21–23]

### Follow up of treated and untreated women

**Frequency of follow up for treated women**
Recommendations for follow-up protocols have to be determined by expert consensus opinion.

- High-risk follow up: Women treated with high-grade disease (CIN2, CIN3, cGIN) require 6–12-month follow-up cytology and annual smears for the subsequent nine years at least, before returning to three to five-yearly smears.
- Low-risk follow up: Women treated for low-grade disease require 6-, 12- and 24-month follow-up cytology. If all are negative, then the patient may be discharged to three to five-yearly routine screening cytology.

There is no clear evidence suggesting that the diagnostic performance of cytology in combination with colposcopy for the detection of persistent disease after treatment for CIN is superior to cytology alone. Women treated for cGIN are at somewhat higher risk of developing recurrent disease than those with high grade CIN.[24] In addition, recurrent disease is more difficult to detect cytologically. Smears should be taken for the same duration with the same frequency as after treatment of CIN2 and CIN3 (minimum standard). Ideally, six-monthly smears would be taken for five years followed by annual smears for a further five years.

**Follow up of untreated women**
Women referred with a smear of mild dyskaryosis or less who have a low-grade lesion on colposcopy may be treated or followed up at six-monthly intervals in the colposcopy

clinic. If the lesion has not resolved within two years of referral, at least a biopsy is warranted. In practice, many women are offered treatment at this point, as persistent surveillance risks default. Approximately 50 per cent of women with a low-grade cytological abnormality who are not treated at first visit will eventually revert to normal cytology and colposcopy. Those who are identified to have a colposcopically low-grade lesion may be followed up. Prospective randomized data suggest that such a policy does not alter the number of women with high-grade lesions who are treated, but does reduce the number of low-grade lesions treated. However, in this study over one-fifth of women defaulted from follow up. Therefore, the decision to follow up rather than treat in the presence of an apparent low-grade lesion must incorporate analysis of the likelihood of default. Furthermore, the positive predictive value for distinguishing low- from high-grade lesions is only 57 per cent. Therefore, follow up is warranted as a result of the inherent poor colposcopic discrimination between high- and low-grade lesions. The ongoing management decisions for this group will often be influenced by the woman's choice.

## Management

### Colposcopy
Further investigation of smear abnormalities is by colposcopy. A colposcope is a low-power binocular microscope that allows magnification from around ×4 to ×25. In the UK, colposcopy is a secondary investigation; in other countries that do not have organized cytological screening, it may be used as a primary tool.

The current indications for colposcopy referral are detailed in Table 67.2.

It is important to recognize that the screening programme has the ability to generate considerable psychological morbidity.[25] Appropriate counselling at the time of or before colposcopy is important, and the vast majority of women can be reassured prior to the examination that they are extremely unlikely to have cancer. This is very important to emphasize.

The cervix is first examined at low magnification (×4–6). A saline-soaked cotton-wool ball is then applied, which moistens the epithelium, allowing the underlying blood vessels to be examined under higher magnification (preferably ×16 or even ×25). A green filter may be used as it makes the capillaries stand out more clearly. The shapes of the capillaries are studied and the intercapillary distances estimated. Acetic acid (3 or 5 per cent) is then applied to the cervix. Areas of CIN will appear as varying degrees of whiteness. This is termed 'acetowhiteness', in contrast to areas of hyperkeratosis or leukoplakia, which appear white before application of acetic acid. The exact reason why CIN tissue turns white with acetic acid is not fully understood. The cytoplasm becomes dehydrated, so in areas of abnormality, where there is a high nuclear:cytoplasmic ratio in

**Table 67.2** Interpretation and management plans for different smear grades

| Smear result | Interpretation | Management plan |
|---|---|---|
| Negative | No cellular abnormalities detected | Routine recall after 3–5 years |
| Borderline changes | Cellular appearances that cannot be described as normal | Repeat smear in 6–12 months and refer for colposcopy if any abnormality persists |
| Mild dyskaryosis | Cellular appearance consistent with underlying CIN1 | Repeat smear within 6 months and refer for colposcopy if any abnormality persists |
| Moderate dyskaryosis | Cellular appearance consistent with underlying CIN2 | Refer for colposcopy |
| Severe dyskaryosis | Cellular appearance consistent with underlying CIN3 | Refer for colposcopy |
| Suspicious of invasive cancer | Possibility of invasive cancer | Refer for colposcopy |
| Glandular neoplasia | Cellular appearance suggests an abnormality in the endocervical canal or endometrium | Refer for colposcopy and gynaecological assessment |
| Inadequate | The smear is unable to be interpreted in the laboratory; it may be poorly prepared at the point of collection, obscured by blood or inflammatory cells or may not contain the right type of cells | Repeat the smear; if infection is suspected as the reason for the inadequate smear, treat this first |

**Table 67.3** Treatment modalities for cervical intraepithelial neoplasia

| Excisional techniques | Ablative techniques |
|---|---|
| **LLETZ** – removal of the transformation zone using an electrodiathermy loop; requires local or general anaesthesia | **Radical electrodiathermy** – burning the transformation zone; usually requires general anaesthesia |
| **Laser cone** – removal of the transformation zone using the laser; requires local or general anaesthesia | **Cold coagulation** – destroying the transformation zone by applying a probe heated to 100–120°C; usually requires local anaesthesia |
| **Knife cone biopsy** – taking a cone with a knife; usually requires general anaesthesia | **Cryocautery** – freezing the tissue; does not require any anaesthesia |
| **Hysterectomy** – may be suitable if the woman has other gynaecological problems | **Laser** – vaporizing the tissue; requires local or general anaesthesia |

the cells, the nuclei become crowded and the light from the colposcope is reflected back. Such areas will therefore appear white. However, not all areas of high nuclear density are abnormal and so not all acetowhiteness necessarily correlates with CIN: areas of regenerating epithelium, subclinical papillomavirus infection and immature metaplasia may also appear acetowhite. One of the challenges facing the colposcopist is to decide which areas of acetowhiteness truly represent pre-malignancy and to avoid treating benign conditions. The classical vessel patterns of CIN are punctation and mosaicism. Bizarre-shaped vessels suggest cancer.

Another test used in colposcopy involves the application of Lugol's iodine solution to the cervix. Normal squamous epithelium contains glycogen and stains dark brown when Lugol's iodine is applied. Conversely, pre-malignant and malignant squamous tissue contains little or no glycogen and does not stain with iodine. This is Schiller's test: areas that are non-staining with iodine are referred to as Schiller-positive and those that take up iodine as Schiller-negative. The test may be used following acetic acid colposcopy.

## Treatment

High-grade lesions (CIN2/3) should be treated, but there is some debate about whether and when CIN1 should be treated, as a proportion will resolve spontaneously. If it is decided that treatment is needed, there are several options. Abnormal tissue can be removed (excisional techniques) or it can be destroyed (ablative techniques) (Table 67.3). Removing the entire transformation zone has the advantage of allowing a large specimen to be examined: the pathologist can comment on the most severe abnormality and can assess whether all the abnormal tissue has been removed. Destroying the transformation zone does not allow this, so it is mandatory to establish the diagnosis by taking a small biopsy before treatment. However, punch biopsy has been shown to be an inaccurate investigation when compared with subsequent loop excision from the same cervix.[26]

The success of treatment is usually defined as negative cytology six months following intervention. Randomized trial data on the different methods of treating CIN do not point to one overwhelmingly superior technique.

Lower genital tract

Cryotherapy is cheap and easy to use, with low morbidity. It should be used as a double freeze–thaw–freeze technique. Success rates for treating CIN3 vary between 77 and 93 per cent. Cryotherapy is a reasonable option for the treatment of low-grade disease, but not of high-grade disease. It may be suitable in resource-poor situations. All of the other ablative and excisional methods achieve cure (or success) rates of 90–98 per cent.[27]

Current treatments rely on the destruction or excision of affected tissue. However, with expanding knowledge about the role of HPV and the body's immune response to it, new immunological methods of disease prevention and therapy have been proposed. These aim to address the cause of the disease (i.e. HPV infection) and to either prevent (prophylactic vaccination) or treat (therapeutic vaccination) it. Prophylactic vaccination targets the viral capsid and aims to prevent infection or the early spread of infection through the production of neutralizing antibody. Therapeutic vaccines aim to boost the host's cell-mediated immune arm to attack established infection.

## Screening for human papillomavirus infection

As HPV infection is so strongly implicated in the genesis of CIN and cervical cancer, it is logical to ask whether viral detection could improve the screening process. Two methods of detecting HPV that are suitable for population screening are the polymerase chain reaction (PCR) and the hybrid capture system. Data from studies using earlier methodology can be disregarded. Applications of HPV testing can be at a primary or secondary level. Most published data refer to HPV testing as an adjunct to cytology and test the hypothesis that HPV detection improves the accuracy of cytology alone.[28,29] Qualitative identification of HPV in women presenting with a high-grade smear is pointless, as the vast majority will be high-risk HPV-positive anyway. It is becoming apparent that the same is true for women who have true mild dyskaryosis (or LSIL). However, in women with a borderline smear, it may be more discriminatory. This is particularly so in situations in which the background prevalence of infection is lower (such as in women over 30 or 35 years of age). Quantitative HPV estimation has been suggested as being more discriminatory than qualitative estimation. Methods of quantification vary and have limited reproducibility. Furthermore, recent data suggest that viral load varies in the natural history of disease and may be of limited predictive value.[30]

## Glandular pre-invasive disease

Adenocarcinoma-*in-situ* (AIS), or high-grade cervical intraepithelial glandular neoplasia (CIGN) of the cervix is a rare condition. It presents a particular challenge to the colposcopist, who may only see one case per year. Cytology screening is unsatisfactory, and the disease has no reliable

colposcopic features. Diagnosis is often made by chance during the treatment of squamous pre-invasive disease, which commonly coexists with AIS. Although the entire endocervical canal can be the site of disease, most lesions lie within 1 cm of the squamo-columnar junction. Skip lesions are rare, making fertility-sparing surgery a possibility, provided that endocervical margins are clear of disease. Recurrent disease occurs in 14 per cent of cases when cone margins are free of disease and rises to more than 50 per cent if the margins are involved. The method of conization is immaterial provided that a large enough specimen is taken and that the endocervical margins can be evaluated by the pathologist. There are no guidelines on the optimal follow up of conservatively managed women; however, most would recommend that regular endocervical cytology be performed in addition to conventional cytology and colposcopy.[31]

### KEY POINTS

- Virtually all cervical cancer is related to HPV infection [B].
- Cervical sampling now utilizes liquid-based cytology.
- The treatment methods (other than cryotherapy) to eradicate CIN are all equally effective [A].
- HPV is an extremely common infection that rarely causes cancer [C].
- Organized cervical cytology programmes have been shown to reduce the incidence of invasive cancer [C].
- The screening of teenagers cannot be justified [E].
- Screening for HPV infection is not yet routinely recommended.
- Neither Pap smear nor colposcopy is a reliable method for detecting glandular disease [D].

## THE VACCINATION PROGRAMME AND THE POTENTIAL FOR PREVENTION

Most, if not all, would now accept the central role played by oncogenic human papillomaviruses in the development of CIN and cervical cancer. Furthermore, there is also some understanding of the role played by the host's immune system in preventing and eradicating infection. It was therefore inevitable that attempts would be made to exploit the virus's immunogenicity and develop vaccines to prevent infection.

There are now two commercially available vaccines, one a quadravalent vaccine directed against HPV6, 11, 16 and 18; the second is a bivalent vaccine directed against HPV16 and 18. The design of both vaccines exploits the ability of viral capsid proteins to self-assemble into virus-like particles (VLP). The VLPs present the same antigenic signature to the host's immune system as 'real' virus, but as they do not contain any internal DNA they are biologically non-infective and non-transforming.

Several large randomized studies have now been completed and published and they have shown that both types of vaccine effectively increase specific IgG, reduce or eliminate infection with type-specific virus and effectively eliminate pre-invasive disease related to the vaccinated subtypes.[32,33] As we believe that up to 70 per cent of cervical cancers are the result of infections caused by either HPV16 or 18, there is an expectation that a vaccination programme, if systematically applied, will result in a significant reduction in the burden of invasive and pre-invasive disease.

There are, however, some unanswered questions. The duration of the effect is unknown, although it would appear that it is at least 4.5 years.[34] There is no guidance as yet as to when and how often booster vaccinations may be required. Although there is some evidence that vaccinating against one subtype may provide cross-resistance with other subtypes, we must still accept that up to 30 per cent of oncogenic subtypes remain potential threats to carcinogenesis and thus it is strongly recommended that despite the introduction of a vaccination programme, women should still be enrolled into the cervical screening programme.[35] Whether the natural spectrum of HPVs will be altered by widespread introduction of the vaccines is also unknown. There does not appear to be any evidence as yet of an increasing prevalence on non-16/18 HPV, although this effect will probably take decades to become noticeable.

The vaccines have not been shown to confer any significant benefit to those who have already been exposed to HPV and the current focus is schoolgirls aged 12 to 13 years with retrograde catch up of older groups. Thus, within the next four years, all girls between the ages of 12 and 17 years will have been offered the vaccine. The vaccination programme commenced in 2008 and is organized through, but not by, schools. The NHS has opted for the bivalent vaccine (Cervarix™), although Gardasil™ can be obtained on a private basis.

Prevention of HPV infection is a desirable goal and now, for the first time, there is clear evidence that at least some cervical cancer can be prevented. Further developments can be expected in this field, particularly in the immunological intervention of those who may already have been exposed and are at risk of developing persistent disease.

## VAGINAL INTRAEPITHELIAL NEOPLASIA

Pre-invasive disease of the vagina is extremely uncommon (about 150 times less common than CIN). In 70 per cent of cases of vaginal intraepithelial neoplasia (VaIN), there will be associated CIN. The average age of the woman with VaIN tends to be higher than for CIN. The major predisposing factor is the same, namely oncogenic HPV, but the reason for the lower incidence is the relative stability of the epithelium compared with the metaplastic cervical epithelium. Women exposed to diethylstilbestrol *in utero* have a higher incidence of VaIN as here the areas of metaplastic transformation extend on to the vagina. Around 25 per cent of women with VaIN will have had a hysterectomy previously, for either CIN

or a benign condition. Like CIN, VaIN is graded 1–3, but in common with vulval intraepithelial neoplasia (VIN), the invasive potential is less than for CIN. Treatment of VaIN3 is by surgical excision, which may necessitate a combined abdomino-vaginal approach to excise the vaginal vault. Chemosurgery using 5-fluorouracil prior to diathermy ablation is an experimental treatment that has shown some promising results. Radiotherapy is an alternative treatment for women who may not be suitable for surgery. Lower grades of disease can be observed. For women who have had a hysterectomy in which VaIN is seen at the vaginal vault, there may still be disease buried above the vault in the cuff that was closed over at hysterectomy. In view of this, if high-grade VaIN is detected at the vault of the vagina, it should be treated by excision rather than destruction.

### KEY POINTS

- VaIN is uncommon and there is little evidence base on the subject.
- It usually coexists with CIN [D].
- The risk factors are similar to those for CIN [D].
- *In-utero* diethylstilbestrol exposure increases the risk of VaIN [D].

## VULVAL INTRAEPITHELIAL NEOPLASIA

Pre-malignant disease of the vulva is much less common than its cervical counterpart. Human papillomavirus infection is recognized as a major factor in the aetiology of some, though not all, vulval intraepithelial neoplasia. The HPV types most commonly associated with VIN are HPV16 and 33. HPV-associated VIN is increasing in incidence, particularly in younger women.[36] This increase may be explained by a number of factors, such as increased awareness amongst medical practitioners leading to improved detection, increased smoking by younger women, or changing sexual attitudes and increased exposure to HPV. These women should be examined for other intraepithelial neoplasia of the anogenital tract.

The pre-malignant potential of VIN has been estimated to range from 4 per cent for treated cases to 80 per cent for untreated cases.[37,38] Most published series estimate a risk of 10 per cent or less.

Vulval intraepithelial neoplasia affects mainly the labia minora and the perineum. It can take a variety of forms and can be difficult to diagnose. Up to 60 per cent of affected women may complain of itching, soreness and burning, but many are asymptomatic and the abnormality can be a chance finding on examination.[39] The lesions may extend to the perianal and anal mucosa. Diagnosis is made by examining the vulva with a good light source, such as the colposcope at low magnification, and by taking representative biopsies. Like CIN, VIN is graded 1–3 in increasing severity of abnormal cell

**Table 67.4** Comparison of characteristics of vulval intraepithelial neoplasia grade 3 (VIN3) and cervical intraepithelial neoplasia grade 3 (CIN3)

|  | VIN3 | CIN3 |
| --- | --- | --- |
| Proportion of cases of disease adjacent to malignancy | 25% | 90% |
| Invasive potential | Low (<10%) | Significant (40%) |
| Time to progress to invasion | 20–30 years | 10–15 years |
| Spontaneous regression | Up to 40% | Low |

maturation and stratification. However, there are some striking differences between VIN and CIN (Table 67.4).

Current treatments for VIN are suboptimal in terms of their poor clinical response rates, high relapse rates and associated physical and psychological morbidities. The high recurrence rates following many therapies may reflect the fact that they fail to remove the reservoir of HPV present in the vulval skin. Low-grade VIN should be observed. VIN3 lesions can be treated by local excision or laser vaporization. Recurrences of 39 and 70 per cent have been described after surgical excision and laser ablation, respectively.[40,41]

A topical immunomodulator called 'imiquimod' may be of use in the management of women with VIN, although it remains experimental at present.

Non-HPV intraepithelial neoplasia is termed 'differentiated VIN' and oncogenesis involves alternative pathways to the HPV model. There appears to be an association with some inflammatory vulval epithelial disorders, such as lichen sclerosus, but the condition is poorly understood.

> ## KEY POINTS
>
> - VIN is uncommon and there is little evidence base on the subject.
> - VIN in younger women is strongly associated with HPV [C].
> - The most common presenting symptom is pruritus [D].
> - Lesions may be multifocal and have a variety of appearances.
> - Multicentric disease should be considered when VIN is diagnosed.
> - Conservative surgery is currently the basis of treatment [E].
> - Long-term follow up is essential as recurrence is common [D].

## MULTICENTRIC INTRAEPITHELIAL NEOPLASIA

There is a small group of women in whom intraepithelial neoplastic changes can be detected at more than one site in the lower genital tract. The sites involved are the cervix,

vagina, vulva, perineum, anal canal and natal cleft. Although the number of women affected by multicentric intraepithelial neoplasia (MIN) is small, the number appears to be increasing, which may be a true reflection of more disease or it may be a result of increased awareness and detection. The aetiology of MIN is a combination of HPV infection and host immunosuppression of varying degrees. Patients in whom cell-mediated immunity is compromised, such as women who have had organ transplantation or who carry the human immunodeficiency virus (HIV), often have recognizable HPV-associated changes in numerous sites in the lower genital tract. Conversely, women with humoral immunodeficiency do not have an increased risk of HPV-associated lesions.

Multicentric intraepithelial neoplasia may be detected in a woman who has repeated abnormal smears despite treatment for CIN, or in a woman being assessed for VIN. Genitourinary physicians who perform colposcopy may also encounter MIN in HIV-positive women under their care.

At the time of writing, there are no national guidelines for the management of women with MIN. Such cases are often complex and become chronic, the women sometimes having repeated surgery over several years. It is therefore important to be aware that these women may suffer adverse psychological sequelae as a result of their condition. As their numbers are small, women with MIN should be managed in large centres to concentrate experience and expertise. Investigations should be individualized, but may include multiple colposcopically directed biopsies, HPV typing, HIV testing and tests of T-cell function. Management aims to exclude invasive cancer and control symptoms while preserving anatomical and functional integrity where possible. The treatments of lesions of the vagina and vulva are described above. Lesions of the perineum and anal canal may require an initial colostomy prior to skin grafting. Such cases require a multidisciplinary team comprising a gynaecologist, colorectal surgeon, plastic surgeon, stoma nurse and possibly a psychologist.

New immunomodulating therapies currently under investigation, such as therapeutic vaccination and imiquimod, hold out some hope for women affected with MIN. Research to date suggests that they are suitable for around 30 per cent of cases and thus upholds the theory that MIN has varied causes.

> ## KEY POINTS
>
> - MIN is a rare condition and there is no evidence base.
> - There is an association with conditions in which cell-mediated immunity is impaired [D].
> - It is often a chronic, relapsing condition [D].
> - The key aim of management is to do the least required to exclude invasion and control symptoms [E].

# SUMMARY

Lower genital tract pre-malignancy is an important area of gynaecology. Most of the pre-cancers in this area have an association with HPV, but HPV infection is extremely common and causes no problems in the majority of individuals affected. Organized national screening seems to have been effective in reducing the incidence and mortality from cervical cancer, but there has been a cost to pay in terms of over-investigation and treatment of women who have very minor changes that are unlikely ever to progress to cancer. Pre-cancers of the vagina, vulva and perineum are much less common, but require specialized skills for accurate diagnosis and appropriate management. Current treatment modalities for the pre-cancers involve destruction or excision. As our knowledge of the aetiology of lower genital tract pre-malignancy expands, it may be possible to target the underlying cause more accurately through the use of therapeutic and prophylactic vaccinations.

## Published Guidelines

National Health Service Cervical Screening Programme. Guideline No. 20. Sheffield: NHSCP, 2004.

National Health Service Cervical Screening Programme. Achievable standards and benchmarks for reporting and criteria for evaluating cervical cytopathology. NHSCSP publication No. 1. Sheffield: NHSCP, May 2000.

National Health Service Cervical Screening Programme. External quality assessment scheme for gynaecological cytopathology: protocol and standard operating procedures. NHSCSP publication No. 15. Sheffield: NHSCP, 2009.

All guidelines from www.cancerscreening.nhs.uk/cervicalpublications.

## Key References

1. Koss LG, Stewart FW, Foote FW *et al.* Some histological aspects of the behaviour of epidermoid carcinoma *in situ* and related lesions of the uterine cervix. *Cancer* 1963; **16**: 1160.
2. McIndoe WA, McLean MR, Jones RW, Mullins PR. The invasive potential of carcinoma *in situ* of the cervix. *Obstet Gynecol* 1984; **64**: 451–8.
3. Richart RM. Natural history of cervical intraepithelial neoplasia. *Clin Obstet Gynecol* 1968; **10**: 748.
4. Cancer Research UK. Cancer incidence statistics 2004. London: Cancer Research UK. Available from: http//info.cancerresearchuk.org/images/excels/cs_inc_t8.2.xls.
5. Cancer Research UK. Cancer incidence statistics 2004. Available from: http//info.cancerresearchuk.org/images/excels/cs_mort_6.6.2.xls.

6. Peto J, Gilham C, Fletcher O *et al.* The cervical cancer epidemic that screening has prevented in the UK. *Lancet* 2004; **364**: 249–56.
7. Sasieni PD, Cuzick J, Lynch-Farmery E. Estimating the efficacy of screening by auditing smear histories of women with and without cervical cancer. The National Co-ordinating Network for Cervical Screening. *Br J Cancer* 1996; **73**: 1001–5.
8. Cervical Screening programme, England 2005–2006.
9. Walboomers JMM. Human papillomavirus is a necessary cause of invasive cervical cancer worldwide. *J Pathol* 1999; **189**: 12–19.
10. Werness BA, Levine AJ, Howley PM. Association of human papillomavirus types 16 and 18 E6 proteins with p53. *Science* 1990; **248**: 76–9.
11. White E. p53 guardian of Rb. *Nature* 1994; **371**: 21–2.
12. Robertson JH, Woodend BE, Crozier EH, Hutchinson J. Risk of cervical cancer associated with mild dyskaryosis. *BMJ* 1988; **297**: 18–21.
13. Soutter WP. The management of a mildly dyskaryotic smear: immediate referral to colposcopy is safer. *BMJ* 1994; **309**: 591–2.
14. Laara E, Day NE, Hakama M. Trends in mortality from cervical cancer in the Nordic countries: association with organised screening programmes. *Lancet* 1987; **I**: 1247–9.
15. National Health Service Cervical Screening Programme. Guideline No. 20. Sheffield: NHSCP, 2004.
16. Herbert A, Stein K, Bryant TN *et al.* Relation between the incidence of invasive cervical cancer and the screening interval: is a five year interval too long? *J Med Screen* 1996; **3**: 140–5.
17. Sasieni P, Adams J. Effect of screening on cervical cancer mortality in England and Wales: analysis of trends with an age cohort model. *BMJ* 1999; **318**: 1244–5.
18. Arbyn M, Kyrgiou M, Simoens C *et al.* Perinatal mortality and other severe adverse pregnancy outcomes associated with treatment of cervical intraepithelial neoplasia: meta-analysis. *BMJ* 2008; **18**: 337.
19. Van Wijngaarden WJ, Duncan ID. Rationale for stopping cervical screening in women over 50. *BMJ* 1993; **306**: 967–7.
20. Soutter WP, Wisdom S, Brough AK, Monaghan JM. Should patients with mild atypia in a cervical smear be referred for colposcopy? *Br J Obstet Gynaecol* 1986; **93**: 70–74.
21. Johnson N, Sutton J, Thornton JG *et al.* Decision analysis for best management of mildly dyskaryotic smear. *Lancet* 1993; **343**: 91–6.
22. Flannelly G, Anderson D, Kitchener HC *et al.* Management of women with mild and moderate cervical dyskaryosis. *BMJ* 1994; **308**: 1399–403.
23. Shafi MI, Luesley DM, Jordan JA *et al.* Randomised trial of immediate versus deferred treatment strategies for the management of minor cervical cytological abnormalities. *Br J Obstet Gynaecol* 1997; **104**: 590–4.

Lower genital tract

24. Teshima S, Shimosato Y, Kishi K *et al.* Early stage adenocarcinoma of the uterine cervix. Histopathalogic analysis with consideration of histogenesis. *Cancer* 1985; **56**: 167–72.

25. Marteau TM, Walker P, Giles J, Smail M. Anxieties in women undergoing colposcopy. *Br J Obstet Gynaecol* 1990; **97**: 859–61.

26. Buxton EJ, Luesley DM, Shafi MI, Rollason T. Colposcopically directed punch biopsy: a potentially misleading investigation. *Br J Obstet Gynaecol* 1991; **98**: 1273–6.

27. Martin-Hirsch PL, Paraskevaidis E, Kitchener H. Surgery for cervical intraepithelial neoplasia *Cochrane Database Syst Rev* 2001; (**4**): CD001318.

28. Bavin PJ, Giles JA, Deery A *et al.* Use of semi-quantitative PCR for human papillomavirus DNA type 16 to identify women with high grade cervical disease in a population presenting with a mildly dyskaryotic smear report. *Br J Cancer* 1993; **67**: 602–5.

29. Cuzick J, Terry G, Ho L *et al.* Type-specific human papillomavirus DNA in abnormal smears as a predictor of high-grade cervical intraepithelial neoplasia. *Br J Cancer* 1994; **69**: 167–71.

30. Woodman CB, Collins S, Winter H *et al.* Natural history of cervical human papillomavirus infection in young women: a longitudinal cohort study. *Lancet* 2001; **357**: 1831–6.

31. Etherington IJ, Luesley DM. Adenocarcinoma *in situ* of the cervix – controversies in diagnosis and treatment. *J Lower Genital Tract Dis* 2001; **5**: 94–8.

32. Paavonen J, Jenkins D, Bosch FX *et al.* Efficacy of a prophylactic adjuvanted bivalent L1 virus-like-particle vaccine against infection with human papillomavirus types 16 and 18 in young women: an interim analysis of a phase III double-blind, randomised controlled trial. *Lancet* 2007; **369**: 2161–70.

33. Joura EA, Leodolter S, Hernandez-Avila M *et al.* Efficacy of a quadrivalent prophylactic human papillomavirus (types 6, 11, 16, and 18) L1 virus-like-particle vaccine against high-grade vulval and vaginal lesions: a combined analysis of three randomised clinical trials. *Lancet* 2007; **369**: 1693–702.

34. Harper DM, Franco EL, Wheeler CM *et al.* Sustained efficacy up to 4.5 years of a bivalent L1 virus-like particle vaccine against human papillomavirus types 16 and 18: follow-up from a randomised control trial *Lancet* 2006; **367**: 1247–55.

35. Jenkins D. A review of cross-protection against oncogenic HPV by an HPV-16/18 AS04-adjuvanted cervical cancer vaccine: importance of virological and clinical endpoints and implications for mass vaccination in cervical cancer prevention. *Gynecol Oncol* 2008; **110** (Suppl. 1): S18–25.

36. Jones RW, Baranyai J, Stables S. Trends in squamous cell carcinoma of the vulva: the influence of vulvar intraepithelial neoplasia. *Obstet Gynecol* 1997; **90**: 448–52.

37. Iversen T, Tretli S. Intraepithelial and invasive squamous cell neoplasia of the vulva: trends in incidence, recurrence and survival in Norway. *Obstet Gynecol* 1994; **6**: 969–72.

38. Jones RW, Rowan DM. Vulvar intraepithelial neoplasia 3: a clinical study of the outcome in 113 cases with relation to the later development of invasive vulvar cancer. *Obstet Gynecol* 1994; **5**: 741–5.

39. Campion MJ, Singer A. Vulvar intraepithelial neoplasia: clinical review. *Genitourinary Med* 1987; **63**: 147–52.

40. DiSaia PJ, Rich WM. Surgical approach to multifocal carcinoma in situ of the vulva. *Am J Obstet Gynecol* 1981; **140**: 136–45.

41. Townsend DE, Levine RU, Richart RM *et al.* Management of vulvar intraepithelial neoplasia by carbon dioxide laser. *Obstet Gynecol* 1982; **60**: 49–52.

# SECTION D
## Gynaecological oncology

# Chapter 68

# Endometrial cancer

*Margaret E Cruickshank*

## MRCOG standards

### Theoretical skills

- Revise your knowledge of pelvic anatomy.
- Understand the epidemiology and aetiology of malignant conditions of the uterus.
- Understand the principles of carcinogenesis and pathology.
- Be able to describe the diagnostic and imaging techniques in the diagnosis of endometrial cancer.
- Be able to describe the role of hysteroscopy and endometrial biopsy in the diagnosis of endometrial cancer.
- Be able to describe the management of endometrial cancer.
- Be able to describe the FIGO classification for endometrial cancer.
- Be able to describe the indications, techniques, complications of outcomes of oncological surgery, radiotherapy and chemotherapy.
- Understand the principles of symptom relief, palliative and terminal care.

### Practical skills

- Be confident to perform outpatient endometrial biopsy.
- Be able to stage endometrial cancer and counsel patients with direct supervision.
- Be able to recognize, assess and manage surgically and non-surgically carcinoma of the endometrium.
- Be able to evaluate response to oncology treatment and counsel regarding prognosis.
- Be able to manage palliative care in liaison with an expert team.

## INTRODUCTION

Endometrial cancer usually arises in post-menopausal women. The incidence continues to increase in many developed countries and it is now the most common gynaecological cancer in the United Kingdom with more than 6500 cases in 2005.[1] Seventy-five per cent of women present with stage I disease and for most of them the management is surgical and the prognosis is very good.

## INCIDENCE

Endometrial cancer is the fourth most common cancer in women in the UK. In 2005, there were 6531 new cases or 17 per 100 000 women per year (European age-standardized). This compares with 4850 new cases (13.8 per 100 000 women per year) in 1997 and 3912 new cases in 1992 (Office of National Statistics), demonstrating an upward trend in the incidence. This increase is most marked in the age group 60–79 years, while the rate in women aged less than 50 years has remained stable. Endometrial cancer is rare in women before the age of 40, at less than 2 per 100 000 women. The incidence increases between the ages of 40 and 55, thereafter reaching a plateau. The incidence of endometrial cancer is four-fold higher in developed countries.

Survival has been improving and the five-year age-standardized relative survival is 77 per cent (CRC Cancer Statistics for England and Wales, 2000–2001) compared with 61 per cent for women diagnosed in 1971–75. For stage I disease, there is an overall five-year survival of 85 per cent, but this falls to 25 per cent for stage IV disease.

## AETIOLOGY

Women with relatively high levels of circulating oestrogens or prolonged oestrogen influence are a recognized high-risk group for endometrial cancer. This is seen in the following situations:

- obesity due to the peripheral conversion of androgens in adipose tissue,
- tamoxifen therapy,
- oestrogen therapy unopposed by progestogens,
- polycystic ovarian syndrome (PCOS),
- early menarche and late menopause.

Endometrial hyperplasia results from protracted oestrogen stimulation. Those cases without atypia are benign, but when cellular atypia is present this is considered to be pre-malignant.

## OBESITY

The rising incidence is associated with the obesity epidemic at a time when the use of HRT has fallen. This suggests that obesity is not responsible for the rising incidence and every day clinical experience confirms the increasing proportion of morbidly obese women amongst women with endometrial cancer. A recent epidemiological study has indicated that the malignancy most strongly associated with obesity is endometrial cancer.[2]

## OESTROGEN REPLACEMENT

The use of unopposed (o)estrogen replacement therapy (ERT) is clearly linked to endometrial cancer and more than doubles the risk (relative risk (RR) 2.3 for users compared with non-users, 95 per cent confidence interval (CI) 2.1–2.5) [A].[3] This meta-analysis of 30 studies found significant heterogeneity between the studies analyzed, which was mostly due to differences in the dose and duration of oestrogen. Higher doses of oestrogen and duration of use of ten or more years have a relative risk of 9.5 (95 per cent CI 7.4–12.3). The risk does reduce after stopping ERT, but interrupted use does not lower the risk compared with daily use. This analysis clearly showed that there is a substantial risk from unopposed ERT and this should only be used for hysterectomized women.

The highest risk of hormone replacement therapy (HRT) is for atypical endometrial hyperplasia, but there is also an effect on advanced cancer and mortality. The concurrent use of a progesterone reduces the relative risk to almost that of a non-ERT-user (RR 0.8, 95 per cent CI 0.6–1.2), but the direction of this effect does vary between case–control and cohort studies. Unopposed ERT increases the rate of irregular bleeding and non-adherence to treatment [A].[4] The addition of progesterone, whether cyclical or sequential, prevents the development of endometrial hyperplasia and improves compliance. Irregular bleeding is more likely with a continuous than a sequential

preparation (odds ratio (OR) 2.3, 95 per cent CI 2.1–2.5), but with longer duration of therapy, continuous is more protective than sequential in preventing endometrial hyperplasia. The UK Million Women study,[5] a prospective cohort study of 716 738 post-menopausal women, confirmed an increased risk in the order of 50 per cent among current users of ERT and 80 per cent in those using tibolone preparations. There was a reduced risk for ever versus never users of continuous combined therapy (relative risk 0.71 (95 per cent CI 0.56–0.90); $p = 0.005$), but no significant difference in risk with combined cyclical preparations (relative risk 1.05 (95 per cent CI 0.91–1.22); $p = 0.5$). Body mass index significantly affected these risks with the adverse effects of tibolone and ERT greatest in non-obese women, and the benefits of combined HRT greatest in obese women. The counteraction of progesterone on oestrogens on the endometrium is greater the more days every month that they are added to oestrogen and the higher the women's BMI [C].

## GENETIC PREDISPOSITION

Endometrial cancer in women under the age of 45 may be associated with Lynch type II familial cancer syndrome, which is known as hereditary non-polyposis colorectal cancer (HNPCC). There does not appear to be a site-specific inherited form of endometrial cancer, but it is associated with a genetic predisposition as a component of the HNPCC syndrome. Families affected with this syndrome have a predisposition to bowel cancer and also to ovarian tumours.

## PATHOLOGY

The uterine corpus lies above the level of the internal cervical os and is composed of the fundus above the tubal ostiae and the body below. The blood supply is the uterine artery, a branch of the internal iliac artery. The lymphatic drainage passes with the artery to the internal, external and common iliac nodes, obturator fossa nodes and para-aortic nodes.

The International Federation of Gynecology and Obstetrics (FIGO) Committee on Gynaecologic Oncology recommends that endometrial cancer is surgically staged.[6] This includes histological verification of the tumour type grading and the extent of tumour. The degree of tumour differentiation has an important impact on the natural history of the disease and on treatment selection. Ninety-five per cent of uterine cancers are adenocarcinomas arising from the endometrium. They are graded with regard to the degree of cell differentiation (Table 68.1).

Notable nuclear atypia that is inappropriate for the architectural grade raises it to the next tumour grade. Nuclear grading

**Table 68.1** Grading of tumour differentiation

| | |
|----|----|
| G1 | 5% or less of a non-squamous or non-morular solid growth pattern |
| G2 | 6–50% of a non-squamous or non-morular solid growth pattern |
| G3 | 50% of a non-squamous or non-morular solid growth pattern |

takes precedence in serous and clear-cell adenocarcinomas. Histopathological reporting should include:

- depth of myometrial invasion,
- tumour grade,
- histological subtype,
- presence or absence of hyperplasia in adjacent non-neoplastic endometrium,
- lymphovascular space invasion,
- lymph node involvement,
- the status of peritoneal washings taken at surgery.

There are clearly recognized risk factors for lymph node involvement, distant metastasis and poor survival. These are tumour grade, non-endometrial tumour and deep myometrial invasion. Papillary serous adenocarcinomas and clear-cell carcinomas are high-risk subtypes and they are associated with about 50 per cent of all relapses. Their five-year survivals are 27 and 42 per cent, respectively. Mucinous, squamous and undifferentiated tumours are rare.

## Histopathology by World Health Organization/International Society of Gynaecological Pathology Classification

- Endometrioid carcinoma.
- Adenocarcinoma.
- Adenocanthoma (adenocarcinoma with squamous metaplasia).
- Adenosquamous carcinoma (mixed adenocarcinoma and squamous cell carcinoma).
- Mucinous adenocarcinoma.
- Papillary serous adenocarcinoma.
- Clear-cell adenocarcinoma.
- Undifferentiated carcinoma.
- Mixed carcinoma.

# PRESENTATION AND DIAGNOSIS

Endometrial cancer usually presents with vaginal bleeding in post-menopausal women. Post-menopausal bleeding (PMB) is defined as bleeding from the genital tract one or more years after a woman's last period. Women who

continue to menstruate after the age of 55 also merit investigation. Up to 10 per cent of women with PMB will have an endometrial carcinoma. The likelihood of an underlying cancer increases with age at presentation.

# INVESTIGATION OF POST-MENOPAUSAL BLEEDING

About 10 per cent of women referred with post-menopausal bleeding will have endometrial cancer and most women with PMB can be investigated effectively and safely as outpatients.

Transvaginal ultrasound scanning (TVS) is an accurate method of excluding endometrial cancer [B]. Women can be assessed quickly and triaged for endometrial biopsy on the basis of their scan findings. TVS limits the need for endometrial biopsy to women with an endometrial thickness of <5 mm, an irregular endometrial outline or fluid within the uterine cavity. The majority of women have a thin, regular endometrium and can be reassured at a first visit without further investigation. A meta-analysis[7] summarized accuracy data using likelihood ratios for various cut-off levels of abnormal endometrial thickness (measuring the thickness of both layers). The most common cut-offs were 4 mm (nine studies) and 5 mm (21 studies). Using the pooled estimates from four studies which used the best quality criteria, a thickness of >5 mm raised the probability of carcinoma from 14.0 per cent (95 per cent CI 13.3–14.7) to 31.3 per cent (95 per cent CI 26.1–36.3) and a thickness <5 mm reduced the risk to 2.5 per cent (95 per cent CI 0.9–6.4) [A]. This reduces the need for further intervention, service costs and patient anxiety, and provides rapid reassurance for those women with a normal result.

There are a number of devices for taking outpatient endometrial biopsies which have been compared in prospective studies. Samples taken by Pipelle are comparable with the Vabra and Novak aspirators in terms of specimen adequacy and diagnostic accuracy. In addition, this method produces less patient discomfort. D&C is no longer recommended for the investigation of PMB.[8]

Hysteroscopy is often used to investigate PMB, as it allows direct inspection of the endometrium. It can detect 95 per cent of intrauterine abnormalities and is a sensitive means of identifying polyps and submucous fibroids [B]. It can be used in the outpatient setting, and outpatient hysteroscopy is highly acceptable to women [B], although general anaesthesia may sometimes be necessary.

## Dedicated post-menopausal bleeding clinic

A dedicated clinic allows rapid assessment and reassurance for women with PMB using a one-stop clinic approach. Most clinics provide TV scanning by appropriately trained staff. Women with a history that meets the criteria of PMB can be fast-tracked to this service, with written information provided in primary care prior to their visit. The diagnosis of cancer can be excluded for most women at their first visit. Endometrial biopsy and outpatient hysteroscopy should be provided for those women with an abnormal scan result at their first assessment. The majority of consultant gynaecologists in a Scottish audit supported such outpatient investigation [C].

---

### EBM: Diagnosis of endometrial cancer

- A meta-analysis of 35 studies found TVS scanning to be an accurate means of excluding endometrial cancer.
- Initial assessment of PMB should be provided as an outpatient service and TVS used to assess the endometrium.
- Seven prospective studies have evaluated TVS in women with PMB, comparing it against D&C or outpatient endometrial biopsy.
- The cost effectiveness and clinical effectiveness of outpatient investigation of PMB have not been evaluated.

---

## WOMEN ON TAMOXIFEN

Tamoxifen is a non-steroidal oestrogen antagonist, which is used widely as adjuvant treatment for post-menopausal women who have breast carcinoma. The absolute improvement in recurrence is greatest during the first five years of treatment [A].[8] Tamoxifen has been shown to decrease the overall progression of the disease and to prevent disease in the contralateral breast. Long-term tamoxifen use is controversial due to its oestrogenic effects on the endometrium. Although it acts as an anti-oestrogen on breast cancer cells, it has a mild oestrogenic effect on the endometrium, bone and cardiovascular system.

Long-term use is associated with proliferative endometrium, and a spectrum of benign and malignant changes of the endometrium has been reported, including hyperplasia, polyps and carcinoma. The incidence of endometrial carcinoma in post-menopausal women taking tamoxifen is significantly higher than in women not on tamoxifen [A].[9] However, the absolute decrease in contralateral breast cancer is twice as large as the absolute increase in endometrial cancer, and overall the benefits of tamoxifen are greater than the risks.

Post-menopausal women who have a uterus and are taking tamoxifen should be advised of these effects. Abnormal bleeding needs to be investigated fully and promptly. A Pipelle biopsy is appropriate as the first line of investigation, but a negative result is not conclusive. Women with a negative result still require hysteroscopy. Transvaginal ultrasound scan can be useful in triaging the urgency of further investigation. The fact that the ultrasonic appearances can be misleading needs to be considered. Tamoxifen has a sono-translucent effect on both the endometrial stroma and myometrium. This can give rise to false-positive reports in cases of cystic atrophy, which appears as thickened cystic endometrium on scan. Histology confirms this to be multiple cystic spaces lined by atrophic epithelium within a dense fibrous stroma. Hysteroscopy may be the investigation of choice in this situation as it allows direct inspection of the endometrium, and full-thickness biopsies can be taken at the same procedure.[7]

There is no evidence that asymptomatic women on tamoxifen should be screened for endometrial changes [C]. Asymptomatic women taking tamoxifen have a greater endometrial thickness on TVS scan. Comparatively, those who present with bleeding have a significantly thicker endometrium and are more likely to have endometrial pathology [B][10] and women with endometrial pathology are also more likely to present with symptoms. Outpatient hysteroscopy, although a good screening tool, is not as useful when biopsies are necessary. A randomized, cross-over study comparing TVS with outpatient hysteroscopy found the former together with sonohysterogram more sensitive, specific and acceptable to women.[11] There is no clinical or cost-effectiveness evidence to support the endometrial screening of asymptomatic women on tamoxifen [B], and the benefit in terms of breast cancer mortality far outweighs the risk to the endometrium. The evidence, however, is less clear for healthy women taking tamoxifen to reduce their risk of breast cancer. The International Breast Cancer Intervention Study (IBIS)[12] reported on the risk:benefit ratio of tamoxifen as preventative treatment in women at increased risk of breast cancer. This trial randomized 7152 women to five years of tamoxifen or placebo. There was a non-significant increase in endometrial cancers in the tamoxifen group. Although there was a 32 per cent risk reduction in breast cancer, the risk:benefit ratio was not clear due to increased deaths from other causes, including thromboembolic disease. An earlier American trial, The Breast Cancer Prevention Trial (BCPT-P-1), was stopped early when a 45 per cent decrease in new breast cancers was reported in the tamoxifen arm. There was also an increase in endometrial cancers. Newer selective oestrogen receptor modulators (SERMs) have a similar profile to tamoxifen without the uterotrophic effects.

---

### EBM: Tamoxifen and the endometrium

- A systematic review of 55 RCTs of adjuvant tamoxifen versus no tamoxifen before recurrence and with at least five years of follow-up data shows that tamoxifen substantially improves the ten-year survival of women with oestrogen-receptor-positive breast cancer. It also found that the incidence of endometrial cancer increases by a factor of 2 at one to two years and by a factor of 4 after five years of tamoxifen treatment.
- There is no evidence to support the screening of asymptomatic women on tamoxifen for endometrial abnormalities.

## STAGING

The staging of endometrial cancer is surgicopathological. Tumour grade and the depth of myometrial involvement are the main determinants of extrauterine spread. These two pathological criteria are often used to determine the risk of recurrence and to select women for post-operative radiotherapy. Metastatic spread occurs characteristically to the pelvic and para-aortic lymph nodes. Distant metastasis is uncommon at presentation. The most common sites of distant spread are the vagina and lungs, but the inguinal and supra-clavicular lymph nodes, liver and brain may also be involved. When surgery is not appropriate or feasible, the clinical staging adopted by FIGO in 1971 is applied (Table 68.2), but selection of this staging system should be noted.

### Radiological imaging

Pre-operative evaluation and planning for treatment require clinical staging. The risk of pelvic and para-aortic lymph node involvement depends on the stage, grade and myometrial invasion. Twelve per cent of women with stage

**Table 68.2** International Federation of Gynecology and Obstetrics (FIGO) classification 2009

| Stage 1[a] | Tumour confined to the corpus uteri |
| --- | --- |
| 1A[a] | No or less than half myometrial invasion |
| 1B[a] | Invasion equal to or more than half of the myometrium |
| Stage II[a] | Tumour invades cervical stroma, but does not extend beyond the uterus[b] |
| Stage III[a] | Local and/or regional spread of the tumour |
| IIIA[a] | Tumour invades serosa of the uterus and/or adnexae[c] |
| IIIB[a] | Vaginal and/or parametrial involvement[c] |
| IIIC[a] | Metastasis to pelvic and/or para-aortic lymph nodes |
| IIIC1 | Positive pelvic nodes |
| IIIC2 | Positive para-aortic lymph nodes with or without positive pelvic nodes |
| Stage IV[a] | Tumour invades bladder and/or bowel mucosa and/or distant metastasis |
| IVA[a] | Invasion of bladder and/or bowel mucosa |
| IVB[a] | Distant metastasis, including intra-abdominal and/or inguinal lymph nodes |

[a]G1, G2 or G3.

[b]Endocervical glandular involvement only should be considered as stage I and no longer as stage II.

[c]Positive cytology has to be reported separately without changing the stage.

I disease will have lymph node metastasis. With grade 3 disease, this rises to 18 per cent, and when there is deep myometrial involvement, to 22 per cent. Without proper assessment and a treatment plan based on the risk of nodal disease, the prognosis is poorer [C].[13]

Endometrial biopsy will already have confirmed the diagnosis and given information on the tumour grade. Myometrial invasion can be assessed by TVS or magnetic resonance imaging (MRI). Transvaginal ultrasound can assess the depth of myometrial invasion and can be used to triage women for appropriate management at a cancer centre or cancer unit. Although TVS is quicker and relatively cheap, it is less accurate than MRI. Magnetic resonance imaging appears to be the optimum method of evaluating the soft-tissue structures of the pelvis, including myometrial invasion and the status of the pelvic lymph nodes with acceptable accuracy and specificity, although micrometastasis will not be detected reducing the overall sensitivity. Computed tomography (CT) scanning is less useful in imaging these soft tissues. The results are similar in predicting nodal disease, but less accurate at assessing the depth of myometrial invasion [B] and cervical involvement, but may be useful for women with high risk histology to detect extra-pelvic disease. A chest x-ray should also be performed for staging, as the lungs are a common metastatic site.

### Endometrial cancer imaging

MRI is the imaging method of choice for pre-treatment staging to assess myometrial invasion, cervical involvement and lymph node status.

## MANAGEMENT

Women with disease localized to the corpus are usually curable by surgery. There are variations in the definition of intermediate and high risk, but the high risk group generally includes deep myometrial invasion and grade 3 tumours including clear cell and papillary serous histological types. High risk features are associated with a poorer prognosis because of the increased risk of nodal disease and recurrence.

Women with endometrial cancer are often elderly with other medical problems, and pre-operative assessment for fitness for an anaesthetic and surgery is essential. Survival rates are reduced by 20 per cent when primary surgery is not feasible.

### Early stage disease

Most women present with early stage disease and primary surgery is fundamental to achieving a cure. The treatment of choice is total abdominal hysterectomy and bilateral salpingo-oophorectomy (TAH/BSO). It is not necessary to remove a vaginal cuff or parametrial tissue [C]. Recurrence at the vaginal vault is related to recognized risk factors and particularly cervical stromal involvement – factors that reflect lymphatic vessel involvement. Endocervical glandular involvement only is now considered as stage 1 disease.

Stage II disease should be treated the same as stage I disease by TAH/BSO. Where there is cervical stromal involvement, the treatment options are radical hysterectomy with pelvic lymphadenectomy or TAH/BSO with or without lymphadenectomy followed by post-operative radiotherapy. The choice of treatment depends on the tumour site and size and the fitness of the patient when considering the feasibility of extirpative surgery. Two meta-analyses[14,15] of laparoscopic assisted hysterectomy for endometrial cancer, while limited by the small size of RCTs and duration of follow up, both found a similar odds ratio for post-operative complications (0.34 (95 per cent CI: 0.13–0.89; $p = 0.03$ and 0.40, 95 per cent CI 0.23–0.70, $p = 0.007$)) for the laparoscopic approach, although the operation time was significantly longer. There was no significant difference between laparoscopic and open approaches to overall (OR = 0.80, 95 per cent CI 0.37–1.70, $p = 0.695$), disease-free (OR = 0.76, 95 per cent CI 0.34–1.72, $p = 0.655$) and cancer-related (OR = 0.89, 95 per cent CI 0.19–4.13, $p = 0.815$) survival [A]. The results of the LAP-2 trial are keenly awaited. This American trial, the largest surgical trial in endometrial cancer, compares laparoscopic and open hysterectomy.

## Role of lymphadenectomy

The role of pelvic lymphadenectomy has been advocated to improve surgical staging, but there is no clear evidence that it improves survival or that it rationalizes the use of radiotherapy by excluding extra-uterine disease. A recently reported RCT (MRC ASTEC trial) on the management of endometrial cancer[16] has shown that lymphadenectomy did not improve recurrence-free, disease-free or overall survival. The hazard ratio (adjusted for baseline characteristics and pathology) was 1.04 (0.74–1.45; $p = 0.83$) and recurrence-free survival 1.25 (0.93–1.66; $p = 0.14$). The rate of reported post-surgical morbidity in ASTEC was low, but there were more cases of ileus, DVT, lymphocyst and major wound dehiscence reported in the women who had been randomized to lymphadenectomy.

Another large RCT of lymphadenectomy in endometrial cancer was reported just prior to ASTEC. In this Italian trial,[17] there was again no evidence of a survival benefit despite improved surgical staging in the lymphadenectomy arm (13.3 versus 3.2 per cent). These trials indicate that routine lymphadenectomy is not beneficial in early stage endometrial cancer.

## Who should perform surgery?

Endometrial cancer categorized as low risk following full pre-operative assessment can be safely treated by TAH/BSO by a general gynaecologist. High-risk disease with a risk of cervical or pelvic node involvement should be referred to a specialist gynaecological oncologist.

## Role of radiotherapy

There have been no RCTs comparing surgery and primary radiotherapy. Women with intermediate- or high-risk early-stage disease considered to be at increased risk of recurrence are often given post-operative adjuvant radiotherapy on tumour histological type, grade and depth of myometrial invasion which predict risk of extra-uterine disease.

The main role for radiotherapy is as adjuvant treatment following surgery to reduce the risk of pelvic relapse. Radiotherapy cure can be achieved in women with early stage disease who are entirely unfit for surgery, but this is suboptimal treatment with risks of intrauterine failure.

Vault brachytherapy is used to prevent vault recurrence, and external-beam therapy to the pelvis is used to treat the parametrium and pelvic sidewalls. It should be remembered that there is no evidence to show that radiotherapy improves survival in an unselected patient population. A meta-analysis of over 2000 patients in RCTs on the management of endometrial cancer (MRC ASTEC/EN.5, PORTEC 1 and GOG 99)[18] has shown no benefit from external beam radiotherapy for early stage endometrial cancer at intermediate and high risk in terms of disease-specific, recurrence-free or overall survival. Although there is a small reduction in isolated local pelvic recurrence, this does not confer any advantage to overall or recurrence-free survival. The isolated local recurrence rate without external beam radiotherapy is small and can be reduced with local brachytherapy which is associated with less toxicity.

The recently reported PORTEC2 trial (REF) has shown that brachytherapy is as effective as external beam radition in high-intermediate risk patients with fewer radiation effects and should be the treatment of choice for these women.[19]

Currently, women are selected with care for post-operative radiotherapy because of the impact of the treatment regime and the associated complications related to quality of life. The incidence of bowel complications is 3 per cent and can be higher after pelvic lymphadenectomy. The post-operative radiation therapy in endometrial carcinoma (PORTEC) trial[20] reported treatment-related complications in 25 per cent of radiotherapy patients, although a fifth of these were grade 1. Most of the complications were associated with the gastrointestinal tract. The symptoms resolved after some years in 50 per cent of women. Grade 1–2 genitourinary symptoms occur in 8 per cent of women treated by surgery and radiotherapy, compared with 4 per cent of women treated by surgery alone. Two per cent of women discontinued radiotherapy due to acute related symptoms. In addition, patients with acute morbidity have an increased risk of late radiotherapy complications, including rectal bleeding, fistulae or radiation damage to the small or large bowel.

The prognosis for most women with endometrial cancer is good, and therefore any impact of radiotherapy on survival will come from salvaging the small number of patients who develop a pelvic recurrence.

## Progesterone therapy

Progesterone therapy for women who have had surgery for early stage endometrial cancer is not recommended, as overall survival is not improved [A].[21] Although deaths from endometrial cancer (OR 0.88, 95 per cent CI 0.71–1.01) and the rate of disease relapse are reduced (OR 0.81, 95 per cent CI 0.65–1.01), non-endometrial cancer-related deaths are more common (OR 1.33, 95 per cent CI 1.02–1.73) [C].

## Hormone replacement therapy

Traditionally, ERT has not been advocated in the first two years following surgery for endometrial cancer because of the concern of activating any residual disease. There is, however, no evidence to support this, and the benefits of ERT may outweigh any theoretical risks [C]. In women aged 45 years or less, treated for early stage disease, ovarian preservation has no effect on cancer-specific survival (hazard ratio 0.58, 95 per cent CI 0.14–2.44) or overall survival (hazard ratio 0.65, 95 per cent CI 0.34–1.35).[22]

## Advanced stage disease

At presentation, only 13 per cent of women have stage III and 3 per cent stage IV disease. In general, women with stage III disease have been treated with surgery and radiation or radiotherapy alone. Treatment with chemotherapy is increasing and is discussed below under Role of chemotherapy. Laparotomy will allow staging and tumour-reductive surgery including hysterectomy if possible. However, sidewall extension will prevent tumour resection. Radiotherapy is used when surgery is inappropriate or incomplete. This may be a combination of intracavity and external-beam radiation, and cure rates of 30 and 20 per cent for stage III and IV disease, respectively, have been reported. If the woman is not fit for either surgery or irradiation, progesterone therapy is appropriate [C]. If radiotherapy achieves significant tumour shrinkage, 'adjuvant' surgery should be considered if the woman is fit.

With stage IV disease, the tumour site and the resultant symptoms will dictate management. Chemotherapy is usually offered first. Bulky pelvic disease or heavy vaginal bleeding may be controlled by radiation, either intracavity or external beam, or in combination. Local radiation can palliate symptomatic metastasis (e.g. to the lung, brain or bone).

## Role of chemotherapy

There is no evidence that chemotherapy has an adjuvant role in primary treatment of low risk disease. There is emerging evidence from phase 2 and 3 trials to support the selection of intermediate or high risk women or those with advanced disease for adjuvant chemotherapy. The diagnosis of advanced endometrial cancer confers a relatively poor prognosis. Traditionally, treatment for women with stage III endometrial cancer has relied on radiotherapy, while women with stage IV disease have been treated with palliative chemotherapy. There has been a gradual shift towards incorporating chemotherapy into the treatment of women with stage III and IV endometrial cancer. There have been a series of GOG phase 1–3 studies to investigate the effectiveness of different combinations of chemotherapeutic agents for systemic control of disease with or without radiotherapy for enhanced locoregional control. Acute and chronic toxicities are higher in women treated with chemotherapy rather than radiotherapy alone, but with improved response rates. The most effective agents for endometrial cancer appear to be doxorubicin and cisplatin. Two prospective randomized trials have demonstrated a superior response rate to doxorubicin and cisplatin as compared with doxorubicin alone; however, survival rates for the two regimens were similar. More recently, paclitaxel has been included into triplet regimes. When combined with a platinum agent, response rates of greater than 40 per cent have been reported. A doublet regime of doxorubicin and paclitaxel has been investigated by the GOG (GOG 163) as an alternative to doxorubicin and cisplatin for women with advanced or recurrent disease. Both regimes had similar response and survival, but there was no difference in progression-free or overall survival. The most recent GOG trial compared doxorubicin and cisplatin to doxorubicin, cisplatin and paclitaxel. The triplet regimen had a statistically significant improved response rate, progression-free and overall survival, but at the cost of higher toxicity. The GOG is currently conducting a trial (GOG 209) comparing paclitaxel and carboplatin to doxorubicin, cisplatin and paclitaxel in women with advanced or recurrent disease because, if equivalent, paclitaxel and carboplatin are less toxic.

PORTEC 3,[23] a randomized phase 3 trial comparing concurrent chemoradiation plus adjuvant chemotherapy with pelvic radiation alone, in high risk and advanced stage endometrial cancer, opened in 2008 and aims to recruit 500 women over five years. For clear cell endometrial cancer, a review by the Society of Gynecologic Oncology[24] recommends comprehensive surgical staging and platinum-based adjuvant chemotherapy with taxol and/or doxorubicin. Radiotherapy has not been shown to be clearly beneficial for clear cell endometrial cancer.

Gynaecological oncology

## EBM: Treatment of endometrial cancer

- Two surgical RCTs relating to early stage endometrial carcinoma with intermediate or high risk features shows that pelvic lymphadenectomy does not increase survival and is not recommended as a routine in addition to TAH/BSO.
- Two meta-analyses show that laparoscopic surgery is as clinically effective as abdominal hysterectomy and is associated with lower post-operative morbidity, although operating time is longer.
- A meta-analysis has shown adjuvant radiotherapy reduces the rate of pelvic recurrence, but without any improvement in overall survival and a 50 per cent increase in moderate and severe complications and late radiotherapy sequelae.
- A meta-analysis of six RCTs and a large RCT have both shown no reduction in death rates for endometrial cancer with progesterone therapy.
- The use of combined chemotherapy appears beneficial in women with high risk histological tumours, but with increased toxicity.

# PROGNOSIS

Survival is related to stage at presentation and grade of tumour (Table 68.3). There is a wide variation in rates of recurrence with early stage disease, from 10 per cent in low-risk women (stage Ia G1 disease) to almost 50 per cent in high-risk women (stage Ic G3 disease). The latest revision of FIGO staging reflects more clearly clinically relevant factors. When the only evidence of extrauterine spread is positive peritoneal washings, the influence on outcome is unclear, and there is no evidence that adjuvant therapy is of value unless extrauterine disease is present [C].[25,26]

## Recurrent disease

Women with recurrence limited to the pelvis who have not previously received radiotherapy may be salvaged by radiotherapy, with a five-year survival of about 25–50 per cent. Para-aortic lymph nodes may be palliated by radiotherapy and, with localized pelvic recurrence; this can be curative when there has been no previous irradiation. The prognosis for distant metastatic endometrial cancer is poor.

**Table 68.3** Five-year survival rates for endometrial adenocarcinoma by stage

| Stage | 5-year survival (%) |
|---|---|
| Stage I | 80 |
| Stage II | 65 |
| Stage III | 30 |
| Stage IV | 10 |

Progesterones will produce a clinical response in about 20 per cent of women with recurrent disease [C] and appear to be more effective in women with a long disease-free interval prior to recurrence. Standard agents are megestrol and medroxyprogesterone. Chemotherapy may have a limited palliative role for women with advanced or recurrent disease not amenable to radiation.

# SUMMARY

Endometrial cancer usually presents with PMB at an early stage. Staging is surgical/pathological, and pre-operative imaging should include a chest x-ray and imaging for depth of myometrial penetration. Early stage disease should be managed by TAH and BSO, with peritoneal washings which is reported separately, but without changing the stage. Pelvic lymphadenectomy is not recommended. While post-operative radiotherapy reduces the rate of local recurrence, as it does not improve overall survival and it is associated with increased toxicity. Brachytherapy is the adjuvant treatment of choice for high-intermediate risk disease with external beam radiation being restricted to high risk early disease.

## KEY POINTS

- Investigation of PMB should be provided as a rapid-access outpatient service.
- The benefits of tamoxifen in breast cancer treatment outweigh the increased risk of endometrial cancer. Any abnormal vaginal bleeding while on tamoxifen requires full investigation.
- Surgery with total abdominal hysterectomy and bilateral salpingo-oopherectomy offers good prognosis in early stage disease, but routine systematic pelvic lymphadenectomy is not recommended as it does not improve survival.
- Endometrial carcinoma is radiosensitive, but the benefits of locoregional control from external-beam radiotherapy do not improve survival and is not recommended for early stage intermediate risk endometrial cancer (<1c, G3).
- Adjuvant radiotherapy should be restricted to early stage high risk disease and advanced disease.
- Combined chemotherapy has an increased role in the treatment of high risk endometrial cancer.

## Published Guidelines

Scottish Intercollegiate Guidelines Network. Investigation of post menopausal bleeding. SIGN Guideline Publication 61. ISBN 1899893 13 X. September 2002.

Royal College of Pathologists. Minimum dataset for the histopathological reporting of atypical hyperplasia and adenocarcinoma in endometrial biopsy and curettage specimens and for endometrial cancer in hysterectomy specimens, 2001. Available from: ‹www.rcpath.org/resources/pdf/datasetreendometrialcancer.pdf›.

Royal College of Obstetricians and Gynaecologists. Recommendations arising from the 37th Study Group: Hormones and Cancer. RCOG Study Group Recommendations. London: RCOG Press, November 1999. Available from: ‹www.rcog.org.uk/study/hormones›.

## Key References

1. CRUK website. UK Uterus (Womb) Cancer incidence statistics. Last accessed August 2009. Available from: http://info.cancerresearchuk.org/cancerstats/incidence/commoncancers/ and http://info.cancerresearchuk.org/cancerstats/types/uterus/incidence/.

2. Renehan A, Tyson M, Egger M *et al*. Body-mass index and incidence of cancer: a systematic review and meta-analysis of prospective observational studies. *Lancet* 2008; **371**: 569–78.

3. Grady D, Gebretsadik T, Kerlikowske K *et al*. Hormone replacement therapy and endometrial cancer risk: A meta-analysis. *Obstet Gynecol* 1995; **85**: 304–13.

4. Lethaby A, Farquhaar C, Sarkis A *et al*. Hormone replacement therapy in postmenopausal women: Endometrial hyperplasia and irregular bleeding. *Cochrane Database Syst Rev* 2000; (**2**): CD000402.

5. Beral V, Bull D, Reeves G. Endometrial cancer and hormone-replacement therapy in the Million Women Study. *Lancet* 2005; **365**: 1543–51.

6. FIGO Committee on Gynecologic Oncology. Revised FIGO staging for carcinoma of the vulva, cervix and endometrium. *Int J Gynaecol Obstet* 2009; **105**: 103–4.

7. Chien PFW, Voit D, Clark TJ *et al*. Ultrasonographic endometrial thickness for diagnosing endometrial pathology in women with postmenopausal bleeding: A meta-analysis. *Acta Obstet Gynecol Scand* 2002; **81**: 799–816.

8. Scottish Intercollegiate Guidelines Network. Investigation of post menopausal bleeding. SIGN Guideline Publication 61. ISBN 1899893 13 X. September 2002.

9. Early Breast Cancer Triallists' Collaborative Group. Tamoxifen for early breast cancer. *Lancet* 1998; **351**: 1451–67.

10. Marconi D, Exacoustos C, Cangi B *et al*. Transvaginal sonographic and hysteroscopic findings in postmenopausal women receiving tamoxifen. *J Am Assoc Gynecol Laparosc* 1997; **4**: 331–9.

11. Timmerman D, Deprest J, Bourne T *et al*. A randomized trial on the use of ultrasonography or office hysteroscopy for endometrial assessment in postmenopausal patients with breast cancer who were treated with tamoxifen. *Am J Obstet Gynecol* 1998; **179**: 62–70.

12. IBIS investigators. First results from the International Breast Cancer Intervention Study (IBIS-I): A randomised prevention trial. *Lancet* 2002; **360**: 817–24.

13. Creasman WT, Morrow CP, Bundy BN *et al*. Surgical pathologic spread patterns of endometrial cancer: a gynecologic oncology group study. *Cancer* 1987; **60**: 2035–41.

14. Lin F, Zhang QJ, Zheng FY et al. Laparoscopically assisted versus open surgery for endometrial cancer – a meta-analysis of randomised controlled trials. *Int J Gynecol Cancer* 2008; **18**: 1315–25.

15. Palomba S, Falbo A, Mocciaro R *et al*. Laparoscopic treatment for endometrial cancer: A meta-analysis of randomized controlled trial. *Gynecol Oncol* 2009; **112**: 415–21.

16. ASTEC Study Group. Efficacy of systematic pelvic lymphadenectomy in endometrial cancer (MRC ASTEC trial): A randomised study. *Lancet* 2009; **373**: 125–36.

17. Panici PB, Basile S, Maneschi F *et al*. Systematic pelvic lymphadenectomy vs no lymphadenectomy in early-stage endometrial carcinoma: Randomized clinical trial. *J Natl Cancer Inst* 2008; **100**: 1707–16.

18. ASTEC/EN.5 Study Group. Adjuvant external beam radiotherapy in the treatment of endometrial cancer (MRC ASTEC abd NCIC CTG EN.5 randomised trails): Pooled trial results, systematic review and meta-analysis. *Lancet* 2009; **373**: 97–9.

19. Nout RA, Smit VTHBM, Putter H for the PORTEC Study Group. Vaginal brachytherapy versus pelvic external beam radiotherapy for patients with endometrial cancer of high-intermediate risk (PORTEC-2): an open-label, non-inferiority, randomised trial. *Lancet* 2010; **375**: 816–23.

20. Creutzberg CL, van Putten WLJ, Koper PC *et al*. Surgery and postoperative radiotherapy versus surgery alone for patients with stage I endometrial carcinoma: Multicentre randomized trial. *Lancet* 2000; **355**: 1404–11.

21. Martin-Hirsch PL, Lilford RJ, Jarvis GJ. Adjuvant progesterone therapy for the treatment of endometrial cancer: Review and meta-analysis of published randomised controlled trials. *Eur J Obstet Gynecol Reprod Biol* 1996; **65**: 2201–7.

22. Wright JD, Buck AM, Shah M *et al*. Safety of ovarian preservation in premenopausal women with endometrial cancer. *J Clin Oncol* 2009; **27**: 1214–19.

23. PORTEC3. Available from: ‹www.clinicalresearch.nl/portec3/›.

24. Olawaiye AB, Boruta DM. Management of women with clear cell endometrial cancer: a Society of Gynecologic Oncology (SGO) review. *Gynecol Oncol* 2009; **113**: 277–83.

25. Kadar N, Homesley HD, Malfetano JH. Positive peritoneal cytology is an adverse factor in endometrial carcinoma only if there is other evidence of extrauterine disease. *Gynecol Oncol* 1992; **46**: 145–9.

26. Benedetti Panici P, Basile S, Maneschi F *et al*. Systematic pelvic lymphadenectomy vs no lymphadenectomy in early-stage endometrial carcinoma: Randomized clinical trial. *J Natl Cancer Inst* 2008; **100**: 1707–16.

Gynaecological oncology

# Cervical cancer

*Pierre L Martin–Hirsch*

## MRCOG standards

### Theoretical skills

- Revise the anatomy of the cervix, blood supply and lymphatics.
- Understand the epidemiology and pathology of disease.
- Know the optimum pre-treatment assessment.
- Know how to manage surgically and non-surgically.

### Practical skills

- Be able to recognize suspicious cervical lesions.
- Be able to take appropriate diagnostic biopsies.
- Be able to counsel patients with regard to diagnosis, management options and prognosis.

## EPIDEMIOLOGY

Cervical cancer is the most common form of cancer in women in developing countries and the second most common form of cancer in women in the world as a whole. Three-quarters of affected women live in developing countries and it is estimated that up to 450 000 new cases of invasive cancer of the cervix occur per year in these countries leading to 275 000 deaths. Cervical cancer accounts for 6 per cent of all malignancies in women. There were an estimated 11 150 new cases of invasive cancer of the cervix and 3670 deaths in the United States in 2007. In the United Kingdom in 2006, there were 2873 registrations, and 941 deaths in 2007. Although cervical screening has been carried out in the UK since the 1960s, the benefits of screening are only now becoming apparent, following the reorganization of the service in 1988. The incidence of cervical cancer has fallen in the UK by 44 per cent since 1975, and mortality from 7.1 per 100 000 in 1988 to 2.4 per 100 000 in 2007. This decrease is almost certainly due to the widespread coverage of screening, which has risen from less than 35 per cent in 1988 to over 80 per cent in 1998 through the introduction of an effective call–recall system for cervical screening. The reduction of deaths is due to a reduction in both incidence and the proportion of advanced disease with around a third of cancers being diagnosed as stage 1. The incidence rate for cervical cancer peaks at 17 per 100 000 women at the age range of 30–40 years, declines in incidence for older age groups but peaks again in the early 80s age band.

Epidemiological studies convincingly demonstrate that the major risk factor, indeed a necessary event for the development of pre-invasive and invasive carcinoma of the cervix, is human papillomavirus (HPV) infection, which far outweighs other known risk factors such as high parity, increasing number of sexual partners, young age at first intercourse, low socioeconomic status and positive smoking history. In an international study consisting of 1000 specimens collected from patients with invasive cervical cancer in 32 hospitals in 22 countries, HPV DNA was present in 99.7 per cent of cervical cancers.[1] HPV 16 was the predominant type in all countries except Indonesia, where HPV 18 was more common.[1] The role of HPV in cervical carcinogenesis is expanded in Chapter 67, Pre-invasive disease. The advent of prophylactic vaccines directed against types 16/18 HPV could reduce the incidence of cervical cancer by 70 per cent in a high coverage population.

## PATHOLOGY

Squamous cell and adenosquamous carcinomas comprise approximately 85 per cent and adenocarcinoma approximately 15 per cent of cervical cancers. Squamous carcinomas are large-cell keratinizing, large-cell non-keratinizing and small-cell types. The rare, but dangerous small-cell neuroendocrine-type typically behaves like similar disease arising from the bronchus. Adenocarcinomas can be pure or mixed with squamous cell carcinomas, the adenosquamous carcinoma. About 80 per cent of cervical adenocarcinomas are made up of cells of the endocervical type with mucin production. The remaining tumours are populated by endometroid, clear, intestinal or a mixture of more than one type of cell.

## KEY POINTS

- Cervical cancer is the most common form of gynaecological cancer in women in developing countries.
- The incidence of and deaths from cervical cancer are decreasing in the UK due to cervical screening.
- HPV DNA is present in virtually 100 per cent of cervical cancers.
- Squamous cell and adenosquamous carcinomas comprise approximately 85 per cent and adenocarcinomas approximately 15 per cent of cervical cancers.

# CLINICAL MANAGEMENT

The goals of the management of cervical cancer are to stage the disease and to treat both the primary lesion and other sites of spread. Cervical cancers spread by direct spread into the cervical stroma, parametrium and beyond, and by lymphatic metastasis into parametrial, pelvic sidewall and para-aortic nodes. Blood-borne spread is unusual. Among the major factors that influence prognosis are:

- stage
- volume
- grade of tumour
- histological type
- lymphatic spread
- vascular invasion.

In a large surgico-pathological staging study of patients with clinical disease confined to the cervix, the factors that predicted lymph node metastases and a decrease in disease-free survival were capillary–lymphatic space involvement by tumour, increasing tumour size and increasing depth of stromal invasion.[2,3] A similar study of 626 patients with locally advanced disease demonstrated that para-aortic and pelvic lymph node status, tumour size, clinical stage, patient age and performance status were all significant prognostic factors for a reduction in progression-free interval and survival.[4] The incidence of para-aortic and pelvic lymph node disease according to stage is illustrated in Table 69.1.

## Staging

Women should be fully staged using the International Federation of Gynaecology and Obstetrics (FIGO) system (Table 69.2). FIGO staging is based largely on clinical assessment, chest x-ray and cystoscopy. Radiological staging, particularly by magnetic resonance imaging (MRI), which permits more accurate determination of disease extent,[11] also permits assessment of lymph node status. Routine use of imaging enhances the selection of women in whom surgery alone is likely to be curative. MRI has become so accurate at staging disease that examination under anaesthetic combined with cystoscopy is often not required. In a limited number of

**Table 69.1** Incidence of nodal disease in cervical cancer according to stage[5-10]

| Stage | No. | Positive pelvic lymph nodes (%) | Positive para-aortic lymph nodes (%) |
|---|---|---|---|
| Ia1 (<1 mm) | 23 | 0 | 0 |
| Ia1 (1–3 mm) | 156 | 0.6 | 0 |
| Ia2 (3–5 mm) | 84 | 4.8 | <1 |
| Ib | 1926 | 15.9 | 2.2 |
| IIa | 110 | 24.5 | 11 |
| IIb | 324 | 31.4 | 19 |
| III | 125 | 44.8 | 30 |
| Iva | 23 | 55 | 40 |

pilot studies, positron emission tomography (PET)-CT has demonstrated enhanced accuracy at diagnosing involved lymph nodes and local invasion, but more robust studies are required.

## Treatment

Specialized gynaecological oncology teams should determine the management of women with cervical cancer. Decisions about how best to treat early disease in young women in particular require considerable experience. Both surgery and radiotherapy are effective in early stage disease, whereas locally advanced disease relies on treatment by chemoradiation. Surgery does provide the advantage of conservation of ovarian function.

Factors that influence the mode of treatment include stage, age and health status. Radiation can be used for all stages, whereas surgery should only be considered an option for early disease, stage I and stage IIa. A large randomized trial reported identical five-year overall and disease-free survival rates when comparing radiation therapy with radical hysterectomy, but women who had surgery and adjuvant radiotherapy suffered significantly higher morbidity than those who had either surgery or radiotherapy alone [B].[12]

There are clear advantages to surgery in women at low operative risk. Surgery permits conservation of ovarian function in premenopausal women and also reduces the risk of chronic bladder, bowel and sexual dysfunction associated with radiotherapy. Complications in the hands of skilled surgeons are uncommon. Surgery also permits the assessment of risk factors, such as lymph node status, that will ultimately influence prognosis. Complications of surgery include fistulae (≤1 per cent), lymphocyst, primary haemorrhage and bladder injury. Chronic bowel and bladder problems that require medical or surgical intervention occur in up to 8–13 per cent of women[13] due to parasympathetic denervation secondary to surgical clamping at the lateral excision margins.

Gynaecological oncology

**Table 69.2** International Federation of Gynecology and Obstetrics (FIGO) staging

| Stage | | |
|---|---|---|
| Stage I | Stage I | Carcinoma strictly confined to the cervix; extension to the uterine corpus does not affect the stage |
| | Stage Ia | Invasive cancer identified only microscopically. All gross lesions, even with superficial invasion, are stage Ib cancers. Invasion is limited to measured stromal invasion with a maximum depth of 5 mm and no wider than 7 mm |
| | Stage Ia1 | Measured invasion of the stroma no greater than 3 mm in depth and no wider than 7 mm diameter |
| | Stage Ia2 | Measured invasion of stroma greater than 3 mm, but no greater than 5 mm in depth and no wider than 7 mm in diameter |
| | Stage Ib | Clinical lesions confined to the cervix or preclinical lesions greater than stage Ia |
| | Stage Ib1 | Clinical lesions no greater than 4 cm in size |
| | Stage Ib2 | Clinical lesions greater than 4 cm in size |
| Stage II | Stage II | Carcinoma that extends beyond the cervix, but has not extended on to the pelvic wall. The carcinoma involves the vagina, but not as far as the lower third |
| | Stage IIa | No obvious parametrial involvement. Involvement of up to the upper two-thirds of the vagina |
| | Stage IIb | Obvious parametrial involvement, but not on to the pelvic sidewall |
| Stage III | Stage III | Carcinoma that has extended on to the pelvic sidewall. On rectal examination, there is no cancer-free space between the tumour and the pelvic sidewall. The tumour involves the lower third of the vagina. All cases with a hydronephrosis or non-functioning kidney should be included, unless they are known to be due to other causes |
| | Stage IIIa | No extension on to the pelvic sidewall, but involvement of the lower third of the vagina |
| | Stage IIIb | Extension on to the pelvic sidewall or hydronephrosis or non-functioning kidney |
| Stage IV | Stage IV | Carcinoma that has extended beyond the true pelvis or has clinically involved the mucosa of the bladder and/or rectum |
| | Stage IVa | Spread of the tumour on to adjacent pelvic organs |
| | Stage IVb | Spread to distant organs |

## Stage Ia disease

Micro-invasive disease is one in which neoplastic cells invade from the epithelium to a maximum depth of 5 mm and a maximum horizontal spread of 7 mm. Any invasion beyond these dimensions upstages the disease to stage Ib. The identification of early disease allows the selection of a group of women who are not at risk of lymph node disease and can be treated with less aggressive and, importantly, fertility-sparing therapy.

Micro-invasive disease comprises 20 per cent of invasive cancers. Stage Ia1 disease (invasion ≤3 mm) is rarely associated with lymph node metastases (see Table 69.1). This disease should be formally diagnosed by cone biopsy or diathermy excision. Knife cone biopsy does not cause any thermal damage, and the extent of disease may be more accurately assessed than on a loop excision specimen. If the disease and any associated intraepithelial neoplasia are removed with clear margins, no further treatment is necessary. If disease is present at the margins, further excision or hysterectomy is required. A simple abdominal total hysterectomy is sufficient, as there is no risk of parametrial involvement. Because invasive disease of ≤3 mm invasion is associated with a very low risk of lymph node disease (see Table 69.1), lymphadenectomy is not indicated. Lymphadenectomy should, however, be considered

for stage Ia2 (invasion 3–5 mm) disease as the rate of node involvement reaches 5 per cent, particularly if the tumour is poorly differentiated.

## Stage Ib–IIa

Stage Ib is divided into Ib1 (≤4 cm diameter) and Ib2 (>4 cm diameter); stage IIa means upper vaginal, but not parametrial involvement.

Surgical therapy for stage Ib and IIa tumours ≤4 cm across usually involves radical hysterectomy and pelvic lymphadenectomy. Radical hysterectomy involves removing the tumour with adequate disease-free margins, by means of excising the parametrial tissue around the cervix and upper vagina, with removal of part or all of the cardinal and utero-sacral ligaments, depending on the extent of the dissection. More radical dissections are associated with a higher incidence of peri-operative morbidity and chronic bladder and bowel dysfunction with no survival advantage [B].[14] The lymph node dissection should include obturator, internal, external and common iliac nodes. In the absence of suspicious pelvic nodes, para-aortic lymphadenectomy is not mandatory, but it should be performed in the presence of involved pelvic nodes or if there is clinical suspicion of para-aortic node involvement. If there is any suspicion about the nature of the para-aortic nodes, they should be removed and subjected to frozen section. Confirmed para-aortic disease at the start of surgery is a contraindication to radical pelvic surgery. Lymphadenectomy may result in lymphocyst formation. Lymphoedema following pelvic lymphadenectomy can occur, although its incidence increases if adjuvant radiotherapy is given.

In cases in which positive nodes are encountered, there are differing views. Some would advocate abandoning surgery in favour of radical chemoradiation. Others would argue that, if possible, radical surgery should be completed to achieve an adjuvant setting for radiotherapy. If suspicious nodes are identified and confirmed to be diseased at frozen section, it is probably best to remove resectable nodes and treat with chemoradiation, including brachytherapy, which requires the uterus to be *in situ*. Radical surgery followed by radical radiotherapy is associated with increased morbidity.

Adjuvant radiotherapy is normally recommended for women with resected positive pelvic nodes to reduce the risk of recurrence. Patients with 'close' vaginal or parametrial margins ($\leq 0.5$ cm) may also benefit from pelvic irradiation.[15] Indirect evidence from non-randomized studies suggests that radiotherapy can improve pelvic control, but there is no firm evidence of increased survival [C].[16,17] Careful pre-operative radiological imaging reduces the risk of encountering unexpected lymphadenopathy or unexpectedly large tumours.

Because bulky Ib tumours have a higher risk of positive nodes and close surgical margins, these are now regarded by many as being better treated with chemoradiation as opposed to surgery or radiotherapy alone. Some women with small-volume stage Ib disease who wish to conserve their fertility might be suitable for trachelectomy (radical excision of the cervix) combined with either laparoscopic or open lymphadenectomy. The most common approach is a vaginal trachelectomy; however, more recently some surgeons are favouring an abdominal approach facilitating greater excision of the parametrium with this technique. Meta-analyses and large UK case series based on the vaginal approach have demonstrated recurrence rates of around 4 per cent, and a 70 per cent term delivery rate.[18,19] Some surgeons recommend the insertion of an abdominal isthmic cervical cerclage to reduce the risk of late miscarriage. Indeed, in selected cases of Ib1 disease that are just greater than 7 mm in horizontal spread, a large cone biopsy may be adequate for central control, even though it may need to be combined with lymphadenectomy.

### Stage IIb and above

It is not feasible to perform surgery with curative intent in these advanced stages of disease. Radical radiotherapy and chemoradiation are the only modalities of treatment that offer the potential for cure. One randomized trial has suggested that pre-operative chemotherapy to shrink disease followed by radical surgery may be superior to radical radiotherapy, but this has not been confirmed.[20] It is inevitable that pre-operative chemotherapy followed by surgery will still require some women to undergo adjuvant or non-adjuvant radiotherapy that is more likely to result in unacceptable toxicity.

## Radical radiotherapy

Radical radiotherapy is indicated for women unfit for surgery, bulky stage Ib2 disease and more advanced disease. The goals of such treatment are to treat primary disease and to control metastatic pelvic lymph nodes. The radical dose is delivered by external-beam (teletherapy) and intracavitary treatment (brachytherapy). The standard technique for the latter is now remote after-loading (e.g. using the Selectron). Intracavitary treatment is designed to give high doses to the primary site. Teletherapy is designed to treat any pelvic spread. The challenge in administering radiotherapy is in achieving an optimal dose throughout the primary tumour and pelvic sidewall without causing high morbidity. The peripheral field of treatment of intracavitary radiotherapy delivers an insufficient dose to treat the pelvic sidewalls. The dose-limiting normal tissues within the pelvis are the rectum posteriorly, the bladder anteriorly and any loops of small bowel within the pelvic radiation fields.

Prescribing rules have been devised for determining the precise dose of radiotherapy within the pelvis, and improved planning by computed tomography (CT) has enabled more accurate targeting of external-beam radiation in particular. An example is the Manchester system. This uses a number of predetermined source sizes and radioactive loadings such that a constant dose rate is delivered to a point A. Point A is defined as a point 2 cm lateral to the central axis of the uterus and 2 cm from the lateral fornix. A second point (B) lying in the same plane 3 cm lateral to point A is used to determine the dose to parametrial tissues. Following the insertion of the sources for each patient, a dose distribution is calculated. The total dose is a product of the dose rate and treatment time. The usual doses delivered are 70–80 Gy to point A and 60 Gy to point B, limiting the bladder and rectal dose to 60 Gy. To achieve this, it is necessary to have adequate packing to keep the bladder and bowel away from the intracavitary source. External-beam radiotherapy is fractionated over 20–30 days treatment, as this technique allows a cancericidal effect while enabling normal tissue recovery between fractions.

Routine extended field radiotherapy designed to include para-aortic nodes has not been proven to improve survival compared with pelvic radiotherapy alone, and it is associated with significantly more gastrointestinal complications [B].[21] While there does not appear to be significant benefit from extended field irradiation for all cases, para-aortic node irradiation is appropriate in cases of proven para-aortic node involvement as indicated by diagnostic imaging or surgical staging.

## Chemoradiation

Five randomized trials from the United States[22–26] have shown an overall survival advantage for cisplatin-based therapy given concurrently with radiation therapy [B]. The patient populations in these studies included women with FIGO stages Ib2–IVa cervical cancer treated with primary radiation therapy and women with FIGO stages I–IIa disease found to have poor prognostic factors (metastatic disease in pelvic lymph nodes, parametrial disease or positive surgical margins) at the time of primary surgery. Although the trials varied somewhat in terms of stage of disease, dose of radiation, and schedule of cisplatin and radiation, they all demonstrate significant survival benefit for this combined approach, the risk of death from cervical cancer being decreased by 30 per cent. These trials reported higher rates of short- and medium-term complications with chemoradiation, and although longer follow up is required to examine the true morbidity of this treatment regimen, there is now international acceptance that chemoradiation is the treatment of choice for advanced cervical cancer.

## Recurrent cervical cancer

Treatment for recurrent cervical cancer depends on the mode of primary therapy and the site of recurrence. Women who have had initial treatment by surgery should be considered for radiotherapy, and those who have had radiotherapy should be considered for exenterative surgery, provided the recurrence is central and there is no evidence of distant recurrence. These women require very careful pre-operative assessment and counselling in order to understand the consequences of defunctioning surgery. Exenterative surgery in carefully selected cases can result in five-year survival of 50 per cent [D]. Positive nodes at the time of attempted salvage surgery and positive resection margins are associated with a poor prognosis. Anterior exenteration requires excision of the bladder and most of the vagina en bloc with the recurrence, and posterior exenteration requires excision of the sigmoid rectum with formation of a colostomy. Sometimes a combination of the two is required. This type of surgery should only be undertaken by teams of highly skilled pelvic surgeons. Relapse within two years of primary treatment, the presence of hydronephrosis and symptoms of pain are all associated with poorer outcomes in terms of exenterative surgery.

## Palliation of progressive cervical disease

Chemotherapy is palliative and should be reserved for patients who are not considered curable by the other two treatment modalities. Urinary tract symptoms are particularly common in advanced cervical disease. Ureteric obstruction with subsequent pain, infection and ultimately impaired renal function are common features. Mechanical diversion by nephrostomy or ureteric stenting is only usually justified as part of treatment with curative intent. Fistulae can occur in late stage disease and can cause intolerable symptoms. If there is a prospect of surviving more than 8 weeks, palliative surgery should be offered in order to divert faeces or urine.

In progressive late stage disease, there is usually ureteric obstruction, which heralds a terminal phase. Pain can be particularly distressing due to infiltration of the lumbosacral nerve plexuses. Meticulous attention to pain control and psychological and emotional support are essential.

### KEY POINTS

- Early micro-invasive disease can be treated by cone biopsy or excisional treatment alone [C].
- Surgery and radiotherapy for stage Ib/IIa disease have similar five-year overall and disease-free survival rates, but women who have had surgery and adjuvant radiotherapy combined have significantly higher morbidity than those who have had either surgery or radiotherapy alone [B].
- Pre-operative imaging with MRI scans reduces the number of women undergoing both modalities of treatment [C].
- Chemoradiation increases survival over radiotherapy alone for advanced disease, but toxicity is increased [B].

## Key References

1. Walboomers JM, Jacobs MV, Manos MM et al. Human papillomavirus is a necessary cause of invasive cervical cancer worldwide. *J Pathol* 1999; **189**: 12–19.

2. Delgado G, Bundy BN, Fowler WC et al. A prospective surgical pathological study of stage I squamous carcinoma of the cervix: a Gynecologic Oncology Group study. *Gynecol Oncol* 1989; **35**: 314–20.

3. Zaino RJ, Ward S, Delgado G et al. Histopathologic predictors of the behavior of surgically treated stage IB squamous cell carcinoma of the cervix. A Gynecologic Oncology Group study. *Cancer* 1992; **69**: 1750–8.

4. Stehman FB, Bundy BN, DiSaia PJ et al. Carcinoma of the cervix treated with radiation therapy. I. A multi-variate analysis of prognostic variables in the Gynecologic Oncology Group. *Cancer* 1991; **67**: 2776–85.

5. Boyce, Fruchter R, Nicastri AD et al. Prognostic factors in stage I carcinoma of the cervix. *Gynecol Oncol* 1981; **12**: 154–65.

6. Inoue T, Okumura M. Prognostic significance of parametrial extension in patients with cervical carcinoma stages IB, IIA, and IIB. A study of 628 cases treated by radical hysterectomy and lymphadenectomy with or without postoperative irradiation. *Cancer* 1984; **54**: 1714–19.

7. Lohe KJ. Early squamous cell carcinoma of the uterine cervix. *Gynecol Oncol* 1978; **6**: 10–30.

8. van Nagell J, Donaldson ES, Wood EG, Parker JC. The significance of vascular invasion and lymphocytic infiltration in invasive cervical cancer. *Cancer* 1978; **41**: 228–34.

9. Tinga DJ, Timmer PR, Bouma J, Aalders JG. Prognostic significance of single versus multiple lymph node metastases in cervical carcinoma stage IB. *Gynecol Oncol* 1990; **39**: 175–80.

10. Nahhas WA, Sharkey FE, Whitney CW *et al.* The prognostic significance of vascular channel involvement and deep stromal penetration in early cervical carcinoma. *Am J Clin Oncol* 1983; **6**: 259–64.

11. Scheidler J, Hricak H, Yu KK *et al.* Radiological evaluation of lymph node metastases in patients with cervical cancer. A meta-analysis. *J Am Med Assoc* 1997; **278**: 1096–101.

12. Landoni F, Maneo A, Colombo A *et al.* Randomised study of radical surgery versus radiotherapy for stage Ib–IIa cervical cancer. *Lancet* 1997; **350**: 535–40.

13. Fujikawa K, Miyamoto T, Ihara Y *et al.* High incidence of severe urologic complications following radiotherapy for cervical cancer in Japanese women. *Gynecol Oncol* 2001; **80**: 21–3.

14. Landoni F, Maneo A, Cormio G *et al.* Class II versus class III radical hysterectomy in stage IB–IIA cervical cancer: a prospective randomized study. *Gynecol Oncol* 2001; **80**: 3–12.

15. Estape RE, Angioli R, Madrigal M *et al.* Close vaginal margins as a prognostic factor after radical hysterectomy. *Gynecol Oncol* 1998; **68**: 229–32.

16. Soisson AP, Soper JT, Clarke Pearson DL *et al.* Adjuvant radiotherapy following radical hysterectomy for patients with stage IB and IIA cervical cancer. *Gynecol Oncol* 1990; **37**: 390–5.

17. Kinney WK, Alvarez RD, Reid GC *et al.* Value of adjuvant whole-pelvis irradiation after Wertheim hysterectomy for early-stage squamous carcinoma of the cervix with pelvic nodal metastasis: a matched-control study. *Gynecol Oncol* 1989; **34**: 258–62.

18. Plante M, Renaud MC, Hoskins IA, Roy M. Vaginal radical trachelectomy: a valuable fertility-preserving option in the management of early-stage cervical cancer. A series of 50 pregnancies and review of the literature. *Gynecol Oncol* 2005; **98**: 3–10.

19. Shepherd JH, Spencer C, Herod J, Ind TE. Radical vaginal trachelectomy as a fertility-sparing procedure in women with early-stage cervical cancer-cumulative pregnancy rate in a series of 123 women. *BJOG* 2006; **113**: 719–24.

20. Sardi JE, Giaroli A, di Paola G *et al.* Long-term follow-up of the first randomized trial using neoadjuvant chemotherapy in stage Ib squamous carcinoma of the cervix: the final results. *Gynecol Oncol* 1997; **67**: 61–9.

21. Haie C, Pejovic MH, Gerbaulet A *et al.* Is prophylactic para-aortic irradiation worthwhile in the treatment of advanced cervical carcinoma? Results of a controlled clinical trial of the EORTC radiotherapy group. *Radiother Oncol* 1988; **11**: 101–12.

22. Whitney CW, Sause W, Bundy BN *et al.* Randomized comparison of fluorouracil plus cisplatin versus hydroxyurea as an adjunct to radiation therapy in stage IIB–IVA carcinoma of the cervix with negative para-aortic lymph nodes: a Gynecologic Oncology Group and Southwest Oncology Group study. *J Clin Oncol* 1999; **17**: 1339–48.

23. Morris M, Eifel PJ, Lu J *et al.* Pelvic radiation with concurrent chemotherapy compared with pelvic and para-aortic radiation for high-risk cervical cancer. *N Engl J Med* 1999; **340**: 1137–43.

24. Rose PG, Bundy BN, Watkins EB *et al.* Concurrent cisplatin-based radiotherapy and chemotherapy for locally advanced cervical cancer. *N Engl J Med* 1999; **340**: 1144–53.

25. Keys HM, Bundy BN, Stehman FB *et al.* Cisplatin, radiation, and adjuvant hysterectomy compared with radiation and adjuvant hysterectomy for bulky stage IB cervical carcinoma. *N Engl J Med* 1999; **340**: 1154–61.

26. Peters WA 3rd, Liu PY, Barrett RJ 2nd *et al.* Concurrent chemotherapy and pelvic radiation therapy compared with pelvic radiation therapy alone as adjuvant therapy after radical surgery in high-risk early-stage cancer of the cervix. *J Clin Oncol* 2000; **18**: 1606–13.

# Benign and malignant ovarian masses

*Sudha Sundar and Karina Reynolds*

## MRCOG standards

- Knowledge of the aetiology and screening involved in gynaecological oncology, including the international perspective.
- Understand presenting symptoms and their management.
- Understand each stage of the diagnostic process, including a comprehension of the different roles and skills required in district lead and gynaeoncologist.
- Knowledge of the prognosis and treatment options of the gynaecological cancers.
- Be able to provide counselling for patients with gynaecological cancer.

## INTRODUCTION

By the age of 65, 4 per cent of women will have been admitted to hospital with an ovarian cyst, making this the fourth most common gynaecological cause for hospital admission in England. Among pre-menopausal patients, more than 90 per cent of surgically managed cases are benign, as opposed to just 60 per cent in the post-menopausal population. Although differentiating malignant from benign disease is critical in optimizing management for the individual, non-invasive diagnosis continues to be elusive. Prompt identification and appropriate treatment of cancer of the ovary are essential if the survival rates are to be optimal. In England and Wales, ovarian cancer is the most common gynaecological cancer and the fourth most common after cancers of the breast, large bowel and lung, representing some 5 per cent of all cancers in women.[1] Although ovarian cancer still continues to kill more women than all other gynaecological cancers together (Table 70.1), five-year survival has increased significantly over the last decade and is now 38 per cent.[1] This may be as a result of improved chemotherapy regimes, treatment by dedicated multidisciplinary teams and surgery by gynaecological oncologists.[2]

**Table 70.1** Five-year age-standardized relative survival for the common gynaecological malignancies in adults (15–99 years) diagnosed during 2001–2006, England

| | Annual number of patients diagnosed (2001–2006) and followed up to 2007 | Five-year survival (%) |
|---|---|---|
| Cervix | 2270 | 64.1 |
| Ovary | 5289 | 38.9 |
| Uterus | 4991 | 75.5 |

- Data from Office of National Statistics.

## HISTOPATHOLOGY AND CLASSIFICATION OF OVARIAN MASSES

An ovarian mass may be neoplastic or physiological, and most adnexal masses are benign. The current edition of *International Classification of Tumours*, published by the World Health Organization (WHO),[3] provides a classification of ovarian tumours that has been universally accepted. Epithelial tumours are derived from the surface epithelium of the ovary and are further classified as benign, borderline or malignant, according to cell type and behaviour (Figures 70.1 and 70.2).

Epithelial tumours account for 60–65 per cent of all ovarian tumours and approximately 90 per cent of those that are malignant. Sex-cord stromal tumours are, as their name suggests, derived from the sex cords and stroma of the ovary and account for approximately 8 per cent of all ovarian tumours. Germ cell tumours, derived from the germ cells, account for 30 per cent of ovarian tumours, largely in the form of mature cystic teratomas (dermoid cysts). Although germ cell tumours account for only 1–3 per cent of all ovarian malignancies, they represent more than 60 per cent of ovarian cancers in children and adolescents.

*Note*: the term ovarian cancer is used in this chapter to include not only epithelial ovarian malignancies, but also malignant sex-cord stromal and germ cell neoplasms.

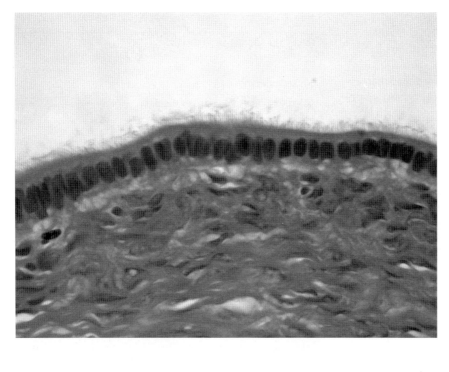

**Figure 70.1** Haematoxylin and eosin staining of a section of tumour demonstrating the typical epithelium of a benign serous cystadenoma – note single layer and bland appearance

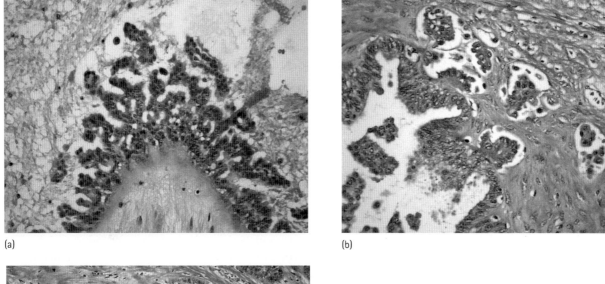

(a)

(b)

(c)

**Figure 70.2** Haematoxylin and eosin sections from borderline, microinvasive and malignant ovarian tumours demonstrating increasing architectural complexity and nuclear pleomorphism. (a) Borderline serous ovarian tumour; (b) borderline serous ovarian tumour with microinvasion; (c) invasive serous cystadenocarcinoma

## Epithelial ovarian tumours

The ovary first appears in fetal life as an aggregation of cells covered with primitive coelomic epithelium. Subsequently, germ cells migrate from the yolk sac into the gonadal area. The coelomic epithelium that covers the ovary also gives rise to a variety of epithelia of Müllerian origin, which line the genital tract structures, including the Fallopian tubes, the uterus and the cervix, and are similar to those found in epithelial tumours of the ovary. Well-differentiated serous carcinoma resembles epithelium of the Fallopian tube, whereas the cell type in endometrioid tumours has a similar appearance to the cells found in endometrial glands. The WHO classification of epithelial ovarian tumours is based on this similarity in cell type (Table 70.2).

The serous tumours are the most common in this group (40–50 per cent). Mucinous tumours (10 per cent) may reach an enormous size and may be associated with pseudomyxoma ovarii and peritoneii. More than 10 per cent of primary endometrioid ovarian carcinomas are associated with carcinoma of the endometrium (coincidental primaries in most cases). Endometrioid carcinomas account for approximately 20 per cent of malignant epithelial tumours, but Brenner tumours make up a very small proportion, as 99 per cent are benign. Clear cell carcinomas account for between 5 and 10 per cent and have a worse prognosis than the other histological types. Bilaterality of epithelial ovarian malignancies is common.

Although endocrine function is most commonly a feature of sex-cord stromal tumours, it may also occur in association with epithelial ovarian tumours. Paraneoplastic syndromes are a rare feature of these tumours.

## Sex-cord stromal tumours

These tumours are composed of granulosa cells, theca cells, Sertoli cells, Leydig cells, fibroblasts or the precursors of these cells in varying proportions. The classification of these tumours (based on the WHO classification) is shown in Table 70.3. They may be associated with an oestrogenic, androgenic or (more rarely) progestogenic effect, but functional activity does not correlate with the appearance of the cell. Many of these tumours are benign and most of

**Table 70.2** Epithelial ovarian tumours – simplified classification

| Serous tumours |
| --- |
| Mucinous tumours |
| Endometrioid tumours |
| Clear cell tumours |
| Transitional cell (Brenner) tumours |
| Mixed epithelial tumours |
| Undifferentiated and unclassified tumours |

**Table 70.3** Sex-cord-stromal tumours – simplified classification

| Granulosa-stromal cell tumours |
| --- |
| Sertoli-stromal cell tumours |
| Gynandroblastoma |
| Sex-cord tumour with annular tubules |
| Unclassified sex-cord tumours |
| Steroid cell tumours |

**Table 70.4** Ovarian germ-cell tumours – simplified classification

| Dysgerminoma |
| --- |
| Teratoma (immature, mature and monodermal) |
| Yolk sac tumour (endodermal sinus tumour) |
| Embryonal carcinoma |
| Polyembryoma |
| Choriocarcinoma |
| Mixed germ cell tumours |

the clinically malignant forms are granulosa cell tumours. Fibromas are well known for their association with ascites and right hydrothorax, reported by Meigs in 1937 (Meigs syndrome).

## Germ cell tumours

Approximately 30 per cent of benign and malignant ovarian tumours are of germ cell origin (Table 70.4). However, as only a small proportion are malignant, they account for less than 5 per cent of all ovarian cancers. Nonetheless, they are the most common ovarian malignancy in the first two decades of life.

Dysgerminoma is the most common germ cell malignancy, and 75 per cent of cases present with stage I disease. In contrast with other malignant germ cell tumours, 10–15 per cent are bilateral, with contralateral involvement usually being microscopic. Five to 10 per cent occur in phenotypic females with abnormal gonads (the androgen insensitivity syndrome or gonadal dysgenesis).

Teratomas are tumours that are composed of tissue derived from two or three embryonic layers. The mature cystic teratoma is the most common ovarian germ cell tumour and is usually benign. Most are unilateral, but 15–20 per cent are bilateral. They are the most common ovarian tumours leading to torsion. Hair and teeth may be present in the cysts, the latter resulting in the classical appearance on plain abdominal x-ray. Malignant transformation is reported in up to 1 per cent, squamous carcinoma being the most common malignancy to develop. A diagnosis of struma ovarii is made when these tumours are predominantly composed of thyroid tissue. Primary ovarian carcinoid tumours are also variants of monodermal teratomas and usually have a favourable prognosis. However, secondary carcinoids (not associated with a monodermal teratoma) are usually metastatic from the gastrointestinal tract and have a poor prognosis.

Immature teratoma is the second most common germ cell malignancy and accounts for approximately 20 per cent of ovarian malignancies in females under 20 years of age. Virtually all immature teratomas are unilateral and they are currently classified according to a grading system that is based on the degree of differentiation and the quantity of immature tissue.

## Embryonic markers

Most patients with ovarian yolk sac tumours have elevated levels of alpha-fetoprotein ($\alpha$FP), but normal levels do not exclude this diagnosis. Embryonal carcinomas are extremely rare. They usually secrete beta-human chorionic gonadotrophin ($\beta$-hCG) and may secrete AFP. Ovarian choriocarcinoma secretes $\beta$-hCG and polyembryoma secretes $\beta$-hCG and $\alpha$FP. These are also very rare tumours. The more common immature teratoma and pure dysgerminoma do not secrete these tumour markers.

## Gonadoblastoma

This rare tumour consists of admixed germ cell and sex-cord stromal elements. This is usually a tumour of the second decade of life and rarely occurs in normal ovaries. Eighty per cent occur in phenotypic females who are virilized, and 20 per cent in phenotypic males with developmental abnormalities of the external genitalia. The most common karyotypes are 46XY and 45XO/46XY (mosaic).

## Secondary ovarian malignancies

Up to 10 per cent of malignant ovarian masses are metastases from some other organ and in many cases the ovarian metastases are detected before the primary tumour. The most common metastatic cancers are those arising from the colon, stomach, breast and, of course, the female genital tract. Bilaterally enlarged ovaries that contain signet-ring cells on microscopic assessment have been named after Krukenberg, who described these ovarian tumours in patients with metastatic gastric or (less commonly) colonic cancer.

## Primary peritoneal carcinoma

Primary peritoneal carcinoma is a highly malignant tumour arising from the peritoneum and resulting in signs and symptoms very similar to those of primary epithelial ovarian cancer. Rare benign and borderline variants have been described. Thus, a patient who has previously had both ovaries removed may develop a condition that clinically simulates ovarian cancer. Management is essentially as for advanced primary epithelial ovarian cancer.

## Primary Fallopian tube cancer

This rare cancer accounts for approximately 0.3 per cent of all female genital tract cancers, and is usually only discovered at surgery. It may be distinguishable from an ovarian cancer metastasis by the presence of associated atypical cytological change elsewhere within the tube. Primary Fallopian tube cancer may be more common than it appears, because it may quickly resemble ovarian cancer.

It is similar to primary epithelial ovarian cancer in histological appearance and clinical behaviour. Management is therefore essentially the same.

## Rare ovarian tumours

Other rare ovarian tumours include primary small-cell carcinoma and various types of sarcoma, all having a poor prognosis. Lymphoma or extramedullary leukaemia may also manifest initially as an ovarian tumour.

---

### KEY POINTS

- Ninety per cent of malignant ovarian tumours are epithelial, but germ-cell tumours account for 60 per cent of ovarian cancers in adolescents and children.
- Bilaterality of epithelial ovarian malignancies is common.
- Up to 10 per cent of ovarian masses are secondary to metastases from some other organ.
- The mature cystic teratoma is the most common ovarian germ cell tumour and the most common ovarian tumour leading to torsion.

---

# EPIDEMIOLOGY, INCIDENCE AND AETIOLOGY OF EPITHELIAL OVARIAN CANCER

In England and Wales, epithelial ovarian cancer is the most common gynaecological malignancy and accounts for more deaths in these countries than the other gynaecological malignancies together (see Table 70.1). The incidence and mortality rates are influenced by country of origin and race. In general, epithelial ovarian cancer is most common and most lethal in industrialized countries (except Japan) and has the lowest rates in the non-industrialized world. In contrast, germ-cell tumours represent up to 15 per cent of ovarian cancers in black and oriental populations, in whom epithelial ovarian cancers are less common.

Approximately 40 per cent of ovarian tumours in post-menopausal women are malignant, but less than 10 per cent are malignant in the pre-menopausal population. Most epithelial ovarian cancers occur in post-menopausal women, with less than 1 per cent affecting females under the age of 21 years. In this age group, more than 60 per cent of ovarian malignancies are of germ cell origin.

## Aetiology

### Environmental factors

The cause of ovarian cancer is unknown. Various associations between environmental factors and the development of ovarian cancer have been reported and reviewed.[4] High-fat diets have been associated with an increased risk of ovarian cancer, as has a diet low in fibre and vitamin A. Perineal dusting with talcum powder has also been shown to increase the risk of subsequent development of this cancer. The risks of a high caffeine intake and of exposure to asbestos or radiation are unclear. The role of certain viral infections (mumps, rubella and influenza) has been studied, with inconclusive results.

### Reproductive and hormonal factors

The effects of reproductive and hormonal factors on ovarian cancer risk have also been extensively documented and summarized.[5,6] It is generally accepted that nulliparity and low parity is associated with a higher risk of ovarian cancer when compared to high parity. It has been postulated that this is at least in part due to an increased risk of ovarian cancer related to nulliparity *per se*. Nonetheless, the published data are consistent, showing that pregnancy is protective, increasing protection occurring with increasing parity. Greatest protection is afforded by the first pregnancy, and breastfeeding also reduces the risk. The data on associations between the timing of menarche and menopause and ovarian cancer risk are less consistent. Tubal ligation has been reported by American and Australian investigators to decrease the risk of ovarian cancer, and all but one European study supports their conclusion that hysterectomy (with ovarian conservation) is also protective (six studies) [C].[5,6]

Based on the results of case–control studies, it is now widely accepted that use of the combined oral contraceptive pill is protective; increasing duration of use increases the level of protection afforded [C]. Factors that limit the number of ovulations are associated with reduced risk of ovarian cancer. Conversely, 'incessant ovulation' is generally associated with increased risk. The association between the use of fertility drugs and ovarian cancer risk has resulted in an international controversy initiated by reports of an increased risk of borderline and malignant ovarian tumours in users. More recent epidemiological studies found an association between the use of fertility drugs and development of borderline and malignant ovarian tumours, but the association was due to the effect of nulliparity alone.

A recent robust cohort study of over 50 000 women attending fertility clinics in Denmark found no evidence of a causal association between the use of ovulatory stimulants and the subsequent development of epithelial ovarian tumours [C].[7]

### Genetic factors

The concept that there is a familial predisposition to ovarian cancer was initially suggested by epidemiological studies that have consistently documented an increased relative risk for ovarian cancer associated with a family history of the disease. Three hereditary ovarian cancer syndromes have been described in which members of these families are at increased risk of developing ovarian cancer:

1  site-specific ovarian cancer, in which ovarian cancer is expressed in multiple female members of the genetic lineage, consistent with the presence of an autosomal dominant gene of high penetrance;
2  hereditary breast–ovarian cancer syndrome, in which breast and/or ovarian cancers are present in family members;
3  Lynch syndrome II (hereditary non-polyposis colon cancer, HNPCC), in which a genetic tendency to develop ovarian, endometrial and colon cancers can be demonstrated in the pedigree.

Hereditary ovarian cancers represent fewer than 10 per cent of all ovarian cancers. The role of hereditary factors in ovarian cancer has been eloquently reviewed.[8]

In 1994, following intense linkage analysis, a large gene was cloned and sequenced and confirmed to be the *BRCA1* (BReast CAncer 1) gene. Confirmatory studies have identified more than 100 mutations. It has been estimated that *BRCA1* mutation is responsible for approximately 5 per cent of ovarian cancers. Although the estimated risk of developing either ovarian or breast cancer by the age of 70 is 82 per cent, most carriers do not develop both diseases, and thus the penetrance for development of ovarian cancer is lower and estimated at 42 per cent. Mutations in the *BRCA2* gene also increase the risk of ovarian cancer in carriers, the site of mutation possibly correlating with risk, as in the case of *BRCA1*.

Hereditary non-polyposis colon cancer has been classified into two syndromes, termed Lynch I and II. The latter has an association with cancers at other sites, including the ovary and endometrium. The genes responsible for HNPCC have now been identified. The lifetime risk of ovarian cancer among gene carriers has not been precisely documented but may be as high as seven times that of non-carriers.[8]

Narod and colleagues[9] have reported in a case–control study that women from families with hereditary ovarian cancer syndromes reduce their risk of developing ovarian cancer by ever use of the combined oral contraceptive pill [II]. Risk-reducing salpingo-oopherectomy (RRSO) has been widely adopted as a key component of breast and gynaecologic cancer risk reduction for women with BRCA1 and BRCA2 mutations.[10]

## KEY POINTS

### Aetiology of ovarian cancer

- Tubal ligation and hysterectomy (with ovarian conservation) is associated with a decreased risk of ovarian cancer [C].
- The use of the combined oral contraceptive pill appears protective, with increasing duration of use increasing the level of protection afforded [C].
- Women from families with hereditary ovarian cancer syndromes may reduce their risk of developing ovarian cancer by ever use of the combined oral contraceptive pill [C].
- Factors which reduce ovulation are associated with a reduced risk of ovarian cancer.
- Evidence of a causal association between the use of ovulatory stimulants and the subsequent development of epithelial ovarian tumours is inconclusive.
- Three hereditary ovarian cancer syndromes have been described.
- Hereditary ovarian cancers represent fewer than 10 per cent of all ovarian cancers.
- Bilateral salpingo-oopherectomy is protective in *BRCA* mutation carriers [B].
- HNPCC has an association with cancer of the ovary and endometrium.

## SCREENING FOR OVARIAN CANCER

The possibility of pre-symptomatic genetic testing raises a number of medical, psychological, ethical, legal and social issues. Due to the limitations of genetic testing at the present time, it is imperative that it is offered only to high-risk individuals in cases for which the result of the test will affect medical management. In this context, it must be remembered that a woman with a single affected relative has a lifetime risk of developing ovarian cancer of only 3–4 per cent (see list of published guidelines p. 827).

Women who are at high risk for developing ovarian cancer (i.e. 10 per cent lifetime risk based on family history) may be offered ovarian screening, though evidence that this is effective is lacking, and participation in the United Kingdom Familial Ovarian Cancer Screening Study (UKFOCSS) prospective, non-randomized trial of ovarian cancer screening should be encouraged. Data regarding the efficacy or potential morbidity of ovarian screening in the asymptomatic general population are also lacking. A prospective multicentre, randomized, controlled trial of asymptomatic women without a significant family history has closed to recruitment (United Kingdom Collaborative Trial of Ovarian Cancer Screening, UKCTOCS). Preliminary results from this trial suggest that screening strategies using ultrasound and Ca 125 levels are feasible, but the key results on the impact of such strategies[11] on mortality are awaited.

Screening this population is contraindicated until results of this study are published. The role of newer tumour markers such as He4 in diagnosis and screening is currently being investigated, but none as yet is being used in clinical practice.

Screening for women deemed to be at high risk of developing ovarian cancer (10 per cent lifetime risk) should be done in the context of familial screening clinics, usually run jointly by a clinical geneticist and a gynaecological oncologist. Women who attend general gynaecological clinics with concerns about their familial risk of ovarian cancer should be referred to such services for an objective calculation of their risk and expert counselling on their options, such as prophylactic surgery or screening.

## MANAGEMENT OF THE ADNEXAL MASS

An adnexal mass may present either as a result of symptoms, which may be severe in the case of a cyst accident, or as an incidental finding when performing a pelvic examination or imaging. Cyst accidents include torsion, haemorrhage and rupture. Pelvic pain radiating down the inner aspect of the leg is a common presenting symptom, and torsion classically presents as severe pain associated with vomiting. Although rupture of a small cyst may be asymptomatic with few associated signs, the abdomen of a patient experiencing a cyst accident is usually tender, with guarding and rigidity. Rupture of a large cyst may produce signs of peritonitis, particularly if the cyst contents are irritant (e.g. endometriotic cyst or dermoid cyst), and the patient may be shocked in cases of extensive rupture or continuing haemorrhage.

### Investigation

A complete history and examination are essential, as the diagnosis is usually based on clinical findings. The history should include information about the duration and growth of the mass. Symptoms, past history or family history increasing the likelihood of malignancy should be sought. The duration of use of combined oral contraception should be noted. General, abdominal, vaginal and rectal examinations are recommended.

Full blood count, group and save, serum amylase, urea, electrolytes and liver function tests should be performed. Tumour markers should be measured if the mass is complex – if this information is not available, serum may be stored until histopathology has been reported. Pregnancy must be excluded and urinalysis performed. A midstream specimen of urine should be sent for culture and sensitivity. Other investigations may be indicated by the patient's condition, for example crossmatch and coagulation screen in cases of haemorrhage.

A pelvic ultrasound, preferably transvaginal, will reveal the dimensions and morphology of the mass and is the single most important investigation in predicting whether an ovarian mass is benign or malignant. Most ovarian masses are cystic, but the presence of solid areas makes a malignancy possible. However, some benign tumours are solid, for example thecoma, fibroma and Brenner tumours. Thickened walls and septae are other features of malignancy. The results of colour Doppler imaging have been disappointing and this technique has not proven superior to morphological assessment. Magnetic resonance imaging (MRI) may have a role in differentiating benign and malignant ovarian tumours, but computed tomography (CT) and positron emission tomography (PET) are not routinely indicated.

Measurement of Ca 125 may be misleading, as normal levels are found in 50 per cent of stage I ovarian cancers and levels are also raised in a number of benign conditions, including endometriosis.

Jacobs and colleagues included ultrasound findings and menopausal status with Ca 125 in an algorithm termed the risk of malignancy index (RMI) and reported 87 per cent sensitivity, 89 per cent specificity and 75 per cent positive predictive value (given an RMI cut-off value of 200).[12] The RMI is the product of the serum Ca 125 level (in units per millilitre), the ultrasound score (0, 1 or 3) and the menopausal status (1 if pre-menopausal, 3 if post-menopausal). The ultrasound score is calculated by giving one point for each of the following findings:

- multilocular cyst
- solid areas
- bilateral lesions
- metastases
- ascites.

The RMI provides a means of triaging women for referral to a gynaecological oncologist (see Table 70.5).

The use of the RMI has been endorsed by both the Royal College of Obstetricians and Gynaecologists (RCOG) and the Department of Health in its *Improving Outcomes Guidance* document (see below under Published guidelines). Since the introduction of this document, most cancer networks deliver gynaecological cancer care using a hub and spoke model and individual cancer networks are responsible for auditing their figures of referral and mortality and morbidity outcomes. With respect to ovarian

cancer, cancer units triage patients with adnexal masses according to the risk of malignancy. As the risk of malignancy increases, the appropriate location for management changes, e.g. a general gynaecologist might manage women with a low risk of malignancy but those at intermediate risk should be managed in a cancer unit and those at high risk in a cancer centre. Surgery by a gynaecological oncologist is recommended when the RMI is over 250 and all women with RMI >250 should be discussed at the cancer centre multidisciplinary team meeting [E].

---

**KEY POINTS**

**Low risk: Less than 3 per cent risk of cancer**

- Management should be in a gynaecology unit.
- Simple cysts less than 5 cm in diameter with a serum Ca 125 level of less than 30 may be managed conservatively.
- Conservative management should entail repeat ultrasound scans and serum Ca 125 measurement every four months for one year.
- If the cyst does not fit the above criteria or if the woman requests surgery, then laparoscopic oophorectomy is acceptable.

**Moderate risk: approximately 20 per cent risk of cancer**

- Management should be in a cancer unit.
- Laparoscopic oophorectomy is acceptable in selected cases.
- If a malignancy is discovered, then a full staging procedure should be undertaken in a cancer centre.

**High risk: greater than 75 per cent risk of cancer**

- Management should be in a cancer centre.
- Full staging procedure as described below under Conservative and surgical management.

---

## Conservative and surgical management

Management depends on the presentation (cyst accident or asymptomatic finding) and the risk of malignancy. Surgical intervention is usually required when an ovarian cyst presents with acute symptoms, although a conservative approach may be taken in mild cases where the findings indicate a low risk of malignancy. Most functional cysts can be managed conservatively and disappear spontaneously within two cycles if managed with combined oral contraceptives or observation alone. Patients with peritonitis or hypovolaemic shock require prompt resuscitation. The RCOG recommends conservative management in post-menopausal women with simple unilateral cysts <5 cm and Ca 125 <30. These cysts can be kept under surveillance with regular transvaginal ultrasound scans and Ca 125 levels and women discharged from follow up if the cyst resolves or remains unchanged at the end of a one year follow-up period.

---

**Table 70.5** An example of a protocol for triaging women using the risk of malignancy index (RMI)

| Risk RMI | Women (%) | Risk of cancer (%) |
|---|---|---|
| Low <25 | 40 | <3 |
| Moderate 25–250 | 30 | 20 |
| High >250 | 30 | 75 |

- See RCOG guideline No 34.

The benefits of laparoscopic surgery are widely reported, and large studies have been published demonstrating the safety and efficacy of this approach (see Published guidelines, p. 827). However, specialized and skilled gynaecologists performed the surgery in these series, and the unfortunate consequences of laparoscopic management of undiagnosed ovarian cancers have been reported. If an adequate pre-operative assessment, including RMI, indicates that the risk of malignancy is low, a laparoscopic approach by a suitably qualified surgeon should be considered. However, laparoscopic aspiration of cysts should not be performed to make a diagnosis of cancer, as the negative predictive value of cyst fluid cytology is low in most departments and aspiration adversely affects the prognosis of a stage I malignancy. Furthermore, therapeutic aspiration of ovarian cysts is usually ineffective, as most recur. In a post-menopausal woman, the appropriate laparoscopic treatment for an ovarian cyst, which is not suitable for conservative management, is oophorectomy, with removal of the ovary intact in a bag without cyst rupture into the peritoneal cavity.

Patients at intermediate risk of malignancy may also be considered for laparoscopic assessment when the operator is skilled, there is a safe method of retrieval of the mass and there are facilities for prompt frozen section analysis. In this situation, access to immediate surgical staging must be available. All patients with obvious malignancy should be referred to a gynaecological oncologist for further management. The role of laparoscopy in the management of ovarian cancer is not proven and is not in routine practice in the United Kingdom [E].

At laparoscopy, a careful assessment is performed and washings taken. If the findings are suspicious of malignancy (e.g. metastases or surface excresences are identified), a biopsy is taken. An appropriate procedure is rescheduled following the results of histopathology (see Surgical and non-surgical management of ovarian cancer, p. 823). If there are no suspicious findings, the surgeon may proceed to cystectomy or oophorectomy as indicated. A recent Cochrane review comprising 796 women reported that in women undergoing surgery for benign ovarian tumours, laparoscopy was associated with a reduction in fever, urinary tract infection, post-operative complications, post-operative pain, number of days in hospital and total cost. These findings should be interpreted with caution, since only a small number of studies were identified.[13]

---

### KEY POINTS

- At the present time, there is no role for ovarian screening in the asymptomatic population.
- All women presenting with vague pelvi-abdominal symptoms warrant a complete history and examination, including vaginal and per-rectal examination.

---

- The RMI is used to stratify cases according to the risk of ovarian cancer and to identify those requiring referral to a gynaecological oncologist [B].
- A proportion of ovarian cysts may be removed laparoscopically by appropriately skilled surgeons.

---

# CLINICAL MANAGEMENT OF OVARIAN CANCER

## Clinical presentation and diagnosis

Primary ovarian cancer is most common in women in the seventh decade of life. Hereditary cancers usually present in younger women, occurring approximately ten years earlier. Most women with ovarian cancer are asymptomatic and when symptoms do occur they are often non-specific and vague. A complete history and examination are essential to make the diagnosis, to identify patients with secondary ovarian malignancy and to assess fitness for surgical and non-surgical management.

## Symptoms

When the tumour is confined to the ovary, the patient may present with pressure symptoms (urinary frequency, constipation, pelvic pain/pressure, dyspareunia) and, rarely, symptoms of a cyst accident. In advanced stage disease, symptoms are usually due to metastases affecting the bowel and mesentery, and ascites. Resulting symptoms (bloating, constipation, early satiety, loss of appetite) may be misinterpreted as irritable bowel syndrome. Symptoms due to pressure effects in the pelvis may also occur. Abnormal vaginal bleeding (in pre-menopausal and post-menopausal women) is a less common presenting feature. As the symptoms of ovarian cancer are vague, delays in presentation and subsequent delays in diagnosis are common. The Department of Health, in conjunction with various ovarian cancer charities, has launched a publicity campaign to encourage earlier self-reporting of symptoms by women, but whether this will have an impact on early diagnosis and mortality rates is unknown.

## Clinical signs

Assessment should include examination of supraclavicular, axillary and inguinal nodes, chest examination (pleural effusion) and abdominal examination, including assessment of liver size. In women presenting with the above symptoms, a pelvic examination is mandatory. The presence of a solid, irregular mass is characteristic, particularly when associated with an upper abdominal mass (omental cake). There is typically a craggy feel in the Pouch of Douglas and rectal examination may reveal a mass impacting on the anterior bowel wall.

Gynaecological oncology

## Investigations

Investigations are performed to assess the likelihood of malignant disease, to assess fitness for anaesthesia and surgery, and to plan the extent of surgery. Ultrasonography (see Screening for ovarian cancer, p. 819) should include assessment not just of the pelvis, but also of the kidneys and liver. Liver parenchymal metastases increase the likelihood of a non-ovarian primary, and significant hydronephrosis should be identified pre-operatively. Chest x-ray is essential. Ca 125 (see above) and carcinoembryonic antigen (CEA) levels should be measured, the latter to identify primary gastrointestinal malignancy. In young women, αFP and β-hCG levels should also be measured, as germ cell tumours are the most common gynaecological malignancy in the first two decades of life. Full blood count, urea, creatinine, electrolytes and liver function tests (including total protein and albumin) should also be performed.

CT scan of the abdomen and pelvis is the investigation of choice to assess the extent of upper abdominal disease. MRI of the pelvis may also assist surgical planning in patients with a fixed pelvic mass. A chest x-ray or CT chest must be performed to assess the possibility of stage IV disease. In patients with abnormal vaginal bleeding, full assessment of the cervix and uterus, including outpatient endometrial biopsy, should be considered – an ovarian mass may be the site of secondary spread from a primary cervical or endometrial carcinoma. Endoscopy of the upper or lower gastrointestinal tract is indicated in women whose symptoms/tumour marker profile or CT suggest a primary gastrointestinal malignancy.

## Staging of primary ovarian cancer

Ovarian cancers are staged according to the International Federation of Gynecology and Obstetrics (FIGO) recommendations (Table 70.6). Staging is based on findings at laparotomy, but pre-operative assessment is required to assess extraperitoneal spread. Accurate staging is of paramount importance as it determines not only prognosis but also to a large extent the requirement for adjuvant treatment. FIGO report the five-year overall survival of patients with stage I disease as 70 per cent, in contrast to survival rates of more than 90 per cent reported in stage I in patients with properly staged disease, which suggests that a significant proportion of women do not undergo careful surgical staging. The Gynaecologic Cancer Intergroup (GCIG) have proposed changes to the current FIGO staging system suggesting that in early-stage disease, grading and in advanced disease, the amount of residual disease should be reported.[14]

**Table 70.6** International Federation of Gynecology and Obstetrics (FIGO) staging and five-year overall survival[a] of ovarian cancer

| Stage | Description | Five-year survival (%) |
|---|---|---|
| **I** | **Confined to one/both ovaries** | |
| Ia | Limited to a single ovary, no ascites, capsule intact with no surface tumour | 89.9 |
| Ib | Limited to both ovaries, no ascites, capsule intact with no surface tumour | 84.7 |
| Ic | One or both ovaries have ruptured capsule or surface tumour, malignant ascites or positive peritoneal washings | 80 |
| **II** | **Extension to pelvic structures** | |
| IIa | Extension to uterus or Fallopian tubes | 69.9 |
| IIb | Extension to other pelvic tissues | 63.7 |
| IIc | As for IIA or IIB, but one or both ovaries have ruptured capsule or surface tumour; malignant ascites or positive peritoneal washings | 66.5 |
| **III** | **As for stage I/II, but also with peritoneal implants outside pelvis or with positive retroperitoneal lymph nodes** | |
| IIIa | Histologically confirmed microscopic seeding of abdominal peritoneal surfaces and negative retroperitoneal lymph nodes | 58.5 |
| IIIb | Histologically confirmed implants of abdominal peritoneal surfaces, <2 cm and negative retroperitoneal lymph nodes | 39.9 |
| IIIc | Histologically confirmed implants of abdominal peritoneal surfaces >2 cm or positive retroperitoneal lymph nodes | 28.7 |
| **IV** | **Distant metastases (including liver parenchyma/positive pleural fluid cytology)** | **16.8** |

[a]FIGO Annual Report on the Results of Treatment in Gynaecological Cancer, 24th volume. International Federation of Gynecology and Obstetrics, Milan 2000.

## Technique for surgical staging

A midline incision is essential to allow adequate access for thorough surgical staging and should be performed whenever an ovarian malignancy is anticipated. A systematic exploration of all peritoneal surfaces and viscera is performed. The staging laparotomy involves the following steps:

- Sending ascites or peritoneal washings for cytological assessment.
- Performing a total abdominal hysterectomy and bilateral salpingo-oopherectomy (TAH/BSO).
- Omentectomy.
- Peritoneal biopsies of all suspicious areas or multiple random sampling if all surfaces are apparently normal.
- Diaphragmatic biopsies or scrapings for cytological assessment.
- Sampling of pelvic and para-aortic lymph nodes.

The rationale for TAH/BSO is the high incidence of bilateral tumours (metastatic or primary) and metastases to the uterus. Furthermore, the endometrium may be the site of a synchronous primary carcinoma, particularly in the case of endometrioid carcinoma of the ovary. The omentum is removed, as it is the major site of abdominal metastases. An infracolic omentectomy is most universally performed, but a supracolic procedure may be preferable and, indeed, is often essential to achieve adequate cytoreduction of gross omental disease. Washings may be positive in apparent stage Ia disease, substantially altering decision making with regard to adjuvant treatment. Table 70.7 illustrates the rate of occult metastases when adequate surgical staging is performed by combining results from 13 published series involving a total of over 1000 cases.

**Table 70.7** Metastases in apparent early stage epithelial ovarian carcinoma presented as percentages

|  | Percentage of cases with occult metastases |
| --- | --- |
| Diaphragm | 7.6 |
| Omentum | 7.1 |
| Cytology | 18.8 |
| Peritoneum | 9.8 |
| Pelvic lymph nodes | 8.9 |
| Para-aortic lymph nodes | 12.3 |

- Adapted with permission from Moore DH. Primary surgical management of early epithelial ovarian carcinoma. In: Rubin CR, Sutton GP (eds). *Ovarian Cancer*, 2nd edn. Philadelphia: Lippincott Williams and Wilkins, 2001, 201–18.

Appendicectomy has not yet been accepted as part of standard procedure. However, the appendix is commonly the site of metastases in advanced stage disease. Furthermore, the ovary may be a site of secondary disease in the rare case of an appendiceal primary and may be associated with pseudomyxoma peritoneii. Appendicectomy is recommended in cases of pseudomyxoma and mucinous tumours to exclude an appendicial primary tumour.

## SURGICAL AND NON-SURGICAL MANAGEMENT OF OVARIAN CANCER

The management of ovarian cancer is discussed below in seven consecutive sections.

## Primary surgery: early epithelial ovarian cancer

In cases of early stage disease, the surgical objective is to identify occult metastases through meticulous systematic exploration. The most common pattern of metastatic spread of epithelial ovarian cancer is transcoelomic. The cells disseminate and implant along the peritoneal surfaces following the circulatory path of peritoneal fluid. Lymphatic dissemination to pelvic and para-aortic nodes is also common and may occur in apparent early stage disease. Haematogenous spread is uncommon at the time of diagnosis, but the liver and lung are the preferred sites. The importance of adequate surgical staging in apparent early disease cannot be overemphasized.

The standard surgical procedure for early stage disease has already been described. However, when operating on a young patient for whom fertility is important, it is advisable to perform an adequate staging procedure while minimizing the risk to future fertility. Although frozen section may be useful if it produces a definitive diagnosis of malignancy, the heterogeneity and size of ovarian malignancies result in under-diagnosis in a considerable proportion of cases. Delaying a sterilizing procedure until the final histopathology is available allows a decision regarding further surgical management to be made in consultation with the patient. An initial procedure in such a case would involve complete surgical staging as described, but the uterus and contralateral ovary would be left *in situ* following careful inspection. A decision regarding completion of surgery and adjuvant treatment should then be made in consultation with the patient and based on the advice of the cancer centre's multidisciplinary team.

Laparotomy is currently the gold-standard surgical procedure for the diagnosis and staging of early ovarian cancer. The role of laparoscopy is undefined and it should only be used as part of well-designed prospective clinical trials.

Gynaecological oncology

## Primary surgery: advanced epithelial ovarian cancer

In contrast with early ovarian cancer, the surgical emphasis in advanced disease is on tumour cytoreduction. Cytoreductive surgery typically involves performing a TAH/BSO, complete omentectomy and resection of any metastases.

The principal goal of cytoreductive surgery is to remove all primary cancer and, if possible, all metastatic disease. If this is not possible, the surgeon aims to reduce the tumour load to achieve 'optimal' status. Griffiths, who suggested in 1975 that residual nodules should be no greater than 1.5 cm in maximum diameter, first introduced this concept. His results have been substantiated by almost every subsequent large series reported. In 1983, Hacker et al. showed that patients with residual disease of 5 mm or less had a median survival of 40 months, compared with 18 months for those with lesions <1.5 cm, and only six months for patients with nodules >1.5 cm.[15] Primary cytoreductive surgery has become established as the standard management of patients with advanced ovarian cancer.

Resectability of disease depends not only on the skill of the surgeon, but also on the site of disease. Optimal cytoreduction is unlikely if there is extensive disease on the undersurfaces of the diaphragms or affecting the liver, porta hepatis or root of the small bowel mesentery. Major morbidity is approximately 5 per cent and operative mortality 1 per cent. Although prognosis depends on the extent of residual disease following surgery, it is also determined by the patient's age, the volume of ascites, performance status comorbidity (independent prognostic variables). In planning management, these factors must be taken into consideration.

Controversy about the role and timing of surgery in advanced ovarian cancer continues. Although it is possible that the biology of the disease determines both resectability and prognosis, recent data show that maximal surgical effort can produce complete cytoreduction and that this has a greater impact on survival than the tumour load at the start of an operation. In earlier systematic review of surgery in advanced ovarian cancer that questioned whether surgical intervention of this type provided the patient with an advantage[16] has now been superseded by a more recent meta-analysis[17] reporting that maximal cytoreduction is one of the most powerful determinants of cohort survival among patients with stage III or IV ovarian carcinoma. Although the evidence for aggressive primary surgery has never been demonstrated in a randomized trial, and is based on retrospective case–control studies [C], the only prospective randomized trial of cytoreductive surgery reported to date [B][18] has demonstrated a survival advantage for patients randomized to a second resection of disease as an interval procedure. Cytoreductive surgery that aims to remove all visible disease remains the current standard of care.

In recent years, it has become relatively common practice to give chemotherapy prior to surgery where the latter is considered unlikely to result in effective cytoreduction, or if the patient is unfit for aggressive surgery.[19] In order to evaluate the effectiveness of this approach, two randomized trials have been performed. The first, an EORTC trial, has reported preliminary data suggesting that survival is equivalent when surgery is delayed after three cycles of chemotherapy compared with surgery up front. Furthermore, surgical morbidity was reduced. Final published results and the results of the other (CHORUS) trial from the UK are awaited.

### KEY POINTS

- The importance of adequate surgical staging in apparent early stage ovarian cancer cannot be overemphasized.
- Cytoreductive surgery to no visible disease plus chemotherapy is the current standard of care for patients with advanced ovarian carcinoma. Although primary surgery followed by chemotherapy has been the standard of care for many years, studies are currently challenging the timing of surgery [A].
- In women for whom initial surgery is unsuitable, chemotherapy can be given initially and surgery performed following tumour shrinkage.

## CHEMOTHERAPY

In general, it is agreed that patients with adequately staged low-grade stage Ia and Ib disease have a very good prognosis and do not require adjuvant treatment [A]. A number of publications and a systematic review of chemotherapy effects in ovarian cancer support this approach [A].[20]

However, patients with early stage disease and poor prognostic factors may benefit from adjuvant treatment, as they have a substantial risk of micrometastases. Two large randomized trials addressing this issue (ICON 1[21] and ACTION[22] – over 900 patients studied) demonstrated a statistically significant improvement in recurrence-free survival and overall survival in women receiving adjuvant chemotherapy. In the ACTION study, women who were fully staged as stage I did not benefit from adjuvant chemotherapy, indicating that those 'stage 1' who did, had possibly been understaged. A multivariate analysis of studies of prognostic variables involving 1545 patients found that degree of differentiation and cyst rupture were independent poor prognostic factors [C].[23] This topic has been the subject of a systematic review by Winter-Roach et al.[24]

Adjuvant radiotherapy for ovarian cancer involves either whole abdominal radiotherapy or the administration of intraperitoneal radiocolloid (P[32]). Whole abdominal radiotherapy is no longer considered the standard treatment for patients with optimal cytoreduction and neither approach has been shown to have an advantage over chemotherapy. Pelvic radiation alone is not as effective as adjuvant chemotherapy but may be used to palliate isolated pelvic recurrence, for example a bleeding mass at the vaginal vault.

Single chemotherapeutic agents active in epithelial ovarian cancer include:

- alkylating agents (e.g. cyclophosphamide);
- platinum compounds (cisplatin and carboplatin);
- anthracyclines (e.g. epirubicin);
- taxanes (paclitaxel and docetaxel) and others.[25]

Alkylating agents were the mainstay of treatment before the 1970s and produced response rates of 40–50 per cent. With platinum-based chemotherapy, response rates rose to more than 70 per cent. Forty-nine trials involving 8763 women have been systematically reviewed. The available evidence suggests that platinum-based therapy is better than non-platinum therapy [B]. There is some evidence that combination therapy improves survival compared with platinum alone [B]. No difference in effectiveness between cisplatin and carboplatin has been shown [B]. In most regimens, carboplatin has now been substituted for cisplatin, as it has the advantage of producing less gastrointestinal, renal and peripheral neurological toxicity.

In two prospective randomized trials in advanced ovarian cancer,[28,29] paclitaxel in combination with cisplatin provided a survival benefit over cyclophosphamide/cisplatin (the previous standard of care). Both studies reported a significant improvement in clinical response rate, median progression-free interval and overall survival in the paclitaxel arm [B]. Based on these trials, paclitaxel and a platinum analogue became the new standard of care. The large ICON 3 study, which involved more than 2000 patients, failed to identify an advantage for the use of paclitaxel/carboplatin over single-agent carboplatin alone, challenging what has become regarded as standard of care.[30] Three randomized trials have compared carboplatin/paclitaxel and cisplatin/paclitaxel, and no differences in outcome have yet been identified.[20]

Standard of care for women with high-risk early stage disease involves adjuvant chemotherapy: usually carboplatin/paclitaxel, though carboplatin alone is acceptable for less fit women, or those who wish to avoid alopecia [B]. For the treatment of advanced stage ovarian cancer, combination chemotherapy with carboplatin and paclitaxel for six cycles is recommended; again carboplatin alone may be preferable in less fit women or in women for whom alopecia is unacceptable.

Although 70 per cent of women receiving adjuvant chemotherapy will respond initially to platinum-based chemotherapy, at least half will relapse within 18 months. Treatment at relapse is essentially palliative in intent, but increasing use of supportive factors such as G-CSF allows women to receive more cycles of chemotherapy and more courses of chemotherapy than previously, and survival for five to six years is now achievable in a large minority. Second-line chemotherapy is indicated in cases

of recurrent or progressive disease. Response rates are much lower than for primary treatment (15–35 versus 70 per cent), and depend on whether the tumour is platinum sensitive, with longer disease-free intervals before recurrence. In patients with platinum-sensitive disease (i.e. women with a progression-free interval of at least six months since platinum-based therapy), retreatment with platinum or paclitaxel is appropriate. In platinum-resistant cases, an agent without cross-resistance is required. These include alkylating agents (liposomal doxorubicin); anthracyclines, topoisomerase inhibitors (etoposide, topotecan) and others (hexamethylmelamine, tamoxifen) and currently, Caelyx® and topotecan are front runners for second-line therapy in women with relapsed ovarian cancer. There is some evidence from observational studies that tamoxifen may produce a response in a modest proportion of women with relapsed ovarian cancer. Single-agent regimens are often adopted due to ease of administration and low toxicity.

At the present time, the role of intraperitoneal chemotherapy is unclear despite the GOG172 trial showing superior survival compared with standard chemotherapy.[26] It has recently been reintroduced in some North American centres; however, this approach is associated with greater morbidity and has not been accepted as routine practice internationally.[27] Further trials are required to demonstrate its feasibility. Routine CA 125 in follow up of ovarian cancer patients needs to be reconsidered following the demonstration that second-line chemotherapy triggered by rising CA 125 does not improve survival when given at clinical relapse (results of MRC OV05/EORTC 55955 randomized trial presented at the plenary session at the American Society of Clinical Oncology (ASCO) 2009 Annual Meeting).[31]

# TARGETED THERAPIES IN OVARIAN CANCER

Given the limitations of chemotherapy and problem of platinum resistance, there is the potential to improve survival from ovarian cancer with targeted therapies. Such agents target specific molecular pathways which are particularly relevant in certain tumours. Two studies of the International Collaborative Ovarian Neoplasm collaborators (ICON) are ongoing: ICON 7 is a multi-centre trial investigating the role of bevacizumab, a monoclonal antibody against VEGF, and ICON 6 is studying the role of EGFR antagonists in ovarian cancer. Other agents that have shown promise in trials are PARP (poly ADP-ribose polymerase) inhibitors, particularly in women with BRCA mutations, and folate receptor antagonists of which several agents are in early phase trials. Scheduling of these agents with conventional chemotherapy and selecting agents to optimize benefits for patients are new challenges that have not yet been addressed.

## KEY POINTS

- Additional therapy may be considered for patients who have early stage disease associated with high-risk factors [B].
- Standard adjuvant therapy for ovarian cancer involves intravenous chemotherapy [B].
- Paclitaxel and a platinum analogue are considered the standard of care for women with respect to chemotherapy for advanced ovarian cancer [B].
- Response rates to second-line chemotherapy are much lower than for primary treatment.
- Patients with low-grade stage Ia and Ib disease do not require adjuvant treatment [B].
- In stage I invasive epithelial ovarian carcinoma, degree of differentiation, capsular penetrance, surface excresences, malignant ascites and cyst rupture are independent poor prognosticators [B].
- Platinum-based therapy is better than non-platinum therapy [B].
- There is some evidence that combination therapy improves survival compared with platinum alone [B].
- No difference in effectiveness between cisplatin and carboplatin has been shown [B].
- Paclitaxel in combination with cisplatin may provide a survival benefit over cyclophosphamide/cisplatin [B].

# SECONDARY CYTOREDUCTIVE SURGERY

As optimal primary cytoreductive surgery is associated with improved outcomes in patients with advanced ovarian cancer, it has been suggested that there is a role for debulking in patients with persistent or recurrent disease. This group of patients is highly heterogeneous, but may be broadly categorized as follows:

- patients with persistent disease following completion of primary treatment;
- patients with recurrent disease after completion of primary treatment.

## Patients with persistent or recurrent disease following completion of primary treatment

Patients whose disease progresses during chemotherapy, those with persistent disease at the completion of chemotherapy and those who develop recurrence early have a limited median survival. Treatment should therefore be directed at optimizing quality of life. As a result, cytoreductive surgery is rarely indicated in these groups. However, patients who have had complete clinical responses to primary treatment

and who develop localized recurrences after a disease-free interval of 12 months or more may benefit from cytoreductive surgery.[32] This approach is best reserved for single site recurrence with good performance status, no ascites and where optimal debulking has previously been achieved. A large prospective multi-centre trial (DESKTOP III) has now been developed to address the issue of whether secondary surgery plus chemotherapy improves survival compared with chemotherapy alone.

# PALLIATIVE SURGERY

The most common indication for palliative surgery is bowel obstruction, which is a relatively common feature of recurrent disease, but may also be the presenting feature in undiagnosed patients. Most patients have small-bowel obstruction, approximately one-third have large-bowel obstruction and a minority have both. However, in many cases of small-bowel obstruction due to ovarian cancer, the site of obstruction is not single and on occasions the entire small bowel is rendered dysfunctional due to extensive peritoneal and mesenteric involvement (carcinomatous ileus). As these latter cases are not amenable to surgery, careful case selection is the essence of good management. Surgery may involve bowel resection, but most commonly intestinal bypass and/or stoma formation is required.

The median survival for patients undergoing palliative surgery for bowel obstruction is 3–12 months. Those who are young, with a good nutritional status (normal albumin levels) and who do not have rapidly accumulating ascites have the best prognosis. Reported morbidity and mortality rates are 30 and 10 per cent, respectively.

# MANAGEMENT OF RARER TUMOUR TYPES

## Borderline ovarian tumours

Approximately 15 per cent of epithelial ovarian tumours are borderline (tumours of low malignant potential). They affect younger women than primary epithelial ovarian cancers and may present in pregnancy. They are usually of low stage and have a very good prognosis. Surgical resection is the primary modality of treatment, as there are no prospective data suggesting that adjuvant treatment prolongs survival. Pre-menopausal women who wish to preserve fertility may be treated by conservative surgery (recurrence rate in the controlateral ovary is at least 10 per cent in these patients). Nonetheless, it should be emphasized that a small subgroup of these patients (those with invasive implants) have rapidly progressive disease and a poor prognosis. Some specialists advise long-term follow up, as late recurrences do occur particularly in cases with invasive implants.

## Germ cell tumours of the ovary

Adequate surgical staging, cytoreduction and adjuvant chemotherapy is current standard therapy for germ cell tumours of the ovary. As these malignancies usually occur in young women, conservation of the contralateral ovary and uterus is appropriate. The importance of a complete and thorough staging procedure cannot be underestimated – patients with stage Ia dysgerminoma and stage I, grade 1 immature teratoma require no further therapy if comprehensively staged. All other patients should be treated with three or more cycles of combination chemotherapy (bleomycin, etoposide and cisplatin). Most patients with these tumours are cured of disease and most survivors can anticipate normal menstrual and reproductive function. Tumour markers such as AFP are often useful in monitoring disease and planning management.

## Sex-cord stromal tumours

Although they are reported to be most common among post-menopausal women, these tumours often affect children and young adults. They are the most hormonally active of all ovarian tumours (hyperoestrogenic) and there is, therefore, an association with hyperplasia and well-differentiated adenocarcinoma of the endometrium. Surgery is the cornerstone of management, but early stage disease may be managed by unilateral oophorectomy and endometrial biopsy when fertility sparing is important. Late recurrence is the hallmark of these tumours.

## Pseudomyxoma peritoneii

This condition involves the accumulation of gelatinous material in the peritoneal cavity. It occurs in association with mucinous tumours of the appendix and/or ovary. It is extremely rare and has a very poor prognosis. Cases should be referred for a specialist opinion as early as possible. A histopathological diagnosis of pseudomyxoma ovarii would warrant such a referral, and appendicectomy is warranted to exclude a primary appendiceal tumour. Radical surgery with peritoneal stripping and hyperthermic chemotherapy has been advocated, but its true benefit has not been proven and trials are needed.

## QUALITY OF LIFE

Most patients with ovarian cancer present late and die of disease. Cure is the ultimate goal of the patient but

realistically, control of the disease for at least 18 months is considered a reasonable initial goal. A careful balance, therefore, must be struck between the pursuit of that goal and optimization of the quality of the period of life remaining. Specific treatments and their potential impact on disease must be weighed against the morbidity of each therapy. The optimum balance between these opposing aims will be different for each patient. The informed patient's voice is critical to finding the best management for her, and should be heard. Management decisions should be made with the balance of probabilities and the patient's desires clearly in focus. With optimal care, mean duration of survival for women with advanced ovarian cancer has gradually lengthened to around three years, which has been accompanied by improved quality of life.

## CONCLUSION

Ovarian cancer survival and associated quality of life are improving with advances in chemotherapy, but rates of cure remain low. It remains to be seen whether targeted therapy such as anti-angiogenics will achieve longer disease-free survival. Over the past ten years, there have been considerable changes in patterns of care and women with ovarian cancer now receive care from dedicated teams of highly specialized individuals. There are considerable challenges ahead, but the next five years will see whether screening is effective in improving survival from ovarian cancer and it will be clearer whether molecular agents are delivering improved survival.

## Published Guidelines

BRCA1 Genetic Screening. Rockville: Kaiser Permanente, 1998: helen.stallings.org.

Drouin P, Dubuc-Lissoir J, Ehlen T *et al.* Guidelines for the laparoscopic management of the adnexal mass. *SOGC Clinical Practice Guidelines* 1998; **76**. Available from: www.g-o-c.org.

Ferrini R. Screening asymptomatic women for cancer. *Am J Prev Med* 1997; **13**: 444–6. Available from: www.acpm.org.

Royal College of Obstetricians and Gynaecologists. Guideline No 34. Management of ovarian cysts in the postmenopausal woman.

Scottish Intercollegiate Guidelines Network. Epithelial ovarian cancer. A national clinical guideline. 2003.

NHS Executive (July 1999) Improving outcomes in gynaecological cancers: Guidance on commissioning cancer services. Available from: http://www.dh.gov.uk/en/Publicationsandstatistics/Publications/PublicationsPolicyAndGuidance/DH_4005385.

# Key References

1. Cooper N, Quinn MJ, Rachet B *et al.* Survival from cancer of the ovary in England and Wales up to 2001. *Br J Cancer* 2008; **99** (Suppl. 1): S70–2.

2. Kitchener HC. Survival from cancer of the ovary in England and Wales up to 2001. *Br J Cancer* 2008; **99** (Suppl. 1): S73–4.

3. Scully RE, Sobin LN. Histological typing of ovarian tumors. In: *World Health Organization International Classification of Tumors*, 2nd edn. Berlin: Springer-Verlag, 1999: 28–36.

4. Daly M, Abrams GI. Epidemiology and risk assessment for ovarian cancer. *Semin Oncol* 1998; **25**: 255–64.

5. Fox H. Origins of ovarian cancer. In: Kavanagh JJ, Singletary SE, Einhorn N, DePetrillo AD (eds). *Cancer in Women*. London: Blackwell Science, 1998: 406–14.

6. Look KY. Epidemiology, etiology and screening of ovarian cancer. In: Rubin SC, Sutton GP (eds). *Ovarian Cancer*. Philadelphia: Lippincott Williams and Wilkins, 2001: 167–80.

7. Jensen A, Sharif H, Frederiksen K, Kjaer SK. Use of fertility drugs and risk of ovarian cancer: Danish Population Based Cohort Study. *BMJ* 2009; **338**: b249.

8. Lynch HT, Casey MJ, Shaw TG, Lynch JF. Hereditary factors in gynecologic cancer. *Oncologist* 1998; **3**: 319–38.

9. Narod SA, Sun P, Risch H. Ovarian cancer, oral contraceptives, and *BRCA* mutations. *N Engl J Med* 2001; **345**: 1706–7.

10. Kauff ND, Domchek SM, Friebel TM *et al.* Risk-reducing salpingo-oopherectomy for the prevention of BRCA1- and BRCA2-associated breast and gynecologic cancer: a multicenter, prospective study. *J Clin Oncol* 2008; **26**: 1331–7.

11. Menon U, Gentry-Maharaj A, Hallett R *et al.* Sensitivity and specificity of multimodal and ultrasound screening for ovarian cancer, and stage distribution of detected cancers: results of the prevalence screen of the UK Collaborative Trial of Ovarian Cancer Screening (UKCTOCS). *Lancet Oncol* 2009; **10**: 327–40.

12. Davies AP, Jacobs I, Woolas R *et al.* The adnexal mass: benign or malignant? Evaluation of a risk of malignancy index. *Br J Obstet Gynecol* 1993; **100**: 927–31.

13. Medeiros LR, Rosa DD, Bozzetti MC *et al.* Laparoscopy versus laparotomy for FIGO Stage I ovarian cancer. *Cochrane Database Syst Rev* 2008; (**4**): CD005344.

14. Petru E, Lück HJ, Stuart G *et al.* Gynecologic Cancer Intergroup (GCIG) proposals for changes of the current FIGO staging system. *Eur J Obstet Gynecol Reprod Biol* 2009; **143**: 69–74.

15. Hacker NF, Berek JS, Lagasse LD *et al.* Primary cytoreductive surgery for epithelial ovarian cancer. *Obstet Gynecol* 1983; **61**: 413–20.

16. Hunter RW, Alexander NDE, Soutter WP. Meta-analysis of surgery in advanced ovarian carcinoma: is maximum cytoreductive surgery an independent determinant of prognosis? *Am J Obstet Gynecol* 1992; **166**: 504–11.

17. Bristow RE, Tomacruz RS, Armstrong DK *et al.* Survival effect of maximal cytoreductive surgery for advanced ovarian carcinoma during the platinum era: a meta-analysis. *J Clin Oncol* 2002; **20**: 1248–59.

18. Van der Burg ME, van Lent M, Buyse M *et al.* The effect of debulking surgery after induction chemotherapy on the prognosis of advanced epithelial ovarian cancer. *N Engl J Med* 1995; **332**: 629–34.

19. Morrison J, Swanton A, Collins S, Kehoe S. Chemotherapy versus surgery for initial treatment in advanced ovarian epithelial cancer. *Cochrane Database Syst Rev* 2007; (**4**): CD005343.

20. Ozols RF, Bookman MA, Young RC. Intraepithelial chemotherapy for ovarian cancer (correspondence). *NEJM* 2006; **354**: 1641–30.

21. International Ovarian Neoplasm (ICON) Collaborators. International Collaborative Ovarian Neoplasm Trial 1: a randomised trial of adjuvant chemotherapy in women with early stage ovarian cancer. *J Natl Cancer Inst* 2003; **95**: 125–32.

22. Trimbos JB, Vergote I, Bolis G *et al.* Impact of adjuvant chemotherapy and surgical staging in early-stage ovarian carcinoma: European Organisation for Research and Treatment of Cancer – Adjuvant Chemotherapy in ovarian Neoplasm Trial. *J Natl Cancer Inst* 2003; **95**:113–25.

23. Vergote I, De Brabanter J, Fyles A *et al.* Prognostic importance of degree of differentiation and cyst rupture in stage I invasive epithelial ovarian carcinoma. *Lancet* 2001; **357**: 176–82.

24. Winter-Roach B, Hooper L, Kitchener H. Systematic review of adjuvant therapy for early stage (epithelial) ovarian cancer. *Int J Gynecol Cancer* 2003; **13**: 395–404.

25. McGuire WP, Harris WL. Chemotherapy of epithelial ovarian cancer. In: Deppe G, Baker VV (eds). *Gynecologic Oncology*. New York: Oxford University Press, 1999: 212–40.

26. Armstrong K, Bundy B, Wenzel L *et al.* Intraperitoneal cisplatin and paclitaxel in ovarian cancer. *N Eng J Med* 2006; **354**: 34–43.

27. Gore M, du Bois A, Vergote I. Intraperitoneal chemotherapy in ovarian cancer remains experimental. *J Clin Oncol* 2006; 24: 4528–30.

28. McGuire WP, Hoskins WJ, Brady MF *et al.* Cyclophosphamide and cisplatin compared with paclitaxel and cisplatin in patients with stage III and stage IV ovarian cancer. *N Engl J Med* 1996; **334**: 1–6.

29. Piccart MJ, Bertelsen K, James K *et al.* Randomized intergroup trial of cisplatin–paclitaxel versus cisplatin–cyclophosphamide in women with advanced epithelial ovarian cancer: three-year results. *J Natl Cancer Inst* 2000; **92**: 699–708.

30. Harper P. A randomized comparison of paclitaxel and carboplatin versus a control arm of single agent

carboplatin or CAP (cyclophosphamide, doxorubicin and cisplatin): 2075 patients randomized into the 3rd International Collaborative Ovarian Neoplasm Study (ICON-3). *Proc Am Soc Clin Oncol* 1999; **18**: A1375.

31. Rustin GJ, van der Burg ME. A randomized trial in ovarian cancer (OC) of early treatment of relapse based on CA125 level alone versus delayed treatment based on conventional clinical indicators (MRC OVO5/ EORTC 55955 trials). *J Clin Oncol* 2009; **27** (18 suppl): 5s (abstract 1).

32. Harter P, du Bois A, Hahmann M *et al.* Surgery in recurrent ovarian cancer: the Arbeitsgemeinschaft Gynaekologische Onkologie (AGO) DESKTOP OVAR trial. *Ann Surg Oncol* 2006; **13**: 1702–10.

# Vulval and vaginal cancer

*John Tidy*

## MRCOG standards

### Knowledge criteria

- Epidemiology, aetiology, diagnosis, prevention, management, prognosis, complications and anatomical considerations of vulval and vaginal cancer.
- FIGO classifications for vulval and vaginal cancer.
- Understand the importance of histological type.
- Indications, techniques, complications and outcomes of surgery and radiotherapy for vulval and vaginal cancer.

### Clinical competency

- Recognize, counsel and plan initial management of vulval and vaginal cancer.

## INTRODUCTION

Vulval and vaginal cancers are rare, accounting for about 1000 new cases per year in the United Kingdom. It is important to recognize the symptoms and signs associated with these cancers to make an early diagnosis. As in all cancers, appropriate treatment at an early stage in the disease will lead to a better outcome for the patient, as reported by a population-based study of a series of 411 women in the West Midlands [D].[1] Most of the evidence for the management of these cancers is derived from case-controlled series, and the rarity of these tumours is a major obstacle in undertaking randomized trials.

## VULVAL CANCER

Vulval cancer is a disease primarily of the older age group, with the majority of cases presenting between the ages of 60 and 75.[2] An increasing proportion with this disease presenting in women below 50 years and therefore this diagnosis must always be borne in mind. Approximately 800 new cases of vulval cancer are diagnosed in the UK each year. The incidence has remained steady over the past three to four decades despite the increasing recognition of patients with vulval intraepithelial neoplasia (VIN) treatment of which will prevent some cancers. The majority (90–95 per cent) of vulval carcinomas are of squamous origin, although adenocarcinomas can arise from the Bartholin's gland and also in conjunction with Paget's disease of the vulva. Melanoma of the vulva is the second most common malignancy arising in the vulva, but is very rare. Basal cell and verrucous carcinomas also occur in the vulva.

## Aetiology

### Pathology

Certain pre-existing vulval dermatoses are known to be associated with the development of vulval carcinoma. Vulval intraepithelial neoplasia is often found in association with vulval cancer and VIN3 is accepted as a pre-invasive condition. The risk of this condition progressing to invasive cancer is highly variable, according to the literature. In women who have previously been treated for VIN, the risk is estimated at between 7 and 8 per cent,[3] whereas in one study in which women remained untreated, the progression rate of VIN to invasive cancer was 80 per cent at 10 years [D].[4] Lichen sclerosus is a common vulval inflammatory dermatosis usually affecting older women and is generally thought to carry a chance of malignant progression, although the exact risk is unknown because the ascertainment of lichen sclerosis is inexact. Women with lichen sclerosus who develop differentiated VIN are at increased risk of progressing to invasive cancer. Extramammary Paget's disease of the vulva is a rare form of VIN and is occasionally associated with cancer of the apocrine gland.

### Molecular biology

Unlike differentiated VIN, so-called basiloid VIN contains high HPV DNA. Approximately 40 per cent of all vulval cancers are associated with human papillomavirus (HPV), usually type 16, and about 80–90 per cent of these vulval cancers develop in women under the age of 50. Variations in the cell-cycle regulatory protein p53 are reported in approximately 30 per cent of cancers and for the remainder, there currently appears to be no aetiological or molecular biological event. Recent studies have shown similar molecular changes, including alterations in p53 expression, to be present in both vulval cancer and surrounding lichen sclerosus.

Smoking may be an important cofactor in the development of HPV-related VIN and is linked to a lower survival rate for women with vulval cancer.

---

## KEY POINTS

### Vulval cancer: epidemiology and pathology

- Vulval cancer is uncommon and most evidence arises from observational studies and case series.
- Population-based observational studies confirm better outcomes with early detection.
- There appear to be different aetiologies: one linked to infection with oncogenic HPV and another linked to pre-existing vulval maturation disorders.
- The reported malignant potential of VIN varies between 5 and 80 per cent. This probably reflects the variations in the observational studies rather than a widely varying biological effect.

---

## Diagnosis

Women with vulval cancer usually present with symptoms, although an asymptomatic mass may be an unusual presentation, occasionally it presents as an enlarged groin lymph node. The associated symptoms are usually vulval soreness and itching and there may be a mass that is painful and bleeds. Investigation of post-menopausal bleeding should always include examination of the vulva. The most common site of involvement is the labium majus (about 50 per cent of cases). The labium minus accounts for 15–20 per cent of cases. The clitoris and Bartholin's glands are less frequently involved. In the majority of cases, a vulval cancer is obvious to the alert clinician, but very early cancers may be clinically indistinguishable from florid warty VIN.

## Investigations

When women present with vulval symptoms, a full clinical examination should be performed, paying particular attention to palpation of the groins for lymphadenopathy. A full-thickness biopsy should be taken from the tumour and should include the interface between the apparent normal surrounding tissue and the cancer. This allows for the most accurate histological interpretation and for the depth of invasion to be assessed, which is important in determining the future management. The cervix should be visualized to exclude a cervical cancer, which may occasionally coexist.

Assessment of the inguinal glands is not absolutely reliable with any imaging technique at present, but should there be a clinical or radiological suspicion of inguinal lymph node enlargement, a computed tomography (CT) or magnetic resonance (MR) assessment of the pelvis should be undertaken to exclude obvious pelvic lymphadenopathy.

## Treatment

There is increasing emphasis placed on the individualization of treatment for women with vulval cancer. In deciding the optimum treatment, it is best to consider early and advanced vulval cancers separately and to manage the primary lesion and the regional lymph glands on individual merit. Because of the rarity of vulval cancer, and the need for careful assessment to optimize both vulval preservation and care, these women should be managed by specialized gynaecological oncologists in cancer centres. In addition to imaging, the pathological assessment of these tumours is extremely important in forming decisions about adjuvant treatment.

### Early stage vulval cancer

#### Primary lesion

Treatment of the primary lesion is in part determined by the risk of local vulval recurrence and the risk of groin node involvement at the time of diagnosis. A retrospective surgical–pathological study of 135 cases found that if a pathological disease-free margin of 8 mm can be achieved, the risk of local recurrence is zero [D].[5] Therefore, the primary lesion should be excised with a 1 cm disease-free margin, including the deep margin. The 1 cm margin will allow for tissue shrinkage due to fixation of the specimen. In most early cancers, this can be achieved by a wide radical local excision and will allow for the preservation of non-involved structures. If the primary lesion is associated with a vulval maturation disorder or VIN, this may be removed as well. However, if the VIN is very widespread, this could necessitate a very large excision requiring myocutaneous flaps. Under these circumstances, it may not be considered essential to remove all VIN as part of the primary surgical procedure to remove a carcinoma.

#### Regional lymph nodes

Depth of invasion is the best predictor of risk of nodal metastasis in vulval cancer.

The most recent staging criteria for vulval cancer (Table 71.1) has recognized the concept of micro-invasive or superficially invasive vulval cancer (Stage Ia), as the risk of nodal involvement in tumours with depth of invasion <1 mm is virtually zero [D].[6] These tumours may therefore be treated by wide local excision alone.

#### Lateral vulval tumours

The management of regional lymph nodes can be modified for patients presenting with lateral vulval tumours. Although

**Table 71.1** FIGO staging of vulval cancer 2009

| FIGO classification | Description |
|---|---|
| Stage I | Tumour confined to the vulva |
| Stage Ia | Lesions ≤ 2cm in size, confined to the vulva or perineum and with stromal invasion ≤ 1mm. No nodal metastasis |
| Stage Ib | Lesions > 2cm in size or with stromal invasion > 1mm confined to the vulva or perineum. No nodal metastasis |
| Stage II | Tumour of any size with extension to adjacent perineal structures (lower 1/3 urethra; lower 1/3 vagina; anus) with negative nodes |
| Stage III | Tumour of any size with or without extension to adjacent perineal structures (lower 1/3 urethra; lower 1/3 vagina; anus) with positive inguinofemoral nodes |
| IIIa | (i) With 1 lymph node metastasis (≥ 5mm), or (ii) 1-2 lymph node metastasis(es) (< 5mm) |
| IIIb | (i) With 2 or more lymph node metastasis (≥ 5mm), or (ii) 3 or more lymph node metastasis(es) (< 5mm) |
| IIIc | With positive nodes with extracapsular spread |
| Stage IV | Tumour invades other regional (upper 2/3 urethra; 2/3 vagina) or distant structures |
| IVa | Tumour invades any of the following (i) Upper urethral and or vaginal mucosa; bladder mucosa; rectal mucosa or fixed to pelvic bone, or (ii) Fixed or ulcerated inguinofemoral lymph nodes. |
| IVb | Any distant metastasis including pelvic lymph nodes |

there is extensive lymphatic crossover in the midline of the vulva, lateral tumours (i.e. those with the medial border at least 2 cm lateral to a line drawn between the clitoris and the anus) require only an ipsilateral inguinal node dissection. If the ipsilateral nodes are negative, the contralateral nodes are rarely involved [D].[7] However, should these nodes be positive, a contralateral node dissection should be undertaken. In a prospective trial, the outcome for 26 women who underwent ipsilateral lateral groin node dissection alone was similar when compared with historical controls [C].[8]

## Inguinal node dissection

Surgical dissection of inguinal nodes is considered mandatory in early-stage vulval cancer when depth of invasion is greater than 1 mm. A randomized trial comparing inguinal node dissection with radiotherapy to the groin in women with clinically normal inguinal nodes found a survival advantage in favour of the surgical arm. However, this trial has been criticized because an inadequate dose of radiotherapy was given to the inguinal nodes.[9] A subsequent systematic review of only three eligible studies suggested that surgery is superior to radiotherapy [A].[10]

Attempts have been made to reduce the morbidity associated with this procedure. Unfortunately, superficial inguinal node dissection, which removes only the lymph nodes above the cribriform fascia, is associated with a higher rate of inguinal recurrence compared with inguinofemoral node dissection, which removes tissue below the cribriform fascia and medial to the femoral vein. In a prospective clinical trial, 155 women underwent a superficial inguinal node dissection and although the overall survival rate was the same compared with a series of historical controls, the rate of inguinal node recurrence was significantly higher.[8] It is therefore recommended that a full dissection should still be performed in cases of early vulval cancer [C]. The routine removal of pelvic lymph nodes in early stage vulval cancer is not recommended. Recent data have suggested that by sparing the long saphenous vein, the short- and long-term morbidity associated with lymphoedema may be reduced [D].

Another approach to reduce morbidity is the identification and removal of the sentinel node. The concept depends on the sentinel node (i.e. the first node to drain the vulval tumour) being identified and, if histologically normal, the remainder of the inguinal lymph node dissection could be omitted. The most reliable technique is probably a hybrid of pre-operative intralesional injection of radiolabelled technetium combined with intralesion injection of blue dye at the time of surgery and scanning of the nodal tissue for a radioactive signal. In the collected series to date, the sentinel node – the anatomical location of which is highly variable – has been identified in almost 100 per cent of cases and there have been only a very few cases reported in which the sentinel node was normal but other nodes were positive for tumour [C].[11] In a recently published report, a sentinel node procedure was performed in 623 groins of 403 women with squamous cancer of the vulva. Out of 259 women with unifocal disease and negative sentinel node, six developed groin recurrence (2.3 per cent). Women who had a positive sentinel node and underwent a full groin excision experienced significantly more morbidity. The current study, GROINSS-VII, is evaluating a protocol in which women with negative nodes have no further groin surgery and those with a positive sentinel node are offered radiation therapy without full groin dissection.[12]

## Advanced vulval cancer

Women in whom the cancer has spread beyond the vulva will benefit from a multimodality approach to their management.

Neoadjuvant chemotherapy and radiotherapy can be used to shrink the tumour and so permit surgery, which may preserve urethral and anal sphincter function. Reconstructive surgery can potentially reduce physical morbidity by filling large tissue defects and may reduce psychological morbidity as well.

## Surgery to the primary lesion

The size and location of the tumour will influence the surgical approach to the primary lesion. The surgical goal is to remove the tumour with at least a 1 cm disease-free margin. In the majority of cases, a triple incision technique can be employed. Several clinical series have shown that the incidence of skin bridge recurrence between the primary lesion and the inguinal node dissection is low, even if there is evidence of lymphatic channel involvement [D].[13] However, if there is evidence of tumour within the skin bridge between the primary tumour and the inguinal nodes at the time of surgery, a radical vulvectomy with en-bloc inguinal node dissection should be considered. If extensive areas of vulval tissue need to be removed, reconstructive surgery with the use of skin grafts or myocutaneous flaps may be required to achieve healing.

## Management of inguinal nodes

In cases in which there is clinical suspicion of inguinal node involvement, an inguinal node dissection should be undertaken. As stated above, if there is concern about lymphatic permeation, an en-bloc dissection should be considered. In cases in which the nodes are fixed or ulcerated, biopsy of these or fine-needle aspiration should be considered, followed by radiotherapy to the inguinal and pelvic lymph nodes. Surgical removal of large inguinal or pelvic nodes should be attempted if feasible, since standard radiotherapy doses to the inguinal nodes may be inadequate to bring about a complete regression.

> ### KEY POINTS
> #### Surgical management of vulval cancer
> - Vulval cancer should be managed in cancer centres.
> - Vulval tumours should be excised with a minimum margin of 10 mm of normal epithelium. This will vary from a wide local excision to radical vulvectomy, depending on the size of the tumour and the nature of adjacent epithelium.
> - Lymphadenectomy is required for all but superficially invasive squamous tumours.
> - Routine lymphadenectomy is not required for basal cell and verrucous carcinomas and melanomas.
> - Lateral tumours initially require only ipsilateral lymphadenectomy.

> - Formal inguino-femoral lymphadenectomy remains the procedure of choice.
> - A triple incision technique will suffice, unless there is evidence of skin bridge involvement at the outset, when an en-bloc approach should be used.
> - Pelvic lymphadenectomy is not routinely used in the treatment of vulval cancer.
> - Advanced disease requires a multimodality approach.

# MANAGEMENT OF OTHER VULVAL CANCERS

Basal cell carcinomas and verrucous carcinomas of the vulva are usually only superficially invasive to a depth of 1 mm and are rarely associated with lymph node metastases. These tumours can be adequately managed by means of a wide local excision. Basal cell carcinomas can be treated with radiotherapy if surgery would compromise the sphincter function, but this is rarely necessary.

Melanomas of the vulva should be managed by wide local excision. Inguinal node dissection does not influence outcome in these cases, and management should be determined as for the criteria for other sites of cutaneous melanoma.

Cancer can develop within the Bartholin's gland and may be either squamous or adenocarcinoma. Its management is the same as for squamous vulval cancer.

## Neoadjuvant therapy

Radiotherapy may be given pre-operatively to the primary lesion to allow for tumour shrinkage. This is particularly useful if primary surgery would necessitate removal of the urethral or anal sphincters. A total maximum dose of 55 Gy may be given with concurrent 5-fluorouracil (5-FU). Subsequent tumour shrinkage may then enable the preservation of sphincters.

## Radical chemoradiotherapy with curative intent

Radical radiotherapy with chemotherapy may be used as an alternative to surgery in the management of advanced squamous vulval carcinomas. There are no published data comparing surgery with chemoradiotherapy in the primary treatment of vulval cancer. Radical radiotherapy alone in the UK has usually been confined to patients who decline surgery or in whom medical morbidity prevents surgery. The recommended dose of radiotherapy is 65 Gy with concurrent 5-FU and cisplatin. In a study of 14 women who were not candidates for standard surgery (nine stage III and five stage IV), nine (64 per cent) had a complete response to radiation (50–65 Gy) in combination with cisplatin (50 mg/m$^2$) and 5-FU (100 mg/m$^2$ per 24 hours for four days).[14]

## Adjuvant radiotherapy

### Surgical margins

Post-operative radiotherapy should be considered in patients with close or positive surgical margins. There is no minimum disease-free margin at which radiotherapy should be considered. However, patients with <8 mm of disease-free margin have a 57 per cent chance of disease recurrence.[4] Where possible, consideration should be given to re-excision of the vulva to improve the disease-free margin rather than radiotherapy [E].

### Inguinal nodes

Post-operative radiotherapy should be considered in patients who have nodal involvement with metastatic disease. Several case series have found that prognosis is only affected when two or more nodes are involved [D]. The presence of extra-capsular spread in any lymph node is an adverse factor and warrants adjuvant treatment [D]. Adjuvant radiotherapy should be confined to the affected side and should also include pelvic nodes. In a randomized trial comparing adjuvant pelvic radiotherapy with pelvic lymphadenectomy, in 114 women with positive inguinal nodes, there was a significant survival advantage (68 versus 54 per cent at two years) in favour of radiotherapy [B].[15] A total dose of radiotherapy between 45 and 50 Gy without 5-FU is recommended.

> ### KEY POINTS
>
> **Non-surgical management of vulval cancer**
>
> - Vulval tumours can be treated by primary radical radiotherapy if surgery is declined or not possible.
> - Adjuvant radiotherapy is recommended when surgical margins are inadequate (<8 mm) if re-excision might compromise function.
> - Radiotherapy to the groin and pelvic node sites is recommended if more than one node is involved or there is evidence of any extracapsular spread.
> - Radiotherapy may be used prior to surgery to attempt to reduce the morbidity and functional loss associated with surgery in large lesions.
> - Radiotherapy with concurrent chemotherapy may improve outcome, but as yet there are no data in support of this approach.

## Treatment-related morbidity

A more conservative approach to the management of vulval cancer and individualization of care have led to a reduction in the treatment-related morbidity. However, there still remains a significant rate of wound infection and wound breakdown. Lymphoedema of the legs is a major cause of long-term morbidity and there are also high levels of psychological and psychosexual morbidity associated with the disfiguring nature of the surgery employed. Radiation can induce long lasting effects and when combined with lymphadenectomy, significantly increases the risk of lymphoedema.

## Morbidity associated with recurrent disease

Recurrent disease affecting the vulva itself should be managed by further surgical excision and, if necessary, radiotherapy. Recurrence involving the inguinal nodes or pelvic nodes should be treated with radiotherapy. However, this can usually only be palliative, and most patients with groin recurrence die of disease.

## Follow up of treated patients

Patients should be followed up on a three-monthly basis for the first two years following treatment, as this allows for the detection of early recurrence and the management of treatment-related morbidity. Once they have completed two years of follow up, they may be seen six monthly for the following three years.

## VAGINAL CANCER

Vaginal cancers are rare gynaecological tumours accounting for only 1–2 per cent of all gynaecological cancers. The majority of vaginal cancers are squamous in origin (about 85 per cent), but adenocarcinoma can also develop in young women and is associated with a higher incidence of metastatic disease to the lymph nodes and lungs. Melanoma and sarcomas are rare causes of vaginal cancer. Clear-cell adeno- carcinomas of the vagina are linked to women with a history of *in-utero* exposure to diethylstilbestrol (DES). An increased incidence of this tumour was first reported in the mid-1970s, but there has been a steady decline in its incidence over recent years with the withdrawal of DES from clinical practice.

## Aetiology

Little is known about the aetiology of vaginal cancer, but it is presumed to share similarities with vulval and cervical cancer and usually contains high risk HPV DNA, especially type 16. Vaginal intraepthelial neoplasia grade 3 (VaIN) is a recognized precancerous condition affecting the vagina and it is frequently seen in combination with cervical intraepithelial neoplasia (CIN). It may occur in one of two ways: as a lateral extension of CIN out on to the vaginal fornices at the time of treatment for CIN, or in women who have previously undergone hysterectomy for CIN, which was incompletely excised by this procedure. In these latter cases, the VaIN is often found within the surgical margin of the vaginal vault. The percentage of women who present with this condition and who subsequently develop vaginal cancer is unknown, but there is a significant risk of invasive disease. Factors that influence the outcome of vaginal cancer are the size of the tumour and the age of the patient.

## Diagnosis

The diagnosis of vaginal cancer may be suspected at the time of colposcopic examination of the vagina. An adequate biopsy, which includes the entire thickness of vaginal epithelium, should be obtained for histological confirmation. This is important, as the depth of invasion of the tumour into the vaginal mucosa and muscle is significant in the staging of the disease (Table 71.2). A diagnosis of cancer of the vagina can only be made with certainty in the presence of a normal cervix or following total hysterectomy, as described above.

## Investigations

The cervix should be carefully examined if still *in situ* to exclude cervical involvement. An MRI of the pelvis will help to determine the extent of any spread from the vagina and also the status of the regional pelvic nodes.

## Treatment

In planning definitive treatment, consideration should be given not only to the stage of disease at presentation, but also to the size and location of the tumour. Surgery in combination with pelvic radiotherapy, when appropriate, can be effective in the management of stage I and II disease, with survival rates of 68 and 48 per cent respectively [D].[15]

**Table 71.2** Staging of vaginal cancer

| FIGO | Description | TNM |
|------|-------------|-----|
| I | Tumour confined to vagina | $T_1N_0M_0$ |
| II | Tumour invades paravaginal tissues, but not to pelvic sidewall | $T_2N_0M_0$ |
| III | Tumour extends to pelvic sidewall | $T_1N_1M_0$ |
| | | $T_2N_1M_0$ |
| | | $T_3N_0M_0$ |
| | | $T_3N_1M_0$ |
| IVa | Tumour invades mucosa of bladder or rectum and/or extends beyond the true pelvis | $T_4$, any N, $M_0$ |
| IVb | All cases with distant metastases | Any T, any N, $M_1$ |

• FIGO, International Federation of Gynecology and Obstetrics classification; TNM, tumour, nodes, metastases; Union Internationale Contre le Cancer (UICC).

## Stage I vaginal cancer

### Tumours <0.5 cm deep
Early vaginal cancer may be managed either by surgery or by intracavity radiotherapy. Surgery should include wide local excision or total vaginectomy with reconstruction of the vagina where possible. Intracavity treatment with 60–70 Gy to the tumour should be given and in cases where the tumour lies within the lower third of the vagina, external beam radiotherapy to the pelvic and inguinal lymph nodes should be considered.

### Tumours >0.5 cm deep
Surgery for this condition should include wide vaginectomy, pelvic lymphadenectomy and reconstruction of the vagina where possible. For lesions in the lower third of the vagina, inguinal lymphadenectomy should be performed as well. Radiotherapy for this condition should be a combination of brachytherapy to the tumour and external beam radiotherapy to the pelvic and inguinal nodes if the tumour is present in the lower third of the vagina.

Although surgery or radiotherapy can be used in the primary management of stage I disease, the usual practice in the UK has been to offer radiotherapy, which has the advantage of vaginal preservation.

## Stage II vaginal cancer

Radical surgery can be considered for this condition and should include radical vaginectomy with lymph node dissection or possibly pelvic exenteration. Radiotherapy may also be used, with a combination of brachytherapy to the tumour and external beam radiotherapy to the pelvic and inguinal lymph nodes.

## Stage III and IV vaginal cancer

These cases should be managed by a combination of brachytherapy to the primary tumour and external beam radiotherapy to the pelvis and inguinal lymph nodes.

## Morbidity

The treatment-related morbidity can be significant. Sexual dysfunction due to vaginal atrophy and damage to the bladder and rectum are not infrequent. Recurrent vaginal cancer can be treated with radical pelvic radiotherapy if recurring after surgery. If disease recurs after radiotherapy, palliative surgery may be possible in selected cases.

## Follow up

Patients should be followed up on a three-monthly basis for the first two years following treatment, as this allows for the detection of early recurrence and the management of treatment-related morbidity. Once they have completed two years of follow up, they may be seen six monthly for the following three years.

## SUMMARY

Vulval and vaginal cancers are rare and affect older women. Individualization of care has led to a reduction in morbidity without affecting cure rates. Multimodality treatment is often required in advanced cases. All vulval and vaginal cancers should be managed at a cancer centre.

## Published Guidelines

Royal College of Obstetricians and Gynaecologists. *Management of Vulval Cancer*. London: RCOG, 2006.

## Key References

1. Rhodes CA, Cummins C, Shafi MI. The management of squamous cell vulval cancer: a population based retrospective study of 411 cases. *Br J Obstet Gynaecol* 1998; **105**: 200–5.
2. Vulval cancer incidence by age. Last accessed 12 April 2010. Available from : ‹http://info.canceresearchuk.org/cancerstats/types/vulva/incidence/index.htm#vulva2›.
3. Herod JJ, Shafi MI, Rollason TP *et al*. Vulvar intraepithelial neoplasia: long term follow up of treated and untreated women. *Br J Obstet Gynaecol* 1996; **103**: 446–52.
4. Jones RW, Baranyai J, Stables S. Trends in squamous cell carcinoma of the vulva: the influence of vulvar intraepithelial neoplasia. *Obstet Gynecol* 1997; **90**: 448–52.
5. Heaps JM, Yao SF, Montz FJ *et al*. Surgical–pathological variables predictive of local recurrence in squamous cell carcinoma of the vulva. *Gynecol Oncol* 1990; **38**: 309–14.
6. Sedlis A, Homesley H, Bundy BN *et al*. Positive groin lymph nodes in superficial squamous cell vulvar cancer: a Gynecologic Oncology Group study. *Am J Obstet Gynecol* 1987; **156**: 1159–64.
7. Homesley HD, Bundy BN, Sedlis A *et al*. Assessment of current International Federation of Gynecology and Obstetrics staging of vulvar carcinoma relative to prognostic factors for survival (a Gynecologic Oncology Group study). *Am J Obstet Gynecol* 1991; **164**: 997–1004.
8. Stehman FB, Bundy BN, Dvoretsky PM *et al*. Early stage I carcinoma of the vulva treated with ipsilateral superficial inguinal lymphadenectomy and modified radical hemivulvectomy: a prospective study of the Gynecologic Oncology Group. *Obstet Gynecol* 1992; **79**: 490–7.
9. Stehman FB, Bundy BN, Thomas G. Groin dissection versus groin radiation in carcinoma of the vulva: a Gynecologic Oncology Group study. *Int J Rad Oncol Biol Phys* 1992; **24**: 389–96.
10. van der Velden J, Ansink A. Primary groin irradiation vs primary surgery for early vulvar cancer. *Cochrane Database Syst Rev* 2006; (**3**): CD002224.
11. Ayhan A, Celik H, Dursun P. Lymphatic mapping and sentinel node biopsy in gynaecological cancers: a critical review of the literature. *W J Surgical Oncol* 2008; **6**: 53–65.
12. Van der Zee AGJ, Oonk MW, De Hulla JA *et al*. Sentinel node dissection is safe in the treatment of early-stage vulval cancer. *J Clin Oncol* 2008; **26**: 884–9.
13. Hacker NF, Leuchter RS, Berek JS *et al*. Radical vulvectomy and bilateral inguinal lymphadenectomy through separate groin incisions. *Obstet Gynecol* 1981; **58**: 574–9.
14. Cunningham MJ, Goyer RP, Gibbons SK *et al*. Primary radiation, cisplatin, and 5-fluorouracil for advanced aquamous carcinoma of the vulva. *Gynecol Oncol* 1997; **66**: 258–61.
15. Homesley HD, Bundy BN, Sedlis A, Adcock L. Radiation therapy versus pelvic node resection for carcinoma of the vulva with positive groin nodes. *Obstet Gynecol* 1986; **68**: 733–9.
16. Tjalma WAA, Monaghan JM, Lopes AB *et al*. The role of surgery in invasive squamous carcinoma of the vagina. *Gynecol Oncol* 2001; **81**: 360–5.

# Gestational trophoblastic disease

*Barry W Hancock*

---

## MRCOG standards

### Theoretical skills

- Understand the pathogenesis.
- Have good knowledge of gynaecological diagnosis and management.
- Have an appreciation of the needs for monitoring and/or medical intervention.

### Practical skills

- Be able to counsel a woman with gestational trophoblastic disease.
- Be able to recognize the clinical features of gestational trophoblastic disease.
- Be able to perform evacuation of molar pregnancy under supervision.

## INTRODUCTION

Gestational trophoblastic disease (GTD) is an uncommon complication of pregnancy. An average consultant obstetrician may deal with only one new case every second year.

The term 'gestational trophoblastic disease' describes a group of inter-related diseases, including complete and partial molar pregnancy, choriocarcinoma and placental site trophoblastic tumour, which vary in their propensity for local invasion and metastasis. Although persistent GTD (now often termed gestational trophoblastic neoplasia (GTN)) most commonly follows a molar pregnancy, it may also be seen after any type of gestation, including term pregnancy, abortion and ectopic pregnancy. Gestational trophoblastic tumours produce human chorionic gonadotrophin (hCG), which is important in the diagnosis, management and follow up of these patients, providing an example of an 'ideal' tumour marker. The first complete responses to methotrexate chemotherapy were described in the 1950s, and presently almost 100 per cent of patients are cured.

## EPIDEMIOLOGY

The incidence of hydatidiform mole is difficult to assess accurately, but appears to be gradually increasing. As GTD follows all kinds of pregnancies, the denominator for the incidence should ideally include all live births, stillbirths, abortions and ectopic pregnancies. The accepted convention, however, has been to report incidence data according to the live-birth rate. Furthermore, reports from different countries often use different denominators, and figures for hospital-based populations are likely to overestimate the incidence compared with community-based figures, particularly in developing countries. Under-reporting may also occur, especially but not uniquely, in communities where medical attention is suboptimal.

Worldwide, the incidence of GTD reportedly varies between 0.5 and 8.3 cases per 1000 live births.[1] The UK figure is approximately 1.5 per 1000 births.[2] In contrast, the incidence is approximately twice as high in some Asian countries and also in native American Indians. There is also a significantly higher incidence in Asian women living in the UK.[3]

Maternal age appears to be the most consistent risk factor associated with molar gestation. Age-specific incidence reports usually reveal a 'J curve', with extremes of reproductive life associated with an increased incidence. Pregnancies below the age of 15 years have a moderately increased risk, whereas those occurring over the age of 50 years are associated with a substantially increased risk. This increased incidence in the youngest and oldest age groups seems to be a consistent finding in all regions and races.

Women who have had a previous mole have an increased risk of further molar pregnancies. Following one mole, the risk is less than 2 per cent, but following two molar pregnancies it increases substantially up to one in six; following three moles the risk may be as high as one in two. Occasionally, family clusters have been seen, implicating an underlying genetic disorder in such cases.

**Table 72.1** Risk factors for gestational trophoblastic disease (GTD)

| Risk factor | |
|---|---|
| Age | ↑ <16 years, ↑↑↑ >45 years |
| Geographic | ↑ Asia |
| Ethnicity | ↑ American Indians, ↑ Asians |
| Previous GTD | ↑ one episode, ↑↑↑ two or more episodes |
| Dietary | ↑ carotene deficiency |
| Genetic | Rare family clusters and repetitive moles |

Nutritional and socioeconomic factors also appear to be risk factors for molar pregnancy in some populations. For example, low dietary intake of carotene and animal fat may be associated with an increased incidence of complete mole (Table 72.1).

In Europe and North America, choriocarcinoma following a complete hydatidiform mole (CHM) is of the order of 3 per cent. Hydatidiform mole is the most common antecedent to choriocarcinoma, with abortion or ectopic pregnancy being the next most common, followed by live births.[2] Although initially the risk of progression of choriocarcinoma from a partial mole was thought to be negligible, recent reports have shown a small but real risk of malignant transformation. In addition, choriocarcinoma occurs more frequently in women of older reproductive years.

## PATHOLOGICAL FEATURES

Hydatidiform mole may be complete or partial and the histopathological features differ (Table 72.2).[4] Complete mole is recognized by the presence of characteristic grape-like structures, which represent swollen chorionic villi, and the absence of a viable fetus. The conceptus is entirely paternally derived and is a total allograft within the mother. The chorionic villi are diffusely hydropic and enveloped by hyperplasic and atypical trophoblast. Complete moles are usually diploid, the most common type being 46XX; in most cases, a haploid sperm divides within an ovum without a nucleus. In contrast, partial moles usually have recognizable embryonic and fetal tissues, with focal hydropic swelling of the chorionic villi and focal trophoblastic hyperplasia. Partial moles are generally triploid, for example 69XXY; they result most often from dispermic fertilization of normal ova. When a fetus is present it often has the features of triploidy, including growth retardation and multiple congenital malformations (Figure 72.1).

In current-day practice, the earlier evacuation of suspected molar pregnancies has meant that there is more likelihood of misdiagnosis. Complete moles are now often characterized by subtle morphological abnormalities that may result in their misclassification as partial moles or non-molar abortions.

**Table 72.2** Pathological features of hydatidiform mole – a comparison between complete and partial mole

| | Complete | Partial |
|---|---|---|
| Macroscopic | Often recognizable, with characteristic grape-like structures | Can resemble hydropic abortion; may have recognizable fetal tissues |
| Microscopic | Diffusely hydropic villi | Focal hydropic swelling of villi |
| | Atypical and hyperplastic trophoblast | Focal trophoblastic hyperplasia |
| | Usually diagnosable from uterine products | Often misdiagnosed as hydropic abortion or complete mole |
| Karyotype | Usually diploid (paternally derived) | Usually triploid (maternal contribution) |

Triploidy is a more common abnormality than androgenetic complete mole and, if most triploids are paternally derived, it would be expected that partial moles should be at least twice as common as complete moles. However, many studies have reported that complete mole is more common than partial mole, suggesting underdiagnosis of the latter. In a UK study, only a third of histologically confirmed moles registered were partial moles.[4] Expert review of referred cases suggested that up to one-half of partial moles are in fact either complete moles or hydropic abortions, which mirrors the experience of others.

The clinical entity of invasive mole occurs when a complete or, less commonly, a partial mole invades deeply into the myometrium (Figure 72.2).

Gestational choriocarcinoma is the malignant form of GTD and may originate from a previous hydatidiform mole or from a normal conception. The definitive histopathological diagnosis of choriocarcinoma requires the demonstration of a dimorphic population of both cytotrophoblast and syncytiotrophoblast without the presence of formed chorionic villi, plus evidence of myometrial invasion. However, because of the availability of a sensitive tumour marker, the majority of patients are treated without the benefit of a histological diagnosis. Gestational choriocarcinoma metastasizes widely, particularly to the lungs, pelvic organs and brain (Figure 72.3).

## CLINICAL FEATURES

The majority of patients with CHM are diagnosed prior to 16 weeks of gestation, or often earlier nowadays. Abnormal vaginal bleeding during pregnancy is the usual means of presentation and this may be associated with anaemia.

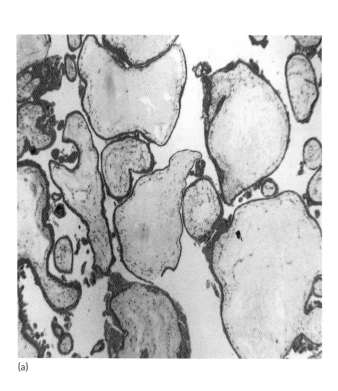

(a)

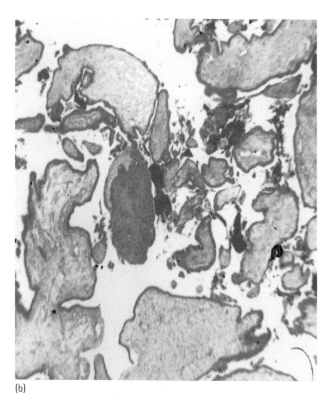

(b)

**Figure 72.1** Histological appearances of complete (a) and partial (b) mole. (a) 46XX, paternal. Haploid sperm fertilizes empty ovum and undergoes cytogenesis; diploid sperm fertilizes empty ovum. (b) Triploid: 69,XXY 69,XXX or 69,XYY. Defective zona pellucidum; dispermic fertilization of haploid ovum

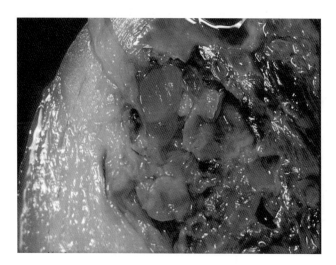

**Figure 72.2** Macroscopic appearance of invasive mole

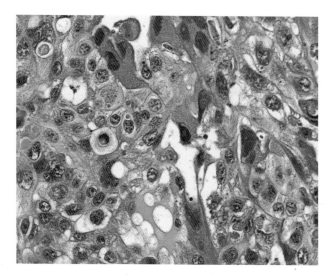

**Figure 72.3** Histological appearance of gestational choriocarcinoma

The clinical presentation of CHM has changed considerably over the past few decades. Excessive uterine size, anaemia, hyperemesis, pre-eclampsia, theca lutein cysts, hyperthyroidism and metastatic disease are seen far less often, except in countries with less well-developed healthcare systems.

Invasive mole can produce heavy bleeding, lower abdominal pain or intraperitoneal haemorrhage. Occasionally, the bladder or rectum is infiltrated, producing haematuria or rectal bleeding. Invasive moles may regress spontaneously or they may embolize, particularly to the lungs, but they do not usually exhibit the progression of true malignancy.

The clinical features of partial mole are less severe than those of complete mole (Table 72.3) and this condition is frequently diagnosed on histological review of curettings

**Table 72.3** Clinical features of hydatidiform mole: a comparison between complete and partial mole

|  | Complete | Partial |
|---|---|---|
| Features | May be severe and/or accompanied by paraneoplastic sequelae | Often mild, resembling spontaneous miscarriage |
| Diagnosis | Usually suspected on clinical or ultrasound scan findings | Often unsuspected and retrospectively diagnosed after uterine evacuation |
| Persistent trophoblastic disease | In up to 20% of cases | In <0.5% of cases |

from what appeared clinically to be a miscarriage. Even in earlier studies, increased uterine size, theca lutein cysts and pre-eclampsia were seen in only a small percentage of cases.[5]

## DIAGNOSTIC INVESTIGATIONS

The increasing use of ultrasound in early pregnancy has probably led to earlier diagnosis of moles. While the ultrasound diagnosis of complete mole is usually reliable, that of partial mole is more difficult. In complete mole, a 'classic' pattern is seen, consisting of multiple small sonolucencies representing the numerous hydropic villi. The finding of multiple cystic spaces in the placenta and a ratio of above 1.5 in the transverse to anteroposterior dimension are suggestive of partial mole.[6] Fetal parts may be seen, but this also occurs in mole with coexistent normal fetus. In over half of cases, the diagnosis of partial mole is not made by ultrasound. In locally invasive moles, increased areas of echogenicity are seen within the myometrium. Transvaginal ultrasound has allowed very early diagnosis in some cases.

Trophoblastic disease is virtually unique in that it produces a specific marker (hCG) which can be measured in urine and/or blood and correlates precisely with the amount of disease present. Human chorionic gonadotrophin is a large placental glycoprotein composed of two peptide subunits and is produced naturally during pregnancy. The alpha subunit is similar to those of other pituitary glycoprotein hormones, but the beta subunit is specific to hCG alone. Higher than normal levels of hCG (particularly when >200 000 IU/L) are suggestive of molar pregnancy, although levels with partial mole are only infrequently above the range for normal pregnancy. As a diagnostic marker for molar pregnancy, hCG measurement is therefore of limited value. It exists in a number of forms (e.g. nicked hCG, hCG missing the beta subunit C-terminal segment, hyperglycosylated hCG and free beta subunit) and

when it is measured in trophoblastic disease it is important that the assay being used detects all main forms of hCG and its beta subunit fragments.[7]

## EVACUATION OF MOLAR PREGNANCY

Suction curettage is the method of choice for evacuation of complete molar pregnancies[8] because of the lack of fetal parts, a suction catheter of up to 12 mm is usually sufficient. Sharp curettage is now not generally recommended because of the possibility of uterine perforation and of increasing the risk of Asherman's syndrome (uterine synechiae). Medical termination of complete mole should be avoided where possible. There is a theoretical concern about the routine use of potent oxytocic agents because of the possibility of forcing trophoblastic tissue into the venous spaces of the placental bed and disseminating disease to the lungs. It is recommended that, when necessary, oxytocic therapy is only commenced once evacuation is complete. If there is significant haemorrhage prior to or during evacuation and some degree of control is needed, such agents may be used according to clinical judgement. It is also suggested that prostaglandin analogues should be reserved for cases for which oxytocic therapy is ineffective. Since evacuation of a large mole is a rare event, advice and help from an experienced colleague should be sought where appropriate. In partial molar pregnancies where the size of fetal parts deters the use of suction curettage, medical termination can be used. Data from the management of molar pregnancies with mifepristone are incomplete; evacuation of complete mole with this agent may be best avoided, as it increases the sensitivity of the uterus to prostaglandins.

The difficulty in making the diagnosis of partial mole before evacuation mandates the histological assessment of material obtained from incomplete miscarriages. Also, since persistent trophoblastic disease may develop after any pregnancy, all products of conception, obtained after evacuation performed for persisting symptoms, should be histologically examined.

---

**EBM**

Though there is much published on evacuation of molar pregnancy, the above text reflects mainly UK expert opinion and practice [C].

---

## REGISTRATION

In the UK, a trophoblastic registration scheme has been in operation since it was initiated by the Royal College of Obstetricians and Gynaecologists in 1973. Three centres – in London (Charing Cross Hospital), Sheffield (Weston Park Hospital) and Dundee (Ninewells Hospital) – co-ordinate the registration and monitoring of all patients. However, only Charing Cross and Weston Park have the specialist facilities to offer appropriate chemotherapy.

Patients with the following should be registered:

- complete hydatidiform mole,
- partial hydatidiform mole,
- twin pregnancy with complete or partial hydatidiform mole,
- limited macroscopic or microscopic molar change judged to require follow up,
- choriocarcinoma, placental-site trophoblastic tumour, and atypical placental-site nodules.

## Twin molar pregnancy

The incidence of twin pregnancy with mole (usually complete) and viable fetus appears to be lower (<1 in 200 molar pregnancies) than twin pregnancy with viable fetuses (about 1 in 100 normal pregnancies). A successful pregnancy outcome occurs in about one-third of cases. Persistent trophoblastic disease requiring chemotherapy may be more frequent, but treatment is invariably successful (as for single molar pregnancies).[9] UK guidance is that 'in the situation of a twin pregnancy where there is one viable fetus and the other pregnancy is molar, the woman should be counselled about the increased risk of perinatal morbidity and outcome for GTN'.

## Ectopic molar pregnancy

As with normal pregnancy, hydatidiform mole may occur in ectopic sites, most often in the fallopian tube.[10] Tubal ectopic moles are rare and over-diagnosed, but strict follow up of confirmed cases is essential, as these are more likely to require chemotherapy for persistent disease [E].

## Persistent trophoblastic disease (gestational trophoblastic neoplasia)

In a proportion of patients (up to 10 per cent in the UK), trophoblastic disease persists, as evidenced by continuing clinical symptoms (particularly vaginal bleeding) and/or elevation of hCG levels. Excessive uterine size, markedly elevated hCG levels and prominent theca lutein cysts may predict persistent trophoblastic disease.

The UK surveillance scheme involves periodic assays of urine and/or serum hCG being performed for six months or longer, depending on when the hCG level reaches normal. This has ensured that the great majority of patients requiring chemotherapy for persistent disease are recognized early. We have been able to adopt a conservative approach using stringent criteria for the initiation of chemotherapy (Table 72.4). For example, whilst it is stressed that 'there is no clinical indication for the routine use of second uterine evacuation in the management of molar pregnancies', this may be recommended in selected cases with persisting mild

**Table 72.4** Defining persistent trophoblastic disease and the need for chemotherapy

| Definitions |
| --- |
| High, static or rising hCG levels after one or two uterine evacuations |
| Persistent uterine haemorrhage with raised hCG levels |
| Pulmonary metastases with static or rising hCG levels |
| Metastases in liver, brain or gastrointestinal tract |
| Histological diagnosis of choriocarcinoma or placental site trophoblastic tumour |

- hCG, human chorionic gonadotrophin.

symptoms and lower levels of hCG. This will reduce the number of patients requiring chemotherapy. We are also prepared to wait for up to six months before initiating treatment for patients whose hCG level continues to fall.

### EBM

The indications for when to use chemotherapy vary internationally. The above guidance relies on retrospective, uncontrolled but substantial data from UK studies [C].

## CHOICE OF CHEMOTHERAPY

Once the decision has been made to initiate chemotherapy, the most appropriate regimen is chosen by assessing the patient's prognostic risk.[11] This involves using a number of factors from the history, examination and investigations to allow the patient to be assigned to a risk group, which in turn facilitates the selection of the least toxic, most effective treatment for that individual (Table 72.5).

Although it is universally recognized that a single accurate and precise staging and classification system is needed, to date there is still a variety of staging and classification

**Table 72.5** Risk factors in patients requiring chemotherapy

| Risk factor |
| --- |
| >40 years old |
| Increasing time since evacuation/diagnosis |
| Increasing level of human chorionic gonadotrophin |
| Postpartum (or unknown origin) |
| Increasing number of metastases |
| Increasing size of metastases |
| Metastases other than in the lungs |
| Previous chemotherapy |

Gynaecological oncology

**Table 72.6** Treatment of persistent gestational trophoblastic disease

| Risk | Treatment |
|---|---|
| Low risk | Methotrexate i.m. (low dose) or dactinomycin i.v. |
| High risk | Etoposide/methotrexate/dactinomycin-cyclophosphamide/vincristine (EMA-CO) (i.v. cyclical, alternating) or methotrexate–etoposide/dactinomycin (M-EA) (i.v. cyclical, alternating) |

systems used by centres treating GTD, and this makes meaningful comparisons of treatment results difficult. In the United Kingdom, we have used a variation of the World Health Organization (WHO) scoring system recently updated by FIGO:[12] 'low-risk' and 'high-risk' groups have been defined and the chemotherapy regimen dictated by risk (Table 72.6). Less than 10 per cent of all registered patients in the UK require chemotherapy. The cure rate approaches 100 per cent. In general, low-risk patients have single agent chemotherapy,[13] whereas high-risk cases require multi-agent treatment.[14] These treatments usually have little effect on subsequent fertility.

---

**EBM**

There is considerable published evidence on the role of chemotherapy in persistent GTD, based mostly on non-randomized, controlled or non-controlled trials [C].

---

## POSTPARTUM CHORIOCARCINOMA

This is a very rare and serious complication with a reported UK incidence of 1 in 50 000 live births. Most cases present with abnormal vaginal bleeding following delivery, and diagnosis may be delayed, with many patients presenting with metastatic disease. Nevertheless, such patients are potentially curable with intensive chemotherapy.[15]

## THE ROLE OF SURGERY

### Indications for hysterectomy in the management of gestational trophoblastic disease

- Choice (older patient, localized disease, family complete).
- Excessive uterine bleeding (before or during treatment).
- Chemoresistant (localized) uterine tumour.
- Placental site trophoblastic tumour.

Older patients who are fit and have completed their family can be offered a hysterectomy, which reduces the risk of persistent disease from 20 per cent to less than 10 per cent. Although hysterectomy eliminates the complications of local invasion, it does not prevent metastatic disease and therefore gonadotrophin follow up is still required.

As GTD is highly chemosensitive, the need for surgical intervention once the diagnosis has been established is small. At present, there are essentially two further indications for hysterectomy, namely to control severe uterine haemorrhage and to eliminate disease that is confined to the uterus and resistant to chemotherapy. In order to minimize the risk of causing trophoblastic emboli, the vessels draining the uterus should be ligated at an early stage and the uterine tissues should be handled as gently as possible. Conservative uterine surgery, whereby local excision of a bleeding invasive trophoblastic tumour is performed, may be reasonable in young women, as their disease may then be cured medically, thus preserving their fertility.

A rare problem is that of vaginal bleeding after completion of successful chemotherapy due to a post-molar arteriovenous malformation. Selective embolization or ligation may preserve fertility, but sometimes hysterectomy is necessary.

Surgery provides the cornerstone of management for the rare placental site trophoblastic tumours. These tumours have a slow growth rate and can present many years after term delivery, non-molar miscarriage or complete mole. The usual presentation is with local disease leading to vaginal bleeding or amenorrhoea, but they may also metastasize, particularly to the lung. Surgery alone is the treatment of choice for localized disease; chemotherapy is needed for metastatic tumour.

---

**EBM**

There is some supporting evidence for the role of hysterectomy in GTD, but the above text relies mainly on retrospective, uncontrolled studies and expert opinion [D].

---

Surgery also has an important role, in selected patients, for the removal of chemotherapy-resistant metastases. Thoracotomy – for which the indications are previous multi-agent chemotherapy, a solitary lung lesion confined to one lung and no other sites of active disease – may achieve remission in over two-thirds of patients. Stereotactic radiosurgery (and less frequently resection) is now recommended in the UK for the treatment of accessible deposits before starting chemotherapy because of the risk of precipitating haemorrhage.

## ROUTINE FOLLOW UP

Patterns of clinical and hCG surveillance for further molar problems vary across the world, determined by local factors and also by knowledge of the difference in risk of sequelae between complete and partial moles. The clinical course of partial mole is almost invariably 'benign'. Persistent trophoblastic disease after partial mole is much less common than after complete mole and almost all cases are low risk. However, it has been confirmed that partial mole can transform into choriocarcinoma.[16] Therefore all patients with confirmed partial mole should undergo hCG follow up.

The risk of molar problems is greatest in the first 12 months following diagnosis, although it is sometimes difficult to decide whether an increase in hCG levels during monitoring is recurrence of the original or occurrence of a second mole; genetic evaluation of the trophoblastic tissue from both episodes may help. It is the convention to ask patients to avoid further pregnancy for six months, or longer, following the molar pregnancy to enable efficient hCG follow up. Some patients either ignore this advice or accidentally become pregnant during this time; fortunately, in the vast majority of cases, the outcome is good. Current advice is therefore to avoid early pregnancy, but, when it does occur, to allow the pregnancy to continue with careful clinical, ultrasound and hCG monitoring.

## CONTRACEPTION

Early studies from London[17] suggested that women who used oral contraceptives after evacuation of a molar pregnancy had a slower rate of hCG decrease and increased risk of developing persistent trophoblastic disease. In the United Kingdom, we therefore still recommend avoiding oral contraception until the hCG level has returned to normal [D]. Numerous studies, however, have noted no increased risk with oral contraceptive use and North American clinicians consider the risks of early further pregnancy greater than the risks of using the oral contraceptive pill. There is agreement that intrauterine contraceptive devices should be avoided until hCG levels are normal, because of the risk of uterine perforation and bleeding.

---

**Auditable outcomes, recommended by the RCOG**

1. The proportion of women with GTD registered with the relevant screening centre
2. The proportion of women with a histological diagnosis of molar pregnancy who have an ultrasound diagnosis of molar pregnancy prior to uterine evacuation.
3. The proportion of women who undergo medical management for evacuation of products of conception with an ultrasound diagnosis of molar pregnancy.

---

**KEY POINTS**

These RCOG recommendations[8] are based on limited but robust evidence that relies on expert opinion and has the endorsement of respected authorities:

- Registration of any molar pregnancy is essential.
- Ultrasound has limited value in detecting partial molar pregnancies.
- In twin pregnancies with a viable fetus and a molar pregnancy, the pregnancy can be allowed to proceed, after appropriate counselling.
- Surgical evacuation of molar pregnancies is advisable.
- Routine repeat evacuation after the diagnosis of a molar pregnancy is not warranted.
- The combined oral contraceptive pill and hormone replacement therapy are safe to use after hCG levels have reverted to normal.
- Women should be advised not to conceive until the hCG level has been normal for six months or follow up has been completed (whichever is sooner).

## Published Guidelines

Royal College of Obstetrics and Gynaecologists. The management of gestational trophoblastic disease, Green-top Guideline No. 38. London: RCOG, 2010.

Hancock BW, Berkowitz R, Seckl M, Cole L. *Gestational Trophoblastic Diseases*, 3rd edn. Sheffield: International Society for the Study of Trophoblastic Disease, 2009. Available from: www.isstd.org

## Key References

1. WHO. World Health Organization Scientific Group on Gestational Trophoblastic Disease. Technical Report Series 692. Geneva: WHO, 1983.
2. Bagshawe KD, Dent J, Webb J. Hydatidiform mole in England and Wales 1973–83. *Lancet* 1986; **ii**: 673–7.
3. Tham BW, Everard JE, Tidy JA *et al*. Gestational trophoblastic disease in the Asian population of Northern England and North Wales. *Br J Obstet Gynaecol* 2003; **110**: 555–9.
4. Paradinas FJ, Browne P, Dent J *et al*. Problems in the histological diagnosis of hydatidiform mole: a survey from the UK. *J Pathol* 1991; **163**: 168A.
5. Berkowitz RS, Goldstein MR, Bernstein MR *et al*. Natural history of partial molar pregnancy. *Obstet Gynecol* 1983; **66**: 677–82.
6. Fine C, Bundy AL, Berkowitz RS *et al*. Sonographic diagnosis of partial hydatidiform mole. *Obstet Gynecol* 1989; **73**: 414–18.

7. Muller CY, Cole LA. The quagmire of HCG and hCG testing in gynaecologic oncology. *Gynecol Oncol* 2009; **112**: 663–72.

8. Royal College of Obstetricians and Gynaecologists (RCOG). *The Management of Gestational Trophoblastic Disease*, Green-top Guideline No. 38. London: RCOG, 2010.

9. Hancock BW, Martin K, Evans CA *et al.* Twin mole and viable fetus. *J Reprod Med* 2006; **51**: 825–8.

10. Burton JL, Lidbury EA, Gillespie AM *et al.* Over-diagnosis of hydatidiform mole in early tubal ectopic pregnancy. *Histopathology* 2001; **38**: 409–17.

11. Fisher PM, Hancock BW. Gestational trophoblastic diseases and their treatment. *Cancer Treat Rev* 1997; **23**: 1–16.

12. Ngan HY, Bender H, Benedet JL *et al.* FIGO Committee on Gynaecologic Oncology. Gestational trophoblastic neoplasia, FIGO 2000 staging and classification. *Int J Gyaecol Obstet* 2003; **83**: 175–7.

13. Alazzam M, Tidy J, Hancock BW, Osborne R. First line chemotherapy in low risk gestational trophoblastic neoplasia. *Cochrane Database Syst Rev* 2009; (**1**): CD007102.

14. El-Helw LM, Hancock BW. Treatment of metastatic gestational trophoblastic neoplasia. *Lancet Oncol* 2007; **8**: 715–24.

15. Dobson LS, Gillespie AM, Coleman RE, Hancock BW. The presentation and management of post-partum choriocarcinoma. *Br J Cancer* 1999; **79**: 1531–3.

16. Seckl MJ, Fisher RA, Salerno G *et al.* Choriocarcinoma and partial hydatidiform moles. *Lancet* 2000; **356**: 36–9.

17. Stone M, Dent J, Kardana A *et al.* Relationship of oral contraception to the development of trophoblastic tumour after evacuation of a hydatidiform mole. *Br J Obstet Gynaecol* 1976; **83**: 913–16.

# Index

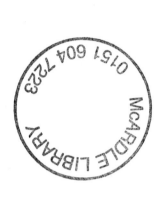